# Bonus Resources
## for
# EXERCISE PHYSIOLOGY

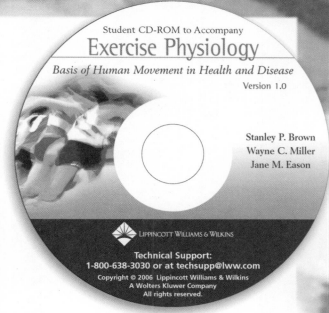

Student CD-ROM to Accompany
**Exercise Physiology**
*Basis of Human Movement in Health and Disease*
Version 1.0

Stanley P. Brown
Wayne C. Miller
Jane M. Eason

LIPPINCOTT WILLIAMS & WILKINS

Technical Support:
1-800-638-3030 or at techsupp@lww.com
Copyright © 2006 Lippincott Williams & Wilkins
A Wolters Kluwer Company
All rights reserved.

## As a bonus for you,
*Lippincott Williams & Wilkins has added two interactive CD-ROMs and online tutoring to provide you additional tools to help you succeed!*

## Student CD-ROM

This CD-ROM offers you a quiz tool with approximately 500 multiple choice and true/false quiz questions so you can test your knowledge or prepare for exams. You can choose study mode or test mode and rationales are given so you can understand the reasoning behind the correct answer. Plus, the CD-ROM contains laboratory exercises, answers to the text's Summary Knowledge questions, and enhancement content, including additional Case Studies, Research Highlights, Biographies, and Perspective boxes not found in the text.

## FOR TECHNICAL SUPPORT,
contact 1-800-638-3030 or at
techsupp@lww.com.

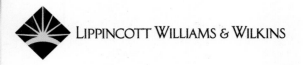

**LIPPINCOTT WILLIAMS & WILKINS**

## Primal Pictures 3D Anatomy CD-ROM

This powerful CD-ROM includes anatomical models of the human body, which you can rotate to gain a full range of insightful perspectives. Layers of anatomy can be added or subtracted, helping you to develop a unique familiarity of the human body. Each body section contains 3-D information on the skeletal system, muscular system, neurovascular system, surface anatomy, and much more.

## LiveAdvise Exercise Physiology

LiveAdvise, powered by Smarthinking™ provides online tutoring and assistance specifically for this text. You can benefit from speaking with an expert educator that intimately knows *Exercise Physiology*. See the attached brochure or http://connection.lww.com/liveadvise for more information.

**Live** Advise

# Exercise Physiology

*Basis of Human Movement in Health and Disease*

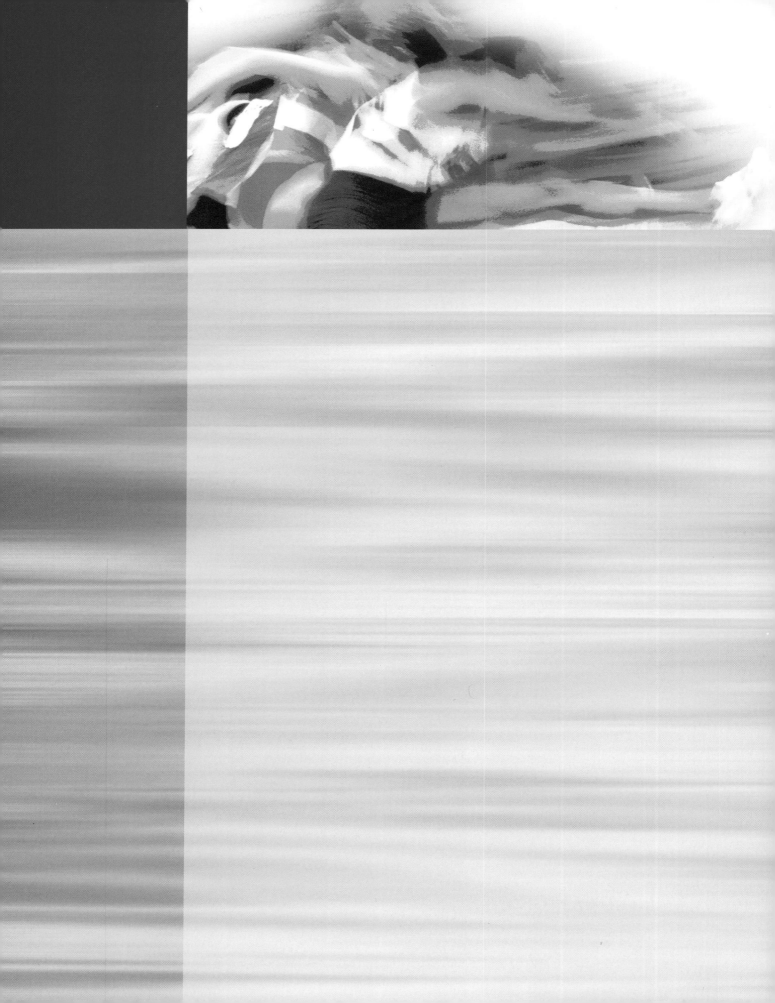

# Exercise Physiology

*Basis of Human Movement in Health and Disease*

**Stanley P. Brown, PhD, FACSM, FSGC**
*Dean, School of Health Sciences*
*Our Lady of the Lake College*
*Baton Rouge, Louisiana*

**Wayne C. Miller, PhD, FACSM**
*Professor, Department of Exercise Science*
*The George Washington University Medical Center*
*Washington, District of Columbia*

**Jane M. Eason, PhD, PT**
*Associate Professor*
*Department of Physical Therapy*
*Louisiana State University Health Sciences Center*
*New Orleans, Louisiana*

◆ LIPPINCOTT WILLIAMS & WILKINS
A **Wolters Kluwer** Company
Philadelphia • Baltimore • New York • London
Buenos Aires • Hong Kong • Sydney • Tokyo

*Acquisition Editor:* Emily Lupash
*Development Manager:* Nancy Peterson
*Managing Editor:* Linda Napora
*Editorial Coordinator:* Katherine Staples
*Marketing Manager:* Christen D. Murphy
*Production Editor:* Kevin Johnson
*Designer:* Risa Clow
*Artist:* Mark M. Miller
*Compositor:* Maryland Composition Inc
*Printer:* RR Donnelley

The publisher is not responsible (as a matter of product liability, negligence, or otherwise) for any injury resulting from any material contained herein. This publication contains information relating to general principles of medical care that should not be construed as specific instructions for individual patients. Manufacturers' product information and package inserts should be reviewed for current information, including contraindications, dosages, and precautions.

*Printed in the United States of America*

**Library of Congress Cataloging-in-Publication Data**

Brown, Stanley P.
   Exercise physiology : basis of human movement in health and disease / Stanley Brown,
Wayne Miller, Jane Eason.
      p. ; cm.
   Includes bibliographical references and index.
   ISBN 0-7817-3592-0
   1. Exercise—Physiological aspects.   I. Miller, Wayne C.   II. Eason, Jane.   III. Title.
[DNLM: 1. Exercise—physiology.   2. Movement—physiology.   3. Exercise Therapy.
4. Physical Fitness—physiology.   WE 103 B8792e 2006]
QP301.B889 2006
612′.04—dc22
                                        2005022533

*The publishers have made every effort to trace the copyright holders for borrowed material. If they have inadvertently overlooked any, they will be pleased to make the necessary arrangements at the first opportunity.*

To purchase additional copies of this book, call our customer service department at (800) 638-3030 or fax orders to (301) 824-7390. International customers should call (301) 714-2324.

**Visit Lippincott Williams & Wilkins on the Internet: *http://www.LWW.com.*** Lippincott Williams & Wilkins customer service representatives are available from 8:30 am to 6:00 pm, EST.

06  07  08  09  10
1  2  3  4  5  6  7  8  9  10

## Dedication

*To Yvonne for her love and uncommon patience—SB*

*Dedicated to all those from whom I have obtained knowledge, wisdom, and understanding throughout my life—WM*

*To my husband, Neil Delude, for his support of my continual involvement in projects that keep me working long hours; to my parents, Claire and Louis, who instilled in me the value of an education and taught me that anything is possible with faith and perseverance; and to my nephews, Adam and Zachary, who remind me of the joy in the simple things of life—JE*

# Foreword

In recent years, the number of resources available to students in the study exercise physiology has been impressive. In many ways, texts have reflected the growth and diversification of exercise physiology as an area of focused study—and possibly a career.

I think of this in the context of my own career path. As an undergraduate and even graduate student at the master's degree level in the mid-1970s, exercise physiology was unique to preparation of physical educators and, to a limited degree in the evolving area of clinical exercise physiology, for newly-emerging treatment programs in cardiac rehabilitation. Beyond the master's degree level at that time, advanced study of basic and applied research of specialized areas within exercise physiology extended the knowledge base of exercise science. As my own career branched into the clinical exercise management of people with cardiovascular, pulmonary, or metabolic disease, studying the variants of normal exercise physiology in the context of these pathologies was essential.

In recent years, research has demonstrated the efficacy of exercise training as an important intervention for numerous other pathologies and conditions. Indeed, there is active debate as to whether exercise physiology is an academic discipline or a profession in its own right.

The purpose of this Foreword is not to engage in that debate, but rather to endorse *Exercise Physiology: Basis of Human Movement in Health and Disease* as a new and excellent resource that embraces the needs of students as they consider the path they may choose to follow in the study of exercise. As we engage the health care challenges of the 21st century, the knowledge of basic and applied physiology is fundamentally important for anyone involved in improved public health—from physical educators to exercise physiologists to physical therapists and, yes, even physicians.

The authors have addressed the contemporary need to appreciate exercise physiology as both a basic and applied science, and have extended their reach to important clinical applications across the life span. Whether the reader is interested in promoting play among children, improving the performance of athletes, resolving physical impairments in the injured, or preventing or rehabilitating people with chronic disease, this text represents the contemporary evolution of preparatory resources available in the broad application of exercise physiology in health and disease.

Reed Humphrey, PT, PhD, FACSM, FAACVPR
Professor of Physical Therapy
Kasiska College of the Health Professions
Idaho State University

# Preface

## Why Study Exercise Physiology?

The answer to the question, *Why Study Exercise Physiology?* differs, even among these three authors, and likely will be different from your answer. We believe that, for exercise science students and students in many of the other health professions, understanding the how's and why's of human movement is essential.

The expansion of exercise physiology as an academic discipline has been very impressive. Consider that only 10 to 15 years ago one would typically find exercise physiology courses taught only to physical education and exercise science students. Today, exercise physiology content is made more relevant and important to students in a wider variety of fields. Students in traditional health professions (physical therapy, occupational therapy, nursing, and dietetics) are finding that knowledge of exercise physiology is necessary in their clinical practice. The subtitle of this book, *Basis of Human Movement in Health and Disease*, conveys the growing importance of exercise physiology to clinical disciplines.

Yet, while this text emphasizes the growing interest clinical disciplines have with exercise physiology, basic exercise physiology content is also fully covered. As exercise physiology itself becomes a more widely recognized clinical discipline, students will continue to find a wider market for their unique clinical services.

The goal of *Exercise Physiology: Basis of Human Movement in Health and Disease* is to merge for the undergraduate student basic exercise physiology content with the clinical aspects of exercise in a much broader way than has been previously accomplished by existing texts. It is offered as a course text not only for the traditional undergraduate physical education, kinesiology, and exercise science students, but to students of other health professions disciplines as well.

We have scaled down the presentation of certain material to allow for a greater scope and breadth of material to the undergraduate student. While this goal has been met, it was also our desire to achieve the appropriate depth to make the text useful for students in professional health professions graduate studies. The tension between breath and depth of content is a healthy one for such texts. Each individual faculty member teaching in the exercise physiology discipline is left with the decision of *how much to cover* and *how deep to go*. Such has always been the case in exercise physiology!

The allowance for choice and flexibility also recognizes that the field has grown tremendously over the past two decades; there is no longer a single course by the title of Exercise Physiology. In reality, numerous courses covering much of the content within this book and with a wide variety of titles are taught at nearly all colleges and universities. This text is designed for any number of these courses, and can be used successfully in your classes.

## Text Organization

The text is organized in four Parts and seven Sections covering 23 chapters.

*Part 1: Energy: The Basis of Human Movement* explains fundamental concepts concerning energy production and utilization. Movement can only occur as energy is changed in the body from one form to another. Since most of our bodily systems are designed to support the processes of cellular energetics, the main theme of Part 1 of the text is energy.

*Part 2: Applied Exercise Physiology* introduces applied concepts, such as the important issues of health, fitness, and performance that are necessary to the study of exercise physiology; concepts of body composition assessment; methods of training for sport performance; and subgroups of the population that require special treatment in an exercise physiology text.

*Part 3: Exercise Physiology for Clinical Populations* centers on clinical issues related to exercise testing and training. This part of the book is especially important for physical and occupational therapy students, and for those students pursuing other health professions. This part of the book is also critical for exercise physiologists who will be working with special populations.

*Part 4: Experiences in Work Physiology* presents a feature unique to exercise physiology texts—laboratory exercises. The best way to learn exercise physiology content is to get into the laboratory and experience these phenomena for yourself. These exercises, which are keyed to content within the text chapters (look for the Lab icon), allow you to systematically test some of the principles you have studied in the text and to correlate what you have learned in the classroom with laboratory data you generate yourself.

## Text Features

Unique chapter features have been designed to assist students' comprehension and retention of information—and to spark interest in instructors and students alike.

### OPEN-ENDED QUESTIONS AND INQUIRY SUMMARIES

Science is a process of investigation that necessarily starts with questioning. Since inquiry is the basis of science, open-ended questions are posed throughout the book, intended to pique interest and inspire further thought about the topic before continuing to read. These questions do not have single, correct answers; rather, they show that science is about making careful observations, asking good questions, and attempting to answer the questions systematically. The goal of this inquiry approach is to spark interest in the process of science.

Each chapter begins with a picture that focuses on the content of the chapter. This image is accompanied by an opening statement, which ends with the first question of the chapter. Then, each main section of text ends with an *Inquiry Summary,* which briefly highlights the preceding content and poses a thought-provoking question. These questions will allow course instructors to explore students' understanding of the section just studied.

### UNIQUE BOXED CONTENT

Several interesting boxes are liberally spread throughout the chapters.

*Perspective Boxes*   These sidebars present interesting, related content that takes the student the extra distance in learning about a specific topic.

*Biography Boxes*   These brief biographies highlight the careers of individuals who have made significant contributions to exercise physiology and related fields.

*Research Highlight Boxes*   These boxes summarize noteworthy research with applications to exercise physiology, and point to implications for future research.

### CASE STUDIES

Ample Case Studies throughout the book provide critical application information for students. They begin with a brief overview of a specific case and then describe the appropriate evaluation and intervention steps.

### LINK-UPS

The Link-Up icon and "teaser" direct the reader to additional Research Highlights, Perspectives, Biographies, and Case Studies found on the Student Resource CD-ROM and the companion website (http://connection.lww.com/go/brownexphys). Students are encouraged to explore this extra material often.

### LAB EXERCISES

Experiences in Work Physiology Lab Exercise, printed in Part 4 of this textbook (and available electronically on the Student Resource CD-ROM and the companion website) are referenced throughout the textbook where appropriate with this icon and a brief note.

### SUMMARY KNOWLEDGE QUESTIONS

At the end of the chapter, additional questions are offered in the *Summary Knowledge* section. These questions are directly tied to the content of the chapter, so their answers should be apparent to the student who has read carefully. Correct answers are supplied in a text appendix.

### REFERENCES AND SUGGESTED READINGS

Key published articles and textbooks are identified for students and faculty to consult for further information on exercise physiology topics.

### ON THE INTERNET

This feature points the student to several web sites that explore chapter content in more depth.

### WRITING TO LEARN

Writing is a critical part of the learning process, and strong writing skills will set students up to succeed in their future careers. These suggested exercises provide students with a thought-provoking writing assignment.

### LAVISH ART PROGRAM

More than 400 full-color illustrations and photographs clarify exercise physiology concepts for the learner.

## Additional Learning Resources

Ancillary content to enhance the student's learning process is included on two CD-ROMs included with this textbook, as well as on a Companion Website.

### STUDENT RESOURCE CD-ROM

This CD-ROM provides extra value to the student, including:

- Quiz Bank with 565 questions and answers
- Laboratory exercises
- Answers to the text Summary Knowledge questions

- Enhancement Content, including more than 75 additional Case Studies, Research Highlights, Biographies, and Perspective boxes not found in the text

## THREE-DIMENSIONAL CD-ROM

This CD-ROM, produced by Primal Pictures, displays anatomical models of the human body that can be rotated and anatomy layers that can be added or removed for real-life, in-depth learning.

## COMPANION WEBSITE

The Student Center on the text's Companion Website (http://connection.lww.com/go/brownexphys) hosts:

- Quiz Bank with 565 questions and answers
- Laboratory exercises
- Answers to the text Summary Knowledge questions
- Enhancement Content, including more than 75 additional Case Studies, Research Highlights, Biographies, and Perspective boxes not found in the text

## Teaching Resources

A strong package of ancillary materials is available to faculty with this edition. These resources include an Instructor Resource CD-ROM and Companion Website.

## INSTRUCTOR RESOURCE CD-ROM

This CD-ROM gives faculty a leg up on preparing for their course. Material is provided in WebCT and Blackboard-ready formats so the content is easy to load into learning management systems. Included are:

- Test Generator with 550 questions and answers
- PowerPoint slide presentations for each text chapter

- Image Collection that allows text art and tables to be imported into PowerPoint presentations and used in other ways to enhance teaching
- Laboratory exercises
- Answers to the text Summary Knowledge questions
- Enhancement Content, including more than 75 additional Case Studies, Research Highlights, Biographies, and Perspective boxes not found in the text

## COMPANION WEBSITE

The Faculty Center of the text's Companion Website (http://connection.lww.com/go/brownexphys) hosts:

- Test Generator with 550 questions and answers
- PowerPoint slide presentations for each text chapter
- Image Collection that allows text art and tables to be imported into PowerPoint presentations and used in other ways to enhance teaching
- Laboratory exercises
- Answers to the text Summary Knowledge questions
- Enhancement Content, including more than 75 additional Case Studies, Research Highlights, Biographies, and Perspective boxes not found in the text

## LiveAdvise

Online teaching advice and student tutoring is also available with this textbook. Our tutors are handpicked exercise physiology educators that we train to help you. They are very familiar with this book and its ancillary package. You can connect live with a tutor during certain hours of the week, or send e-mail style messages to which the tutor will respond quickly—often within 24 hours. *This service is free with the purchase of your textbook!*

Instructors—to use this service, please visit http://connection.LWW.com/liveadvise

# User's Guide

*This User's Guide shows you how to the put the features of*
*Exercise Physiology: Basis of Human Movement in Health and Disease*
*to work for you.*

## CHAPTER OPENING ELEMENTS

**Each chapter begins with the following elements, which**
**will help orient you to the material:**

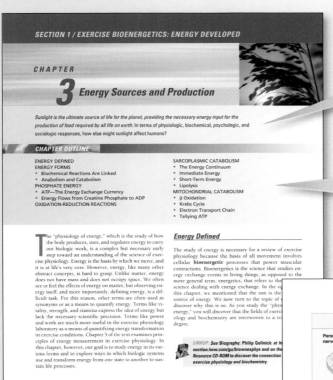

**Chapter Opening.** Chapters open with a picture that focuses on the content of the chapter, accompanied by an opening statement and a thought-provoking question.

**Chapter Outline.** This serves as your "roadmap" to the chapter content.

## SPECIAL FEATURES

**Unique chapter features will aid readers' comprehension**
**and retention of information—and spark interest in**
**students and faculty:**

**Inquiry Summaries.** These sections highlight the preceding content and pose critical-thinking questions.

**Box 12.3**

### PERSPECTIVE

## Protein/Amino Acid Supplements

The goal of many athletes and fitness enthusiasts is to increase muscle mass. Fitness centers, web sites, magazines, and professionals often cater to the athlete's desire to increase muscle mass by selling protein and/or amino acid supplements. You have learned in this chapter that protein supplements do not increase exercise performance nor increase muscle mass if there is not a deficiency already. You have also learned that most athletes consume adequate amounts of protein in their every-day diet. Nonetheless, protein and/or amino acid supplements are "big business."

Shown below is a copy of the label that was posted on a container of Joe Weider's Weight Gainer. The amino acid supplement was to be consumed with 2 cups (0.47 L) of milk. We have added to the label what the amino acid content would be for 2.5 cups (0.59 L) of milk by itself. You can see from the nutrition information that you can get more of each amino acid listed for Joe Weider's supplement by just ingesting 0.5 cups (120 ml) of milk. This becomes a "no brainer." Forget the expensive amino acid supplement and drink an extra half-cup (120 ml) of milk.

| Joe Weider's Weight Gainer | | |
| --- | --- | --- |
| Amino Acids (mg) | Gainer + 2 cups milk | 2.5 cups milk |
| Histidine | 944 | 1085 |
| Isoleucine | 1968 | 2275 |
| Leucine | 3364 | 3810 |
| Lysine | 2756 | 2893 |
| Methionine | 870 | 985 |
| Phenylalanine | 1600 | 1905 |
| Threonine | 1653 | 1718 |
| Tryptophan | 540 | |
| Valine | 2244 | |

- How is the supplement being marketed? (e.g., drug store, internet, sports club, "underground")
- Why would you (or client) be interested in taking the supplement? (e.g., improve performance, rehabilitation, gain a competitive edge)

Subjective information alone should not be used to determine whether a dietary supplement is safe and efficacious, but the information can be compared to more detailed factual information. Sometimes factual information is sparse, however, and decisions must be made based primarily on subjective information. Listed below are some questions that can be asked that will help you gather factual scientific information about a supplement.

- Objective (detailed scientific or medical information)
  - Is the supplement generally safe? (e.g., side effects, risks, inherent dangers?)
  - What is the reputation of the company who produces the supplement? (e.g., well-established com-

**Perspective Boxes.** Look here for interesting content that gives extra information about a related topic.

**Biography Boxes.** These stimulating biographies highlight historical and contemporary pioneers in exercise physiology.

**Box 1.3**

### BIOGRAPHY

## Hans Selye: "The Einstein of Medicine"

Hans Selye was born in Vienna in 1907. As early as his second year of medical school (1926), he began developing his theory of the influence of stress on individuals' ability to cope with and adapt to the pressures of injury and disease. He discovered that patients with a variety of ailments manifested many similar symptoms, which he ultimately attributed to their bodies' efforts to respond to the stresses of being ill. He called this collection of symptoms the general adaptation syndrome. For his efforts, he gained international acclaim as the acknowledged "father" of the stress field and later was referred to as "the Einstein of medicine."

Since publishing the first scientific paper to identify and define "stress" in 1936, Selye wrote more than 1700 scholarly papers and 39 books on the subject. At the time of his death in late 1982, his work had been cited in more than 362,000 scientific papers, in countless popular magazine stories, in most major languages, and in all countries worldwide. He is still by far the world's most frequently cited au-

thor on stress topics. Two of his books, *The Stress of Life* (1956) and *Stress Without Distress* (1974) were best-sellers (the latter in 17 languages). A physician and endocrinologist, Selye held three earned doctorates (MD, PhD, DSc) plus 43 honorary doctorates. He also served as a professor and director of the Institute of Experimental Medicine and Surgery at the Université de Montréal. In his work he demonstrated the role of emotional responses in causing or combating much of the wear and tear experienced by human beings throughout their lives. He died in 1982 in Montréal, where he had spent 50 years studying stress.

Hans Selye

3. Cutting a lawn with a push mower or a riding mower
4. A hand therapist manipulating the fingers of a patient in a therapy session (again, focus on the patient)

These activities probably require some thought before classification, and there may be two right answers for Figure 1.9B. It is conceivable that a person may cut his/her lawn as an exercise activity, i.e., to achieve a fitness benefit! The classification of an activity should be tied directly to the definitions, which in turn, are linked to the idea of purposeful intention. If the intention of the activity is to increase physical fitness, performance, health, or appearance (e.g., decrease body fat), then it is an exercise. If the activity is physical in nature and related to other activities besides exercise, it can be classified as a physical activity. *Can some work-related occupations produce physical fitness?* The answer to this question is yes if the activity is strenuous enough, performed frequently enough, and for a long enough duration to result in an increase in physical fitness. Individuals may become fit from a number of different job-related activities or from more traditional exercise programs. As you progress through this book, the reasons for this should become more apparent. The key ingredient is the level of physical stress involved in the physical activity

is cons ...
initio ...

**EXER ...**

Exerci ...
tion o ...
physic ...
tivity a ...
or psy ...
forces ...
homeo ...
respon ...
the str ...
der str ...
ability ...
proven ...
quire a ...
the abs ...
a certa ...
ate, in ...

Thi ...
lye, wh ...
he ter ...

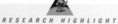

**Box 6.1**

### RESEARCH HIGHLIGHT

**McKenzie DC, Lama IL, Potts JE, Sheel AW, Coutts KD. The effect of repeat exercise on pulmonary diffusing capacity and EIH in trained athletes. Med Sci Sports Exerc 1999;31:99–104.**

**RESEARCH SUMMARY**

Highly trained endurance athletes experience the phenomenon of exercise-induced arterial hypoxemia (EIH), a widening of the alveolar−arterial $O_2$ difference ($\Delta A - aO_2$) that results in a lowered $PaO_2$. EIH may limit maximal exercise performance of these athletes by reducing their maximum $O_2$ uptake ($\dot{V}O_{2max}$) secondary to a lower arterial $O_2$ content and reduced maximal arterial−venous $O_2$ difference ($\Delta a - \dot{v}O_2$). However, the exact mechanism that produces hypoxemia in these individuals is being debated. Two hypotheses that explain EIH are a diffusion limitation across the alveolar pulmonary capillary membrane and a ventilation-perfusion mismatch. Both of these conditions could result from interstitial edema which itself may result from a stress failure of the capillary endothelium which has been demonstrated after intense exercise in human and animal research models. Evidence for a failure of the alveolar-capillary membrane and the development of interstitial edema comes from the observation of a decrease in pulmonary diffusing capacity (DL) below that of pre-exercise levels which persists for a minimum of 6 hours into recovery. A decreased DL is used in these studies as an indirect indicator of interstitial edema.

Therefore, the purpose of this research study was to examine the effect of two bouts of heavy exercise on the development of EIH and to assess the corresponding changes in diffusing capacity and pulmonary capillary volume. Subjects ($\dot{V}O_{2max}$ = 67.0±3.6 mL·kg$^{-1}$·min$^{-1}$) completed two maximal exercise bouts ($\dot{V}O_{2max}$ tests) separated by 60 minutes of seated rest. At the end of each rest period (60 minutes post-exercise), a carbon monoxide diffusing capacity

test ($DL_{CO}$) was performed. DL decreased by 11% from pre-exercise values after the first exercise test and decreased by 6% further after the second exercise test. The first decrease in DL was accounted for by a concomitant decrease in both membrane-diffusing capacity (−11%) and pulmonary capillary volume (VC, −10%). However, after the second maximal exercise bout, the decrease in DL was accounted for by a decrease in VC only (−10%). These findings show that DL is limited after an initial heavy exercise bout by pulmonary interstitial edema, but the limiting factor changes after a second heavy exercise bout to a redistribution of pulmonary capillary blood. Although of physiologic significance, these findings are of limited clinical significance because the outcome of the second maximal exercise test was not influenced, i.e., there was no significant reduction in minute ventilation, maximal aerobic capacity, maximal heart rate, or respiratory frequency. Percent saturation of arterial $O_2$ ($\%SaO_2$) decreased from pre-exercise levels after each exercise bout, but there was no difference between the minimal saturation achieved in test 1 and test 2. Therefore, even though there was a progressive decrease in DL with the second heavy exercise bout, $\%SaO_2$ was not affected and no increase in EIH was observed, leading the researchers to conclude that pulmonary fluid accumulation during exercise was not of clinical significance. Therefore, the meaning of post-exercise measures of $DL_{CO}$ is questioned. The occurrence of hypoxemia during maximal exercise is not related to diffusing capacity.

**IMPLICATIONS FOR FURTHER RESEARCH**

Exercise-induced hypoxemia has been demonstrated in a subset of highly trained male athletes. Further research is needed to demonstrate whether there is an effect based on the gender of the athlete, and, if so, to identify the important physiologic characteristics accounting for this difference.

throughout the body provide feedback to control respiration. Mechanoreceptors are strategically placed in the lungs and chest wall. There are three types of lung and chest wall receptors, each functioning in the control of ventilation. These proprioceptors are activated through mechanical sensory information. Chest wall mechanoreceptors are:

- Joint receptors that are activated by movement of the ribs in relation to their relative position with the vertebral column and sternum
- Golgi tendon organs that are located in the intercostal

muscles and diaphragm to monitor the force of muscle contraction and inhibit inspiration

- Muscle spindles that are also in the intercostal and abdominal wall muscles (but more scarce in the diaphragm) to help coordinate breathing during changes in posture and speech, and to stabilize the rib cage in times of increased airway resistance or decreased lung compliance when breathing is impeded

The lung mechanoreceptors are:

- Stretch receptors that respond to increasing lung volumes by turning off inspiratory neurons, thereby

**Research Highlight Boxes.** These boxes summarize noteworthy research with applications to exercise physiology.

**Case Studies.** Cases show real-life application of concepts and integrate clinical topics for further comprehension.

**Stunning Art Program.** More than 400 full-color illustrations and photographs clarify exercise physiology concepts for the learner.

**Link-Up.** This section directs you to Enhancement Content found on the Student Resource CD-ROM and Companion Website.

**Lab Exercise.** The barbell icon directs you to a related Experiences in Work Physiology Lab Exercise, printed in Part 4 of the book.

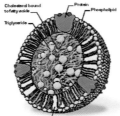

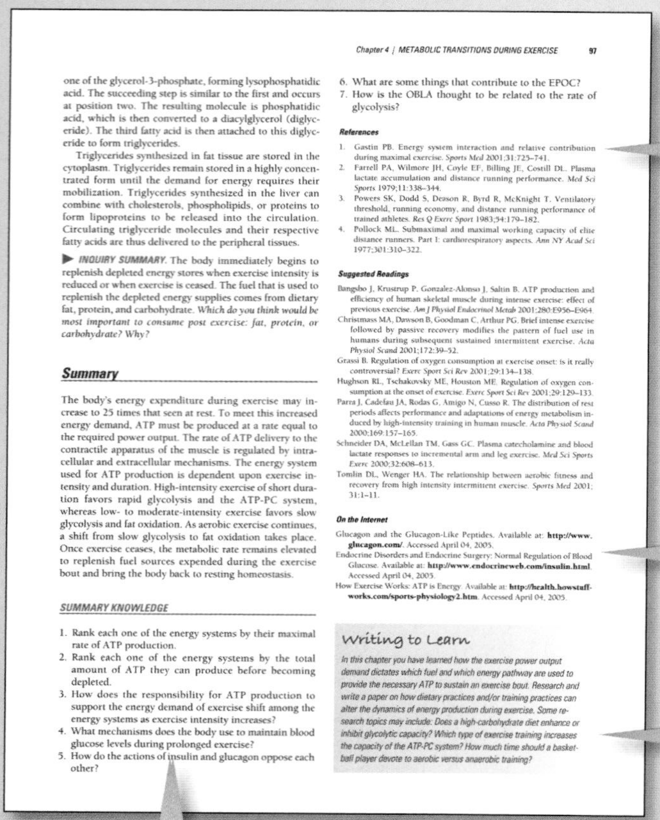

The page shows a sample textbook page (Chapter 4 | METABOLIC TRANSITIONS DURING EXERCISE, page 97) with callout annotations.

**References and Suggested Readings.** Key published articles and textbooks are identified for further information on exercise physiology topics.

**On the Internet.** This feature points the student to several web sites that explore chapter content in more depth.

**Writing to Learn.** These suggested exercises provide students with thought-provoking writing assignments.

**Summary Knowledge Questions.** Chapter review questions, with correct answers supplied in a text appendix.

---

## ADDITIONAL LEARNING RESOURCES

### This powerful learning tool also includes:

**Live**Advise
Exercise Physiology

**LiveAdvise Exercise Physiology.** Online tutoring service offers access to live help from experienced exercise physiology tutors. You can chat with expert educators and get help while studying for tests or working on assignments. Visit **http://connection.lww.com/liveadvise** for more information and to try this free service.

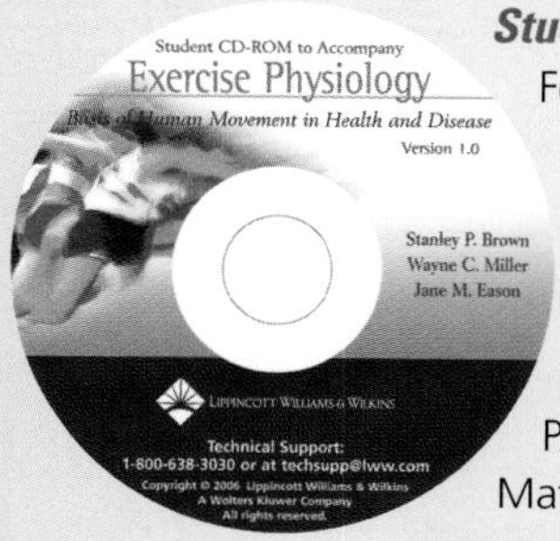

**Student Resource CD-ROM.** Features a Quiz Bank with 565 questions and answers; Laboratory Exercises; Answers to the text Summary Knowledge questions; and additional Case Studies, Research Highlights, Perspectives, and Biographies. Materials also available on companion website: **http://connection.lww.com/go/brownexphys.**

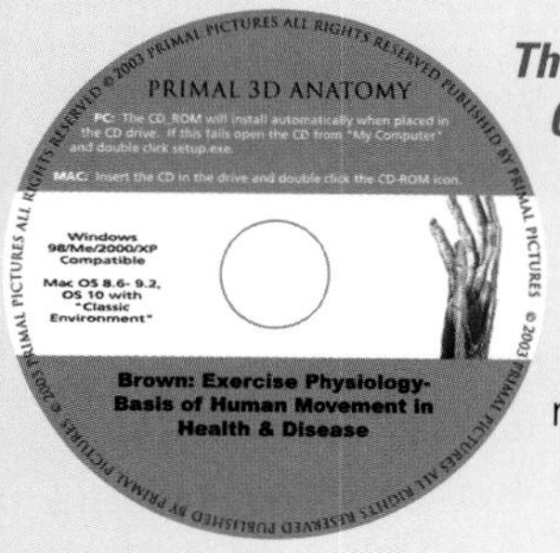

**Three-dimensional Anatomy CD-ROM from Primal Pictures.** Displays anatomical models of the human body that can be rotated and anatomy layers that can be added or removed for real-life, in-depth learning.

# Acknowledgments

The authors would like to first express their appreciation and thanks to the exercise science publishing group at Lippincott Williams & Wilkins for their expert insight and guidance of this project from its inception four years ago to its completion in 2006. Special thanks go out to Pete Darcy (original Acquisition Editor) who believed in us and let us be creative in what we wanted to achieve in this work. Also, without the day-to-day help of Linda Napora (Managing Editor) and Nancy Peterson (Development Manager), work on this project would not have been as smooth or as enjoyable as it has been. The assistance of Kevin Johnson (Production Editor) has also been appreciated.

Thank you, also, to Nicholas DiCicco, of Camden County College in Blackwood, New Jersey, who wrote the Student Quiz Bank and Instructor Test Generator, and Stasinos Stavrianeas, of Willamette University in Salem, Oregon, who wrote the PowerPoint slides.

The Authors

My contact with the editors and staff at Lippincott Williams & Wilkins goes back further than the inception of this project, and I would like to thank them again at this point. They made my venture into book publishing so enjoyable that I wanted to try again; thus, the creation of the work before you. I also want to thank a few individuals who guided me in professional development over the years: Drs. Ron Byrd (Master's) and Walter Thompson (Doctoral) served as excellent academic advisors and teachers of the clinical basis of exercise physiology. Drs. Don Cheek and Gene Anderson (University of Mississippi) and Dr. Dot Hash (Southwest Baptist University Department of Physical Therapy) encouraged my scholarly endeavors from their positions as Department Chairs. Finally, Dr. Beverly Farrell, Vice President for Academic Affairs at Our Lady of the Lake College, has provided an excellent example of academic leadership.

Stanley P. Brown, PhD

I would like to express my appreciation to all those people who, in one way or another, helped me become a scholar of exercise science. Although I cannot acknowledge each one of their contributions in a personal manner, I would like to pay a special tribute to a few individuals who have been particularly influential throughout my academic life:

I want to thank my high school coach, Fred Lusso, for setting me off into my college career in exercise science. I thank my undergraduate mentor, Doctor Lunt, for teaching me that exercise science is a true academic discipline. I thank my Master's degree advisor, Dr. Lanny Nalder, for introducing me to the scientific basis of exercise. I thank Dr. Robert Conlee for mentoring me through my doctoral program and teaching me the rigors of scientific research. Finally, I thank Drs. Larry Oscai, Warren Palmer, and Bob Hickson for refining my research skills and teaching me how to critically evaluate the exercise science literature.

Wayne C. Miller, PhD

There are two people who were instrumental in my professional development. First, I would like to thank my doctoral advisor, Dr. Steven Dodd at the University of Florida, for his excellent mentorship and guidance as I learned the process of scientific research. I also give thanks to my post-doctoral mentor, Dr. Arthur English at Emory University, for his guidance in further refinement of my research and writing skills.

Jane M. Eason, PhD, PT

# Reviewers

The publisher and authors gratefully acknowledge the many professionals who shared their expertise and assisted in refining our plan, developing this textbook, appropriately targeting our marketing efforts, creating useful ancillary products, and setting the stage for subsequent editions. These individuals include:

**Christina Beaudoin, PhD**
Assistant Professor
Department of Sports Medicine
University of Southern Maine
Gorham, Maine

**Dale Brown, PhD**
Associate Professor
Exercise Physiology
Illinois State University
Normal, Illinois

**David E. Cundriff, PhD**
Head of ERLS Department
University of Tennessee at Chattanooga
Chattanooga, Tennessee

**Joshua A. Dobbs, MS Ed**
Associate Coordinator
Adult Fitness and Cardiac Rehabilitation Program
Director
Undergraduate EXSCI Laboratory
Ball State University
Muncie, Indiana

**Jim Mansoor, PhD**
Associate Professor
Physical Therapy Department
University of the Pacific
Stockton, California

**Laurie Milliken, PhD**
Assistant Professor
Human Performance and Fitness Department
University of Massachusetts Boston
Boston, Massachusetts

**Marian A. Minor, PhD, PT**
University of Missouri
Columbia, Missouri

**Geri A. Moore, MA, ACSM-Exercise Specialist, NSCA-CPT**
Director
Fitness Testing Laboratory
Creighton University Exercise Science Department
Omaha, Nebraska

**Rick L. Sharp**
Interim Chair
Department of Health and Human Performance
Iowa State University
Ames, Iowa

**Brad Stockert, PhD, PT**
Associate Professor
Exercise Physiology
University of the Pacific
Stockton, California

# Contents

## PART 4  EXPERIENCES IN WORK PHYSIOLOGY / 577

## APPENDICES

# Expanded Contents

## APPENDICES

# PART

# 1

# Energy:
# The Basis of Human Movement

*Although this text necessarily focuses on physiological principles as the basis of human movement, underlying these concepts are more fundamental ideas concerning energy production and utilization. Movement can only occur as energy is changed in the body from one form to another. Since most of our bodily systems are designed to support the processes of cellular energetics, the main theme of Part 1 of the text is energy.*

*Section 1 centers on principles of bioenergetics and helps us discover how energy is developed in the body. The logical place to start this discussion is in the cell. After an introductory chapter, we begin our discussion of the basic science of nutrient assimilation in Chapter 2. In Chapter 3, we learn how the energy from dietary nutrients is transformed and liberated to perform cellular work, such as muscular contraction. From there we explore how energy production is upregulated to meet the demands of exercise and how exercise physiologists measure energy production in Chapters 4 and 5.*

*The energy processes of the cell, however, must be supported by systems designed to deliver $O_2$ to the tissues. Section 2 covers the cardiopulmonary system (Chapter 6 & 7) and temperature regulation during exercise (Chapter 8). These chapters teach us how other bodily systems are used to support the energy demands of exercise, and how the environment affects exercise capacity.*

*Section 3 ends Part 1 by focusing on the neuromuscular system, which is designed to produce movement. In Chapter 9 we explore how the nervous system is organized to control other body systems, including the apparatus to produce bodily movement: the muscles. Finally, Chapters 10 and 11 present an in-depth understanding of muscle structure and mechanics.*

CHAPTER

# 1 Introduction to Exercise Physiology

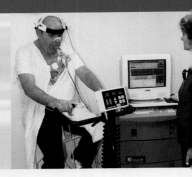

*"Exercise physiology is to a high degree an integrated science that has as its goal the revelation of the mechanisms of overall bodily function and its regulation" (Per-Olof Åstrand, 1992). The word integrated is highly instructive regarding the nature of the field of exercise physiology. Think of ways in which exercise physiology integrates other scientific disciplines and answer this question:* In what way does the clinical situation shown here demonstrate the integrative nature of exercise physiology?

## CHAPTER OUTLINE

A FUTURE PERSPECTIVE ON EXERCISE
WHAT IS EXERCISE PHYSIOLOGY?
- The Academic Setting
- A Unified Vision of Exercise Science as a Discipline
- Exercise Physiology and the Disablement Model
- Movement, Physical Activity, and Exercise
- Exercise and Physical Activity as Stressors

A BRIEF HISTORY OF EXERCISE IN MEDICINE
- The "Laws of Health" from Ancient Medicine to the 19th Century
- 19th Century Foundation and the Rise of Exercise Physiology

Today, more than ever before, it is necessary for individuals to recognize the vital role exercise plays in their well being. Since the 1970s, exercise has become inculcated into the culture of our society, and the importance of exercise as a preventive and rehabilitative measure is widely recognized. Owing to this fact, a wide variety of health professionals should understand how to implement exercise and why it is important *(Fig. 1.1)*. Students interested in a career in health or physical activity professions must be committed to the study of exercise physiology. Without this knowledge appropriate counseling about healthy lifestyles falls short of the mark.

The opening chapter of this book explores how exercise physiology is taking a giant leap into the future by the incorporation of research techniques that will allow scientists to ask and answer important questions related to performance and health. Exercise physiology is then defined according to its relationship to the wider field of exercise science and to the health professions. The chapter next presents a brief historical perspective that sets the stage for the present day utilization of the content of exercise physiology in the practice of various health

professions. The material in Chapter 1 forms a foundation for the remaining chapters in this book, which integrate scientific knowledge about exercise and allow the successful practice of your chosen health care or physical activity profession.

## A Future Perspective on Exercise

The decade of the 1960s was a turning point in our culture. From social unrest to breakthroughs in *science* (laser-invented in 1960; first cloning of a vertebrate in 1967), *technology* (first commercial minicomputer equipped with a keyboard and monitor in 1960; first man in earth orbit in 1962; first man on the moon in 1969), and *medicine* (first transplants: lung in 1963, liver in 1967, and heart in 1967), the 1960s was a decade that had a tremendous influence on those that have followed. The social and political upheaval of the 1960s was the causative agent for change in the last third of the 20th century in many different spheres of human endeavor. Education in general did not escape change, nor did the field of **physical education**, which experienced

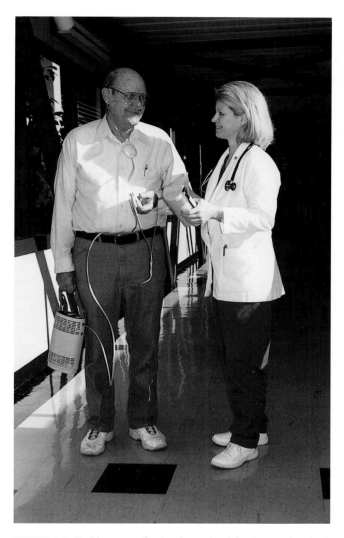

**FIGURE 1.1.** Health care professionals need training in exercise physiology to work with a wide array of individuals. Shown in the photograph is a respiratory therapist assisting a patient with pulmonary disease during a brief walk.

its own upheaval, out of which sprang the integrative discipline of **exercise science** (1).

Undoubtedly, the impetus for change in the field of physical education in this era was the seminal criticism in 1963 of teacher education by James Conant, former president of Harvard University. His call before a congressional committee for the abolishment of graduate programs in physical education, a particular focus of his attack, led to an introspective movement that eventually strengthened curricular science content within physical education. This led to a large-scale change in department titles from physical education to others that accentuated the exercise sciences. These new departmental titles were not a cosmetic gloss but were indicative of a real refocusing toward an emphasis on research. Thus, the Conant report was a particularly important event in the development of exercise physiology as an academic discipline, allowing those physical educators with training in the physiologic basis of

exercise and sport to become focused on research. As the oldest and most established of the exercise sciences, exercise physiology is still undergoing a tremendous amount of development due to contemporary technologic advancement. These advances are truly of epic proportion and in many ways validate the saying, "*The science fiction of today becomes the science of tomorrow.*"

Before the introduction of exercise physiology in the context of modern medicine and health care in this opening chapter, the changing times in which we live are explored. In one episode of the science fiction television series *Star Trek*, which premiered in 1966, the captain of the starship, the *U.S.S. Enterprise*, is shown in the sick bay of the ship performing an exercise test using a type of leg ergometer to verify his physical fitness for continual command. The console behind him is awash with blinking lights, all indicating the functioning of some aspect of his physiology, yet there is no apparent connection to the patient by any instrumentation. Obviously, being able to gather physiologic data during exercise without placing any device on the patient to generate the data is not yet possible, but current day medical "viewing" has taken on proportions which, in the decade of the 1960s, would have been regarded as science fiction (*Fig. 1.2*).

In this 40-year span of time, medical technology has progressed to a level of noninvasiveness that is truly remarkable and has greatly impacted the field of exercise physiology. Physiologic instrumentation today has made certain routine exercise physiology measurements, once very difficult, far easier. Students of exercise physiology can today measure variables like energy expenditure with an ease that would have been considered science fiction just one generation ago. For example, *Figure 1.3* shows oxygen consumption ($\dot{V}O_2$) being measured with minimal instrumentation. Once the "bread-and-butter" measurement of exercise physiology, the measurement of $\dot{V}O_2$ has now become almost anachronistic in more advanced exercise physiology laboratories that focus their research on measurement at the molecular level. Technologic advances have also aided health care practice, allowing practitioners to easily monitor physiologic measurements.

*Experiences in Work Physiology Lab Exercise 1: Tests and Measures Used in Exercise Physiology (in Part 4 of this text) provides a partial list of the many tests and measures used by exercise physiologists, physical therapists, and other health professionals who have been aided by advanced technology. Provided with each test is the variable being quantified, the tools used in measuring the variable, and the data gathered.*

How the earlier example from the annals of science fiction relates to the study of contemporary exercise physiology is evident when one recognizes that the progress in physiologic measurement during various exercise paradigms has advanced at an alarming rate in one generation.

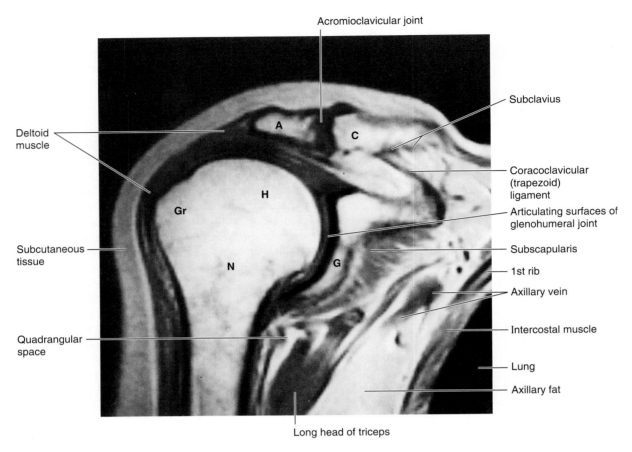

**FIGURE 1.2.** Medical imaging using magnetic resonance imaging (MRI) technology has greatly aided researchers in exercise physiology, notably in the areas of body composition, muscle hypertrophy, and muscle metabolism. This coronal MRI is of the glenohumeral and acromioclavicular joints. (Reprinted with permission from Moore KL, Dalley AF. *Clinically oriented anatomy.* 4th ed. Baltimore: Lippincott Williams & Wilkins, 1999.)

Like the previous saying which compares science fiction to science future, Ernest Starling's oft-used quote, "*the physiology of today is the medicine of tomorrow,*" establishes the importance of physiologic measurement. The progress in physiologic measurement has greatly aided exercise physiology by allowing investigators to ask heretofore unanswerable research questions related to performance and health issues.

The technologic advances of the last third of the 20th century have greatly influenced the direction exercise physiology has taken. For instance, from about the late 1960s to the early 1970s, exercise physiology research was focused at the organ level through the ability to measure physiologic variables in exercising animals and humans connected to the measuring instrumentation by invasive technology (i.e., studying arterial blood flow while exercising). The experimental subjects thus "instrumented" could be monitored for extended time periods.

The next stage in the development of exercise physiology that ended approximately in the mid-1980s allowed for research questions at the subcellular level. The "biochemistry of exercise" period was possible because of the ability

to track energy substrates through different parts of the body by radioisotope technology, which allowed a more precise glimpse into exercise metabolism.

"State of the art" science in exercise physiology is currently in the so-called "molecular" period because of the explosion of the tools of **molecular biology** (e.g., **gene cloning**, DNA sequencing, and **transgenic animal models**) that allow researchers to probe genetic makeup (2). A case in point is the recent advance in **gene-chip microarray** technology. Box 1.1 provides an example of research in the field of molecular biology. After reading this Research Highlight, answer the following question: *Do you think physical activity produces a similar kind of reprogramming of the genetic makeup which might affect the aging process?* Don't expect to be able to answer this question any time soon because the answer is still being unraveled in the research arena. Where this kind of research will take exercise physiology in the upcoming years is speculative, but technologic breakthroughs will continue to open new avenues of research that will produce the science of tomorrow.

Exercise physiology research in the 21st century is also likely to follow the health challenges of the early 21st

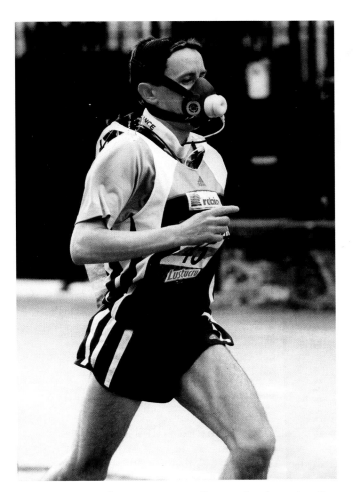

**FIGURE 1.3.** Far easier to measure now than was true in previous time periods, the photograph shows the measurement of gas exchange during the Paris Marathon in 2000. A participant is being tested during the event. Photo courtesy of Cosmed, Pavona di Albano, Rome, Italy and Véronique Billat, Université Lille 2-France.

century and the growing realization that exercise and physical activity are vital to healthy living. Exercise is a key environmental factor that likely impacts specific sets of genes (gene families) influencing the etiology of various disease processes and even aging itself (2). Identifying which of these gene families linked to specific diseases, or even to aging, might be affected by exercise will be a key avenue of research in the coming years, truly bringing science fiction into the real world. It is because of this strong future connection to questions of clinical significance that this text focuses on the clinical aspects of exercise physiology.

▶ *INQUIRY SUMMARY.* Exercise physiology expanded greatly following the well-publicized suggestion that graduate programs in physical education be abolished. Since this episode in the early 1960s, exercise physiology

has developed into a major scientific discipline by incorporating technologic advances that have impacted physiologic and biomedical science in general. *What are likely to be the health challenges of tomorrow and where might exercise physiology fit in?*

## *What is Exercise Physiology?*

As the nature of exercise physiology is explored in this section, a good starting point is the earlier quote from Åstrand to understand why exercise physiology is an integrated science. For a scientific field to become integrative, an approach to research that draws upon many other science specialties and new technologies is necessary to provide answers to complex research questions related to the acute and chronic effects of exercise. An integrative science, such as exercise physiology, approaches a problem by incorporating many perspectives (including the physical sciences and engineering), bringing together a diversity of disciplines that complement one another to unravel the complex question at hand. For example, conventional medical research focuses on particular aspects of specific subsystems of the body, while integrative medical research takes a more interactive viewpoint and works with the concept that the whole is more than the sum of its parts.

In exercise physiology, integrative research necessitates a focus on both basic and applied areas but also incorporates other fields of study, like molecular biology, to ask and answer questions that were once impossible from a nonintegrative approach (Box 1.2). Clearly, complicated research questions with exercise as a central focus are going to be answered in the future by scientists working in disciplines that are able to integrate a broad knowledge base concerning those degenerative diseases which are influenced heavily by activity/inactivity factors. Integration within exercise physiology and other disciplines is needed to answer some of the more pressing health care concerns of the 21st century (2).

### THE ACADEMIC SETTING

To define exercise physiology, the context within which it is studied in academia needs to be explored briefly. Exercise physiology is part of a larger, more general academic discipline, termed exercise science, which is concerned with studying movement and physical activity from biophysical, sociocultural, and behavioral standpoints. Movement and physical activity, in all of their varied forms and meanings, are explored from diverse starting points using the methods of many different academic disciplines. Exercise physiology is one of the chief biophysical subdisciplines of exercise science through which movement and physical activity are studied. Therefore, to have a better

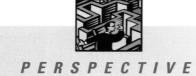

Box 1.1

*P E R S P E C T I V E*

# Molecular Biology and Exercise Science

In the past two decades, the discipline of molecular biology has revolutionized our understanding of living organisms. Molecular biologists study the structures that ultimately determine the physical appearance and function of cells. All human cells contain between 75,000 to 100,000 genes and in each cell, about 500 to 1000 of these genes are expressed. Each gene participates in the synthesis or expression of a single type of protein, which performs some critical function for the cell. Signals, either internal or external to the cell, regulate the amount of protein synthesized in concert with the metabolic and environmental demands placed upon the cell. Understanding those factors, which regulate the expression of genes, is a major goal of modern molecular biology. The "signaling pathways" which regulate gene expression are also of enormous importance to physiologists and exercise scientists.

Exercise training causes well-described adaptations to a host of cells, which allow better tolerance of the imposed metabolic stress. It is known that endurance training increases the intracellular density of the energy-producing organelle called the mitochondrion. Hence, the molecular biologist working in conjunction with an exercise scientist can unravel the question of how exercise regulates the expression of genes that make the mitochondrial proteins. Results from this type of scientific collaboration might allow the exercise scientist to design the most effective training regimen to achieve a desired performance benefit (the dose-response relationship is an important concept in exercise prescription).

Recent studies have shown that physical activity is associated with a decreased incidence of certain diseases. The mechanism by which this potential health benefit is acquired is not yet clear. One of the more revolutionary tools available to the molecular biologist is called the polymerase chain reaction (PCR), for which its developer, Kary Mullis, won the 1995 Nobel prize. With this technique, differences in the concentration of messenger RNA (mRNA, an index of gene expression) can be determined by how fast it takes (number of cycles) to make a certain amount of mRNA. The use of PCR has made it possible to measure minute levels of mRNA in difficult-to-obtain populations of immune cells in lung tissues. Following exercise, there is a greater amount of mRNA for beta interferon (IFN-β) after 60 cycles, compared to the control. IFN-β is a cytokine protein that improves the defense against infections when expressed at higher levels in the lung immune cells. Thus, with the help of molecular biologists, exercise scientists may one day be able to explain how regular physical activity may improve the functioning of the immune system as well as other physiologic systems.

*Used with permission from: Durstine JL, Brown SP. Future of exercise science. In Brown SP, ed. *Introduction to exercise science.* Baltimore: Lippincott Williams & Wilkins, 2000:409–418.

understanding of exercise physiology, it is important at the outset to see clearly how exercise physiology *intersects* with the other subdisciplines of exercise science and with the other academic fields of study.

## A UNIFIED VISION OF EXERCISE SCIENCE AS A DISCIPLINE

The biophysical, sociocultural, and behavioral perspectives of which exercise science is concerned are composed of approximately 11 separate subdisciplinary fields, yet they are all concerned with understanding movement and physical activity, the common knowledge base shared by these subdisciplines. Though the knowledge base is shared, these subdisciplines have a tendency to be only loosely related to one another, giving the conglomerate field of exercise science a certain amount of fragmentation (3). Therefore, the prevailing *multidisciplinary* nature of exercise science is derived from this fragmentation, resulting in the potential loss of overall integrity within the discipline base. As the discipline of exercise science matures, a more favorable *interdisciplinary* (i.e., integrative) relationship between the subdisciplines will evolve and is likely to result in greater growth in the knowledge base through a more integrative approach to research (3) (*Fig. 1.4*). In time, when interdisciplinary relatedness is established,

**Box 1.2**

## R E S E A R C H   H I G H L I G H T

**Lee CK, Kloop RG, Weindruch R, et al. Gene expression profile of aging and its retardation by caloric restriction. *Science* 1999;285:1390–1393.**

### RESEARCH SUMMARY

The molecular basis for physiologic aging is unknown, but it may include damage to DNA leading to instability in the genome, altered gene expression patterns, and oxidative damage to critical macromolecules (damaged or misfolded proteins). The only intervention that seems to slow the intrinsic rate of aging-related pathology in mammals is caloric restriction. This has worked in laboratory rodents by extending the maximum lifespan. Aside from possibly reversing the three factors related to physiologic aging, caloric restriction may also extend life by depressing the metabolic rate. In this study, genes responsible for normal aging were analyzed via GeneChip technology (Affymetrix) in mice following a calorie-restricted diet (25% fewer calories throughout adulthood) that normally extends the lifespan by 30%. The normal genetic changes due to aging in the older mice that were given their regular diet were present (~55 genes were

downregulated and 58 genes were upregulated), but these changes were ameliorated in mice that were calorie restricted, and the mice underwent what the authors called "metabolic reprogramming." The results indicated that mitochondrial dysfunction (i.e., energy metabolism) plays a central role in aging. There is likely a stress response during aging that results from proteins damaged by oxidative stress. Caloric restriction slows metabolism, resulting in a lower production of toxic byproducts of metabolism, but at the same time causes a metabolic shift toward increased biosynthesis.

### IMPLICATIONS FOR FURTHER RESEARCH

Exercise training also regulates the mitochondrial system of striated muscle. Therefore, questions related to the role of physical activity (or inactivity) in the aging process are critical as the new technology advances. Is aging associated with defects in the mitochondrial genome that are either exacerbated or improved by activity? In other words, what role does exercise training play in the mechanisms responsible for increasing lifespan by caloric restriction?

---

exercise science will have acquired the status of a truly integrative discipline.

*Figure 1.5* illustrates the conceptual framework through which knowledge about movement and physical activity is acquired (the chief work of the disciplines) and practiced (the chief work of the professions). Exercise science, as an

integrative academic discipline, rests upon the knowledge base of the various cognate sciences and the humanities, presented at the bottom of the figure. Specific academic disciplines are situated below each of the four cognate areas. These academic disciplines serve as the parent fields for the 11 subdisciplines of exercise science, shown imme-

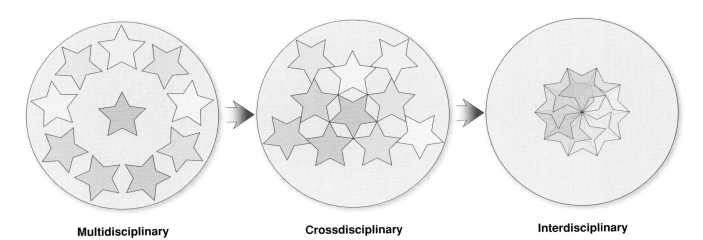

**Multidisciplinary**      **Crossdisciplinary**      **Interdisciplinary**

**FIGURE 1.4.** Evolutionary progression of exercise science towards an interdisciplinary relationship between the subdisciplines (represented by small stars). The more interdisciplinary a field becomes, the more integrated it is.

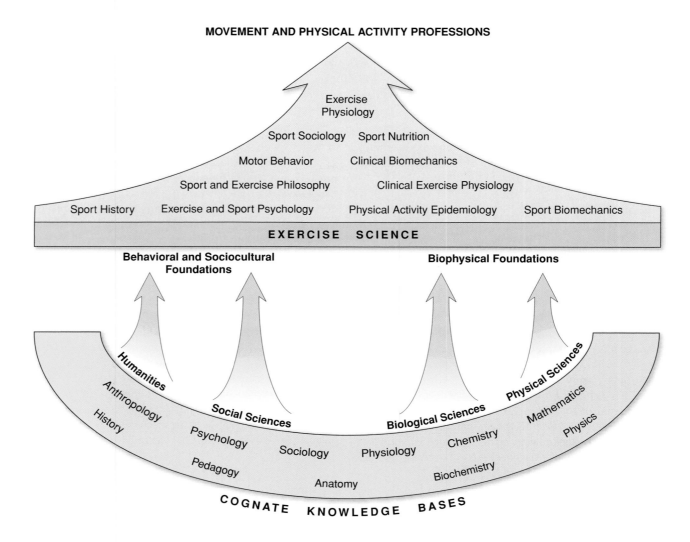

**FIGURE 1.5.** Conceptualization of the interdisciplinary field of exercise science shown in relation to the movement and physical activity professions (the topmost region) and the foundational cognate disciplines (lower regions). The professions are founded upon and are tied to the various knowledge bases.

diately under the professions. These subdisciplines are, in turn, foundational to one or more of the *movement and physical activity professions* shown at the top of the figure.

Because of the importance of movement and physical activity to the human condition, it is not surprising that these professions have developed. *Figure 1.6* shows some of these professionals at work. Though some of these professional fields are quite different, they all share movement and physical activity as a knowledge base.

*LINKUP: Access* **Perspective: Discipline and Profession** *at* **http://connection.lww.com/go/brownexphys** *and on the Student Resource CD-ROM for insight on the topic of professionalism. Look for definitions and explanations of the terms discipline and profession, and answer this question:* **Is exercise physiology a discipline or a profession?**

## EXERCISE PHYSIOLOGY AND THE DISABLEMENT MODEL

Exercise physiology is concerned with at least two general goals:

1. Use of physical activity and exercise as research tools to explore physiologic responses and adaptations
2. Use of physiologic measurements to understand physical activity and exercise

These general goals establish the boundaries around which basic and applied scientists explore physical activity and physiology from different vantage points. The first goal is accomplished whenever researchers use physical activity or exercise to study physiologic responses and adaptations of organs and systems to activity and exercise training. A question related to this goal might be: *How does exercise training affect the immune system?* The second goal is achieved when physiology itself becomes the tool to better understand and improve performance. Within this goal, three major interests of exercise physiology include sports performance, **physical fitness**, and health benefits of physical activity. The latter two components are especially important given the prevalence of **hypokinetic diseases** in the population.

 *LINKUP: See* **Perspective: Basic and Applied Research** at ***http://connection.lww.com/go/brownexphys** and on* **the Student Resource CD-ROM** *for a viewpoint on basic*

*and applied research. While reading this feature, ponder questions such as:* **How might the integration of basic and applied exercise physiology with other fields of study be necessary to solve health problems associated with complex disorders such as obesity and type 2 diabetes?**

Hypokinetic diseases are caused by chronic, long-term sedentariness (a habitual lack of physical activity), and the long-term effect is a systems-wide deterioration in function, which may lead to **disability**. Disability is the direct

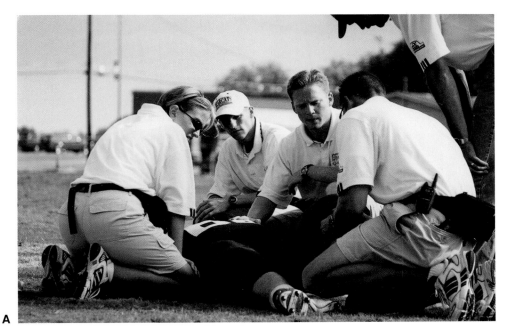

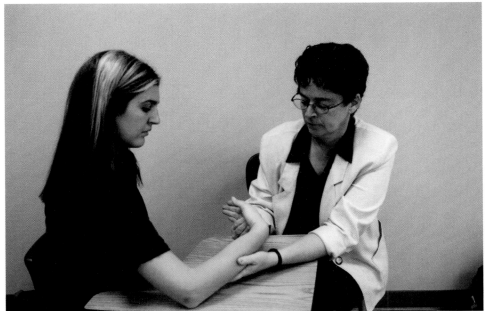

FIGURE 1.6. Movement and physical activity professionals at work. **A.** Athletic training (photo courtesy of Amanda Rutherford, Southwest Baptist University, Bolivar, Missouri). **B.** Occupational therapy (photo courtesy of Katherine Krieg, Our Lady of the Lake College, Baton Rouge, Louisianna).

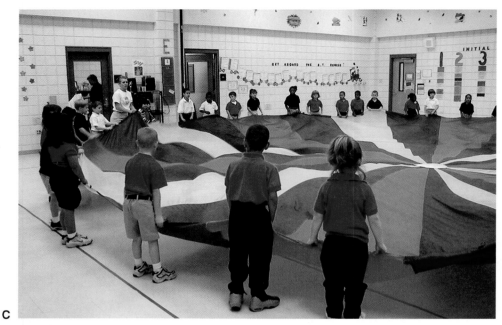

C

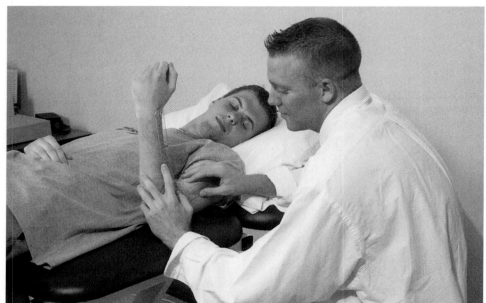

D

**FIGURE 1.6 *(continued)* C.** Physical education (photo courtesy of Charles Duncan, University of Louisiana at Lafayette and Ossun Elementary School, Lafayette Parish, Louisianna). **D.** Physical therapy (photo courtesy of Dorothy Hash, Southwest Baptist University, Bolivar, Missouri).

consequence of **functional limitations**, which are defined as difficulties in performing activities of daily living (ADL); refer to Table 1.1 for some examples. Functional limitations are due to a loss of function in the neuromusculoskeletal, cardiopulmonary, or other systems of the body.

With advancing age, the gradual loss of functional capacity exacerbated by inactivity may not be apparent until the individual is suddenly unable to perform a crucial function. These functional limitations are the result of **impairments**. An example of an impairment is a loss in joint range of motion (ROM) as a result of arthritis. This is associated with difficulty in performing ADL tasks, and the inevitable

increase in sedentariness that brings with it a generalized decrease in physical fitness. *Figure 1.7* shows the smallest ROM at which older subjects with arthritis could perform several ADLs with no difficulty. As knee (part A) and shoulder (part B) ROM increases (level of impairment is not as great), more difficult ADL tasks can be performed with greater ease. For instance, more vigorous activity (i.e., going up and down stairs) can be tolerated without difficulty when subjects' knee impairments due to arthritis are not as great (i.e., 110 degree vs. 70 degree ROM capability). Subjects with movement ranges less than those shown for specific tasks experienced at least some difficulty in these tasks.

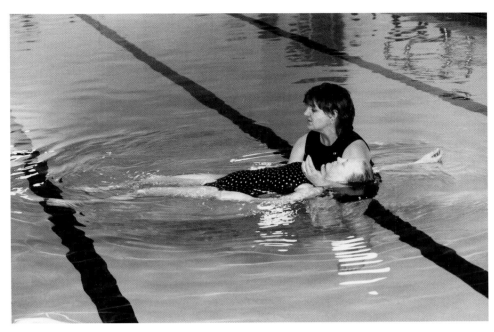

**FIGURE 1.6. *(continued)* E.** Therapeutic recreation (photo courtesy of D. Laree Shanda, Constellate Aquatic Therapy Services, Spokane, Wash).

Disablement is a complicated process impacted by many factors (*Fig. 1.8*). The major categories shown are biologic, demographic, lifestyle, psychosocial, and physical/social environment. Each of these factors that interact to create a person's disability may be impacted by prevention and the promotion of health, wellness, and fitness by the health care community. With knowledge of exercise physiology, health practitioners are better able to promote healthy lifestyle choices to their clientele through scientifically sound **primary**, **secondary**, and **tertiary prevention** schemes. Many of the concepts and principles covered throughout this text can be applied to these prevention schemes. Case Study 1.1 provides a definition of physical fitness and provides an early glimpse into the exercise prescription process, which will be fully developed in Part 3 of this text.

## MOVEMENT, PHYSICAL ACTIVITY, AND EXERCISE

At this point, basic terms like *movement*, *physical activity*, and *exercise* need to be defined for clarification. These terms are often used interchangeably, but they are not synonymous. Semantic differences between these terms are important because many individuals have misconceptions related to these concepts. For example, individuals working different manual labor jobs may consider their particular job-related functions to be physically taxing, yet these job-related activities are not often associated with a great enough caloric expenditure or do not produce enough of the right kind of bodily movement to cause positive health outcomes. Comments like the following are often heard, "*I work hard on my job, why do I need to exercise?" What are some examples of job activities about which people may express this attitude?*

How you view the terms *movement*, *physical activity*, and *exercise* often depends on the particular exercise science discipline or movement and physical activity profession you are studying. Remember that the knowledge base of all the exercise sciences is movement and physical activity. This common knowledge base is studied through the

| **Table 1.1** | **EXAMPLES OF ACTIVITIES OF DAILY LIVING** |
|---|---|
| **Categories** | **ADL** |
| Eating | Eat with spoon, eat with fork, cut with knife, open milk carton, pour liquid, drink from cup |
| Bathing/grooming | Turn on faucet, wash hands, dry with towel, manage cosmetics, brush teeth |
| Bed/bathroom | Get out of bed, transfer to toilet, reach objects on nightstand, sit up in bed |
| Dressing and undressing | Reach clothes in closet, put on shoe, manage zippers, remove coat |
| Transfer/ambulatory activities | In and out of bus, in and out of car, safe outdoor ambulation, endurance |
| Other activities | Propel wheelchair forward, propel wheelchair backward, manage elevator, hold book, dial telephone, use scissors |

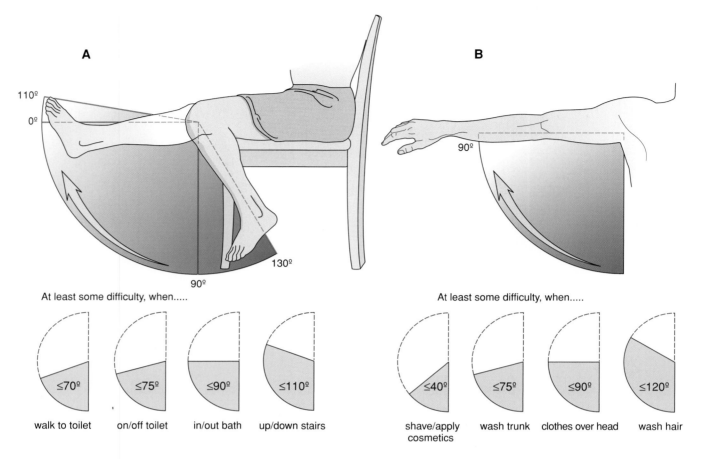

**FIGURE 1.7.** Smallest ROM for the knee **(A)** and shoulder **(B)** joints at which a subject had no difficulty at performing specific ADL tasks.

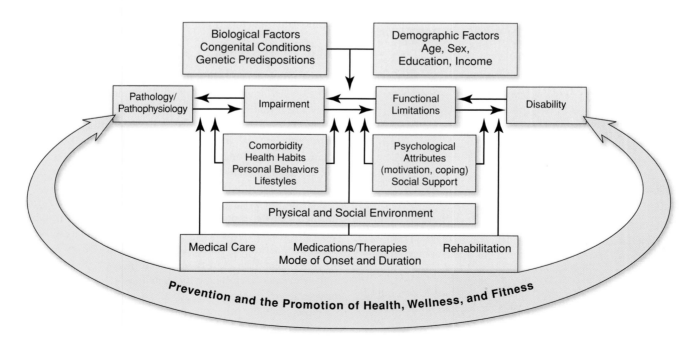

**FIGURE 1.8.** The disablement model. The model shows the progression to disablement as impacted by interactions among individual and environmental factors, prevention, and the promotion of health, wellness, and fitness. (Adapted with permission from *Guide to physical therapist practice*. 2nd ed. Alexandria, Va: American Physical Therapy Association.)

## CASE STUDY 1.1: *PHYSICAL FITNESS IN REHABILITATION PRACTICE*

### CASE

Michael is a 52-year-old tax accountant with coronary artery disease; he received coronary angioplasty two years ago. Recently Michael has complained of exertional chest pain that subsides when activity ceases (usually yard work involving a combination of upper body static contractions while ambulating). Michael presents with a body weight 40 pounds over what is recommended for his height (% body fat is 30%) and is mildly hypertensive (145/95). His only other risk factor is a positive family history of coronary artery disease (father died of MI at age 55). He was very sedentary prior to receiving the angioplasty procedure and has not complied with exercise recommendations given at the time of the procedure.

### DESCRIPTION

Michael is very anxious concerning his age and the demise of his father of approximately the same age. Michael's physician has decided to continue to manage him medically and with lifestyle adjustments. Michael has been referred to the cardiopulmonary rehabilitation program at the local hospital. A comprehensive exercise program was devised that seeks to improve all of the components of physical fitness.

### EVALUATION/INTERVENTION

Personnel in the rehabilitation program, in consultation with the medical director and with Michael's goals for improvement in mind, devised a well-ordered exercise therapy program that addresses the following components of physical fitness:

1. Cardiorespiratory endurance: the capacity of the cardiopulmonary system to deliver oxygen to the working muscles during endurance exercise. Michael's test outcome revealed a very low score from the graded exercise test with electrocardiographic indication of ischemic heart disease. Michael experienced chest pain during the test. He will be started on a low-level regimen of endurance exercise three mornings a week and progressed accordingly.

2. Flexibility: the capacity of a joint to move through a full ROM. An initial workup in this area revealed limited ROM through the low back area with extreme tightness in the rear thigh and gluteal region. Initial attention will be given to these areas.

3. Body composition: the relative fatness of the body. This component takes into consideration Michael's age and gender and will be followed based on activity and dietary recommendations that seek to move Michael to a level of energy expenditure commensurate with a steady and safe weight loss.

4. Muscular strength: the capacity of muscle groups to exert maximal force over one contraction. Though Michael was assessed for muscle strength, this component will be downplayed to address the other component of neuromuscular fitness.

5. Muscular endurance: the capacity of muscle groups to exert force repeatedly over many contractions. Activity in this component will be delayed for approximately one month until Michael's responses to exercise can be adequately studied and a baseline level of cardiovascular fitness can be established.

This general plan is associated with outcome criteria for discharge (*functional limitations, disability, primary or secondary prevention, and patient/client satisfaction*). Part III of the text defines and develops more specific examples of these terms in other case studies. In most cases, the rehabilitation team of physical therapists, exercise physiologists, psychologists, and nutritionists seeks to improve the patient's overall well-being within the confines of his disease. Part of this process involves a well-conceived plan of exercise therapy that is individualized to the patient and that follows the principle of specificity of physical fitness.

---

various subdisciplines of exercise science. As one of these subdisciplines, exercise physiology exists to attach *physiologic* (pertaining to body function) meaning to the study of movement.

However, strictly speaking, exercise physiology is usually concerned with only those movements that can be classified as physical activity. Consider, for example, a comparison between exercise physiology, an academic discipline that exists to expand knowledge about movement, and **physical therapy** and **occupational therapy**, two health professions also concerned with movement and activity but from different perspectives than that of exercise physiology. Physical therapy is concerned with such areas as *arthrokinematics* (the study of surface joint motion), *pathomechanics* (how improper mechanics due to pathology detract from normal joint motion), *proprioception* (sensing the position of a joint or body part in motion), and *kinesthesia* (total body awareness of movement). Physical therapy is also more focused on gross movement pathologies that may involve the whole individual or just a single joint (i.e., improper shoulder joint mechanics), and seeks to correct these by applying exercise (and other physical means) and/or therapeutic agents.

While some overlap exists, occupational therapy is more interested in fine motor processes that dictate movement ability, especially in ADL (e.g., tying shoelaces, putting on makeup, etc.). Physical therapy is more concerned with the science of clinical biomechanics (one of the 11 subdisciplines of exercise science; see Fig. 1.5) and neurology/neuroscience in the treatment of joint motion abnormalities and other forms of movement dysfunction; occupational therapy also uses this same science foundation to help people move more efficiently in ADL.

The following are three examples in which exercise physiology can intersect with these two professions:

1. Determining the energy cost of abnormal gait mechanics following stroke
2. Determining the heart rate response to arm exercises in an individual with paraplegia compared with a healthy individual
3. Determining the energy cost required to perform various ADL tasks

While exercise physiology and the professions of physical therapy and occupational therapy (among others) are concerned with movement, the examples cited above illustrate that movement is a broad term, encompassing whole-body physical activity and exercise or the movement of a body part. Physical activity and exercise are subclassifications of movement, and some of the differences between these two terms and movement relate to the voluntariness of the motion involved and the cognitive goal intended. Study the following definitions carefully, and try to relate these terms and definitions to specific movement and physical activity professions or to the different subdisciplines of exercise science.

- Movement: voluntary or involuntary motions performed by the whole person or any body part (as in a joint); the movement may be abnormal (pathokinesiology) or normal
- Physical activity: voluntary, intentional movement performed by the person to achieve a desired goal as related to sport, exercise, leisure, or work activity
- Exercise: intentional physical activity performed for the purpose of improving performance, health, fitness, and/or appearance

Understanding the differences and similarities in these terms will help you differentiate among the exercise science subdomains and the movement and physical activity professions themselves. It will also allow you to counsel individuals about the nature of exercise.

Also inherent in these definitions is the idea that exercise is a subclassification of physical activity. Not all physical activity is exercise, but all exercise is physical activity. A corollary to this is that exercise usually has very positive health outcomes for most people. However, the same cannot be said for all physical activities. In fact, some forms of physical activity are particularly unhealthy. Both physical activity and exercise are purposeful, but exercise relates directly to a more narrowly defined outcome. Because of the nature of exercise, the outcome will involve an improvement in physical fitness, while the same cannot be

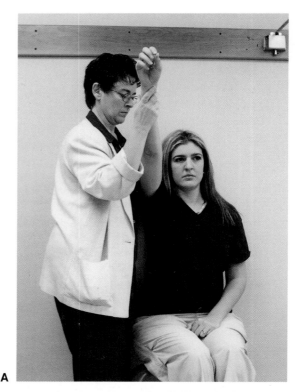

A

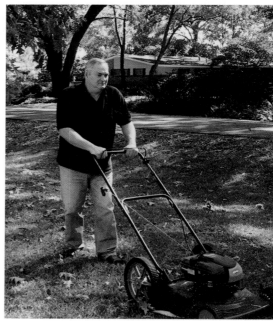

B

**FIGURE 1.9.** Examples of physical activity **(A)** testing ROM, and exercise **(B)** pushing a lawn mower.

said for all forms of physical activity. Consider the following examples and answer this question for each: *Is this an example of a physical activity or an exercise?* Two of the answers are provided in *Figure 1.9.*

1. A NASCAR driver participating in a race
2. A physical therapist helping a patient move her arm through a full ROM (focus on the patient)

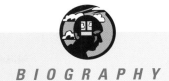

**Box 1.3**

## B I O G R A P H Y

# *Hans Selye:* *"The Einstein of Medicine"*

Hans Selye was born in Vienna in 1907. As early as his second year of medical school (1926), he began developing his theory of the influence of stress on individuals' ability to cope with and adapt to the pressures of injury and disease. He discovered that patients with a variety of ailments manifested many similar symptoms, which he ultimately attributed to their bodies' efforts to respond to the stresses of being ill. He called this collection of symptoms the general adaptation syndrome. For his efforts, he gained international acclaim as the acknowledged "father" of the stress field and later was referred to as "the Einstein of medicine."

Since publishing the first scientific paper to identify and define "stress" in 1936, Selye wrote more than 1700 scholarly papers and 39 books on the subject. At the time of his death in late 1982, his work had been cited in more than 362,000 scientific papers, in countless popular magazine stories, in most major languages, and in all countries worldwide. He is still by far the world's most frequently cited author on stress topics. Two of his books, *The Stress of Life* (1956) and *Stress Without Distress* (1974) were bestsellers (the latter in 17 languages).

A physician and endocrinologist, Selye held three earned doctorates (MD, PhD, DSc) plus 43 honorary doctorates. He also served as a professor and director

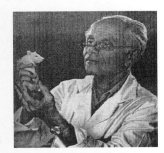

Hans Selye

of the Institute of Experimental Medicine and Surgery at the Université de Montréal. In his work he demonstrated the role of emotional responses in causing or combating much of the wear and tear experienced by human beings throughout their lives. He died in 1982 in Montréal, where he had spent 50 years studying stress.

---

3. Cutting a lawn with a push mower or a riding mower
4. A hand therapist manipulating the fingers of a patient in a therapy session (again, focus on the patient)

These activities probably require some thought before classification, and there may be two right answers for Figure 1.9B. It is conceivable that a person may cut his/her lawn as an exercise activity, i.e., to achieve a fitness benefit! The classification of an activity should be tied directly to the definitions, which in turn, are linked to the idea of purposeful intention. If the intention of the activity is to increase physical fitness, performance, health, or appearance (e.g., decrease body fat), then it is an exercise. If the activity is physical in nature and related to other activities besides exercise, it can be classified as a physical activity. *Can some work-related occupations produce physical fitness?* The answer to this question is yes if the activity is strenuous enough, performed frequently enough, and for a long enough duration to result in an increase in physical fitness. Individuals may become fit from a number of different job-related activities or from more traditional exercise programs. As you progress through this book, the reasons for this should become more apparent. The key ingredient of the level of physical stress involved in the physical activity is considered in the next section, which rounds out the definition of exercise physiology.

## EXERCISE AND PHYSICAL ACTIVITY AS STRESSORS

Exercise physiology is the discipline that studies the function of the body under the *stress* of **acute** and **chronic** physical activity. Exercise physiology studies physical activity and exercise as a form of **stress**, defined as physical or psychologic forces experienced by individuals. These forces (**stressors**) are external stimuli that disrupt body homeostasis and produce automatic and instantaneous responses that increase the body's capacity to cope with the stressor. Unlike a simple machine that breaks down under stress over a period of time, the human body has the ability to adapt to appropriate stress levels with an improvement in function. Generally, biologic organisms require a certain amount of stress to maintain well-being. In the absence of appropriate stress, the human body may lose a certain amount of its function. If the stress is inappropriate, injury or disease can easily be manifested.

This biologic concept of stress was developed by Hans Selye, who related exposure to a stressor over time to a process he termed the **general adaptation syndrome** (Box 1.3). According to Selye, the general adaptation syndrome covers three stages. The physiologic responses and adaptations experienced with specific kinds of exercise training are key to the study of exercise physiology and will be covered throughout the rest of the book.

## Alarm Stage

In the *alarm reaction* stage, the body acutely recognizes the stressor by activating the pituitary-adrenocortical axis, which in turn produces the necessary hormonal responses that activate diverse physiologic systems to prepare the organism for "fight or flight." For instance, when blood is drawn, epinephrine levels rise, which cause heart rate and blood glucose levels to increase (among other acute responses). With each successive exposure to the stressor, the stressor is deemed as less a threat and the alarm reaction may be reduced. When exercise is the stressor, the alarm reactions are the acute responses of the body to exercise. These responses, while of a general nature, are somewhat specific to the type of exercise being applied.

## Resistance Stage

In the *resistance* (adaptive) stage, the body begins to repair the effects of the alarm reaction by making favorable physiologic adaptations. In the context of exercise as a stressor, this stage is best viewed from a chronic standpoint. Resistance in this context represents the attainment of physical fitness, developed over time with repeated exposure to the stressor (exercise). One goal of rehabilitative exercise training is to apply an appropriate level of exercise stress at a critical threshold level to affect resistance-stage adaptations in the patient or client. Many individual differences are seen in resistance-stage adaptations (and alarm reactions for that matter). Resistance-stage adaptations can also be viewed in the acute sense, as when a stressor is inappropriately applied. The body can acutely maladapt. For instance, when a cardiac patient is overstressed by too much exercise in a therapy session, myocardial infarction (MI) is a real possibility. While the example of an acute MI may be oversimplifying the possible outcome of too much exercise for a susceptible patient, it does serve to illustrate the exhaustion-stage reaction, which is presented next. (Actually MI is a multifactorial outcome of many causative factors functioning together).

## Exhaustion Stage

In the *exhaustion* stage, the body responds inappropriately to an intolerable stress level. The acute MI mentioned earlier is one possible exhaustion-stage response to inappropriate exercise (stressor) in a cardiac patient. Other examples may be acute or chronic orthopedic problems or injuries. The exhaustion stage may also manifest in serious diseases. In this view, when the body can no longer respond to the stress in the resistance stage, exhaustion-stage response may be a lifestyle-related disease. The etiology of lifestyle diseases involves, at some level, a maladapted stress response. Overtraining syndrome is another likely maladaptive exhaustion stage response. Symptoms of overtraining are listed below:

- Decline in physical performance that is unexplained and persistent

- Decreased appetite and loss of body weight
- Painful muscles
- Susceptibility to upper respiratory infections
- Insomnia
- Occasional nausea
- Elevated resting pulse and blood pressure
- Disturbed mood states
- Overuse injuries

Many forms of physical activity can be considered stressors. When **exercise training** is prescribed, the goal is to apply appropriate levels of the stimulus for the purpose of increasing physical fitness. To be successful, programs must work within the principles of the general adaptation syndrome to effect appropriate adaptive changes in clients. A general philosophy of exercise training for athletic competition called **periodization** incorporates the principles of the general adaptation syndrome by including training cycles designed around stimulus (stressor/exercise)–response (adaptations) cycles for the purpose of peak performance (maximizing training sessions) and to avoid overtraining. In the example of a periodization schedule illustrated in *Figure 1.10*, there are two 26-week cycles in which training volume (total weight lifted as reflected by sets and repetitions) starts high and finishes low, and training intensity (amount of weight lifted per repetition) starts low and finishes high. The general adaptation syndrome applied to physical training in which there is an appropriate training stimulus illustrates the biologic principle of stimulus and response ending in improvements in physiologic systems.

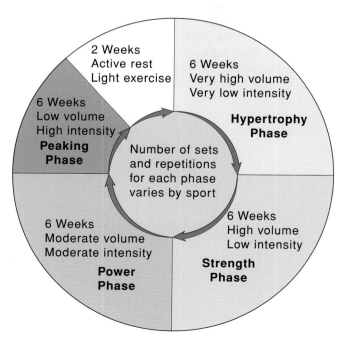

**FIGURE 1.10.** Periodization for strength/power sports shown in a 26-week cycle. Hypertrophy refers to the physiologic process of adding tissue, in this case, muscle.

▶ *INQUIRY SUMMARY.* Exercise physiology is the science that seeks to understand movement, physical activity, and exercise from a purely physiologic standpoint while integrating other basic sciences in the effort. Through exercise physiology, we are able to understand how the body responds to physical stress in the form of exercise and other kinds of physical activity. *How might this science be of value to health professions such as medicine, physical therapy, occupational therapy, and nursing?*

## A Brief History of Exercise in Medicine

The use of exercise and physical activity to achieve health has its roots in ancient medical practice. The writings of the Greek physician Herodicus (ca. 480), himself an athlete, influenced the most famous of the Greek physicians, Hippocrates (460–370 BC), the "father of preventive medicine." Later the Roman physician Galen (131–201 AD) studied exercise in a sophisticated and scientific manner. These individuals connected exercise and other "lifestyle factors" with the maintenance of good health and as a treatment for specific diseases (4). The classical Greek preventive hygiene, or "laws of health," was subsequently popularized in the 19th century through the developing field of physical education, and it is embodied today by the term "wellness" (4). In the modern era, the concept that exercise is valuable in both prevention and treatment is substantiated by at least a century of sound experimental and epidemiologic research, establishing the place of exercise in modern health care practice. In this section, we now turn to the past to gain an understanding of and appreciation for the place exercise has in modern culture and to learn of the roots of exercise physiology. In doing this, we will be better able to answer the question posed by Åstrand, "*Why has a subdiscipline entitled 'exercise physiology' developed?*" (5)

### THE "LAWS OF HEALTH" FROM ANCIENT MEDICINE TO THE 19TH CENTURY

A quote from Edward Stanley, Earl of Derby (1799–1869), typifies the thought of those ancient practitioners of medicine who applied scientific thought to its practice: "*Those who think they have not time for bodily exercise will sooner or later have to find time for illness.*" As understood by ancient physicians, especially following the path laid down by Hippocrates and Galen, good health rested in *natural* (qualities of an innate or physiologic origin) and *nonnatural* (noninnate or hygienic lifestyle factors which individuals may choose to follow) principles. The innate qualities predisposing one to illness may be influenced to one degree or another by proper lifestyle modifications around the nonnatural tradition. The nonnaturals, or "laws of health" in the 19th century, and what we refer to today simply as "wellness," have remained unchanged and represent good advice through the centuries:

1. Breathe fresh air
2. Eat proper food and drink proper beverages
3. Exercise
4. Get adequate sleep
5. Have a daily bowel movement
6. Control your emotions (4)

Used, or adhered to, in moderation, Galen thought these factors would produce good health, and if an imbalance or overindulgence in any one ensued, it could also lead to disease.

Galen's practice of the "art of health," through adherence to the nonnaturals (i.e., scientific hygiene), ties him closely to what we think of today as applied exercise physiology. He recorded his views through numerous writings, but his book *On Hygiene* is representative of his best writing on health and exercise. It might be described in today's vocabulary as a self-help book on personal wellness since it was written for the educated layman. *On Hygiene* served as a precursor to an avalanche of self-help lay literature that began appearing in about the 16th century. An excerpt from *On Hygiene* shows how closely Galen's thought is to modern understanding:

> "To me it does not seem that all movement is exercise, but only when it is vigorous. But since vigor is relative, the same movement might be exercise for one and not for another. The criterion of vigorousness is change of respiration; those movements, which do not alter the respiration, are not called exercise. But if anyone is compelled by any movement to breathe more or less or faster, that movement becomes exercise for him. This therefore is what is commonly called exercise or gymnastics." (6)

Galen left a substantial amount of written work and, along with the works of other ancient Greek physicians who followed Hippocrates' tradition of scientific medicine, influenced thought on health and medical practice during the period in history leading to the enlightenment in Europe. Beginning in about the 18th century, some physicians even began to replace dubious medical practices (e.g., purging, bleeding, and drugging) with the nonnatural or "laws of health" tradition, recapturing sound practice once again. In addition, at the time of the enlightenment, discoveries were being made in the field of physiology which greatly aided medical practice and added to the scientific content of medicine. Two prominent examples are important to mention from this period. Antoine Lavoisier, the "father of chemistry," proved that atmospheric air provides oxygen for animal respiration and quantified the effects of muscular work on metabolism. Lavoisier also conducted the first exercise physiology experiment in France in 1789 on the measurement of oxygen consumption at rest, after a meal, and during exercise. Robert Boyle showed that combustion and respiration required air and discovered the laws governing the properties of gases. Later in the 19th century Claude Bernard's concept of the *milieu interior* (the concept that the internal environment is unchanging) and work in regulatory physiology greatly aided medical science. These are but a small sample of the scientific discoveries that helped establish a stronger science base for the practice of medicine, which maintained a close connection to exercise due to the influence of Herodicus, Hippocrates, and Galen.

## 19TH CENTURY FOUNDATION AND THE RISE OF EXERCISE PHYSIOLOGY

The proliferation of the biomedical sciences, which led to a stronger scientific base for the practice of medicine in the 19th century, had a major influence on the beginnings of exercise physiology. The early 19th century saw the use of a new term, physical education, come into vogue by physicians who used the term to represent the task of teaching children the "laws of health" (4). Physicians throughout the 19th century, especially those who had enjoyed athletic careers as students, also aligned themselves with emerging physical education societies. As pointed out by Roberta J. Park, of the 49 individuals present at the 1885 founding of the American Association for the Advancement of Physical Education (AAAPE), 11 were physicians (7). The 600 members in this organization at the beginning of the 20th century were still comprised of nearly 15% physicians. The membership of AAAPE was not substantially different in makeup from that of the American Physiological Society, formed in 1887. Physical education and the field of medicine were, therefore, very early on "connected" through the close philosophical ties they both had with the nonnatural tradition of the classical concept of preventive medicine. Physical education, and later, exercise physiology, would eventually develop into the academic discipline that most aptly perpetuated the classical "laws of health" embodied in the nonnatural tradition. However, beginning in the early 20th century, the emphasis within the profession of physical education shifted away from health and fitness aspects to games and sports. Further development of the discipline of exercise physiology in the 20th century continued the nonnatural tradition by scientific studies on the connection between exercise and health.

The importance of physicians and the rise of biomedical science to the infant field of exercise physiology cannot be overly stressed. Early research investigations on athletic endurance were performed by physicians. One example was Austin Flint who in 1870 analyzed the food and drink consumed by a professional long-distance walker during a 400-mile walk. Flint's findings that food contained the "force" (i.e., potential energy) that is subsequently liberated in muscle contraction were reported in 1871. Flint's extensive writings influenced another American physician, Edward Hitchcock, Jr., who was the first medically trained and scientifically oriented professor of physical education. By the beginning of the 20th century, many studies had been conducted on athletes to gain a better understanding of physiology. Along with this early research effort, a curriculum connecting physical education to the sciences was begun at

Harvard University in the newly created Department of Anatomy, Physiology, and Physical Training (1892–1896), headed by another physician, George Fitz. Fitz holds the distinction of being the first person to teach a formal course in exercise physiology. The exercise physiology course taught by Fitz included experimental investigations and six hours of laboratory study; its prerequisite was a course in general physiology at the medical school. This department, though short lived, represented the formal connection between the more established biomedical sciences and the infant field of exercise physiology. It also housed the first exercise physiology laboratory in the United States. After the degree program was closed in 1896, it would take more than 30 years before the opening of the Harvard Fatigue Laboratory in 1927, and its subsequent closure in 1947 had the effect of perpetuating the field of exercise physiology across America. Out of the Harvard Fatigue Laboratory, newly formed curricula were developed by science-oriented physical educators who were trained physiologists (4). The laboratory's director for its 20-year existence was David Bruce Dill, who made contributions in the fields of exercise and environmental physiology during the laboratory's existence and thereafter. Most notable were his expeditions to high-altitude, tropical, and desert environments to study the effects of environmental extremes under natural as well as laboratory conditions. Dill continued his research in the Nevada desert until the age of ninety-five.

 *LINKUP: **Access** Biography: Harvard Fatigue Laboratory at http://connection.lww.com/go/brownexphys and on the Student Resource CD-ROM for a profile of the importance of this laboratory to the rise of exercise physiology.*

While this section of the chapter has stressed the origins of exercise physiology, it should be pointed out that several movement and physical activity professions have a common historical origin. For an example, refer to the suggested reading list for an excellent history of physical therapy.

As we did in opening this section, we again quote Åstrand to end the section: *"It is regrettable that so few pages in standard textbooks of physiology for medical students are devoted to discussions of the effects of exercise on different functions and structures. That may explain why a majority of physicians do not recommend regular physical activity."* (8) Certainly the medical profession has been at the forefront of promoting such health care practices as cardiac rehabilitation. As of yet, however, exercise physiology is generally not included in medical curricula. This was borne out in an earlier study investigating final-year medical students' knowledge of exercise physiology. Though this research is old and may not be representative of all medical students, the 1980 survey of British medical students indicated that 57% did not know that physical training reduces an elderly person's heart rate response to exercise (9). While there is no current research like this available about the knowledge level of present-day medical students, hopefully this state of affairs has changed or is changing rapidly. Likewise, equally important is the inclusion of courses in exercise physiology in curricula for other health professions. In reality, what is needed is a paradigm shift that sees individuals engaging in regular physical activity as representing a condition of normal physiology and the sedentary state as initiating a cascade of pathologic changes. In modern health science, the study of physiology has too often relegated exercise to an exceptional condition with little relevance to basic biology.

▶ *INQUIRY SUMMARY.* We have seen that exercise has been at the center of sound medical advice from the very founding of the practice of medicine. Thus, the modern era, with its frenzied fascination with exercise, has regained old truths instead of discovering new ones. Think about the advice or medical counsel you have received from your personal physician. *What are ways in which physicians or other health professionals can promote exercise to all patients?*

## Summary

Exercise physiology is the science that explains the functioning of the human body during periods of acute and chronic exercise. This science has been of interest for millennia but was refined as an academic discipline in the late 19th century. A further refinement took place in the late 20th century, making it possible for exercise physiology to enjoy a reputation in the academic community it did not have formerly. The content of exercise physiology has exploded in recent years owing to advances in technology that are allowing new insights into human function. This will lead inexorably to future breakthroughs as the tools of molecular biology are brought to bear in the scientific study of exercise. Because of these developments, exercise physiology continues to be a valuable science course for the education of health practitioners who are better able now, more than ever before, to provide proper counseling about exercise.

### SUMMARY KNOWLEDGE

1. How will improved technology alter the future course of exercise physiology as a field of study?
2. What is the difference between exercise science and exercise physiology?
3. Why do exercise physiologists study acute and chronic exercise?
4. Devise two research questions: one of an applied and one of a basic nature.
5. Explain the relationship of stress to exercise.

6. Differentiate between movement, physical activity, and exercise by providing several examples that are exclusive of the others.
7. List the "laws of health" and correlate these to your concept of wellness.
8. Explain why the content of exercise physiology is gaining increasing recognition in the health care community.

### References

1. Byrd RJ, Brown SP. The emergence of exercise science. In Brown SP, ed. *Introduction to exercise science.* Baltimore: Lippincott Williams & Wilkins, 2000:1–25.
2. Baldwin KM. Research in the exercise sciences: where do we go from here? *J Appl Physiol* 2000;88:332–336.
3. Abernethy B, Kippers V, Mackinnon LT, et al. *The biophysical foundations of human movement.* Champaign, Ill: Human Kinetics, 1997.
4. Berryman JW. The tradition of the "six things non-natural:" exercise and medicine from Hippocrates through ante-bellum America. *Exerc Sport Sci Rev* 1989;17:515–559.
5. Åstrand P-O. Why exercise? *Med Sci Sports Exerc* 1992;24:153–162.
6. Green RM. *A translation of Galen's hygiene* (de sanitate tuenda). Springfield, Ill: Charles C. Thomas, 1951:53–54.
7. Park RJ. High-protein diets, "damaged hearts," and rowing men: antecedents of modern sports medicine and exercise science, 1867–1928. *Exerc Sport Sci Rev* 1997;25:137–169.
8. Åstrand P-O. From exercise physiology to preventive medicine. *Ann Clin Res* 1988;20:10–17.
9. Young A, Gray JAM, Ennis JR. "Exercise medicine:" the knowledge and beliefs of final-year medical students in the United Kingdom. *Med Educ* 1983;17:369–373.

### Suggested Readings

Åstrand P-O. From exercise physiology to preventive medicine. *Ann Clin Res* 1988;20:10–17.
Baldwin KM. Research in the exercise sciences: where do we go from here. *J Appl Physiol* 2000;88:332–336.
Byrd RJ, Brown SP. The emergence of exercise science. In: Brown SP, ed. *Introduction to exercise science.* Baltimore: Lippincott Williams & Wilkins, 2001:1–25.
Buskirk E, Tipton CM. Exercise physiology. In: Massengale JD, Swanson RA, eds. *The history of exercise and sport science.* Champaign, Ill: Human Kinetics, 1997:367–438.
Murphy W. *Healing the generations: a history of physical therapy and the American Physical Therapy Association.* Alexandria, Va: American Physical Therapy Association, 1995.
Pagliarulo MA. *Introduction to physical therapy.* St. Louis: Mosby-Year Book, Inc, 1996.
Park RJ. High-protein diets, "damaged hearts," and rowing men: antecedents of modern sports medicine and exercise science, 1867–1928. *Exerc Sport Sci Rev* 1997;25:137–169.
Robergs RA, Roberts SO. In: *Fundamental principles of exercise physiology for fitness, performance, and health.* St. Louis: McGraw-Hill, 2000.
Tipton CM. Contemporary exercise physiology: fifty years after the closure of Harvard Fatigue Laboratory. *Exerc Sport Sci Rev* 1998;26:315–339.
*Guide to physical therapist practice.* 2nd ed. Alexandria, Va: American Physical Therapy Association, 2001.

### On the Internet

National Aeronautics and Space Administration. Space station science: why do research off the planet? Available at: **http://spaceflight.nasa.gov/station/science/index.html**. Accessed March

25, 2005. Learn more about how NASA is researching movement in space.

The University of Kansas School of Medicine—Wichita. Kansas health careers. Available at: **http://wichita.kumc.edu/KHC/careers.html**. Accessed March 25, 2005. List of careers in health care.

The University of Texas System Digital Library. Available at: **http://tilt.lib.utsystem.edu/**. Accessed March 25, 2005. How to use library/web resources in doing research.

American College of Sports Medicine. Careers in sports medicine and exercise science. Available at: **http://www.acsm.org/health+fitness/pdf/careers011302.pdf**. Accessed March 25, 2005. List of careers in exercise science.

## Writing to Learn

*In this chapter we have presented the idea of "movement and physical activity professions," which may be a new concept for you. Research and write a paper that demonstrates a common historical origin for the discipline of exercise physiology and any of the movement and physical activity professions. You might also find it worthwhile to research and write a paper on a person important in the historical development of exercise physiology.*

# CHAPTER

# 2 Nutrients for Physical Activity

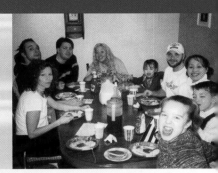

*The sight and smell of food brings about varied thoughts for all individuals, depending upon their own personal experiences. Food is associated with everything from religious rituals to physical health. Although the science of nutrition is relatively young, much is known about what is needed for and where to get an adequate diet; however, much less is known about how our eating patterns affect our ability to exercise in both health and disease.* In what ways are food and eating habits related to exercise performance, physical health, emotional health, well-being, self-concept, and personal relationships?

## CHAPTER OUTLINE

NUTRIENTS: BUILDING BLOCKS OF ENERGY
CARBOHYDRATES
- Monosaccharides
- Disaccharides
- Polysaccharides
- Digestion and Absorption of Carbohydrates
- The Role of Carbohydrates in the Body
FATS
- Triglycerides and Fatty Acids
- Phospholipids
- Lipoproteins
- Glycolipids
- Sterols
- Digestion and Absorption of Fats
- The Role of Fats in the Body
PROTEINS
- Digestion and Absorption of Proteins
- The Role of Proteins in the Body
VITAMINS
- Fat-Soluble Vitamins
  - Vitamin A
  - Vitamin D

- Vitamin E
- Vitamin K
- Water-Soluble Vitamins
  - Thiamine
  - Riboflavin
  - Niacin
  - Vitamin $B_6$
  - Folate
  - Vitamin $B_{12}$
  - Pantothenic Acid
  - Biotin
  - Vitamin C
MINERALS
- The Major Minerals
- The Trace Minerals
WATER
DIETARY GUIDELINES
- Food Guide Pyramid
- Vegetarianism

nergy is the key factor in all physiologic processes in the body. To maintain the functional integrity of the body, expended energy must be replenished and fundamental materials that are lost must be replaced. Food provides the body with the energy to perform work as well as the materials necessary to build and repair tissues. You may have heard the old saying, "*You are what you eat.*" What you eat not only determines what you are, but it also determines what you can do. The substances in the food you eat are vital to every physiologic process in the body. Thus, to study the physiology of exercise, one also needs a basic understanding of nutrition. The goal of this chapter is to introduce the basics of nutrition and to provide an understanding of how the nutrients we consume affect our ability to exercise and be physically active.

## Nutrients: Building Blocks of Energy

Substances obtained from food that are used for growth, maintenance, and repair of tissues are called **nutrients**. Nutrients are organized into six different classes: carbohydrates, fats, proteins, vitamins, minerals, and water. The first three—carbohydrates, fats, and proteins—are energy-yielding nutrients that provide the energy for all energy-dependent processes of the body, including exercise. These energy-yielding nutrients constitute a major portion of most foods. The last three nutrients—vitamins, minerals, and water—do not provide the body with energy, but they are necessary to assist the body in utilizing the energy from fats, proteins, and carbohydrates.

Carbohydrates and proteins are **polymers**, which means they consist of many identical or similar single units, with each unit (monomer) being a smaller molecule. Each monomer can be combined with other monomers to form the larger polymer (mono means one; poly means many). Polymers are important in exercise physiology because the energy-yielding nutrients are often stored in the body as polymers. Polymers are also added to sport drinks or power bars, which may help improve exercise performance. More on the effectiveness of polymers as ergogenic aids is discussed in Chapter 12.

The energy-yielding nutrients have a physiologic fuel value (i.e., available energy to do cellular work) associated with them termed **metabolizable energy**. This is the amount of energy actually made available to the body when the energy-yielding nutrient is "burned" in the cell. The metabolizable energy, expressed as **kilocalories** (kcal), contained in these nutrients—*4 kcal per gram for dietary carbohydrate, 4 kcal per gram for dietary protein, and 9 kcal per gram for dietary fat*—is calculated after accounting for the nutrient's **gross energy** and **digestible energy**. Gross energy is the energy liberated as the "heat of combustion" when the food source is consumed in a **bomb calorimeter**, a device used to measure the heat energy given off when a food product is completely burned (measured in kcal).

Gross energy is the energy content of food before ingestion. *Figure 2.1* demonstrates how the gross energy originally available in the nutrients is degraded by the process of digestion due to energy loss in feces and urine. In addition, not all dietary food items are digested with the same degree of efficiency. Digestibility refers to the percent of the food ingested that is actually absorbed from the intestinal lumen. Digestibility of major foodstuffs averages about 96% for ingested carbohydrates, 96% for fats, and 92% for proteins. Thus, the digestible energy of these three nutrients is 96%, 96%, and 92%, respectively, of their gross energy value. As Figure 2.1 shows, gross energy is reduced by approximately 4% in carbohydrates and fats, and by 8%

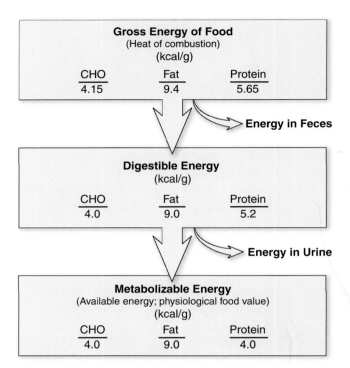

**FIGURE 2.1.** The energy content of food as it becomes available for physiologic processes. The energy available to the body from carbohydrates, fats, and proteins degraded by the process of digestion.

in proteins once absorption takes place. Once in the body, the energy available for cellular activity (metabolizable energy) remains constant for fats and carbohydrates, while the energy available from protein metabolism is reduced by an additional 23%. These values for metabolizable energy have been widely used and are averages based on a number of different kinds of foods for each nutrient class. For fats and carbohydrates, these energy variables are related according to the following equation:

$$\text{Metabolizable Energy (kcal·g}^{-1}\text{)} = \text{Digestible Energy (\%)} \times \text{Gross Energy (kcal·g}^{-1}\text{)}$$

Protein metabolism by the cell releases less energy than burning proteins completely in a bomb calorimeter. This is true because energy is "lost" as the nitrogen products of protein metabolism are lost in the feces and urine. These waste products account for the rather large difference in the metabolizable energy of proteins.

▶ *INQUIRY SUMMARY.* Carbohydrates, fats, and proteins are energy-yielding nutrients. *Why do you suppose nutritionists say dietary fat is more energy-dense than carbohydrate or protein?*

## Carbohydrates

Carbohydrates are composed of three elements: carbon, hydrogen, and oxygen. The term carbohydrate actually

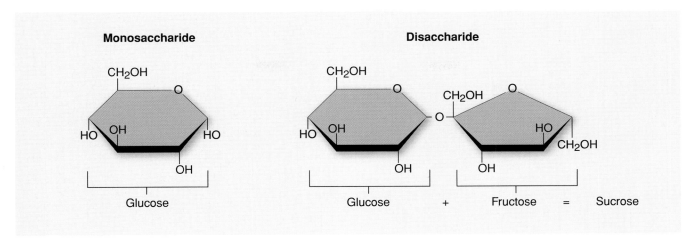

**FIGURE 2.2.** The structures of two common simple sugars, glucose and sucrose (table sugar). Glucose is a monosaccharide, whereas sucrose is a disaccharide consisting of one glucose unit and one fructose unit.

means hydrated carbon. The number and arrangement of these three elements in the carbohydrate molecule differentiate one carbohydrate from another. The simpler forms of carbohydrates are called sugars, and the more complex forms are called starches and dietary fiber. The simple carbohydrates, or simple sugars, are divided into two categories, monosaccharides and disaccharides. The complex carbohydrates are also divided into two categories, polysaccharides and fiber.

## MONOSACCHARIDES

The basic carbohydrate unit is composed of 6 carbons, 12 hydrogens, and 6 oxygens. Notice that if you divide the chemical formula for the basic carbohydrate unit $C_6H_{12}O_6$ by 6, you get $CH_2O$, or a hydrated carbon. This simple carbohydrate or simple sugar unit is also referred to as a **monosaccharide** because it consists of only one (mono) simple sugar (saccharide). Glucose is the major monosaccharide (*Fig. 2.2*). Glucose is either derived from foods in its natural state or produced in the body as a result of digestion of other carbohydrates. Under physiologic conditions in which carbohydrate supplies are limited, such as exercise, glucose can be synthesized from other compounds, a process called **gluconeogenesis**. For example, protein can be partially broken down and its constituents used to form glucose.

Fructose is a monosaccharide that is primarily found in fruits and honey. Fructose is the sweetest of the simple sugars and therefore is often refined and added to foods to enhance their taste. Galactose is the last of the single sugars, and it does not exist free in nature to any appreciable extent. Once inside the body, fructose and galactose are easily converted into glucose. Hence, when referring to blood sugar, we are always speaking about blood glucose.

## DISACCHARIDES

A **disaccharide** is formed when two monosaccharides combine chemically through a reaction called condensa-

tion (a water molecule is released from this combination). Sucrose, or table sugar, is the most common disaccharide. This double sugar is composed of one glucose molecule and one fructose molecule. Sucrose is found naturally in beets and cane and is easily refined and added to food products. Maltose is a disaccharide consisting of two glucose molecules. Maltose is found in malt products and germinating cereals. However, maltose does not contribute substantially to the average person's diet. A more common dietary disaccharide is lactose, which is a combination of glucose and galactose. Lactose is found in milk and dairy products and is often referred to as milk sugar.

## POLYSACCHARIDES

**Polysaccharides** are made when three or more monosaccharides form linkages among themselves (*Fig. 2.3*). For this reason, polysaccharides are often referred to as complex carbohydrates or complex sugars when compared to the simple sugars (mono- and disaccharides). Although the possibility exists for innumerable different polysaccharides, there are very few that are found in the common diet. Dietary polysaccharides are basically either starch or fiber. Starch is simply a straight or branched-chain polysaccharide containing hundreds of glucose molecules linked together (Fig. 2.3). Starch is the storage form of carbohydrates in plants and is the major constituent in foods such as potatoes, rice, breads, cereals, and pasta. Starch is our most abundant source of dietary carbohydrate.

Another type of polysaccharide is **glycogen**, which is the storage form of carbohydrate in animals. When there is an abundance of glucose in the liver and muscles, glucose molecules link together to form the polysaccharide glycogen. Most meat products contain only small amounts of glycogen, and some of the glycogen stored in meat is lost during cooking. Therefore, meats are not considered a dietary carbohydrate source. The role of glycogen in the body

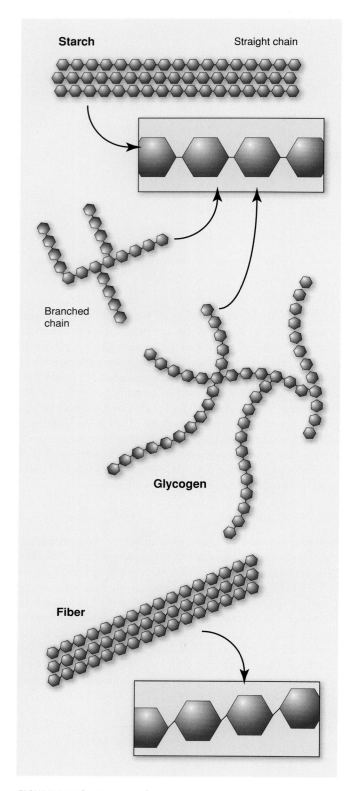

**FIGURE 2.3.** The structure of complex carbohydrates, starch, glycogen, and fiber. Each of these complex carbohydrates is a polysaccharide, consisting of many single sugars linked together by chemical bonds. The chemical bonds in fibers are not broken by digestive enzymes and render the energy from the fiber unavailable to the body.

is to provide energy for muscle contraction and to serve as a glucose reserve when blood glucose levels are reduced.

*Can you now deduce an important difference in the function of liver versus muscle glycogen for energy metabolism?* During short periods of strenuous activity, energy is released in the muscles by the breakdown of glycogen to glucose monomers that can be used for energy production. This process will be explained in Chapter 3. The liver is also able to readily convert its glycogen stores to free glucose molecules for release into the general circulation to maintain blood glucose levels and to provide a supply of glucose to be taken up for energy use by various tissues like the kidneys, heart, and skeletal muscle. The amount of stored glycogen we have is affected by our dietary and exercise habits. Glycogen formation is increased when our diets are rich in carbohydrates and is decreased when dietary carbohydrate intake is low.

There are several types of glycogen storage diseases, which are caused by missing enzymes in the affected organ. Symptoms result from the accumulation of glycogen or its byproducts or from an inability to produce glucose when needed. Two common symptoms are severe muscle cramps during exercise or unaccustomed activity and low blood sugar levels. Diagnosis is made when the examination of a tissue biopsy, usually muscle or liver, determines that a specific enzyme is missing. Treatment depends on the type of disease. For many people, treatment consists of eating several small carbohydrate-rich meals throughout the day to prevent blood glucose levels from dropping. Glycogen storage diseases tend to cause the waste product uric acid to accumulate, which can cause gout or kidney stones. Drug treatment to prevent this accumulation is often necessary.

In some types of glycogen storage diseases, exercise intensity must be limited to prevent muscle cramps. An example is seen with one of the most common glycogen storage diseases, **McArdle disease**. The enzyme muscle phosphorylase is missing in McArdle disease. Phosphorylase is the enzyme that breaks apart the glycogen molecule into its glucose units so that glucose can be used for energy during exercise. Hence, the outward symptom of McArdle disease is muscle cramping during exercise.

Dietary fiber, which is derived from plants, is another type of polysaccharide. However, the human digestive system cannot break down dietary fiber. The chemical bonds that bind glucose molecules together in dietary fiber are different from those that bind glucose molecules together in starch and glycogen (Fig. 2.3). When starch and glycogen are digested, chemical bonds are split through a reaction called hydrolysis. In hydrolysis reactions, molecules are split as they either take up or give up water. Dietary fibers are resistant to hydrolysis by the digestive enzymes, and this indigestibility of dietary fibers may be the key to their health-promoting effects. Dietary fibers have been associated with a lower occurrence of obesity, type 2 diabetes, intestinal disorders, and cardiovascular disease. Dietary fibers are classified into two categories. **Soluble fibers** are those fibers that dissolve or swell when put into water and can be broken down by intestinal bacteria. Pectins, gums, and mucilages are soluble fibers that are easily found in citrus fruits, beans, barley, legumes, rye, seeds, vegetables, oats, and oat bran. These fibers delay stomach emptying, slow glucose absorption, and can lower blood cholesterol levels. The **insoluble fibers** consist of celluloses, hemicelluloses, and lignins. These fibers do not dissolve in water and are not broken down by intestinal bacteria. Insoluble fibers assist in digestion and can be found in all plants, particularly brown rice, fruits, legumes, seeds, vegetables, wheat bran, and whole grains.

## DIGESTION AND ABSORPTION OF CARBOHYDRATES

Carbohydrates from most foods cannot be absorbed until they are broken down into monosaccharides. This process of digestion begins in the mouth with the secretion of saliva (*Fig. 2.4*). Saliva contains various enzymes, protein molecules that regulate chemical reactions but are not consumed in the reactions, that break apart the polysaccharides into smaller pieces and the disaccharide maltose. The reactions regulated by salivary enzymes are the breaking of the linkages between single sugar units of a polysaccharide. As food passes to the stomach, stomach enzymes and acids destroy the salivary enzymes. This temporarily halts the digestion of the polysaccharide. Digestion resumes in the small intestine where more polysaccharide splitting enzymes from the pancreas break the carbohydrate down completely into disaccharides. Disaccharides that are consumed, along with the maltose from the partially digested polysaccharide, undergo one more split on the membranes of the intestinal mucosal cells. Maltose is split into two glucose molecules; lactose is split into one glucose and one galactose; and sucrose into one glucose and one fructose. These monosaccharides traverse the cells of the small intestine lining and enter the circulation. The blood then carries the monosaccharides to the liver where they are taken up and converted into either glucose, glycogen, or fat. Glucose and fat are released from the liver and circulated to other tissues in the body. Cells in the body tissues can either utilize circulating glucose and fat for energy or store them in the form of glycogen (storage form of glucose) and triglycerides (storage form for fat and glucose).

As mentioned earlier, dietary fiber is not digested in the body because humans do not have the necessary enzymes to break it down during the digestive process. Hence, dietary fiber remains in the digestive tract and travels to the colon where it provides bulk, holds water, and binds minerals and acids. The binding of acids like bile assists in the digestion of fats. In the colon, fiber encounters resident bacteria that release small amounts of nutrients from the fiber along with some gas.

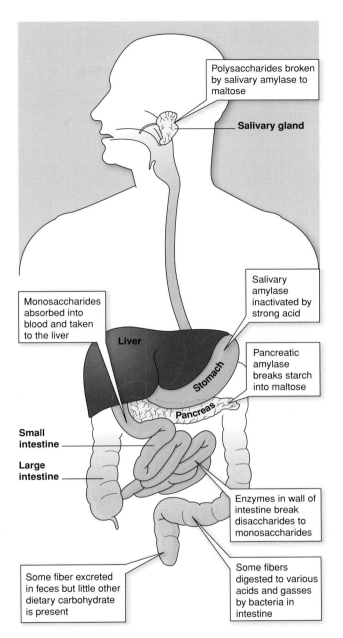

**FIGURE 2.4.** Digestion and absorption of carbohydrates. Polysaccharides are sequentially broken down into monosaccharides before they are absorbed in the small intestine.

## THE ROLE OF CARBOHYDRATES IN THE BODY

The primary function of carbohydrates in the body is to serve as an energy source. At rest, approximately half of the energy utilized by the body is derived from carbohydrate, whereas the other half comes from fat. During heavy exercise, virtually all of the energy for muscular contraction can be derived from carbohydrate, so fat becomes only a small contributor to the energy pool.

The liver is the organ that regulates the availability of carbohydrate (glucose) to all of the body tissues. Under normal conditions, blood glucose levels are regulated within a narrow range (70 to 110 mg·dL$^{-1}$ or 3.9 to 6.1 mmol·L$^{-1}$). When blood glucose levels drop below a critical level, a person feels nervous, irritable, and hungry. This condition is called hypoglycemia (low blood sugar). Under this condition, the hormone glucagon causes the liver to combat hypoglycemia by breaking down liver glycogen and releasing its glucose residues into the bloodstream. Other symptoms of hypoglycemia may include acute fatigue, lightheadedness and nausea. The symptoms may be severe, as in the case of an individual with diabetes, who may experience delirium, coma, and possibly death. Case study 2.1 presents information on management of blood glucose during exercise for the person with diabetes.

An elevated blood glucose level is called hyperglycemia (high blood sugar). In this case, the liver stores glucose in the form of glycogen and converts excess glucose into fat for storage in the fat cells. The hormone insulin, which is released from the pancreas, assists the liver in removing glucose from the bloodstream. In contrast, when blood sugar levels become low (hypoglycemia), the hormone glucagon is released from the pancreas. Glucagon causes liver glycogen to be broken down into its glucose units, which can then enter the circulation to raise blood sugar levels. Muscle glycogen, however, cannot be released into the circulation. Glucose from broken down muscle glycogen can only be used to

---

## CASE STUDY 2.1: *DIABETES*

### CASE

John is a 45-year-old businessman who has been sedentary since the age of 20. John reported feeling fatigued and very irritable over the past few months. He made an appointment with his primary care physician after noting symptoms of blurred vision and excessive urination. The physician orders an oral glucose tolerance test, which is preceded by a fasting glucose measurement. Fasting plasma glucose measured 215 mg·dL$^{-1}$ and glucose levels were 300 mg·dL$^{-1}$ following the glucose tolerance test.

### DESCRIPTION

Type 2 diabetes is a metabolic disease involving carbohydrate, fat, and protein metabolism. The disease results from hyposecretion or hypoactivity of insulin, and it affects 14 million Americans. It is estimated that half of all persons meeting the clinical criteria for diabetes are unaware of their condition. The immediate threat of uncontrolled diabetes is the risk of diabetic coma, resulting from hyperglycemia. Chronic risks associated with diabetes include stroke, cardiovascular disease, kidney disease, and peripheral vascular disease. All of these ill effects can be prevented or attenuated through blood glucose monitoring and regular physical activity.

People with type 1 diabetes are born with a genetic predisposition for diabetes, but the symptoms may not manifest for several years. During the asymptomatic period, the body's immune system destroys the beta cells of the pancreas. Destruction of the beta cells places the body in a condition of insulin shortage, and insulin injections are necessary to facilitate glucose entry into the cells.

Type 2 diabetes generally affects adults and obese individuals. Insulin insensitivity or impaired glucose tolerance, which may affect 70 to 80 million Americans, is a precursor to type 2 diabetes. Impaired glucose tolerance will progress into type 2 diabetes in those persons who develop relative insulin

deficiency. Nutrition intervention and exercise participation are the predominant tools in management of type 2 diabetes.

For a diagnosis of diabetes to be confirmed, a patient must meet one of the following criteria on two separate test days:

1. Fasting plasma glucose level ≥126 mg·dL$^{-1}$
2. Symptoms of diabetes such as excessive urine production, excessive thirst, and unexplained weight loss with a random plasma glucose level of ≥200 mg·dL$^{-1}$
3. Two-hour plasma glucose level ≥200 mg·dL$^{-1}$ during an oral glucose tolerance test using 75 g of glucose

The goal of diabetes treatment is to help the patient gain knowledge, competence, and motivation, which will empower the patient to self-manage the disease. Effective nutrition intervention in diabetes results in improved self-monitoring of blood glucose, blood lipids, glycated hemoglobin, blood pressure, renal function, and weight management; reduction in medications; reduction in frequency of hypoglycemia; reduction in hospitalization; reduction in cost of overall health care; and improved quality of life. Effective exercise intervention results in increased insulin sensitivity.

### DIAGNOSIS:

Type 2 diabetes

### THERAPEUTIC RECOMMENDATIONS

John was instructed to meet with a dietitian for nutritional counseling. He was also enrolled in a diabetes education course to be conducted at the outpatient care center. John made an appointment with an exercise physiologist for an exercise prescription. John's blood glucose levels will be monitored daily throughout the diabetes education course and exercise programming. If his plasma glucose levels come within an acceptable range, he will continue with diet and exercise as primary therapies. If plasma glucose does not come under control, John will be placed on an oral hypoglycemic.

support muscle contraction because intracellular glucose cannot escape from inside the muscle cell. More about the role of glucose in energy production will be discussed in Chapter 3. The body has three energy sources of carbohydrate, the so-called glucose pools: blood glucose, liver glycogen, and muscle glycogen. Energy stored in these sites totals approximately 1850 kcal, which may be readily depleted with only one day of fasting or a couple hours of vigorous exercise!

▶ *INQUIRY SUMMARY.* The major role of carbohydrate is to provide energy for the body. *Recognizing that the total amount of carbohydrate stored in the body is less than 2000 kcal, where does the body get energy in times of fasting or prolonged endurance exercise?*

# Fats

Fat is the second energy-yielding nutrient in the diet. Fat refers to the class of lipids that are solid at room temperature, whereas lipids that remain liquid at room temperature are termed oils. In health care settings, the term fat is commonly used when referencing both fats and oils. Similarly, the terms fat and lipid will be used in this book when referencing all lipids. Fats are normally classified into groups: simple fats (fatty acids and triglycerides), compound fats (fats in combination with other chemical groups—phospholipids, lipoproteins, glycolipids), and derived fats (sterols), as listed in Table 2.1.

## TRIGLYCERIDES AND FATTY ACIDS

Fats, like carbohydrates, are composed of carbon, hydrogen, and oxygen, but fats contain a lower ratio of oxygen atoms to carbon atoms when compared to carbohydrates. Since 95% of dietary fats and body fats are in the form of **triglycerides**, an understanding of triglyceride metabolism (formation and degradation) is essential to the comprehension of fat's nutritional role.

Although triglycerides come in many sizes and varieties, they all share a common structure. The "backbone" of the triglyceride molecule is a molecule of glycerol (*Fig. 2.5*). Glycerol is a carbohydrate derivative that contains three carbon atoms. Three fatty acids are attached to the glycerol molecule. Fatty acids can vary considerably in size and composition, but the basic structure of all fatty acids is a chain of carbon atoms bonded to hydrogen atoms and possibly oxygen atoms (*Fig. 2.6*). An acid or carboxyl group lies on one end of the fatty acid, while there is a methyl or omega group on the other end.

Two types of notation have been established to identify the chain length of a fatty acid as well as the number and position of any double bonds. The basic difference in the two types of notation is which end of the fatty acid is used to start counting carbons. For example, the fatty acid α-linolenic acid (Fig. 2.6), which contains three double bonds, is labeled 18:3 ω-3. This notation starts counting carbons at the carboxyl end of the fatty acid. The notation identifies the total number of carbons, the number of double bonds, and the location of each double bond. The second system of notation for α-linolenic acid starts counting carbons at the methyl end of the fatty acid. This system of notation identifies the total number of carbons, the number of double bonds, and the location of the first double bond. Using the second system of notation, α-linolenic acid is labeled 18:3 ω-3.

The fatty acid portion of the triglyceride molecule is the dominant type of fat used by the muscle cells for energy.

| Table 2.1 | CLASSIFICATION AND CHARACTERIZATION OF FATS | | |
|---|---|---|---|
| **Fat classification** | **Basic structure** | **Primary function** | **Dietary source** |
| **Simple fats** | | | |
| Saturated fatty acids | String of carbon atoms bound together with single bonds | Energy for cell functions and muscular work | Animal products, vegetables, nuts, grain products |
| Unsaturated fatty acids | String of carbon atoms bound together with at least one double bond | Energy for cell functions and muscular work | Vegetables, nuts, grain products |
| Triglycerides | Glycerol molecule bound to 3 fatty acids | Energy for muscular work, energy storage | Animal products, vegetables, nuts, grain products |
| **Compound fats** | | | |
| Phospholipids | Glycerol molecule, 2 fatty acids, plus a phosphate group | Membrane structure | Egg yolks, liver, soybeans, peanuts |
| Lipoproteins | Triglyceride and cholesterol core, phospholipid shell | Transport of lipids in liquid environments | Not consumed, assembled in liver and intestine |
| Glycolipids | Carbohydrate in combination with a lipid | Cell membrane structure | Not consumed, assembled in cells |
| **Derived fats** | | | |
| Sterols | Multiring structure | Hormone structure | Animal products |

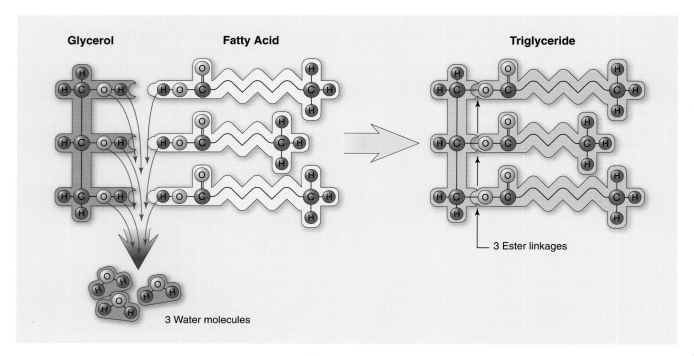

**FIGURE 2.5.** The structure of a triglyceride molecule. Three molecules of water are released as three fatty acids condense with the glycerol backbone when the triglyceride molecule is formed.

This fat energy is primarily stored in adipocytes (fat cells) and is liberated in times of energy need by the process called **lipolysis**. Lipolysis splits the triglyceride molecule into a glycerol unit and three fatty acids. The fatty acids are then taken up into the circulation and used as an energy source by contracting muscles. Triglycerides are also found in the sarcoplasm of muscle cells where they undergo lipol-ysis, and the respective fatty acids can be used for energy during muscle contraction.

Carbon atoms have four bonding sites. If all of the carbon atom bonds within a fatty acid are single bonds, then the fatty acid is saturated with hydrogen atoms (Fig. 2.6). If a fatty acid has one double bond, then it is monounsaturated. If two or more double bonds are found within a fatty

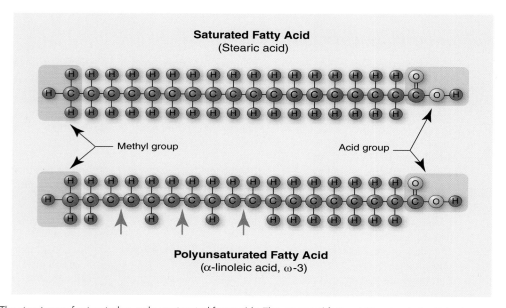

**FIGURE 2.6.** The structures of saturated vs. polyunsaturated fatty acids. The saturated fatty acid is saturated with hydrogens and there are no double bonds between carbons. The polyunsaturated fatty acid has a double bond between carbons numbered 3, 6, and 9 from the methyl end or carbons numbered 9, 12, and 15 from the carboxyl end.

acid, it is polyunsaturated. The positions of the double bonds within a fatty acid affect its chemistry. A polyunsaturated fatty acid with its endmost double bond situated three carbons away from the methyl end of the fatty acid is called an omega-3 fatty acid. Similarly, a polyunsaturated fatty acid with its endmost double bond situated six carbons away from the methyl end of the fatty acid is called an omega-6 fatty acid.

The human body can only synthesize fatty acids with double bonds coming after the ninth carbon atom counted from the methyl end of the fatty acid. This means that omega-3 (linolenic acid) and omega-6 (linoleic acid) fatty acids must be ingested since their double bonds come after the third and sixth carbon atoms, respectively. Those fatty acids that are available to the body only through ingestion are called **essential fatty acids**. Omega-3 and omega-6 fatty acids are essential fatty acids that are important for cell structures, certain immunities, vision, and hormone-like compounds. Box 2.1 provides a perspective on the different types of dietary fats containing various degrees of saturation.

**Box 2.1**

*PERSPECTIVE*

# Labeling Fats

The food that we eat today, with little exception, is highly processed. This processing involves the use of saturated fats, mostly from oils from tropical plants such as palms and coconuts. These oils contain mostly palmitic acid, a 16-carbon saturated fat. Saturated fats in the diet raise blood cholesterol levels more than do monounsaturated and polyunsaturated fats, or even dietary cholesterol itself. Since high blood cholesterol is a risk factor for heart disease, dietary guidelines have been developed to limit fat intake to a total of 30% of your total energy intake; of the 30%, less than one-third or 10% of total fat intake should be saturated fat.

It is nearly impossible not to consume processed foods in our culture. Therefore, saturated fats usually appear in our diets in quantities that could do harm in the long term. However, due to educational efforts and cooperation from the food industry, the use of tropical oils in processing is declining, with some manufacturers opting to print the words "no tropical oils" on packaged food labels. Consumers are well advised to avoid overconsumption of saturated fats by simply reading the ingredient lists on all food labels placed on packaged goods because saturated fats in the form of hydrogenated vegetable oils may still be used. Hydrogenation is a process that adds hydrogen to the double bonds of a polyunsaturated fat, thus making it saturated. So manufacturers may legitimately place the "no tropical oils" sign on the label while still putting forth a food product containing an abundance of saturated fat in the form of palmitic acid. The table below lists those oils common in the American diet and the relative percentage of different types of fats. The fats low in polyunsaturated fat can be seen clearly, making them the better choices in the marketplace. For heart health, therefore, we should all become label readers and strive to maintain a minimum of saturated fats in our diets.

| Fats | % Saturated | % Monounsaturated | % Polyunsaturated |
|---|---|---|---|
| Coconut oil | 90 | 8 | 2 |
| Palm kernel oil | 85 | 12 | 3 |
| Dairy fats | 65 | 30 | 5 |
| Palm oil | 50 | 40 | 10 |
| Meat fat | 50 | 45 | 5 |
| Poultry fat | 30 | 45 | 25 |
| Margarine, soft | 20 | 35 | 45 |
| Cottonseed oil | 28 | 20 | 52 |
| Soybean oil | 15 | 25 | 60 |
| Corn oil | 12 | 28 | 60 |
| Sunflower oil | 12 | 20 | 68 |
| Safflower oil | 10 | 15 | 75 |

Fats are not soluble in water and therefore do not mix well in body fluids. Because of this insolubility, fatty acids usually do not exist in a free form in the body. Circulatory free fatty acids are bound to albumin proteins in the bloodstream while they are transferred from their storage sites in adipose cells to other tissues in the body. Intracellular fatty acids are also bound to fatty-acid–binding proteins, although the exact function of these binding proteins has not yet been determined.

## PHOSPHOLIPIDS

Another class of lipids is the **phospholipids**, the most common of which come from the lecithin family. Similar to triglycerides, lecithins have a glycerol backbone with attached fatty acids (*Fig. 2.7*). However, only two fatty acids are attached to the glycerol molecule of a lecithin rather than three fatty acids (as with a triglyceride). In the place of the third fatty acid is a phosphate group attached to a choline molecule. Lecithin is the major constituent of cell membranes and helps maintain the integrity of the cell. Lecithins are not essential nutrients because all of the lecithins needed for building cell membranes and other body functions are synthesized in the liver.

## LIPOPROTEINS

In order for lipids to be transported in the circulation, they need to be packaged into lipoprotein carriers. **Lipoproteins** consist of a core of triglycerides and cholesterol that is surrounded by a shell made up of phospholipids with embedded proteins and cholesterol (*Fig 2.8*). There are many classes and subclasses of lipoproteins that are distin-

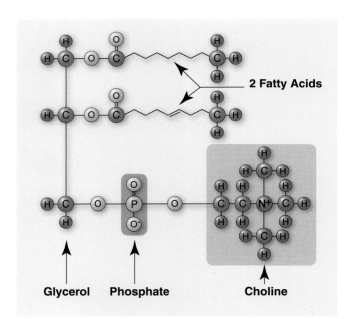

**FIGURE 2.7.** Structure of a phospholipid molecule. The structure of a phospholipid molecule is similar to that of a triglyceride molecule except that the third fatty acid of the triglyceride is replaced by a phosphate and choline group.

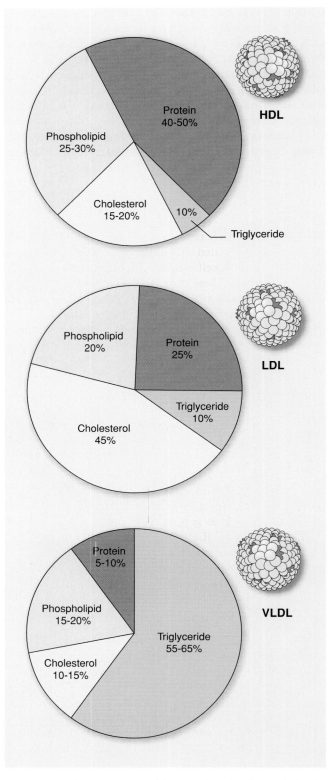

**FIGURE 2.8.** The composition of lipoprotein molecules. High-density lipoproteins have a higher concentration of protein than do low-density lipoproteins. As the lipoprotein becomes denser, the proportion of protein increases as the proportion of lipid (triglyceride, cholesterol, phospholipid) decreases. HDL, high-density lipoprotein; LDL, low-density lipoprotein; VLDL, very-low-density lipoprotein.

guished mainly by the size, density, and composition of their lipid core. Generally as the percentage of triglycerides in the core drops, the density of the lipoprotein increases. A lipoprotein with little triglyceride and a small core is denser than one with much triglyceride and a large core. A large amount of circulating lower-density lipoproteins has been associated with cardiovascular disease, whereas a greater amount of high-density lipoproteins has been associated with cardiovascular health. High-fat diets are believed to increase the amount of circulating low-density lipoproteins, whereas exercise is known to increase concentrations of high-density lipoproteins.

## GLYCOLIPIDS

Carbohydrates that serve a function in the cell membrane structure are associated with either proteins or lipids. Only about 10% of these cell membrane carbohydrates are associated with lipids. These carbohydrate-bound lipids, called **glycolipids**, reside on the cell membrane surface and are most often part of receptor sites that interact with hormones or other substances and allow for transport of materials across the cell membrane.

## STEROLS

The **sterols** are the last class of lipids in the body. Sterols are different from triglycerides, phospholipids, lipoproteins, and glycolipids in that they have a multiringed structure and lack the long-chain fatty acids of triglycerides and phospholipids (*Fig. 2.9*). However, sterols are synthesized from a derivative of acetic acid, a small fatty acid. Some of the most common sterols are cholesterol, testosterone, estrogen, cortisol, and vitamin D. Cholesterol is found only in animal foods, but it can be synthesized in the body if dietary sources are inadequate. Testosterone and estrogen are hormones, which regulate growth, development, and metabolic processes. Vitamin D is a separate nutrient that will be discussed later in this chapter.

## DIGESTION AND ABSORPTION OF FATS

Fats are difficult to digest because of their insolubility. Since fats do not mix with stomach fluids, fats are separated from other compounds in the stomach and little digestion takes place (*Fig. 2.10*). Once fat enters the small intestine, bile, which is made in the liver and stored in the gallbladder, assists with fat digestion. Bile is a yellow-green pasty material consisting of water, salts, acids, pigments, cholesterol, phospholipids, and electrolytes. The presence of fat in the intestine stimulates the release of bile from the gallbladder. The bile acids and phospholipids help mix fats and water so that the digestive enzymes can act upon the fats. This process of emulsification suspends the fats in tiny particles so that fat-digesting enzymes can digest the triglycerides. Once bile has done its job, it is recycled through the liver and stored again in the gallbladder.

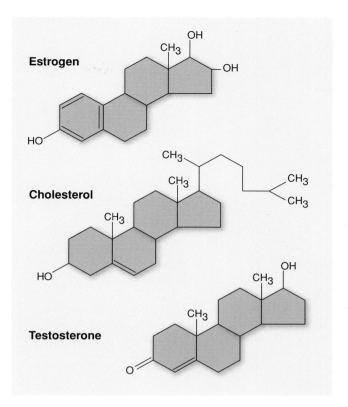

**FIGURE 2.9.** The common steroid structure as found in cholesterol, testosterone, and estrogen.

After the fatty acids are removed from the glycerol backbone, absorption can take place. Free fatty acids, glycerol, and even monoglycerides are small enough to pass through the cell membranes of the small intestine. These fat fragments are then reassembled into triglycerides within the intestinal cells. Most of the triglycerides, as well as cholesterol and phospholipids, join proteins to form lipoproteins. The lipoproteins are then packaged into **chylomicrons** (*Fig. 2.11*). Chylomicrons are released into the lymph system and thereafter are emptied into the veins of the neck.

## THE ROLE OF FATS IN THE BODY

Like carbohydrates, triglycerides have a primary role in the body to serve as an energy source. Unlike carbohydrates though, triglycerides are better storage compounds because they have a higher energy yield per gram and do not require water for storage. From a dietary standpoint, triglycerides provide satiety (feeling satisfied after eating) because they delay the emptying of the stomach after eating. Triglycerides also add texture and flavor to foods—this is the reason high-fat foods are very palatable. Fat-soluble vitamins are carried to the intestine by triglycerides where triglycerides assist in vitamin absorption. Triglycerides stored in adipose tissue insulate the body and provide protection. Subcutaneous fat insulates the whole body while fat pads surrounding internal organs provide protection to those organs.

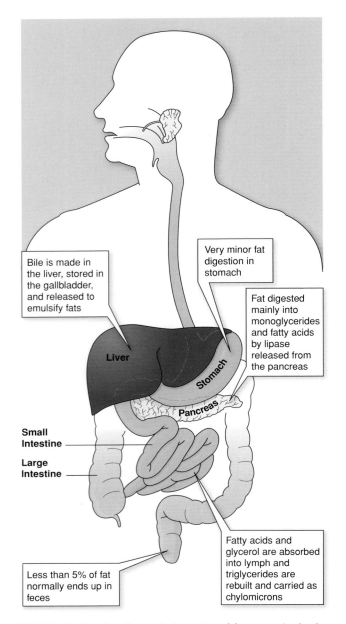

Bile is made in the liver, stored in the gallbladder, and released to emulsify fats

Very minor fat digestion in stomach

Fat digested mainly into monoglycerides and fatty acids by lipase released from the pancreas

Liver

Stomach

Pancreas

Small Intestine

Large Intestine

Fatty acids and glycerol are absorbed into lymph and triglycerides are rebuilt and carried as chylomicrons

Less than 5% of fat normally ends up in feces

**FIGURE 2.10.** The digestion and absorption of fats. In order for fats to be digested, they need to become soluble. Bile that is formed in the liver and stored in the gallbladder is released into the small intestine to help emulsify or solubilize the fat so enzymes can break it down.

Lecithin is a major constituent of cell membranes, and it helps emulsify fat in the intestine before digestion. Sterols found in bile acids also act as emulsifiers. Other sterols are found in hormones like testosterone and estrogen. Sterols are also incorporated into cell membranes. Vitamin D, which is a fat-soluble vitamin, has a steroid structure. Although phospholipids and sterols constitute only 5% of the total lipids, their physiologic role is critical.

▶ *INQUIRY SUMMARY.* Fat is not only a primary source of energy for the body but is also necessary for the formation

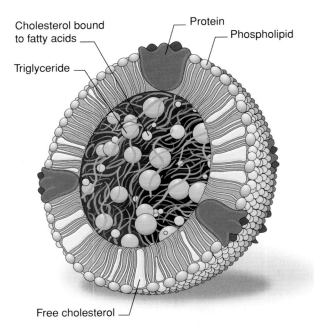

Cholesterol bound to fatty acids

Triglyceride

Protein

Phospholipid

Free cholesterol

**FIGURE 2.11.** The chylomicron. Digested fats are packaged into chylomicrons so they can be transported in the blood to tissues in the body. Chylomicrons are composed of 80%–90% triglycerides, 2%–7% cholesterol, 3%–6% phospholipids, and 1%–2% protein.

of membrane structures and hormones and for insulation and protection of vital organs. *If fat is so essential to bodily functions, why do you suppose many people in our society have become fearful of eating fat?*

## Proteins

Proteins are chemical compounds that contain carbon, hydrogen, oxygen, nitrogen, and sometimes sulfur, phosphorus, and iron. Just as carbohydrates and fats are made up of simpler subunits, proteins are made up of subunits called **amino acids**. There are 20 different types of amino acids in the diet. Nine of the amino acids cannot be synthesized by the body and are therefore essential to the diet. These are called essential amino acids. The remaining amino acids are nonessential because they can be synthesized in the body if the proper components are available.

Although each amino acid is characteristically distinct from all other amino acids, there is a common structure that distinguishes amino acids from other chemical compounds. An amino group ($NH_2$) and acid group (COOH) are both attached to a central carbon in every amino acid (*Fig. 2.12*). The remaining amino acid side chain is what differentiates one amino acid from another.

Proteins are constructed by linking amino acids to each other to form a chain. One amino acid is joined to another by a **peptide bond**. The peptide bond is formed by connecting the carboxyl group (−COOH) from one

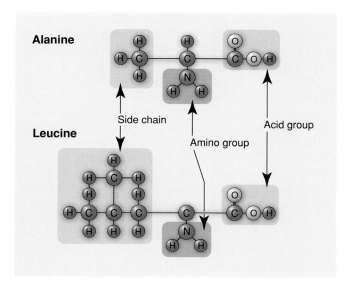

**FIGURE 2.12.** The basic amino acid structure. The side chain of amino acids distinguishes one amino acid from another. Each amino acid, however, has an amino group and an acid group.

amino acid to the amino group ($-NH_2$) of another amino acid. Two amino acids, joined together by a peptide bond, form a **dipeptide** (*Fig. 2.13*), whereas a **tripeptide** contains three amino acids. An **oligopeptide** describes a chain of 4 to 10 amino acids, and a **polypeptide** contains more than 10 amino acids. The sequence of amino acids in a protein chain is what individualizes that particular protein. As there are 20 amino acids that can be combined and replicated in any fashion to form a protein, the possible number of proteins the body can synthesize is enormous.

Protein synthesis in the body is dependent upon the availability of the amino acid building blocks for the specific proteins to be constructed. Dietary protein nutrients that contain the proper quantity and ratio of essential amino acids to maintain proper protein turnover in the body, as well as allow for growth and repair, are known as **complete proteins**. Incomplete proteins are either deficient in one or more of the essential amino acids or lack the proper ratio of the essential amino acids necessary for proper protein balance.

Disorders of amino acid processing can be defects in either the breakdown of amino acids or their transport into cells. The most common of these disorders is **phenylketonuria** (PKU), a disorder in which the enzyme that processes the amino acid phenylalanine is missing. Most phenylalanine is converted to tyrosine, another amino acid, and eliminated from the body. Without the enzyme that converts phenylalanine to tyrosine, phenylalanine builds up in the blood and becomes toxic to the brain, causing mental retardation. Early diagnosis is made when a high phenylalanine level and low tyrosine level are detected during the screening of a newborn. If not treated, affected infants soon develop severe mental retardation.

Treatment consists of severely restricting the intake of phenylalanine. Since phenylalanine is common to all protein sources, consuming enough protein without exceeding the acceptable amount of phenylalanine is impossible. Consequently, a person must eat a variety of synthetic foods that supply the other amino acids. Low-protein natural foods, such as fruits, vegetables, and restricted amounts of certain grain cereals, can be eaten.

## DIGESTION AND ABSORPTION OF PROTEINS

Digestion of proteins begins in the stomach (*Fig. 2.14*). Cells lining the stomach walls secrete a protein digestive enzyme called pepsinogen. Pepsinogen itself is not active in breaking down proteins but becomes active through contact with the hydrochloric acid in the stomach. The active pepsinogen is now called pepsin. Pepsin breaks the protein into individual amino acids and polypeptides of varying lengths. When these polypeptides enter the small intestine, other enzymes split them into smaller peptides and amino acids. Some of these enzymes come from the intestine, and some come from the pancreas. The pancreatic enzymes are released into the small intestine in response to protein being present in the intestine. The amino acids,

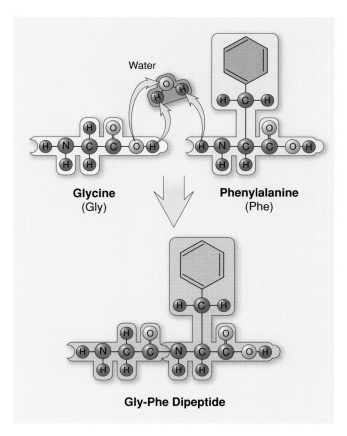

**FIGURE 2.13.** The formation of a peptide through a hydrolysis reaction. The amino group from one amino acid combines with the acid group from another amino acid to form a peptide bond. The resulting structure is a protein fragment called a peptide.

even during moderate intensity exercise. During very intense exercise, the contribution of protein to the energy pool can be 10% to 20%. A small portion of this protein-derived energy is obtained by utilizing amino acids directly as an energy source. The major portion of protein-derived energy, however, is obtained by converting amino acids, like alanine, to glucose and then metabolizing the glucose. Under these conditions and those of starvation or carbohydrate depletion, protein is converted into glucose through the process of gluconeogenesis (making new glucose).

A major function of protein is regulatory. This includes the actions of some hormones, which are derivatives of amino acids; enzymes, which regulate chemical reactions; antibodies, which are integral parts of the immune system; and transport receptors, such as lipoproteins in the blood and receptor proteins in cell membranes. Box 2.3 provides an explanation of the role enzymes play in the regulation of chemical reactions in the body.

Another major function of proteins is structural. Muscles, connective tissue, and bone matrices are all composed of proteins. Most proteins are highly specialized, like the visual pigments in the eyes or the blood clotting factor proteins. A more general role for proteins is to maintain fluid balance. Large proteins that cannot traverse cell membranes help maintain **osmotic pressure** and hence fluid balance. Other proteins assist in the acid-base balance by buffering strong acids.

▶ *INQUIRY SUMMARY.* Proteins play a role in regulating every chemical reaction that occurs in the body. Proteins also are used for muscle structure, muscle contraction, hormone structure, immunity, transport of other molecules, blood clotting, vision, and maintaining fluid balance. *If proteins have such a major role in the body, why is it recommended that only 15% of our daily energy intake be in the form of protein?*

## Vitamins

Vitamins are carbon-containing compounds that are needed for important biochemical reactions in the body. There are 13 different vitamins that have been isolated, classified, and analyzed. Sources and functions of these vitamins are shown in Table 2.2. Recommended dietary intake has been established for these vitamins because the human body cannot synthesize them. Vitamins are not energy-yielding nutrients, but they facilitate energy-yielding chemical reactions and promote growth and development. Vitamins A, D, E, and K dissolve in fat and are called the **fat-soluble vitamins**. **Water-soluble vitamins** are thiamine ($B_1$), riboflavin ($B_2$), pyridoxine ($B_6$), cobalamin ($B_{12}$), niacin (nicotinic acid), folate (folacin or folic acid), pantothenic acid, biotin, and vitamin C.

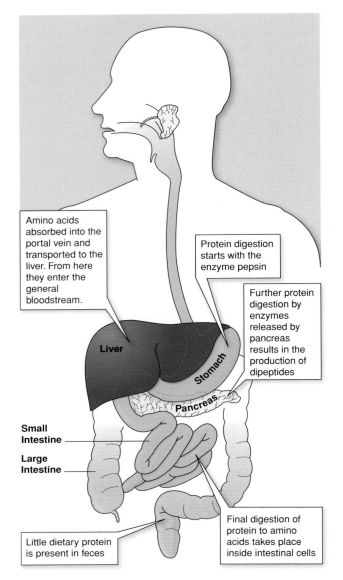

Amino acids absorbed into the portal vein and transported to the liver. From here they enter the general bloodstream.

Protein digestion starts with the enzyme pepsin

Further protein digestion by enzymes released by pancreas results in the production of dipeptides

Liver

Stomach

Pancreas

Small Intestine

Large Intestine

Little dietary protein is present in feces

Final digestion of protein to amino acids takes place inside intestinal cells

**FIGURE 2.14.** Protein digestion and absorption. Digestion and absorption of protein follows a process of breaking bonds among amino acids and forming fragments called peptides. The peptides are sequentially broken down into individual amino acids before they are absorbed by the small intestine.

along with some tripeptides and dipeptides, are taken up by active pumps on the cell membranes of the small intestine. These pumps carry the amino acids into the intestinal cells where they can be passed on further to the blood. The dipeptides and tripeptides that enter the intestinal cells are broken down into individual amino acids before being released into the blood.

### THE ROLE OF PROTEINS IN THE BODY

Unlike carbohydrates and fats, the main function of proteins is not energy supply. The contribution of protein to energy production at rest is negligible and minimal

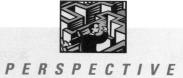

*PERSPECTIVE*

# Proteins as Enzymes

The dry weight of animal cells is nearly half protein, and almost 90% of this weight is enzymes. In fact, cells have been called "bags of enzymes" to emphasize the importance of enzymes in cellular processes. Single cells may contain as many as 1000 to 4000 different enzymes, each specifically suited for catalytic activity with a particular substrate molecule. Enzymes work by lowering the activation energy required to start the reaction process. This *catalytic* activity is important to maintain life processes; without it, cellular activity would proceed too slowly for life to be sustainable.

The amount of energy needed to speed chemical reactions to biologically useful rates is termed the energy of activation. An example of how enzymes work to control the rate of metabolism is seen in the following example:

$$\text{Glucose} + O_2 \xrightarrow{\text{enzymes}} CO_2 + H_2O + ATP + \text{energy} + \text{heat}$$

Without enzymes, this breakdown of glucose might take decades to occur instead of a fraction of a second. Though the equation depicts glucose breakdown in one step, this summary formula actually represents approximately 24 separate chemical reactions (three metabolic pathways in two main compartments of the cell), each catalyzed by a specific enzyme.

Generally, an enzyme binds to a substrate (e.g., glucose) to produce products (e.g., $CO_2$, $H_2O$, and ATP). If metabolism is like a series of roads, the enzymes are the traffic controllers that control the flow of energy (ATP formation) in the cell.

Solubility bestows on vitamins many of their characteristic behaviors such as how they are absorbed, transported, stored, and utilized. Since fat-soluble vitamins are stored in fat and oily parts of foods, these vitamins are absorbed like dietary fat—with the assistance of bile acids. Once absorbed, the fat-soluble vitamins enter the lymphatic system before circulating in the blood, where they are transported by protein carriers. Excess fat-soluble vitamins are stored in the liver and adipose tissue and remain there until needed. This

### Table 2.2    SOURCES AND FUNCTIONS OF THE VITAMINS

| Vitamin | Primary role | Dietary source |
|---|---|---|
| **Fat-soluble vitamins** | | |
| A | Vision, immunity, growth, reproduction | Cooked carrots, sweet potato, spinach, mango, cantaloupe |
| D | Bone development, growth | Fortified milk, fortified cereals |
| E | Antioxidant | Wheat germ oil, safflower oil, cottonseed oil, sunflower oil |
| K | Blood clotting | Turnip greens, raw spinach, raw cauliflower, raw cabbage |
| **Water-soluble vitamins** | | |
| Thiamine | Energy production | Wheat germ, pork, ham, oatmeal |
| Riboflavin | Energy production | Yogurt, cereals, milk |
| Niacin | Energy production | Meat, poultry, fish-fortified cereals |
| Pantothenic acid | Energy production, biosynthesis | Chicken, beef, potatoes, oats, tomato products |
| Biotin | Biochemical reactions involving $CO_2$ | Cauliflower, peanuts, cheese |
| $B_6$ | Protein metabolism, blood cell synthesis, nervous system | Oatmeal, banana, chicken breast, bran cereals |
| Folate | DNA synthesis, cell division, protein metabolism | Fortified cereals, raw spinach, lentils, pinto beans, black beans |
| $B_{12}$ | Folate metabolism, nerve integrity | Clams, oysters, crab, salmon, fortified foods, tuna |
| C | Antioxidant, iron absorption, immunity, collagen formation | Orange juice, citrus fruits, tomatoes, strawberries, cantaloupe, mangos |

storage ability also differentiates the fat-soluble from the water-soluble vitamins, which are excreted through the urine when in excess. Storage of fat-soluble vitamins also allows the body to go for months and even years without intake of these vitamins, compared to only days or weeks for the water-soluble vitamins. However, the risk of **toxicity** is greater for the fat-soluble vitamins than for the water-soluble ones.

Therefore, when comparing the characteristics of fat-soluble versus water-soluble vitamins, you can think in terms of **deficiency** and toxicity. Water-soluble vitamins need to be consumed more frequently than fat-soluble ones because excess water-soluble vitamins will be excreted in the urine. This means a greater risk of deficiency with the water-soluble vitamins with a low risk of toxicity. On the other hand, excess intake of the fat-soluble vitamins can result in toxicity easier than with water-soluble ones because fat-soluble vitamins are stored more readily in the body; however, the risk of fat-soluble vitamin deficiency is low. The key is to make sure that the diet includes enough water-soluble vitamins but not too much of the fat-soluble ones. Think about this as you read through the following sections that describe the individual vitamins and some of their dietary sources.

## FAT-SOLUBLE VITAMINS

Except for vitamin K, the fat-soluble vitamins are not readily excreted from the body. The risk of toxicity from vitamins A and D is greater than that of vitamins E and K. A toxic effect from vitamin D can be seen when one consumes only ten times the body's need. In contrast, consuming just three times the body's need for vitamin A can lead to toxicity, particularly in pregnant women. Therefore, taking highly potent supplements of vitamins A and D can lead to health problems. On the other hand, since most multivitamins contain only one to two times the recommended intake, supplementation with a multivitamin generally will not lead to adverse effects. Deficiency in the fat-soluble vitamins is not commonly seen in the United States and Europe, whereas it is seen more often in third world countries where starvation and poverty are more prevalent.

### Vitamin A

Vitamin A was the first fat-soluble vitamin to be recognized. It comes in three forms which are somewhat interconvertable: retinal, retinol, and retinoic acid. Retinol is the active form of vitamin A and has a yellow color. Carotene is the precursor of retinol and is a bright orange. The conversion of carotene to retinol is not a one-for-one exchange—three units of carotene are required to synthesize one unit of retinol. Therefore, nutritionists express the nutrient content of foods as retinol equivalents rather than units of carotene since retinol is the active form of vitamin A.

Vitamin A is the most versatile of the fat-soluble vitamins because of its role in many physiologic processes. The most recognized role of vitamin A is in vision, especially night vision. Vitamin A allows for light perception at the retina and clearness of vision at the cornea. Other functions of Vitamin A include:

- Maintenance of cell membrane stability
- Assistance in the synthesis of cortisol
- Assistance in the production of red blood cells
- Assistance in immune reactions
- Maintenance of nerve impulse transmission capacity
- Regulation of thyroxin secretion from the thyroid gland

Dietary sources for vitamin A or its precursor, carotene, include beef liver, carrots, sweet potatoes, green vegetables, milk, butter, cheese, and fortified margarines and spreads.

### Vitamin D

Vitamin D is different from all of the other vitamins in that it is not an essential nutrient. Skin cells exposed to sunlight can make all the vitamin D necessary for the body in the absence of dietary sources. Ultraviolet rays from the sun hit 7-dehydrocholesterol, the precursor of vitamin D, which over the next 36 hours will undergo a series of reactions that ultimately convert it to active vitamin D.

Vitamin D is somewhat like a hormone in that it is synthesized in one part of the body, is secreted into the blood, and exerts its action on a specific tissue. The function of vitamin D is to regulate blood calcium levels. When blood calcium levels are low, the parathyroid gland releases parathyroid hormone. This stimulates the kidney to release calcitriol, the active form of vitamin D. The rise in blood parathyroid hormone and calcitriol (vitamin D) will elevate the blood concentration of calcium by increasing its absorption from the intestines, withdrawing calcium from the bones into the blood, and stimulating calcium retention by the kidneys. High blood calcium levels cause the thyroid gland to release calcitonin and the parathyroid gland to stop releasing parathyroid hormone. Calcitonin reverses the release of calcium from the bones, shifting the flux of calcium toward bone synthesis. Decreased parathyroid levels inhibit the release of calcitriol (vitamin D) from the kidney, slowing calcium absorption.

The recommendation for vitamin D in children is twice that of mature adults to promote proper growth and development. For this reason, milk is highly fortified with vitamin D. Other dietary sources of vitamin D include cod-liver oil, eggs, dairy products, and fortified margarines or spreads.

### Vitamin E

Vitamin E is actually a family of compounds known as the tocopherols and tocotrienols. Vitamin E is one of the body's **antioxidants**. An antioxidant donates electrons or hydrogen ions to an electron-seeking compound and thereby protects other molecules from being oxidized. Vitamin E protects polyunsaturated fats and other fat-soluble substances, such as vitamin A, from destruction by oxygen. Vitamin E has an especially important role in the lungs, where cells are exposed to high concentrations of oxygen which can destroy their membranes. Red and white blood cells that pass through the lungs are protected by vitamin E. Within the mitochondria of the cell, vitamin E protects the process of transferring fuel energy to ATP. Overall, vitamin E exerts its protective role by:

- Detoxifying oxidizing radicals that are byproducts of normal metabolism
- Stabilizing cell membranes
- Regulating oxidation reactions
- Preventing unwanted oxidation of vitamin A and polyunsaturated fatty acids

Vitamin E is found in a variety of foods, but its major source is from vegetable oils found in salad dressings, margarines or spreads, and shortening. A smaller portion of vitamin E comes from fruits, vegetables, and grains. Animal fats such as milk, butter, and other dairy products have only negligible amounts of vitamin E.

## Vitamin K

The family of compounds known as vitamin K include phylloquinone from plants and menaquinones found in fish oils and meats. The K in vitamin K stands for koagulation (Danish spelling), which adequately describes the vitamin's role in the body. Vitamin K is essential for the synthesis of at least four proteins necessary for blood clot formation, including prothrombin. This vitamin also assists in the use of calcium by giving the proteins in bones, muscles, kidneys, and blood their calcium-binding potential. The major source of vitamin K is green leafy vegetables, while minor amounts are derived from cereals, meats, and fruits.

## WATER-SOLUBLE VITAMINS

The American diet generally contains adequate amounts of the water-soluble vitamins. Many common foods are fortified with B vitamins, and several beverages are fortified with vitamin C. However, some of the water-soluble vitamins are destroyed by heat during cooking, and all of them are subject to leaching into cooking water. The best way to retain the water-soluble vitamins during food preparation is to steam, stir-fry, or microwave. Since the first stages of thiamine deficiency can be seen after 10 days of exclusion and vitamin C deficiency after 20 to 40 days of exclusion, a consciousness of one's dietary intake of water-soluble vitamins is prudent.

## Thiamine

Recall that an enzyme is a protein that regulates the rate of a chemical reaction without being consumed itself in the reaction. Most of the B vitamins serve as coenzymes—they work with enzymes to regulate the rate of chemical reac-

tions. Enzymes are usually inactive unless their counterpart, the coenzyme, is present.

The coenzyme thiamine pyrophosphate participates in reactions in which $CO_2$ is lost from a larger molecule. The most common of these reactions occurs in the metabolism of carbohydrates (glucose). When pyruvate, which is a derivative of glucose, is converted into acetyl coenzyme A, $CO_2$ is released. Acetyl coenzyme A is the focal point of all energy-producing pathways in the body. Therefore, thiamine is vital to energy production in the cells. Foods containing large amounts of thiamine are pork products, organ meats, whole grains, and seeds.

## Riboflavin

The coenzymes of riboflavin are also important in the cellular metabolic reactions that produce energy. The specific metabolic role of the riboflavin coenzymes is to act as electron and hydrogen ion acceptors and donors. The active form of riboflavin is flavin adenine nucleotide (FAD), which can either receive hydrogen ions and the accompanying electrons from other entities (FADH) or donate the ions to other entities (FAD). Milk products, meats, and vegetables are the primary sources of riboflavin in the diet.

## Niacin

The niacin vitamin is found in two forms, nicotinic acid and nicotinamide. Nicotinic acid can easily be converted into nicotinamide, which is the active form of the vitamin. Niacin exists in two coenzyme forms, nicotinamide adenine dinucleotide (NAD) and nicotinamide adenine dinucleotide phosphate (NADP). NAD and NADP are like the riboflavin coenzymes in that they accept (NADPH, NADH) and donate (NADP, NAD) electron and hydrogen ions in chemical reactions. Hence, niacin is important in the energy-producing pathways of metabolism. Food sources of niacin include liver, lean meats, and legumes.

## Vitamin B6

The active coenzyme of vitamin $B_6$ is pyridoxal phosphate (PLP). Vitamin $B_6$ is necessary for the activity of more than 50 enzymes involved in carbohydrate, fat, and protein metabolism. The most important function of vitamin $B_6$ is in protein metabolism. As mentioned earlier, all amino acids have an $NH_2$ attached to a central carbon atom. The initial reaction in the breakdown of amino acids is the removal of $NH_2$ from the amino acid. The PLP coenzyme is necessary for this reaction to occur. Fruits and vegetables such as bananas, cantaloupe, broccoli, and spinach are rich in vitamin $B_6$. However, vitamin $B_6$ found in foods like meat, fish, and poultry is more absorbable than that found in plant sources.

## Folate

Folate is also known as folic acid and folacin. The primary coenzyme form of folate is tetrahydrofolic acid (THFA), which is a constituent of an enzyme complex that handles 1-carbon units that arise during normal metabolism. THFA is necessary for the synthesis of deoxyribonucleic acid (DNA) that occurs in rapidly growing cells. Most of the dietary folate is found bound to a string of amino acids, particularly glutamic acid (polyglutamate). Absorption of free folate or monoglutamate is performed in the intestine. Intestinal enzymes break the polyglutamate into its monoglutamate forms for absorption. Once absorbed, polyglutamate can be reconstructed in the liver and stored, or the monoglutamate can be methylated and sent to the gallbladder. From there, excess folate can be excreted or recycled. The methylated monoglutamate is recycled with the assistance of vitamin $B_{12}$. Folate is found in abundance in legumes, green vegetables, whole wheat products, fish, and poultry.

## Vitamin $B_{12}$

The coenzyme of vitamin $B_{12}$ has an integral relationship with folate in that vitamin $B_{12}$ assists the enzyme that removes the methyl group from methyl folate so the folate coenzyme THFA can be regenerated. Vitamin $B_{12}$ also maintains the myelin sheath that surrounds and protects nerve fibers and promotes their normal growth. Other metabolic processes seem to depend upon vitamin $B_{12}$. Vitamin $B_{12}$ is the only vitamin that is found almost exclusively in animal products. Therefore, people who consider themselves strict vegetarians (vegans) need to supplement their diet with vitamin $B_{12}$. Muscle meats, eggs, and dairy products contain adequate amounts of this vitamin.

## Pantothenic Acid

Pantothenic acid is a constituent of coenzyme A. Coenzyme A plays a vital role in fat, protein, and carbohydrate metabolism. Acetyl coenzyme A is a common factor in all aerobic metabolism. Typical diets seem to provide an adequate amount of pantothenic acid because it is abundant in a variety of foods including meat, fish, poultry, cereals, and legumes.

## Biotin

Biotin exists in two forms, biotin itself and biocytin. Biocytin is the inactive form of biotin that contains the amino acid lysine. The coenzymatic role of biotin is to assist in adding $CO_2$ molecules to other compounds. Metabolically, biotin helps to metabolize 3-carbon fatty acids, provide oxaloacetate for gluconeogenesis, synthesize fatty acids, and break down some amino acids. Legumes, egg yolks, cauliflower, peanuts, and cheese are rich in biotin.

## Vitamin C

Vitamin C, or ascorbic acid, is a 6-carbon compound with a structure similar to glucose. It is found in all living tissues, and most animals form their own vitamin C from glucose. However, humans cannot synthesize vitamin C, which makes it an essential vitamin. Vitamin C performs many

functions, the most common being that of an antioxidant. Vitamin C is important for iron absorption because of its antioxidant property. Vitamin C keeps the iron in its $Fe^{2+}$ form, which promotes its solubility and absorption. Vitamin C is important for the synthesis of many compounds that are necessary for metabolism and maintaining integrity of the biologic system. Some of the compounds are thyroxine, epinephrine, norepinephrine, carnitine, serotonin, bile acids, steroids, and collagen. Vitamin C is also vital to the proper functioning of the immune system.

Dietary requirements for vitamin C are easily met with a diet containing fruits and vegetables. Citrus fruits, tomatoes, cantaloupe, broccoli, green peppers, potatoes and strawberries all contain large amounts of vitamin C. Box 2.2 highlights what is believed to be the first scientific research experiment performed in nutrition, conducted by James Lind.

▶ *INQUIRY SUMMARY.* Vitamins are nutrients that do not provide us with energy and are only needed in very small amounts in the body. However, vitamins are necessary for everything from growth and development to energy production to protection against cellular destruction and disease. *Since vitamins are so important to our health, what are the pros and cons a person must consider prior to taking a vitamin supplement?*

## *Minerals*

Minerals are classified as either major or trace minerals according to the amount humans need each day. A mineral with a requirement of 100 or more mg per day is considered a **major mineral**, while a mineral with a requirement of less than 100 mg per day is considered a **trace mineral**. The terms major and trace refer to the required amount of a certain mineral, not its importance. For example, the daily iron requirement for a young woman is 15 mg. Iron is a vital component of hemoglobin, which is the protein in the blood that carries oxygen to the tissues. One can easily see that an iron deficiency can greatly compromise oxygen delivery to the tissues. Hence, iron is classified as a trace mineral, but it plays a major physiologic role.

### THE MAJOR MINERALS

The typical American diet tends to be too high in sodium. Thus, no **recommended dietary allowance** (RDA) has been established for sodium. This means that sodium is not a major mineral. Notwithstanding, the estimated minimum requirement for adults is 500 mg (1).

Sodium is a positively charged **ion** (or cation) that is a key factor in water retention. Sodium also helps maintain acid-base balance and proper nerve conduction. Depletion of body sodium is very unlikely because of the high amount of sodium in the typical diet. Even in extreme conditions, when a person loses several pounds of water

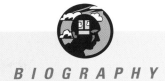

**Box 2.2**

*B I O G R A P H Y*

# James Lind

The physician James Lind can probably be credited with conducting the first clinical trial in nutrition. In the 15th and 16th centuries many European sailors, on long voyages to the Americas, developed the disease scurvy. These sailors ate very few fruits and vegetables during these voyages, and Lind discovered that citrus fruit cured the scurvy. The report that was published in London during 1758 describes the same scientific method that is used in clinical trials today.

On May 20, 1747, twelve sailors were taken with scurvy (*Observation: sailors on long voyages become ill with scurvy*). Lind was suspicious that some dietary mechanism was responsible for the disease because he noted that the diets of these sailors were all similar (*Hypothesis: lack of a certain food or the contents of a food causes scurvy*). All 12 of these sailors were housed together, and six pairs were given different diets (*Controlled experimental design*). Each pair of sailors received one of the following dietary supplements; 1 quart of cider per day, 25 gutts of elixir vitriol 3 times per day, 2 spoonfuls of vinegar 3 times a day, one-half pint or more of sea water per day, a concoction of nutmeg with other spices, or two oranges and one lemon per day.

Within only six days, one of the sailors eating the fruit was well enough to return to duty. By the time the boat arrived at Plymouth (June 16th), the other sailor who ate fruit had become well and was appointed to nurse the remaining ten sick sailors.

Soon after this discovery, British scientists discovered that lime juice prevented or cured scurvy. Subsequently British sailors were given a daily ration of lime juice, which earned them the nickname "limeys." It was not until 200 years later that scientists discovered that it was vitamin C, found in fruits and vegetables, which prevents scurvy.

---

through perspiration, sodium losses can be replaced through a normal diet.

The concentration of sodium in perspiration is about 0.2% compared to 0.3% in the blood. Accordingly, periods of heavy perspiration actually increase the concentration of sodium in the blood. Therefore, replacement of water lost through perspiration is much more important than conscientiously replacing the sodium. *How does this information affect the practice of taking sodium tablets after a hard athletic practice?*

Chloride is the ionic form of chlorine and forms an important negative ion (or anion) in extracellular fluids. Chloride is usually found in association with sodium (sodium chloride or table salt), but it is also a part of the hydrochloric acid found in the stomach. Most of the body's chloride is excreted by the kidneys, but some is lost in perspiration. Analogous to sodium, chloride deficiency is rare because of the high salt content of the American diet.

Potassium is a positively charged ion like sodium that serves the same function on the inside of the cell as sodium does extracellularly. In addition to regulating water content of the cell, potassium helps maintain membrane integrity of nerve fibers during impulse transmission. Potassium depletion or **hypokalemia** is also rare because fruits, vegetables, and legumes contain large amounts of this mineral. However, people who are using **diuretics** may be at risk for hypokalemia because some diuretics cause excessive potassium excretion.

Calcium is the most abundant mineral in the body. Although all cells need calcium, more than 99% of the body's calcium is found in the bones and teeth. Forming and maintaining bone structure is the most important function of calcium, but it is also necessary for muscle contraction, blood clotting, nerve transmission, and metabolic regulation of certain hormones and enzymes. Calcium requires an acidic environment to be absorbed; therefore, its absorption occurs primarily in the upper part of the small intestine where acidic stomach contents enter the intestinal tract. Calcium absorption also depends upon active vitamin D. For this reason, milk, which is rich in calcium, is fortified with vitamin D.

Poor calcium intake is not manifested for several years because the hormonal system maintains blood levels of calcium by leaching calcium from the bones. The bones, however, pay the price of chronic calcium deficiency. Osteoporosis, which occurs when bone mass is decreased with no evident external cause, is the most common problem associated with poor bone structure. Related effects of aging, poor diet, and hormones of menopause in women culminate to cause osteoporosis. A plan for prevention of osteoporosis is a lifestyle that includes moderate sun exposure (to promote synthesis of vitamin D), weight-bearing exercise (to promote bone growth), and a diet adequate in calcium.

Phosphorus is less of a concern in diet planning than calcium because it is absorbed very easily and is available in many foods. Vitamin D assists in phosphorus absorption as it does for calcium. Approximately 85% of the phosphorus in the body is found in the bones and teeth. The remaining phosphorus circulates in the blood and has specific functions in the cells. Phosphorus plays a part in one of the body's major buffering systems, the phosphate buffer system, in the kidney and intracellular fluids, where there is a high concentration of phosphates. It is part of DNA and ribonucleic acid, which contain the genetic material in every cell and are responsible for growth and development. Phosphorus is a part of ATP (adenosine triphosphate), which is the "energy currency" of the body. Many enzymes and B vitamins become active only when phosphorylated (phosphate attached). Phosphorus is also a part of the phospholipids that are constituents of cell membranes. Milk, cheese, bakery products, and meats are major contributors of phosphorus in the diet. Cereals, bran, eggs, and nuts also contain phosphorus. In addition to these natural sources, processed foods, such as soft drinks, are high in phosphorus.

Magnesium is another mineral that is found primarily in the bones and is absorbed with the assistance of vitamin D. The most prominent role of magnesium is as a cofactor in chemical reactions. More than 300 enzymes use magnesium as a cofactor. Many metabolic reactions require magnesium, including muscle contraction, cardiac function, nerve function, and protein synthesis. Good food sources of magnesium are whole grains, broccoli, squash, beans, nuts, seeds, chocolate, cocoa, and legumes.

The body does not use sulfur itself as a nutrient but uses it as part of other compounds. Sulfur is found in nutrients such as thiamine and all proteins. Protein structure is largely determined by sulfur-sulfur bonding within the protein molecule. Sulfur also helps with acid-base balance and with detoxifying drugs in the liver. Sulfur does not need to be consumed directly since it is naturally part of a healthy diet. Sulfur is also used in some food preservatives.

## THE TRACE MINERALS

The importance of trace minerals to humans has been recognized only within the past 40 years. Knowledge about trace minerals and their significance is probably the most rapidly growing area in nutrition. Researching the role of trace minerals is difficult because they are required in such small amounts. In addition, producing trace mineral deficiencies in laboratory animals requires sophisticated technology and much work. Human deficiencies in trace mineral intakes are rare, considering all of our mineral sources in food, air, and water. There are RDAs for only a few of the trace minerals, and most of these RDAs are just estimates.

Iron forms a part of the hemoglobin in red blood cells and the myoglobin in muscle cells. Both of these proteins (hemoglobin and myoglobin) assist in transporting oxygen throughout the body and within the cell. Iron is also important for the synthesis of certain metabolic enzymes, as well as some enzymes of immunity. Regulating iron absorption is important because the body does not excrete

excess iron that is absorbed. However, iron deficiency is rather common, whereas iron toxicity is rare.

*LINKUP:* **Research Highlight: Effects of Iron Repletion on Blood Volume and Performance Capacity in Young Athletes,** *found at http://connection.lww.com/go/ brownexphys and on the Student Resource CD-ROM, hightlights an investigation into how iron supplements affect* $\dot{V}O_{2max}$ *and exercise performance.*

Several factors augment the absorption of iron, including vitamin C, stomach acid content, demand for red blood cells, low body stores, and heme iron. Iron that is still a part of the hemoglobin or myoglobin molecule when consumed is called heme iron. Heme iron is absorbed twice as easily as nonheme iron. The greatest sources of heme iron in the American diet are animal products, particularly red meats.

When neither diet nor the body stores can supply the necessary iron for hemoglobin production, the number of red blood cells in the circulation is reduced. Anemia is the clinical term to describe the condition in which the red blood cell number falls low enough to affect the oxygen-carrying capacity of the blood. The greatest periods of risk for iron-deficient anemia are during infancy, preschool years, puberty, and childbearing years when menses occurs. Case study 2.2 illustrates how iron-deficiency anemia can affect women and their exercise performance.

It is beyond the scope of this book to detail the functions of all the trace minerals. Iron has been described in some detail due to its importance during exercise. Table 2.3 lists the trace minerals and briefly describes their functions along with examples of food sources rich in those minerals.

▶ *INQUIRY SUMMARY.* Minerals are nutrients that do not provide the body with energy. The recommended daily intake of minerals helps categorize them as either major ($\geq 100$ mg·day$^{-1}$) or trace ($< 100$ mg·day$^{-1}$). Although iron is considered a trace mineral, it serves a major metabolic role. *Why do you suppose a person with iron-deficiency anemia is often heard to say "I just don't have any energy"?*

## Water

Approximately 60% of an individual's body weight is water (*Fig. 2.15*). Water constitutes about 75% of the weight of muscle and 25% or less of the weight of body fat. Although different tissues in the body have different concentrations of water, total body water is in dynamic equilibrium. This means that whatever affects one compartment of water in the body will more or less affect all water compartments. A real-life example of this movement in body water can be demonstrated by a construction worker laying asphalt on the roads of South Carolina in the middle of August. This worker will lose a tremendous amount of body water by perspiring throughout the day. The water in the perspiration will come from all body water compartments,

## CASE STUDY 2.2: IRON-DEFICIENCY ANEMIA

### CASE

Jane is a 20-year-old college athlete who runs long distance for the track team. Over the past several months, Jane's running performance decreased substantially. She reported feeling fatigued with shortness of breath even during low-intensity exercise. These symptoms became more prevalent over the past month. Jane went to the sport nutritionist working with her track team and reported a history of heavy menstrual bleeding. Jane stated that she recently decided to become a vegetarian and stopped consuming meat 3 months ago. Jane also reported that she reduced her caloric intake in an effort to lose weight. The nutritionist performed an intake evaluation and referred Jane to her primary care physician. The physician ordered a complete blood cell count lab workup. The lab report showed the following:

| Blood Measure | Jane's Value | Normal Value |
|---|---|---|
| Hemoglobin | 8 g·100 mL$^{-1}$ | >11 g·100 mL$^{-1}$ |
| Hematocrit | 30% | 38%–47% |
| Transferrin | 7% saturated | ≥10% saturated |
| Ferritin | 15 μg·L$^{-1}$ | ≥20 μg·L$^{-1}$ |

### DESCRIPTION

The body recycles iron by taking it in red blood cells and recycling it to bone marrow to be used again in the formation of new red blood cells. The body loses large amounts of iron only when red blood cells are lost through bleeding, causing a deficiency of iron. Iron deficiency is one of the most common causes of anemia, and iron-deficiency anemia is usually indicative of gastrointestinal bleeding in men and postmenopausal women. Monthly menstrual bleeding may cause iron deficiency in premenopausal women. Iron deficiency is often found in adult and adolescent females, especially in female athletes who perform regular endurance training.

Iron-deficiency anemia usually develops gradually. The symptoms that usually develop in the later stages include fatigue, shortness of breath, inability to exercise, and dizziness upon standing (orthostatic hypotension). The stages of iron-deficiency anemia are:

1. Iron reserves are depleted because iron loss exceeds intake. Iron content in the bone marrow is reduced, and blood levels of ferritin progressively decrease.
2. Red blood cell production is diminished because depleted iron reserves cannot meet the needs of newly formed red blood cells.
3. Anemia begins to develop. Initially the red blood cells appear normal, but the concentration of them in the blood is low. Hemoglobin levels and hematocrit are reduced.
4. Cell division is accelerated in the bone marrow in an attempt to compensate for lack of iron. This results in the production of small red blood cells.
5. As iron deficiency and anemia progress, the symptoms of iron deficiency become more pronounced and the symptoms of anemia worsen.

### DIAGNOSIS

Stage 3 iron-deficiency anemia

### THERAPEUTIC RECOMMENDATIONS

Since iron supplements increase ferritin levels, transferrin saturation, and hemoglobin or red blood cell count, Jane was prescribed daily oral supplements of ferrous sulfate. She will meet with the dietitian for nutritional guidance on how to ensure adequate intakes of iron, vitamin B$_{12}$, and folate. Counseling will also cover the pros and cons of vegetarianism. The patient is to refrain from heavy exercise for one month. At one month, the patient will receive a complete blood cell count lab workup, and her prescription will be modified according to the results.

At her 1-month review, Jane's blood values improved: hemoglobin is 10 g·100 mL$^{-1}$, hematocrit is 40%, transferrin is 9% saturated, and ferritin is 20 μg·L$^{-1}$. She will continue with treatment for another month, at which time her blood chemistry will be tested again.

---

including the blood and different tissues. When the worker goes home at night and drinks plenty of fluids, the body water that was lost during the day is replaced. This replacement occurs in all the tissues of the body. Through this dynamic equilibrium, water content of the body remains relatively stable within an individual over time.

Rapid changes in body water content that cause an imbalance are quickly adjusted with either appropriate fluid intake or elimination. Thus, the proper balance of body water is maintained through fluid intake and output. Table 2.4 shows how much water is taken in and eliminated from the body throughout the day under normal conditions, as well during exercise in a hot environment. Obviously, fluid intake must be increased significantly during exercise in the heat to avoid dehydration and heat disorders. More information on fluid balance during exercise in extreme conditions can be found in Chapters 8 and 12.

**LINKUP:** *See* **Perspective: Water and Exercise** *at* **http://connection.lww.com/go/brownexphys** *and on the Student Resource CD-ROM for guidelines from the American College of Sports Medicine on fluid replacement during exercise.**

| Table 2.3 | TRACE MINERAL FUNCTIONS AND DIETARY SOURCE | |
|-----------|---------------------------------------------|---|
| **Mineral** | **Function** | **Dietary source** |
| Chromium | May assist insulin in regulating blood glucose | Vegetable oils, pork, egg yolks, whole grains |
| Copper | Part of enzymes regulating protein metabolism and hormone synthesis, aids in iron metabolism | Meats, liver, beans, legumes, whole grains, nuts |
| Fluoride | Increases resistance of teeth to decay | Fluoridated water, tea, toothpaste, dental treatments |
| Iodide | Part of thyroid hormone, regulates metabolism | Iodized salt, fish, dairy products, white bread |
| Iron | Part of hemoglobin, myoglobin, immune system, and cytochromes | Red meats, peas, broccoli, bran, seafood, enriched breads |
| Manganese | Part of some enzymes involved in carbohydrate metabolism | Rice, nuts, oats, beans |
| Molybdenum | Part of enzymes | Beans, grains, nuts |
| Selenium | Peroxide metabolism | Meats, eggs, milk, organ meats, seafood |
| Zinc | Part of enzymes that regulate growth and metabolism | Sea foods, meats, green vegetables, whole grains |

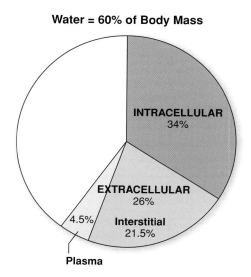

**Water = 60% of Body Mass**

**FIGURE 2.15.** The body water compartments. Approximately 60% of the body mass is water, which is distributed between the intracellular and extracellular spaces. Only a small fraction of the extracellular water is found in the plasma.

| Table 2.4 | HUMAN WATER BALANCE | | | | |
|-----------|---------------------|---|---|---|---|
| **Daily water intake** | | **Daily water output** | | | |
| **Normal conditions** | | **Normal conditions** | | **Heat and exercise** | |
| **Source** | **Amount (mL)** | **Source** | **Amount (mL)** | **Amount (mL)** | |
| Fluids | 1400 | Urine | 1500 | 500 | |
| Food | 800 | Skin | 600 | 5000 | |
| Metabolism | 350 | Lungs | 350 | 700 | |
| | | Feces | 100 | 100 | |
| Total | 2550 | | 2550 | 6300 | |

The body actually makes water during metabolism as carbohydrates, fats, and proteins are oxidized for energy (see Chapter 3). Since the formation of water during metabolism is minimal, the intake of water through the diet is critical to fluid balance in the body.

Body water serves various functions in the biologic system. One of these functions is to help regulate body temperature. This is done in two ways. Within the body, water can absorb a considerable amount of heat with only a small change in temperature. Outside the body, perspiration helps remove heat from the skin surface when it evaporates. Water also provides the proper environment for the biochemical reactions that occur inside the cells. The rates of many of these reactions are increased during exercise.

Another function of body water is to help maintain tissue structure and integrity. Since water is incompressible, tissue cells can maintain form and shape under various conditions. Finally, water is the basis for the transportation and communication systems of the body. Through the circulatory system, gases, nutrients, and waste products are transported throughout the body to and from every cell in every tissue. Hormones, which act to communicate messages between body parts, are also transported by the circulatory system.

Sweating during exercise of a moderate intensity can cause a water loss of about 0.5 to 1.5 L·hour$^{-1}$, whereas vigorous exercise can produce a water loss as high as 3.0 L·hour$^{-1}$. Water loss can be significant even when the exercise environment is not considered challenging (e.g., swimming, winter sports). Nonexercise-induced water loss can also occur when athletes are attempting to aggressively reduce or maintain a reduced body weight, such as that which occurs in sports like wrestling.

Just about any degree of dehydration will impair physiologic processes and impede body temperature regulation. A body water loss of just 1% of body mass (700 to 1000 mL) can significantly raise core temperature. Greater water losses (3% to 5% body mass) can impair sweating ability, decrease VO$_{2max}$, and decrease exercise capacity. As dehydration occurs, heat dissipation is reduced, heat tolerance is diminished, cardiovascular function is compromised, and exercise capacity is hampered. Exercise-induced water losses of 1.5% of body mass or more should be followed by a period of recovery and rehydration.

▶ *INQUIRY SUMMARY.* Water is probably the most important nutrient we consume. Not surprisingly, water is also the easiest nutrient to obtain. If it weren't for water, none of the other nutrients could exert their effects. *Describe how water is necessary for each of the other nutrient types to exert their effects.*

## *Dietary Guidelines*

By now you should be aware that different foods contain different nutrients and that no single food can provide all

of the nutrients in the amounts required. Nutrient deficiencies can cause disease, but overconsumption of certain nutrients can also be unhealthy. *How is it then that a person can plan their diet to get the proper amount of each one of the dietary nutrients? The answer to that question may not be as complex as it seems.*

The United States Department of Agriculture and Department of Health and Human Services have published guidelines to help Americans eat a healthy diet. *Nutrition for Your Health: Dietary Guidelines for Americans* is their 40-page booklet that outlines the basics of good nutrition; it can be downloaded from the website http://www.usda.gov/cnpp/dietary_guidelines.html. The overall message of the Dietary Guidelines is as simple as the ABCs (Table 2.5).

### FOOD GUIDE PYRAMID

The Food Guide Pyramid is the starting point for planning eating around foods you enjoy while being proactive in preserving your health (*Fig. 2.16*). Although you may have already seen the Food Guide Pyramid, you may not be aware of how its design so eloquently illustrates the fundamentals of good nutrition. Starting with the structure, the two-dimensional triangle and three-dimensional pyramid are the strongest geometric shapes that can be used in architectural design. Thus, the visual of the pyramid itself represents nutritional strength and solidarity.

The pyramid is divided into six segments, each representing a specific food group. The largest segment is the Bread, Cereal, Rice & Pasta group. This food group is placed at the bottom of and provides the foundation for the pyramid. Likewise, foods from this group should form the foundation of the diet. You should consume more servings each day from this group than any of the other food groups.

| Table 2.5 | THE ABC'S OF NUTRITION FOR AMERICANS |
|---|---|
| A | Aim for fitness<br>Aim for a healthy weight<br>Be physically active each day |
| B | Build a healthy base<br>Let the Food Guide Pyramid guide your food choices<br>Choose a variety of grains daily, especially whole grains<br>Choose a variety of fruits and vegetables daily<br>Keep food safe to eat |
| C | Choose sensibly<br>Choose a diet that is low in saturated fat and cholesterol and moderate in total fat<br>Choose beverages and foods to moderate your intake of sugars<br>Choose and prepare foods with less salt<br>If you drink alcoholic beverages, do so in moderation |

Adopted from: United States Department of Agriculture, Department of Health and Human Services. *Nutrition for your health: dietary guidelines for Americans.* Washington, DC: U.S. Government Printing Office; 2000.

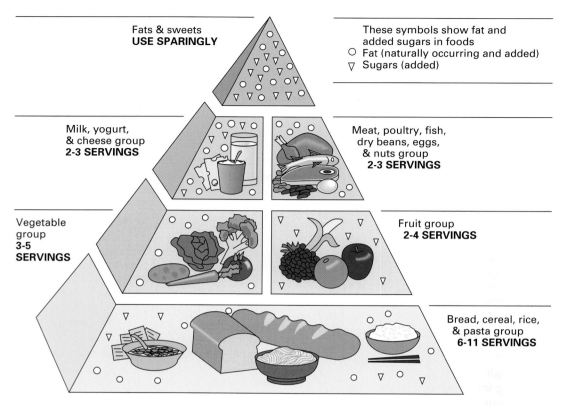

**FIGURE 2.16.** The Food Guide Pyramid. The Food Guide Pyramid provides a visual on how a healthy diet could be constructed. Source: United States Department of Agriculture and United States Department of Health and Human Services.

According to the guidelines, you should choose a variety of grains daily, especially whole grains. Whole-grain products contain more vitamins, minerals, and fiber than refined white grain products.

You build upon the grain base of the pyramid with foods from the Fruit and Vegetable groups. Americans are currently not eating enough fruits and vegetables daily. Programs like the "Five a Day" program have been promoted to encourage Americans to consume the minimum of three vegetable and two fruit servings a day. Fruits and vegetables should be eaten with the peel, if possible. The peel is high in fiber, and Americans are only consuming about 15 g of fiber per day, about half the recommended amount.

Notice that the bottom two tiers of the pyramid (grain, fruit, and vegetable groups) consist predominately of carbohydrates and make up about 60% of the volume of the pyramid. Similarly, it is recommended that 55% of your energy intake be carbohydrates (*Fig. 2.17*). Although Americans are currently consuming about 50% of their energy in the form of carbohydrates, a large portion of this carbohydrate intake is refined sugar. The daily intake of refined sugar in the United States amounts to approximately 100 g per day, or about one-half cup of sugar per day. It is easy to see that if Americans were to reduce their consumption of sweets and replace the sweets with fruits and vegetables, they would have adequate amounts of carbohydrate and fiber in their diet.

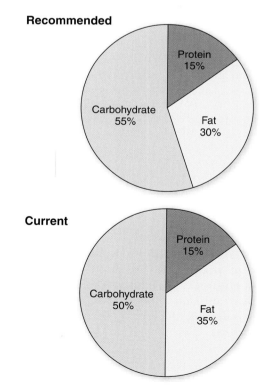

**FIGURE 2.17.** A comparison of what Americans are eating now with what is recommended. A shift away from fat and toward carbohydrate is all that is needed to bring our diet to what is recommended.

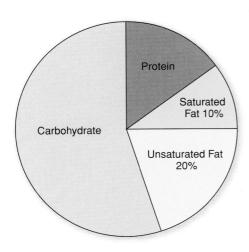

**FIGURE 2.18.** Recommended dietary intake for fat. The United States Department of Agriculture and the United States Department of Health and Human Services recommend that 30% or less of our energy intake be fat, with only 10% being saturated fat.

Much has been said over the past two decades about the health risks of a high-fat diet. Federal health agencies recommend reducing intake of total fat, saturated fat, and cholesterol. Indeed, much progress has been made over the past few decades. During the mid 1960s, 45% of our energy intake was derived from fat. Today the amount is approximately 35%. Although the proportion of our energy intake from fat has been reduced, our total energy intake (kcal·day$^{-1}$) has risen. This means that we are actually consuming more total g of fat per day. Hamburgers, French fries, and desserts contribute the most to our fat intake. Based on a 2000-kcal·day$^{-1}$ intake, it is recommended that total fat intake be limited to 65 g, saturated fat to 20 g, and cholesterol to 300 g (*Fig. 2.18*).

This recommendation brings us back to the Food Guide Pyramid. Notice the triangles and circles dispersed throughout all the food groups in the pyramid. The circles represent fat concentration, while the triangles represent sugar content. Also note how the two bottom tiers of the pyramid contain only small concentrations of sugar and fat, while the top two tiers contain a high concentration of sugar and fat. Focus now on the Milk, Yogurt & Cheese group and Meat, Poultry, Fish, Dry Beans, Eggs & Nuts group. These two food groups contain substantial amounts of fat. Food from these food groups can also contain substantial amounts of cholesterol. On the other hand, foods in the bottom two rungs of the pyramid contain polyunsaturated fats. By building the base of your diet on the bottom rungs of the pyramid, you can reduce the amount of total fat, saturated fat, and cholesterol in the food you eat. This concept is also emphasized in the ABCs of the Dietary Guidelines.

Do not interpret these recommendations to mean that foods from the upper portion of the pyramid should be removed from your diet; they just mean that smaller amounts of these foods should be consumed in comparison to foods in the lower portion of the pyramid. In fact, there are many foods in the upper portions of the pyramid that provide nutrients which cannot be obtained easily from foods found in the bottom of the pyramid. Foods in the Milk, Yogurt & Cheese group and Meat, Poultry, Fish, Dry Beans, Eggs & Nuts group are high in protein. Although both animal and plant foods contain protein, the quality of protein in these foods is different. As stated previously, proteins that contain the proper quantity and ratio of essential amino acids that are needed to maintain proper protein turnover in the body are complete proteins. Animal foods are rich in complete proteins, whereas plant proteins are incomplete. The only plant protein that is complete is soy. Although the protein in one plant food may lack certain amino acids, the protein in another plant food may be a complementary protein that contains the essential amino acids the first plant food is missing (*Fig. 2.19*). For example, the protein in milk can complement the protein found in breakfast cereal. The protein in legumes, such as kidney beans, complements the protein in pasta.

 *Experiences in Work Physiology Lab Exercise 2: Analyzing Your Diet outlines a lab experience in which you will evaluate the nutritional quality of your diet.*

## VEGETARIANISM

The number of vegetarians in the United States has doubled in the past 10 years. People often chose a vegetarian diet because of religious beliefs, concern for the environment, philosophies about animal rights, or concerns about health. Critics contend that vegetarian diets do not provide enough protein and other essential nutrients. However, with careful planning, a diet that contains no animal products can be nutritionally balanced and provide

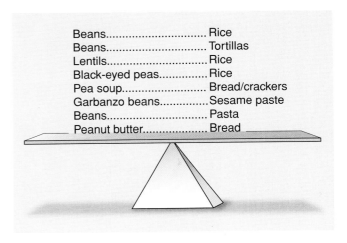

**FIGURE 2.19.** The balancing of complementary proteins in the diet. Protein in one plant food may be complementary to the protein contained in another plant protein. Balancing of complementary proteins can result in a diet adequate in complete proteins.

| Table 2.6 | TYPES OF VEGETARIAN DIETS | |
|---|---|---|
| **Type** | **Excluded Foods** | **Animal Foods Included** |
| Vegan | All animal products | None |
| Lacto-vegetarian | Eggs, all animal flesh | Dairy products |
| Ovo-vegetarian | Dairy products, animal flesh | Eggs |
| Lacto-ovo-vegetarian | Any animal flesh | Dairy products, eggs |
| Fruitarian | All foods except raw fruits, nuts, and green foliage | None |
| Pesco-vegetarian | Beef, pork, poultry | Dairy products, eggs, fish |
| Semi-vegetarian | Red meats (beef, pork) | Dairy products, eggs, poultry, fish |

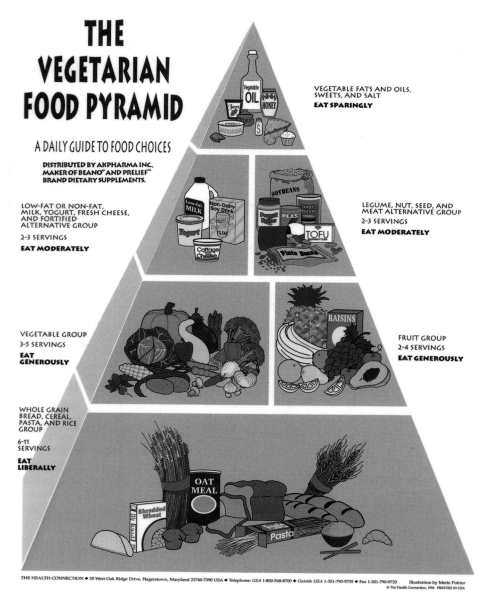

**FIGURE 2.20.** The Vegetarian Food Guide Pyramid. The Vegetarian Food Guide Pyramid provides a visual on how to construct a healthy diet without consuming animal products. Printed with permission from The Health Connection, Hagerstown, Maryland.

additional health benefits. Young adults frequently decide to become vegetarians because of their desire to lose weight or because of concerns about animal cruelty. Unfortunately, these inexperienced youth think that all they have to do to become a vegetarian is to stop eating animal products. If they do this without supplementing their diet or replacing the essential amino acids from animal food with high-quality complete proteins from plant food, they put themselves at risk for protein malnutrition.

The general rule is that the more limited the vegetarian diet, the more likely are the nutritional deficiencies (Table 2.6). Some people reduce this risk by becoming a semivegetarian—avoiding red meat but consuming small amounts of chicken, fish, or dairy products. This type of approach can ensure that they receive enough iron, zinc, calcium, vitamin D, vitamin $B_6$, and vitamin $B_{12}$— nutrients that are lacking in plant foods but found in abundance in animal foods. Vegans, who avoid all animal products, must supplement their diets with vitamin $B_{12}$ because it is not found in plant foods. The Vegetarian Food Guide Pyramid (*Fig. 2.20*) follows the same pattern as the Food Guide Pyramid and can be used similarly to help vegetarians plan a healthful diet.

▶ *INQUIRY SUMMARY.* The United States government has established dietary guidelines for Americans. These guidelines have been outlined in the Food Guide Pyramid and elaborated upon in the ABCs of good health. By following these guidelines, Americans can obtain all of the nutrients in the proper quantities and proportions necessary for optimal health. The foundation of our diet should be grains, fruits, and vegetables. Foods in these groups are rich in carbohydrates, fiber, vitamins, and minerals. Foods in the upper portion of the pyramid are also rich in vitamins and minerals, and they contribute high-quality protein to our diet. Vegetarian diets can provide all of the essential nutrients if they are carefully planned. *List some of the pros and cons of vegetarianism.*

## Summary

Nutrients are substances obtained from food that are used for growth, maintenance, and repair of tissues. Nutrients are organized into six different classes: carbohydrates, fats, proteins, vitamins, minerals, and water. The first three— carbohydrates, fats, and proteins—are energy-yielding nutrients that provide the energy for all energy-dependent processes of the body, including exercise. These energy-yielding nutrients constitute a major portion of most foods. The primary role of carbohydrates is to provide energy. Fats provide energy, insulation, protection, and assistance with vitamin absorption. Proteins provide a limited amount of energy, but they help regulate all chemical reactions in the body.

The last three nutrients—vitamins, minerals, and water—do not provide the body with energy, but these nutrients are necessary because they assist the body in using the energy from fats, proteins, and carbohydrates. Vitamins are used as cofactors in many metabolic processes, and they assist in the maintenance of health and protection against disease. Minerals are also cofactors in metabolic processes, but they have structural roles as well. Water provides the medium for all the biochemistry and communication in the body, and it plays a critical role in regulating body temperature. Although most of the nutrients have specific functions, many of them need to work in cooperation with other nutrients to perform their own functions.

The Food Guide Pyramid and the ABCs of health provide helpful advice on how to plan a healthful diet. By following these guidelines, you can promote good health and reduce the risk of chronic diseases such as heart disease, cancer, type 2 diabetes, stroke, and osteoporosis. The guidelines focus on building a healthy base and choosing sensibly. Although these guidelines are easily understood and available, some thought and planning is needed to derive the benefits of a healthy diet.

## SUMMARY KNOWLEDGE

1. What are the six classifications of nutrients?
2. What is the physiologic energy value for one g of carbohydrate, fat, or protein?
3. What are the differences among monosaccharides, disaccharides, and polysaccharides?
4. What are the different ways in which fats are classified?
5. What is the difference between a saturated and polyunsaturated fatty acid? Which of these is healthiest for you to consume?
6. What is a complete protein?
7. What are the primary roles for carbohydrates, fats, and proteins?
8. Describe the characteristics of fat-soluble and water-soluble vitamins.
9. What is the general role of vitamins in the body?
10. Are trace minerals any less important physiologically than major minerals? Why or why not?
11. Which minerals serve primarily metabolic functions and which serve primarily regulatory and structural functions?
12. Why is water the most critical nutrient of all?
13. Describe how the balance of water in the body changes during exercise.
14. Describe the six food groups in the Food Guide Pyramid.
15. What are the ABCs for health, and how do they relate to the Food Guide Pyramid?

### References

1. Whitney EN, Hamilton EMN, Rolfs SR. *Understanding nutrition.* 5th ed. St. Paul, Minn: West Publishing, 1990.

### Suggested Readings

Berning J, Steen SN. *Nutrition for sport & exercise.* 2nd ed. Gaithersburg, Md: Aspen Publishers, 1998.

Brown JE. *Nutrition now.* 4th ed. New York: Wadsworth Publishing, 2005.

Insel P, Turner RE, Ross D. *Nutrition.* 2nd ed. Boston: Jones and Bartlett Publishers, 2004.

Wardlaw GM, Hampl JS, Disilvestro RA. *Perspectives in nutrition.* 6th ed. Boston: McGraw-Hill, 2003.

### On the Internet

American Dietetic Association. Available at: **http://www.eatright.org**. Accessed March 25, 2005.

Society for Nutrition Education. Available at **http://www.sne.org**. Accessed March 25, 2005.

KidsHealth from the Experts at the Nemours Foundation. Available at: **http://www.kidshealth.org**. Accessed March 25, 2005.

National Center for Education in Maternal & Child Health. Available at **http://www.ncemch.org.** Accessed May 24, 2005.

American Society for Nutritional Sciences. Available at: **http://www.nutrition.org**. Accessed March 25, 2005.

International Food Information Council Foundation. Available at: **http://www.ific.org**. Accessed March 25, 2005.

Sports, Cardiovascular & Wellness Nutritionists (SCAN). Available at: **http://www.scandpg.org**. Accessed March 25, 2005.

USDA Center for Nutrition Policy and Promotion. Available at: **http://www.usda.gov/cnpp**. Accessed March 25, 2005.

## Writing to Learn

In this chapter we discussed the importance of each one of the six dietary nutrients. The Food and Nutrition Board of the National Academy of Sciences determines recommended nutrient intake levels that apply to healthy individuals. Research and write a paper about how Dietary Reference Intakes for the nutrients are determined.

## CHAPTER

# 3 Energy Sources and Production

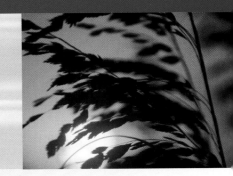

*Sunlight is the ultimate source of life for the planet, providing the necessary energy input for the production of food required by all life on earth.* In terms of physiologic, biochemical, psychologic, and sociologic responses, how else might sunlight affect humans?

## CHAPTER OUTLINE

ENERGY DEFINED
ENERGY FORMS
- Biochemical Reactions Are Linked
- Anabolism and Catabolism

PHOSPHATE ENERGY
- ATP—The Energy Exchange Currency
- Energy Flows from Creatine Phosphate to ADP

OXIDATION-REDUCTION REACTIONS

SARCOPLASMIC CATABOLISM
- The Energy Continuum
- Immediate Energy
- Short-Term Energy
- Lipolysis

MITOCHONDRIAL CATABOLISM
- β Oxidation
- Krebs Cycle
- Electron Transport Chain
- Tallying ATP

The "physiology of energy," which is the study of how the body produces, uses, and regulates energy to carry out biologic work, is a complex but necessary early step toward an understanding of the science of exercise physiology. Energy is the basis by which we move, and it is at life's very core. However, energy, like many other abstract concepts, is hard to grasp. Unlike matter, energy does not have mass and does not occupy space. We often see or feel the effects of energy on matter, but observing energy itself, and more importantly, defining energy, is a difficult task. For this reason, other terms are often used as synonyms or as a means to quantify energy. Terms like vitality, strength, and stamina express the idea of energy but lack the necessary scientific precision. Terms like power and work are much more useful in the exercise physiology laboratory as a means of quantifying energy transformation in exercise conditions. Chapter 5 of the text examines principles of energy measurement in exercise physiology. In this chapter, however, our goal is to study energy in its various forms and to explore ways in which biologic systems use and transform energy from one state to another to sustain life processes.

## Energy Defined

The study of energy is necessary for a review of exercise physiology because the basis of all movement involves cellular **bioenergetic** processes that power muscular contractions. Bioenergetics is the science that studies energy exchange events in living things, as opposed to the more general term, energetics, that refers to the physical science dealing with energy exchange. In the opening of this chapter, we mentioned that the sun is the ultimate source of energy. We now turn to the topic of energy to discover why this is so. As you study the "physiology of energy," you will discover that the fields of exercise physiology and biochemistry are interwoven to a remarkable degree.

*LINKUP: See Biography: Philip Gollnick at http://connection.lww.com/go/brownexphys and on the Student Resource CD-ROM to discover the connection between exercise physiology and biochemistry.*

At the outset, it is necessary to think of energy in two important ways: *inactive* (stored) and *active* (working) energy. **Potential energy** is stored energy, ready at any moment to do **work**. Examples of potential energy include an unlit firecracker, table sugar, or a rock at the top of a hill. In contrast, **kinetic energy** is energy working. Examples of kinetic energy include an exploding firecracker, burning sugar, and a rock rolling down the hill (*Fig. 3.1*). The boulder atop a hill has a large amount of potential energy because of its position, but it begins to transfer this potential energy to kinetic energy as it rolls down the hill. If you find it hard to imagine a rock rolling down a hill as transferring its potential (stored) energy to kinetic (working) energy, envision what would happen if that large boulder were to strike a wall after rolling down the hill. Kinetic energy *works* on that which it affects. In the case of the boulder hitting the wall, a change (effect) has occurred in the wall. Fortunately, energy exchange or transfer in the body does not involve such destructive change!

Energy is the basic necessity of all life. We need energy not only to move, but to perform the simplest of cellular functions. The term *work* is particularly suited to express the idea of energy because work is also synonymous with life itself. To live is to do work, even for the laziest of couch potatoes. In fact, if you were to lie motionless in bed for 24 hours, roughly the same amount of energy would be used as during an 18-mile race. The term work takes on significance at this point because from a physiological standpoint, our cells and organ systems never cease to work, even while we are at rest. This can be seen in the following examples:

- Cells "work" in pumping substances across membranes and in synthesizing new compounds
- The heart "works" by pumping large amounts of blood throughout the body continually
- Skeletal muscles "work" to maintain our erect posture even when we are not moving

Energy, therefore, is related to the ability to perform work. A release of energy is necessary to perform useful work, and it also generates heat in the process. In fact, virtually all of the energy spent by the body eventually ends up as heat.

Kinetic energy is energy working. This work affects matter by a transfer of motion to other objects, such as happens when flowing water turns a turbine. The term work, though, can be confusing because we must know the precise energy form involved to know the type of work being performed. Work, in its mechanical form, is defined as the product of a given force acting through a given vertical distance. Mechanical work is performed, for example, when the forearm mass is rotated at the elbow. Our cells perform both chemical and electrical work more often than mechanical work, with energy conversions taking place in the process. The following are examples of biologic work:

- Glandular secretion
- Tissue synthesis
- Vitamin D production
- Muscle contraction
- Digestion
- Nerve function
- Sight
- Cell growth and repair

At this point, two principles of bioenergetics (the laws of thermodynamics) are important to understand before moving on with the definition of energy.

The **first law of thermodynamics** states that energy is neither created nor destroyed but can only be converted from one form to another. The couch potato mentioned earlier would soon encounter this law if he/she continued to live an inactive lifestyle and continued to eat a normal amount of food. Weight gain or loss conforms to the first law in the following equation:

$$\text{Energy intake (food consumption)} = \text{Energy output} \ \text{(work} + \text{heat)} + \text{Energy stored (as fat)}$$

In a practical sense, the average overweight individual is all too familiar with this principle. Examining the equation closer, we can readily see the first law in action. If energy intake exceeds energy output, the result is a transformation of the energy originally in the food to the chief storage form of energy in our body—fat. In this example, energy has been conserved in the form of energy-rich matter, but new energy has not been created. Likewise, a power plant does not create energy; it merely transforms energy from one form (fossil fuel) to another (electricity). If you want to lose weight, you have to convert stored energy (fat) to heat and mechanical energy (work). Losing weight is a matter of losing excess energy.

The **second law of thermodynamics** states that the process of energy transformation leads to a large amount of energy, usually in the form of heat, being lost. All forms of biologic work (including muscle contraction) are notoriously inefficient since most of the energy in cellular activity is lost as heat. Efficiency is an important

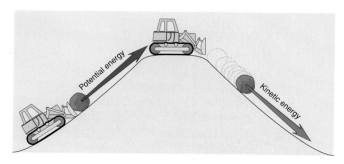

**FIGURE 3.1.** As the rock ascends the hill, it gathers more potential energy. From its position at the hilltop, the large amount of potential energy can be converted easily to kinetic energy. The rock performs work as it rolls down.

concept in everyday life because we all want, for instance, the most mileage for a given gallon of gas in our cars. Yet, most internal combustion engines are less than 25% efficient. That is, only 25% of the energy released when gasoline is burned in the engine is transformed to useful mechanical energy that allows the car to move. In fact, our body is not much more efficient than this during various kinds of activities! The second law states that in these energy conversions most of the energy will not be available to perform useful work but instead will be lost. The ultimate effect of this "lost" energy is an increase in randomness and disorder, called **entropy** in the science of energetics. Using the car example, the heat released cannot perform work since it is in random molecular motion, not a useful form of energy. The heat released represents the inherent inefficiency in any form of energy transformation. In our bodies the heat released from the breakdown of energy nutrients, while not usable by the cell, does accomplish at least two important purposes: maintains body temperature and helps to increase the rate of chemical reactions within the body.

Along with these concepts, it is also important to know that a release of energy directly results in a change in a system (a cell, an organ, a muscle group, or an individual). Energy release always involves change, but we must have an understanding of energy forms to understand energy transformations. The heat given off by the body during exercise can be measured and partitioned into evaporative and a combination of radiative, convective, and conductive heat loss (refer to Chapter 8).

 *Experiences in Work Physiology Lab Exercise 3: Temperature Regulation During Exercise presents a simple experiment you can perform in most exercise physiology laboratories to measure heat loss during exercise.*

▶ **INQUIRY SUMMARY.** Energy is the ability to do work or cause change. Potential energy is available to do work, and kinetic energy is energy being used to do work. The laws of thermodynamics govern energy transformations in the universe, whether on a planetary scale or inside our cells. The first law states that energy cannot be created or destroyed but only converted from one form to another. The second law states that systems (our bodies or cells) naturally tend toward increasing entropy (disorder). *How do the laws of thermodynamics relate to energy flow in our bodies or to your everyday life? In what ways do we use energy to survive?*

## Energy Forms

The six forms of energy are: (1) atomic, (2) radiant, (3) thermal, (4) chemical, (5) electrical, and (6) mechanical. According to the first law of thermodynamics, any of these six forms can be converted to another form. For example,

our bodies transform the chemical energy in food (i.e., sugar) to electrical and mechanical energy and heat. Common household appliances convert electrical energy to light and heat.

The order in which these six forms are listed above is meant to relay the direction in which energy transformation affecting life on our planet takes place. All of the energy processes on earth are "driven" first by energy transformations on the sun in the form of nuclear fusion reactions (atomic energy), which convert more than 120 metric tons of solar matter into radiant energy each minute. The resultant release of heat and light into space warms the planet and drives chemical processes in plant life. Only a small fraction (about two-billionths) of this energy release ever hits the earth's upper atmosphere. About one-third of the energy hitting the atmosphere is reflected back into space, and of the remaining, only about 1% of the light "harvested" on the planet is transformed into chemical energy in plants.

### BIOCHEMICAL REACTIONS ARE LINKED

Virtually all life depends on this amount of light energy (contained in "packets" called photons) bombarding the earth and producing chemical changes in plants. Using this light energy, plants convert $CO_2$ and water ($H_2O$) into the food molecules (carbohydrates, fats, and proteins) we consume. This process, called photosynthesis, involves a "coupling" of energy reactions—the nuclear reactions of the sun with photosynthesis on the planet. This linking of one kind of energy transformation (nuclear to light) to another kind (light to chemical) on a planetary scale is mirrored on a much smaller scale inside every living cell on earth. That is, coupled reactions are paired for the purpose of driving biosynthesis—the building up of large biomolecules from smaller ones (also called **anabolism**). In one reaction the free energy liberated is used to make other reactions proceed. *Figure 3.2* illustrates this point. As reactants high in energy are broken down to products in one set of reactions, the release of free energy "drives" another set of reactions to form products. In the second set of reactions, products with a higher energy content are formed through a process of **endergonic** (energy adding) reactions. These anabolic reactions are biosynthetic, whereas **catabolic** (breaking down) reactions involve the degradation of larger biomolecules to smaller ones.

Coupled reactions involve a linking of **exergonic** reactions, those resulting in a net loss of free energy (the sun's loss of energy into space), with endergonic reactions, those resulting in a net gain in free energy (plants "trapping" this light energy and increasing their total energy content in the process). In the case of biologic systems, the coupling that occurs in the cells is designed to facilitate movement through the constant resupply of important energy carrier molecules—the high-energy phosphates, of which adenosine triphosphate (ATP) is the most important (*Fig. 3.3*).

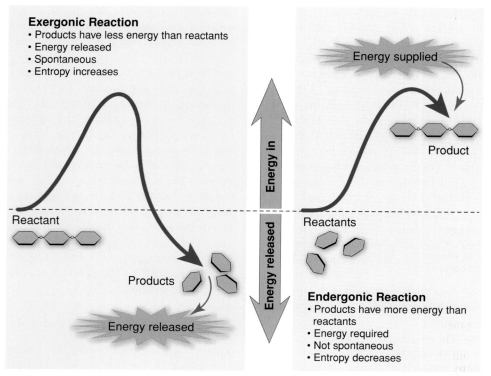

**FIGURE 3.2.** Illustration of coupled reactions: exergonic and endergonic reactions. In chemical reactions the exergonic release of free energy in one set of reactions powers the endergonic formation of new products that have a higher energy yield than the original reactants. The laws of thermodynamics dictate that a reaction will not proceed spontaneously unless the molecules that result from the reaction, the products, have lower energy than the molecules that began the reaction, the reactants.

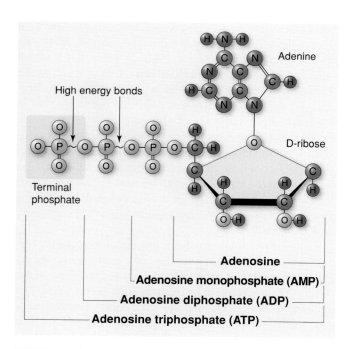

**FIGURE 3.3.** The structure of ATP. The terminal phosphate bond is hydrolyzed in coupled reactions, and the resultant free energy release is the "cause" of many cellular activities, including muscle contraction.

In this biologic cycling of energy, both free energy (the energy available at any moment to do cellular work) and potential energy (the energy stored in chemical form) are constantly depleted and resupplied in cellular processes with the goal to maintain a **steady-state** phosphate supply in the cell. Bioenergetics uses many other important substances, both at rest and in exercise, in chemical processes known as **metabolism**.

## ANABOLISM AND CATABOLISM

Anabolism and catabolism, the two components of metabolism, are related to each other through energy coupling. *Figure 3.4* depicts a simplified version of this relationship in which the cellular breakdown of energy nutrients (left side) allows for the transfer of free energy to "energy carrier" compounds whose subsequent breakdown powers biosynthesis. All of these reactions are enzymatically controlled. The rate at which they proceed is dependent on **substrate** and enzyme availability, energy need of the cell, and physical conditions like temperature and acidity of the cell. Cellular **energy charge** is particularly controlling, as indicated in *Figure 3.5*, which shows that ATP-generating metabolic pathways in the cell are inhibited by a high-energy charge,

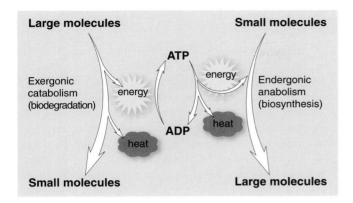

**FIGURE 3.4.** The design of metabolism showing that energy derived from catabolic reactions cannot be used directly by anabolic reactions but must first go through an intermediary process (synthesis of ATP) through which the free energy from food sources enables cellular "work," such as muscle contraction.

while ATP-utilizing metabolic pathways are stimulated by a high-energy charge. The energy charge of the cell can have a value ranging from 0 (all adenosine monophosphate [AMP]) to 1 (all ATP). When the energy charge of the cell is low (towards 0 on the X-axis of the plot), as is the case in exercise, the relative rate of generating ATP is high in an effort to maintain muscular ATP concentrations. As shown in Figure 3.5, processes which utilize ATP for biosynthesis are relatively less active at this point. However, as the energy charge increases (towards 1 on the X-axis), a reversal of this situation occurs. Energy charge is thus maintained within narrow limits. These processes represent a "balancing act" between catabolism and anabolism upon which cell function is dependent.

Enzymes are protein molecules that serve as biologic catalysts. That is, they accelerate the rate of chemical reac-

tions but remain largely unchanged in the process while reactants change into products. The rate of chemical reactions typically increases by many thousand-fold to million-fold when catalyzed by enzymes. Enzymes make it possible for "spontaneous" reactions to proceed at rates fast enough to be physiologically useful. They accomplish this by lowering an energy barrier, called the **energy of activation**, which tends to impede the rate of spontaneous reactions. Once the activation energy is lowered, the probability of the reaction occurring is greatly increased. If movement has a bioenergetic origin, then enzymes are key ingredients in this equation.

**Metabolic pathways** are controlled by enzymes in step-by-step sequences in which the product of one reaction becomes the starting point (substrate) for another. The chemical reactions of metabolism either absorb or release energy. For example, the complete breakdown of glucose in a cell releases energy as ATP (available to do work) and heat (unavailable to do work). The chemical equation below demonstrates this simple concept:

$$Glucose + O_2 \Leftrightarrow CO_2 + H_2O + ATP + Heat$$

▶ *INQUIRY SUMMARY.* Some of the predominant activities of our cells involve changing energy from one form to another. In the process, entropy is increased and a tremendous amount of energy is lost as heat. To "resist" entropy, we need a constant input of energy, which is regulated by metabolic processes. Metabolism occurs in stepwise sequences called metabolic pathways, some of which are anabolic and some catabolic. These pathways occur in different parts of the cell. The steps in these pathways are catalyzed by enzymes, which speed up reactions by lowering the energy of activation. The pathways that catabolize the energy nutrients "reinvest" the energy in these nutrients in the form of ATP in a coupling of exergonic to endergonic processes. *Why is this coupling process important in human movement?*

## *Phosphate Energy*

Metabolism (from the Greek word meaning "change") is defined as the sum total of all the chemical reactions that take place in the cells. One goal of metabolism is to sustain the energy charge of the cell by maintaining adequate concentrations of phosphate compounds, which act as *energy carriers*. ATP, a key compound in metabolism, is maintained by the exergonic breakdown of energy nutrients (primarily fats and carbohydrates but a small percentage of protein as well) in the presence of $O_2$.

### ATP—THE ENERGY EXCHANGE CURRENCY

The coupling of energy reactions in cells is designed for the purpose of maintaining adequate concentrations of phosphates, especially ATP, the *energy currency* of the cell. The

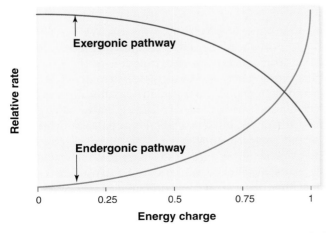

**FIGURE 3.5.** The energy charge of the cell governs the rates at which endergonic and exergonic pathways proceed.

| Table 3.1 | FREE ENERGY RELEASE OF SOME IMPORTANT PHOSPHORUS MOLECULES | |
|---|---|---|
| **Compound** | | **Free energy available*** |
| Phosphoenolpyruvate | | −14.8 |
| Creatine phosphate | | −10.3 |
| ATP (to ADP) | | −7.3 |
| Glucose-1-phosphate | | −5.0 |
| Glucose-6-phosphate | | −3.3 |

*These values relate to the standard energy release under conditions of pH = 7.0 and temperature = 25°C.

reason why ATP is the preferred energy exchange currency for biologic activity relates to its position among other phosphate energy carriers in its ability to donate free energy (Table 3.1). Under standard conditions (standard acidity and temperature) when the terminal, high-energy phosphate bond of ATP is hydrolyzed (broken by water), forming adenosine diphosphate (ADP) and inorganic phosphate ($P_i$), 7.3 kilocalories (kcal)/mol of free energy is released to power many different kinds of biologic processes. The high-energy phosphate bond is depicted in Figure 3.3 as a wavy line (∼). The 7.3-kcal/mol value represents the amount of free energy transferred to endergonic reactions in the cell.

*What is the immediate source of energy during exercise?* This key question often befuddles students who typically think too much in terms of the energy nutrients. The right answer to the question is ATP because its breakdown (an exergonic process) represents an instantaneous source of energy for muscle contraction (an endergonic process). Answers such as carbohydrate or fat are wrong because energy liberated from the splitting of the covalent (carbon to carbon) bonds of these nutrients cannot be used directly to perform cellular activity. The chemical equation depicting ATP breakdown is:

$$ATP + H_2O \Leftrightarrow ADP + P_i + \text{Free energy} + \text{Heat}$$

The free energy and heat release depicted in this equation represent caloric expenditure. A kcal is the amount of heat energy required to raise 1 kg of water by 1°C. ATP donates 7.3 kcal of free energy from its own hydrolysis, while ADP and AMP readily receive free energy from the breakdown of other energy carriers. This makes ATP intermediate (see ATP's relative position in Table 3.1) among other phosphate compounds in terms of its potential to transfer energy in the cell. The other phosphate energy carrier important in contracting muscle, **creatine phosphate** (CP), is unable to perform this role simply because its potential for transferring energy is higher, making it more unstable in solution. It functions as a ready donor of free energy but not a ready acceptor.

## ENERGY FLOWS FROM CREATINE PHOSPHATE TO ADP

The vital processes of the cell involve a multitude of chemical reactions. Consider that the average person uses approximately 360 L of $O_2$ each day to "burn" several hundred g of carbohydrates and fats and that about 3000 kcal of heat are generated. Cells are able to maintain a high concentration of ATP by using food (energy substrate) nutrients (in the case of animals) or light (in the case of plants) as free energy sources. However, these sources of energy cannot directly donate their energy to perform cellular work (muscle contraction or other kinds of cellular activity). Notice that in Table 3.1, both glucose-1-phosphate and glucose-6-phosphate have lower energy states than ATP. These relatively stable molecules can accept free energy transfers in the form of donated phosphoryl groups. ATP/ADP serves both functions, allowing free energy to flow through these molecules. ATP accomplishes much of its work by transferring its phosphate group to another molecule in a process called **phosphorylation**, energizing the organic molecules receiving the phosphate group, which are then used in later reactions. Phosphorylation may be shown schematically by the following chemical equation:

$$ATP + \text{C-C-C-C-C-C} \Leftrightarrow \text{C-C-C-C-C-C-P} + ADP$$
Glucose   Hexokinase          Glucose-6-phosphate

The amount of ATP turnover in the cell on a daily basis is tremendous. A typical adult uses the equivalent of about 200 kg of ATP daily, but at any given time only a few g of ATP are available. Instead of making this daily amount of ATP from scratch, we turn over our total body supply every minute or so by recycling chemical energy from other forms. This means that the amount of ATP we have at any moment is very small. We do not increase the amount of stored ATP; rather, when we have a positive energy balance (from too much eating and/or too little physical activity), the excess energy is stored as fat and glycogen.

Understanding the process of metabolic production of energy requires knowledge of other molecules that are important in energy-yielding pathways. While ATP is the energy currency of the cell, there are other molecules produced from catabolism that function in the process of transferring energy. These molecules are collectively termed high-energy intermediates because they are produced in intermediary metabolism and must undergo further breakdown, often in a different cellular compartment. Cellular compartmentalization is an important concept in energy metabolism. *Figure 3.6* shows that the reactions of the major metabolic pathways are housed in the cytosol, mitochondria, or both compartments.

Although ATP is the energy currency for cellular activity, we nevertheless have a very small bank account. The muscle storage capacity for ATP is approximately 80 to 100 g (approximately 5.0 mmol/kg wet weight), an amount that is readily depleted after only a few seconds of maximal

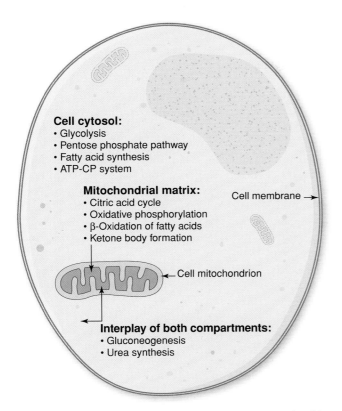

**FIGURE 3.6.** The pathways of metabolism are compartmentalized into different areas of the cell.

exercise (e.g., sprinting). Later in the chapter we will discover how the cell is able to break down energy nutrients to resynthesize ATP at rest and during exercise. It is important to know now, however, that another phosphate compound exists to serve as a reservoir of phosphate units for the purpose of maintaining adequate concentrations of ATP. CP (*Fig. 3.7*) provides this function in muscle cells. In a reaction catalyzed by the enzyme creatine kinase, a phosphate group from CP is added to ADP to form ATP (1). CP can serve in this role for two reasons: its concentration in muscle is approximately five times greater than

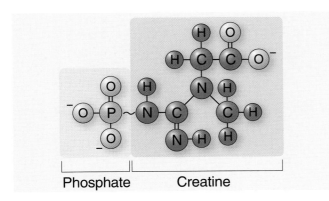

**FIGURE 3.7.** The creatine phosphate molecule. The phosphate group can be added to ADP to form ATP.

that of ATP and its ability to donate phosphate is greater than that of ATP (its potential energy of hydrolysis is higher). The concentration of CP is approximately 25 mmol/kg wet weight. This amount of CP allows for a ready transfer of phosphate to ADP during rapidly depleting ATP stores, as in periods of heavy muscular effort. Beyond that, CP is more unstable than ATP in solution. Its available free energy release actually signifies its potential (called transfer potential) to provide (transfer) phosphate units to compounds of lower energy. Notice that its position in Table 3.1 indicates the direction in which the phosphate transfer proceeds (from CP to ADP).

▶ *INQUIRY SUMMARY.* The work being done in the body is fueled by the potential energy available in the ATP molecule, which is produced and maintained in our cells by complicated metabolic processes that use the energy nutrients studied in Chapter 2. ATP is the energy currency of cells. Cells make ATP to be able to perform different kinds of functions, and when subsequently hydrolyzed, the right amount of energy is released to drive cellular reactions, including muscle contraction during exercise. Thus, the "coupling" of ATP hydrolysis (an exergonic process) to muscle contraction (an endergonic process) is a key event in metabolism. *How are coupled reactions important in metabolism?*

## Oxidation-Reduction Reactions

Oxidation and reduction are chemical reactions in metabolism that harness electrons and protons. Protons are hydrogen atoms that have lost their electrons. This cellular activity is vital because proton movement is the driving force that provides the majority of ready energy (ATP) for the cell as nutrients are broken down. Reduction, so named because it involves the addition of negatively charged electrons, is an example of an endergonic reaction because it takes the compound to a higher energy state. In reduction, the electrons added to a molecule may be either alone or in combination with protons (molecular hydrogen [$H_2$]). $H_2$ consists of two protons and two electrons; however, when hydrogen is stripped of its electrons, it is referred to as a proton and symbolized as $H^+$. As we will see later in the chapter when we discuss acid buildup in blood and muscle during exercise, a proliferation of protons ($H^+$) in solution determines its acidity (pH), an important factor in fatigue during exercise.

Since electrons are negatively charged, their addition to a molecule "reduces" it. Reduction and oxidation work in concert, and because of this are referred to as *redox* reactions. In redox reactions one molecule is oxidized, and the oxidizing agent is another molecule, which also serves as the electron acceptor. The molecule that is oxidized serves in these kinds of reactions as the reducing agent because it donates its electrons to the molecule that is reduced. The reducing agent is itself oxidized, and the oxidizing agent is reduced. The following generic equation serves to illustrate these concepts:

$$A{:}e \quad + \quad B \quad \rightarrow \quad A \quad + \quad B{:}e$$

| Reducing agent | Oxidizing agent | Oxidized molecule | Reduced molecule |

Examples of oxidation reactions are those that are involved in the degradation of glucose to $CO_2$ and $H_2O$. The products ($CO_2$ and $H_2O$) have far less energy than does the original, unoxidized compound (glucose). Reduction can be seen in the near reversal of this process. Oxidized compounds such as $CO_2$ contain less potential energy than do reduced compounds such as methane. Carbon compounds can be made via biosynthetic reactions (anabolism) into glucose. Both degradative and synthetic processes in the cell use reduction and oxidation at various points.

*Why are oxidation and reduction reactions important in metabolism?* The answer to that question requires knowledge of two other "energy carrier" compounds, **nicotinamide adenine dinucleotide ($NAD^+$/NADH)** and **flavin adenine dinucleotide (FAD/FADH$_2$)** (*Fig. 3.8*). These molecules are specialized hydrogen carriers. They transport hydrogens and their associated energy to be used in specialized metabolic pathways that generate energy (ATP) via the use of $O_2$. Both FAD and NAD exist in the cell in two forms: oxidized ($FAD^+$, $NAD^+$) and reduced ($FADH_2$, NADH). *Can you explain the difference between these two alternative forms in the language of oxidation-reduction reactions?* In all cells, the oxidized forms of these compounds are reduced, via a reduction reaction, when they accept electrons and a proton during a chemical reaction. Free energy release and its reharnessing in the form of ATP is only one important motif of energy metabolism. The other important theme is the release and reharnessing, in the form of NADH and FADH$_2$, of electrons and protons. The harnessing of electrons and protons occurs during the catabolism of the energy-yielding nutrients.

▶ *INQUIRY SUMMARY.* Many different kinds of chemical reactions are involved in metabolic processes. Oxidation-reduction reactions occur simultaneously and involve stripping electrons off molecules (oxidation) and adding electrons to other molecules (reduction). The overall processes of metabolism involve both anabolic and catabolic reactions. *Which part of metabolism is reductive and which is oxidative, and why?*

## *Sarcoplasmic Catabolism*

This section considers the energy-releasing "downhill" portion of metabolism. After studying this section, you will be able to describe how the muscle cell produces ATP during different kinds of exercises, sports events, and activities. This section will also introduce the rationale behind the concept of **metabolic specificity** and why, from a

metabolic standpoint, some exercise training regimes may be appropriate for a given participant while others may not, depending on the goal to be achieved.

Three systems provide the energy for cellular work (*Fig. 3.9*). Discussion of these systems in this text is limited to ATP generation in the muscle, which is compartmentalized into metabolic processes occurring in the **sarcoplasm** and **mitochondria**. These processes are either true pathways, that is, they end in the formation of a product(s), or *cycles*, which return molecules to the first events in the series. Pathways occurring in the sarcoplasm are **anaerobic** (do not involve $O_2$), while mitochondrial pathways and cycles are **aerobic** (involve $O_2$). A key to understanding how the three energy systems work is to approach them from the standpoint of how quickly ATP can be generated by each. When viewed this way, the three systems have other descriptive terms, such as immediate (phosphagen), short term (glycolytic), and long term (mitochondrial respiration/aerobic).

Two of the three ATP-generating pathways occur in the sarcoplasm, and none of the sarcoplasmic pathways use $O_2$ in their sequential steps. The **phosphagen system** is the simplest because it uses few enzymes (and therefore has few steps in its catalytic sequence). Glycolytic metabolism is much more complex because it has more steps, and it involves two separate pathways, glycogen degradation (glycogenolysis) and glucose breakdown (**glycolysis**). Another key sarcoplasmic catabolic activity is **lipolysis**, the breakdown of triglyceride to fatty acids. Lipolysis does not produce ATP directly, but serves to free the carbons in fatty acids for subsequent generation of ATP in mitochondrial respiration. When exercise is sustained, as in aerobic activities such as jogging, the sarcoplasmic products from glycolysis (**pyruvate**) and lipolysis (fatty acid) are shuttled into the mitochondria and are more completely broken down to the low-energy end products of **cellular respiration**, $CO_2$ and $H_2O$. Cellular (i.e., mitochondrial) respiration is an aerobic process that couples $O_2$ to the regeneration of ATP via **oxidative phosphorylation**. The two main stages of cellular respiration are the **Krebs cycle** and **electron transport chain**. Fatty acid breakdown to acetyl coenzyme A (CoA) via *β* **oxidation** also occurs in the mitochondria. The key catabolic pathways (and cycles) important in ATP generation during exercise are summarized in Table 3.2. The next few sections will briefly detail these processes. For a more detailed understanding, review the Suggested Readings.

### THE ENERGY CONTINUUM

The way in which particular energy-delivering pathways generate ATP has important consequences for athletic/exercise performance. The pathways that generate ATP in the muscle can be placed along a time-energy system continuum, with each pathway exhibiting characteristic ATP-generating *power* and *capacity*. In maximal exercise lasting only a few seconds, ATP production is primarily from

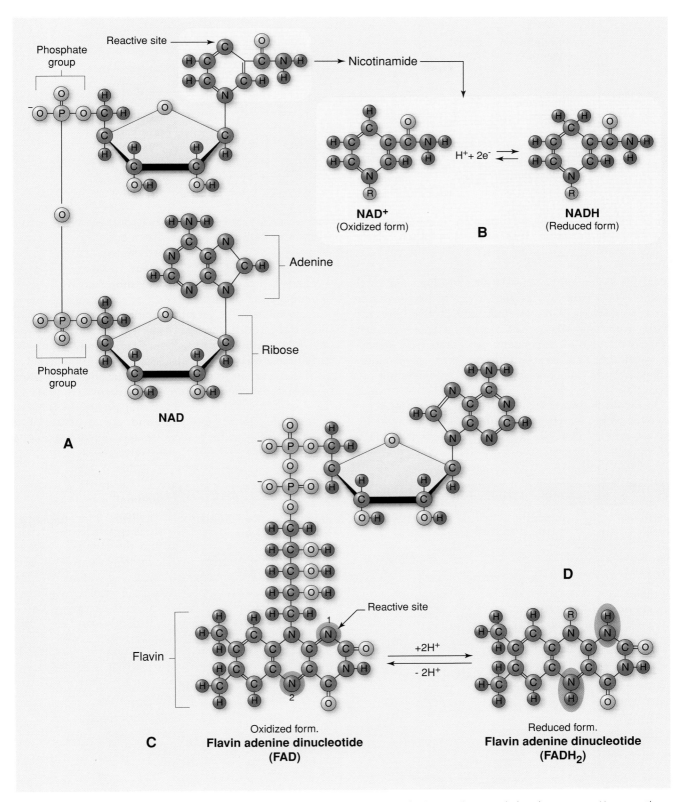

**FIGURE 3.8.** The chemical structure of NAD **(A)** and FAD **(C)**. NAD, like ATP, consists of adenine, ribose, and phosphate groups. However, the active part of NAD$^+$ **(B)** is a nitrogen-containing ring called nicotinamide, which is a derivative of nicotinic acid (niacin, a B vitamin). Niacin is one of the compounds added to breakfast cereals to make them "vitamin fortified." The one reactive site (where H$^+$ is added) is shown. FAD is like NAD, but contains the molecule flavin, which contains two reactive sites **(D)** for the addition of H$^+$.

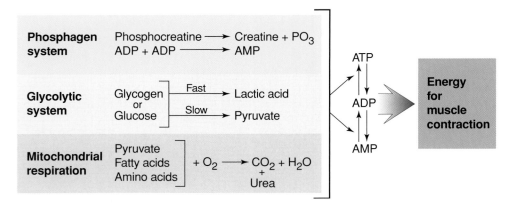

**FIGURE 3.9.** Three energy systems produce ATP: phosphagen system, glycolytic system, and mitochondrial respiration. Each system has particular substrate molecules and produces particular end products as ATP is generated for muscle contraction.

metabolic systems that generate ATP at a high rate (high power). These pathways are anaerobic. For maximal exercise lasting longer than 2 minutes, ATP production is primarily from metabolic systems that have a large capacity to produce ATP but produce it at a slower rate (low power). These pathways are aerobic. Capacity refers to an amount independent of time, and power refers to an amount in a given time.

Metabolic pathways are relatively more powerful if they have the ability to very rapidly supply ATP during highly intense activity. Power relates to the rate at which ATP is

generated by a pathway. Capacity, however, refers to the amount of ATP made over time. Power and capacity are inversely related; the metabolic pathway that is the most powerful also has the least capacity, and vice versa. The anaerobic pathways are therefore far more powerful, but they have a very limited capacity for ATP production.

It is important to understand that no single exercise or sport activity relies solely on one energy system to the exclusion of others. There is an overlapping of the three energy systems in ATP production for any given activity at any time, whether the activity is short and very intense or

| Table 3.2 | SUMMARY REVIEW OF KEY CATABOLIC PROCESSES IN MUSCLE CELLS THAT FORM ATP | | | | | |
|---|---|---|---|---|---|---|
| Pathway/ cycle | Substrate | Key enzymes | Number of enzymes | Key product formed | Power | Capacity |
| $\beta$ oxidation (aerobic) | Fatty acids | $\beta$ ketothiolase | 5 | Acetyl CoA, $FADH_2$, NADH | Included in ETC rating | Included in ETC rating |
| Electron transport chain (aerobic) | NADH, $FADH_2$ | ATPSYN | 1 | ATP, $H_2O$ | Very low | Very high |
| Glycogenolysis (anaerobic) | Glycogen | Phosphorylase | 3 | Free glucose | Included in glycolysis rating | Included in glycolysis rating |
| Glycolysis (anaerobic) | Glucose | PFK, PK, LDH | 10 or 11 | Pyruvate, lactate, ATP, NADH | High | Low |
| Lipolysis (aerobic) | TG | Type L HSL | 1 | Free fatty acids | Included in ETC rating | Included in ETC rating |
| Krebs cycle (aerobic) | Acetyl CoA from fat, protein, CHO | PDH, IDH | 8 (9) | NADH, $FADH_2$, $CO_2$, ATP | Included in ETC rating | Included in ETC rating |
| Phosphagen system (anaerobic) | Creatine phosphate, ADP | CK MK | 1 1 | ATP ATP | Very high | Very low |

ATPSYN, ATP synthetase; CHO, carbohydrate; CK, creatine kinase; ETC, electron transport chain; HSL, hormone-sensitive lipase; IDH, isocitrate dehydrogenase; LDH, lactate dehydrogenase; MK, myokinase; PDH, pyruvate dehydrogenase; PFK, phosphofructokinase; PK, pyruvate kinase; TG, triglyceride.

long and very easy. The four basic patterns below can ultimately be used for the determination of a precise exercise training program:

1. For any exercise duration, all three energy systems function simultaneously
2. The phosphagen system is the predominant energy system for maximal activities lasting 15 seconds or less, and it contributes 8% of the ATP generated for maximal activities up to 2 minutes in length (thereafter, as duration increases, it contributes proportionately less energy)
3. The glycolytic system is the predominant energy system for activities lasting less than 2 minutes, but this system still contributes 15% of the ATP generated for activities lasting as long as 10 minutes
4. By 5 minutes of continuous exercise, mitochondrial respiration is the dominant system, and the longer the duration of the exercise, the more important mitochondrial respiration becomes in supplying ATP to contracting muscle

The ability to rapidly transfer phosphate from substrate to form ATP is due to the fact that the sarcoplasmic pathways are independent of $O_2$. When exercise itself is rapid and intense, there is no time for the cardiorespiratory system to respond with increased $O_2$ delivery to contracting muscle to accommodate the muscle's increased demand for ATP. When ATP cannot be adequately supplied via oxidative means, phosphate is added to ADP by the process of substrate-level phosphorylation. These reactions take place in the sarcoplasm, where there is a high concentration of glycolytic enzymes and substrate (glycogen). However, the substrate-level phosphorylation involved in glycolytic metabolism is too *slow* to be of value when an ultra–short-term intense burst of activity is needed. For this, we rely on the immediate energy system, the phosphagen system, for the development of ATP. Glycolytic metabolism is slightly less powerful than the phosphagen system but is tremendously important because it provides an additional 1.5 minutes of very intense muscular activity beyond exhaustion of the phosphagen system (<15 seconds).

## IMMEDIATE ENERGY

CP and ATP represent immediate sources of energy for muscular contraction during intense activities. The reasons for this are because the phosphates in this system are stored directly with the contractile mechanism of muscles, this system does not rely on a long series of chemical reactions, and $O_2$ is not required. Intense activities (e.g., sprinting) will deplete CP, the phosphate reservoir, in <15 seconds. When this occurs, cellular ATP concentrations begin to diminish (Fig. 3.10). Both CP and ATP are maintained at resting levels in muscle cells (time 0 in Fig. 3.10). When intense activity is initiated and sustained, ATP breakdown powers contracting muscles, and its concentration is maintained as long as there is suffi-

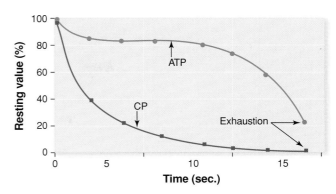

**FIGURE 3.10.** Example of how ATP and creatine phosphate are used in very intense activity.

cient CP concentration. When the concentration of CP decreases significantly, ATP concentration also diminishes. The phosphagen system reaches the point of exhaustion shortly after. For intense activity to continue, ATP *must* subsequently be supplied by another ATP-generating pathway.

The phosphagen system, which utilizes two separate enzymatic reactions to produce ATP, is often referred to by the more limiting term, ATP-PC system (PC is an abbreviation for the compound phosphocreatine, but CP, for creatine phosphate, is the synonymous term used in this text). These reactions involve the coupling of ATP hydrolysis via myosin ATPase to either the myokinase or the creatine kinase reactions (Fig. 3.11). The myokinase reaction catalyzes the formation of ATP using two ADP molecules as substrate. While this reaction is important, it is the CP concentration that serves as the principle phosphate reservoir, governing the rate (i.e., power) of the phosphagen system. Thus, the creatine kinase reaction dominates the phosphagen system. In the ATP-PC system, the creatine kinase reaction occurs simultaneously with the ATPase reaction and is preeminent because CP serves as the phosphate reservoir. However, as ADP concentration increases, the catalytic activity of myokinase increases, making this reaction important as well.

The creatine kinase reaction is reversible in that ATP can be used to phosphorylate creatine and replenish the muscle's CP stores. During exercise, the reaction proceeds in the direction of ATP formation so that muscular work can continue. When exercise intensity is reduced to a low level or during recovery from exercise, the reaction will be reversed and ATP derived from fat, carbohydrate, and protein metabolism will be used to replenish the muscle's CP stores. Hence, ATP is recycled at the expense of either CP or dietary nutrients, while CP is recycled only at the expense of dietary nutrients. Therefore, the only expendable items are the dietary nutrients.

The phosphagen system supplies ATP for muscle contraction when the rate of ATP production from glycolysis and mitochondrial respiration is inadequate for a given

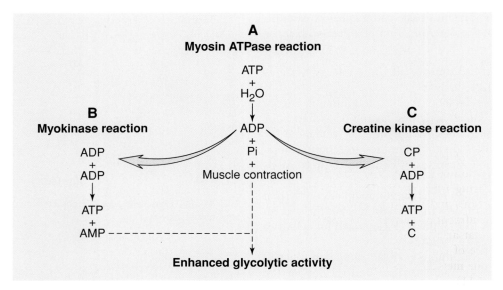

**A**
**Myosin ATPase reaction**

ATP
+
H$_2$O
↓
ADP
+
Pi
+
Muscle contraction

**B**
**Myokinase reaction**

ADP
+
ADP
↓
ATP
+
AMP

**C**
**Creatine kinase reaction**

CP
+
ADP
↓
ATP
+
C

**Enhanced glycolytic activity**

**FIGURE 3.11.** The phosphagen system involves the near simultaneous catalytic activity of three enzymes: **(A)** myosin ATPase, which liberates free energy from ATP to produce muscle contraction; **(B)** myokinase, which rephosphorylates ADP and also produces AMP, a stimulator of glycolytic activity; and **(C)** creatine kinase, which uses creatine phosphate to drive the rephosphorylation of ADP to maintain ATP concentrations in the cell.

activity. At this time the muscle's sudden demand for ATP cannot be met by adequate ATP supply from any other energy system. The time frame of the activity is an important consideration. Existing phosphagen stores are used almost exclusively when very intense activity lasts <15 seconds. *Think of activities that would meet these criteria.* Figure 3.10 shows the ATP depletion rate during such an activity. Activities such as sprinting exhibit a high dependence on phosphagens during maximal effort. Heavy resistance exercise has also been shown to produce a significant increase in P$_i$ concentration when the effort is short lasting (<10 seconds) and intense. As shown in *Figure 3.12*, muscle lactate (a product of fast glycolysis or the short-term energy pathway) is relatively unchanged during this type of weightlifting. The fact that muscle P$_i$ concentration is increased when lactate concentration is unchanged means

that fast glycolysis was not active to a great extent. Resistance exercise is a good example of an activity/exercise that can be performed in a manner that stresses the phosphagen system to the exclusion of the glycolytic system so that lactate is not produced in the muscle. The resistance exercise is to be completed in less than approximately 10 to 15 seconds, and fairly long rest periods (2 to 3 minutes) between exercise sets are needed. If the number of repetitions is sufficient to carry the set beyond 10 to 15 seconds, the glycolytic system is progressively stressed, and more and more lactate accumulates in the muscle. The production of lactate in this form of resistance exercise and in other forms of intense exercise lasting longer than 15 seconds represents a backup source of ATP production to power intense, prolonged activity. Without this backup, our complete repertoire of exercises and activities would be more limited.

### SHORT-TERM ENERGY

The glycolytic energy system is composed of two separate pathways: glycogenolysis, the pathway that liberates glucose molecules from glycogen, and glycolysis, the partial breakdown of glucose to generate ATP. During exercise, these pathways work in concert to deliver ATP energy to the contractile machinery of muscles.

The storage form of carbohydrate in the body is glycogen, which makes up about 1% to 2% of wet muscle weight (400 g total) and about 6% to 10% of wet liver weight (100 g total). Muscle glycogen is used in glycolysis to produce ATP during muscular contraction, whereas liver glycogen is used to maintain blood glucose levels during fasting or the latter stages of endurance exercise. As you saw in Chapter 2, glycogen is a branched-chain polysaccharide

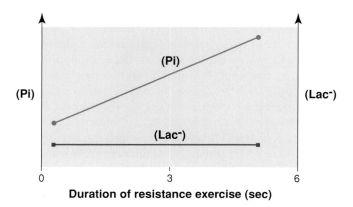

(Pi)

(Pi)                                          (Lac⁻)

(Lac⁻)

0                    3                    6

**Duration of resistance exercise (sec)**

**FIGURE 3.12.** When resistance exercise is very short lasting (<10 seconds), little lactate formation occurs while an increase in cellular P$_i$ occurs from creatine phosphate breakdown.

consisting of only glucose molecules linked together by chemical bonds. The degradation of glycogen is controlled by the initial reaction in which **phosphorylase** cleaves the bonds between the glucose residues of the glycogen chain. A few of the residues are released as free glucose, but the greatest majority is released as glucose-1-phosphate, which is quickly converted to glucose-6-phosphate. The free glucose and glucose-6-phosphate can now enter into the glycolytic pathway.

The catalytic rate of glycogenolysis is directed by an increased concentration of calcium ($Ca^{2+}$) and $P_i$ in contracting muscle. Rising intracellular $Ca^{2+}$ (the stimulus for muscle contraction) and $P_i$ concentrations (the direct result of muscle contraction) activate the enzyme phosphorylase. Recall that an increase in $P_i$ concentration is a direct consequence of CP breakdown so that the product (i.e., $P_i$) from one metabolic pathway helps to activate another (see Fig. 3.11). The role of phosphorylase is to cleave glucose in the form of glucose-1-phosphate from glycogen in periods of low cellular energy, allowing the muscle to have access to carbohydrate carbons in the metabolic "pool." In addition, the end product of glycogenolysis is a phosphorylated glucose (glucose-6-phosphate), which is the first intermediate in glycolysis, connecting glycogenolysis with glycolysis. Glycogenolytic activity starts immediately upon initiation of muscle contraction and is sustained as long as the two stimulating factors are present.

*Figure 3.13* shows that glucose for glycolytic metabolism can come from many sources. During exercise, the preferred source is muscle glycogen. This makes sense from a bioenergetic standpoint. Glucose may also enter from the blood as "free" glucose. Under normal circumstances, the blood glucose pool is supplied from liver glycogen. However, an exogenous source may also add to the blood glucose pool in times of muscle and liver glyco-gen depletion as in long-duration exercise. *From where might this exogenous source of glucose come?*

Substrate for glycolysis comes preferably from muscle glycogen in all forms of exercise. Glycogenolysis provides the glycolytic substrate in the form of glucose-6-phosphate, a phosphorylated form of glucose that is trapped in the cell due to the negative charge contained on the phosphate unit. Using glycogen as a starting point is more bioenergetically efficient. This is true because ATP is not used to phosphorylate the glucose produced in glycogenolysis. However, when blood glucose is used in the initial step of glycolysis, ATP serves as the phosphate donor via the **hexokinase** reaction. When muscle glycogen is depleted, the only other available source of glucose is the circulating blood pool. Using "free" glucose from this source starts the energy pathway from an energetically disadvantaged standpoint (*Fig. 3.14*, Step 1). The reason for this is because the glucose-6-phosphate generated from free glucose through the activity of hexokinase uses ATP to phosphorylate the glucose molecule. The result is that when beginning glycolytic energy production from the starting point of free glucose, the net energy production is one less molecule of ATP; that is, using muscle glycogen results in three ATP molecules produced versus two when a free glucose molecule is the starting point. Hexokinase, bound to the intracellular side of the sarcolemma, is an enzyme specific to glucose that has been transported across the cell membrane to undergo either storage (glycogenesis) or breakdown for energy derivation (glycolysis). However, to see how ATP is produced in glycolysis, we need to take a closer look at this system.

Glycolysis is a 10- or 11-step process that produces pyruvate or lactate, respectively. The importance of glycolysis as an energy system is that it is the only way ATP can be produced from the breakdown of an energy nutrient

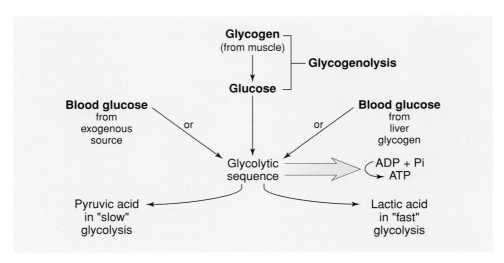

**FIGURE 3.13.** Source of muscle glucose for glycolytic metabolism. Notice that glycogenolysis is not an energy pathway but merely serves to release stored glucose for the energy pathway, glycolysis.

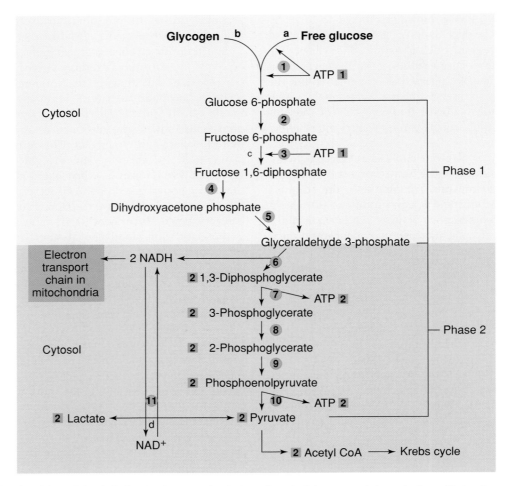

**FIGURE 3.14.** Abbreviated view of glycolysis showing important beginning substrates (glycogen and glucose), phases (first and second), and end products (pyruvate and lactate). Also shown is how glycolysis intersects with mitochondrial activity via pyruvate formation. The letters indicate key enzymes at the beginning of glycolysis: a = hexokinase; b = phosphorylase; c = phosphofructokinase; d = lactate dehydrogenase. The circled numbers refer to the steps of glycolysis—10 total steps from glucose to pyruvate and 11 total steps from glucose to lactate. The numbers in green boxes signify the number of end product or ATP produced per reaction.

molecule in the absence of $O_2$. Figure 3.14 presents an abbreviated review of glycolysis. The following points are important to remember about glycolysis:

- Phase 1 of glycolysis readies the glucose molecule for the production of ATP in phase 2 of glycolysis when a net increase of two ATPs are generated in the cell. Starting with glucose-6-phosphate, phase 1 consists of four enzymatic reactions that end in the production of two molecules of glyceraldyhyde-3-phosphate. To get to that point, phase 1 uses two ATP (steps 1 and 3), resulting in a decrease in cellular ATP concentration. The phosphofructokinase (PFK) reaction (step 3 of phase 1) is the most important step of glycolysis since this enzyme is rate limiting (i.e., it regulates the flux of all the reactions in glycolysis). Once the kinetic barrier in the PFK reaction is overcome, the remaining reactions in glycolysis proceed without interruption.
- Phase 2 of glycolysis starts with a redox reaction, which increases cellular NADH + H⁺ formation (i.e.,

two NADH + H⁺ are formed at the beginning of phase 2). This product formation is an important reaction since NADH will be shuttled to the mitochondria and participate in mitochondrial respiration in the aerobic production of ATP. Note that at this point the glycolytic "stream" has doubled since phase 1 ends with the production of two molecules of glyceraldyhyde-3-phosphate, each one participating in glycolytic energy production. Therefore, from this point on, there will be two intermediates formed in each of the remaining steps of glycolysis (notice the 2 in green boxes in front of each molecule in phase 2). In phase 2, four ATP molecules are formed, resulting in a net intracellular increase of two ATPs (three when starting with glycogen).
- If activity is slow, glycolysis is said to be slow, and the end-product is pyruvate, which participates in mitochondrial respiration by serving as a substrate molecule for the Krebs cycle by forming acetyl CoA in the mitochondrial matrix.

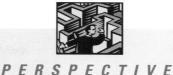

Box 3.1

## PERSPECTIVE

# Is Glycolysis Aerobic or Anaerobic?

While the ATP-generating pathways in the sarcoplasm do not utilize oxygen, at times glycolytic metabolism is referred to as aerobic and at other times anaerobic. This confusing use of the terms *aerobic* and *anaerobic* in relation to glycolytic metabolism has led to an incorrect understanding of the exact nature of the glycolytic generation of ATP during different kinds of exercise. The mistaken perception is that there are two forms of glycolysis active in exercise conditions; aerobic glycolysis and anaerobic glycolysis. The current confusion over terms can be traced to the 19th century and the work of scientists investigating glycolysis in unicellular organisms (i.e., yeast). In these "test-tube" experiments scientists either withdrew or permitted an oxygen environment and studied the subsequent development of two different glycolytic end products in the organism—*lactate* and *pyruvate*. They also studied the speed with which the end products developed. It was found that lactate accumulated very rapidly in the absence of oxygen, and the cell became acidic (increased concentration of $H^+$); however, when oxygen was present, glycolysis was slow and pyruvate accumulated. Glycolysis was then classified as either aerobic or anaerobic. This pattern later began to be applied to muscle contraction during exercise of differing intensities, and it was assumed that if lactate appeared anaerobiosis was present in the muscle. However, today we know that lactate acid appears in the blood even under resting conditions, and that its appearance under any condition does not automatically connote production, but may be a consequence of a reduced removal rate from blood. In short, applying terminology developed long ago to exercising mammalian systems is not warranted and leads to confusion.

- If activity is fast, glycolysis is said to be fast, and the end-product is lactate (in an eleventh step), the reduced form of pyruvate, which diffuses out of the cell and into the general circulation.

Glycolysis is considered to be fast or slow depending on the rate (i.e., intensity) of exercise (i.e., sprinting vs. jogging). However, in the case of intense exercise, there is no necessary connection to anaerobic conditions in muscle even when lactate accumulates because glycolysis actually has little to do with the presence of $O_2$ in contracting muscle. Instead, during intense exercise, fast glycolysis is associated with a discontinuity between sarcoplasmic and mitochondrial metabolism, a condition that allows for lactate development even when $O_2$ tension in muscle is adequate. In moderate exercise, when glycolysis is slow, metabolism between the two cellular compartments is linked (see the section on mitochondrial pathways below). Though the terms aerobic and anaerobic may be used to describe the metabolic consequences and responses of particular activity forms, these terms are not properly descriptive of glycolysis during exercise and are not used to describe glycolysis in the text. *Is glycolysis aerobic or anaerobic?* The terms aerobic and anaerobic applied to glycolytic activity in contracting muscle has led to confusion among students. Box 3.1 provides an example from history and clears up the use of these misapplied terms.

For sustained intense performance, the production of lactate in glycolysis is necessary. This may come as a shock to students who have read too much popular exercise literature which credits lactate with everything from muscle fatigue and soreness to the development of pain during exercise. Lactate has unquestionably received "bad press" because of the supposed negative consequences of its development. However, you should remember that the negative consequences of the development of acidosis is only "associated" with lactate, not caused by it. *Invariably this leads to the question, is lactate "good or bad"?* The answer is that without lactate, intense exercise cannot continue, making lactate production an absolute necessity.

The formation of lactate depends upon the relative activities of both the sarcoplasmic and mitochondrial pathways. Lactate production is prevalent under exercise conditions such as: (a) transitioning from rest to exercise, (b) transitioning from one level of exercise to a higher level, and (c) exercising at levels that are higher than that which can be sustained by mitochondrial respiration. In addition, some lactate is probably always developed from pyruvate regardless of the rate of exercise because of the mass action effect, which dictates the development of lactate when pyruvate production exceeds its rate of entry into the mitochondria. There is always a basal level of lactate production in the cell that results in a resting muscle lactate concentration of 1 mmol/kg wet weight.

*LINKUP: Access* **Perspective: Lactate or Lactic Acid?** *at http://connection.lww.com/go/brownexphys and on the Student Resource CD-ROM. This feature explores new theories on the role of lactate in metabolism, as well as its role during intense exercise.*

From a bioenergetics standpoint, how can a person continue to sprint (or perform other forms of intense exercise) beyond 15 seconds if the phosphagen system has been exhausted? This is a key question because we are capable of intense exercise well beyond this time frame. *Is ATP further developed by mitochondrial respiration at this point?* The answer to this question is no because mitochondrial respiration is not powerful enough (cannot produce ATP rapidly enough) to sustain the intense muscle contractions required of continued intense exercise. The production of lactate permits the rapid development of ATP in contracting muscles beyond 15 seconds. This is an added source of rapid ATP development that would not normally be available if not for the mechanism of lactate formation.

Recall that phase 2 of glycolysis starts with the reduction of $NAD^+$ and produces a net increase of two to three ATP molecules in the cell. Under normal conditions (resting or light to moderate exercise), the NADH that is developed is transported to the mitochondria to participate in oxidative phosphorylation. However, when intense exercise is sustained, there is an increased need for ATP development through substrate-level phosphorylation in the sarcoplasm. Under rapid exercise conditions, this is only possible when a high sarcoplasmic **redox potential** is maintained. The redox potential is the ratio of oxidizing agent ($NAD^+$) to reducing agent (NADH). For glycolysis to continue under fast conditions, enough $NAD^+$ must be available for the first step of phase 2 of glycolysis (see Fig. 3.14), otherwise the ATP-generating second half of glycolysis would be hampered, and repeated intense muscle contractions would be reduced in intensity due to the lack of sarcoplasmic ATP generation. In view of this, lactate is a necessary product that allows for the rapid development of ATP that enables glycolysis to continue when CP levels have severely diminished. Molecules of NADH produced in the first step of phase 2 of glycolysis are used to convert pyruvate to lactate in the last step of fast glycolysis. This step frees $NAD^+$ to serve in a cyclic manner in the first redox reaction of glycolysis (first step of phase 2). Production of lactate then serves to maintain a fast rate of phase 2 of glycolysis when there is a net increase in ATP concentration. *What would happen if you were unable to produce lactate in your muscles?*

Case study 3.1 addresses this by describing the medical consequences of someone with a glycogen storage disease brought on by an enzyme deficiency. The ability to produce lactate in the muscles is essential for engaging in strenuous activity. McArdle disease patients have difficulty utilizing glycogen, the predominant fuel for fast glycolysis, because of an enzyme deficiency. *If glucose can be delivered* from an exogenous source and enter the glycolytic pathway, thereby bypassing the need to use glycogen as the preferred substrate, might this increase the tolerance of these individuals for strenuous activity?

*LINKUP:* See **Research Highlight: McArdle Disease** *at http://connection.lww.com/go/brownexphys and on the Student Resource CD-ROM for information about a study on McArdle disease and glucose infusion as a means to enhance these patients' abilities to tolerate heavy work.*

*What causes the problems that have been commonly associated with lactate formation?* In short, there is an associated developing acidosis that interferes with the process of muscle contraction and with the catalytic rate of several metabolic enzymes that is ultimately related to fatigue.

## LIPOLYSIS

The last sarcoplasmic metabolic pathway considered in this chapter provides the fatty acids essential for energy transformations in long-term sustained exercise. Fats can be oxidized only in the mitochondria, making fat a fuel source available during aerobic activity and not fast, anaerobic activity. This has important consequences in exercise metabolism for weight loss.

Intramuscular lipolysis is possible because triglycerides are stored on a limited basis within muscle sarcoplasm, but the vast majority are deposited in adipose cells where the major part of total body lipolysis takes place (2). Therefore, this section also contains a discussion on mobilizing fat from adipocytes. Though the muscle takes up fatty acids from the circulation for energy derivation, intramuscular stores of fat are also an important source of energy for contracting muscles.

Whether lipolysis occurs in muscle or adipocytes, the breakdown of triglycerides into free fatty acids to be taken up by mitochondria for β oxidation is the first step in the process of degrading fats. Using fats is a process that involves the following steps: (1) mobilization, (2) translocation, (3) β oxidation, and (4) mitochondrial respiration. We will briefly consider mobilization and translocation at this point. The breakdown of fats through β oxidation and mitochondrial respiration will be covered as part of the section on mitochondrial respiration.

Mobilization is a three-fold process. The first step in mobilization is triglyceride degradation via lipolysis, whereby triglycerides are degraded to their constituent parts, fatty acids and glycerol (*Fig. 3.15*). Lipolysis in adipose and muscle uses two enzymes, lipoprotein lipase (in the capillary walls of adipose and muscle) and hormone-sensitive lipase (an intracellular lipase). These lipolytic enzymes have different focal points for their catalytic activity. The capillary wall enzyme hydrolyzes triglycerides that are carried in blood-borne **lipoproteins**, and the released fatty acids are subsequently taken up by the

## CASE STUDY 3.1: McARDLE DISEASE

### CASE

KS is a 39-year-old male who was diagnosed at age 27 with myophosphorylase deficiency or McArdle disease. McArdle disease is an autosomal-recessive deficiency of the muscle phosphorylase enzyme, resulting in the inability of the muscle to break down glycogen and provide fuel for oxidative metabolism. KS has a lifelong history of exercise intolerance, and he described his physical education classes as "a nightmare." He typically avoided strenuous physical activity, as his legs would tire and feel heavy with running. He tried wrestling in the eighth grade but was unable to continue due to exertional fatigue without cramping. At age 16, he had a prominent episode of exertional muscle cramps when trying to swim across a pond. He has had many episodes of exertional muscle cramps or contractures. After some of these episodes, his urine would be dark or the color of cola. His level of creatine kinase has risen to greater than 80,000 units/L. He rapidly fatigues initially with exercise; however, if he continues with low-intensity exercise, his exercise capacity increases after approximately 10 minutes. His exercise capacity is improved if he eats something prior to exercise. He has tried to adapt to his situation by avoiding strenuous activity and warming up slowly prior to exertion. His initial muscle biopsy at age 25 was interpreted as normal. A subsequent muscle biopsy at age 27 confirmed the diagnosis of McArdle disease when special stains for the myophosphorylase enzyme revealed its absence. He has one sister also affected by McArdle disease and an unaffected brother. He has two sons who are unaffected. His neurologic exam demonstrates no abnormalities at rest. Exercise testing demonstrated a typical response with no increase in lactate production during ischemic forearm exercise.

### DESCRIPTION

While rarely encountered, McArdle disease is estimated to have a prevalence of 1 in 100,000. Often the disease is not detected until the patient is in his or her twenties or thirties as it is less severe in children. Health professionals should recognize the acute symptoms of this metabolic disease:

- Exertional fatigue and weakness with moderate exercise
- Muscle cramps resulting as a direct consequence of exertion are characterized by shortened, hard muscles, and are usually intensely painful—the muscles are unable to be lengthened for minutes to hours (i.e., the limb is "locked up")
- Myoglobinuria (presence of myoglobin in the urine) usually is similarly triggered by brief maximal exercise (sprinting, wrestling, attempting to water ski), and pigmenturia (urine that has the color of cola) is noted within hours

- Progressive muscle weakness that occurs later in life (fifth decade and beyond, but occasionally affecting younger patients)
- Rhabdomyolysis (muscle necrosis or breakdown) producing skyrocketing creatine kinase levels
- Myalgia (muscle pain, usually intense)

Because these acute attacks can be very painful and may produce significant muscle injury and myoglobinuria-induced kidney damage, a major goal in living with this form of metabolic myopathy is to prevent attacks. In response, many people have learned to avoid activities that they know will trigger an attack and have made dietary modifications designed to circumvent the blocked metabolic pathway.

The major long-term consequence of McArdle disease is muscle weakness. A likely mechanism is recurrent muscle injury, which ultimately exceeds the regenerative capacity of skeletal muscle. Muscle magnetic resonance imaging sensitively identifies focal muscle injury and decreased mass. For patients with focal muscle atrophy, special attention should be given to eliminating patterns of exercise which promote muscle injury, augmenting substrate availability and improving the capacity to oxidize available substrates, and providing adequate dietary protein to promote protein synthesis.

### EVALUATION/INTERVENTION

A diet rich in protein and adequate in carbohydrates is recommended and has improved exercise capacity. Regular aerobic exercise increases mitochondrial density and enhances the activity of rate-limiting oxidative enzymes, thus increasing fat oxidation and reducing the requirement for carbohydrate utilization to supply muscle energy needs. Exercise recommendations that encourage health outcomes in normal individuals are also necessary for these patients. However, precautions are recommended. Intensity of aerobic exercise should be individualized on a day-by-day (sometimes minute-to-minute) basis because of acute variation of patterns of substrate mobilization. Serum creatine kinase should be monitored to ensure that the exercise program is not producing increased muscle injury. The most devastating acute consequence of McArdle disease is massive exertional muscle injury with myoglobinuria.

The treatment management for KS consists of 20 to 30 minutes of sustained aerobic activity 3 to 4 days per week at moderate intensity (maximum heart rate at 60% to 70% of the predicted maximum). Exercise should begin at even less intensity for the first 5 to 10 minutes to allow for a warming-up period to produce the second-wind phenomenon (i.e., enhanced work tolerance). He is to avoid isometric or anaerobic exercise. This protocol has been demonstrated to improve

---

### Case Study 3.1, continued

exercise and muscle oxidative capacity by improving availability and utilization of blood-borne glucose and free fatty
acids. Dietary therapy is suggested to support muscle regeneration. Fifty percent of the total calories should come from
carbohydrates; however, an excessive caloric intake should be
avoided to reduce the risk of obesity. A glucose-containing
meal 30 minutes prior to exercise is recommended. Exercise
should be terminated with any evidence of muscle cramping

or contracture, and the patient should immediately increase
fluid intake. Should home urine testing demonstrate myoglobin, he is to go to the hospital for more intensive treatment
to avoid myoglobinuria-induced renal failure.

Used with permission from Alan W. Martin, MD and
Ronald G. Haller, MD, Neuromuscular Division, Institute for
Exercise and Environmental Medicine, Presbyterian Hospital
of Dallas, TX.

---

muscle. The intracellular lipase hydrolyzes those triglycerides stored in the fat and muscle cells. These enzymes
are regulated in that they allow for the breakdown of fat
in times of energy need as in exercise (intracellular lipase
is activated) and for the storage of fat after eating (intracellular lipase is inhibited by insulin). Other hormones
such as epinephrine, norepinephrine, and growth hormone stimulate lipolysis during exercise.

Mobilization of free fatty acids from adipocytes is also
related to the dual processes of circulation and uptake.
These two factors refer to the transport via the blood and
entry of free fatty acids into muscles from blood of lipids
liberated from adipocytes and not intramuscular stores. An
increased entry rate of free fatty acids into muscle is the result of three factors: (1) increased adipose lipolysis, (2) increased rate of blood flow through muscle, and (3) number
of sarcolemmal fatty acid receptor sites.

Translocation of fatty acids from the sarcoplasm to the
interior of the mitochondria is the first step of intracellular
fatty acid oxidation in the mitochondrial matrix. Translocation involves activation of the fatty acid molecule by the
attachment of sarcoplasmic CoA. A coenzyme is a low-
molecular-weight organic molecule that allows enzymes to
perform their function. *Figure 3.16* shows the structure of
CoA and acetyl CoA. In translocation, the fatty acid and
CoA combination forms a fatty acyl-CoA molecule, the
activated fatty acid. The fatty acyl-CoA is subsequently
transported into the mitochondria by a transport mechanism involving the molecule carnitine, which is the fatty
acyl carrier bound to the mitochondrial membrane. In this
process the fatty acid is exchanged between the CoA molecule in the sarcoplasm and carnitine in the mitochondrial
membrane. The CoA is stripped from the fatty acyl, and the
fatty acid is accepted by carnitine. Once accepted by carnitine, the acyl-carnitine complex is dissociated with the release of the fatty acid to the mitochondrial matrix. Once in
the matrix, the fatty acid can undergo $\beta$ oxidation to produce acetyl CoA, $FADH_2$, and NADH molecules. The acetyl
CoA then serves as substrate in the Krebs cycle in which
additional hydrogen carriers are produced. These high-energy carriers undergo mitochondrial oxidation in the aerobic development of ATP. For each NADH produced, three
ATPs are resynthesized, and for each $FADH_2$ produced,

two ATPs are resynthesized. The reason for this disparity is
explained in the summary of the electron transport chain.

**LINKUP:** *See* **Case Study: Systemic Carnitine Deficiency** *at* **http://connection.lww.com/go/brownexphys**
*and on the Student Resource CD-ROM. This case de-
scribes a lipid storage disease that can cause exercise
intolerance.*

▶ *INQUIRY SUMMARY.* Several of the pathways of catabolism occur in the sarcoplasm. These sarcoplasmic pathways do not utilize $O_2$ and are therefore anaerobic. Because
$O_2$ processes are excluded in sarcoplasmic reactions, ATP
is derived quickly from these pathways, making them important in intense muscular events. While all the catabolic
reactions are always used to one extent or another, it is
possible to study the systems that predominate during particular events, sports, or exercises. *Can you explain why you
experience a burning sensation in your muscles when you perform an intense bout of resistance exercise? Which sarcoplasmic pathways discussed do not directly participate in ATP
formation?*

## *Mitochondrial Catabolism*

Our focus now shifts to a discussion of cellular energy
processes that function when exercise intensity is low
enough to allow continuity between sarcoplasmic pathways and mitochondrial function. In this case there is an
effective transport of substrate and hydrogen carriers
from the sarcoplasm to the mitochondria. Mitochondrial
metabolism is *aerobic* in that it depends on the coopera-
tive interaction of two systems: the Krebs cycle and electron transport chain. However, $O_2$ does not come into
play until oxidative phosphorylation in the electron transport chain. Mitochondrial respiration can be "backed up"
when there is a failure at any step in supplying substrate
or if $O_2$ tension declines. In fact, the presence of $O_2$ inside the mitochondria enables the continued functioning
of not only the electron transport chain, but all other mitochondrial reactions as well.

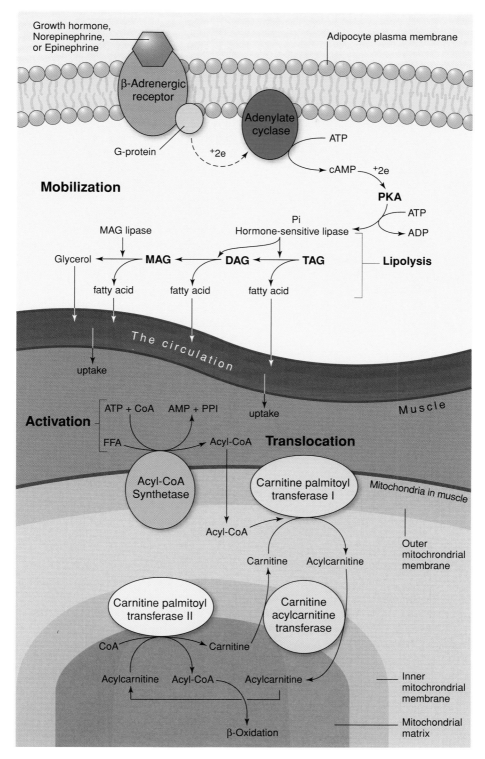

**FIGURE 3.15.** Mobilization and translocation of fatty acids into the mitochondria.

Mitochondrial respiration involves the coordinated activity of the Krebs cycle (*Fig. 3.17*) and electron transport chain (*Fig. 3.18*). In resting conditions or conditions of low to moderate exercise, intermediate products of carbohydrate (pyruvate), fat (acetyl CoA), and protein (various amino acids) metabolism enter a common catabolic process in the mitochondrial matrix. *Figure 3.19* depicts metabolism in three stages. In the first stage large molecules are broken down into smaller units, and no useful energy in generated. In the second stage the smaller molecules are degraded to a few simple units that play key roles in metabolism, most being converted to acetyl CoA. A

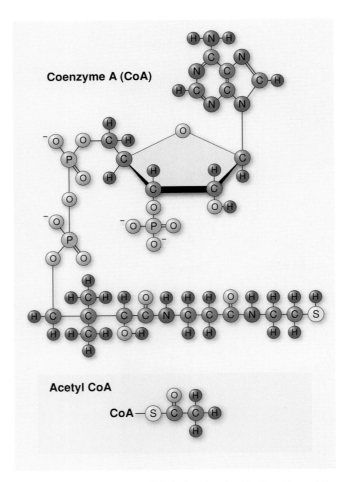

**FIGURE 3.16.** The structure of CoA showing the binding site, and the structure of acetyl CoA.

small amount of ATP is generated in this stage. In the third stage the Krebs cycle and oxidative phosphorylation are the final common pathways in the oxidation of molecular fuel. Most ATP generation occurs in this stage.

The Krebs cycle catalyzes reactions that produce $CO_2$, NADH, $FADH_2$, and ATP from carbon intermediate compounds that started out as energy nutrients. The ATP is formed by substrate-level phosphorylation in the Krebs cycle, and it accounts for only a small fraction of the total ATP production in the mitochondria. The $CO_2$ produced in the Krebs cycle diffuses out of the mitochondria and the cell and is carried to the lungs for delivery into the atmosphere via external respiration. Measurement of the volume of $CO_2$ produced in metabolism is a major topic of Chapter 5. The hydrogen carriers produced in $\beta$ oxidation and the Krebs cycle undergo mitochondrial oxidation in a process that removes protons from NADH and $FADH_2$ and passes them through specialized proton channels in a way that transfers the potential energy from the hydrogen carriers to ADP in the formation of ATP. This process uses the enzyme ATP synthetase and requires that protons be continually removed by combination with molecular $O_2$ in the

formation of water. Chapter 5 is also concerned with measuring this volume of $O_2$ consumed as an index of the level of aerobic metabolism during exercise. A brief summary of $\beta$ oxidation, the Krebs cycle, and the electron transport chain is presented next.

## $\beta$ OXIDATION

$\beta$ oxidation is so named because it degrades fatty acyl CoA in a cyclic process that cleaves two carbons off the fatty acid molecule at a time (*Fig. 3.20*). In a four-step process that takes place in the mitochondrial matrix, the fat molecule is cleaved between the $\alpha$ and $\beta$ carbons. The fat is completely oxidized, which usually takes between seven and eight turns of $\beta$ oxidation since fats are usually composed of 16 or 18 carbon chains (the last cycle produces 2 acetyl CoA molecules). For example, when stearic acid (an 18-carbon fat) undergoes $\beta$ oxidation, nine acetyl CoA molecules are formed in eight cycles. Each round of the cycle also produces one $FADH_2$ and one NADH molecule. $\beta$ oxidation is controlled at the last step by $\beta$ ketothiolase, which is inhibited by adequate acetyl CoA.

## KREBS CYCLE

The Krebs cycle has also been descriptively labeled the citric acid cycle because the organic acid citrate is involved in the cycle as an intermediate (see Fig. 3.18). The purpose of this cycle is to oxidize acetyl CoA, the common degradation product from fat, carbohydrate, and protein metabolism. Only three amino acids enter the Krebs cycle as acetyl CoA, while the majority of amino acids enter as Krebs cycle intermediates or their precursors (*Fig. 3.21*) (3). While not of major importance during exercise (only 2% to 15% of the fuel utilized during exercise comes from protein), carbon skeletons from amino acids may play a significant role during prolonged exercise when muscle glycogen and blood glucose concentrations are low. In this scenario amino acid conversion to Krebs cycle intermediate compounds helps maintain the integrity of Krebs cycle function and a high rate of mitochondrial respiration. The Krebs cycle functions primarily to reduce $NAD^+$ and FAD to NADH and $FADH_2$.

Pyruvate formed in glycolysis enters the mitochondria via a transport protein located on the outer mitochondrial membrane. Notice that pyruvate is not used in the Krebs cycle directly. Once in the matrix, the mitochondrial enzyme pyruvate dehydrogenase oxidizes pyruvate and decarboxylates it (removes $CO_2$). The two-carbon compound (acetate) that remains condenses with CoA to form acetyl CoA, which then combines with the end product of the just-completed round of the Krebs cycle (oxaloacetate, a four-carbon compound) to form the initial substrate (citrate) of the cycle. The cycle then begins another round (see Fig. 3.17). Glycolysis and the Krebs cycle are linked by the conversion of pyruvate to acetyl CoA in mitochondria. While pyruvate is the product of glycolysis that enters a

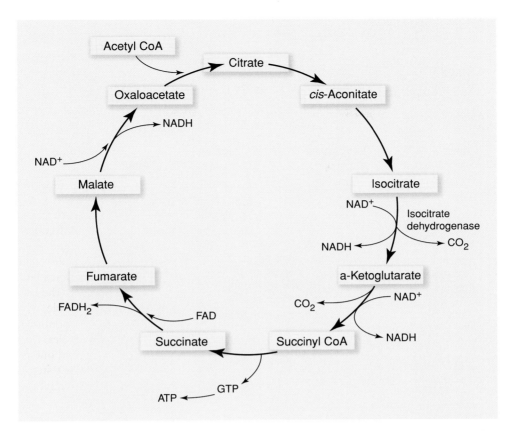

**FIGURE 3.17.** The Krebs cycle shows how $CO_2$, NADH and $FADH_2$ are produced in the mitochondria. This is an important intermediate step in energy transduction. The Krebs cycle processes pyruvate from glucose breakdown and acetyl CoA from fat breakdown.

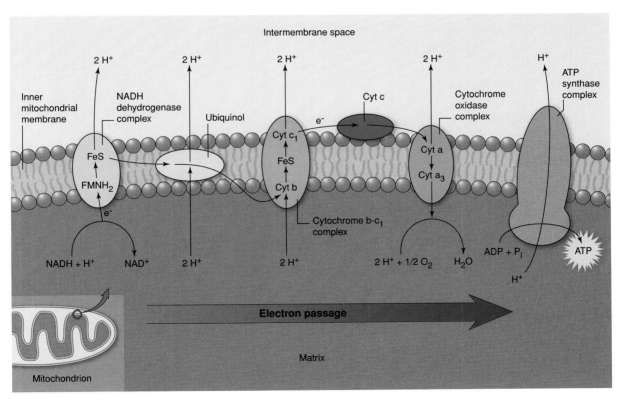

**FIGURE 3.18.** Overview of the electron transport chain (ETC). Having been developed in glycolysis, $\beta$ oxidation, and the Krebs cycle, NADH and $FADH_2$ donate their electrons to the ETC. As electrons pass from the carrier in or on the membrane, the energy of electron flow is used to concentrate (pump) protons into the intermembrane space. As the electrons flow to the final acceptor, $O_2$, the protons flow back through the ATP synthetase complex, and in doing so, synthesize ATP in the process of oxidative phosphorylation.

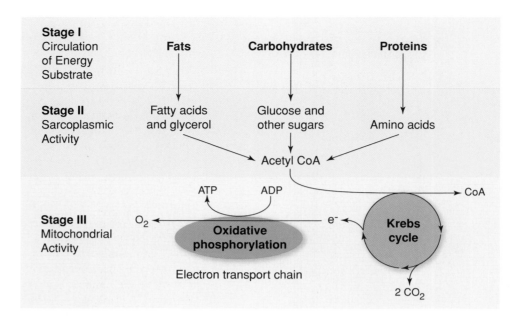

**FIGURE 3.19.** An overview of how nutrients enter the common degradative pathway, the Krebs cycle. From the Krebs cycle, high-energy reduced compounds gain entry to the beginning of the electron transport chain.

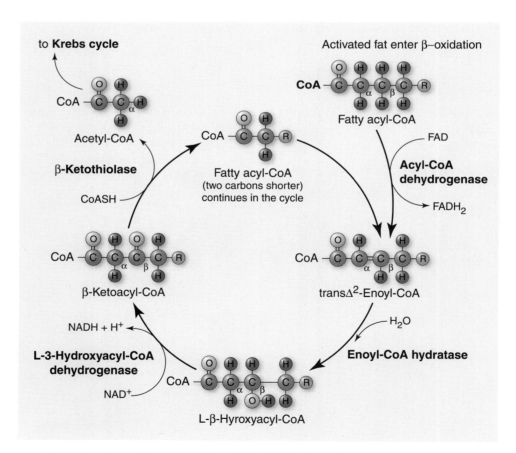

**FIGURE 3.20.** $\beta$ oxidation is a cyclic pathway that processes fatty acid (acyl) chains by producing acetyl CoA with each cycle. Each cycle results in a fatty acid chain that is shortened by two carbons, which is processed again through $\beta$ oxidation. The acetyl CoA produced with each round enters the Krebs cycle. In the illustration of this cycle, the bolded terms are the enzymes.

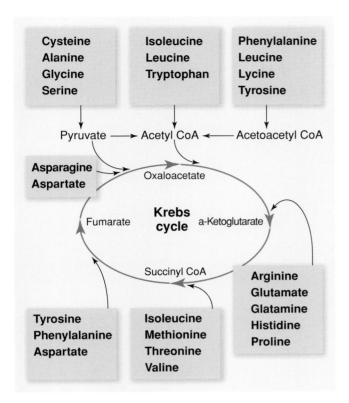

**FIGURE 3.21.** Amino acid metabolism. Carbon skeletons from deaminated amino acids are metabolized by entry into the Krebs Cycle. These amino acids, shown in the rectangles, gain access to the Krebs cycle by various pathways.

mitochondrion, it is the acetyl group of acetyl CoA that actually enters the Krebs cycle. The following is a brief stepwise summary of the Krebs cycle:

1. Acetyl CoA condenses with oxaloacetate to form citrate (a six-carbon compound), the entering substrate of the Krebs cycle.
2. The cycle itself involves eight enzymes. The isocitrate dehydrogenase (IDH) step is rate limiting, being sensitive to the redox potential of the cell. The other dehydrogenases are sensitive to this factor as well, but the position of IDH in the cycle as the first dehydrogenase makes this the rate-limiting step.
3. Each turn of the cycle produces three NADH, one FADH$_2$, one ATP, and two CO$_2$ molecules. One additional NADH and one CO$_2$ are produced from the oxidation of pyruvate prior to entering the cycle.
4. In summary, glucose metabolism results in two pyruvate molecules produced, each undergoing one turn of the Krebs cycle, entering as acetyl CoA. The acetyl CoA may come from fatty acid, carbohydrate, or amino acid oxidation and thus is considered a common degradation product.

Although CO$_2$ is released from the reactions in the mitochondria, no O$_2$ is involved yet in respiration. Most of the energy derived from the steps of the Krebs cycle is temporarily contained in the high-energy electrons of NADH and FADH$_2$. This energy is "mobile" and is harvested via oxidative phosphorylation in the second phase of mitochondrial respiration, the electron transport chain.

Although protein is not a major source of energy during exercise, amino acids in excess of those needed for synthesis of proteins must be metabolized because they cannot be stored or excreted. Amino acid metabolism can be divided into two phases, disposal of the α amino group of the amino acid and catabolism of the remaining skeleton. Urea is the disposal form of the α amino groups derived from amino acids. The process of urea formation is called the urea cycle. In this process, the α amino group from the amino acid is transferred to α ketoglutyrate to form glutamate, which is then deaminated (removal of the amino group) to yield ammonia (NH$_3$). The ammonia is then converted to urea to be excreted through the kidneys. The carbon skeletons of the remaining α amino acids are converted to common intermediates of intermediary metabolism. When the energy state of the cell is low, amino acids will be catabolized to support the energy demand of exercise. The energy yield from each amino acid depends on its entry point in the Krebs cycle. Alanine, for example, enters the cycle through pyruvate and yields 15 ATP molecules.

## ELECTRON TRANSPORT CHAIN

The Krebs cycle produces CO$_2$, NADH, and FADH$_2$ from the breakdown of acetyl CoA. NADH and FADH$_2$ in turn release their hydrogens and electrons to flow to O$_2$ in the electron transport chain. ATP is produced as O$_2$ is used during the formation of water. It is important to note, however, that ATP and O$_2$ are not directly coupled. Aerobic respiration is cellular respiration in the presence of O$_2$, and compared to glycolysis and the Krebs cycle, the electron transport chain is a bonanza for ATP synthesis.

The electron transport chain is located in the mitochondria along the inner membrane, which folds into cristae. It is along these structures that the actual sites for electron transport chain redox and phosphorylation reactions are located. Along these sites, hydrogens and electrons start a series of oxidation-reduction reactions that move electrons and hydrogens through several carriers, which are proteins in or on the inner membrane. The movement of electrons is called electron flow, and it is the actual sequence of the electron and hydrogen carriers that is termed the electron transport chain. The term oxidative phosphorylation refers to the combination of the redox reactions of electron transport that enable the cell to use the energy in NADH and FADH$_2$ to convert ADP plus P$_i$ to ATP. Therefore, the term oxidative phosphorylation is a "hybrid" term, signifying the coupling of different biochemical activities into a unified process.

The electron transport chain is like a series of tiny, successively stronger magnets, each of which has a higher potential than its predecessor. Each component of the chain pulls electrons away from the weaker neighbor and gives

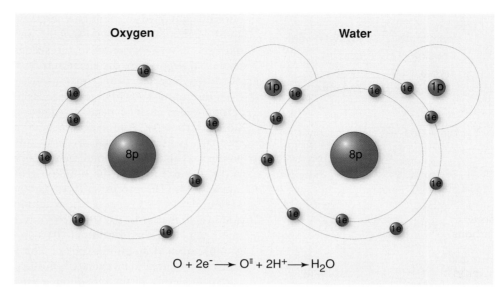

**FIGURE 3.22.** $O_2$ is the final electron acceptor in mitochondrial respiration. The outer shell of oxygen has room for eight electrons but contains only six. It can accept two electrons in electron transport. Accepting two electrons at the end of the respiratory chain increases oxygen's negative charge by two, allowing two hydrogen ions to be attached and forming water.

them up to the stronger one, which has a higher *affinity* for electrons. Affinity refers to the potential to attract electrons and its measure is called the **reduction potential**. The electron transport chain eventually ends with a terminal electron acceptor, $O_2$. $O_2$ accepts two electrons, which increases its negative charge, making it attract the positively charged hydrogen ion (*Fig. 3.22*). In biochemical terms, $O_2$ has the largest reduction potential. In the chain, the hydrogens and electrons flow from NADH toward $O_2$, and electrons are stripped from hydrogens, which then continue along the chain.

There are approximately nine electron carriers in the chain along the inner membrane. These carriers are proteins or protein complexes and pigments, some of which accept the hydrogens and release them into the intermembrane space. Refer to Figure 3.18, which shows the model for the sequence of steps in the chain. According to the model, as electrons continue down the chain between carriers, the energy from electron flow drives the transport of protons from one side of the inner mitochondrial membrane to the other.

The chain starts at the flavin mononucleotide and electrons flow to cytochrome a/a3, which in turn passes the electrons to $O_2$. $O_2$ combines with electrons from the chain and with protons from the matrix, producing water:

$$O_2 + 4\,e^- + 4H^+ \Leftrightarrow 2\,H_2O$$

Note that the transport of protons from one side of the inner membrane to the other requires energy, which is provided by the movement of electrons through the electron transport chain.

Notice that ATP is produced in the chain (right side of Fig. 3.18). *A key question at this point is: how do protons that are pumped by the electron transport chain provide en-*

*ergy for ATP synthesis?* The answer to this question was provided by Peter Mitchell, British scientist and Nobel prize winner, who suspected that the inner mitochondrial membrane must have a role in ATP synthesis. Mitchell proposed the chemiosmotic theory to explain ATP synthesis in mitochondria.

Recall that the flow of electrons provides the energy to actively pump protons across the membrane. Once across the membrane, relatively few of the protons leak back across, with the consequence that there is a much higher concentration of protons in the intermembrane space. A proton gradient is achieved which provides the potential for free energy to be harnessed from the controlled release of protons down the gradient. Referring to Figure 3.18, ATP synthetase, the enzyme that makes ATP, protrudes into the matrix at thousands of locations throughout the membrane, making the mitochondrial membrane a "powerhouse" for making ATP. As the proton gradient builds pressure in the intermembrane space, the gradient is relieved as protons escape through ATP synthetase. The energy provided by this proton flow is used to make ATP (4). This is analogous to water from the bottom of a reservoir rushing out through a drainpipe in the dam and turning a turbine that makes electricity. ATP synthetase can be considered a spinning turbine as protons pass through, providing the energy to make ATP.

Notice that $O_2$, which is essential to most life, comes into the energy-producing process only at the very end of mitochondrial respiration. $O_2$ is necessary to act as a final electron acceptor. Without $O_2$, hydrogen would equilibrate on either side of the inner membrane and flow would stop. ATP production would grind to a halt as the chemiosmotic energy produced by flowing hydrogen dissipated. In humans, think of all the anatomic and biochemical adapta-

| Table 3.3 | ATP TALLY FROM CATABOLISM OF GLUCOSE AND STEARIC ACID IN SKELETAL MUSCLE | |
|---|---|---|
| **Glucose** | **Energy carrier produced** | **ATP subtotal** |
| Glycolysis | 3 ATP (glycogen as substrate) | 3 ATP |
| | 2 NADH | 3 ATP (mitochondrial membrane shuttle exchanges $H^+$ from NADH to $FADH_2$) |
| Pyruvate to acetyl CoA | 2 NADH | 5 ATP |
| Krebs cycle | 2 ATP (substrate level phosphorylation) | 2 ATP |
| | 6 NADH (2 pyruvate enters each turn) | 15 ATP |
| | 2 $FADH_2$ | 3 ATP |
| | | 31 total ATP from the complete breakdown of glucose molecule taken from glycogen |
| **Stearic acid (18 carbons)** | **Energy carrier produced** | **ATP subtotal** |
| Activation of the fatty acid in sarcoplasm after lipolysis | −2 ATP | −2 ATP |
| $\beta$ oxidation (8 turns | 8 NADH | 20 ATP |
| produces 9 acetyl CoA) | 8 $FADH_2$ | 12 ATP |
| Krebs cycle | 27 NADH | 68 ATP |
| | 9 $FADH_2$ | 14 ATP |
| | 9 ATP | 9 ATP |
| | | 121 total ATP from the complete breakdown of stearic acid |

tions that are necessary to deliver $O_2$ to the end of the electron transport chains in our cells. Noses, lungs, arteries, red blood cells, and hemoglobin are among some of the necessary parts.

## TALLYING ATP

*What kind of capacity does this electron and proton gradient have? Put another way, how much ATP can be generated in the electron transport chain?* Each NADH drives the synthesis of three ATPs, while each $FADH_2$ drives the synthesis of two ATPs. These values are the ATP equivalents for the hydrogen carriers. The difference in ATP count from these high-energy carriers is due to the fact that $FADH_2$ enters the electron transport chain just below the entry point for NADH bypassing one of the sites for ATP formation. The effect of this entry point is that each $FADH_2$ results in pumping two pairs of protons across to the intermembrane space, instead of the three pairs pumped by NADH. With this knowledge, it is now possible to calculate the number of ATP molecules generated in catabolism. Table 3.3 presents these numbers for glucose and stearic acid.

▶ *INQUIRY SUMMARY.* Respiration is the major form of energy transformation of the cell. In the presence of sufficient $O_2$, pyruvate from glycolysis moves into mitochondria and is converted to acetyl CoA, which enters the Krebs cycle.

Acetyl CoA from lipolysis and a small amount from protein catabolism also enter the Krebs cycle. Each "turn" of this cycle uses one molecule of acetyl CoA and produces $FADH_2$, NADH, and $CO_2$. $\beta$ oxidation also produces $FADH_2$ and NADH. Electrons from NADH and $FADH_2$ are subsequently donated in the electron transport chain in which electron carriers in the inner mitochondrial membrane pass electrons along to $O_2$ and pump protons into the intermembrane space. The resulting proton gradient produced by electron transport provides the energy necessary for making ATP by the process of oxidative phosphorylation. The complete aerobic respiration of one molecule of glucose can produce as many as 38 molecules of ATP, while an 18-carbon fatty acid can produce as many as 121 molecules of ATP. *Explain the significance for weight loss in "burning" fat versus carbohydrate.*

## Summary

Energy is the ability to do work or cause change. All of life's activities require that energy be transformed from one form to another, and these transformations are governed by the laws of thermodynamics. In our body these energy transformations are summed up in the process of metabolism, and they occur in step-by-step sequences called metabolic pathways, some of which are catabolic (breaking down) and some anabolic (building up). The metabolic transformations are designed to ensure that adequate amounts of ATP are produced so that cells can perform a myriad of activities. ATP is constantly resupplied in cells by catabolic processes that move free energy from one form (energy nutrients) to another (ATP). The metabolic processes in the cell produce ATP at different rates during exercise of differing intensities. During high-intensity exercise, sarcoplasmic pathways produce ATP at a fast rate but have a very limited capacity for total ATP production. At low to moderate exercise intensities, sarcoplasmic pathways are linked to the mitochondrial pathways, and ATP is produced at a slower rate but with a far greater total capacity, owing to the fact that more energy nutrients come into play. Energy metabolism can be thought of in these terms: *immediate* production of ATP in the sarcoplasm by catabolism of phosphagen stores, *short-term* production of ATP in the sarcoplasm by catabolism of glucose, and *long-term* production of ATP by catabolism of all three energy nutrients in both sarcoplasmic and mitochondrial processes.

## SUMMARY KNOWLEDGE

1. What is the difference between potential and kinetic energy?
2. Why are the laws of thermodynamics important in the study of exercise physiology?
3. What is metabolism? What two major components does it include?
4. Why is some exercise considered anaerobic and some aerobic?
5. How are coupled reactions important in metabolism?
6. Why is lactate produced in skeletal muscle during exercise? Is its production good or bad for exercise performance?
7. Explain the role of glycogen during exercise.
8. Explain the concepts of power and capacity as these terms relate to metabolism during exercise.
9. Why are there different ATP production totals from different catabolic pathways of skeletal muscles?
10. At the onset of exercise, why are ATP and CP the preferred energy sources over carbohydrate and fat?
11. What is aerobic respiration and how does it depend on $O_2$?

### References

1. Greenhaff PL, Timmons JA. Interaction between aerobic and anaerobic metabolism during intense muscle contraction. *Exerc Sport Sci Rev* 1998;26:1–30.
2. Martin WH III. Effects of acute and chronic exercise on fat metabolism. *Exerc Sport Sci Rev* 1996;24:203–231.
3. Wagenmakers AJM. Muscle amino acid metabolism at rest and during exercise: role in human physiology and metabolism. *Exerc Sport Sci Rev* 1998;26:287–314.
4. Houston M. *Biochemistry primer for exercise science.* Champaign, Ill: Human Kinetics, 1995.

### Suggested Readings

Gilbert HF. *Basic concepts in biochemistry: a student's survival guide.* 2nd ed. New York: McGraw-Hill, 2000.

Hargreaves M. Interactions between muscle glycogen and blood glucose during exercise. *Exerc Sport Sci Rev* 1997;25:21–39.

Nicklas BJ. Effects of endurance exercise on adipose tissue metabolism. *Exerc Sport Sci Rev* 1997;25:77–103.

Berg JM, Tymoczko JL, Stryer L. *Biochemistry.* 5th Ed. San Francisco: WH Freeman & Co, 2002.

Tonkonogi M, Sahlin K. Physical exercise and mitochondrial function in human skeletal muscle. *Exerc Sport Sci Rev* 2002;30:129–137.

Wagenmakers AJM. Muscle amino acid metabolism at rest and during exercise: role in human physiology and metabolism. *Exerc Sport Sci Rev* 1998;26:287–314.

### On the Internet

Metabolic Pathways of Biochemistry. Available at: **http://www.gwu.edu/~mpb/**. Accessed March 31, 2005.

The 20 Amino Acids. Available at: **http://www.people.virginia.edu/~rjh9u/aminacid.html**. Accessed March 31, 2005.

Carbohydrate Chemistry. Available at: **http://cvu.strath.ac.uk/lorna/chemistry/home.html**. Accessed March 31, 2005.

Forms of Energy. Available at: **http://edugreen.teri.res.in/explore/n_renew/energy.htm**. Accessed March 31, 2005.

Adenosine Triphosphate—ATP. Available at: **http://www.bris.ac.uk/Depts/Chemistry/MOTM/atp/atp1.htm**. Accessed March 31, 2005.

Major Roles of Biological Lipids. Available at: **http://web.indstate.edu/thcme/mwking/lipids.html**. Accessed March 31, 2005.

McArdle Disease. Available at: **http://members.aol.com/itsgumby/**. Accessed March 31, 2005.

## Writing to Learn

*Mammalian species, humans included, are able to engage in a wide range of physical activities, from long duration (low power) activities to short duration (high power) burst of activity. This is due to the nature of the biochemical pathways responsible for energy transduction. Write a paper answering the following question. What are the advantages and disadvantages of aerobic versus anaerobic respiration and how do these relate to exercise performance?*

# CHAPTER

# 4 Metabolic Transitions During Exercise

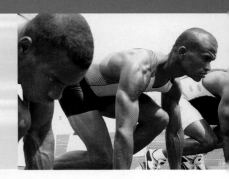

*The instant exercise begins, the body has to adjust its metabolic rate so that enough adenosine triphosphate (ATP) is available to support the energy demands of the exercise. During heavy exercise, the body's energy expenditure may increase to 25 times that at rest. Most of this energy (ATP) is used within the exercising muscles, which can increase their metabolic rate by 200-fold. A small amount of the increased energy demand is for sustaining the systems that indirectly support the exercising muscles, such as the cardiovascular system. In this chapter, we will discover how several systems of the body communicate with each other during transition from rest to exercise, in sustained exercise, and in recovery from exercise. Which systems of the body do you think need to communicate with each other as an athlete begins a race?*

## CHAPTER OUTLINE

**REST-TO-EXERCISE TRANSITIONS**
- Energy Accessibility
- Energy Systems Stressed by Exercise
- Response to Exercise Energy Demands: Hormonal Regulation
  - Regulation of Hormone Secretion
  - Hormone-Receptor-Cell Interaction
  - Major Hormones Involved with Exercise
  - Hormonal Response to Exercise
- Results of an Exercise-Induced Rise in Metabolism

**MAINTAINING ENERGY SUPPLY DURING EXERCISE**
- Exercise Intensity and Fuel Selection
- Exercise Duration and Fuel Supply

**RECOVERY FROM EXERCISE: RESYNTHESIS OF FUELS**
- Regeneration of ATP and PC
- Reformation of Glucose
- Synthesis of Glycogen
- Synthesis of Fatty Acids and Triglycerides

We learned in Chapter 3 that ATP is the energy currency of the body, and that when energy demand increases, the body has the capacity to increase its ATP production to meet those demands. Chapter 3 also presented three primary biochemical pathways that supply ATP to the exercising muscles: the adenosine triphosphate-phosphocreatine (ATP-PC) system (phosphagen system), rapid glycolysis (lactic acid system), and mitochondrial respiration (aerobic system). The rate of ATP production, or power output, of these pathways varies dramatically. When the rate of ATP production is insufficient to meet the demand from exercise, the muscles become fatigued. Therefore, muscular fatigue

and endurance can be expressed in terms of either exercise intensity or energy source.

This chapter will help you understand how the muscles adjust their metabolic activity as the transition from rest to exercise occurs, how the muscles sustain exercise for prolonged periods of time, and how energy supplies in muscles are restored following an exercise bout. In order to meet these objectives, we will learn about the physiologic markers exercise scientists use to evaluate the energy state of the muscles. When the exercise professional knows how the energy systems function, interact, and adapt as they supply energy for exercise, he/she will be better able to predict the results of exercise training, control the

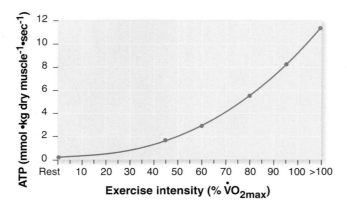

FIGURE 4.1. Rest-to-exercise transitions in ATP production. As the relative intensity of exercise increases, the rate of ATP production rises concurrently to meet the exercise energy demand.

conditioning process, and gain the most physiologically for the time invested during exercise training.

## Rest-to-Exercise Transitions

At rest, the muscles are in a state of energy balance or homeostasis. The amount of energy (ATP) used to sustain cellular activity at rest is derived almost exclusively from aerobic metabolism, with a mixture of fat and carbohydrate fuels used to meet the energy demand. The power output of the muscles at rest is very low, and it is easy for the muscles to maintain this state of energy balance. The instant exercise begins, the muscles must increase their ATP production to that which is required to sustain the exercise intensity (*Fig. 4.1*). At this point in time, the body adjusts the rate at which ATP supplies the exercising muscles according to exercise intensity. The relative intensity of exercise that can be supported by each energy system is shown in Table 4.1.

A clear relationship exists between maximal power output of an energy system and the relative exercise intensity that system can support. When the rate of ATP production is insufficient to meet the demand from exercise, the muscles become fatigued. Very–high-intensity exercise can only be supported by the ATP-PC energy system for about

15 seconds before fatigue sets in and exercise must cease unless the intensity is reduced (*Fig. 4.2*). Rapid glycolysis cannot support very–high-intensity exercise but will support high-intensity exercise for up to 1 minute. Exercise longer than 1 minute will be supported by slow glycolysis, but only at a lower intensity than rapid glycolysis. Within 2 hours, at this low-intensity level of exercise, glycogen depletion will occur and the muscles will become fatigued. Fat stores must now be the primary source for ATP supply, but the power output from fat is lower still. The energy reserve stored in fat can support very–low-intensity exercise for several days, but the rate of ATP production is extremely low. Only in the state of starvation, however, will a marked reduction in body fat stores occur due to exercise.

In reality, there is some overlap among the different energy systems (Fig. 4.2). Energy required for exercise below 40% to 50% of the maximum $O_2$ consumption ($\dot{V}O_{2max}$) is derived primarily from oxidation of fat with some contribution from carbohydrate oxidation (slow glycolysis). As the intensity of exercise increases to 50% to 70% of $\dot{V}O_{2max}$, additional oxidation of carbohydrate must occur because there is a requirement for higher power output. At about 70% of $\dot{V}O_{2max}$, the higher rate of energy production necessitates that rapid glycolysis play a greater role in ATP production. If the exercise intensity is further increased to near or above maximal aerobic capacity, ATP and PC stores will be utilized for producing the energy necessary for muscular contraction. Box 4.1 highlights research investigating how the ATP:PC ratio and metabolic concentration affects physiologic functioning in cardiac patients.

### ENERGY ACCESSIBILITY

Accessibility is another important factor that comes into play as fuel sources are mobilized for ATP production. The energy systems with the highest capacity for power output also have the most readily available fuel sources. The most readily available fuel source of all is the phosphagens. The next most readily available fuel source for ATP production is carbohydrate. Glycogen is stored in close proximity to the contractile mechanism of the muscle, and glucose can rapidly be mobilized from it to produce ATP through rapid glycolysis. Once

| Table 4.1 | ATP PRODUCTION FROM DIFFERENT ENERGY SYSTEMS | | | | |
|---|---|---|---|---|---|
| Energy system | Moles ATP available (mmol ATP·kg$^{-1}$) | Maximal power (dry muscle·sec$^{-1}$) | Relative exercise intensity supported | Exercise time | Exercise or event |
| ATP stores | 0.02 | 11.2 | very high | 1–2 sec | hitting a baseball |
| PC stores | 0.34 | 8.6 | very high | 10–15 sec | tennis rally |
| Rapid glycolysis | 5.20 | 5.2 | high | 30–60 sec | 400-M sprint |
| Slow glycolysis | 70.00 | 2.7 | moderate | 90–120 min | marathon |
| Fat oxidation | 8,000.00 | 1.4 | low | 350 hr | Tour de France |

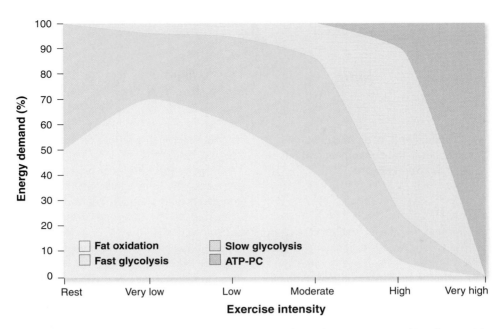

**FIGURE 4.2.** Relative contributions of the energy systems to the exercise energy demand. As a person transitions from rest to very intense exercise, the relative contributions of the different energy systems shift to meet the power output demand.

the rate-limiting reactions in glycolysis are disinhibited, glycolytic ATP production can proceed at capacity.

Slow glycolysis and fat oxidation are the least readily available fuel sources in the contracting muscle for a few reasons. Oxygen is needed to produce ATP aerobically, and $O_2$ must be transported into the mitochondria for the electron transport chain to be functional. Some intracellular $O_2$ is available, but most of the $O_2$ needed for aerobic metabolism must be transported from the atmosphere to the muscles through the cardiovascular system. It takes time to increase the rate of cardiovascular $O_2$ delivery to the muscles. Once $O_2$ is available, slow glycolysis can proceed at capacity. Before fat oxidation can occur, triglycerides must be broken down to glycerol and fatty acids, and the fatty acids must be transported across the mitochondrial membrane and then broken down to their acetyl coenzyme A (CoA) subunits through β oxidation to enter the Krebs cycle.

Thus, the energy systems with the highest capacity for power output also have the most readily available fuel sources. The significance of this is that regardless of the intensity of exercise, all energy systems will be called upon to deliver ATP to the contracting muscles. As exercise continues for several seconds to several minutes, the priority will be to derive ATP from the energy system that can endure the longest and still meet the power output demand.

## ENERGY SYSTEMS STRESSED BY EXERCISE

As energy systems are called upon to produce ATP when exercise begins, they work cooperatively to ensure a smooth metabolic transition from rest to exercise. Three scenarios illustrate when each of the three energy systems are called upon to provide the major portion of ATP needed to sustain

exercise at a given intensity. The risk of this type of presentation is that you can easily digress into thinking that each of the energy systems is independent, and that as one system produces ATP, the other systems become dormant. Remember that all of the systems are producing ATP simultaneously throughout exercise, but the proportional contribution of ATP to the metabolic demand from each system will shift according to exercise intensity.

The first example of the rest-to-exercise transition in the energy systems is given for very–high-intensity exercise. The ATP-PC energy system is the only system with the capacity to meet the power output demand of very–high-intensity exercise (Table 4.1 and Fig. 4.2). All other systems and fuel sources are mostly excluded. Although the other energy systems will produce ATP at much slower rates during very–high-intensity exercise, their proportional contribution to the energy supply is minimal.

Once the ATP-PC stores become depleted, exercise intensity has to be reduced to continue exercise. The primary responsibility for supporting power output demand shifts from the ATP-PC system to rapid glycolysis as the exercise intensity is reduced from very high intensity to high intensity. A similar scenario occurs when exercise is initiated at a high intensity rather than a very high intensity.

After several minutes of exercise at this level, the intensity must be shifted again to a low or moderate level if exercise is to continue. Now the aerobic pathways become almost exclusive providers of ATP to support the exercise. Oxidation of fat will become more predominant than oxidation of carbohydrate as the exercise bout goes beyond minutes into hours.

Chronic exercise training focused on stressing each of the energy systems will cause them to increase their

**Box 4.1**

## RESEARCH HIGHLIGHT

**Okita K, Yonezawa K, Nishijima H, et al. Muscle high-energy metabolites and metabolic capacity in patients with heart failure.** *Med Sci Sports Exerc* **2001;33:442–448.**

### RESEARCH SUMMARY

The major limiting symptom in patients with chronic heart failure (CHF) is exercise intolerance. The traditional line of thinking is that exercise intolerance in persons with CHF is caused by a reduced perfusion to the skeletal muscle during exercise. This reduction in muscle perfusion has been attributed to an impaired vasodilator reserve and diminished cardiac output. Morphologic, histologic, and biochemical analyses of resting skeletal muscle of patients with CHF have shown a reduction in muscle fiber size, increased proportion of fast-twitch fibers, and reduced aerobic enzyme capacity. Skeletal muscle abnormalities in persons with CHF are described by a rapid depletion of phosphocreatine (PC), reduction in pH, and early onset of fatigue. These characteristics suggest that high-energy metabolite concentration (HEMC) is altered in persons with CHF.

Subjects for this study were 27 male and 7 female patients with CHF, and 10 male and 3 female age- and size-matched controls. Exercise capacity (peak $VO_2$) was determined through a graded exercise test to symptom-limited maximum on a cycle ergometer. Resting HEMC data were obtained by the use of $^{31}P$-magnetic resonance spectroscopy ($^{31}P$-MRS). Plantar flexion was performed 40 times per minute, and muscle energy metabolism was evaluated by $^{31}P$-MRS. Metabolic capacity of the muscle was calculated through a regression equation using the exercise $^{31}P$-MRS data.

The peak heart rate, peak workload, anaerobic threshold, and peak $VO_2$ were significantly lower in the CHF patients compared with controls. The muscle metabolic capacity, evaluated as the PC slope, was significantly steeper in patients with CHF than in normal subjects, indicating that muscle metabolism was impaired during exercise in patients with CHF. Muscle pH at maximal workload was significantly lower in patients with CHF than in the controls. The PC:ATP and inorganic phosphate:ATP were significantly greater in patients with CHF than in the healthy controls.

The major finding of this study is that HEMC is altered in patients with CHF. The PC:ATP ratio seems to be a valid marker for the capacity of the ATP-PC energy system. The increased PC:ATP ratio seen in the patients with CHF is probably caused by an imbalance in the energy supply systems. The lower aerobic capacity in the CHF patients may be compensated by an alteration in the ATP-PC system, as well as an increase in rapid glycolysis, as seen by a more rapid decline in muscle pH during exercise.

### IMPLICATIONS FOR FURTHER RESEARCH

The results of this study imply that the HEMC in skeletal muscle of CHF patients is altered because of the inability of the aerobic energy system to provide an adequate energy supply during exercise. If this is the case, it will be necessary to discover the mechanism that induces the elevation in PC:ATP seen in CHF patients and if there is a way to induce this change without any negative side effects.

---

capacity to produce ATP. The exercise professional should be familiar with how to design an appropriate training regimen to increase the capacity of whichever system is called upon during any specific type of exercise performance.

## RESPONSE TO EXERCISE ENERGY DEMANDS: HORMONAL REGULATION

We have already discussed how the metabolic rate of the different energy systems adjusts to meet the increased energy demand of exercise at varying intensities. *How does the body know that there is an increased need for energy? How are metabolic fuels mobilized from different tissues so that energy steady state can be maintained during exercise?* This section provides the answers to these questions.

The two major systems that regulate communication about the energy status of tissues, organs, and organ systems of the body are the endocrine and nervous systems. Both of these systems are designed to receive information, interpret that information, and elicit the desired response through the appropriate tissue or organ. These two systems frequently work together, communicating similar messages to the same tissue or organ. The two systems differ, however, in the way they communicate information. For instance, the nervous system uses neurotransmitters to relay messages from one nerve to another or from nerve to tissue. The endocrine system releases hormones into the blood to circulate to the tissues. The nervous system is presented in detail in Chapter 9.

Communication within the endocrine system is initiated when a host tissue, usually an endocrine gland, secretes minute quantities of a chemical messenger called a hormone (*Fig. 4.3*). The hormone interacts with receptors on a target organ or tissue. The response will subsequently be propagated by the target tissue or organ. A hormone, therefore, is a chemical substance that is synthesized by a specific host tissue or gland, is secreted into the blood, is circulated throughout the body, and subsequently exerts an effect on a specific tissue or organ. Its function is to alter the rate of specific cellular reactions within the receptor cells.

Hormones can be classified into three types: amine, peptide, and steroid. Amine hormones are derived from amino acids and exert their action by binding to specific receptors on the cell membrane of target cells. Epinephrine, norepinephrine, and thyroxine are examples of amine hormones. Peptide hormones are similar to amine hormones in that they cannot pass through the cell membrane so they bind to receptor proteins on the cell membrane. Insulin and antidiuretic hormone (ADH) are examples of peptide hormones. Both amine and peptide hormones are water soluble and are transported in solution in blood plasma. Steroid hormones are different from amine and peptide hormones in that they have a chemical structure similar to cholesterol, and as such, are lipid soluble. These hormones can diffuse through cell membranes and are received by protein receptors found in the cell cytoplasm or on the nuclear membrane. Testosterone and estrogen are the most notable of the steroid hormones.

Most hormones are carried in the blood and circulated to all the tissues of the body. However, only cells of the targeted tissues interact with the hormone. The interaction between hormone and target cell occurs because the target cell contains protein receptors, which are usually embedded in the cell membrane. Some of these protein receptors will interact with the hormone and then transmit a signal into the cell that propagates the desired effect, while other protein receptors will allow the hormone itself to transverse the membrane and enter the cell to exert its effect.

The magnitude to which the cell is activated by the hormone depends upon the concentration of the hormone in the blood, relative number of cell receptors, and sensitivity of the receptors to the hormone. The state in which the concentration of the hormone in the blood is high and all the receptors of a cell are bound to the hormone is called **saturation**.

The sensitivity of hormone receptors sometimes changes under varying circumstances. The number of receptor molecules may decrease in a cell when the cell is chronically exposed to a high concentration of the hormone. This is called **downregulation**, a protective mechanism that prevents the target cell from overresponding to the persistently high hormone levels. On the other hand, **upregulation** occurs when the cell produces a greater number of receptors in response to hormone stimulation. The greater the number of cell receptors, the greater the sensitivity of the cell to the hormone. Each cell typically has 2000 to 10,000 receptors.

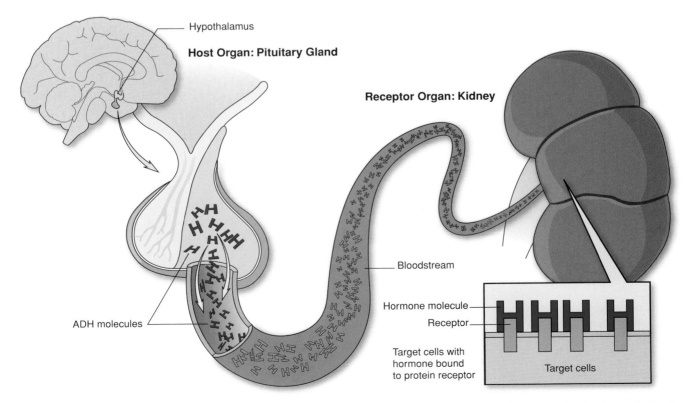

**FIGURE 4.3.** The endocrine system communicates messages to the body tissues. In this example, antidiuretic hormone (H) that is secreted by the pituitary gland acts on the kidney to cause the reabsorption of water.

The concentration of a hormone in the blood is affected by three factors: the quantity of hormone produced by the host gland, rate at which the hormone is secreted into the blood, and rate at which the hormone is removed from the blood. The quantity of hormone produced by the host gland is generally stable in healthy persons. The rate at which the hormone is secreted is dependent upon the magnitude of stimulation or inhibition of the host gland. In either stimulation or inhibition, secretion is affected by chemical input to the host gland. This input can come in three forms; hormonal, humoral, and neural. Most endocrine glands are under the influence of more than one type of input.

## Regulation of Hormone Secretion

Hormonal input occurs when one hormone influences the release of another hormone. Many of the hormones released from the anterior pituitary gland stimulate the release of other hormones. In effect, when a chemical signal is received by the pituitary gland, it prompts the secretion of a pituitary hormone; the secreted hormone is received by a target gland, which responds by secreting another hormone. Increasing blood levels of the target hormone provide feedback to the pituitary gland, which inhibits the release of the pituitary hormone and ultimately further secretion of the targeted hormone.

Circulating levels of nutrients, ions, bile, and other fluids also provide input to endocrine glands. This is called humoral input. The control of blood sugar levels by the hormone insulin is an example of humoral input. Elevated blood sugar levels stimulate the release of insulin from the pancreas, and insulin then promotes the uptake of glucose from the blood into cells. As glucose is removed from the blood and blood glucose levels decline, the humoral stimulus of the pancreas is diminished, ending the secretion of insulin. The pancreatic cells sometimes become less responsive to insulin. Decreased insulin sensitivity is commonly seen in overweight or obese individuals. The result is that these individuals cannot metabolize glucose effectively. If insulin sensitivity is reduced dramatically, type 2 diabetes is diagnosed. Box 4.2 explains why insulin resistance is becoming a major health problem in the United States.

**Box 4.2**

## *PERSPECTIVE*

# *Insulin Resistance*

Diabetes mellitus is a metabolic disease in which the body is not able to metabolize glucose correctly. There are two general classifications of diabetes. Type 1 diabetes, or insulin-dependent diabetes, occurs when the pancreas does not secrete enough of the hormone insulin. Consequently, there is not enough circulating insulin to interact with the receptors in the target tissues, primarily the muscles. The result is that blood glucose levels rise because the tissues cannot extract the glucose from the blood.

The second general classification of diabetes is called type 2 diabetes, or noninsulin-dependent diabetes mellitus (NIDDM). In these cases, the pancreas secretes normal insulin amounts, but the tissues are not responsive to the circulating insulin. Similar to type 1 diabetes, blood glucose levels rise in NIDDM because the glucose cannot enter the tissues. NIDDM accounts for 80% to 90% of all diabetes cases in the United States. NIDDM is the form of diabetes that is most responsive to diet and exercise behaviors.

It is estimated that 80 million adult Americans (25% of the population) have a subdiagnosable form of NIDDM called insulin resistance. In these cases, the tissues have a reduced ability to take up glucose at any given blood insulin concentration. The receptors, in other words, do not respond to insulin. This nonresponsiveness to insulin causes blood glucose levels to remain elevated. The high blood glucose levels continue to stimulate the pancreas to secrete more insulin. If the pancreas cannot secrete enough insulin to reduce blood glucose levels, NIDDM develops.

There are other detrimental effects of insulin resistance. The hyperinsulinemia (high blood insulin) seen with insulin resistance can lead to hypertension (high blood pressure). The theory is that insulin resistance affects sympathetic nervous activity, causing elevated secretions of the hormones epinephrine and norepinephrine. These catecholamines cause blood pressure to rise due to their effects on cardiac output. Furthermore, elevated insulin increases water retention, which increases blood volume and subsequently blood pressure. Lastly, it is suspected that elevated insulin causes smooth muscle cells in the blood vessels to proliferate, restricting blood flow and increasing blood pressure. The resulting conditions from hyperinsulinemia due to insulin resistance are hypertension, arteriosclerosis, and nerve disease.

Regular physical activity can greatly reduce one's risk for developing NIDDM. The majority of persons who are insulin resistant can prevent the development of NIDDM and other complications associated with hyperinsulinemia when they participate in a regular exercise program.

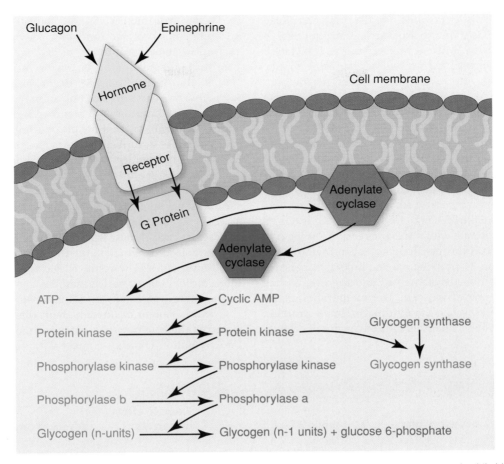

**FIGURE 4.4.** Epinephrine- and glucagon-stimulated glycolysis. The red color indicates an inactive enzyme or compound, while blue indicates an active enzyme or compound. Through hormone-receptor interaction, the enzyme adenylate kinase is activated. Active adenylate kinase converts ATP to cyclic AMP. The cyclic AMP sets off a series of cascading enzymatic events that shut down glycogen synthesis and stimulate glycogen breakdown.

The third way in which hormone secretion is regulated is through neural stimulation. *Were you ever anxious prior to an athletic competition and felt your heart racing?* This is an example of neural input. In this case, the **sympathetic nervous system** stimulates the adrenal medulla to secrete hormones called **catecholamines**. For example, the catecholamine epinephrine causes the elevation in heart rate seen during anxiousness or stress.

Another example of neural control is seen during exercise. Activation of the **hypothalamus** and sympathetic nervous system during exercise causes a reduction in the secretion of insulin from the pancreas. This results in a decrease in blood insulin levels during exercise and ensures that blood glucose levels will be maintained so that the central nervous system is not starved of nutrients. Even though circulating insulin levels are diminished during exercise, contracting muscles are not robbed of glucose because exercise itself has an insulin-like effect on the muscles.

 *LINKUP: More about the effects of exercise in glucose transport can be found in Perspective: Exercise Facilitates Glucose Uptake into the Cells at http://connection.lww.com/go/brownexphys and on the Student Resource CD-ROM.*

## Hormone-Receptor-Cell Interaction

It was stated earlier that hormones are carried by the circulation to all the body tissues and that only certain tissues are affected by hormones through hormone receptor interaction. Many cell receptors for hormones are protein molecules that reside in the cell membrane. These proteins are not fixed in the membrane but are fluid or mobile within the membrane structure. Other receptors reside in the cytoplasm of the cell and interact with the hormone after it enters the cell. The number of receptors in a cell varies from a few hundred to a hundred thousand, depending on the type of receptor. It is the chemical structure of the protein receptor that makes that receptor specific for a certain hormone.

An example of how a hormone interacts with a receptor protein in a cell membrane is shown in *Figure 4.4.* This example is particularly important because it illustrates the following basic concepts about hormonal control of metabolism during exercise: receptor-hormone interaction, enzyme activation, cyclic 3′,5′-adenosine monophosphate (cyclic AMP) formation, and amplification of the hormone signal. The events that are illustrated in Figure 4.4 are specific to glycogenolysis (catabolism of glycogen) but are typical of general events that regulate many metabolic processes.

Glycogenolysis is controlled by the phosphorylase enzyme, which exists in two isoforms, phosphorylase b and phosphorylase a. Muscle phosphorylase b is active only in the presence of high levels of adenosine mono-phosphate (AMP). However, under most physiologic conditions, phosphorylase b is inhibited by ATP and glucose-6-phosphate. Phosphorylase b can be converted into phosphorylase a, the more active isoform, simply by phosphorylating it. The sequence of events leading to the **phosphorylation** of phosphorylase b may seem complex at first, but it is a classic example of the principle of signal amplification in the biologic system.

Glycogenolysis is activated primarily by two hormones: glucagon and epinephrine (Fig. 4.4). Circulating levels of these hormones interact with a specific receptor in the cell membrane. The receptor then activates a G protein within the cell membrane. G proteins are the links between the hormones on the outside of the cell and the events that follow on the inside of the cell. The membrane-bound enzyme, adenylate cyclase, is stimulated by G protein. Adenylate cyclase then catalyzes the conversion of ATP to cyclic AMP.

The newly formed cyclic AMP activates a protein kinase enzyme that serves two functions: activation of phosphorylase kinase and inhibition of glycogen synthase. This coordinated regulation of glycogen synthesis and degradation is important so that ATP is not wasted in two opposing pathways. The activated phosphorylase kinase enzyme works upon phosphorylase b and converts it to the more active a form by a phosphorylation reaction. The phosphorylase in turn stimulates glycogenolysis.

You might wonder why such a complicated series of events is necessary just to stimulate one enzyme (phosphorylase b). The purpose of the sequential steps is to amplify the hormonal signal. One epinephrine molecule received by a receptor will cause activation of several protein kinase molecules. Each of these will activate several phosphorylase kinase molecules, which in turn activate many phosphorylase b molecules. The result is that many more glycogen molecules will be degraded by the enzyme cascade than if the hormone interacted only with phosphorylase b.

The other point of interest about this series of cellular events is the role of cyclic AMP. Hormones released into the circulation come in contact with every tissue of the

| Table 4.2 | SUMMARY OF THE MAJOR HORMONES INVOLVED IN EXERCISE | | | |
|---|---|---|---|---|
| **Hormone** | **Secretory gland** | **Metabolic Effect** | **Exercise effect on secretion** | **Affected organ or tissue** |
| Glucagon | Pancreas | Glycogenolysis, gluconeogenesis, lipolysis | Increased | Most cells, particularly muscles, fat, and liver |
| Insulin | Pancreas | Promotes glucose, fatty acid, and amino acid transport into cells | Decreased | Most cells, particularly muscles and fat |
| Epinephrine | Adrenal | Glycogenolysis, gluconeogenesis, lipolysis | Increased | Most cells, particularly muscles, fat, and heart |
| Norepinephrine | | Gluconeogenesis, lipolysis | | Most cells, particularly blood vessels and fat |
| Cortisol | Adrenal | Gluconeogenesis promotes fatty acid and protein catabolism; conserves blood sugar | Increased | Most cells, particularly muscles |
| Aldosterone | Adrenal | Increased potassium secretion and sodium reabsorption | Increased | Kidneys |
| Antidiuretic hormone | Pituitary | Promotes water reabsorption | Increased | Kidneys and blood vessels |
| Corticotropin | Pituitary | Gluconeogenesis, fatty acid mobilization, protein catabolism, causes release of cortisol and aldosterone | Increased | Adrenal cortex |
| Growth Hormone | Pituitary | Gluconeogenesis, promotes fatty acid mobilization and protein synthesis | Increased | All cells, particularly muscles and bone |

body. On a smaller scale, the cyclic AMP that is formed within the cell in response to the hormonal message comes in contact with everything in the cell. Cyclic AMP is, therefore, called the second messenger, communicating to the intracellular components the signal delivered by the first messenger, the hormone.

At the same time, cyclic AMP activates other proteins which affect cellular metabolism. Cyclic AMP stimulates hormone-sensitive lipase, the enzyme that breaks down triglycerides into glycerol and fatty acids. Here again we can see that the energy systems are not independent of each other. Cyclic AMP causes the breakdown of glycogen to be used in either fast (anaerobic) or slow (aerobic) glycolysis at the same time it causes the breakdown of triglycerides, which can only be metabolized aerobically.

## Major Hormones Involved with Exercise

Several hormones come into play as you exercise (Table 4.2). Some of them affect the energetics of muscle contraction, whereas others affect physiologic processes related to exercise such as water balance, temperature regulation, and cardiorespiratory control. The hormones that affect the energetics of muscular contraction are glucagon, insulin, epinephrine, norepinephrine, cortisol, corticotropin (also known as adrenocorticotropic hormone [ACTH], and growth hormone (GH). ADH and aldosterone prolong the onset of fatigue by regulating fluid balance and ion exchange. The overall goals of the endocrine system during exercise are to:

- Mobilize fuel for the production of ATP necessary to support muscle contraction
- Maintain blood glucose levels
- Enhance cardiac output
- Increase blood supply to the active tissues
- Maintain blood pressure by stabilizing fluid and electrolyte balance

These goals are met by coordinating the magnitude of effect the hormones have on the cardiovascular system and the storage depots for fuel (liver, muscles, and adipocytes).

Glucagon is a hormone secreted by the alpha cells of the pancreas. Its function is to maintain blood glucose levels by stimulating glycogenolysis in the liver (*Fig. 4.5*). Glucagon exerts its gluconeogenic (producing glucose from noncarbohydrate sources) effect by promoting amino acid uptake by the liver. These amino acids are subsequently converted to glucose and released into the circulation. Glucagon also stimulates lipolysis (triglyceride breakdown) and mobilization of fatty acids from the fat cells. The free fatty acids are released into the circulation and can be taken up by the muscles and used to support aerobic metabolism.

A reduction in blood glucose levels is the primary stimulus for glucagon secretion. At rest this occurs during periods of fasting, starvation, or inadequate carbohydrate intake. However, epinephrine released either during exercise

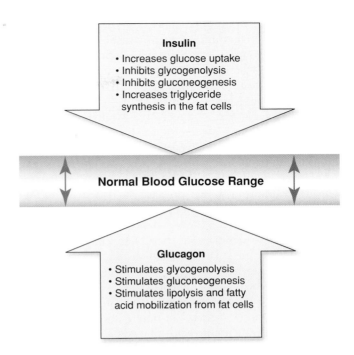

**FIGURE 4.5.** The reciprocating actions of insulin and glucagon in blood glucose control.

or in anticipation of exercise stimulates glucagon release regardless of circulating levels of blood glucose. During the initial stages of exercise, the effect of glucagon is most pronounced in skeletal muscle where glycogenolysis directly supports the energy demand. Glucagon's effect during the latter stages of exercise is shifted toward glycogenolysis in the liver so that blood glucose levels are maintained.

Insulin is secreted by the beta cells of the pancreas and functions in direct opposition to glucagon (Fig. 4.5). Insulin controls blood glucose metabolism of most tissues by regulating glucose transport into the cells. When blood glucose levels are elevated, insulin inhibits glycogenolysis and gluconeogenesis by counteracting the stimulation of adenylate cyclase seen with epinephrine and glucagon (Fig. 4.4). Insulin secretion is also affected by plasma amino acid concentrations as well as sympathetic and **parasympathetic** nerve stimulation. Triglyceride synthesis is elevated in the fat cells when insulin provides more substrates for fatty acid synthesis by increasing the transport and metabolism of glucose in the cells. Insulin secretion is reduced when glucose levels drop and when epinephrine levels rise during exercise.

Comparing the actions of insulin and glucagon to each other, one can consider glucagon to be the "*energy release hormone*" and insulin to be the "*energy storage hormone.*" Hence, in the resting state when glucose supplies are abundant, insulin levels are elevated and glucagon levels are reduced to encourage energy storage and discourage energy breakdown. In contrast, when energy supplies are needed to support muscle contraction during exercise, insulin levels fall while glucagon levels rise.

Epinephrine and norepinephrine are part of a group of biologically active amines called catecholamines. These two hormones are released from the adrenal glands in response to low blood glucose concentration and exercise or its anticipation. The adrenal glands are part of the sympathetic nervous system, and most of the actions of the adrenal catecholamines are mediated through cyclic AMP or other second messenger systems (Fig. 4.4). The actions of these hormones include stimulation of glycogenolysis, lipolysis, and gluconeogenesis. In addition to the energetics of muscle contraction, the catecholamines affect cardiac output, respiration, blood pressure, and neuromuscular transmission during exercise. The catecholamine response generated in a target tissue depends on the receptor type and whether epinephrine or norepinephrine is involved. The response may be stimulatory in one case and inhibitory in another.

Cortisol is the major **glucocorticoid** secreted by the adrenal cortex. It reduces glucose catabolism and stimulates glycogen synthesis. Cortisol promotes the breakdown of tissue proteins into amino acids that can be utilized by the liver for gluconeogenic reactions. Cortisol also stimulates gluconeogenesis by increasing synthesis of the amino acid **deaminating** enzymes, which help remove nitrogen from amino acids before they can be converted to glucose. The gluconeogenic effects of glucagon are supported by cortisol. The secretion of cortisol also depresses liver lipogenesis while accelerating the mobilization and use of fat for energy production during exercise. Cortisol blocks the entry of glucose into the exercising muscles, forcing the muscles to use fatty acids for fuel.

Aldosterone is a **mineralocorticoid** responsible for the reabsorption of sodium and excretion of potassium in the kidney. Aldosterone acts by regulating sodium reabsorption in the distal tubules of the kidney. When aldosterone is secreted, sodium ions are reabsorbed into the blood, drawing large amounts of fluid with them. Each sodium ion that is reabsorbed is counterbalanced by the excretion of either a potassium or hydrogen ion. The effect of aldosterone on fluid retention helps maintain blood pressure and cardiac output during exercise. Proper potassium and hydrogen ion balance, due to the effects of aldosterone, helps maintain neuromuscular function and plasma pH. Hence, aldosterone supports exercise by maintaining integrity of the neuromuscular and cardiovascular systems.

ADH is another key hormone secreted during exercise, and it acts on the kidneys to stimulate the reabsorption of water. Two stimuli are responsible for the secretion of ADH. Receptors in the hypothalamus sense plasma osmolality (plasma water concentration). If the plasma osmolality is high (low water content) due to excessive sweating during exercise, these receptors shrink and neural feedback to the hypothalamus causes ADH release. Another mechanism that stimulates ADH secretion is low plasma volume. If plasma osmolality is normal but plasma volume is low, stretch receptors in the left atrium of the heart initiate neural communication that causes ADH secretion.

ACTH regulates the release of hormones secreted by the adrenal cortex. Although ACTH does not directly affect metabolism, the indirect effects are seen in the metabolic pathways, nervous system, muscular system, and cardiovascular system. The indirect action of ACTH on metabolism is to enhance fatty acid mobilization from the fat cells, stimulate gluconeogenesis, and increase protein catabolism. This effect is achieved by the ACTH-stimulated release of cortisol from the adrenal cortex. During exercise, ACTH also stimulates the production and release of aldosterone, which helps decrease fluid excretion from the kidney.

GH exerts some metabolic effects during and after exercise. During exercise, GH opposes the action of insulin by decreasing the use of blood glucose for fuel. GH also helps stimulate gluconeogenesis in the liver and promotes the mobilization of fatty acids from fat cells. These actions assist in maintenance of blood glucose levels during exercise. Post-exercise GH promotes cell division and protein synthesis throughout the body by facilitating amino acid transport through plasma membranes and activating the ribosomes. The post-exercise effects of GH are seen in muscle hypertrophy, connective tissue growth, and skeletal growth.

## Hormonal Response to Exercise

The magnitude of hormonal response to exercise depends upon the intensity of exercise and its duration. Most of what is known about the hormonal response to exercise has come from research on extended-duration submaximal aerobic exercise and incremental aerobic exercise to $VO_{2max}$. The hormonal response to exercise has been determined by measuring the concentration of circulating hormones. However, changes in blood concentration of hormones may not indicate an increase in secretion because blood hormone levels are also affected by clearance rate, blood volume, receptor turnover, as well as other factors.

Except for insulin, the blood levels for all the aforementioned hormones increase during an acute bout of exercise. The rise in concentration of the metabolic hormones in the blood is gradual with increasing intensities of exercise up until between 50% and 75% of $VO_{2max}$ (Fig. 4.6). Thereafter, the concentration of hormones in the blood rises exponentially. This is not surprising as we have already seen how exercise intensity dictates the rate of ATP hydrolysis in the exercising muscles. Thus, as the exercise intensity increases and the demand for ATP rises, the endocrine system is called into play so that fuel sources from all locations can be recruited to supply the energy demand.

The pattern of hormonal response to exercise duration is not as uniform as that seen with exercise intensity (Fig. 4.7). Stimulation of the sympathetic nervous system causes an immediate rise in norepinephrine and epinephrine concentrations as exercise is anticipated and initiated. The continual rise in these catecholamines, thereafter, is due to their release from the adrenal glands. The immediate rise in

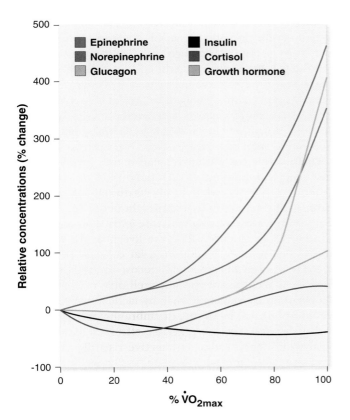

**FIGURE 4.6.** Blood levels of metabolic hormones during incremental exercise. The blood concentrations of the metabolic hormones change dramatically from resting values to those seen when VO$_{2max}$ is achieved.

epinephrine concentration causes glucagon levels to rise concurrently.

As exercise duration proceeds, glucagon levels remain elevated in response to increased epinephrine and decreasing blood glucose levels. Since insulin is an antagonist to glucagon, the concentration of insulin decreases immediately as exercise begins and remains depressed throughout the entire exercise bout. Unlike the other metabolic hormones, cortisol and GH are slow acting hormones. The blood concentration of cortisol may not reflect its true secretion rate because the clearance rate of the hormone often exceeds secretion. Blood concentration of growth hormone, on the other hand, remains at baseline level during the first several minutes of exercise. Thereafter, concentration rises dramatically. This delay between the onset of exercise and changes in blood levels of GH is shortened with higher intensities of exercise.

Visualize what happens as a person goes from the resting state through a 60-minute exercise bout at a constant speed requiring an energy output of 75% of VO$_{2max}$. Anticipation of the exercise bout stimulates the sympathetic nervous system, which causes an immediate rise in epinephrine and norepinephrine levels. Glucagon is released from the pancreas in response to rising epinephrine levels. At the same time, insulin levels begin to decline.

The effects of these initial hormonal changes are increased glycogenolysis, increased lipolysis, increased gluconeogenesis, and decreased glucose uptake. The metabolic result is that liver glucose is free to enter the circulation, muscle glycogen is free to enter glycolysis, and fatty acids are released into the circulation. The initial stages of exercise see a continued rise in epinephrine and norepinephrine due to stimulation of the adrenal glands. Glucagon continues to rise, while insulin drops and is maintained at about 50% of resting levels.

As the duration of exercise continues, ACTH begins to exert its effects on the adrenal cortex. The result is that the glucocorticoid cortisol is released and the mineralocorticoid aldosterone is secreted. Cortisol increases gluconeogenesis and retards entry of glucose into the muscles, forcing the muscles to rely more heavily upon fatty acids for fuel. Aldosterone, on the other hand, helps maintain blood volume by increasing sodium reabsorption in the kidney. At the same time, ADH assists in maintaining blood volume by restricting water excretion. GH comes into play during the latter part of the exercise bout and helps maintain blood glucose levels by inhibiting glucose uptake by the muscles, increasing gluconeogenesis, and promoting mobilization of fatty acids from the fat cells. Altogether, the hormonal milieu seen during exercise increases the availability of metabolic substrates for muscular ATP production,

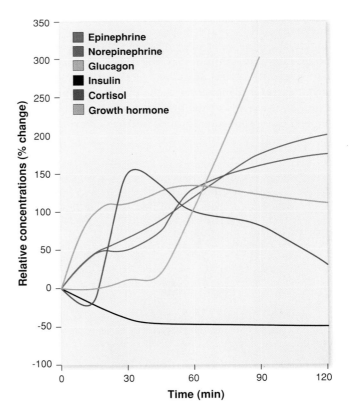

**FIGURE 4.7.** Blood levels of metabolic hormones during steady state exercise. The blood concentrations of the metabolic hormones shift during 120 minutes of continuous steady-state exercise at 60% to 70% of VO$_{2max}$.

maintains glucose supply to the nervous system, and maintains the integrity of the circulatory system.

## RESULTS OF AN EXERCISE-INDUCED RISE IN METABOLISM

Earlier in this chapter we discussed how each of the energy systems responds to an immediate demand for increased energy when exercise begins. You learned that the contribution of each energy system to the total power output during exercise is determined by the intensity and duration of the exercise. Although very insightful, the previous discussion only presented a qualitative representation of the rest-to-exercise transitions in metabolism that occur with exercise. We now focus our attention on methods that help quantify how much of the power output during exercise is contributed by each of the energy systems (*Fig. 4.8*).

Aerobic energy production from the oxidation of carbohydrate and fat is easily quantified because there is a direct relationship between $O_2$ uptake ($\dot{V}O_2$) measured at the mouth and whole-body production of ATP. This relationship does not hold true for protein; however, since the contribution of protein to the aerobic energy supply during exercise is minimal, protein's contribution is generally ignored. Each L of $O_2$ consumed yields approximately 5 kcal (20 kJ) of energy. The exact energy yield per L of $O_2$ consumed varies slightly, depending on whether the fuel source for aerobic energy production is carbohydrate or fat.

The relative contribution of carbohydrate and fat to the energy supply can be quantified by measuring the production of $CO_2$ as well as $\dot{V}O_2$. The ratio of $CO_2$ produced to the amount of $O_2$ consumed is called the **respiratory quotient** when measured at the cellular level and the **respiratory exchange ratio** if measured at the mouth. The process of determining energy expenditure by measuring $O_2$ consumption and $CO_2$ production is called **indirect calorimetry**.

Table 4.3 contains the caloric values for $O_2$ consumed depending on the ratio of carbohydrate to fat in the fuel mix. The respiratory exchange ratio (RER) is 0.70 when fat is the sole fuel source, while the RER is 1.00 when carbohydrate is the only fuel source. The RER of 0.85 is achieved when the fuel mix of carbohydrate and fat is approximately equal. *According to what you have learned so far, where in the RER scale (high or low) would a person be if he/she were performing high-intensity exercise that primarily taxed glycolysis?* You may want to refer again to Figure 4.2 before answering this question.

Indirect calorimetry can be used in the clinical setting to estimate the fuel source used during exercise. For example, if a person was exercising when the ratio of $O_2$ consumption to $CO_2$ production (RER) was 0.79, he/she would be utilizing fat sources to support approximately 70% of the exercise energy demand and carbohydrate sources to support 30% of the energy demand (Table 4.3). Similarly, if a person was exercising when the RER was 0.92, he/she would be utilizing fat to support approximately 26% of the energy demand and carbohydrate to support about 74% of the demand. These estimates hold true regardless of fitness level or exercise intensity. Nonetheless, at any given RER, a trained person can produce ATP at a faster rate than an untrained person, even though the fuel mix for each person is comparable.

To calculate the exact caloric expenditure for any given exercise intensity, the RER value is needed as well as the absolute value for $\dot{V}O_2$. For example, if a person was exercising at a RER value of 0.82 and his/her absolute $\dot{V}O_2$ value were 2.0 L·min$^{-1}$, the energy expenditure would be 9.65 kcal·min$^{-1}$ (2.0 L·min$^{-1}$ × 4.825 kcal·L$^{-1}$ $O_2$). Thus, indirect calorimetry can be used to estimate energy expenditure as well as fuel source contribution during any intensity of aerobic exercise.

> ◭ *Experiences in Work Physiology Lab Exercise 4: Measuring Metabolic Transitions from Rest to Exercise provides a lab experience in which you measure and calculate energy expenditure and substrate utilization during exercise.*

Note that the measurements used to quantify aerobic metabolism are made in the cardiorespiratory system, not within the muscles themselves. This is possible because oxidative metabolism is an open system that depends on communication and exchange between the exercising muscles and other systems of the body (e.g., cardiorespiratory system). On the other hand, anaerobic metabolism is closed and self-contained (all the necessary ingredients are in the cell).

Methods to quantify anaerobic energy production are less precise than those for aerobic energy production because measurements of metabolites made in the blood do not accurately reflect metabolism within the muscles (1). Furthermore, measurements and estimations of

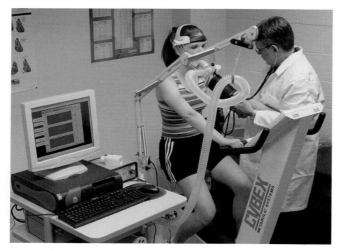

**FIGURE 4.8.** Measuring exercise energy expenditure through indirect calorimetry. Analysis of respiratory gases allows the exercise scientist to indirectly measure aerobic energy production during exercise.

| | | | | | | | |
|---|---|---|---|---|---|---|---|
| **Table 4.3** | **CALORIC EQUIVALENT OF $O_2$ AND RATIO OF FAT:CARBOHYDRATE CALORIES PROVIDED FOR EACH RESPIRATORY EXCHANGE RATIO VALUE** | | | | | | |
| **RER** | **kcal·L$^{-1}$ O$_2$** | **% Carbohydrate** | **% Fat** | **RER** | **kcal·L$^{-1}$ O$_2$** | **% Carbohydrate** | **% Fat** |
| 0.70 | 4.686 | 0.0 | 100.0 | 0.86 | 4.875 | 54.1 | 45.9 |
| 0.71 | 4.690 | 1.1 | 98.9 | 0.87 | 4.887 | 57.5 | 42.5 |
| 0.72 | 4.702 | 4.8 | 95.2 | 0.88 | 4.899 | 60.8 | 39.2 |
| 0.73 | 4.714 | 8.4 | 91.6 | 0.89 | 4.911 | 64.2 | 35.8 |
| 0.74 | 4.727 | 12.0 | 88.0 | 0.90 | 4.924 | 67.5 | 32.5 |
| 0.75 | 4.739 | 15.6 | 84.4 | 0.91 | 4.936 | 70.8 | 29.2 |
| 0.76 | 4.751 | 19.2 | 80.8 | 0.92 | 4.948 | 74.1 | 25.9 |
| 0.77 | 4.764 | 22.3 | 77.2 | 0.93 | 4.961 | 77.4 | 22.6 |
| 0.78 | 4.776 | 26.3 | 73.7 | 0.94 | 4.973 | 80.7 | 19.3 |
| 0.79 | 4.788 | 29.9 | 70.1 | 0.95 | 4.985 | 84.0 | 16.0 |
| 0.80 | 4.801 | 33.4 | 66.6 | 0.96 | 4.998 | 87.2 | 12.8 |
| 0.81 | 4.813 | 36.9 | 63.1 | 0.97 | 5.010 | 90.4 | 9.6 |
| 0.82 | 4.825 | 40.3 | 59.7 | 0.98 | 5.022 | 93.6 | 6.4 |
| 0.83 | 4.838 | 43.8 | 56.2 | 0.99 | 5.035 | 96.8 | 3.2 |
| 0.84 | 4.850 | 47.2 | 52.8 | 1.00 | 5.047 | 100.0 | 0.0 |
| 0.85 | 4.862 | 50.7 | 49.3 | | | | |

Data derived from Lusk G. *Science of nutrition.* 4th ed. Philadelphia: WB Saunders, 1928.

metabolite production derived from muscle biopsy techniques are not accurate because of inherent weaknesses in the technique itself (1).

The instant exercise begins, the muscles must increase their ATP production from that required at rest to that which is required to sustain the exercise intensity. The fact that $\dot{V}O_2$ does not increase instantly to a level that meets the $O_2$ demand of submaximal exercise indicates that an anaerobic energy contribution makes up the difference. The difference between the amount of energy contributed from aerobic ATP production and that required to sustain the exercise is called the **$O_2$ deficit** (*Fig. 4.9*). Within 1 to 4 minutes of starting light or moderate exercise, and after several more minutes for high-intensity exercise, the amount of energy produced aerobically will meet the demands of the exercise workload.

The point at which aerobic energy supply equals the exercise energy demand is called **steady state**. The term steady rate is also used to describe the same phenomenon when the rate of aerobic ATP production meets the rate of ATP demand. When exercise is terminated, the power

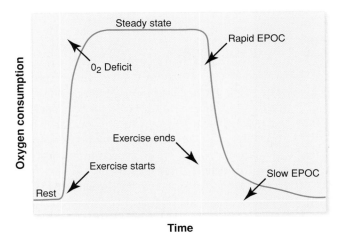

**FIGURE 4.9.** Transitions in $O_2$ consumption from rest to steady state and through recovery during submaximal exercise. As exercise begins, the increased energy demand is met by contributions from the anaerobic as well as the aerobic system. After several minutes, the body reaches a steady-state level at which the exercise energy demand is met by the aerobic energy system. Aerobic metabolism above the resting level following exercise is called excess post-exercise $O_2$ consumption.

output demand drops immediately. $O_2$ uptake, however, remains elevated for several minutes post-exercise. The amount of $O_2$ consumed post-exercise above the resting metabolic rate is called the **excess post-exercise $O_2$ consumption** or EPOC. Box 4.3 highlights some of the contributions of Sir Archibald Vivian Hill, one of the first scientists to study metabolism during exercise.

Originally, it was thought that the EPOC was a payback for the $O_2$ deficit incurred during the onset of exercise. Later studies revealed that the volume of EPOC was actually greater than the volume of the $O_2$ deficit. The theory of EPOC was then modified to delineate two phases of EPOC (Fig. 4.9). The rapid EPOC phase was defined as the phase in which elevated $O_2$ consumption was used to regenerate depleted ATP and PC stores and restore depleted $O_2$ stores in the blood and tissues. The slow EPOC phase was defined as the phase in which elevated $O_2$ consumption was used for the oxidative conversion of lactic acid back to glucose. Research again showed that the volume of EPOC during the slow phase was greater than the volume of $O_2$ required to convert lactic acid to glucose.

The theory has been further modified to suggest that slow EPOC serves other functions than heretofore described. The current theory suggests that the slow phase of EPOC is also used to support elevated heart rate and respiration post-exercise. Increased body temperature and elevated hormones that remain in the circulation post-exercise are responsible for elevated slow EPOC. Table 4.4 summarizes all of the factors that may contribute to the EPOC.

Let's see how these principles are applied in a clinical or laboratory setting. Suppose you wanted to determine the exact energy cost of a steady-state (steady-rate) aerobic exercise bout. *What would you need to know?* You would need to measure the energy cost of the exercise bout itself plus the energy expended during the EPOC period. The energy expenditure during the exercise bout can easily be measured through indirect calorimetry. However, the metabolic measurements taken will only be accurate once the subject reaches steady-state exercise since indirect calorimetry cannot measure $O_2$ deficit. The energy expended during the EPOC period can similarly be measured through indirect

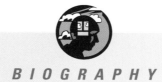

**Box 4.3**

## BIOGRAPHY

# Sir Archibald Vivian Hill

One of the most notable scientists who pioneered the field of modern-day exercise physiology was Sir Archibald Hill (1886–1977). Dr. Hill combined the disciplines of physiology, physics, mathematics, and biology in his research career that spanned several decades. Hill was recognized early in his career when he shared the Nobel Prize in Medicine with German scientist Otto Meyerhof. Both of these scientists were investigating the chemical and mechanical properties of muscle contraction. Hill was awarded for his pioneering work that enabled him to measure heat production in contracting muscle, while Otto was awarded for his work on the relationship between $O_2$ consumption and the production of lactic acid in contracting muscle.

In addition to his work related to heat production in muscle, Hill also researched the kinetics of $O_2$ uptake during exercise and recovery. Hill and his coworker Hartley Lupton were the first to introduce the concept of $O_2$ debt. These men proposed that $O_2$ debt was the excess $O_2$ consumption (above rest) that was necessary to pay back the $O_2$ deficit incurred at the onset of exercise. Their theory was that during exercise recovery, 80% of the lactic acid produced was reconverted to glycogen, while the remaining 20% was

oxidized to $CO_2$ and $H_2O$. Further work by Hill and others delineated the two phases of the $O_2$ debt or excess post-exercise $O_2$ consumption.

Along these same lines of research, Hill's work led to the hypothesis that lactic acid causes fatigue. His early work on lactic acid kinetics provided the base upon which scientists today study the anaerobic threshold or onset of blood lactate accumulation.

In addition to studying the relationships among glucose, lactic acid, and glycogen during exercise and recovery, Hill also studied how the other energy systems relate to glycolysis. Hill was particularly interested in discovering how the aerobic energy system was used to replenish energy stores that were depleted in the anaerobic systems following exercise.

Hill was the one to introduce the term maximal $O_2$ consumption ($\dot{V}O_{2max}$). It was primarily the work of Hill in the 1920s and 1930s that lead to the publication of a significant amount of data on $\dot{V}O_{2max}$ or peak $\dot{V}O_2$ for athletes performing various types of maximal exercise.

Although many of Hill's theories have been reexamined and modified, his work provided a sound foundation for what exercise scientists are studying today.

| Table 4.4 | SUMMARY OF THE PHYSIOLOGIC FACTORS THAT CONTRIBUTE TO EXCESS POST-EXERCISE $O_2$ CONSUMPTION |
| --- | --- |
| **EPOC phase** | **Contributing factors** |
| Rapid | Rephosphorylation of depleted phosphagen stores; restoration of depleted $O_2$ stores |
| Slow | Conversion of lactic acid, pyruvic acid, and partially metabolized glucose back to glucose; support metabolic cost of elevated cardiorespiratory function following exercise; support metabolic cost of elevated body temperature following exercise; support catecholamine-stimulated metabolic rate due to elevated hormone levels; support metabolic cost of redistributing ions across membranes |

calorimetry. Once these two values are determined, you can add them to find the total cost of the exercise bout. Remember, though, that in order to obtain the true cost of the exercise bout, you will need to subtract the resting energy expenditure from the total energy expenditure during both the exercise and EPOC periods. Case Study 4.1 shows the details of how all of this is done.

The preceding dialogue explained how measurements of $\dot{V}O_2$ and $CO_2$ production ($\dot{V}CO_2$) can be used to learn how the aerobic energy systems contribute to the energy demand during steady-state exercise. Aerobic metabolism can be quantified by measuring $\dot{V}O_2$ and $\dot{V}CO_2$ because there is a direct relationship between aerobic metabolism and the exchange of these two gases (see Chapter 5). *How do you think exercise scientists measure the anaerobic contribution to the energy supply during exercise?*

Methods to quantify anaerobic energy production are less precise than those for aerobic energy production because anaerobic metabolism is a closed and self-contained system. The end product of the ATP-PC system is creatine. However, creatine is converted back to PC within seconds of reducing the exercise intensity or the cessation of exercise, and blood levels of creatine are not indicative of muscle creatine concentration. Therefore, it is currently not possible to quantify ATP-PC activity during whole-body exercise.

Quantification of the contribution of rapid glycolysis to the energy supply during exercise is not as problematic as with the ATP-PC system, but it is still somewhat elusive. The end product of rapid glycolysis is lactic acid. Many scientists believe that the rapid rise in blood lactic acid levels represents the point of increasing reliance on rapid glycolysis for energy. Terms that have been used to describe this systematic rise in blood lactic acid are the **anaerobic threshold**, **lactate threshold**, and **onset of blood lactate accumulation** (OBLA). The inflection point at which OBLA occurs is found at approximately 50% to 60% of $VO_{2max}$ in untrained subjects and at approximately 65% to 80% of $VO_{2max}$ for trained subjects (*Fig. 4.10*).

The OBLA has been used, in combination with other measures, to predict success in distance running and to set guidelines for exercise training intensity for athletes (2,3). However, use of the OBLA for estimating the contribution of rapid glycolysis to the exercise energy supply has been criticized because blood lactate concentrations do not truly reflect muscle lactic acid production (1). Muscle biopsies determine lactic acid concentrations but not its production rates and therefore cannot be used to accurately quantify rapid glycolysis. There is also a dissociation between OBLA and EPOC so measurements of EPOC cannot be used to accurately reflect lactic acid production (1).

The fact that all of the energy systems are called into play as soon as exercise begins makes it impossible to distinguish between the alactic and lactic energy components. At present, the muscle biopsy technique and gas-exchange methods provide the best insights into anaerobic energy production during exercise (1). Only by combining the measurements and interactions of several techniques can a relative contribution of the energy systems to varying intensities and durations of exercise be quantified.

▶ *INQUIRY SUMMARY.* Once a person begins to exercise, metabolic adjustments are made so that the energy requirement of the exercise bout can be met. The selection of a fuel source and energy system used to provide the necessary ATP for exercise is dependent upon the exercise power output demand or exercise intensity. The endocrine system regulates the need for additional ATP supply to be provided to the musculature during exercise. If the exercise energy requirement is met by aerobic metabolism, a steady state is achieved. The $O_2$ deficit describes the anaerobic contribution to the energy supply during the initial stages of exercise before steady state is achieved. EPOC refers to the elevated metabolic rate seen during exercise recovery. *What measurements or estimations do you think need to be made before the total energy cost of an exercise bout can be calculated?*

## Maintaining Energy Supply During Exercise

The sources for ATP in exercising muscles are stored ATP, stored PC, carbohydrate, fat, and protein. The amount of ATP supplied for exercise from stored ATP and PC is limited to the preexercise content of these substances found in the muscles because the ATP-PC energy system is a closed, self-contained system. The only way exercising

## CASE STUDY 4.1:  *ENERGY COST OF EXERCISE*

### CASE

Sarah is a 28 year-old woman who is moderately fit but wants to lose some of the excess weight she gained during her recent pregnancy. Sarah comes to the clinic for an exercise test to determine the energy cost of her newly designed exercise program. Her program consists of walking for 30 minutes a day at a pace of 4 miles per hour (15-minute miles).

### DESCRIPTION

Energy expenditure through aerobic metabolism is easily quantified because there is a direct relationship between whole-body $O_2$ consumption ($\dot{V}O_2$) and ATP production. Each L of $O_2$ consumed yields approximately 5 kcal (20 kJ) of energy. The exact energy yield per L of $O_2$ consumed varies slightly, depending on whether the fuel source for aerobic energy production is carbohydrate or fat. The relative contributions of carbohydrate and fat to the energy supply can be quantified by measuring the production of $CO_2$ as well as $\dot{V}O_2$. The ratio of $CO_2$ produced to the amount of $O_2$ consumed is called the respiratory exchange ratio (RER). The RER is 0.70 when fat is the sole fuel source, while the RER is 1.00 when carbohydrate is the only fuel source. An RER of 0.85 is achieved when the fuel mix of carbohydrate and fat is approximately equal. Table 4.3 contains the energy values for $\dot{V}O_2$ depending on the ratio of carbohydrate to fat in the fuel mix.

Modern technology has allowed for the interfacing of specialized pieces of equipment with computers so that clinicians can easily measure gas exchange in the respiratory system and calculate metabolic parameters. The result is that clinicians can almost instantaneously measure metabolism in any client under various controlled conditions. This case study shows you how this is done by giving insight into how the metabolic measurements and calculations are performed.

### EVALUATION

The first thing to do is measure Sarah's resting metabolic rate using the principle of indirect calorimetry and the metabolic system. The metabolic measurements show the following readout for Sarah's resting metabolism:
- $\dot{V}O_2$ = 0.300 L·min$^{-1}$
- RER = 0.84

- Caloric equivalent of $O_2$ = 4.85 kcal·L$^{-1}$ $O_2$
- Resting energy expenditure = 1.46 kcal·min$^{-1}$

You next begin the exercise testing. Treadmill speed is set at 4 miles per hour, and Sarah begins to walk. Although the metabolic system calculates Sarah's energy expenditure on a minute-by-minute basis, you realize that during the first several minutes of exercise the numbers are lower than her actual energy expenditure because the equipment can only measure her aerobic energy expenditure, and she has not yet reached steady-state (steady-rate) exercise. In other words, some of the energy demand is met by contributions from the anaerobic energy systems (Fig. 4.9). Sarah continues at the same speed until she completes 30 minutes of exercise. At 30 minutes she rests while you continue to measure her energy expenditure. Her energy expenditure does not come back to the resting state until 20 minutes post-exercise.

Using the metabolic system's computer, you average the numbers for Sarah's steady-state exercise and obtain the following:
- $\dot{V}O_2$ = 1.125 L·min$^{-1}$
- RER = 0.89
- Caloric equivalent of $O_2$ = 4.911 kcal·L$^{-1}$ $O_2$
- Exercise energy expenditure = 5.53 kcal·min$^{-1}$
- 30-minute exercise energy expenditure = 166 kcal (5.53 kcal·min$^{-1}$ × 30 min)

However, the analysis is not complete. You must subtract the resting energy expenditure from the total energy expenditure during the exercise bout to derive the true energy cost of the exercise. Sarah's resting energy expenditure for the 30 minutes of exercise would have been 44 kcal·min$^{-1}$ (1.46 kcal·min$^{-1}$ × 30 min). Subtracting 44 kcal from 166 kcal gives 122 kcal for the 30-minute exercise bout. But, you still are not finished. You must add the excess post-exercise $O_2$ consumption (EPOC) to that value. Summing the minute-by-minute energy expenditure values for the 20 minutes post-exercise, you see that Sarah expended 42.2 kcal post-exercise. Subtract her resting metabolic rate for the 20-minute post-exercise period (29.2 kcal) and you get 13.0 kcal as her EPOC. Add this to her energy cost of exercise (122 kcal) and you get 135 kcal for the total cost of her daily exercise bout. If Sarah relies solely on her exercise program without changing her diet, she will lose approximately 1 pound a month.

---

muscles can generate more ATP than what is available from the ATP-PC system is through catabolism of protein, carbohydrate, and fat.

The role of protein as a fuel source for exercising muscle is minimal because protein contributes only about 2% of the energy supply for exercise lasting less than 1 hour.

Protein may contribute up to 15% of the exercise energy supply but only during the final minutes of an exercise bout that lasts for several hours. Therefore, carbohydrate and fat predominate as the fuels used for exercise under most conditions. The determination of whether carbohydrate or fat is the selected fuel choice depends on the

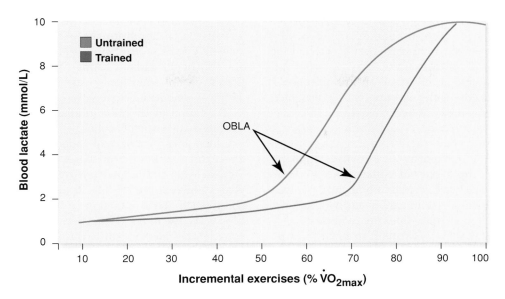

**FIGURE 4.10.** Onset of blood lactate accumulation or the lactate threshold in trained and untrained persons. The trained person can exercise at a greater relative intensity than the untrained before lactate begins to accumulate in the blood.

intensity of exercise, duration of exercise, and nutritional state of the individual. The way in which the nutritional state of an individual affects exercise performance and fuel selection in the energy systems is presented in Chapter 12. The next section covers the process in which exercise intensity and duration determine the amount of carbohydrate or fat that is used to support the exercise workload.

## EXERCISE INTENSITY AND FUEL SELECTION

The primary fuel for exercise at intensities below 30% to 40% of $\dot{V}O_{2max}$ is fat, whereas the primary fuel for exercise at intensities above 60% to 70% of $\dot{V}O_{2max}$ is carbohydrate. At intensities between 40% to 60% of $\dot{V}O_{2max}$, the fuel mix is somewhat balanced. The relative exercise intensity at which the shift from fat to carbohydrate metabolism occurs varies somewhat depending upon the state of training and nutritional status of the individual. An endurance athlete derives more energy from fat at a higher percent of his or her $\dot{V}O_{2max}$ than does an untrained person. A person on a high-fat diet will derive more energy from fat at a given submaximal workload than a person consuming a high-carbohydrate diet, and a person who consumes carbohydrates shortly before starting to exercise will derive more energy from carbohydrate than a person who refrains from carbohydrate consumption prior to exercise.

In spite of individual variation, the pattern of fuel selection during exercise of increasing intensities looks similar to what is presented in *Figure 4.11*. The point at which the energy derived from carbohydrate exceeds that of fat is called the **crossover point**. Again, the crossover point will vary among individuals, depending on their state of training and dietary practices.

There are three physiologic factors other than nutrient supply that cause the shift from carbohydrate to fat as the exercise intensity increases. All of these factors are directly related to the power output demand of the exercise. As previously shown in Table 4.1, when the power output demand is high, fat metabolism contributes very little to the energy supply. *A key question is: what happens physiologically in the exercising muscle that allows for this shift in fuel selection?*

The answer is three-fold. The first has to do with the physiologic makeup of skeletal muscle. As you will learn in Chapter 10, skeletal muscle is composed of three predominant types of muscle fibers (cells). Two of these fiber types (types IIa and IIb) are highly glycolytic, meaning they have a high capacity for rapid glycolysis. The other fiber (type I) has a high capacity for fat oxidation but a lesser capacity for glycolysis. As the intensity of exercise increases, more and

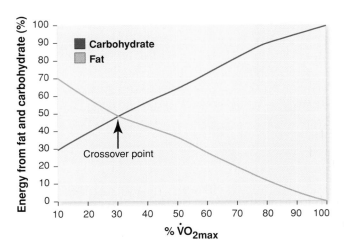

**FIGURE 4.11.** Relative contribution of fat vs. carbohydrate to the energy supply as exercise intensity increases.

more of the fibers with high glycolytic capacity will be recruited to support the exercise bout. Therefore, by fiber type recruitment, carbohydrate becomes the selected fuel source during high-intensity exercise.

The second physiologic influence on fuel selection at increasing exercise intensities is hormonal. It was mentioned previously that the hormone epinephrine is secreted into the blood in anticipation of and during exercise. As exercise intensity increases, there is a progressive rise in the concentration of epinephrine in the blood. Epinephrine does stimulate lipolysis, but epinephrine is a more potent stimulator of glycogenolysis. Epinephrine's glycogenolytic effect provides an abundant quantity of carbohydrate to the muscles as exercise intensity increases.

The third factor that forces the shift from fat to carbohydrate metabolism at increasing exercise intensities is lactic acid. As carbohydrate is being metabolized in rapid glycolysis, lactic acid is being produced. This increased lactic acid production inhibits fat metabolism by reducing the availability of fatty acids to the muscle for fuel. A diminished fatty acid supply to the exercising muscle promotes the further use of carbohydrate as the fuel source.

## EXERCISE DURATION AND FUEL SUPPLY

We have already seen that the amount of fuel available to the exercising muscle limits the metabolic capacity of the muscle. This is the absolute case for the ATP-PC system because that system is closed and self-contained during exercise. Fat supply to the exercising muscle is inexhaustible because it is not possible for a person to exercise for 350 hours without eating (Table 4.1). Carbohydrate stores, on the other hand, can become depleted within 2 hours at a moderate exercise intensity.

Depletion of carbohydrate stores reduces the rate of glycolysis in exercising muscle. As glycolysis slows, the production of pyruvic acid is decreased. Pyruvic acid is a precursor for the intermediates of the Krebs cycle (e.g., oxaloacetate, citrate, malate). When Krebs cycle intermediates are reduced, the level of Krebs cycle activity is diminished. This reduction in Krebs cycle activity precludes the use of fat for fuel because the entry point of fat into aerobic metabolism is through the condensation of acetyl CoA (the product of β oxidation of fatty acids) with oxaloacetate, a Krebs cycle intermediate. The result of this reduction in Krebs cycle intermediates is a shift from fat to carbohydrate as the selected fuel source. If exercise continues, the depletion of carbohydrate stores will cause fatigue. However, as discussed below, the body has mechanisms that can be used to regenerate carbohydrate supplies for the exercising muscles.

As the duration of exercise continues from initiation to minutes and hours, the body has several mechanisms designed to maintain energy supplies. The first mechanism exists in the ATP-PC system. As ATP is used for muscle contraction, adenosine diphosphate (ADP) is formed. PC

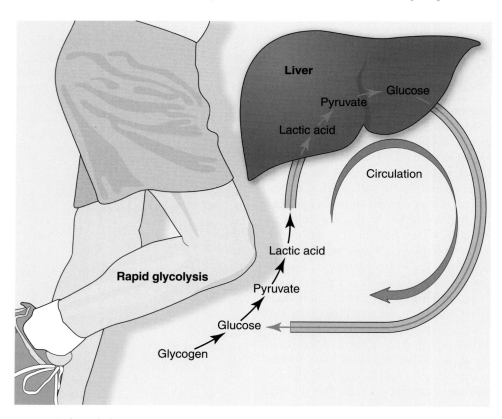

**FIGURE 4.12.** Gluconeogenesis through the Cori cycle. Lactic acid formed during rapid glycolysis is circulated to the liver where it is converted back to glucose. The new glucose can be returned to the tissues to meet metabolic demands.

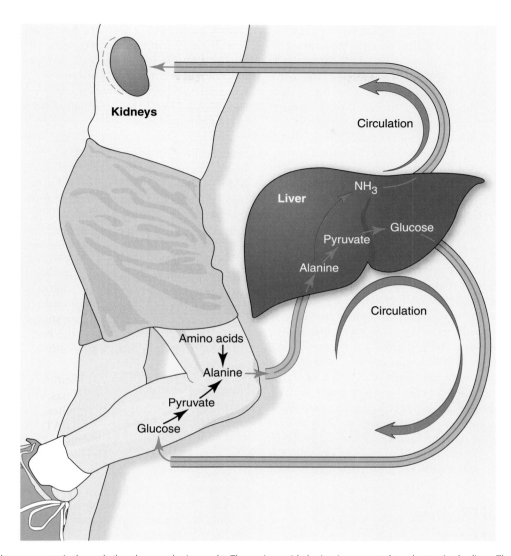

**FIGURE 4.13.** Gluconeogenesis through the glucose-alanine cycle. The amino acid alanine is converted to glucose in the liver. The new glucose can be returned to the tissues to meet metabolic demands.

will donate a phosphate to the ADP to regenerate ATP. However, PC stores are limited. When PC stores begin to decline, ADP begins to accumulate in the cell. A method exists that can convert two ADP molecules into one ATP and one adenosine monophosphate (AMP) molecule. The reaction is commonly called the myokinase reaction because it is regulated by the enzyme myokinase (also called adenylate kinase). The reaction follows the path: ADP + ADP ↔ ATP + AMP. The myokinase reaction cannot delay fatigue indefinitely, but it will add a few more seconds to the time the ATP-PC system can support the exercise bout.

**Gluconeogenesis** mechanisms are used to maintain carbohydrate supplies. One of these gluconeogenic mechanisms is the Cori cycle (*Fig. 4.12*), a biochemical pathway that occurs in the liver and involves the recycling of lactic acid. Lactic acid is produced by exercising muscles undergoing rapid glycolysis energy metabolism. Lactic acid is

subsequently released into the circulation and transported to the liver. Inside the liver the lactic acid is converted back to glucose and released again into the blood, where the newly formed glucose can be taken up by the exercising muscles, but more importantly, it can be used to maintain the integrity of the central nervous system.

A second gluconeogenic mechanism used for maintaining carbohydrate supplies is called the glucose-alanine cycle (*Fig. 4.13*). In this cycle, amino acids in the muscle are converted into alanine, which is then released to the circulation. The carbon fragments from the side chain of the amino acid that was converted to alanine can be oxidized for energy within the specific muscle cell. The liver takes the circulating alanine and removes the amino acid radical ($NH_3$). The remaining carbon skeleton is converted into glucose and then released back into the blood. The newly formed glucose can be extracted by the working muscles and catabolized to support muscular contraction.

Recent research on protein metabolism during exercise has shown that protein contributes much more to the energy supply than was originally concluded. Early research assumed that protein metabolism was directly related to urinary nitrogen excretion. However, we now know that nitrogen excretion in the sweat can increase during exercise without a parallel increase in urinary nitrogen excretion. We also know that exercising in a carbohydrate-depleted state causes more metabolism of protein than when carbohydrate supplies are plentiful, particularly in endurance exercise. After 4 hours of continuous light exercise, the liver's output of alanine-derived glucose can reach 45% of its total glucose output (*Fig. 4.14*). In fact, it has been estimated that as much as 10% to 15% of the total exercise energy requirement can be generated from the glucose-alanine cycle.

▶ *INQUIRY SUMMARY.* Exercise intensity and duration are the two primary factors that determine whether carbohydrate or fat will be the dominant fuel source during exercise. As exercise intensity increases, fat contributes less to the energy supply, while carbohydrate contributes more. Blood glucose levels must be sustained during exercise to maintain the integrity of the central nervous system. The body has several gluconeogenic pathways which are used for this purpose. The Cori cycle converts lactic acid to glucose, while the glucose-alanine cycle converts the amino acid alanine to glucose. *How would exercise performance be affected if there was not constant communication and feedback among the energy systems within the muscle cells and the extracellular systems of the body that support exercise?*

# Recovery from Exercise: Resynthesis of Fuels

Once the power output demand to sustain exercise is reduced, by either decreasing the exercise intensity or

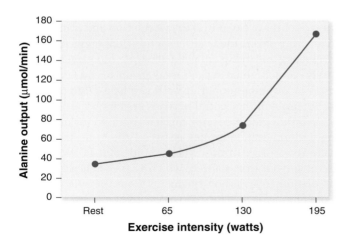

**FIGURE 4.14.** Amino acid metabolism during exercise. Influence of 40 minutes of cycle ergometer exercise at various workloads on alanine output from the legs. Data from Felig P, Wahren J. Amino acid metabolism in exercising man. *J Clin Invest* 1971;50:2703–2714.

stopping exercise, a shift in the metabolic contribution from the different energy systems to the overall metabolic rate begins. We have previously investigated some of the physiologic factors that contribute to EPOC. Now we will focus on what occurs biochemically to regenerate energy supplies and bring the musculature back to a resting state of energy homeostasis.

The phosphagens of the ATP-PC system are not totally expended in the production of ATP but are brought to a lesser energy state by **dephosphorylation**. Therefore, AMP, ADP, and creatine only need to be rephosphorylated into ATP and PC to bring the energy state of the cell back into resting homeostasis. Lactic acid and pyruvic acid formed in glycolysis are partially metabolized glucose molecules and will either be further metabolized aerobically or be converted back to glucose and glycogen in the recovery process. In contrast, the end products of aerobic metabolism are $CO_2$ and $H_2O$. These molecules do not have any inherent energy value to the body, and thus there is no real recovery of aerobically metabolized carbohydrate and fat.

## REGENERATION OF ATP AND PC

The ATP and PC stores are replenished within a couple minutes of cessation of exercise. As the energy demand of the body decreases, ATP produced from the metabolism of carbohydrate and fat can be diverted from the contractile mechanism of the muscle to the regeneration of ATP and PC. The process follows the pattern shown in *Figure 4.15*:

1. Stored ATP is hydrolyzed to provide immediate energy for muscle contraction
2. As ATP stores become depleted, the high-energy bond from PC is used to regenerate ATP
3. The ATP produced from dietary nutrients replenishes the ATP and PC stores only when exercise intensity is reduced or during recovery from exercise

In the whole process, ADP is converted to ATP at the expense of either PC or ATP derived from dietary nutrients (carbohydrate and fat). PC, however, can only be recycled at the expense of the ATP formed from the metabolism of dietary nutrients.

AMP can be converted back to ATP by reversal of the myokinase reaction (ADP + ADP ↔ AMP + ATP). When the demand for energy is reduced, the myokinase reaction reverses its direction, forming ADP that can ultimately be converted to ATP at the expense of either PC or dietary-derived ATP.

## REFORMATION OF GLUCOSE

Substrates for gluconeogenesis are primarily lactic acid and α-ketoacids such as pyruvate, oxaloacetate, and α-ketoglutarate, derived from either amino acids or rapid glycolysis. Glycerol, or any intermediate of the Krebs cycle, can also give rise to the synthesis of glucose. Acetyl CoA cannot be converted to glucose because it cannot be converted into pyruvic acid. Thus, an important point to

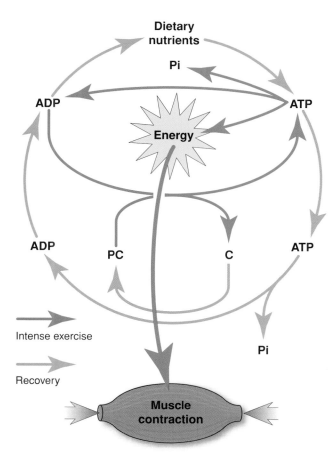

**FIGURE 4.15.** The ATP-PC energy system during exercise and recovery. Red indicates the closed functioning of the ATP-PC system during intense exercise when ATP and PC sources are limited to those stored in the muscle. Green indicates how ATP and PC stores are replenished by the metabolism of dietary nutrients when immediate energy demand is low. ATP, adenosine triphosphate; ADP, adenosine diphosphate; PC, phosphocreatine; C, creatine; $P_i$, inorganic phosphate.

hydrolysis. Gluconeogenic formation of glucose is favored because these three bypassed reactions of glycolysis are also irreversible. The net cost of gluconeogenesis is six high-energy phosphate bonds so glycolysis and gluconeogenesis are not in equilibrium.

## SYNTHESIS OF GLYCOGEN

Glycogen is a branched chain polysaccharide (*Fig. 4.17*) consisting of glucose molecules linked together by a 1–4 or 1–6 **glycosidic bond**. Glycogen is made by adding one glucose unit at a time to an existing molecule by forming a 1–4 glycosidic bond and then rearranging the glycogen chains to make branches. Branching is necessary because it increases the solubility of the glycogen molecule. Theoretically, a glycogen polysaccharide chain could be built of

remember with respect to energetics is that fat cannot be converted to carbohydrate, only catabolized or stored as body fat.

The starting point for gluconeogenesis is pyruvic acid. Eight of the gluconeogenic reactions are actually reversals of glycolytic reactions (*Fig. 4.16*). However, there are three glycolytic reactions that are irreversible. These irreversible reactions are bypassed by three new gluconeogenic reactions that favor glucose synthesis. The first barrier to overcome in the synthesis of glucose from pyruvic acid is the irreversible glycolytic pyruvate kinase reaction. This barrier is bypassed by converting pyruvic acid to oxaloacetate and then converting oxaloacetate to phosphoenolpyruvate. ATP is necessary in this reaction, but the ATP can be obtained from several sources since the body is recovering from exercise. The second barrier to overcome is the irreversible glycolytic phosphofructokinase reaction, which is overcome by the **hydrolysis** of fructose-1,6-diphosphate with the enzyme fructose-1,6-diphosphatase. The third irreversible glycolytic reaction, the hexokinase reaction, is also overcome through

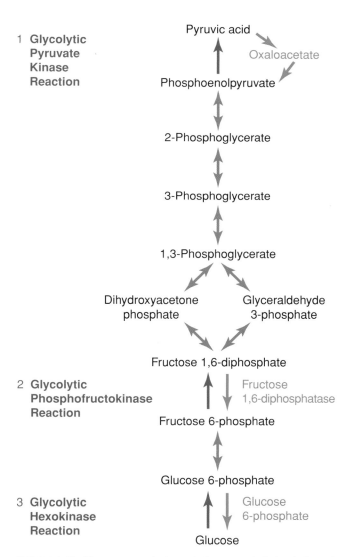

**FIGURE 4.16.** Gluconeogenesis through the reversal of glycolysis. Red indicates unidirectional reactions that are specific only to gluconeogenesis. Blue indicates unidirectional reactions that are specific only to glycolysis. Purple indicates reversible reactions that are common to both glycolysis and gluconeogenesis. Sites numbered 1–3 are reaction sites in glycolysis that must be bypassed during gluconeogenesis.

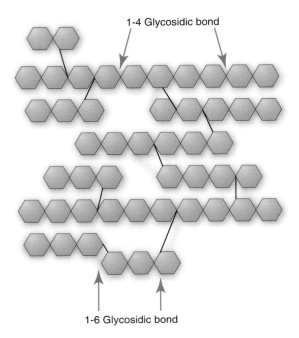

**1-4 Glycosidic bond**

**1-6 Glycosidic bond**

**FIGURE 4.17.** The glycogen molecule. Glycogen is a polysaccharide made up of numerous glucose units bound together at either the 1–4 or 1–6 carbons.

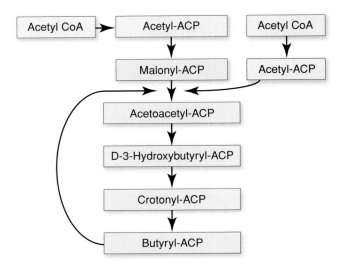

**FIGURE 4.18.** Fatty acid synthesis. Fatty acid synthesis can be described as the sequential addition of two-carbon units (acetyl CoA) to a growing fatty acid chain (butyryl-ACP). CoA, coenzyme A; ACP, acyl-carrying protein.

indefinite length. However, when the chain reaches a length of about 7 units, the chain is transferred to another smaller chain four units away from another branch. The transfer forms a 1–6 glycosidic bond.

It is not clear what limits the actual size of a glycogen molecule or the total amount of glycogen stored within a tissue. Even under a heavy glucose load, excess glucose will be stored as fat rather than glycogen. In spite of the liver having a higher concentration of glycogen (400 $\mu$mol·g$^{-1}$ wet weight) than does muscle (85 $\mu$mol·g$^{-1}$ wet weight), the muscles contain the bulk of the body glycogen stores because of their larger tissue mass.

## SYNTHESIS OF FATTY ACIDS AND TRIGLYCERIDES

The path for the synthesis of fat is distinct from that of degradation. The first step in fat synthesis is the formation of fatty acids. Fatty acid formation occurs in the cytosol, whereas fatty acid degradation occurs in the mitochondria. The overall synthetic process is an elongation of the growing fatty acid chain by the sequential addition of two-carbon units derived from acetyl CoA (*Fig. 4.18*). Acetyl CoA is converted to acetyl-acyl carrying-protein (ACP) and then into malonyl-ACP. The malonyl-ACP combines with another acetyl-ACP molecule to form a four-carbon unit called acetoacetyl-ACP. The three subsequent reactions convert acetoacetyl-ACP to butyryl-ACP. The butyryl-ACP combines with another acetyl-ACP, adding two carbons to the growing fatty acid chain. The product is another acetoacetyl-ACP with two more carbons than the original acetoacetyl-ACP. The reactions then proceed to form butyryl-ACP as before, but with two additional

carbons. The process continues to repeat itself by sequentially adding two carbons to the growing butyryl-ACP chain until the fatty acid achieves full length. Once fatty acids are formed, they can be attached to a glycerol molecule to form a triglyceride.

The synthesis of the triglyceride molecule starts with the formation of glycerol-3-phosphate, the "backbone" upon which the newly synthesized fatty acids are attached (*Fig. 4.19*). Glycerol-3-phosphate can be formed in either the liver or fat cells. Triglyceride synthesis proceeds by the transfer of a fatty acid from its CoA derivative to position

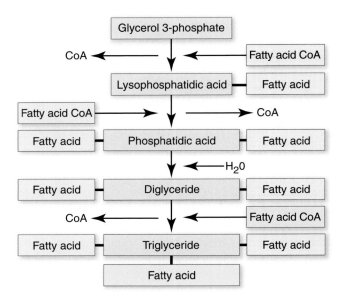

**FIGURE 4.19.** Triglyceride synthesis. Fatty acids (yellow, green, pink) are sequentially attached to a glycerol backbone (blue) to form the triglyceride molecule.

one of the glycerol-3-phosphate, forming lysophosphatidic acid. The succeeding step is similar to the first and occurs at position two. The resulting molecule is phosphatidic acid, which is then converted to a diacylglycerol (diglyceride). The third fatty acid is then attached to this diglyceride to form triglycerides.

Triglycerides synthesized in fat tissue are stored in the cytoplasm. Triglycerides remain stored in a highly concentrated form until the demand for energy requires their mobilization. Triglycerides synthesized in the liver can combine with cholesterols, phospholipids, or proteins to form lipoproteins to be released into the circulation. Circulating triglyceride molecules and their respective fatty acids are thus delivered to the peripheral tissues.

▶ *INQUIRY SUMMARY.* The body immediately begins to replenish depleted energy stores when exercise intensity is reduced or when exercise is ceased. The fuel that is used to replenish the depleted energy supplies comes from dietary fat, protein, and carbohydrate. *Which do you think would be most important to consume post exercise: fat, protein, or carbohydrate? Why?*

## Summary

The body's energy expenditure during exercise may increase to 25 times that seen at rest. To meet this increased energy demand, ATP must be produced at a rate equal to the required power output. The rate of ATP delivery to the contractile apparatus of the muscle is regulated by intracellular and extracellular mechanisms. The energy system used for ATP production is dependent upon exercise intensity and duration. High-intensity exercise of short duration favors rapid glycolysis and the ATP-PC system, whereas low- to moderate-intensity exercise favors slow glycolysis and fat oxidation. As aerobic exercise continues, a shift from slow glycolysis to fat oxidation takes place. Once exercise ceases, the metabolic rate remains elevated to replenish fuel sources expended during the exercise bout and bring the body back to resting homeostasis.

### SUMMARY KNOWLEDGE

1. Rank each one of the energy systems by their maximal rate of ATP production.
2. Rank each one of the energy systems by the total amount of ATP they can produce before becoming depleted.
3. How does the responsibility for ATP production to support the energy demand of exercise shift among the energy systems as exercise intensity increases?
4. What mechanisms does the body use to maintain blood glucose levels during prolonged exercise?
5. How do the actions of insulin and glucagon oppose each other?
6. What are some things that contribute to the EPOC?
7. How is the OBLA thought to be related to the rate of glycolysis?

### References

1. Gastin PB. Energy system interaction and relative contribution during maximal exercise. *Sports Med* 2001;31:725–741.
2. Farrell PA, Wilmore JH, Coyle EF, et al. Plasma lactate accumulation and distance running performance. *Med Sci Sports* 1979;11:338–344.
3. Powers SK, Dodd S, Deason R, et al. Ventilatory threshold, running economy, and distance running performance of trained athletes. *Res Q Exerc Sport* 1983;54:179–182.
4. Pollock ML. Submaximal and maximal working capacity of elite distance runners. Part I: cardiorespiratory aspects. *Ann NY Acad Sci* 1977;301:310–322.

### Suggested Readings

Bangsbo J, Krustrup P, Gonzalez-Alonso J, et al. ATP production and efficiency of human skeletal muscle during intense exercise: effect of previous exercise. *Am J Physiol Endocrinol Metab* 2001;280:E956–E964.

Christmass MA, Dawson B, Goodman C, et al. Brief intense exercise followed by passive recovery modifies the pattern of fuel use in humans during subsequent sustained intermittent exercise. *Acta Physiol Scand* 2001;172:39–52.

Grassi B. Regulation of oxygen consumption at exercise onset: is it really controversial? *Exerc Sport Sci Rev* 2001;29:134–138.

Hughson RL, Tschakovsky ME, Houston ME. Regulation of oxygen consumption at the onset of exercise. *Exerc Sport Sci Rev* 2001;29:129–133.

Parra J, Cadefau JA, Rodas G, et al. The distribution of rest periods affects performance and adaptations of energy metabolism induced by high-intensity training in human muscle. *Acta Physiol Scand* 2000;169:157–165.

Schneider DA, McLellan TM, Gass GC. Plasma catecholamine and blood lactate responses to incremental arm and leg exercise. *Med Sci Sports Exerc* 2000;32:608–613.

Tomlin DL, Wenger HA. The relationship between aerobic fitness and recovery from high intensity intermittent exercise. *Sports Med* 2001; 31:1–11.

### On the Internet

Glucagon and the Glucagon-Like Peptides. Available at: **http://www. glucagon.com/**. Accessed April 04, 2005.

Endocrine Disorders and Endocrine Surgery: Normal Regulation of Blood Glucose. Available at: **http://www.endocrineweb.com/insulin.html**. Accessed April 04, 2005.

How Exercise Works: ATP is Energy. Available at: **http://health.howstuff works.com/sports-physiology2.htm**. Accessed April 04, 2005.

### Writing to Learn

*In this chapter you have learned how the exercise power output demand dictates which fuel and which energy pathway are used to provide the necessary ATP to sustain an exercise bout. Research and write a paper on how dietary practices and/or training practices can alter the dynamics of energy production during exercise. Some research topics may include: Does a high-carbohydrate diet enhance or inhibit glycolytic capacity? Which type of exercise training increases the capacity of the ATP-PC system? How much time should a basketball player devote to aerobic versus anaerobic training?*

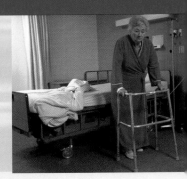

## CHAPTER

# 5 Ergometry and Calorimetry: The Measurement of Work and Energy

*Ambulation-assistive devices elevate the $O_2$ cost of walking.* What are the implications of this fact for the individual pictured?

I n Chapters 2 through 4, we examined nutrient availability, principles of cellular energy conversion, and metabolic processes during exercise that are fundamental to our understanding of movement. Chapter 5 ends Section 1 of the text by discussing measurement principles and the energy requirements of physical activity.

While we participate in cross-country cycling, running on a treadmill, hiking over rugged terrain, gardening, or various activities of daily living (ADL), energy is being expended at a rate dictated by the intensity of our physical effort. This energy requirement is related to metabolic rate; therefore, measurement of the $O_2$ cost of various physical activities provides a picture of the energy requirement of the activity. The exact magnitude of the energy expenditure during exercise is often determined (for research studies) or at least closely estimated (for clinical purposes). In rehabilitation programs, for example, patients are often prescribed exercise according to the desired oxygen consumption ($\dot{V}O_2$) response. The material presented in this chapter will help you understand how $\dot{V}O_2$ responses

during physical activities can be equated to energy expenditure. Therefore, the purpose of this chapter is to present principles of ergometry and calorimetry and to show how these principles are important to a solid understanding of measurement in exercise physiology.

## Ergometry: The Measurement of Work

Measuring work produced or power generated during exercise involves the use of devices to quantify these two factors with exacting precision. These devices, called **ergometers**, are necessary in exercise physiology research and rehabilitation programs. For example, ergometers are used in exercise physiology research to accurately quantify training adaptations at particular workloads. Without the ability to accurately apply a desired workload and reapply these workloads from day to day, researchers would not be able to document the physiologic cost of exercise at a particular ergometer workload or the way in which training improves performance. Ergometer exercise also provides the accuracy and reliability necessary for clinicians in rehabilitation programs to repeat work bouts without fear of misapplying a prescribed workload for a patient. Units of measurement derived from these devices can be converted to whatever energy or metabolic unit of measurement is desired, thus allowing the researcher or clinician to express exercise intensity in measurement units suitable to a given situation.

Measurement of work in exercise physiology involves an accurate determination of the force (mass of the object to be moved) and distance (vertical displacement) over which the force is applied. This can be done using human subjects in several ways. First, a subject can perform work on a cycle (leg or arm) ergometer by pedaling/cranking at a constant rate against a constant resistance. Second, a subject can walk or run up a grade using a motorized treadmill. Finally, a subject can perform work by moving his/her body mass vertically, as in bench stepping. Several of these devices are shown in *Figure 5.1*. These are some of the traditional ergometers used in exercise physiology laboratories and clinical exercise programs, but they do not represent all of

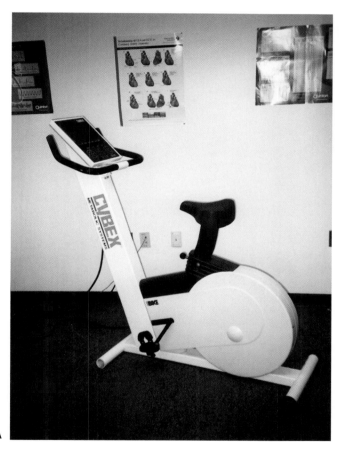

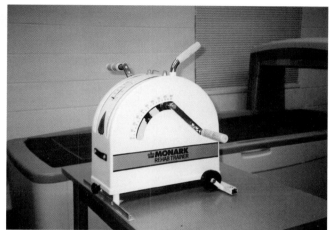

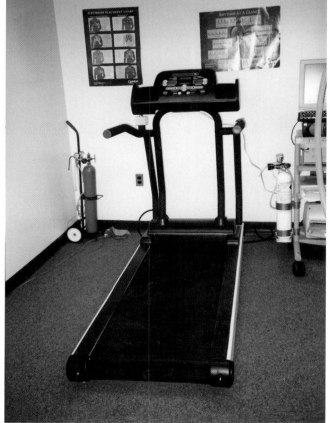

**FIGURE 5.1.** Traditional ergometers used in exercise physiology and clinical laboratories. **A.** Cycle (leg) ergometer. **B.** Cycle (arm) ergometer **C.** Treadmill ergometer.

the ways in which exercise conditions can be imposed on subjects for the purpose of studying physiologic responses to exercise or for rehabilitation. *What are some other exercise or activity forms that can be used to study exercise responses?*

## UNITS OF MEASUREMENTS

Ergometry entails the use of specific terminology and types of equipment with which health care students should become familiar. This familiarity will lead to competence in the research laboratory or rehabilitation clinic. Common units of measurement used to quantify human exercise are listed in Table 5.1. It is important to become familiar with both the metric system and Système Internationale d'Unités (International System of Units, SI). SI units, based on the metric system, were adopted in 1960 at the Eleventh General Conference of Weights and Measures. Table 5.2 presents guidelines to help with the use of SI units. Metric and SI units are the standard measurement systems used by the scientific community, and they have been adopted by most medical and scientific journals. Although this list is complete for our purposes here, it is not a comprehensive listing of all possible measurement terms used in exercise physiology, allied health, or medicine.

| Table 5.1 | COMMON MEASUREMENT TERMS AND CONVERSIONS* | | |
|---|---|---|---|
| **Quantity** | **Unit** | **Symbol** | **Common conversions** |
| Area | *square meter* | m$^2$ | |
| Mass | *kilogram* | kg | |
| Length | *meter* | m | |
| Time | *second* | s | |
| Force | *Newton* | N | |
| | kilopond | kp | = 9.80665 N |
| | kilogram | kg | = 9.80665 N |
| Work | *joule* | J | = 1 N·m |
| | kilogram meter | kg·m | = 9.797 J or 0.009797 kJ |
| | kilocalorie | kcal | = 4186.8 J or 4.1868 kJ |
| Heat | *joule* | J | |
| | kilocalorie | kcal | |
| Energy | *joule* | J | |
| | kilocalorie | kcal | |
| Power | *watt* | W | = 6.118 kg·m·min$^{-1}$ |
| | kilogram meter per minute | kg·m·min$^{-1}$ | = 0.16345 W |
| | | | = 1 J·s$^{-1}$ or 0.0098068 kJ·min$^{-1}$ |
| Velocity | *meters per second* | m·s$^{-1}$ | |
| Torque | *Newton-meter* | N·m | |
| Volume | *cubic meter* | m$^3$ | |
| | liter | L | = 10$^{-3}$ m$^3$ |
| Pressure | *Pascal* | Pa | = 0.007501 mm Hg |
| | millimeters of mercury | mm Hg | = 133.322 Pa |
| | torr | torr | = 133.322 Pa or 1.0 mm Hg |
| Temperature | *Kelvin* | K | |
| | degree Celsius | °C | = 1 K |
| **Substance** | | | |
| Concentration | *mole per liter* | mol·L$^{-1}$ | |
| Molality | *mole per kilogram* | mol·kg$^{-1}$ | |

*Terms in italics are Système Internationale d'Unités units and are placed first in the list, followed by common units often used in exercise physiology laboratories. After this, when appropriate, common conversions are given. English units are not included in the table but are included in the problems placed in the text for students to gain experience in converting from these units, which are still in common usage in the United States.

| Table 5.2 | BASE UNITS OF SYSTÈME INTERNATIONALE NOMENCLATURE | | | | | | |
|---|---|---|---|---|---|---|---|
| **Unit & definition** | **Physical quantity & SI base unit** | **SI symbol** | | **SI style guidelines** | **Example** | **Not correct** | **Correct** |
| Degree Celsius (°C) 0°C = 273.15 K | | | | Lowercase for unit symbols except when derived from a person's name | kilogram Kelvin Newton Watt *Exceptions* Liter | Kg k n w | kg K N W L |
| Joule (J) Work done by a force of 1 Newton acting to move an object a distance of 1 m in the direction of the force | | | | Do not pluralize unit symbols | Kilograms | kgs | kg |
| | | | | Do not put periods after unit symbols except at the end of a sentence | Meter Mole | m. mol. | m mol |
| Kelvin (K) Fraction 1/273.16 of the thermodynamic temperature of the triple point of water | T Kelvin | K | | Product of units is indicated by a dot above the line | | N × m | N·m |
| | | | | Space or hyphen is used to separate the names of individual units when spelled out | Torque | Newton × meter | Newton meter or Newton-meter |
| | | | | Symbols for units formed from other units by division are indicated by means of a solidus (/), negative exponents, or horizontal line | Velocity | | m/s; $m \cdot s^{-1}$; $\dfrac{m}{s}$ |

*(continues)*

| Table 5.2 | BASE UNITS OF SYSTÈME INTERNATIONALE NOMENCLATURE *(Continued)* | | | | | | |
|---|---|---|---|---|---|---|---|
| Unit & definition | Physical quantity & SI base unit | SI symbol | SI style guidelines | Example | Not correct | Correct |
| Kilogram (kg) Unit of mass equal to the mass of the international prototype of the kg | Mass Kilogram | kg | Unit names and unit symbols are not to be combined | Power | kilo gram· meter·s$^{-1}$ | kg·m·s$^{-1}$ |
| Meter (m) Path length traveled by light in a vacuum during a time interval of 1/299,792,458 of a second | Length Meter | m | When numbers are printed, symbols are preferred | | 100 meters | 100 m |
| Newton (N) Force required to accelerate a body with the mass of 1 kg by one m·s$^{-1}$·s$^{-1}$ | | | Space between number and symbol | | 50mL | 50 mL |
| Pascal (Pa) Pressure produced by a force of 1 N applied, with uniform distribution, over an area of 1 m$^2$ | | | Place zero before decimal | | .01 | 0.01 |
| Second (s) The duration of 9,192,631,770 periods of the radiation that corresponds to the transition between two hyperfine levels of the ground state of the cesium-133 atom | Time Second | s | Decimal numbers are preferable to fractions | | 3/4 | 0.75 |
| Watt (W) Power that in 1 second gives rise to the energy of 1 J | | | | | | |

| Table 5.2 | BASE UNITS OF SYSTÈME INTERNATIONALE NOMENCLATURE (Continued) | | | | | | |
|---|---|---|---|---|---|---|---|
| Unit & definition | Physical quantity & SI base unit | SI symbol | SI style guidelines | Example | Not correct | Correct |
| Mole (mol) Amount of substance of a system which contains as many elementary entities as there are atoms in 0.012 kg of carbon-12. | Amount of substance Mole | mol | | | | |

For SI units in exercise physiology, the term body weight is properly referred to as mass (kg), height should be referred to as stature (m), second is s, minute is min, hour is h, week is wk, month is mo, year is y, day is d, gram is g, liter is L, joule is J, kilocalorie is kcal, Pascal is Pa, revolutions per minute is rpm, and Watt is W. These abbreviations or symbols are used for the singular or plural form. T, temperature.

*LINKUP: In the course of your studies in exercise physiology, you will likely be required to write laboratory reports and research papers that require a solid understanding of ergometry. See Perspective: Writing Laboratory Reports at http://connection.lww.com/go/ brownexphys and on the Student Resource CD-ROM for guidance through this process.*

## Energy

In Chapter 3, energy was defined as the capacity or ability to do work. Energy is manifested in various forms: motion (kinetic energy), position (potential energy), atomic, radiant, thermal, chemical, electrical, and mechanical. Energy in the body is not tangible and does not lend itself readily to direct measurement. While a very common laboratory unit of energy is the kilocalorie (kcal), energy may also be expressed in other units such as **kilogram-meter** (kg·m). Therefore, the units used to express energy are interconvertible. The American College of Sports Medicine (ACSM) prefers the use of kilojoules (kJ) as the unit of choice for energy and work. A joule (J) represents the application of a force of 1 Newton (N) through a distance of 1 meter (m).

## Work

Work is the result of an expenditure of energy. Stated another way, it is the outcome of a release of energy. It is also defined in physics as the product of a force and its vertical displacement.

Work = Force (or mass)
$\qquad$ × Distance (vertical displacement)

In exercise physiology, the most common laboratory unit for work is the kg·m, but it may also be expressed in other units such as the kcal. Unlike energy, work can be measured simply and directly.

## Power

**Power** (work rate) denotes the amount of work or energy per unit of time. The time frame is usually in minutes, but power may also be expressed per second. Common units of power are $kg·m·min^{-1}$, $kcal·h^{-1}$, and $kcal·min^{-1}$. The watt is the SI unit of power output. The kilopond (kp, a unit of force) is often used interchangeably with kilogram (kg, a unit of mass) for the purpose of calculating work and power for cycle ergometry. These units, though not technically the same, can be used interchangeably when measuring work or power at the normal acceleration of gravity. Thus, 1 kp is the force acting upon a mass of 1 kg at the normal acceleration of gravity.

Note that the work equation may be applied to positive work (as when an object is moved vertically to a higher position, i.e., using concentric muscular contractions) or negative work (as when an object is moved vertically to a lower position, i.e., using eccentric muscular contractions). Although the same value for work would be calculated when a 2-kg mass is moved 2 m vertically, either up or down, the energy involved per unit of work is different. The $\dot{V}O_2$ response for positive work is two to four times higher than for negative work, increasing as power output increases (*Fig. 5.2*).

The slope for negative, eccentric work of leg cycling is essentially flat (0.28), indicating a very slight increase in $\dot{V}O_2$ over resting levels even at high power outputs. This has implications for rehabilitation practice as cardiovascular responses are generally less for eccentric muscular contractions (see Chapter 7).

*LINKUP: Perspective: Practice Problems at http:// connection.lww.com/go/brownexphys and on the Student Resource CD-ROM provides many practice problems using the equations in this section and throughout the remainder of the chapter.*

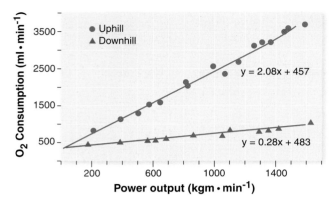

**FIGURE 5.2.** $O_2$ consumption responses from individuals bicycling "uphill" (O) and "downhill" (▲) on a motor-driven treadmill plotted against power output. The metabolic demand of the positive, concentric work is greater than for the negative, eccentric work. The regression equation for each type of work is included. Data from Asmussen E. Ergonomics Society Symposium on Fatigue, 1953.

## COMMON ERGOMETERS

Work and energy can be measured in the laboratory by treadmills, leg and arm cycles, and stepping ergometers. Because the external power output can be adjusted easily and is precisely known, these instruments are invaluable aids in the study of the physiologic effects of exercise and are used quite often in exercise physiology experimentation and clinical settings. You should become familiar with all four types of ergometers and be able to calculate work and work rate (power output); you should also be proficient at calibrating these devices to ensure that their settings (e.g., resistance on the cycle flywheel, treadmill speed and grade) are providing accurate readings. Uncalibrated ergometers give erroneous work and power measures, which introduce measurement error in research and invalidate exercise prescriptions in clinical practice.

### Cycle Ergometer

There are two major types of cycle ergometers used in clinical and research practice: electrically braked and friction braked. Electrically braked cycle ergometers are designed to maintain a constant power output even when the cycling speed is altered. The electrically braked cycle does this by varying the resistance (force) that the built-in electronic resistance mechanism applies to the flywheel as the pedaling speed changes during a work bout. Calibration of electrically braked cycle ergometers is typically performed by the manufacturer. Friction-braked cycle ergometers apply force to the rotating flywheel via a friction belt wrapped around the flywheel. Braking force is added to the flywheel, and this force is measured by way of a weighted pendulum that is calibrated in kg resistance. As force is applied, the pendulum is displaced in units of kp (or kg) (*Fig. 5.3*).

The following brief procedure is useful for properly testing a subject on a friction-braked cycle (leg) ergometer. When the subject is pedaling, a force (calibrated in kg) is applied to the flywheel to add resistance. Exercising subjects on the cycle ergometer usually follow these basic steps:

1. Adjust the seat height to allow one leg to almost extend completely with the foot on the pedal. Detecting the proper seat height (i.e., whether the leg is extended enough) may best be accomplished by having the subject briefly pedal against a light resistance.
2. Set the metronome (device to maintain cadence) at 100 beats·min$^{-1}$ (other speeds are just as suitable, e.g., 120, 140). In 1 minute of pedaling at this rate, the wheel will turn 50 revolutions. *What is the rpm when pedaling at metronome settings of 120 and 140 beats·min$^{-1}$? Why is it important to track pedal rate?*
3. When the subject begins pedaling, adjust the resistance by turning the resistance knob. This should be done only while the wheel is in motion. It is important to keep in time with the beat of the metronome or to monitor pedal rate via the onboard frequency device to maintain pedal frequency, otherwise the power output will rise or fall in accordance with increasing or decreasing pedal speed. Do not allow subjects to stop pedaling when you are changing the resistance.

Current models of friction-braked ergometers come with an onboard device that measures pedal frequency so that metronome control of pedal rate may not be necessary.

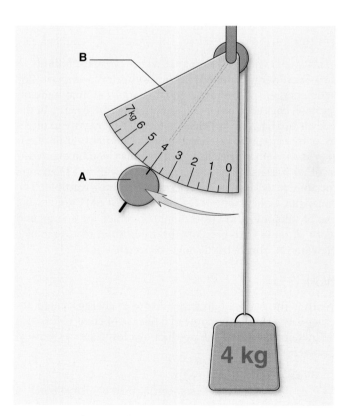

**FIGURE 5.3.** The Monark cycle ergometer scale calibrated in kp (kg) showing the pendulum (A) and scale (B). A calibration weight of 4 kg has been attached, and the pendulum has been deflected to the 4-kp mark on the scale, indicating correct calibration.

However, research studies require the very precise measurements of power output; therefore, it is advisable to control the pedal rate of subjects with a calibrated metronome.

Common friction-braked cycle ergometers (e.g., Monark) have flywheel diameters that allow 6 m of horizontal distance traveled per flywheel revolution (6 m·rev$^{-1}$). Other cycle ergometers (Tunturi and Bodyguard) have flywheels that are one-half this diameter, making the distance traveled 3 m·rev$^{-1}$. The Monark Rehab Trainer is a friction-braked arm ergometer with a flywheel diameter that allows 2.4 m·rev$^{-1}$. Work can easily be calculated on these ergometers as the product of distance traveled times the force applied to the flywheel. Note also that body mass is not a factor in calculating work on the cycle. The force is determined by the amount of resistance on the flywheel. The distance of displacement depends on the number of revolutions of the flywheel and is calculated as follows for the Monark cycle ergometer:

rev·min$^{-1}$ × 6 m·rev$^{-1}$ pedaled
= Horizontal distance traveled

For the Monark, a pedal frequency of 50 rev·min$^{-1}$ results in a horizontal distance of 300 m for each minute of pedaling. *What is the distance using the Monark Rehab Trainer?* Once the distance is known (as based on pedal speed and flywheel size), it is an easy matter to calculate power output using the following equation:

Power output (kg·m·min$^{-1}$) = rev·min$^{-1}$
× m·rev$^{-1}$ × kg resistance

This equation is simply an expression of the power output formula presented earlier. Power output calculated this way uses the metric unit kg·m·min$^{-1}$. To change kg·m·min$^{-1}$ to SI units (W), multiply by 0.16345.

The introduction of the Monark cycle ergometer to the United States market paralleled the fast rise of exercise physiology as an academic discipline in America through the 1960s and 1970s. Box 5.1 chronicles Per-Olof Åstrand and the beginning of the Monark cycle ergometer.

## Step Ergometer

A simple platform with no moving parts on the device can serve as an ergometer (*Fig. 5.4*). Work is measured on this device in the same manner as presented in the lifting problems earlier. The only difference now is that the force (mass) being lifted is the individual's body mass and the distance is the height of the step or platform. Therefore, work is measured by using the work equation applied to bench stepping.

Work = Force (body mass) × Distance (step height)

Using bench stepping as the exercise mode, however, involves repeatedly stepping up and down over several minutes. Therefore, this formula, which provides the work produced in one cycle of stepping (once up and once down), must be modified by including the stepping rate in

steps per minute to determine the power output according to the following equation:

Power output = Force (body mass)
× Distance (step height) × Step rate

Note that the work of stepping down is ignored in this calculation.

The metronome is first set at the desired cadence when a subject is exercising using a step ergometer. For instance, if a cadence of 132 beats·min$^{-1}$ is selected, 33 repetitions (stepping cycles) will be performed in 1 minute since subjects synchronize their foot placement with the beats of the metronome. Stepping is done in time with the metronome—two beats up, two beats down. This gives four steps per repetition or 33 repetitions per minute. The next consideration is the height of the bench being used. If the bench can be adjusted, 10, 20, 30, and 40 cm are common step heights. Because work and power in exercise physiology laboratories are often converted to kg·m and kg·m·min$^{-1}$, respectively, the heights will have to be converted from cm to m.

## Treadmill Ergometer

No external work is being performed when walking or running horizontally (on a level grade) because there is no translation of a force against gravity. In the classic definition of work, only vertical displacement is considered. Therefore, technically no mechanical work is accomplished at a zero percent grade. The slight vertical elevation of the body's center of gravity during the push-off phase after each foot plant during running is not considered because it is not easily measured and differs among individuals. Also when positive work is done as the center of gravity of the body rises during the push-off phase, negative work is performed when the body's center of gravity falls. Thus, these two opposite vertical displacements cancel each other, and no work is performed for horizontal movement.

In contrast to horizontal walking or running, walking or running on a treadmill set at an angle (grade walking or running) allows the calculation of work on the treadmill ergometer. In grade walking or running, subjects move their body mass at a vertical distance that is a function of the angle at which the treadmill is set. The vertical displacement can be estimated in the following manner. For example, if a 70-kg subject walks for 15 minutes at a rate of 100 m·min$^{-1}$ and a 10% grade, he will walk 1500 m and have a vertical displacement of 150 m. Consider the following:

Distance (d) = Rate × Time (e.g., 100 m·min$^{-1}$
× 15 min = 1500 m)

Displacement = 1500 m × 0.10 = 150 m

Therefore, work is calculated with the following equation:

Work = Force × Displacement (e.g., 70 kg
× 150 m = 10,500 kg·m)

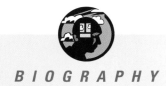

*B I O G R A P H Y*

# Per-Olof Åstrand and the Monark Ergometer

A milestone in ergometry occurred in 1913 when Nobel Laureate (awarded in 1920 for physiology or medicine) August Krogh published an article describing a very precise cycle ergometer. This early, electrically powered ergometer was incorporated into the laboratory research of Erik Hohwu Christensen (Department of Physiology, College of Physical Education, Stockholm). In 1954 another milestone occurred when aviation doctor Wilhelm von Döbeln and equipment maker Harry Hagelin constructed a cycle ergometer in which the wheel was braked mechanically by a belt running around the rim. Both ends of this belt were attached to a revolving drum to which a pendulum was fixed. The device thus acted as a pendulum scale. A member of the faculty in the College of Physical Education at this time was Per-Olof Åstrand, who later became a professor at the Karolinska Institute in Stockholm. Åstrand had graduated from the College of Physical Education in 1946 and Karolinska Institute Medical School in 1952. He is most famous for his work on physical working capacity of men and women from childhood to adulthood and the physiologic responses to intermittent exercise. Åstrand discusses what occurred in the 1950s in the evolution of the Monark cycle ergometer:

"At that time our department was involved in a program of education with a fixed aim: to teach teachers of physical education and biology, athletic coaches, and interested 'amateurs' the foundations required to be able to inform and instruct in many health-related questions. With the help of this cycle ergometer, it was natural to teach interested people to construct tests of heart function and to inform them on state of physical fitness. In doing this, we were able to move the ergometer from the traditional laboratory and hospital environment to schools, clubs, and other enterprises. It was such a success that the existing resources to manufacture the cycle ergometer were inadequate. The popularity of the athletics movement, and to some extent our institution, persuaded Monark to take up the production of the cycle ergometer."

This cycle ergometer proved so revolutionary and groundbreaking that the Monark ergometers became the world's most widely used clinical and research ergometer. Åstrand, recognized as one of the mainstays of the fledging science of exercise physiology in the mid-20th century, was influential in the export of this cycle ergometer to exercise physiology laboratories in America. This was perhaps a result of the scientific reputation of Swedish exercise physiology research in general and because Åstrand's book, *Textbook of Work Physiology* became a best-selling graduate text in America. The works of Åstrand and some of his students, such as Bengt Saltin and Björn Ekblom, have been cited a phenomenal number of times in the scientific literature over the last 35 years.

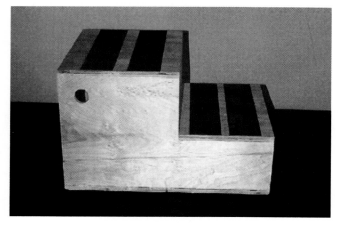

**FIGURE 5.4.** The step test is the oldest of the exercise protocols used in clinical cardiology to screen for heart disease.

## Ergometer Calibration

Calibration refers to procedures in which measurement instruments are standardized. Calibration is necessary in research and clinical practice so that the results obtained are *valid* and *reliable*. For example, if exercise devices are incorrectly calibrated prior to data collection, the resulting data being gathered for research and/or clinical purposes would not accurately reflect the exercise state imposed and, therefore, validity would be lost. Validity in this sense means the extent to which an instrument measures what it is intended to measure.

For instance, if you want a patient to exercise on a cycle ergometer at 300 kg·m·min$^{-1}$ but the actual power output is closer to 350 kg·m·min$^{-1}$ because the cycle's calibration was off, validity suffers. If you were also measuring $\dot{V}O_2$

during exercise at an invalid work output, the metabolic response would be indicative of an incorrect workload. Therefore, validity addresses what we are able to do with test results.

 *LINKUP:* **Perspective: Treadmill and Cycle Ergometer Calibration Procedures,** *found at http://connection. lww.com/go/brownexphys and on the Student Resource CD-ROM, briefly describes how these ergometers can be calibrated. Also see* **Perspective: Laboratory Guidelines** *for general guidelines to observe during laboratory sessions.*

Another important concept is the reliability of measurement. Reliability relates to an instrument producing the same or nearly the same score with repeated tests. An ergometer that is properly calibrated ensures that the measurement of work output is at the same time valid (correct work output is actually determined) and reliable (measurement of work output is stable upon subsequent work bouts). A testing instrument such as an ergometer, if correctly calibrated, gives valid and reliable measures. However, just because a test is reliable does not mean that it is valid. *Can you think of an example in which this would be true?*

The measurement of various physiologic variables during exercise in either research or clinical practice presupposes that the exercise device is correctly calibrated to ensure validity and reliability. Of the three standard types of ergometers used in exercise physiology, the cycle and treadmill ergometers (because of moving parts) have the potential to periodically lose their calibration, albeit infrequently. With repeated use, the calibration of these devices must be checked so applied workloads accurately match the intended workloads.

▶ *INQUIRY SUMMARY.* Ergometric devices provide valid and reliable measures of work and power. The ability to quantify work and power is essential for both clinical and research applications. Think about what separates an ergometer from any other exercise device. *Do you think nonergometric exercise devices have a place in research and/or clinical programs? Explain your answer.*

## Calorimetry: The Measurement of Energy

The process of cellular respiration consumes energy nutrients and $O_2$ and produces ATP. The ATP is subsequently consumed to power cellular activity, such as muscle contraction. Heat is released in each of these processes, and each process is coupled to the other in the following manner:

Cellular respiration        Cellular work
Energy nutrients + $O_2$ → ATP → Muscle contraction + ADP
           ↓                  ↓
       Heat produced      Heat produced

In the chemical equations above, the energy in nutrient chemical bonds is transformed to a mechanical form, i.e., muscle contraction, and heat is a byproduct as these energy transformations are coupled. The process of measuring this heat release is termed **calorimetry** (from *calorie*, meaning heat). Note that the rate of heat release is proportional to the rate of metabolism ($\dot{V}o_2$), a relationship whose importance to exercise physiology laboratory measurement will become apparent.

Energy expenditure (heat release) in humans can be measured by several techniques:

- Direct calorimetry: measurement of the heat emission of a subject enclosed in a chamber
- Indirect (respiratory) calorimetry: measurement of respiratory gas exchange
- Indirect (doubly labeled water) calorimetry: measurement of integral oxygen consumption ($\dot{V}o_2$) from the difference in the elimination rate of $^2H$ and $^{18}O$ from labeled body water
- Indirect ($^{13}CO_2$ breath test) calorimetry: measurement of $^{13}C$ enrichment of breath $CO_2$ after the administration of $^{13}C$ sodium bicarbonate
- Noncalorimetric methods, including monitoring heart rate (HR) and the use of accelerometers

The gold-standard techniques for measuring energy expenditure are the first two listed above. These techniques provide information on energy expenditure during time periods lasting less than 4 hours. The doubly labeled water technique is useful over prolonged periods of time in free-living conditions and has an accuracy of 3% to 5%, an error rate of sufficient magnitude to preclude its inclusion among the gold-standard tests (1). The $^{13}CO_2$ breath test has also been shown to be a valid and reliable indirect method to measure energy expenditure over short periods of time, but it is not yet considered among the gold-standard tests (2).

The noncalorimetric tests provide *estimates* of energy expenditure through data that are closely correlated with energy expenditure values derived from indirect calorimetry methods. For example, HR is linearly related to $\dot{V}o_2$ through a wide range of aerobic exercise intensities. This relationship is discussed in a separate section below. For our purposes in this chapter and because the technique is common in research and clinical programs, only the respiratory method of indirect calorimetry will be presented in detail.

### DIRECT CALORIMETRY

As the name implies, direct calorimetry determines heat release by measuring a change in temperature. For example, heat is liberated when food particles are oxidized in a bomb calorimeter, a small device shaped like a chamber or box. The calorimeter is referred to as a bomb for a reason— food samples combust in 30 atmospheres of pure $O_2$ in a few seconds.

Pictured in *Figure 5.5A* is the Parr Oxygen Bomb Combustion Calorimeter, which is used to measure the

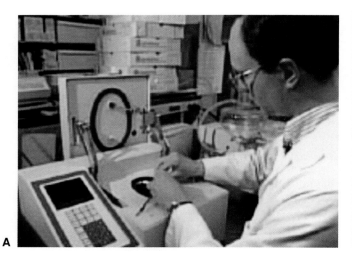

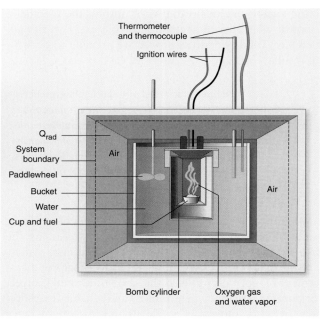

**FIGURE 5.5.** Calorimeter technician preparing a sample for combustion **(A)**. The internal mechanisms of the calorimeter **(B)**.

chemical potential energy in food by burning the food inside a strong, sealed container and measuring the temperature rise of the surrounding water in a carefully isolated thermal chamber. The sample of food (about 2 g) is placed inside the steel "bomb" container, which is then filled with pure $O_2$. This "bomb" is immersed in a water chamber surrounded by an insulated (nonconducting) shell (schematic shown in Fig. 5.5B). A sensitive electronic thermometer is used to measure the temperature of the water. Two wires pass through the shell to the inside of the "bomb." When an electric current heats the small igniter, the sample burns rapidly. The combustion process releases chemical potential energy of the food in the form of heat. Since the food is in a pure $O_2$ environment, it burns completely. The heat is transferred to the water bath, causing a rise in temperature that is measured by the thermometer. Because the water bath is well insulated, the energy cannot escape, and the rise in the water's temperature can be used to calculate the energy that was trapped in the food sample before it was burned. Each increase in water temperature of 1°C per kg of water equals an input of heat (energy) of 1 kcal. The kcal is the common laboratory unit of energy and is used for describing the energy content of food (e.g., a 300-kcal candy bar) and energy expenditure during exercise (e.g., a 300-kcal work bout). Since 1 kcal is equal to 1000 calories, the term *calorie* and *kilocalorie* are not equivalent. This difference is often overlooked when the terms are used interchangeably.

Since the change in temperature (heat content) is measured directly, the technique is referred to as *direct* calorimetry. These calorimeters are of several types, all related to the type of material to which the heat is conducted: airflow (temperature change in air), water flow (temperature change in water), and gradient layer (temperature change in a sheet of solid material). Several types of direct calorimeters have been utilized in studying human metabolism: room-sized chambers, booth or closet-sized chambers, and suit calorimeters. Room-sized direct calorimeters allow for the study of energy expenditure in "freely living" subjects. Pictured in *Figure 5.6* is the United States Department of Agriculture's direct calorimeter in Beltsville, Maryland, a device measuring $3.05 \times 2.74 \times 2.44$ m (representing a total physical volume of 20.39 m$^3$ or 20,390 L). This calorimeter uses combined direct and indirect techniques to measure 24-hour energy expenditure.

The practice of studying the metabolic rate of animals enclosed in a chamber is more than 100 years old. Current-day direct calorimetry methods (room, closet, or suit) are used to study thermal equilibrium and heat exposure, heat regulation during exercise and sleep, thermic effect of food, and oxidation rates of energy substrate (fat, protein, and carbohydrate). However, a complicating factor in research using direct calorimetry and freely living subjects is the need to control other sources of heat besides that which the subject produces. For example, if the subject is performing ergometric exercise inside a room-sized direct calorimeter, there is always some heat being generated from the ergometer (unless the ergometer has no moving parts, as in stepping). Although small, this heat produced from ergometers, largely as a result of friction, may need to be taken into account in determining the total heat production.

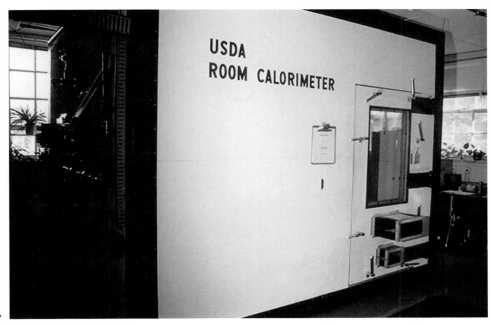

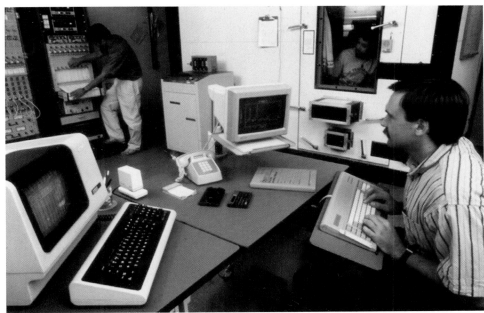

**FIGURE 5.6.** United States Department of Agriculture's direct (room) calorimeter **(A)** in Beltsville, Maryland is part of the Human Nutrition Research Center. **B.** Control room.

## INDIRECT CALORIMETRY

The heat liberated from the body is the result of the metabolic consumption of food substrate in mitochondrial respiration:

$$\text{Energy nutrients} + O_2 \rightarrow \text{Heat} + CO_2 + H_2O$$

Therefore, $\dot{V}O_2$ and energy (heat) expenditure are directly related, i.e., as energy expenditure increases, $\dot{V}O_2$ increases as well. It is not possible for most laboratories to directly measure energy expenditure (heat production) since the direct calorimetry method is not universally available and is very expensive. Therefore, a technique called indirect calorimetry is more commonly employed in exercise physiology laboratories and clinical programs to measure $O_2$ metabolism and estimate energy expenditure during resting and exercise conditions. This form of calorimetry directly measures the $O_2$ consumed in metabolism through the measurement of respiratory gases. The $\dot{V}O_2$ data are then converted to an equivalent energy cost in kcal. The indirect calorimetry technique, which provides energy expenditure data via the direct measurement of $O_2$

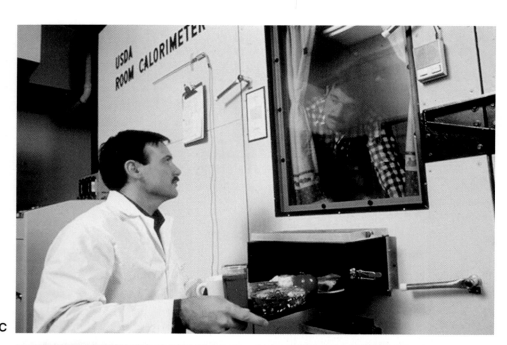

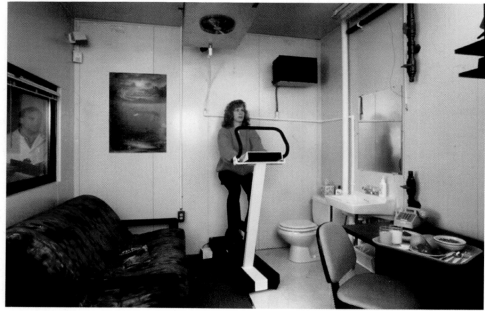

**FIGURE 5.6.** *(continued)* **C.** Providing subject meals, and **(D)** subject exercising. The calorimeter allows simultaneous measurement of heat production and metabolism. Oxygen consumption (respiratory calorimetry) equals heat production (direct calorimetry measurement) by the person living in the calorimeter.

metabolism, yields results comparable to direct methods. That is, when results from direct and indirect calorimetry are compared, there is no significant difference in the measured energy expenditure.

Heat production is derived indirectly in respiratory calorimetry by first measuring the metabolic consumption of $O_2$ and converting this value to energy expenditure. This is possible because the $O_2$ consumed can be converted to heat equivalents when the type of nutrients undergoing metabolism is known. As was shown in Chapter 4, the energy liberated when only fat is oxidized is 4.7 kcal·$L^{-1}$

$O_2$ consumed, and there is an energy release of 5.05 kcal·$L^{-1}$ $O_2$ consumed when only carbohydrate is oxidized (see Table 4.3). Since substrate utilization is rarely exclusively fat or carbohydrate during steady-state exercise, the caloric expenditure during exercise is usually estimated as 5 kcal·$L^{-1}$ $O_2$ consumed. For instance, when a person exercises at a steady-state $O_2$ cost of 1.0 L·$min^{-1}$, the approximate energy expenditure would equal 5 kcal·$min^{-1}$.

Respiratory calorimetry may be performed by either a **closed-circuit spirometry** or an **open-circuit spirometry** method. Closed-circuit systems have subjects breathing

100% $O_2$ from a prefilled spirometer connected to a recording apparatus to account for the $O_2$ removed from the spirometer and $CO_2$ produced and collected by an absorbing material. This technique is most commonly used to measure resting energy expenditure in clinical laboratories. Its usefulness during exercise conditions is limited because of the resistance to breathing offered by the closed circuit, making it uncomfortable to exercising subjects.

To accommodate exercising subjects, the open-circuit technique is most commonly used (*Fig. 5.7*). In respiratory calorimetry involving open-circuit apparatuses, subjects inspire directly from the atmospheric air and measurements of the fractional amounts of $O_2$ and $CO_2$, symbolized as $FEO_2$ and $FECO_2$, respectively, are made from the expired air. Breathing frequency and tidal volume are also measured directly by the open-circuit apparatus to acquire the expired minute ventilation ($\dot{V}E$, the product of breathing frequency and tidal volume). These variables constitute the "raw" data being measured in open-circuit spirometry, which is a relatively simple and easy way to assess energy expenditure. From these direct (raw) measures, $\dot{V}O_2$, $\dot{V}CO_2$, and the respiratory exchange ratio (RER) are calculated and provided in "real time" by interfacing electronic gas analyzers to a computer.

## MEASURING $\dot{V}O_2$ AND $\dot{V}CO_2$ BY OPEN-CIRCUIT SPIROMETRY

The open circuit spirometry technique makes it possible to measure $\dot{V}O_2$ and $\dot{V}CO_2$ by making use of the following relationships:

$\dot{V}O_2$ = Volume of $O_2$ inspired − Volume of $O_2$ expired

$\dot{V}CO_2$ = Volume of $CO_2$ expired
                    − Volume of $CO_2$ inspired

The fractional concentrations of $O_2$ ($FIO_2$) and $CO_2$ ($FICO_2$) in the inspired air are constant and are 0.2093 and 0.0003, respectively. Therefore, the term *volume of $O_2$ inspired* is equal to $FIO_2$ times the volume of inspired air

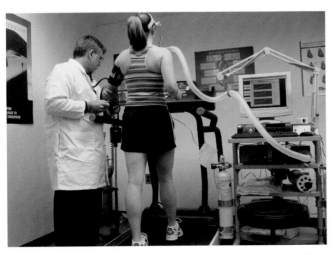

**FIGURE 5.7.** Open-circuit spirometry system with computer interface.

($\dot{V}I$), and the term *volume of $O_2$ expired* is equal to $FEO_2$ times the volume of expired air ($\dot{V}E$). When we exhale, the amount of $O_2$ in the exhaled air is smaller than that which was inhaled. The difference is the amount of $O_2$ consumed in metabolism. Likewise, when measuring $\dot{V}CO_2$, the term *volume of $CO_2$ expired* is equal to $FECO_2$ times $\dot{V}E$, and the term *volume of $CO_2$ inspired* is equal to $FICO_2$ times $\dot{V}I$. When we inhale, the amount of $CO_2$ in the inhaled air is smaller that that which is present in exhaled air. The difference is the amount of $CO_2$ produced in metabolism. We can now derive the following equations for $\dot{V}O_2$ and $\dot{V}CO_2$:

$$\dot{V}O_2 = (\dot{V}I \times FIO_2) - (\dot{V}E \times FEO_2)$$
$$\dot{V}CO_2 = (\dot{V}E \times FECO_2) - (\dot{V}I \times FICO_2)$$

Of the variables in the above equations, two are assumed to be constant values and are not measured ($FIO_2$ and $FICO_2$) and two are measured by the gas analyzers ($FEO_2$ and $FECO_2$). Depending on the design of the open-circuit spirometric device, either $\dot{V}E$ or $\dot{V}I$ is also measured. Most open-circuit spirometers are designed to measure only expired gas volumes ($\dot{V}E$), since it is not necessary to measure both $\dot{V}E$ and $\dot{V}I$. Rather than measuring both $\dot{V}E$ and $\dot{V}I$, these devices make use of a concept referred to as the **Haldane transformation** (John Haldane is highlighted in a biographic sketch at http://connection.lww.com/go/brownexphys and on the Student Resource CD-ROM for Chapter 6). In the following equation, $\dot{V}I$ can be calculated when $\dot{V}E$ is measured, and vice versa, because $N_2$ is neither used nor produced in metabolism. Therefore, the volume of $N_2$ we inhale must equal the volume we exhale. The Haldane transformation presents the relationship of gaseous nitrogen to inspired and expired pulmonary ventilation as follows:

$$\dot{V}I \times FIN_2 = \dot{V}E \times FEN_2$$

To solve for $\dot{V}I$ when $\dot{V}E$ is known, a simple algebraic rearrangement results in the following:

$$\dot{V}I = (\dot{V}E \times FEN_2) \div FIN_2$$

To use the Haldane transformation, the values for $FEN_2$ and $FIN_2$ must also be obtained. Fortunately, $FIN_2$, known to be 0.7904, is constant in the atmosphere. The value for $FEN_2$ is derived in the following manner from the measured values of $FEO_2$ and $FECO_2$:

$$FEN_2 = 1.0 - (FEO_2 + FECO_2)$$

$O_2$ and $CO_2$ fractions are subtracted from 1.0 because the sum of the fractions of these three gas species must add up to 1.0 since they represent 100% of the gases in the atmosphere. $\dot{V}CO_2$ is also calculated by applying the value already derived for $\dot{V}I$ to the proper equation.

## STANDARDIZING GAS VOLUMES

Because gas volumes such as $\dot{V}O_2$ and $\dot{V}E$ are influenced by temperature and pressure, these gas volumes must be standardized to reference conditions. Standardization means that the values are adjusted to standard temperature and pressure conditions that are different from the conditions under which the measurements were made. Standardization must also remove the effect on the gas of water vapor tension (humidity). Without standardization, measurements made in different laboratories in different parts of the country or world could not be compared directly, because differences would reflect environmental conditions (i.e., laboratory temperature, **barometric pressure**, and humidity).

Barometric pressure (PB) is the force per unit area exerted by the earth's atmosphere. This force equals 14.7 pounds per square inch, which is equal to 760 mm Hg (one atmosphere of pressure). In most instances laboratory temperature is not drastically different between facilities (most research laboratories are maintained at around 21°C). However, PB may be drastically different (e.g., sea-level regions compared with mountainous regions). Room humidity may also fluctuate. Standardization, therefore, allows the results of your research experimentation or clinical findings to be directly compared with those of others in locations remote from your own.

The effect of temperature on a gas volume is described by **Charles' Law**, which states that temperature and gas volume are directly proportional. As temperature increases, gas volume increases and as temperature decreases, gas volume decreases. Therefore, to make comparisons between gas volumes collected at different laboratories, temperature must be corrected so that differences are not merely that of temperature variations. The same thing is true of pressure variations between laboratories.

The second gas law, **Boyle's Law**, states that gas volumes vary inversely with pressure. As PB increases, gas volume decreases and as pressure decreases, volume increases. PB decreases as we ascend in altitude because the column of gas above us progressively shortens (*Fig. 5.8*). For instance, going from sea level to 15,000 feet decreases the PB to about 429 mm Hg. When comparing equal exercise responses (i.e., at the same ergometric workload) at these two extremes of altitude, a correction must be made for the effect on gas volume of the different barometric pressures from one altitude to the next. The effect on gas volume is drastic. There is an increase in volume at the higher altitude, which renders comparisons of volume measurements useless unless gas volumes collected under different temperature and pressure conditions are corrected to standard conditions. Therefore, procedures have been developed to adjust gas volume measures to standard conditions (Table 5.3).

Although corrections from ambient (ATPS) to standard (STPD) conditions are the most common, other conversions are also possible for a given situation, as Table 5.3 shows. By definition, a gas volume measured under ATPS conditions is subject to the ambient conditions of the laboratory, whereas the STPD condition refers to the reference condition of standard temperature (0°C) and pressure (760 mm Hg).

Table 5.3 shows correction factors under the "Multiply By" column. The gas volume to be corrected (i.e., from ATPS to STPD) is then multiplied by numerical values

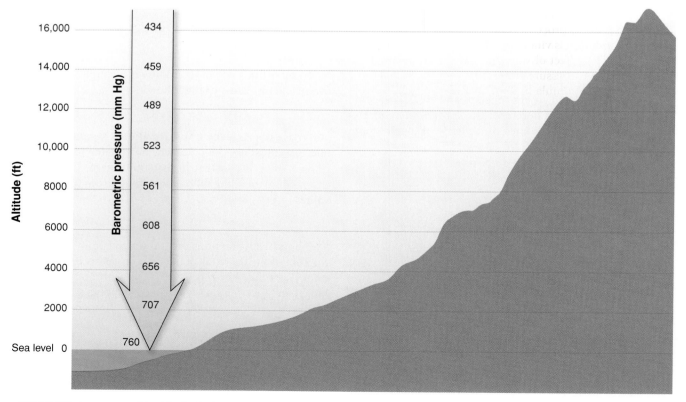

**FIGURE 5.8.** As you ascend in altitude, PB decreases, causing gas volumes to expand when they are measured at progressively higher altitudes.

| Table 5.3 | CONVERSION EQUATIONS FOR GAS VOLUMES | | |
|---|---|---|---|
| **To convert from** | **To** | **Multiply by** | |
| ATPS | STPD | $[(P_B - P_{H_2O}) \div 760] \times [273 \div (273 + T)]$ | |
| | BTPS | $[(P_B - P_{H_2O}) \div (P_B - 47)] \times [310 \div (273 + T)]$ | |
| | ATPD | $(P_B - P_{H_2O}) \div P_B$ | |
| ATPD | STPD | $(P_B \div 760) \times [273 \div (273 + T)]$ | |
| | BTPS | $[P_B \div (P_B - 47)] \times [310 \div (273 + T)]$ | |
| | ATPS | $P_B \div (P_B - P_{H_2O})$ | |
| BTPS | STPD | $[(P_B - 47) \div 760] \times (273 \div 310)$ | |
| | ATPS | $[(P_B - 47) \div (P_B - P_{H_2O})] \times [(273 + T) \div 310]$ | |
| | ATPD | $[(P_B - 47) \div P_B] \times [(273 + T) \div 310]$ | |
| STPD | BTPS | $[760 \div (P_B - 47)] \times (310 \div 273)$ | |
| | ATPS | $[760 \div (P_B - P_{H_2O})] \times [(273 + T) \div 273]$ | |
| | ATPD | $(760 \div P_B) \times [(273 + T) \div 273]$ | |

ATPS, ambient temperature and pressure, saturated with water vapor; ATPD, ambient temperature and pressure, dry; BTPS, body temperature and atmospheric pressure, completely saturated with water vapor at body temperature; STPD, standard temperature and pressure, dry; $P_B$, barometric pressure (mm Hg); T, ambient temperature (°C); $P_{H_2O}$, ambient vapor pressure of water (See Table 5.4). Conversions from BTPS assume a body temperature of 37°C and $P_{H_2O}$, 47 mm Hg.

produced by these formulas. For instance, to correct a $\dot{V}_E$ measure from the ATPS to STPD condition, the ATPS gas volume measured in the laboratory is multiplied by the appropriate correction factor. In all cases, when correcting from the ATPS to the STPD condition, the resultant gas volume corrected to STPD will be smaller. This is true because the calculated correction factor, in this instance, is a value less than 1.0. The following example illustrates this point, and also indicates why gas volumes become smaller when corrected from ATPS to the STPD condition.

However, before proceeding with the example, another piece of information is vital. The STPD reference condition also removes the effect of water vapor pressure ($P_{H_2O}$) by subtracting vapor pressure from the ambient or initial $P_B$ (refer to the first formula in Table 5.3). Vapor pressure is dependent only on temperature according to the following equation:

$$P_{H_2O} = 13.955 - 0.6584T + 0.0419T^2 \text{ (T is the ambient temperature)}$$

When the ambient temperature in our example below is applied to this equation, $P_{H_2O}$ is 18.61 mm Hg.

During open-circuit spirometry, the measured $\dot{V}_E$ (ATPS) is $110 \text{ L·min}^{-1}$ at an ambient $P_B$ of 758 mm Hg and temperature of 21°C. The ambient pressure and temperature are used to calculate a correction factor which is then used to adjust $110 \text{ L·min}^{-1}$ to a standardized value based on 0°C and 760 mm Hg (the STPD reference conditions). We are now ready to calculate the correction factor using the ATPS to STPD formula provided in Table 5.3, as follows:

$$\dot{V}_{E\ STPD} = 99.373 = 110 \times [(758 - 18.61) \div 760] \times [273 \div (273 + 21)]$$

In the calculation above, $110 \text{ L·min}^{-1}$ is the measured ATPS gas volume, $[(758 - 18.61) \div 760]$ is the standard

pressure correction, $[273 \div (273 + 21)]$ is the standard temperature correction, and $99.373 \text{ L·min}^{-1}$ is the measured gas volume corrected to the STPD condition when the correction factors are multiplied by 110. The combined correction factor is calculated to be 0.9034. Even though the volume of gas is smaller (compare $99.374 \text{ L·min}^{-1}$ with $110 \text{ L·min}^{-1}$), the same number of gas molecules is present, the difference being the effect of decreasing the temperature to 0°C (which constricts the volume) and increasing the $P_B$ (which also constricts the volume). For these reasons, converting from ATPS to STPD conditions always constricts the original gas volume. To convert the ATPS gas volume to other conditions besides the STPD condition, simply apply the appropriate formula to the ATPS volume. Once the measured $\dot{V}_E$ has been standardized to STPD conditions, $\dot{V}_E$ STPD is used in all other calculations, including $\dot{V}_I$, $\dot{V}_{O_2}$, and $\dot{V}_{CO_2}$. In this way, the other gas volumes (i.e., $\dot{V}_I$, $\dot{V}_{O_2}$, and $\dot{V}_{CO_2}$) are automatically calculated as STPD volumes. Using the following data and the $\dot{V}_E$ STPD example just provided ($99.373 \text{ L·min}^{-1}$), calculate $\dot{V}_{O_2}$, $\dot{V}_{CO_2}$ and RER (in your calculations use $F_{EO_2}=0.1762$ and $F_{ECO_2}=0.0311$).

▶ **INQUIRY SUMMARY.** Calorimetry is the process in which the heat produced (energy expended) in metabolism is measured. Energy expenditure can be measured by direct or indirect means, or both simultaneously. When indirect calorimetry is used, the most common method is respiratory calorimetry in which the fractional $O_2$ and $CO_2$ components of expired air are measured. Current-day spirometric techniques use sophisticated gas analyzers interfaced with computers which have the capability to provide $\dot{V}_{O_2}$ and $\dot{V}_{CO_2}$ data in real time as the subject is exercising. *Why is knowledge of calorimetry important for health personnel involved with exercise rehabilitation programs?*

## Energy Expenditure

Clinical practice in programs such as cardiopulmonary rehabilitation requires some competence in converting metabolic variables from one form to another. For example, these calculations greatly expedite formulation of an exercise prescription.

### EXPRESSING $\dot{V}O_2$

Knowledge of how to convert $\dot{V}O_2$ to heat equivalent units (J or kcal) is essential in exercise physiology. $\dot{V}O_2$ may be expressed in a variety of units. Options include $L \cdot min^{-1}$, $mL \cdot min^{-1}$, $mL \cdot kg^{-1} \cdot min^{-1}$, metabolic equivalents (METs), and $mL \cdot kgLBM^{-1} \cdot min^{-1}$ (LBM is the lean body mass of the individual). The first two units mentioned are "absolute" units since they are dependent on the subject's body mass. $\dot{V}O_{2max}$ expressed in absolute units is influenced by body size and cannot inform us about the relative fitness level of individuals since $\dot{V}O_{2max}$ may be large solely due to body mass and not because of fitness (*Fig. 5.9*). To get a much better indication of the fitness level of individuals, $\dot{V}O_{2max}$ should be expressed in $mL \cdot kg^{-1} \cdot min^{-1}$, METs, or $mL \cdot kgLBM^{-1} \cdot min^{-1}$. These units are relative to body mass, which neutralizes the effect of body mass so that a better understanding of the individual's cardiorespiratory fitness level is possible.

Becoming proficient in converting $\dot{V}O_2$ from absolute to relative units and vice versa helps in using regression equations that predict submaximal $\dot{V}O_2$.

The following is an example of how $\dot{V}O_2$ units may be manipulated. A 50-kg individual is exercising on a cycle ergometer at a $\dot{V}O_2$ of $1.839$ $L \cdot min^{-1}$. This absolute unit can be converted easily to $mL \cdot min^{-1}$ (the other absolute unit) by multiplying by 1000, resulting in a value of $1,839$ $mL \cdot min^{-1}$. To convert this absolute unit to $mL \cdot kg^{-1} \cdot min^{-1}$ (a relative unit), simply divide 1839 by body mass (50 kg) and find that the individual is exercising at a $\dot{V}O_2$ of $36.8$ $mL \cdot kg^{-1} \cdot min^{-1}$. Also, if the individual has 18% body fat, the 41 kg of lean body mass would give a $\dot{V}O_2$ of $44.9$ $mL \cdot kgLBM^{-1} \cdot min^{-1}$.

We also know something about the individual's resting $\dot{V}O_2$ prior to this workout. Resting $\dot{V}O_2$ (or resting metabolic rate [RMR]) is equivalent to the basal metabolic rate (BMR) plus the metabolic cost of arousal. RMR is the metabolic rate approximately 3 to 4 hours after a light meal but with no prior physical activity. Resting $\dot{V}O_2$ can be estimated for any healthy subject as $3.5$ $mL \cdot kg^{-1} \cdot min^{-1}$. *What is the RMR in absolute units ($mL \cdot min^{-1}$)?* To answer this question, multiply $3.5$ $mL \cdot kg^{-1} \cdot min^{-1}$ by body mass (50 kg). This negates the kg expression in the relative term and leaves $175$ $mL \cdot min^{-1}$, the expression of resting $\dot{V}O_2$ in absolute units for a 50-kg individual. *Why is it necessary to know resting $\dot{V}O_2$?* The reason is that $\dot{V}O_2$ is measured as

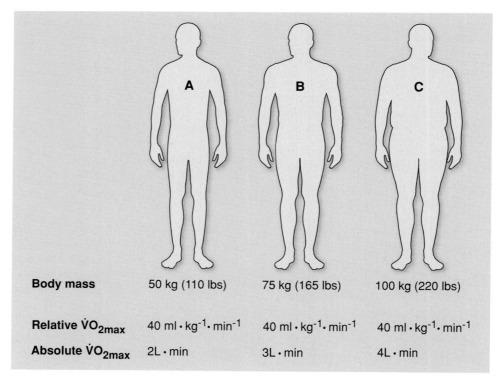

| | A | B | C |
|---|---|---|---|
| **Body mass** | 50 kg (110 lbs) | 75 kg (165 lbs) | 100 kg (220 lbs) |
| **Relative $\dot{V}O_{2max}$** | 40 ml · kg⁻¹· min⁻¹ | 40 ml · kg⁻¹· min⁻¹ | 40 ml · kg⁻¹· min⁻¹ |
| **Absolute $\dot{V}O_{2max}$** | 2L · min | 3L · min | 4L · min |

**FIGURE 5.9.** Comparison of $\dot{V}O_{2max}$ measured in $L \cdot min^{-1}$ in individuals of progressively larger body mass: A. 50 kg. B. 75 kg. C. 100 kg. Each individual has a relative $\dot{V}O_{2max}$ of 40 $mL \cdot kg^{-1} min^{-1}$, which indicates a similar cardiovascular fitness level for each individual. As you see, if their degree of cardiovascular fitness was judged by absolute $\dot{V}O_{2max}$, we would falsely assume that person (C) was the most fit, but such is not the case.

gross $\dot{V}O_2$ when it is measured in the laboratory. Gross $\dot{V}O_2$ can be expressed as follows:

$$\text{Gross } \dot{V}O_2 = \text{Resting } \dot{V}O_2 + \text{Exercise (or net) } \dot{V}O_2$$

When $\dot{V}O_2$ is displayed by an open-circuit spirometric measurement device, it is always expressed as gross $\dot{V}O_2$ (the addition of the resting value plus the effect of exercise). Later we will calculate variables in which an understanding of the exercise $\dot{V}O_2$ (or net = gross $\dot{V}O_2$ − resting $\dot{V}O_2$) is important. When we subtract resting $\dot{V}O_2$ from gross $\dot{V}O_2$, the $O_2$ cost of the exercise itself is left. In the example this is calculated to be 1664 mL·min$^{-1}$ or 1.664 L·min$^{-1}$. As you do these calculations, you should always take the $\dot{V}O_2$ value in L·min$^{-1}$ out to three significant decimal places. *Why do you think this is important?*

The individual's exercise level, expressed as METs, is the next unit commonly used to report $\dot{V}O_2$. METs relate to multiples of resting $\dot{V}O_2$, one MET being equivalent to 3.5 mL·kg$^{-1}$·min$^{-1}$. Therefore, to convert $\dot{V}O_2$ values to METs, the original unit of measurement must be in mL·kg$^{-1}$·min$^{-1}$. In this example the individual is working at an $O_2$ cost of 36.6 mL·kg$^{-1}$·min$^{-1}$, which is then divided by 3.5 to convert it to 10.5 METs. We have now expressed our subject's exercise level using five common units of measurement for $\dot{V}O_2$. Once $\dot{V}O_{2max}$ is known, we can also express the exercise intensity as a percentage of $\dot{V}O_{2max}$. If the $\dot{V}O_{2max}$ is 50 mL·kg$^{-1}$·min$^{-1}$, the current exercise intensity would be 73% of $\dot{V}O_{2max}$ (36.6 ÷ 50), a moderate exercise intensity.

## RESPIRATORY EXCHANGE RATIO

*How much energy is being expended at 10.5 METs?* Converting from $\dot{V}O_2$ to kcal depends on the relative contribution of fat versus carbohydrate metabolism in supplying ATP to the working muscle during steady-state (submaximal) exercise. That is, the relative contribution of energy substrate utilized depends on the RER. Knowledge of the steady-state RER gives the caloric value per L of $O_2$ consumed when carbohydrate and fat are being oxidized during steady-state exercise. These values are listed in Table 4.3. In the example above, the individual exercising at 1.839 L·min$^{-1}$ is also producing an RER of 0.85. As Table 4.3 also shows, equal amounts of fats and carbohydrates are being oxidized on the basis of 4.862 kcal liberated for each liter of $O_2$ consumed. This means that at 1.839 L·min$^{-1}$, the individual is expending 8.94 kcal per minute (1.839 × 4.862) during steady-state exercise.

The RER is an important metabolic variable because it provides knowledge of the relative contribution that fats and carbohydrates make to energy expenditure during exercise (protein oxidation during exercise is ignored because of its minor role). Fats and carbohydrates differ in the amount of $O_2$ used and $CO_2$ produced during oxidation. As a variable of external respiration, the nonprotein

RER is easily measured at the mouth by open-circuit spirometry, as we saw in the last section. The RER is also roughly equivalent to the term respiratory quotient (RQ), which refers to internal (cellular) respiration. The two terms, although used synonymously, are not exactly the same. At the cellular level when $O_2$ consumption is maximal, $CO_2$ production matches the rate of $O_2$ consumption, resulting in a one-to-one exchange of $O_2$ and $CO_2$. This produces a RQ of 1.0 (the numerator and denominator in the $\dot{V}CO_2 / \dot{V}O_2$ ratio are identical).

Since the cell does not have the ability to produce $CO_2$ at a greater rate than its maximal $\dot{V}O_2$ (there is one $CO_2$ produced for each $O_2$ consumed), the upper limit of RQ remains at 1.0. This corresponds to the following chemical equation:

$$1 \text{ mol } C_6H_{12}O_6 + 6 \text{ mol } O_2 \rightarrow 6 \text{ mol } CO_2 + 6 \text{ mol } H_2O$$

In the equation, six mol of $O_2$ are consumed and six mol of $CO_2$ are produced, a ratio of 6/6 or an RER of 1.0. The same relationship would hold at rest if an individual consumed only carbohydrates in the diet. However, if only fats are consumed in the diet, more $O_2$ is needed as $O_2$ combines with carbon to form $CO_2$ and with $H_2$ to form water. Therefore, fat oxidation requires more $O_2$ than carbohydrate oxidation. This necessitates a larger $\dot{V}O_2$ (the denominator), which reduces the ratio below 1.0. This corresponds to the following equation:

$$1 \text{ mol } C_{16}H_{32}O_2 + 23 \text{ mol } O_2 \rightarrow$$
$$16 \text{ mol } CO_2 + 16 \text{ mol } H_2O$$

Twenty-three mol of $O_2$ are consumed and 16 mol of $CO_2$ are produced, a ratio of 16/23 or 0.70. At this RER, 4.686 kcal is liberated for every L of $O_2$ consumed (see Table 4.3). Since we never consume only one type of fuel in the diet, the ratio falls between 0.7 and 1.0 at rest and during steady-state exercise. However, in periods of transition when we go from the rest to exercise state, too much $CO_2$ is blown off (hyperventilation), falsely elevating RER above the RQ. Hyperventilation also occurs in heavy to maximal exercise, when $\dot{V}CO_2$ is greater than $\dot{V}O_2$ and RER exceeds 1.0.

It is important to note that for RER to be used as an estimate of substrate utilization during exercise, a steady-state condition must be present. Steady state is present after a period of adjustment during exercise when the energy demand of the exercising musculature is met fully by $O_2$ metabolism. However, this is not the case when transitioning from rest to steady-state exercise. As was discussed in Chapter 4, this transition period is referred to as a nonsteady-state condition because there is an imbalance between the supply of $O_2$ to the working muscles and the demand of these muscles for $O_2$. Therefore, the muscle must receive its energy supply from anaerobic sources. The difference between the $O_2$ required during exercise and the $O_2$ supplied and utilized is called the $O_2$ deficit. The amount of metabolic energy being met by anaerobic sources during this rest to exercise transition depends on exercise intensity at the start of exercise, fitness level, age, and health status of the individual.

The time period during which there is a transition from exercise to rest, $\dot{V}O_2$ remains elevated while $\dot{V}CO_2$ quickly declines, causing RER to drop below 0.70. As in the previously discussed transition period, this situation is not reflective of the actual metabolic state (RQ). Therefore, RQ and RER are not well correlated under either transition period conditions. The exercise to rest transition is called $O_2$ recovery or excess post-exercise $O_2$ consumption (see Chapter 4). This represents a period of elevated metabolism during which several physiologic and metabolic perturbations caused by acute exercise are adjusted back to their original resting levels. As discussed in Chapter 4, the elevated $\dot{V}O_2$ is due to a number of factors:

- Restoration of ATP-PC stores
- Restoration of $O_2$ stores
- Elevated cardiorespiratory function
- Elevated catecholamines
- Elevated body temperature
- Lactate removal

## BASAL AND RESTING METABOLIC RATES

The amount of energy the body uses each day (total daily energy expenditure) is dependent on three factors: the BMR; the *thermic effect of feeding* (food and drug intake); and the *thermic effect of physical activity* (increase in metabolism due to physical activity, as directly dictated by the duration and intensity of the activity) (*Fig. 5.10*). BMR is different from RMR in that it is the minimum energy requirement needed to sustain life processes (i.e., respiration, circulation, and other vital cellular functions). BMR can only be measured under certain strict conditions:

- Morning after a restful night of sleep
- 12 to 18 hours after a meal to avoid thermogenesis due to digestion of food

- Supine position
- State of wakefulness
- Thermoneutral environment (20°C to 23°C)
- No strenuous exercise 24 hours before testing
- Free of all psychic and physical disturbances (i.e., medications, drugs, depression, excessive stress)

Unless the measurement of BMR is required for research or clinical purposes, RMR is usually measured in exercise physiology laboratories as an alternative since the measurement of RMR is not as stringent. For RMR measurements, the individual reports to the laboratory or clinic about 4 hours after eating a light meal and rests for up to 1 hour prior to the measurement of RMR, usually by open-circuit spirometry.

BMR accounts for about 60% to 75% of the total energy expenditure for an average sedentary individual. As the major component of RMR, BMR is dependent on factors such as body size and composition, gender, health status, and age. For example, individuals with chronic obstructive pulmonary disease (COPD) may have a BMR that is 40% to 50% greater than normal, owing to the increase energy cost (work) of breathing. Because of this, the prediction of BMR makes use of **regression equations** that are gender and age specific. However, these equations may be invalid in certain disease populations and with the use of certain medications.

$$\text{Females: BMR (kcal·day}^{-1}) = 665 \\ + (9.6 \times \text{kg [body mass]}) + (1.7 \times \text{cm [height]}) \\ - (4.7 \times \text{age [years]})$$

$$\text{Males: BMR (kcal·day}^{-1}) = 66 + (13.7 \times \text{kg}) \\ + (5.0 \times \text{cm}) - (6.9 \times \text{age})$$

▶ *INQUIRY SUMMARY.* Energy expenditure calculations involve converting $\dot{V}O_2$ into various units of measurement. Gross $\dot{V}O_2$ represents the addition of resting and exercise $\dot{V}O_2$. The $O_2$ cost of submaximal exercise can be converted to caloric cost when the RER is known. The RER also provides knowledge of the fuel substrate used during exercise. Basal and resting metabolism are important components of the total daily energy requirement. *Why does a decrease in basal metabolism usually signal impending weight increase?*

## *Efficiency and Economy*

**Efficiency** and **economy** are important concepts to consider in fields as disparate as coaching and therapeutic rehabilitation. To become more economic or efficient, individuals must be able to sustain a given mechanical work rate at a lower percentage of $\dot{V}O_{2max}$. This has been shown to be advantageous for performing prolonged physical activity, whether the activity is an international cycling competition or yard work. Economy and efficiency are especially important for the elite athlete with a comparatively modest $\dot{V}O_{2max}$ compared to their peers. For these

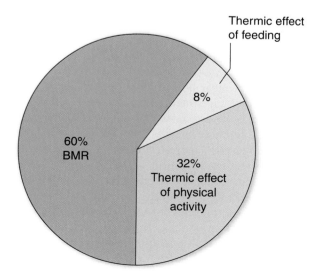

Thermic effect
of feeding

8%

60%
BMR

32%
Thermic effect
of physical
activity

FIGURE 5.10. Components of the total energy expenditure.

individuals to compete successfully in high-level competition despite a $\dot{V}O_{2max}$ significantly lower than the competition, a superior running economy or cycling efficiency is essential. An inverse relationship between $\dot{V}O_{2max}$ and running or cycling economy or efficiency has been demonstrated in highly trained runners and cyclists. This demonstrates that a high $\dot{V}O_{2max}$ is not the main determinant of endurance performance success. Although a sufficiently high $\dot{V}O_{2max}$ is still needed for such competition, a high efficiency/economy for these individuals allows them to sustain a lower $\dot{V}O_2$ at a given race pace, thus allowing them to competitively match the pace of individuals with higher $\dot{V}O_{2max}$ values. The concept of economy and efficiency is also important for people performing everyday physical tasks and for individuals with chronic disabilities. The goal of training, whether for athletic competition or physical rehabilitation, is often to increase economy or efficiency of effort. This allows the athlete or patient to perform a given task at the lowest possible energy expenditure, which also means that **energy reserve** is maximized for any given task.

## EFFICIENCY

Efficiency is the ratio between useful work produced and the energy expended during the work. Efficiency is expressed as a percentage; therefore, the units for work and energy expended must be identical in the numerator and denominator in the following equation:

$$E\ (\%) = (\text{Work output} \div \text{Energy expended}) \times 100$$

Since the measurement units for work and energy are interconvertible, at least one conversion (either in the numerator or denominator) must be made when using this equation. For example, if the work output is 300 kg·m·min$^{-1}$ and the energy expended is 1.0 L·min$^{-1}$, the terms have to be equated. One method is to convert both terms to kcal (300 ÷ 427 = 0.703 kcal; 1.0 × 5 = 5.0 kcal). In this example efficiency is 14% ([0.703 ÷ 5] × 100). After you derive answers for problem 2, plot two graphs (between workload [X-axis] and efficiency [Y-axis]; and between workload [X-axis] and energy expenditure [Y-axis]) and answer the following questions. *Is efficiency constant with changing workloads?* Before reading on, can you suggest a reason for your answer. *What is the relationship between work rate and energy expenditure?*

In a completely efficient process, all the energy utilized is converted to useful work and the numerator and denominator are equal. However, no machine is completely efficient since some energy is lost because of friction. The efficiency of human work varies tremendously with the task, probably never being higher than about 40%. Swimming, a notoriously inefficient process, converts less than 10% of the energy expended into forward motion in the water. The portion of the energy expenditure not being used to produce the work output is released as heat. The

following are some important factors governing muscle efficiency or economy:

- Anthropometric factors (e.g., body mass and body mass distribution, body structure, gender)
- Mechanical factors (e.g., performance skill, flexibility, stride length)
- Ergometric factors (e.g., work rate, speed of movement, resistance or drag applied to the movement, cycle seat height)
- Physiologic factors (e.g., muscle fiber type, fitness level)
- Calculation methods (the type of efficiency being calculated)
- Disease state (patients with disease-related alterations in movement patterns have an increased energy expenditure of movement, e.g., anterior cruciate ligament deficiency, cerebral palsy)

One of the most important considerations in understanding efficiency is the relationship between energy expenditure and work rate. *Figure 5.11* shows that as work rate increases, energy expenditure also increases but at a greater incremental rate beyond the moderate exercise intensity. This means that the relationship between work rate and energy expenditure is not linear, but curvilinear. The curvilinear nature of the relationship between work rate and energy expenditure results in efficiency ratios that are lower at higher workloads than they were at lower workloads. This effect is caused as energy expenditure at higher workloads rises out of proportion to the incremental increase in work rate at these workloads. This means that there is a greater energy cost of exercise at higher workloads than is reflective merely of the increased workload. Therefore, efficiency is lowered at these greater workloads.

### Calculating Efficiency

The way in which efficiency is calculated produces variations in the efficiency ratio. There are two classic methods used to calculate efficiency. The first is termed *gross* efficiency because it incorporates gross $\dot{V}O_2$ in the denominator of the equation. However, we know that resting $\dot{V}O_2$ is intrinsic to gross $\dot{V}O_2$, which increases the size of the denominator of the gross efficiency ratio, driving efficiency down. This is problematic because resting energy expenditure does not contribute to exercise performance. Efficiency ratios thus produced are artificially lower than normal.

The second classic method used to calculate efficiency is termed *net* efficiency because resting $\dot{V}O_2$ is subtracted out of the denominator, resulting in net $\dot{V}O_2$ being used to calculate efficiency.

$$E\ (\%) = \text{Work output} \div (\text{Gross energy expended} - \text{Resting } \dot{V}O_2) \times 100$$

However, net efficiency is difficult to ascertain due to problems in precisely measuring the appropriate resting energy expenditure. Gross and net efficiency calculations

**Box 5.2**

*R E S E A R C H    H I G H L I G H T*

**Jacobs PL, Mahoney ET. Peak exercise capacity of electrically induced ambulation in persons with paraplegia. *Med Sci Sports Exerc* 2002;34:1551–1556.**

### RESEARCH SUMMARY

Individuals with spinal cord injuries are limited to performing daily tasks and beneficial exercise using those motor units that remain intact following injury. Because these tasks may be severely limited, depending on the location of the injury, these individuals' activity levels are lower, which leads to deconditioning and increases in the risk of secondary disabilities and medical complications such as heart disease or other maladies. One goal of therapy is to increase the activity level of these individuals enough to reduce the risk of chronic illness. While the use of arm ergometry is prevalent in this population, the energy expenditure of arm exercise is low compared to leg exercise, and arm cranking in this population has been associated with increased incidences of musculoskeletal pain in the shoulders, elbows, and wrists that further limits daily activity. A recently developed therapeutic intervention for individuals with paraplegia is to produce patterns of functional movement in the paralyzed limbs in the form of recumbent bicycling or ambulation via functional electrical stimulation (FES). Recumbent bicycling using FES has been shown to not engage the cardiovascular system with enough intensity to allow beneficial physiologic adaptations. More recently FES technology has allowed some individuals with paraplegia to attain upright stance and control independent stepping actions, thereby allowing functional locomotion. The use of ambulatory gait training may involve high enough energy expenditure to produce cardiovascular adaptations. The purpose of this study was to test whether electrically stimulated walking produces greater work levels or greater endurance capabilities than voluntary arm exercise. In this investigation peak physiologic responses of persons with spinal cord injury were measured during arm ergometry and FES ambulation.

Fifteen subjects with complete spinal cord injury at the level of T4–T11 participated by completing two peak exercise tests performed in random order and separated by 48 to 96 hours. In one test, subjects utilized arm cranking using a Monark arm ergometer (881) while seated in their own wheelchairs. The test was performed to volitional fatigue. Peak heart rate response and peak metabolic variables, such as $\dot{V}O_2$, $\dot{V}CO_2$, RER, and $\dot{V}E$, were measured. The second test was an incremental peak ambulation test performed using a commercial FES system (Parastep-1). This device applies six channels of transcutaneous electrical stimulation at a frequency of 24 Hz to the quadriceps and gluteal/spinal erector muscles (bilaterally). This stimulation produces an upright standing position. To produce stepping movements, the area near the common

peroneal nerve is stimulated. Subjects controlled the Parastep-1 system manually during ambulation. Ambulation testing began with subjects seated before a 10-m runway and resting for 20 minutes. Respiratory gases and heart rate data were collected. After the resting period was over, subjects activated the Parastep-1 system to attain the upright position. After remaining stationary for 1 minute, subjects were told to use the FES system and begin stepping along the 10-m path at a very slow and controlled pace. The metabolic measurement cart was pushed alongside the subjects as they ambulated. At the end of the runway, subjects paused so that their heart rates could be taken manually; subjects also recorded their perceived exertion level. Subjects continued to make passes down the runway at a gradually faster pace each time to produce a graded effect in metabolic, heart rate, and perceived exertion responses. This process continued to the point of volitional exhaustion or until the subject could no longer increase the pace of controlled FES ambulation. Five to eight walking bouts were performed. The same metabolic data as collected during arm ergometry were measured during ambulation testing.

Test durations of FES and arm ergometry were 12.5±4.0 and 17.8±5.2 minutes, respectively. Peak heart rate response was significantly higher during FES ambulation (191 beats·min⁻¹) than during arm ergometry (179 beats·min⁻¹). However, none of the metabolic variables tested were significantly different between tests. In particular, peak $\dot{V}O_2$ was very similar between trials (arm: 22.9 mL·kg⁻¹·min⁻¹ and FES: 22.7 mL·kg⁻¹·min⁻¹). These exercise modes, therefore, allow similar peak aerobic capacity. This investigation was the first to show that FES ambulation allows comparable cardiorespiratory demands as those elicited by volitional arm ergometry. Because of these high metabolic and cardiac responses, FES ambulation has been shown elsewhere to increase cardiorespiratory capacity and produce positive peripheral adaptations within the paralyzed limbs. Therefore, FES ambulation seems to be an alternative for endurance conditioning of individuals with paraplegia, especially since this exercise spares musculoskeletal complications of the shoulder joint.

### IMPLICATIONS FOR FURTHER RESEARCH

FES ambulation appears promising as a therapeutic exercise mode for individuals with incomplete or complete spinal cord injury. Future studies should investigate the use of treadmill FES ambulation as compared to traditional overground FES walking. In addition, a more complete investigation of the central cardiac responses to FES ambulation is warranted. *For example, are the stroke volume and cardiac output responses to FES ambulation similar to those of healthy individuals doing similar motor activity?* This and other related questions are important to investigate.

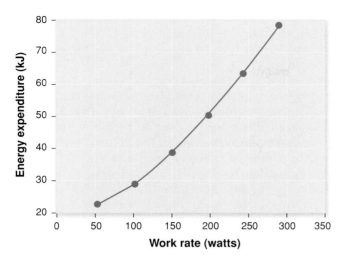

**FIGURE 5.11.** As the work rate increases, energy expenditure increases in a curvilinear fashion.

produce efficiency ratios that are lower than usual and that increase with increasing workloads. The fact that gross and net efficiency increase as workload increases is clearly indicative of an artifactual error in calculating these efficiency ratios. We know this is true because efficiency must remain constant or decline with increasing work rates since energy expenditure and workload have a curvilinear relationship.

Two alternative equations (methods) have been proposed to overcome this problem, and they have both been studied extensively. The first is termed *work* efficiency because it subtracts the energy cost of unloaded pedaling out of the denominator.

$$E\ (\%) = \text{Work output} \div (\text{Gross energy expended} - \text{Unloaded pedaling } \dot{V}_{O_2}) \times 100$$

The second is called *delta* (change in) efficiency, which makes two subtractions: one in the numerator and one in the denominator. For the numerator, the previous work output (i.e., in the prior stage of a multi-stage test) is subtracted from the current work output; for the denominator, the previous energy expenditure is subtracted from the current energy expenditure:

$$E\ (\%) = \Delta \text{ Work output} \div (\Delta \text{ Energy expended}) \times 100$$

Work and delta efficiency produce higher initial (and all subsequent) efficiency ratios than those of gross and net efficiency, and, more importantly, as work rate increases, work and delta efficiency decrease. This is the desired result because it is congruent with the known curvilinear relationship between work rate and energy expenditure.

*Experiences in Work Physiology Lab Exercise 5: Measuring Cycling Efficiency provides a laboratory exercise in determining exercise efficiency.*

## ECONOMY

To determine muscle efficiency during exercise, power output must be calculated. However, this is not always possible. For instance, no work is performed during horizontal running; therefore, other terminology has been adopted to describe movement efficiency in these circumstances. In situations when work is not quantifiable, the term *economy* is used. Economy is defined as the steady-state $\dot{V}_{O_2}$ needed to maintain a given velocity of movement or a given activity. For example, a runner with a lower $\dot{V}_{O_2}$ response at a given velocity is more economic.

This was shown in a classic study of trained and untrained men and women, which demonstrated that there is a gender and training effect on running economy (*Fig. 5.12*) (3). In this study trained men and women ran with a lower $\dot{V}_{O_2}$ response at a given running velocity than untrained men and women, respectively. Moreover, the untrained men had a lower $\dot{V}_{O_2}$ response than the untrained women. For example, Figure 5.12 shows that at 200 m·min$^{-1}$, the $\dot{V}_{O_2}$ response of trained men was about 37 mL·kg$^{-1}$·min$^{-1}$, while the untrained men and trained women were about equal ($\sim$ 40 mL·kg$^{-1}$·min$^{-1}$), and the untrained women about 41.5 ml·kg$^{-1}$·min$^{-1}$. A lower $\dot{V}_{O_2}$ at a given speed indicates a more economic runner.

Factors that appear to be involved in the variability in running economy with respect to gender include anthropometric/structural differences between the sexes (e.g., body mass and its distribution, femur angle) and/or mechanical differences in **gait** related to running experience (e.g., too much vertical displacement during running

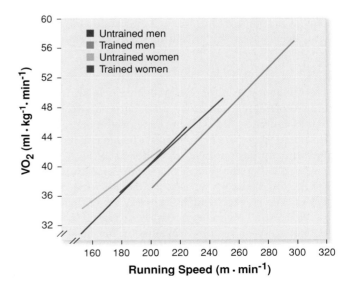

**FIGURE 5.12.** The relationship between $O_2$ consumption and running speed in trained and untrained men and women. Notice that in this study the trained women and untrained men had similar slopes for their respective lines indicating that running economy is comparable. Data from Bransford DR, Howley ET. Oxygen cost of running in trained and untrained men and women. *Med Sci Sports* 1977;9:41–44.

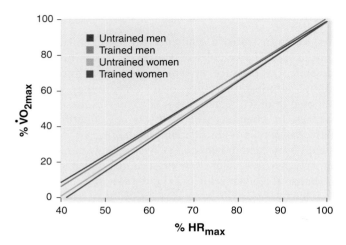

**FIGURE 5.13.** The relationship between $\%\dot{V}O_{2max}$ and $\%HR_{max}$ during deep-water running in trained and untrained men and women. The relationship was not affected by age, but both female groups exercised at a lower $\%\dot{V}O_{2max}$ for a given $\%HR_{max}$ compared with the male groups. Data from Brown SP, Jordan JC, Chitwood LF, et al. Relationship of heart rate and oxygen uptake kinetics during deep water running in the adult population—ages 50 to 70 years. *J Aging Phys Act* 1998;6:248–255.

in novice versus subelite or elite athletes). Recent work has confirmed the effect of gender on running economy (4).

By comparing $\dot{V}O_2$ responses, economy can also be ascertained for any form of exercise or physical activity in which work is not quantifiable. Water exercise is another example. At any intensity level, pictured in *Figure 5.13* as $\%HR_{max}$, $\%\dot{V}O_{2max}$ is lower in the female groups during deep-water running, making these individuals more economic in the water. The reason for this is probably related to the increased buoyancy afforded women by their increased body fat percentage (5,6). Also, it appears that age is not a factor in exercise economy during deep-water running.

## CLINICAL APPLICATIONS

Like efficiency, economy of movement is an important clinical concept. For instance, ambulation-assistive devices such as crutches and walkers increase the energy cost of movement (*Fig. 5.14*). Patients with movement dysfunctions already have a lower than normal $\dot{V}O_{2max}$, and any increase in the energy cost of movement because of gait dysfunction or the use of assistive devices further reduces their **energy reserve**, which is already lower than normal. The degree to which energy cost is increased in these patients depends on the physical ailment. For instance, paraplegia necessitates a higher energy cost than do lower extremity fractures while ambulating. Spasticity, for example, doubles the energy cost of simple physical activities. Ambulation energy cost also increases in sedentary aging due to the following changes in gait:

- Mild rigidity leading to less body motion
- Decrease in amplitude and speed of arm swing
- Less ability to use gravity (increases muscle work)
- Less accuracy and speed in use of hip muscles
- Shorter steps to ensure safety
- Stride width broader to ensure more stable base to ensure safety
- Decrease in swing-to-stance ratio (improves safety by allowing more time in the phase of double support)
- Decrease in vertical displacement secondary to stiffness
- Decrease in excursion of leg during swing phase (free leg extends to a lesser degree)
- Decrease in heel-to-floor angle
- Slower gait to ensure safety
- Decrease in rotation of the hip and shoulder
- Decrease in the velocity of limb motion

These changes as a result of sedentary aging reduce movement economy during gait secondary to a loss of the base of support as a result of poor posture and reduced balance, flexibility, and strength. In addition, energy expenditure has been shown to be 55% greater in elderly patients with above-knee prostheses compared to normal elderly individuals (7). See Case Study 5.1 for an example.

Individuals with conditions that result in an altered gait, such as cerebral palsy, arthritis, or stroke, typically chose an ambulation speed at a velocity that produces the lowest $\dot{V}O_2$ response (i.e., they move at a pace that produces the best economy for them). Because abnormal gait causes an increased energy cost of movement, physical therapists often work to retrain patients' gait patterns in an attempt to increase their economy of effort. However, because patients have already self-selected a gait pattern that produces the best economy of effort for them, altering this pattern by retraining the gait will further increase energy expenditure and may result in an increased incidence of

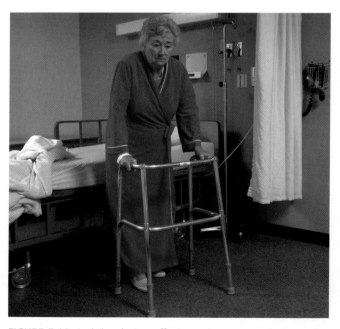

**FIGURE 5.14.** Assistive devices affect exercise economy by increasing the $O_2$ cost of ambulation.

## CASE STUDY 5.1: *GERIATRIC AMPUTEE*

### CASE

Byron is a 75-year-old individual with a recent lower extremity amputation. To assess his aerobic endurance, he performed a 500-foot ambulation test with his prosthesis on. At the conclusion of the test, he had elevated heart rate (120 beats·min$^{-1}$) and blood pressure (170/105 mm Hg) responses. To confirm these adverse physiologic responses, a second ambulation test was given for the purpose of measuring ambulatory $\dot{V}O_2$. This test produced similar cardiovascular responses and a $\dot{V}O_2$ of 16.3 mL·kg$^{-1}$·min$^{-1}$.

### DESCRIPTION

The geriatric amputee patient presents with problems in addition to an altered gait resulting in poor movement economy. Ninety percent of amputees over the age of 55 undergo lower extremity amputation as a result of a disease process. Seventy percent of these patients received their amputations because of peripheral arterial disease. Therefore, it is important for physical therapists to consider concurrent diagnoses when evaluating and implementing rehabilitation programs. The most critical phase in the gait cycle of the geriatric amputee is the point of heel contact and the period immediately following heel contact. This phase of gait relates to the stability of the knee in the prosthesis. Accordingly, there are two factors that should be addressed by the therapist: the loss of hip and/or knee extensor power and too much ankle plantar flexion.

### EVALUATION/INTERVENTION

The $\dot{V}O_2$ response recorded with the second ambulation test is higher than that which a healthy individual with a normal gait would produce when ambulating at the speed Byron achieved on the test. Byron has a reduced movement economy (higher $\dot{V}O_2$ response at a given ambulation speed). Therefore, one goal of therapy is to reduce the $O_2$ cost of ambulation. Therapists may assist older individuals to

improve their exercise economies in the following manner:
- Recommend proper fitting shoes and orthotics to maximize foot stability
- Address muscle imbalance and loss of flexibility, especially the tight and weak hip flexor muscles
- Advise a daily routine of exaggerated hip extension, hip rotation, and arm movements

An example of an activity that addresses shortened hip flexors is to stand in a position of exaggerated hip extension. This helps increase the range of hip extension in the push-off phase of the gait cycle. To compensate for the loss of extensor power, the following should be considered by the therapist:
- Prescribe exercises to increase quadriceps strength
- Work with a prosthetist to adjust the prosthesis
- Change the body alignment
- Attach elastic to the prosthesis to help pull the knee into extension
- Use a knee lock to lock the prosthetic knee in extension
- Use a soft-sach heel or a single-axis heel to compensate for too much plantar flexion

The increased energy expenditure during gait is an important therapeutic consideration. Therapeutic intervention should stress attaining a more normal gait to avoid the use of assistive devices as much as possible. Assistive devices increase the energy cost of ambulation (i.e., decreased movement economy). Lastly, cardiovascular exercise training helps to reduce heart disease risk factors, a particular problem in amputees, and increase Byron's energy reserve by increasing $\dot{V}O_{2max}$. Training also promotes an increase in movement economy by reducing the $O_2$ cost of ambulation at a given speed, regardless of whether a person is ambulating with only a prosthesis or with an assistive device in conjunction with a prosthesis. This will also widen the patient's energy reserve during activity. In this case, 2 months of cardiovascular conditioning resulted in a $\dot{V}O_2$ response to the 500-foot ambulation test of 12.4 mL·kg$^{-1}$·min$^{-1}$. In activities requiring walking, Byron now has widened his $\dot{V}O_2$ reserve.

---

fatigue. *Why do you think walking with a four-point walker increases the $\dot{V}O_2$ response in individuals who need this type of ambulation assistance?*

Also important to clinical practice is the fact that efficiency and economy decline with arm work. The $O_2$ cost of arm ergometry is about 40% greater than that of leg ergometry (3 mL·kg$^{-1}$·min$^{-1}$ per kg·m·min$^{-1}$ versus 1.8 mL·kg$^{-1}$·min$^{-1}$ per kg·m·min$^{-1}$, respectively). Thus, the denominator of the efficiency ratio with arm ergometry is automatically higher, resulting in a lower efficiency ratio. This extra $O_2$ cost is due to the recruitment of extra muscles which function to stabilize the torso during arm

cranking. These muscles contract statically in this form of exercise, adding to the overall $O_2$ cost. The cardiovascular effect of this extra energy expenditure is greater blood pressure and HR responses.

In healthy persons, mechanical efficiency during leg ergometry ranges from 23% to 25% (8). This is about 5% to 10% higher than arm mechanical efficiency in healthy individuals (8). Leg and arm efficiency ratios in individuals with chronic disease tend to follow this same pattern (i.e., arm efficiency lower than leg efficiency). However, mechanical efficiency of the legs and arms in these individuals is lower when compared to healthy individuals. A

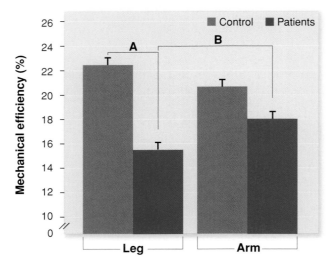

FIGURE 5.15. The mechanical efficiencies (mean±SEM) of arm and leg ergometry performed at 50% of the individually measured peak loads of an incremental leg and arm ergometry test. Significant differences are: ** $p < 0.001$ for COPD patients vs. controls and # $p < 0.05$ for arm vs. leg efficiency. Data from Franssen FME, Wouters EFM, Baarends EM, et al. Arm mechanical efficiency and arm exercise capacity are relatively preserved in chronic obstructive pulmonary disease. *Med Sci Sports Exerc* 2002;34:1570–1576.

notable exception to the above pattern is that individuals with COPD tend to preserve mechanical efficiency of the arms but not the legs. As shown in *Figure 5.15*, arm efficiency in clinically stable patients with COPD was higher than leg efficiency and not significantly different than arm efficiency in healthy controls. The reason for the difference in upper versus lower limb mechanical efficiency of COPD patients is speculative at this time but may be related to the following:

- Unlike leg efficiency, arm efficiency is not affected by decreased pulmonary function (i.e., increased $O_2$ cost of breathing)
- Differences in the training status of the upper versus lower limbs in COPD patients due to decreased physical activity patterns involving leg work
- Through the course of their disease, COPD patients may selectively preserve type I muscle fibers in the upper versus lower extremities, which would tend to also preserve mechanical efficiency of arm work

The finding of a preserved mechanical efficiency of upper extremities in COPD patients is clinically important and could influence the type of exercise intervention chosen. For example, because COPD patients preserve their arm mechanical efficiency, it may be disadvantageous to focus their training on inefficient muscle groups during pulmonary rehabilitation. The reason for this is that a focus on inefficient leg exercise in these patients might contribute to increased energy expenditure during exercise because of low leg efficiency. This could have the effect of

promoting catabolism and negatively influencing these patients' responses to nutritional therapy. Nutritional therapy is often sought for COPD patients because of the commonly observed dual problem of weight loss and depletion of fat-free mass (a consequence of disturbed protein balance), secondary to increases in the total daily energy expenditure, particularly the thermic effects of physical activities (see Fig. 5.10). Therefore, exercise intervention should be preferentially aimed at the efficient muscle groups, i.e., the arms (8).

Another patient group in which arm work is a focus of exercise therapy is individuals with paraplegia. A recent study investigated the physiologic effects of peak arm ergometric exercise compared with incremental electrically stimulated peak gait training (Box 5.2) (9). While the focus of this study was functional electrical stimulation gait training, the results demonstrated that individuals with paraplegia (complete thoracic spinal cord injury at levels T4–T11) are able to utilize arm ergometry for aerobic training (*Fig. 5.16*). In this study adults (mean age = 28 years) were able to perform arm ergometry exercise to a peak power output of 380 kg·m·min$^{-1}$ and peak $\dot{V}O_2$ response of 1570 mL·min$^{-1}$. This is compared to older pulmonary patients (mean age = 61 years; 306 kg·m·min$^{-1}$ peak power; 851 mL·min$^{-1}$ peak $\dot{V}O_2$) and control subjects (mean age = 61 years; 661 kg·m·min$^{-1}$ peak power; 1637 mL·min$^{-1}$ peak $\dot{V}O_2$).

▶ *INQUIRY SUMMARY.* Efficiency and movement economy can be used to understand how individuals respond to a bout of exercise. This has important implications for individuals with movement dysfunctions, as these individuals must learn to budget their energy output due to a reduced energy reserve. *Why do stroke patients often experience*

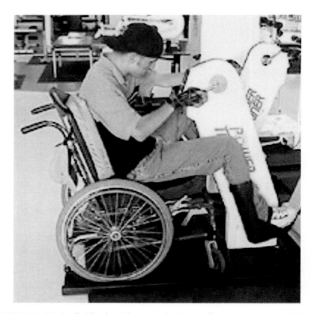

FIGURE 5.16. Individual with paraplegia performing arm-cranking exercise.

*shortness of breath with post-event ambulation speeds that are equal to pre-event ambulation speeds?*

## Energy Cost of Physical Activity

Since physiologic responses are dependent, to a large degree, on relative energy expenditure, it is important to understand the energy cost of various activities. Energy expenditure during physical activities is related to the type and intensity of the activity. We will focus here on traditional forms of exercise as a subset of physical activity and apply this material to rehabilitative settings. Without a doubt, other forms of physical activity such as vigorous yard work also have rehabilitative value, but the energy cost of these is less stabile.

Endurance exercise activities may be placed in two categories: weight supported and weight bearing. Cycling is representative of the former, and walking or running of the latter. Weight-bearing exercise activates a larger muscle mass; therefore, the rate of caloric expenditure during weight-bearing activity tends to be greater. In the next section these activities are discussed with regard to the vital relationship between HR and $\dot{V}O_2$, a relationship that helps us estimate energy expenditure.

### RELATIONSHIP BETWEEN HEART RATE AND $\dot{V}O_2$

HR and $\dot{V}O_2$ are linearly related across a wide range of aerobic exercise intensities. However, when using absolute units of measurement for each variable (i.e., beats·min$^{-1}$ for HR and L or mL·min$^{-1}$ for $\dot{V}O_2$), this relationship varies considerably among individuals and is influenced by the following factors:

- Individual aerobic fitness level (i.e., $\dot{V}O_{2max}$)
- Mode of exercise
- Environmental temperature

- Psychologic factors
- Previous food intake
- Body position
- Muscle groups exercised
- Continuous or discontinuous exercise
- Dynamic or static muscle contraction

For example, a problem in using HR to predict $\dot{V}O_2$ occurs when the HR from a static exercise form, such as weightlifting, is applied to a HR— $\dot{V}O_2$ regression line that was developed during cycling. A typical outcome is that HR in this situation would overpredict the level of $\dot{V}O_2$ response. This is true because HR and $\dot{V}O_2$ are not closely related in resistance exercise, and the $\dot{V}O_2$ response during resistance exercise is lower than would be predicted from HR response. For a discussion of the $\dot{V}O_2$ response to resistive exercise see Chapter 7. A way around the problem presented by most of the items listed above is to estimate $\dot{V}O_2$ (energy expenditure) as a percentage of its maximal value (% $\dot{V}O_{2max}$) from HR as a percentage of its maximal value (%HR$_{max}$).

When using these relative terms, the ACSM suggests that 50%, 60%, 80%, and 85% of $\dot{V}O_{2max}$ represent 60%, 70%, 85%, and 90% of HR$_{max}$, respectively, for the general population. However, these corresponding values have been shown to be inaccurate (10). Table 5.4 lists representative regression equations for weight-bearing and weight-supported exercise. *Figure 5.17* shows the regression lines from these equations.

There is no homogeneous equation, i.e., one that fits all modes. In general, these regression equations are distinguishable between weight-bearing and weight-supported land-based exercises, and between land-based and water-based exercises. Therefore, the relationship between HR and $\dot{V}O_2$ appears to be mode specific and is based on the differential responses of weight-bearing and weight-supported exercises. For example, water-based exercise, a

| Mode | Regression equation | Comments |
|---|---|---|
| **Table 5.4** | | **REPRESENTATIVE REGRESSION EQUATIONS FOR THE RELATIONSHIP BETWEEN HEART RATE AND $\dot{V}O_2$** |
| WB | % $\dot{V}O_{2max} = 1.26(\%HR_{max}) - 31.9$ | The WB combined equation includes treadmill, skiing, shuffling, and stepping modes from seven different studies |
| WS | % $\dot{V}O_{2max} = 1.36(\%HR_{max}) - 42.3$ | The WS combined equation is generated from five studies of cycle ergometry |
| Rower | % $\dot{V}O_{2max} = 1.18(\%HR_{max}) - 21.0$ | This equation comes from only one study |
| DWR | % $\dot{V}O_{2max} = 1.50(\%HR_{max}) - 52.1$ | This equation combines the data from young and older men from two studies |
| DWR | % $\dot{V}O_{2max} = 1.63(\%HR_{max}) - 65.2$ | This equation combines the data from young and older women from two studies |

These equations do not include data from studies using chronically ill individuals, and the WB, WS, and rower equations are generated from data collected from men. WB, weight bearing; WS, weight supported; DWR, deep-water running.

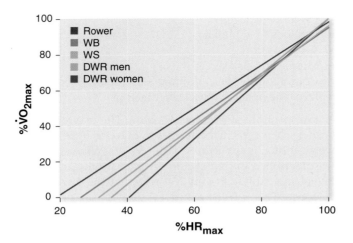

**FIGURE 5.17.** Linear regression lines from the equations presented in Table 5.4. WB = weight bearing; WS = weight supported; DWR = deep-water running.

form of weight-supported exercise, has a uniquely different response than other exercise modes. Note that compared to land-based weight-supported exercise, weight-bearing exercise (treadmill, skiing, shuffle skiing, and stepping from Table 5.4) has a lower **slope** and higher **intercept**.

For the most part, the slopes and intercepts from all weight-bearing exercises tend to be similar. However, weight-supported exercises do not follow this pattern, producing much different regression coefficients, for example, between the rower and leg ergometer. This is not the case for deep-water running for which the relationship between %HR$_{max}$ and %$\dot{V}O_{2max}$ is different between the sexes but not between age groups. Therefore, these equations have been grouped by sex in Table 5.4. No sex differences for land-based exercise have been reported for the relationship between %HR$_{max}$ and % $\dot{V}O_{2max}$.

The corresponding values for %$\dot{V}O_{2max}$ and %HR$_{max}$ using these equations are slightly different from those published by the ACSM. At 60% HR$_{max}$ the average deviation from the ACSM corresponding value for %$\dot{V}O_{2max}$ (i.e., 50%) was −12%. Deviation from the ACSM value tends to be reduced as the %HR$_{max}$ increases. The only exception to this is the rowing equation, which produces nearly identical corresponding values to the ACSM equation.

Determining energy expenditure using these equations involves determining the steady-state HR as a percentage of the maximal HR (220 − age = HR$_{max}$). For example, if a 30-yr-old individual's HR$_{max}$ is 190, a steady-state training HR of 162 beats·min$^{-1}$ (85% of 190) gives an estimated %$\dot{V}O_{2max}$ of 75% using the weight-bearing equation from Table 5.4. If this individual has a $\dot{V}O_{2max}$ of 40 mL·kg$^{-1}$·min$^{-1}$ and is 70 kg, the exercise metabolic rate equals 30 mL·kg$^{-1}$·min$^{-1}$ or 2.1 L·min$^{-1}$. This represents an estimated energy expenditure of 10.5 kcal·min$^{-1}$, predicted on the basis of HR response. An obvious drawback to this method is that HR$_{max}$ and $\dot{V}O_{2max}$ need to be known to make these calculations.

## ESTIMATING SUBMAXIMAL $\dot{V}O_2$: THE METABOLIC EQUATIONS

The energy expenditure of submaximal physical activity can also be estimated with accuracy by using predictors indicative of physical effort. These predictors relate mechanical measures of work rate to their metabolic equivalent in regression equations that are arranged in the same fashion as the gross $\dot{V}O_2$ equation presented earlier. That is, these equations estimate gross $\dot{V}O_2$ using three components:

- A component that relates to forces moving horizontally
- A component that relates to forces moving vertically
- A resting component (i.e., resting $\dot{V}O_2$).

The first two of these three components equate to the exercise or net $\dot{V}O_2$ response from the equation depicting gross $\dot{V}O_2$. Exercise $\dot{V}O_2$ has been factored into two components for the purpose of predicting $\dot{V}O_2$ response because there is a metabolic (energy) cost in moving horizontally *and* vertically. These two energy costs are added together to produce the net $\dot{V}O_2$ response.

*LINKUP:* **Case Study: Using Metabolic Equations** *at http://connection.lww.com/go/brownexphys and on the Student Resource CD-ROM shows how metabolic equations can be used for clinical purposes. It is necessary to become proficient in the use of the equations because they are important in formulating exercise prescriptions for clinical populations.*

For walking or running, the O$_2$ requirement is a function of speed (*Fig. 5.18*). However, walking requires less energy than running. The amount of energy required for horizontal walking is 0.1 mL·kg$^{-1}$·min$^{-1}$ for each m·min$^{-1}$ of horizontal movement, compared to 0.2 mL·kg$^{-1}$·min$^{-1}$ for horizontal running. Also, these factors

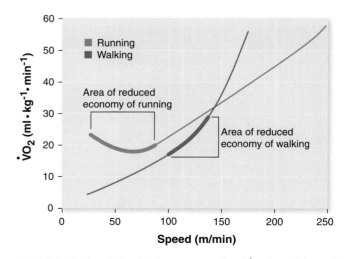

**FIGURE 5.18.** The relationship between speed and $\dot{V}O_2$ for walking and running. Economy decreases for both as a function of higher $\dot{V}O_2$ responses when walking or running outside of an optimal speed zone.

| Table 5.5 | THE ACSM METABOLIC EQUATIONS PREDICTING GROSS $\dot{V}O_2$ IN ML·KG$^{-1}$·MIN$^{-1}$ | | | | |
|---|---|---|---|---|---|
| | | **Equation components** | | | |
| **Exercise mode** | **HC** | **+** | **VC** | **+** | **RC** |
| Walking | $\dot{V}O_2 = (0.1 \cdot S)$ | + | $(1.8 \cdot S \cdot G)$ | + | 3.5 |
| Treadmill and outdoor running | $\dot{V}O_2 = (0.2 \cdot S)$ | + | $(0.9 \cdot S \cdot G)$ | + | 3.5 |
| Leg ergometry | $\dot{V}O_2 = 0$ | + | $(10.8 \cdot W \cdot M^{-1})$ | + | 7.0 |
| Arm ergometry | $\dot{V}O_2 = 0$ | + | $(18.0 \cdot W \cdot M^{-1})$ | + | 3.5 |
| Stepping ergometry | $\dot{V}O_2 = (0.2 \cdot f)$ | + | $(1.33 \cdot 1.8 \cdot H \cdot f)$ | + | 3.5 |

HC, horizontal component; VC, vertical component; RC, resting component; $\dot{V}O_2$, gross oxygen consumption in ml·kg$^{-1}$·min$^{-1}$; S, speed in m·min$^{-1}$; G, percent grade expressed as a fraction; W, power in Watts (when starting with kg·m·min$^{-1}$, multiply by 0.16345 to convert to Watts); M, body mass in kg; f, stepping frequency in steps·min$^{-1}$; H, step height in meters. To convert from mph to m·min$^{-1}$, multiply by 26.8. Modified with permission from American College of Sports Medicine. *ACSM's guidelines for exercise testing prescription.* 6th ed. Baltimore: Lippincott Williams and Wilkins, 2000.

are only valid for a narrow range of walking and running speeds. For instance, walking between 50 and 100 m·min$^{-1}$ (1.9 to 3.7 mph) requires 0.1 mL·kg$^{-1}$·min$^{-1}$ $O_2$ consumption, but the loss of economy walking at speeds greater than 100 m·min$^{-1}$ due to stride lengthening and other exaggerated body movements increase $O_2$ requirements. In a like manner, running at speeds less than 80 m·min$^{-1}$ (3.0 mph) causes a similar loss of economy. Table 5.5 lists the metabolic equations published by the ACSM for estimating $\dot{V}O_2$ response using ergometrically determined workloads.

 *LINKUP: Research on the accuracy of the ACSM equations is still being conducted. One of the most recent studies is summarized in* Research Highlight: The Accuracy of the ACSM Stair-Stepping Equation, *featured on http://connection.lww.com/go/brownexphys and on the Student Resource CD-ROM.*

▶ *INQUIRY SUMMARY.* The linear relationship between HR and $\dot{V}O_2$ provides an alternative method for estimating energy expenditure during exercise. This relationship is best viewed as a percentage of each variable's maximal value. When viewed this way, HR can be used to estimate $\dot{V}O_2$ response and, thus, energy expenditure. Ergometric workloads can also be used to estimate energy expenditure since workload and $\dot{V}O_2$ response are linearly related. *Why is knowledge of the $O_2$ cost of exercise important?*

## Summary

Ergometers such as treadmills, stationary cycles, and step ergometers are used for the purpose of measuring work. The measurement of work output is important in exercise physiology because the ability to quantify work has both clinical and research implications. When work is done, metabolic heat is released. This heat is quantifiable through the process of calorimetry. Direct calorimetry measures heat directly as a change in the temperature of a fluid circulating around a device. Indirect calorimetry measures $O_2$

consumption, which can be converted to heat equivalent units. The rate of energy expenditure in exercise is dependent on the fuel substrate utilized. This can be determined by knowing the RER during a steady-state work bout. The RER is the ratio of $\dot{V}CO_2$ to $\dot{V}O_2$. These values can be determined by open-circuit spirometry by measuring expiratory gas volumes and fractional components of $O_2$ and $CO_2$ in the expiratory air. During ergometric exercise, efficiency of movement can be measured as the ratio of work output to energy input. Movement economy is an important clinical concept because as patients become more economic in ADL, they impinge less on their energy reserves. Energy expenditure can be estimated by the relationship between HR and $\dot{V}O_2$. Energy expenditure can also be estimated from ergometric workloads.

### SUMMARY KNOWLEDGE

1. How is the process of measuring work different for treadmill, cycle, and step ergometry?
2. What is the relationship between work and power?
3. How do the principles of direct and indirect calorimetry differ?
4. Why is the Haldane transformation important in open-circuit spirometry measurement?
5. Is it possible for $F_{EN_2}$ to be different than $F_{IN_2}$? Explain.
6. Why are Charles' and Boyle's laws important in gas volume measures?
7. What is the difference between the respiratory quotient and the respiratory exchange ratio?
8. What is the difference between basal and resting metabolic rates?
9. What is the relationship between energy expenditure and workload, and why is this relationship important in the concept of efficiency
10. What is the difference between gross and net $\dot{V}O_2$, and how does this difference relate to efficiency?
11. What is the difference between efficiency and economy?
12. Why is the concept of movement economy clinically relevant?
13. How does exercise intensity affect efficiency?

14. Is the relationship between $\%\dot{V}O_{2max}$ and $\%HR_{max}$ linear or curvilinear? Explain.
15. Why are there different $O_2$ costs of exercise for the various ergometers discussed in this chapter?

### References

1. Westerterp KR, Brouns F, Saris WH, et al. Comparison of doubly labeled water with respirometry at low-and high-activity levels. *J Appl Physiol* 1988;65:53–56.
2. Richards ML, Davies PSW. Energy cost of activity assessed by indirect calorimetry and a $^{13}CO_2$ breath test. *Med Sci Sports Exerc* 2001;33:834–838.
3. Bransford DR, Howley ET. Oxygen cost of running in trained and untrained men and women. *Med Sci Sports* 1977;9:41–44.
4. Kyröläinen H, Belli A, Komi PV. Biomechanical factors affecting running economy. *Med Sci Sports Exerc* 2001;33:1330–1337.
5. Brown SP, Chitwood LF, Beason KR, et al. Deep water running physiologic responses: gender differences at treadmill-matched walking/running cadences. *J Strength Cond Res* 1997;11:107–114.
6. Brown SP, Jordan JC, Chitwood LF, et al. Relationship of heart rate and oxygen uptake kinetics during deep water running in the adult population—ages 50 to 70 years. *J Aging Phys Act* 1998;6:248–255.
7. Lewis CB. Musculoskeletal changes with age: clinical implication. In: Lewis CB, ed. *Aging: the health care challenge*. Philadelphia: FA Davis Co, 1996.
8. Franssen FME, Wouters EFM, Baarends EM, et al. Arm mechanical efficiency and arm exercise capacity are relatively preserved in chronic obstructive pulmonary disease. *Med Sci Sports Exerc* 2002;34:1570–1576.
9. Jacobs PL, Mahoney ET. Peak exercise capacity of electrically induced ambulation in persons with paraplegia. *Med Sci Sports Exerc* 2002;34:1551–1556.
10. Swain DP, Abernathy KS, Smith CS, et al. Target heart rates for the development of cardiorespiratory fitness. *Med Sci Sports Exerc* 1994;26:112–116.

### Suggested Readings

American College of Sports Medicine. *ACSM's guidelines for exercise testing and prescription*. 6th ed. Baltimore: Lippincott Williams & Wilkins, 2000.

Seale JL, Rumpler WV. Synchronous direct gradient layer and indirect room calorimetry. *J Appl Physiol* 1997;83:1775–1781.

Lang PB, Latin RW, Berg KE, et al. The accuracy of the ACSM cycle ergometry equation. *Med Sci Sports Exerc* 1992;24:272–276.

Latin RW, Berg K, Kissinger K, et al. The accuracy of the ACSM stair-stepping equation. *Med Sci Sports Exerc* 2001;33:1785–1788.

### On the Internet

Beltsville Agricultural Research Center: The Diet and Human Performance Laboratory. Available at: **http://www.barc.usda.gov/bhnrc/dhpl/**. Accessed April 07, 2005.

Cycling Performance Tips. Available at: **http://www.cptips.com/**. Accessed April 07, 2005.

Physics of Bicycling. Available at: **http://www.physicsofbicycling.homestead.com/**. Accessed April 07, 2005.

The Effects of Tire Pressure on Wheeling Efficiency. Available at: **http://www.seatingandmobility.ca/Iss2002/ToSunnyHill2/iss2002html/024_THEEFFECTSOFTIREPRESSUREONWHEELINGEFFICIENCY.htm**. Accessed April 07, 2005.

The University of Sydney, Faculty of Health Sciences, Rehabilitation Research Centre: The Shake-a-Leg FES Research Project. Available at: **http://www2.fhs.usyd.edu.au/ess/rrc/shakeleg.htm**. Accessed April 07, 2005.

## Writing to Learn

*Research the following question and write a paper using current scientific literature. How much greater is gait energy expenditure in patients with movement dysfunctions compared with control subjects, and does the increased energy expenditure vary with the severity and type of pathologic involvement? Use at least three pathologic conditions in which gait mechanics are altered. In your paper, also investigate the increase in the energy cost of movement with different assistive devices and with different stepping techniques, such as step-to versus another walking technique aided by an assistive device.*

# CHAPTER

# 6 Respiratory Exercise Physiology

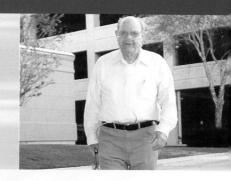

*The mechanical process of respiration is automatic and rhythmic and does not require a healthy individual to consciously decide when or how deeply to breathe. Instead, respiration is constantly adjusted to meet the daily requirements of life, such as during exercise and speech. While exercise causes an increase in respiration, this increase may be labored in certain patient groups. Notice the nasal cannula in place on the pulmonary patient.* Do you think the extra $O_2$ supply helps improve exercise performance in individuals with respiratory disorders?

## CHAPTER OUTLINE

I n Section 1 we discovered that the energy needed for normal activities is mainly derived from the oxidative breakdown of energy nutrients in a process termed *cellular (internal) respiration*. In this gas exchange process, $O_2$ is taken up from blood and utilized by mitochondria, and the $CO_2$ produced in the mitochondria diffuses into the blood. The $O_2$ used to combust nutrients is ultimately derived from the atmosphere, while the $CO_2$ produced is eliminated from the body to the atmosphere during *external respiration*. To facilitate external respiration, the lungs are structured to maximize the interface between the atmosphere outside of the body and blood circulating through the lungs. The chief component of external respiration, there-

fore, is gas exchange between the air in the lungs and the blood perfusing them.

The material in this chapter is essential content for a well-rounded understanding of the physiology of rest and exercise and is foundational for much of the remainder of the book. Some questions you will encounter and answer in this chapter are:

- *Where does the rhythmic process of breathing originate?*
- *How is breathing generated?*
- *How is the transport of the respiratory gases facilitated?*

The chapter begins with the mechanics of breathing and gas exchange. Pulmonary blood flow is then considered in a discussion of the match between ventilation and perfusion. Finally, the chapter is rounded out with a discussion of respiratory control. Through the presentation of these topics, function during exercise is stressed. While you read, consult Table 6.1 frequently as important abbreviations are introduced. You will find that there is an extensive use of standard symbols in respiratory physiology, thus the table provided should prove helpful.

## Exchange of Respiratory Gases at the Alveolar-Capillary Interface

A person may live for several days without liver, kidney, or higher brain function, but death will ensue in only about 5 minutes without breathing and circulating blood. Accordingly, the primary function of the lungs is to distribute inspired air and pulmonary blood flow so that there can be an adequate exchange of the respiratory gases ($O_2$ and $CO_2$) between the alveoli and pulmonary capillary beds.

Since failure in the process of gas exchange is a common abnormality in clinical care, physical therapists, exercise physiologists, and other health care workers who monitor patient exercise should pay particular attention to the cardiorespiratory system. The respiratory system is of prime importance since it is where $O_2$, the respiratory gas necessary for life, is "acquired." Ventilating the lungs is an efficient process in the healthy person with the exchange of air ranging from a resting level of 6 $L \cdot min^{-1}$ to a maximal level during high-level endurance competition that may approach or even exceed 198 $L \cdot min^{-1}$. This wide range adequately demonstrates that the lungs are indeed built for exercise.

The lungs perform a number of functions, most of them respiratory in nature. In addition to their role in gas exchange, the lungs have these other important functions:

- Trapping blood-borne particles (small traveling blood clots called emboli) and degrading them by the release of heparin from lung mast cells
- Metabolism of a variety of **vasoactive** substances

| Table 6.1 | **SYMBOLS IN RESPIRATORY PHYSIOLOGY** | | |
|---|---|---|---|
| **Variable** | **Symbol Used** | **Variable** | **Suffix** |
| Content or capacity | C | Alveolar | A |
| Diffusion | D | Arterial | a |
| Fractional concentration of dry gas | F | Airway | aw |
| Conductance | G | Barometric | B |
| Pressure, partial pressure, or gas tension | P | Capillary | c |
| Mean pressure | $\bar{P}$ | Dead space | DS |
| Volume of blood | Q | Expired | E |
| Flow of blood (i.e., $L \cdot min^{-1}$) | $\dot{Q}$ | End-tidal air (= alveolar gas) | ET |
| Resistance | R | Elastic | el |
| Saturation | S | Frequency of breathing | f |
| Volume of gas | V | Inspired | I |
| Flow of gas, ventilation (i.e., $L \cdot min^{-1}$) | $\dot{V}$ | Lung | L |
| | | Left atrial | la |
| | | Pulmonary artery | pa |
| | | Pleural space | pl |
| | | Pulmonary venous | pv |
| | | Resistive | res |
| | | Tidal | T |
| | | Tissue | t |
| | | Total | tot |
| | | Upper Respiratory Passages | U |
| | | Venous | v |
| | | Mixed venous | $\bar{v}$ |
| | | Chest wall | w |

The primary variables in these symbols are given as capital letters (e.g., pressure [P] or volume [V]), while the location to which they apply is given by a suffix (e.g., $Ppaco_2$ is the partial pressure of $CO_2$ in the pulmonary artery).

- Removal of air-borne foreign material by the **mucociliary** mechanism
- Warming and hydration of the atmospheric air entering the lungs
- Regulating hydrogen ion ($H^+$) concentration in blood

While these functions are significant, in this chapter we focus on the four main functional events of respiration: the exchange of gases between the alveoli and the blood circulating through the lungs, ventilating the lungs (breathing), transport of the respiratory gases, and ventilatory regulation. The lungs distribute inspired air and pulmonary blood flow in a way that facilitates gas exchange between alveoli and pulmonary capillary blood. In **ventilation**, an optimal composition of alveoli gas is maintained so that a unidirectional flow of $O_2$ (into the body) and $CO_2$ (out of the body) is achieved. These important functions must be carried out with minimal energy expenditure so that the work of breathing is minimized. Pulmonary circulation, gas exchange, and respiratory control are discussed later in the chapter. First we investigate the lungs' primary role, the mechanical aspects of breathing and gas exchange.

## RESPIRATORY GASES MOVE BY DIFFUSION

Before discussing **pulmonary ventilation**, it is important to understand the laws of gas diffusion. Gas diffusion in the lungs is the movement of air from one location to another as precipitated by the inherent kinetic motion of each gas species following its concentration gradient across the alveolar-capillary interface (*Fig. 6.1*). That is, diffusion is the passive thermodynamic flow of molecules between regions of different **partial pressures** of the respiratory gases. This process is highly efficient, producing a rapid equilibrium of $O_2$ and $CO_2$ concentrations between alveoli and the blood leaving the lungs (*Fig 6.2*), even in periods of heavy exercise stress. A number of factors favor the ready diffusion of gas across the alveolar-capillary interface:

- A large partial pressure difference (the "driving" pressure)
- The thickness of the respiratory membrane (a short distance to travel from a region of high gas concentration to one of lower gas concentration)
- A high **diffusivity** (respiratory gases are of small molecular size and are highly soluble in water)
- A large total alveolar-capillary surface area
- The number of red blood cells and the **hemoglobin** concentration
- The amount of time red blood cells spend in the pulmonary capillary (transit time)

## DRIVING PRESSURE AND GAS DIFFUSION

Understanding the partial pressure of a gas is crucial to understanding gas movement by diffusion. Partial pressure is a measure of the total number of molecules of a particular gas species resident in a container (like an alveolus). An individual gas species exerts pressure by the summated forces of all the molecules of that gas striking the walls of the container at any given instant. This makes the pressure directly proportional to the concentration of gas molecules for a given gas species. **Dalton's law** states that the total pressure exerted by a gas mixture (all of the individual gas species taken together) equals the sum of the partial pressures exerted by each gas species. The term partial pressure means that each of the respiratory gas species ($N_2$, $O_2$, and $CO_2$) exerts a pressure independent of any others in the container.

The partial pressure (P) of any gas is a function of its fractional concentration (F) and the absolute barometric pressure ($P_B$). If the concentration of the gas or $P_B$ is low, the partial pressure exerted by that gas is also low. The opposite is also true. The following calculations show the partial pressures of atmospheric, inspired (I) $O_2$ ($P_{IO_2}$), $CO_2$ ($P_{ICO_2}$), and nitrogen ($P_{IN_2}$) at sea level ($P_B = 760$ mm Hg) using the generally accepted composition of atmospheric air (20.93% $O_2$, 0.03% $CO_2$, 79.04% $N_2$). Notice that the sum of the three partial pressures equals the -absolute barometric pressure at the altitude being considered:

$$P_{IO_2} = 760 \text{ mm Hg} \times 0.2093 = 159.1 \text{ mm Hg}$$
$$P_{ICO_2} = 760 \text{ mm Hg} \times 0.0003 = 0.2 \text{ mm Hg}$$
$$P_{IN_2} = 760 \text{ mm Hg} \times 0.7904 = 600.7 \text{ mm Hg}$$

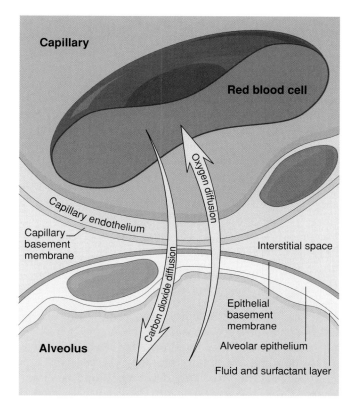

**FIGURE 6.1.** Cross-sectional schematic of the microstructure of the alveolar-capillary interface (membrane). The thickness of the membrane averages about 0.6 μm.

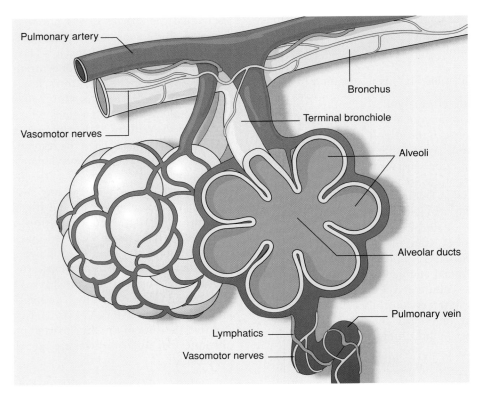

**FIGURE 6.2.** The respiratory (gas exchange) units, numbering approximately 300 million in two lungs, contain many alveoli, each having a diameter of 0.2 mm. Within the thin walls of the alveoli is an extensive network of interconnecting capillaries (capillary plexus) that allows blood flow through the alveolar wall. Because of the anatomy of the capillary plexus, the pulmonary capillary blood flow has been described as a thin stream or "sheet" of flowing blood.

As atmospheric air enters the upper respiratory passages, the air becomes totally humidified with water vapor, which reduces the partial pressure of each respiratory gas. This is so because the total pressure in the lungs cannot rise to more than the atmospheric pressure. In the upper respiratory passages at a normal body temperature of 37°C, the $P_{H_2O}$ is 47 mm Hg. The water vapor dilutes the partial pressures of the respiratory gases in the upper respiratory passages (U) to values lower than those of atmospheric air:

$$P_{UO_2} = (760 \text{ mm Hg} - 47 \text{ mm Hg}) \times 0.2093$$
$$= 149.2 \text{ mm Hg}$$

$$P_{UCO_2} = (760 \text{ mm Hg} - 47 \text{ mm Hg}) \times 0.0003$$
$$= 0.2 \text{ mm Hg}$$

$$P_{UN_2} = (760 \text{ mm Hg} - 47 \text{ mm Hg}) \times 0.7904$$
$$= 563.6 \text{ mm Hg}$$

Notice that the $P_{O_2}$ difference between the atmosphere and upper respiratory passages is 10 mm Hg, while the $P_{CO_2}$ remains fairly constant. From a $P_{O_2}$ of about 149 mm Hg in the upper respiratory passages, the $P_{O_2}$ falls to a lower level in the alveolar and **venous blood** compartments. However, $P_{CO_2}$ is greater in the alveoli compared to the upper respiratory passages and higher still in the mixed venous blood compartment. *Figure 6.3* demonstrates the direction of the $P_{O_2}$ and $P_{CO_2}$ gradients. The values for the alveolar partial pressures of $O_2$ and $CO_2$ ($P_{AO_2}$ and $P_{ACO_2}$, respectively) are typically about 102 mm Hg and 40 mm Hg, respectively. This sudden reduction in $P_{O_2}$ (from upper respiratory passages to alveoli) of about 47 mm Hg is primarily due to the rapid rate of diffusion of $O_2$ out of the alveoli into pulmonary capillary blood as venous blood from the pulmonary artery passes through the pulmonary capillaries. The sudden increase in $P_{CO_2}$ (from pulmonary artery blood to alveoli) of about 6 mm Hg is primarily due to the rapid rate of diffusion of $CO_2$ out of pulmonary capillary blood and into the alveoli as venous blood passes through the pulmonary capillaries.

The driving pressure for $O_2$ entering the aqueous state is actually greater when considering the partial pressure of $O_2$ in the venous blood ($P_{O_2}$) entering the pulmonary capillary at the arterial end (see Fig. 6.3). This pressure difference, the "driving pressure," is 102 mm Hg − 40 mm Hg = 62 mm Hg. *Figure 6.4* shows the effect on the $P_{O_2}$ of this blood as it passes through the pulmonary capillaries. A rapid equilibration is reached at approximately 102 mm Hg. However, only about 98% of the blood entering the left atrium from the lungs has passed through the pulmonary capillaries. The other 2% of the blood passing through the lungs bypasses the alveoli where gas exchange takes place (pulmonary shunt blood). This blood instead passes from the systemic circulation (through the bronchial arteries) and nourishes lung structures that do not participate in gas exchange.

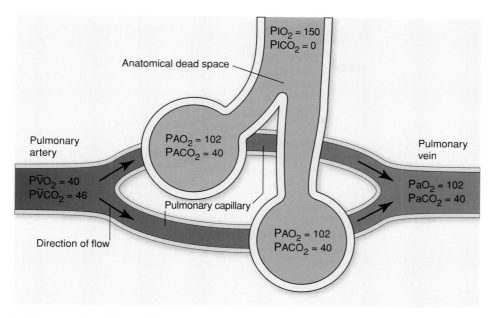

**FIGURE 6.3.** Schematic of the normal ventilation/perfusion process showing two parallel respiratory units. The values represent normal adult resting values for gas partial pressures (P) in inspired (I) air, alveolar gas (A), and mixed venous ($\bar{v}$) blood arriving at the pulmonary capillaries from the right ventricle via the pulmonary artery.

Most of this blood flows into the pulmonary veins, combining with oxygenated blood that has just passed through the pulmonary capillaries. This flow of blood, called the "right-left shunt" flow, has a $P_{O_2}$ equal to that of normal venous blood (40 mm Hg) and mixes (the venous admixture of blood) with the oxygenated blood of the pulmonary veins to reduce the $P_{O_2}$ of the blood in the left ventricle to about 95 mm Hg. Thus, the $O_2$ cascade resulting from ventilatory and diffusional factors ends in the pulmonary capillaries where an equilibration occurs with $P_{AO_2}$, but the $P_{O_2}$ is lower in arterial blood pumped by the left side of the heart because of the right-left shunt leading to an admixture of blood. The venous admixture always lowers

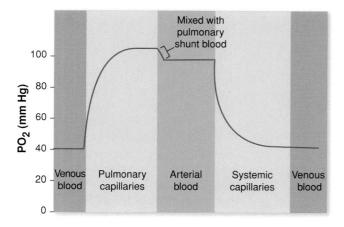

**FIGURE 6.4.** Change in $P_{O_2}$ in several blood compartments as the blood moves in the venous system from the body to the lungs and in the arterial system from the lungs to the body.

the systemic arterial partial pressure of $O_2$ ($P_{AO_2}$) and hemoglobin **saturation**, thereby reducing the efficiency of cellular gas exchange.

As stated previously, each respiratory gas species diffuses along its partial pressure gradient (from high to low concentration) independently of the movement of any other respiratory or anesthetic (e.g., ether, nitrous oxide) gas. Figure 6.1 showed that the direction of diffusion of $O_2$ and $CO_2$ is opposite and in line with their concentration gradients. Thus, $O_2$ is literally "driven" into capillary blood because of the partial pressure difference of 47 mm Hg. This partial pressure difference represents a measure of the net tendency of $O_2$ to move out of the alveoli and into blood. In moderate to heavy exercise the *driving pressure* for putting $O_2$ into capillary blood actually increases, because $P_{AO_2}$ increases from its approximate resting level of 102 mm Hg. The increase in $P_{AO_2}$ during this level of exercise is because of a greatly increased rate in the entry of new $O_2$ into the lungs due to the marked increase in ventilation that occurs in moderate to heavy exercise.

*Figure 6.5* demonstrates that beyond the moderate exercise point ($\dot{V}_{O_2} > 50\%$ to 60% of $\dot{V}_{O_{2max}}$), **minute ventilation** ($\dot{V}_E$) increases out of proportion (curvilinear increase) to increases in $\dot{V}_{O_2}$. However, the fixed level of $P_{IO_2}$ limits the maximal level that $P_{AO_2}$ can attain. *Figure 6.6* shows that even in moderate exercise ($\dot{V}_{O_2} = 1000$ mL·min$^{-1}$), **alveolar ventilation** ($\dot{V}_A$) must increase from a resting level of about 5 L·min$^{-1}$ to about 20 L·min$^{-1}$ just to maintain $P_{AO_2}$ at the resting level of 102 mm Hg. In actuality, as alveolar hyperventilation occurs, $P_{AO_2}$ increases to levels greater than 102 mm Hg but remains below 149 mm Hg ($P_{IO_2}$). The driving pressure is thus

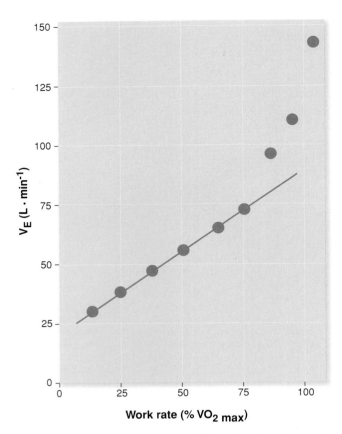

**FIGURE 6.5.** The increase in minute ventilation plotted against exercise intensity ($O_2$ consumption, $\dot{V}O_2$) showing the initial linear increase in $\dot{V}E$ with increasing $\dot{V}O_2$, and the switch to a curvilinear response (i.e., greater increase in $\dot{V}E$ per unit increase in $\dot{V}O_2$) at higher metabolic rates.

increased in heavy exercise, facilitating diffusion of $O_2$ to blood. *What do you think would happen to any of these gas partial pressures at an altitude greater than sea level, or if you were to breathe air with a higher or lower $O_2$ content? Also, speculate on the clinical consequences arising from any of these circumstances.*

*LINKUP: Access* **Perspective: Gas Partial Pressures, Gas Percentages, and Altitude** *at http://connection. lww.com/go/brownexphys and on the Student Resource CD-ROM to find answers to some of these questions.*

## SHORT DISTANCES ENHANCE DIFFUSION

In general, random thermal motion of gas molecules dictates that a dynamic equilibrium (zero net gas movement between compartments) will be established as the gas is dispersed due to the kinetic energy of the molecules. This process is especially rapid over microscopic distances (as exist in the alveolar-capillary interface), but it occurs more slowly across membranes that have been thickened by disease processes. For example, in clinical conditions such as pulmonary fibrosis and congestive heart failure, patients

become hypoxic (**hypoxia** is a condition of low $P_{O_2}$) because the diffusion of $O_2$ from the alveolus to the capillary is reduced by increasing the distance $O_2$ has to travel. In the case of fibrosis, an abnormal thickening of the alveolar-capillary interface occurs. In the case of congestive heart failure, the distance is increased due to pulmonary edema (fluid accumulating at the interface). In these two clinical conditions, the developed **hypoxemia** is pathologic.

The time/distance relationship for molecular diffusion is 1 millisecond to diffuse 1 $\mu$m. However, this relationship is altered by the square of the distance over which diffusion occurs. For example, a 100-fold increase in diffusion distance requires about a 10,000-fold increase in the time to reach a given degree of completion. The average distance between alveolar gas and red blood cells in the capillaries, for instance, is 1.5 $\mu$m, which represents a very short diffusion pathway. The red blood cell is usually so close to the capillary membrane that at times it may literally touch the capillary wall, which aids diffusion by lowering the amount of plasma respiratory gases have to traverse to get to the red blood cell (*Fig. 6.7*). In addition, the red blood cell passes through the capillary in single file because of the extremely small diameter of the capillary.

## DIFFUSIVITY DETERMINES RAPIDITY OF DIFFUSION

The size of the diffusing molecule and the medium through which it is diffusing dictate a molecule's diffusion coefficient (*D*). The diffusion coefficient is inversely related to both the size of the molecule and viscosity of the medium. Molecular size also helps determine the diffusivity of the molecule. The greater solubility of $CO_2$ in water, compared to $O_2$, allows $CO_2$ to diffuse about twice as fast as $O_2$ across the alveolar-capillary interface. This is so even though $O_2$ is a smaller molecule and has a much greater partial pressure difference (62 mm Hg for $O_2$ versus 6 mm Hg for $CO_2$) between venous blood (pulmonary artery) and

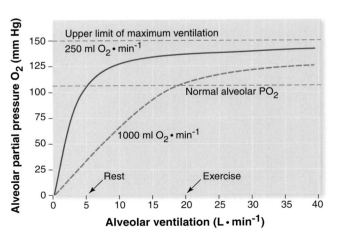

**FIGURE 6.6.** The $P_{O_2}$ is plotted against alveolar ventilation at two rates of $O_2$ absorption from the alveoli (at rest: 250 mL·min$^{-1}$ and at moderate exercise: 1000 mL·min$^{-1}$). (Courtesy of Guyton AC, Hall JE, University of Mississippi Medical Center, Jackson, Mississippi.)

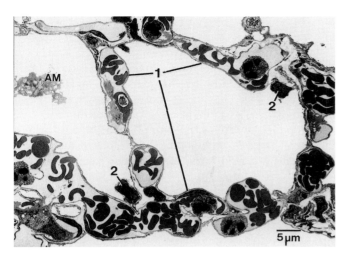

**FIGURE 6.7.** Low-power transmission electron micrograph of a human lung alveolus. The capillaries fill most of the alveolar walls so that $O_2$ and $CO_2$ exchange can be processed efficiently. The main, type 1 (1), alveolar lining epithelium covers nearly all of the alveolus. The type 2 (2) cells are small but are very active in producing, packaging, secreting, and recycling the air-liquid surfactant. Black objects in the capillaries are the erythrocytes. At the left margin is a portion of an alveolar macrophage (AM). (Courtesy of Albertine KH, University of Utah Health Sciences Center, Salt Lake City, Utah.)

alveolar gas (Fig. 6.3). Fick's first law of diffusion describes the relationships among the variables governing diffusion across a membrane:

$$J = -DA(\Delta c \div \Delta x)$$

J is the net rate of gas transfer in g per unit time, *D* is the diffusion coefficient of the gas, A is the area of the membrane, $\Delta c$ is the concentration difference across the membrane, and $\Delta x$ is the thickness of the membrane.

This equation shows that diffusion rate is proportional to the area of the membrane and to the difference in the concentration of the diffusing gas on the two sides of the membrane (the partial pressure difference). However, as membrane thickness increases in pathologic conditions (but not normal physiology), diffusion is impeded. In the lung, diffusion is aided by the thinness of the alveolar-capillary interface and the large total surface area available for diffusion. In humans, the actual total surface area for gas exchange at the alveolar-capillary interface is extremely large, estimated at $\geq 70$ m$^2$. This provides a great amount of space for diffusion to occur. Diffusion is further enhanced over this large area because of the relatively small capillary blood volume that exists at any given instant in the gas exchange vessels of the lung (about 60 to 140 mL in resting men). The small blood volume spread over a large area allows for a rapid gas equilibration over the space of one cardiac cycle.

Diffusing capacity is the volume of gas that diffuses through a membrane each minute for a pressure difference of 1 mm Hg. This value is approximately 21 mL·min$^{-1}$·mm Hg$^{-1}$ and 400 mL·min$^{-1}$·mm Hg$^{-1}$ for $O_2$ and $CO_2$, respectively, at rest. Diffusion capacity increases during

moderate to heavy exercise to a value of approximately 65 mL·min$^{-1}$·mm Hg$^{-1}$ for $O_2$ and about 1180 mL·min$^{-1}$·mm Hg$^{-1}$ for $CO_2$. The exercise response is nearly linear for untrained and trained males and females; however, the absolute values are lower for females. The three-fold increase in diffusion capacity during exercise for $O_2$ and $CO_2$ is due to the opening of pulmonary capillaries that were closed at rest, the greater dilatation of already partially opened capillaries, and a better match between the ventilated alveoli and perfused capillaries (the ventilation-**perfusion** ratio).

## DIFFUSION AND TRANSIT TIME

Diffusion is not limited during exercise in normal sedentary and moderately trained individuals but can be hampered because of a decrease in **transit time** that sometimes occurs in elite athletes during very heavy endurance exercise. In the resting state the red blood cell normally spends about 0.75 seconds in the pulmonary capillary in its transit from the pulmonary arterial side to the pulmonary venous side of the capillary bed. At rest this represents more than twice the time necessary to oxygenate the blood (normally about 0.3 seconds). Exercise causes an expansion of the pulmonary capillary bed and an increase in cardiac output. The expanded size of the pulmonary capillary bed during exercise ensures that the increased cardiac output can be accommodated with a minimal increase in blood velocity through the capillaries. If not for this increased expansion, the time of exposure of the red blood cell to gas exchange structures would be too short for effective gas exchange to occur (*Fig. 6.8*). This is true because transit

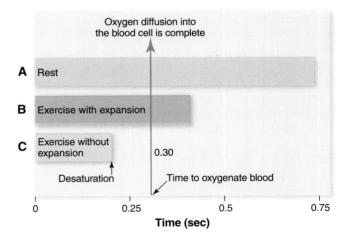

**FIGURE 6.8.** The arrow shows the normal time (0.30 seconds) that it takes to equilibrate $O_2$ into the red blood cell as venous blood passes through the pulmonary capillaries. Bar A shows that red blood cells stay in the capillary bed for about 0.75 seconds at rest. As the capillary bed is expanded (increased recruitment) with exercise (B), the red blood cells spend less than half the time in the capillary bed, but still enough time to equilibrate. However, without capillary bed expansion (C), the flow rate would be too fast to allow complete equilibration and gas exchange is compromised. (Courtesy of Cerny FJ, Burton HW, State University of New York at Buffalo.)

time would be markedly decreased owing to the increased flow rate through a vascular bed that had not expanded. Bar C in Figure 6.8 demonstrates this phenomenon.

▶ *INQUIRY SUMMARY.* Since gas molecules diffuse following pressure gradients, proper **external respiration** is dependent on the physics of gas movement along concentration gradients from ambient air to the individual alveolus. Gas, therefore, is literally "driven" from one compartment to the next by a pressure head, but the rapidity of diffusion is also dependent on other factors such as the chemical property of the gas species, diffusion distance, and transit time through the pulmonary capillary bed. *If some athletes become hypoxic due to the interaction of high cardiac output with decreased transit time, how do you think diffusivity would have to change to balance this out and eliminate the hypoxemia?*

## Ventilating the Lungs

Ventilation maintains an optimal composition of alveolar gases so that $P_{AO_2}$ remains above the venous $O_2$ tension ($P_{VO_2}$), and venous $CO_2$ tension ($P_{VCO_2}$) remains above $P_{ACO_2}$. In this way gas molecules diffuse along their respective concentration gradients, $CO_2$ being released to the atmosphere while $O_2$ is transported to body tissues. When we engage in exercise, $P_{O_2}$ decreases and $P_{CO_2}$ increases in venous blood. This necessitates an increase in ventilation in an effort to maintain $O_2$ and $CO_2$ **homeostasis**.

### VENTILATORY PARAMETERS

Ventilation is measured as the frequency of breathing multiplied by the volume depth of each breath, the **tidal volume** ($V_T$). Respiratory frequency and depth and other lung volumes and capacities are measured with a technique known as spirometry. During quiet breathing, respiratory depth is normally about 0.5 L, with a frequency of about 12 breaths (br)·min$^{-1}$. This results in a normal resting ventilation rate of 6 L·min$^{-1}$. This rate of ventilation, also called minute ventilation, increases during maximal exercise to as much as 198 L·min$^{-1}$ (45 br·min$^{-1}$ × 4.4 L·br$^{-1}$) in a well-trained endurance athlete. Regardless of whether an individual is at rest or exercise, minute ventilation is the total volume of air entering (inspiratory, $\dot{V}_I$) or leaving (expiratory, $\dot{V}_E$) the lungs each minute.

*Figure 6.9* is a spirogram showing the measurement of $V_T$ during quiet breathing and other lung volumes and capacities. A spirogram is a graphic output of the spirometric technique. Notice that the **total lung capacity** (TLC) is the maximum lung volume that can be achieved, usually about 5 to 6 L in normal adults. However, to measure TLC, **residual volume** (RV) (normally 1 to 1.2 L) must also be measured. The RV represents a reserve air supply in the lungs. TLC minus RV produces the **vital capacity** (VC), which is the largest breath that can be taken (about 4 to 5 L in adults depending on body size, especially height).

Figure 6.9 also shows that normal tidal breathing is close to the midrange of the TLC.

Other important pulmonary capacities are also shown in Figure 6.9. The **inspiratory capacity** (IC) is the volume between the end expiration of a tidal breath and the upper limits of the TLC. The limits of the IC can be defined in mechanical terms by the maximal limits of thoracic cage expansion in the anterior/posterior dimensions and also in the lateral and inferior/superior dimensions of the thorax. Individuals with **restrictive lung disease** have smaller ICs (restrictions to inspiration). Thoracic changes, such as kyphoscoliosis (rounding of the spine), can reduce thoracic excursion, thereby causing lung restriction by mechanical means. If the restriction is pulmonary in origin (e.g., interstitial fibrosis), lung **compliance** and diffusing capacity are reduced. Inspiratory capacity might also be smaller in mid- to end-stage emphysema because of the barrel-chest deformity which is characteristic of this form of **chronic obstructive pulmonary disease** (COPD) (*Fig 6.10*). In normal lifespan development of the chest structure, there is a rounded appearance in infancy, progressing to an elliptical appearance in adulthood and returning to a rounded appearance in normal aging. With COPD, the ribs become more horizontal and the antero-posterior diameter of the chest increases.

In end-stage emphysema, the barrel-shaped deformity of the chest limits the amount of real excursion (movement) remaining to allow a deep breath to be taken (and therefore the volume of air maximally inhaled). Diaphragmatic excursion is also decreased in individuals with COPD. Typically these patients have increased muscle activity of the respiratory accessory muscles and decreased diaphragmatic contribution to quiet breathing. Normal diaphragmatic excursion is 3 to 5 cm, but diaphragmatic

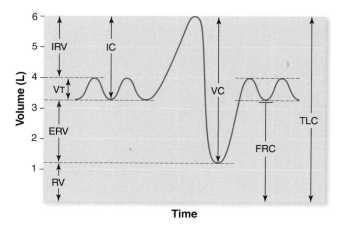

**FIGURE 6.9.** The spirometric tracing begins with lung volume changes during two normal tidal breaths (VT). After the two normal tidal breaths (~ 0.7 L), the subject made a maximal inspiration and maximal expiration to the residual volume (VC). After this maximal breath, the tracing ends with two more tidal breaths. IC, inspiratory capacity; FRC, functional residual capacity; IRV, inspiratory reserve volume; VT, tidal volume; ERV, expiratory reserve volume; RV, residual volume; VC, vital capacity; TLC, total lung capacity.

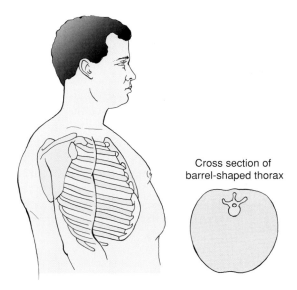

**FIGURE 6.10.** *Barrel chest* is the prominent chest wall configuration in chronic obstructive pulmonary disease (COPD) characterized by a loss of the normal elliptical thoracic architecture seen in normal adults. (Reprinted with permission from Weber J, Kelly J. *Health assessment in nursing.* 2nd ed. Philadelphia: Lippincott Williams & Wilkins, 2003.)

flattening is present in obstructive disease due to over-inflated lungs. The work of breathing is more difficult for individuals with COPD than for healthy individuals.

The **functional residual capacity** (FRC) is the volume of gas that remains in the lung after passive expiration. Normally FRC represents a volume that is 40% of TLC (2.0 to 2.4 L in adults). The inspiratory reserve volume is the difference between lung volume at the end of normal inspiration and the VC, and the amount of air that can be forced from the lung after normal expiration is the expiratory reserve volume (ERV) (Fig. 6.9). ERV is influenced by muscle strength and is smaller in those patients who cannot mount sufficient thoracic and abdominal muscle effort to expel air from the lungs. Individuals with advancing Guillain-Barre syndrome, polio, and other neuromuscular diseases have smaller FRCs than unaffected persons. However, in persons with COPD, FRCs are larger and lead to a series of other problems. *Figure 6.11* shows the proportional changes that occur in obstructive and restrictive lung diseases compared with the normal lung. In these diseases, exercise is limited by respiration as more energy is expended to breathe at rest compared with unaffected persons. Also, the breathing effort can be disproportionally increased with even minimal activity.

*LINKUP: Values for the various lung volumes and capacities are individually determined because lung volumes are affected by age and health status.* **Perspective: Lung Volumes and Capacities Between Sexes,** *featured at http://connection.lww.com/go/brownexphys and on the Student Resource CD-ROM, shows that lung volumes are also different between the sexes by virtue of the anthropomorphic differences between males and females.*

When defining lung ventilation, it is important to recognize that minute ventilation is always greater than alveolar ventilation, which is the amount of air ventilating the alveoli. $\dot{V}_A$ is the volume of air that enters the alveoli each minute, and its size is dependent on the size of the **anatomic dead space** (DS) and the $V_T$. The anatomic DS represents the volume of air in the conducting airways that does not participate in gas exchange (about 2 mL·kg$^{-1}$ body mass in adults). Alveolar ventilation, calculated as the difference between $V_T$ and DS multiplied by breathing frequency, is about 4.2 L·min$^{-1}$ ($0.5 - 0.15 \times 12$) in the normal resting adult. This represents 30% less air reaching the alveoli in the resting state than that which enters the lungs each minute. Using the example of minute ventilation during maximal exercise, 198 L·min$^{-1}$ (45 br·min$^{-1}$ $\times$ 4.4 L·br$^{-1}$), the air ventilating the alveoli in this example [$\dot{V}_A = (4.4 - 0.15) \times 45$] is 191.25 L·min$^{-1}$ or approximately 3% less air reaching the alveoli than entering the lungs at maximal exercise. The difference is due the fact that DS remains constant.

Another important pulmonary DS is the **physiologic dead space**, calculated as the sum of the anatomic DS and the **alveolar dead space**. Since air in the lungs is of little use unless the alveoli are adequately perfused with blood, the alveolar DS represents the volume of air in an alveolus that has no perfusion (i.e., respiratory gas exchange is not operative in these regions). The physiologic DS is normally 30% of the $V_T$, or about 0.15 L at rest. If the ratio of the

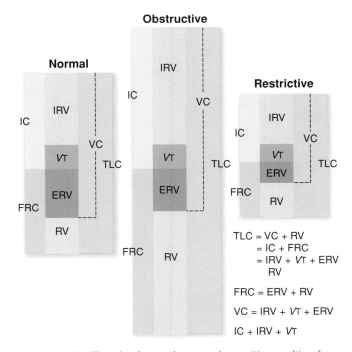

**FIGURE 6.11.** Changing lung volumes and capacities resulting from obstructive or restrictive lung disease compared to the normal lung. IC, inspiratory capacity; FRC, functional residual capacity; IRV, inspiratory reserve volume; VT, tidal volume; ERV, expiratory reserve volume; RV, residual volume; VC, vital capacity; TLC, total lung capacity.

physiologic DS to VT increases to 0.50 (0.25 ÷ 0.50) or greater, there is an extra ventilatory demand. This results in marked **dyspnea** (shortness of breath), as is the case, for example, in emphysema or pulmonary embolus.

In some cases or stages of emphysema, the $CO_2$ tension in the arterial blood is slightly elevated and is associated with increased ventilation. This is important in that it is the $Pa_{CO_2}$ and not the $Pa_{O_2}$ that regulates $\dot{V}_A$. Alveolar ventilation and $Pa_{CO_2}$ are inversely related. When ventilation is normal, $Pa_{CO_2}$ is approximately 40 mm Hg. This value either increases or decreases in states of hypo- or hyperven-

tilation, respectively. Hyperventilation (overbreathing), in which $\dot{V}_A$ is excessive for metabolic needs, is associated with a $Pa_{CO_2}$ of less than 35 mm Hg. In hypoventilation (underbreathing), $\dot{V}_A$ is too low for metabolic needs and less $CO_2$ is eliminated, resulting in a $Pa_{CO_2}$ greater than 45 mm Hg. *What effect do you think emphysema would have on gas exchange between the lungs and the blood passing through them?*

Figure 6.3 depicts the normal ventilation and perfusion matching process in the lungs with respect to $P_{O_2}$ and $P_{CO_2}$. In ideal conditions, when the $Pa_{CO_2}$ is 40 mm Hg, the

---

## CASE STUDY 6.1: *AIRWAY CONGESTION CAUSED BY ACUTE PNEUMONIA*

### CASE

Tom, a 50-year-old male, was admitted with acute **community-acquired** pneumonia. Signs and symptoms upon admittance were: body temperature 39.7°C, heart rate 115 beats·min$^{-1}$, respiratory rate 22 br·min$^{-1}$, dyspnea, pleuritic right-sided chest pain, hypoxia, and cough producing sputum. A chest x-ray after admission showed signs of consolidation (engorgement of the lungs) over the right middle and lower lobes, and the following arterial blood gases: $Pa_{O_2}$ = 70 mm Hg, $Pa_{CO_2}$ = 37 mm Hg, and $Sa_{O_2}$ = 88%. Diagnosis of the $O_2$ transport system reveals altered $O_2$ transport and gas exchange, airway obstruction, ventilation-perfusion mismatch, and ineffective breathing pattern due to edema and mucous buildup.

### DESCRIPTION

Several pulmonary conditions lead to a buildup of secretions that ultimately cause breathing difficulties. Pneumonia is the acute inflammation of the lung **parenchyma**, characterized by hypertrophy of the mucous membranes of the lung, respiratory acidosis, inflamed pleura, impaired gas exchange, and excess fluid in the interstitial spaces. Excess sputum production is a common symptom.

### INTERVENTION

The primary concern for correcting the altered cardiopulmonary function is to optimize alveolar volume and ventilation. Promotion of airway clearance is a main goal of therapy. Goals of management by the physical therapist include the following:

1. Reverse alveolar hypoventilation
2. Increase perfusion
3. Increase diffusion
4. Increase ventilation-perfusion matching
5. Ensure lymphatic drainage
6. Minimize the effects of increased mucous production

A total approach is advocated, and a combination of physical therapy interventions, especially postural drainage and mobilization, should be vigorously pursued. Intervention

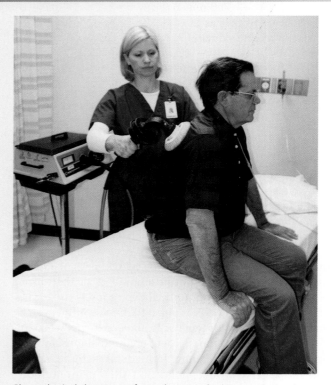

Chest physical therapy performed on a pulmonary patient using a mechanical percussor. Photo courtesy of Robert Clements, Our Lady of Lourdes Regional Medical Center, Lafayette, La.

is paced according to patient tolerance. Mobilization may include any of the following as tolerated by the patient: ambulation, cycle ergometry, activities of daily living, standing, transferring, dangling, turning in bed, and bed exercises. Proper rest is advocated between activities coordinated with deep breathing and coughing. Airway clearance treatment focuses on mucociliary clearance, reducing excess mucous accumulation, and reducing mucous stasis. Gravity-assisted passive postural drainage techniques allow the bronchopulmonary tree to be drained according to the specific lobe of the lung affected. While in this position, the patient can then be treated with other airway clearance techniques, such as percussion (see illustration).

PAO₂ is 102 mm Hg in subjects at sea level. These values and the others shown represent normal human adult resting values for gas partial pressures in inspired (I) air, alveolar (A) gas, and mixed venous ($\bar{v}$) blood arriving at the capillaries from the right ventricle via the pulmonary artery. The pulmonary veins carry oxygenated blood (a) to the left heart. When hypo- or hyperventilation alters PaCO₂, a necessary corollary is that PAO₂ is also affected. The relationship between PAO₂ and PaCO₂ is demonstrated in the alveolar gas equation:

$$PAO_2 = PIO_2 - PaCO_2[FIO_2 + (1 - FIO_2)/RER]$$

In this equation PIO₂ is determined by subtracting the partial pressure of water (seen earlier as 47 mm Hg) from the PB at sea level (760 mm Hg) and multiplying the result by FIO₂ (seen earlier as 20.93%). For example, at a PB of 730 mm Hg (approximately 1000-foot elevation), the PIO₂ = 143.0 mm Hg [(730 − 47) × 0.2093]. In Chapter 5 we saw that the respiratory exchange ratio (RER) was calculated as the ratio of CO₂ production to O₂ consumption (V̇CO₂ ÷ V̇O₂), approximately 0.8 at rest. Using the alveolar gas equation and these values, PAO₂ is calculated to be 95.1 mm Hg. In hypoventilatory conditions (increased PaCO₂), PAO₂ decreases; however, during hyperventilation (decreased PaCO₂), PAO₂ rises because total alveolar gas pressure cannot exceed PB. The most common cause of hypoventilation is respiratory failure, as happens in severe lung disease or nervous system depression. Hyperventilation can occur in hypoxia or anxiety. *Can you estimate the alveolar-arterial O₂ pressure gradient based on the following data from a man with smoke inhalation rescued from a fire? (Hint: he was put on 100% O₂.) PaCO₂ = 36 mm Hg; PB = 732 mm Hg.* Case Study 6.1 demonstrates the importance of these variables in clinical practice.

## THE VENTILATORY PUMP

The lungs together with the structures of the thoracic cavity, which include the rib cage, intercostal muscles, diaphragm, and other accessory breathing muscles collectively, act as a kind of breathing pump in external respiration. For a 70-kg adult, lung mass amounts to about 1 kg, or about 1.5% of a person's body mass, with the actual lung tissue amounting to about 60% and pulmonary blood volume accounting for the rest. Besides the lungs, however, the other structures of the breathing pump represent a considerably larger mass. These accessory structures include the diaphragm, chest wall, and airways. The diaphragm is the primary muscle of respiration and is responsible for about 75% of inspiration during quiet breathing. *Figure 6.12* shows the diaphragm in relation to the structures of the chest wall, as well as the intercostal muscles.

The accessory muscles in the neck region (sternocleidomastoids and the scaleni) assist in inspiration during exercise by pulling up on the upper ribs. The accessory muscles may also contract and help inspiratory movements as when inward airflow is limited in the case of respiratory failure (see *Fig 6.13*). The abdominal muscles assist in expiration during exercise as they contract, reducing the cross-sectional area of the abdominal cavity and increasing intraabdominal pressure, thereby providing an additional drive to help the diaphragm rebound toward the thoracic cavity. With the exception of the abdominal muscles, these structures form the thoracic cavity, a structure capable of changing its dimension in a rhythmic fashion to achieve the two phases of ventilation: *inspiration* and *expiration*.

The chest wall is lined by the parietal pleura. An intrapleural space occupied by a thin layer of liquid (approximately 20 μm thick, amounting to about 10 mL of plasma ultrafiltrate) that reduces friction and allows the pleura to glide over each other separates the parietal pleura from the visceral pleura (external lining of each lung). This liquid coupling of the pleura allows the lungs to slide along the chest wall during breathing. The lungs are separated from the chest wall only by these pleural membranes, which are in turn divided into right and left halves (i.e., right and left lung) by the mediastinum. Gas is not present in the intrapleural space until pathology or trauma produces a pneumothorax.

The diaphragm is dome-shaped, physically separates the thoracic and abdominal cavities, and is innervated by the two phrenic nerves arising out of the third to fifth cervical segments of the spinal cord (*Fig. 6.14A*). When stimulated to contract, the diaphragm moves downward, protruding into the abdominal cavity, and rotates the lower ribs toward the horizontal plane when in inspiration, which increases the cross-sectional area of the thoracic cavity (Fig. 6.14B). In expiration the opposite effect occurs; there is rib motion away from the horizontal plane

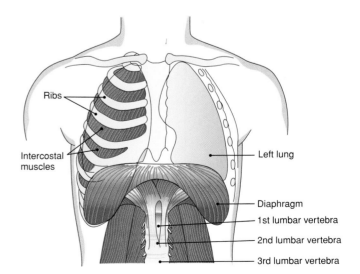

**FIGURE 6.12.** The diaphragm and respiratory muscles of the chest. The angle of the external intercostal muscles allows them to lift the rib cage when they contract and expand the chest, whereas the internal intercostal muscles act to lower the rib cage. (Reprinted with permission from Cohen BJ. *Memmler's the human body in health and disease.* 10th ed. Baltimore: Lippincott Williams & Wilkins, 2005.)

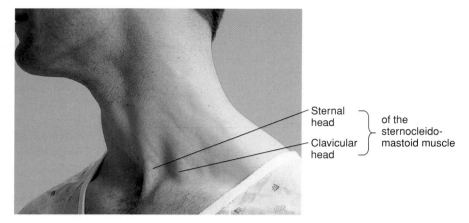

Sternal head ⎫
Clavicular head ⎬ of the sternocleido-mastoid muscle
⎭

**FIGURE 6.13.** Pulmonary patients with end-stage pulmonary disease must use the accessory breathing muscles even in resting ventilation. (Reprinted with permission from Bickley LS, Szilagyi P. *Bates' guide to physical examination and history taking.* 8th ed. Philadelphia: Lippincott Williams & Wilkins, 2003.)

and the thoracic cavity reduces in size as the diaphragm and ribs rebound to their original positions.

There must be a pressure differential between the atmosphere (ambient pressure) and the alveoli (alveolar pressure, PA) for airflow to be achieved. Therefore, in inspiration PA becomes subatmospheric, causing air to rush into the lungs; during expiration PA exceeds PB,

driving air out of the lungs. Achieving the cyclic inflow and outflow of air requires the cyclic alteration of PA produced by a change in pleural pressure. During inspiration, a reduction in the pressure in the pleural space surrounding the lungs is achieved as the thoracic cavity expands as a direct consequence of central nervous system stimulation of the diaphragm and intercostal

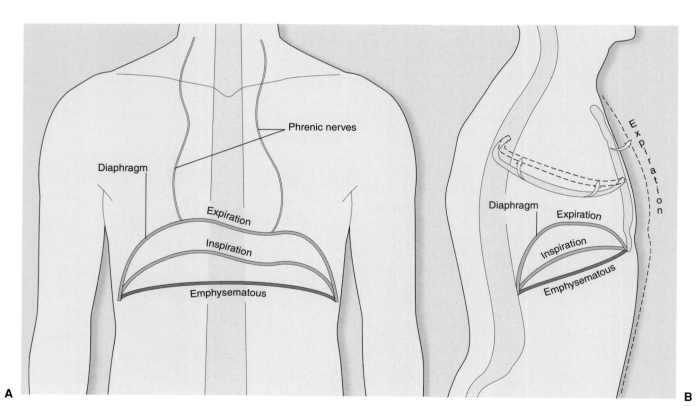

**A**

**B**

**FIGURE 6.14.** Diaphragm in the frontal **(A)** and lateral **(B)** views in the upright posture. In the frontal view, the diaphragm is shown in its expired and inspired positions. As it contracts downward in inspiration, the lower ribs flare (*arrows*) and the chest wall moves outward. In the lateral view, the chest and abdominal walls bulge in inspiration as the diaphragm shortens and moves downward. The ribs are shown rotating (I, pail-handle effect) as caused by diaphragmatic movement. The bottom solid line in both views shows the chronic (flattened) position of the diaphragm in severe emphysema.

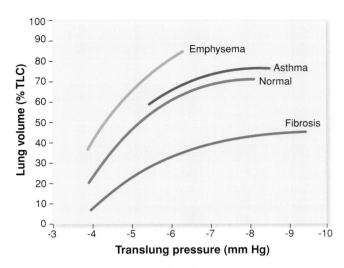

**FIGURE 6.15.** Distensibility (compliance) curves representing lungs with various chronic diseases.

muscles to contract. Because the lungs have an elastic quality, their volume changes as pleural pressure changes. In the case of inspiration, as the pleural pressure decreases, the distensible lungs expand passively, decreasing the P$_A$ and drawing air movement inward. Inward airflow stops when P$_A$ = P$_B$. During the passive process of expiration, the elastic recoil of the lungs and movement of the thoracic cavity back to its original shape

reverse the process of inward airflow. Pleural and alveolar pressures increase and air flows out of the lungs.

Compliance refers to the ease (or difficulty) with which the lungs (or chest wall) can be distended. Decreased compliance affects lung function by making it more difficult to fill (as in restrictive disease), and increased compliance affects lung function by making it more difficult to recoil and thus empty (as in obstructive disease). *Figure 6.15* shows the relationship of lung pressure to lung volume in normal and diseased lungs. In emphysema, an obstructive disease, air remains trapped in the lungs during exhalation. At any level of **translung pressure**, lung volume is greater in emphysema. In fibrosis, the decreased compliance leads to less filling at any given level of translung pressure.

▶ *INQUIRY SUMMARY.* The movement of gas molecules into and out of the lungs and across the alveolar-capillary interface requires the coordinated contraction of muscles of the thoracic cage that creates pressure differentials. *What do you think accounts for the approximately 10% greater lung volumes in athletes?*

## The Respiratory Tree

The upper respiratory passages consist of structures that perform important functions in ventilation: the nose, nasopharynx, oropharynx, oral cavity, and laryngopharynx (*Fig. 6.16*). The upper airways have several general

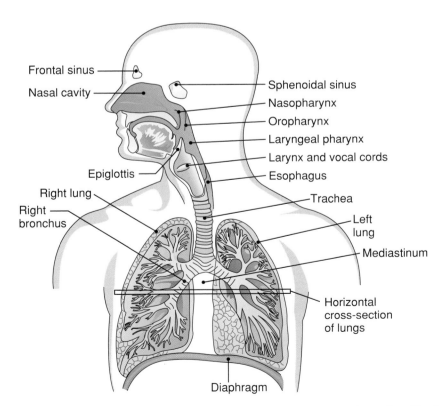

**FIGURE 6.16.** Sagittal section of the head and neck showing how the upper air passages connect to the trachea. (Reprinted with permission from Cohen BJ. *Memmler's the human body in health and disease*. 10th ed. Baltimore: Lippincott Williams & Wilkins, 2005.)

functions, which make ventilation much easier. The general functions of the upper airways are three-fold:

1. Conducting system for air to enter the lower airways
2. Protective barrier to prevent foreign objects or material from entering the respiratory tree
3. "Air conditioner" of the inspired air, with the mucous membranes warming and humidifying the air passing into the lungs

The upper airway is richly endowed with blood vessels which are located very close to the inner surface of the air passages, an anatomic arrangement that is necessary for the efficient exchange of heat. Additionally, the water/mucin blanket that covers the membrane surface of the upper airways humidifies the air as it passes over the membranes. The water/mucin blanket adds a large quantity of water to the inspired air, especially if the ambient air is dry. Several hundred mL of water per day are lost from the surface of the mucous membranes in the upper airways solely for the purpose of humidifying the inspired air. By the time inspired air has passed into the trachea, it is nearly 100% humidified and is warmed to the body's core temperature. However, during exercise when respiratory minute volumes are large, the air may not be fully humidified or warmed by the time it reaches the trachea. The lower airways are then involved in the task of conditioning the inspired air.

The larynx connects the pharynx with the trachea, and the trachea links the larynx to lungs. The larynx is the narrowest structure of the upper airway and its opening (the glottis) is protected from passage of solid objects during swallowing by the epiglottis, a leaf-shaped elastic cartilage. The larynx provides a significant amount of resistance to airflow, which is exploited in vocalization.

The upper airways have the sole purpose of conducting the inspired air to the alveolar-capillary interface where ventilation occurs. No $O_2$ or $CO_2$ exchange takes place in the upper respiratory passages; therefore, the total cross-sectional area of the conducting zone is much smaller than in the respiratory zone (*Fig. 6.17*). The portion of each breath residing in these divisions is wasted ventilation and constitutes the anatomic DS. This amounts to about 30% of each normal breath. *Figure 6.18* shows that the trachea is the first component (generation) of the respiratory tree, the branching set of tubes that link the respiratory surface to the atmosphere. The trachea branches after 12 cm (at about the sternal angle) into the two main-stem cartilaginous bronchi (second generation)—one for each lung. In turn these main bronchi branches give rise to two smaller branches (left lung) and three smaller branches (right lung). These branch divisions correspond to the number of different lobes of each lung (3 for the right and 2 for the left) and represent the third generation of the respiratory tree. The bronchi decrease in number and length with each successive branching, and the cartilaginous support gradually disappears until it is absent in tubes smaller than about 1 mm in diameter.

The upper portions of the respiratory tree are ciliated. The cilia beat rhythmically in a thin liquid layer and help to transport secreted mucus and inhaled particles out of the lung via the trachea. The cilia also gradually disappear with each successive generation. When there is no longer any cartilage or cilia in the smooth muscle of the airway, the term *bronchiole* is used. The bronchioles continue to divide until they become the last generation (terminal bronchioles) of the conducting (nonrespiratory) airways. The bronchioles constitute all the airways smaller than 1 mm in diameter. In all, there are 20 to 25 generations of conducting passages. Distally, the bronchioles develop outpouchings, which are the alveoli, and the first of the bronchioles to have alveoli are called respiratory bronchioles since they participate in gas exchange.

The lung **parenchyma** consists of the remaining divisions of the lung from division 17 to 23. This region of the lung is frequently called the peripheral lung and is the site at which emphysema occurs, a COPD. This portion of the lower airway is responsible for gas exchange.

The working unit of the lung—the area involved in gas exchange—is called the *acinus* and is comprised of the following divisions: the respiratory bronchiole, alveolar duct, alveolar sac, and alveoli. These structures all have $O_2$ and $CO_2$ exchange capabilities. However, the amount of gas exchange increases as air travels down the acinus toward the alveolus. For example, the respiratory bronchiole accounts for less than 5% of the total $O_2$–$CO_2$ exchange, whereas the alveolar sac and alveoli account for 70% or

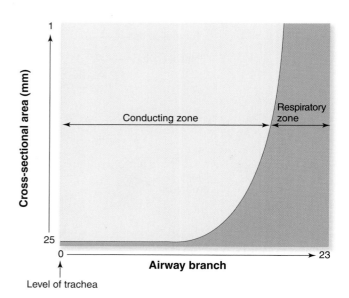

**FIGURE 6.17.** The increase in the cross-sectional area of the parts of the lung is seen in the transition from the conducting to respiratory zones. Airway branch refers to the successive generation of airway divisions, which become progressively smaller in diameter from about 25 mm for the diameter of the trachea to about 1 mm or less for the diameter of the bronchioles that terminate the conducting zone (branches 1–16). Beginning in the last few divisions of the conducting zone, the cross-sectional area increases exponentially.

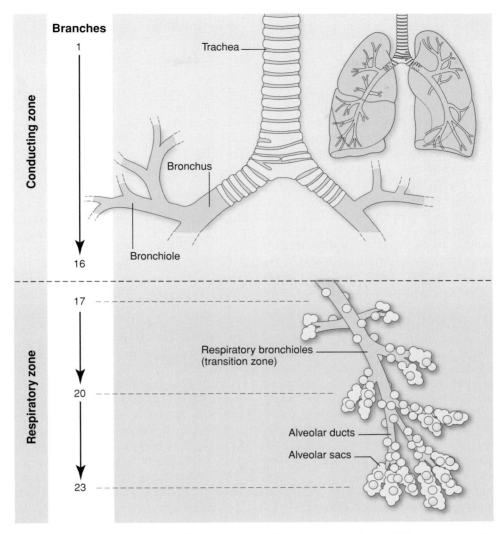

**FIGURE 6.18.** The trachea initiates the respiratory tree, which begins as a conducting zone (branches 1–16) but quickly transitions to the respiratory zone (branches 17–23).

more of all $O_2$–$CO_2$ exchange. The upper respiratory passages may become laden with secretions that make airflow leading to the gas exchange areas difficult. Case Study 6.2 provides an example of the kind of treatment often needed in patients demonstrating breathing difficulties.

▶ *INQUIRY SUMMARY.* A myriad of pathologic and physiologic situations may cause a disruption in external respiration. The challenge for the body is to overcome these disruptions so that breathing is maintained and life is sustained. *After reviewing case study 6.1, answer the following: How might clearance techniques differ for obstructions in different areas of the lungs?*

## Ventilation/Perfusion Matching

Ventilation is the process of gas exchange and pulmonary perfusion is the pulmonary arterial blood flow. These are almost but not identically matched in the normal lung. A useful index of how well this matching is occurring is the ventilation/perfusion ratio ($\dot{V}/\dot{Q}$; both values are expressed in like units, usually $L \cdot min^{-1}$). An adequate match between ventilation and perfusion maintains $Pa_{O_2}$ and $Pa_{CO_2}$ near their ideal levels (see Fig. 6.3).

### PULMONARY PERFUSION

As in other vascular beds, blood flow through the lungs is dependent on the perfusion pressure and **pulmonary vascular resistance** (defined as R = $\Delta P/\dot{Q}$). Blood flow is shown in the following equation:

$$\dot{Q} = \Delta P \div R$$

$\dot{Q}$ is blood flow rate (cardiac output), $\Delta P$ is the change in pressure from one end of the **pulmonary circuit** to the other, and R is the pulmonary vascular resistance (these variables are also discussed for the **systemic circuit** in

## CASE STUDY 6.2: *HYPOXEMIA*

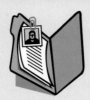

### CASE

Mark is a 16-year-old boy diagnosed with cystic fibrosis at the age of 2 years. He was recently hospitalized with a lower respiratory tract infection. He presented with green sputum, labored breathing, and cyanosis. Pulmonary function test results were: forced expiratory volume in one second: 45% of predicted, forced vital capacity: 58% of predicted, and midexpiratory flow rate: 56% of predicted. The arterial blood gases on 2 $L \cdot min^{-1}$ of $O_2$ were: $Pao_2$ = 65 mm Hg, $Paco_2$ = 51 mm Hg, $[HCO_3^-]$ = 31 $mEq \cdot L^{-1}$, and $Sao_2$ = 87%. A physical therapy diagnosis revealed altered cardiopulmonary function via an impaired gas exchange caused by alveolar hypoventilation secondary to cystic fibrosis. The patient was in acute respiratory acidosis with renal compensation, as indicated by the increased $[HCO_3^-]$.

below:

| PaO2 | SIGNS AND SYMPTOMS |
| --- | --- |
| 80–100 mm Hg | Normal |
| 60–80 mm Hg | Moderate tachycardia and possible onset of respiratory distress |
| 50–60 mm Hg | Malaise, lightheadedness, nausea, vertigo, impaired judgment, incoordination, restless, increased $\dot{V}E$ |
| 35–50 mm Hg | Marked confusion, cardiac arrhythmias, labored breathing |
| 25–35 mm Hg | Cardiac arrest, decreased renal blood flow, decreased urine output, lactic acidosis, poor oxygenation, lethargy, maximal $\dot{V}E$, loss of consciousness |
| <25 mm Hg | Decreased $\dot{V}E$ secondary to depression of the respiratory center |

### DESCRIPTION

Hypoxemia is low $Pao_2$, which can result from several causes: hypoxia, hypoventilation, ventilation/perfusion mismatching, right-to-left shunts, and diffusion problems across the alveolar-capillary membrane. $Pao_2$ ranges in the young adult from 90 to 100 mm Hg in the upright position, 85 to 95 mm Hg in the supine position, and 70 to 85 mm Hg during sleeping. In normal aging, $Pao_2$ decreases as a result of reduced alveolar surface area, pulmonary capillary blood volume, and diffusing capacity. The value for $Pao_2$ in normal older individuals can be calculated as 110 − 0.5(age). In older people, smokers, and individuals with pathology, the positional and sleep effects on $Pao_2$ are accentuated. Chronically low $Pao_2$ results in impaired cognitive function, constriction of the pulmonary capillary bed, increased pulmonary artery pressure, right-sided heart failure, cardiac arrhythmia, and eventually death. Common signs and symptoms of low $Pao_2$ are provided in the table

### INTERVENTION

Interventions should include mucous transport and maximizing alveolar ventilation (optimizing pulmonary gas exchange). **Deconditioning** is a major problem in these patients; therefore, their ability to transport $O_2$ should be optimized as well. A regular exercise program should help mobilize airway secretions, and with improved aerobic conditioning, further acute exacerbations of the condition may limit compromise of the $O_2$ transport system. In patients with an acute episode, restricted mobility should be minimized to lessen the deconditioning effect on the $O_2$ transport system. A long-term exercise training effect may also be an improved immune response, which will minimize the risk and severity of infection. As tolerated by the patient, treatment should include gradual and paced low-intensity mobilization (see Case 6.1) and frequent body position changes. Exercise as tolerated should be monitored for further $O_2$ desaturation as these patients become hypoxemic and distressed readily. Furthermore, a therapeutic exercise program to improve any postural malalignment or weak trunk and shoulder girdle muscles should be instituted as needed.

---

Chapter 7). Notice that P in Table 6.1 refers to pressure, whether the pressure resides in the pulmonary circuit, as in this example, or is the partial pressure of a gas.

Compared with pumping blood through the systemic circulation, about 85% less effort is required of the heart to pump blood through the pulmonary circuit. The difference is due to the large cross-sectional area of the pulmonary circulation, which results in a very low pulmonary vascular resistance ($\Delta P/\Delta \dot{Q}$). During exercise there is a considerable rise in cardiac output ($\dot{Q}$), which would normally dictate a large rise in pulmonary perfusion (driving) pressure. However, the pressure increase in the lungs is small, owing to

falling resistance of the pulmonary vessels. The falling resistance is due to two events: the recruitment of additional vessels and the passive distension of vessels that were already open. This phenomenon is illustrated in *Figure 6.19*, which shows a pressure-flow curve for the pulmonary circulation. The bend in the curve towards the flow axis as flow increases means that pulmonary vascular resistance decreases. If this did not occur, the pulmonary driving pressure would be greater. It is interesting to note that when a lung is partially removed (as is often necessary in cancer treatment), there is less vascular recruitment reserve remaining when the postoperative patient exercises. *What do you think would be the*

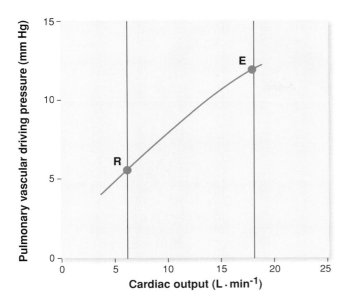

**FIGURE 6.19.** Representative pressure-flow curve theoretically obtained in the pulmonary circulation of a supine normal human. The curve is the pressure-flow plot at cardiac outputs of 6 and 18 L·min⁻¹ during rest (R) and steady-state exercise (E), respectively. The bend in the curve as flow rises demonstrates falling resistance in the pulmonary circuit with exercise.

*effect on pulmonary pressure during exercise in this situation and on the exercise capacity of this patient?*

Adequate perfusion of the lungs is based on the working pressures in the pulmonary venous and arterial systems. *Figure 6.20* shows the phasic and mean vascular pressures of the pulmonary and systemic circuits and those of the cardiac chambers. A distinction of the pulmonary circuit is the low resident pressures, which reduce the work of right cardiac pumping to approximately 16% (14 ÷ 90 = 0.16) of that required for the systemic circulation (left heart). This value corresponds roughly to the low level of resistance offered to blood flow in the pulmonary circuit compared with the rest of the body. This can be seen in the following comparison calculations for pulmonary vascular resistance (PVR) and systemic vascular resistance (SVR) using the values from Figure 6.20. In these calculations, resistance in a circuit is the ratio of $\Delta P$ (the change in vessel pressure from one end of the circuit to the next) to blood flow:

$$PVR = 6 \text{ mm Hg} \div 5 \text{ L·min}^{-1} = 1.2 \text{ mm Hg·L}^{-1}\text{·min}^{-1}$$

$$SVR = 87 \text{ mm Hg} \div 5 \text{ L·min}^{-1} = 17.4 \text{ mm Hg·L}^{-1}\text{·min}^{-1}$$

These calculations show that resistance in the pulmonary circuit is approximately 7% of the systemic circuit. Blood flow in this calculation is the typical resting value for cardiac output, or 5 L·min⁻¹

## PHYSIOLOGY OF $\dot{V}/\dot{Q}$ MATCHING

Lung perfusion refers to the pulmonary blood flow (the product of pulse rate and right ventricular stroke volume), which is typically 5 L·min⁻¹ at rest. Ventilation and perfusion are distinct physical processes that are closely matched so that, in the normal lung, a near ideal ventilation/perfusion ratio ($\dot{V}/\dot{Q}$) can exist. This ideal ratio would equal 1.0 if all parts of the lungs were equally ventilated and perfused, leading to an optimal gas exchange. For the lungs as a whole, however, the average value for the $\dot{V}/\dot{Q}$ ratio is about 0.84 ($\dot{V}A$ = 4.2 L·min⁻¹ and $\dot{Q}$ = 5.0 L·min⁻¹). This value does not hold true for all areas of the lung. Due to the effects of gravity, the upright lung is better perfused at the base than at the apex. Three pressures govern the flow of blood to different parts of the lung:

1. Hydrostatic pressure in the pulmonary arteries in different parts of the lungs, rising from base to apex
2. Pressure in the pulmonary veins
3. Pressure of the air in the alveoli

For the base of the lung, the higher blood flow (denominator of the $\dot{V}/\dot{Q}$ ratio) means that $\dot{V}/\dot{Q}$ is low (estimated at approximately 0.6). As you advance up the upright lung, local blood flow falls about three times faster than ventilation, ensuring that the $\dot{V}/\dot{Q}$ ratio will increase progressively. The increase is gradual at first, but then at a point beyond two-thirds of the way up, the ratio rises steeply to a value greater than 3 at the apex (*Fig. 6.21*). In the upper quadrant of the lung during exercise, the $\dot{V}/\dot{Q}$ ratio will be still higher because ventilation increases disproportionately more than pulmonary blood flow. In fact, ventilation-perfusion matching is improved during exercise, indicating that the blood entering the pulmonary circuit is more than adequately ventilated at the alveoli.

Neither ventilation nor blood flow is uniformly distributed throughout the entire lung, and mismatching alveolar ventilation to alveolar blood flow most commonly causes systemic arterial hypoxemia in patients with cardiopulmonary disease. In optimal matching ($\dot{V}/\dot{Q}$ = 1.0), as in the mid-regions of the lung, the alveoli are well perfused and ventilated, allowing blood to equilibrate with the alveolar air and become arterialized. In alveoli that are poorly ventilated but well perfused ($\dot{V}/\dot{Q}$ < 1.0), as in the lower lung, $PO_2$ and $PCO_2$ in alveolar air equilibrate with the blood, resulting in lower $PO_2$ but almost normal $PCO_2$. Lastly, in the upper regions of the lung, the alveoli are well ventilated but poorly perfused ($\dot{V}/\dot{Q}$ > 1.0), resulting in a lowering of the $PCO_2$ as more $CO_2$ is lost from the blood due to a favorable pressure gradient. This situation also occurs in heavy exercise.

The following is a brief clinical example illustrating ventilation-perfusion mismatching in a 35-year-old healthy man who fainted while running up an incline. The following values were recorded subsequent to this episode: mean pulmonary pressure: 45 mm Hg; mean right atrial pressure: 16 mm Hg; mean right ventricular pressure: 17 mm Hg; mean left atrial pressure: 15 mm Hg; cardiac

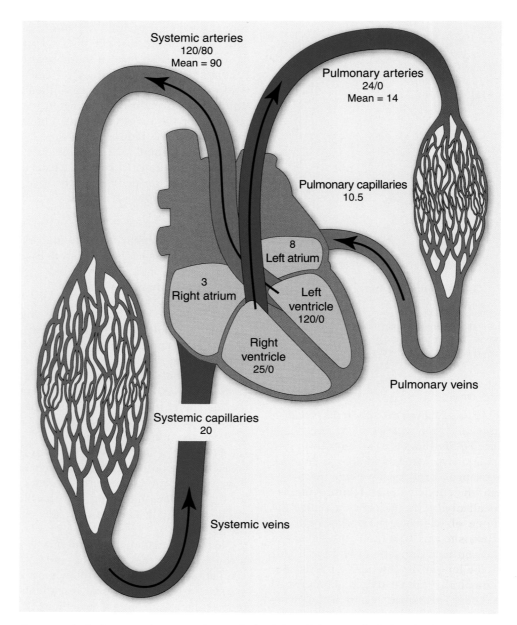

**FIGURE 6.20.** Normal pressures in the human pulmonary and systemic circulations. Values are phasic (systolic/diastolic) and mean pressures in mm Hg. At rest the driving pressure in the systemic circuit (Pa − Pra) is 87 mm Hg (90 − 3), but it may rise during moderate exercise to 100 mm Hg (considering an increase in the mean pressure of systemic arteries from 90 to 103 mm Hg). This is compared with the driving pressure in the pulmonary circuit of 6 mm Hg (14 − 8). Since cardiac output has to remain the same in both circuits because the circuits are in series, the resistance to flow through the lungs is less than 10% that of the systemic circuit.

output: 3.0 L·min⁻¹. Based on these values, the pulmonary vascular resistance can be calculated, which permits an answer to each of the following questions:

1. *What is the relationship of the calculated PVR in this case to the normal SVR and what are the physiologic implications?*
2. *If this individual's V̇ is 4.2 L·min⁻¹, what is the V̇/Q̇ ratio?*
3. *Given the value for V̇/Q̇ in this example, do you think this individual's blood gases are normal or abnormal (comment further if abnormal)?*

▶ **INQUIRY SUMMARY.** The ventilation-perfusion ratio is not uniform, and it deviates markedly with postural position and disease states. In exercise, ventilation-perfusion matching is improved, indicating that the blood entering the pulmonary circuit will be more than adequately ventilated at the alveoli. *What would be the effect on ventilation-perfusion matching and exercise performance if ventilation during exercise only increased in proportion to lung perfusion? Be sure that there is a physiologic basis for your answer.*

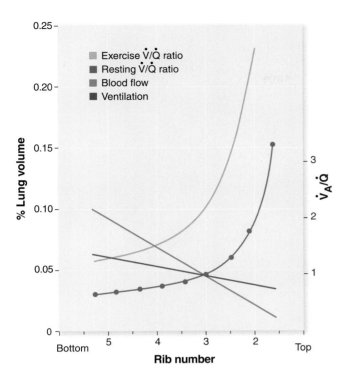

**FIGURE 6.21.** The distribution of ventilation, blood flow, and the ventilation-perfusion ratio in the normal upright lung at rest and during exercise.

## *Transport of Oxygen and Carbon Dioxide*

Respiratory gas exchange occurs at the alveolar-capillary level in the lung and the capillary-tissue level systemically (*Fig. 6.22*). Since all organ systems depend on $O_2$ to varying degrees, one of the primary functions of the cardiovascular system is to transport $O_2$ from the lungs to systemic capillaries and to transport $CO_2$ from systemic capillaries back to the lungs. Understanding this interaction is essential to a well-rounded appreciation of the physiology of exercise in health and disease.

### OXYGEN TRANSPORT

The $O_2$ content of blood equals both dissolved $O_2$ and $O_2$ bound to hemoglobin. The solubility of $O_2$ in blood is low, and the amount of dissolved $O_2$ at a $PaO_2$ of 100 mm Hg is equal to just 3 mL $O_2 \cdot L^{-1}$ of blood. This is only about 1.5% of the total $O_2$ carried in blood at rest, and this amount decreases even more during maximal exercise. However, in the clinical care of patients on supplemental $O_2$ ($FIO_2 = 1$), dissolved $O_2$ represents 30% to 40% of the total $O_2$ carried at rest and about half this value during maximal exercise. Resting whole-body metabolism requires about 250 mL $O_2 \cdot min^{-1}$; therefore, if dissolved $O_2$ was the only means by which the blood was able to carry $O_2$ to the tissues, the heart would have to pump more than 80 L of blood each minute to supply the $O_2$ required to sustain metabolism. These facts mean that dissolved $O_2$ plays a minor role in $O_2$ transport, which leads to the question: *What is the physio-*

*logic role of dissolved $O_2$?* First, it is the $O_2$ dissolved in plasma not $O_2$ bound to hemoglobin that determines the $PO_2$ in venous and arterial blood. Second, as we will see, the $PO_2$ dictates how much $O_2$ is bound to hemoglobin, making $PO_2$ determinative in the process of loading and unloading $O_2$ at different locations (lungs versus tissues) of the body.

### Role of Hemoglobin

Fortunately, the majority of the $O_2$ carried in blood is in combination with hemoglobin, an $O_2$-binding protein contained within red blood cells. Each hemoglobin molecule contains a protein part (globin) consisting of four polypeptide chains and four nitrogen-containing pigment molecules (hemes). The hemoglobin molecule depicted in *Figure 6.23* shows that each of the four polypeptide groups is combined with one heme group.

The center of each heme group contains one atom of ferrous iron ($Fe^{2+}$), which combines loosely with one molecule of $O_2$. Therefore, the $O_2$-binding capacity of one

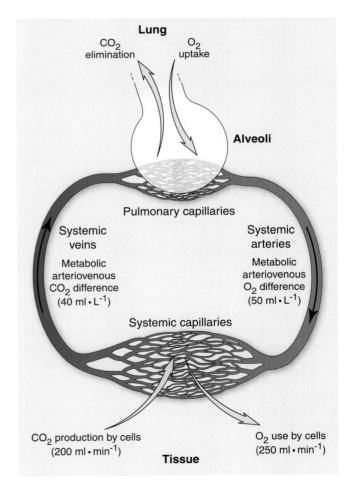

**FIGURE 6.22.** The process of external and internal respiration at rest, showing that $O_2$ is carried from the pulmonary capillaries to the systemic capillaries by the systemic arteries, and $CO_2$ is carried from the systemic capillaries to the pulmonary capillaries by the systemic veins.

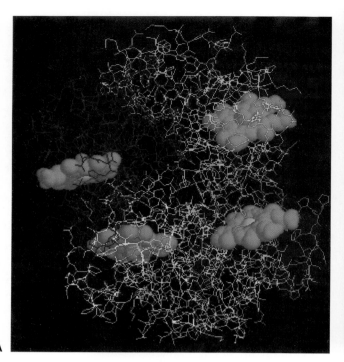
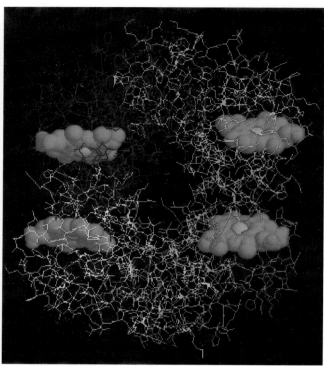

**FIGURE 6.23.** The quaternary structure of the hemoglobin molecule showing the four peptide chains (two α and two β chains). Each peptide chain has a single heme group which binds a single $O_2$ molecule, allowing one molecule of hemoglobin to carry four molecules of $O_2$. **A.** The oxy form (note the collapsed central cavity due to extrusion of 2,3-BPG upon oxygenation), and the deoxy form (note the empty central cavity occupied by 2,3-BPG) of the molecule **(B)**.

molecule of hemoglobin is four $O_2$ molecules. When bound to $O_2$, hemoglobin is designated as oxyhemoglobin ($HbO_2$); when $O_2$ dissociates from $HbO_2$, the resultant molecule is referred to as *deoxyhemoglobin*. Hemoglobin fully saturated with $O_2$ is bright red. However, when hemoglobin progressively loses its $O_2$ molecules, the bright red color becomes more and more dull in appearance. The molecule becomes a deep purple when most of the $O_2$ is lost, producing the darker color associated with venous blood compared to arterial blood. If deoxyhemoglobin exceeds 5 $g \cdot dL^{-1}$ of blood, the skin and mucous membranes appear blue, signaling the onset of **cyanosis**, a condition encountered in people with breathing and/or circulatory problems.

The amount of hemoglobin bound to $O_2$ is described in two ways: the $O_2$ *content* measured in $mL \cdot L^{-1}$ of blood and the $O_2$ *capacity* measured as the relative percentage ($O_2$ saturation, $SO_2$) of the maximum amount that can be bound. *Figure 6.24* shows these two measures (one on each Y-axis) of the $HbO_2$ dissociation curve, and *Figure 6.25* demonstrates the exercise response.

Referring to the right Y-axis of Figure 6.25, the $HbO_2$ dissociation curve can be used to determine an important variable in cardiovascular physiology, the arterial to mixed venous $O_2$ difference ($\Delta a - \bar{v}O_2$), described in greater detail in Chapter 7. Figure 6.25 shows that under resting conditions ($PaO_2 = 100$ mm Hg and $PvO_2 = 40$ mm Hg), the difference in $O_2$ content between arterial and venous

blood, that amount unloaded to the tissues, is 4.5 mL $O_2 \cdot dL^{-1}$ of blood flow through the tissues. This value is increased during exercise due to the rightward shift in the curve and the lower $PO_2$ as a result of the increase in active muscle metabolism.

Hemoglobin is essential for the transport of $O_2$, with which it combines *rapidly* (speed is essential as blood remains in the pulmonary and systemic capillaries less than 1 second) and *reversibly* (hemoglobin must be able to both receive and give up $O_2$ readily to serve as an effective $O_2$ carrier in metabolism). The extent to which the transported $O_2$ is dependent on hemoglobin is illustrated by the fact that hemoglobin increases the $O_2$-carrying capacity of blood by 65 times. Therefore, almost all of the $O_2$ transported in arterial blood is chemically bound to hemoglobin.

Hemoglobin is an **allosteric** compound. This means that it changes its structure based on the $PO_2$ in the blood. Hemoglobin changes shape slightly as the $SO_2$ of blood changes. For example, as hemoglobin arrives at the alveolar-capillary interface in the lung where it can take up $O_2$, it is folded in such a way that most of the $O_2$ binding sites are covered. As one site takes on an $O_2$, hemoglobin slightly reconfigures itself, uncovering another site to bind $O_2$. As the hemoglobin takes on more $O_2$ molecules, the hemoglobin molecule progressively unfolds and assumes its saturated shape—a shape that is characteristic of hemoglobin when it is maximally bound with four $O_2$ molecules.

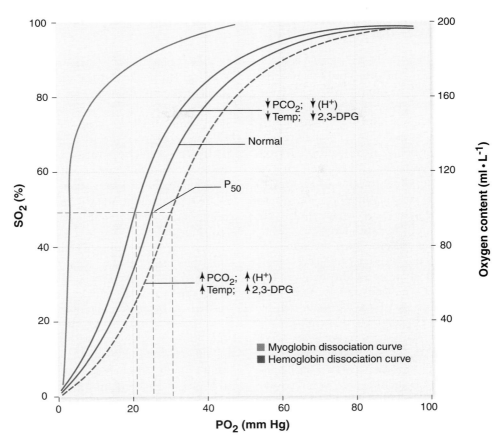

**FIGURE 6.24.** The $HbO_2$ dissociation curve for a $Pco_2$ of 40 mm Hg at 37°C (center curve). Under these conditions the $P_{50}$ is 26 mm Hg (the partial pressure at which hemoglobin is 50% saturated). When any of the four physiologic factors shown on the illustration is increased, the curve is shifted to the right and downward (dashed line). This shift leads to a decreased affinity of hemoglobin for $O_2$ ($O_2$ is bound more loosely). When any of the four physiologic factors is decreased, the curve shifts to the left of normal and the hemoglobin molecule binds more tightly to the $O_2$ molecule. Also shown is the oxymyoglobin dissociation curve, with a $P_{50}$ of 5 mm Hg (the normal intracellular $Po_2$ of muscle).

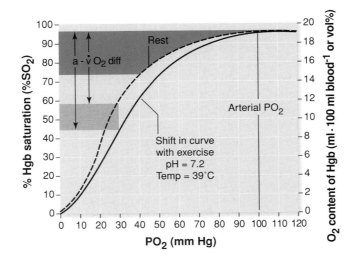

**FIGURE 6.25.** The $HbO_2$ dissociation curve during rest and exercise showing the shift to the right under exercise conditions (solid S-shaped curve) and the attendant increase in $\Delta a - \bar{v}O_2$. The red area shows the extent of $O_2$ extraction (19.5 − 15.0 = 4.5 mL $O_2 \cdot 100$ mL$^{-1}$ blood) at rest (venous $Po_2$ = 40 mm Hg and arterial $Po_2$ = 100 mm Hg). The yellow area shows that there is an extra 3 mL of $O_2$ per 100-mL blood extraction owing to the steep part of the curve as the $Po_2$ drops an additional 10 mm Hg. As the curve shifts to the right with exercise, the green area shows that even when $Po_2$ is maintained at 30 mm Hg, $O_2$ extraction is increased further by 3 mL $O_2 \cdot 100$ mL$^{-1}$ blood.

The progressive ease with which the molecule can add an additional $O_2$ after receiving the previous $O_2$ is referred to as *cooperativity*. This causes the molecule to display sigmoidal (S-shaped) $O_2$ kinetics. The S shape of the dissociation curve reflects the alterations in hemoglobin's affinity for $O_2$ as partial pressure is varied in the circulatory system. The sigmoidal nature of the dissociation curve is physiologically significant because as $PO_2$ falls from 100 mm Hg to about 60 mm Hg, the saturation of the hemoglobin molecule decreases by only about 10%. However, as the $PO_2$ falls below 60 mm Hg, the curve becomes relatively steep so that small changes in $PO_2$ cause large changes in the degree of hemoglobin saturation. When the hemoglobin molecule releases $O_2$ in the periphery to a cell, the allosteric or conformational changes in the hemoglobin structure reverse as it loses $O_2$ molecules to the cell.

The allosteric binding and release of $O_2$ is affected by the concentrations of $O_2$ and hemoglobin in the blood. We have already discussed how concentration gradients effect $O_2$ movement across membranes. The presence of an $O_2$ gradient also affects the allosteric changes seen in hemoglobin. This means that hemoglobin is able to receive $O_2$ when it is in the pulmonary capillaries where there is a high $O_2$ tension in the alveolus. If it were not for hemoglobin's ability to change its conformational shape according to the $SO_2$ of the blood, $O_2$ would be irreversibly bound to hemoglobin and would never cross over into the cells of the body.

Four other physiologic factors also cause conformational changes in hemoglobin's tertiary structure. These are: $H^+$ concentration $[H^+]$, $PCO_2$, temperature, and 2,3-bisphospho-glycerate (2,3-BPG). The position of the dissociation curve shifts as these factors vary; therefore, a standard position for the curve has been set at a pH of 7.4, $PCO_2$ of 40 mm Hg, and T of 37°C. At these conditions, hemoglobin is 50% saturated with $O_2$ at a $PO_2$ of 26 mm Hg, the $P_{50}$. The $P_{50}$ increases (decreased affinity, shift to the right of the dissociation curve) when any of these factors increase. For instance, when local metabolism increases (as in exercise), local temperature and $[H^+]$ rise and hemoglobin dissociates from $O_2$ more easily, liberating more $O_2$ to the cells that need it to sustain the increase in aerobic metabolism. The opposite happens when any of the four factors decrease ($P_{50}$ decreases, increased affinity for $O_2$ and there is a shift to the left of the dissociation curve). Shifting of the dissociation curve under differing physiologic conditions is referred to as the *Bohr effect*. The shift in the curve has a significant effect on tissue $O_2$ extraction. Referring again to Figure 6.25, an extra unloading of $O_2$ on the order of about 29% is demonstrated by the shift in the curve. *Can you determine this percent increase for yourself by reading across the right Y-axis of the figure? How does this shift help individuals when performing maximal exercise?*

The effect of changing $[H^+]$ is caused by the greater affinity hemoglobin has for $H^+$ than for $O_2$, causing a lower $SO_2$ at any given $PO_2$. The principle effect of $CO_2$ is through its ability to release $H^+$ (increasing $[H^+]$) as carbonic acid is formed in plasma in the carbonic anhydrase reaction (explained in the following section). Lastly, the compound 2,3-BPG is present in red blood cells in higher amounts than in other cells because red blood cell metabolism is 100% glycolytic (the cells being void of mitochondria). 2,3-BPG is produced in red blood cells as a side reaction to anaerobic glycolysis, and 2,3-BPG binds more strongly to deoxyhemoglobin, reducing the affinity of hemoglobin for $O_2$. The production of 2,3-BPG increases during hypoxic conditions, and its role in exercise training has been extensively studied.

Oxymyoglobin stores $O_2$ in skeletal muscle and is structurally similar to a single globin chain of $HbO_2$ with its heme group. Oxymyoglobin's dissociation curve lies far to the left of the $HbO_2$ curve, and it is also distinguished by its hyperbolic shape (Fig. 6.24). Myoglobin has a higher affinity for $O_2$ than does hemoglobin, allowing it to *irreversibly* bind with $O_2$, giving directionality to the molecule and allowing $O_2$ to be transferred to the mitochondria in muscle fibers. Since intramuscular $PO_2$ may be as low as 5 mm Hg during heavy exercise, there is an increased tendency for the molecule to give up $O_2$ at these low partial pressures.

The factors affecting arterial blood gas tension are important in clinical care. For instance, in the geriatric patient, cardiac output (Q), residual volume (RV), and maximal breathing capacity gradually decrease from age 60 to 90 years. This affects the $PaO_2$ by reducing it by 1 mm Hg per year over this timespan. Oxygen saturation is important to monitor in patients with cardiopulmonary dysfunction because **desaturation** may occur to a further extent during periods of increased physical activity or exercise.

## Effects in Exercise

The concentration of hemoglobin in blood is about 15.0 $g \cdot dL^{-1}$ in males and 13.5 $g \cdot dL^{-1}$ in females. Each g of hemoglobin can combine with 1.34 mL of $O_2$, giving the hemoglobin in 1 L of blood the capacity to combine with about 200 mL of $O_2$ at 100% hemoglobin saturation. Thus, for a normal adult female, when the $PO_2$ is close to 100 mm Hg, as in the arterial blood, the hemoglobin is 97% saturated and the $O_2$ content of the blood is $13.5 \times 1.34 \times 0.97 = 17.5$ mL $O_2 \cdot dL^{-1}$ bound to hemoglobin *plus* 0.3 mL of $O_2$ dissolved in physical solution, giving a total $O_2$ content of 17.8 mL $O_2 \cdot dL^{-1}$ blood. *Calculate the value of this variable for the average male. Also, speculate on the degree to which these disparate values for males and females differentially affect maximal aerobic exercise performance.*

This value is representative of the average untrained female. With aerobic exercise training, the absolute quantity of $O_2$ in the blood increases by about 12% owing to the increase in blood volume, which occurs rapidly with training at any age (1,2). Since blood volume is directly related to the amount of $O_2$ transported to tissues, the increase in blood volume not only increases the absolute quantity of $O_2$ carried but also contributes to the increase in aerobic power of the individual as well. Using the example of the average untrained female previously cited, starting from a typical absolute blood volume of 4 L, an extra 0.5 L can be added with exercise training. This represents an extra 87.5 mL of $O_2$ (175 mL $O_2 \cdot L^{-1}$ blood $\times$ 0.5 L) transported after training. This increase in absolute blood volume and $O_2$ carried tracks well the increase in peak $\dot{V}O_2$ experienced with exercise training.

In addition to the increase in absolute $O_2$ content of blood following exercise training, there is an increase in the relative $O_2$ content during acute exercise caused by **hemoconcentration**. Hemoconcentration causes a 10% increase in hemoglobin concentration in blood. In our earlier example using a female subject, this would increase the hemoglobin concentration from 13.5 g·dL$^{-1}$ to 14.9 g·dL$^{-1}$. *Calculate the increase in the relative and absolute $O_2$-carrying capacity of blood that occurs from acute hemoconcentration.*

 *LINKUP: $O_2$ is continually being used and as such, there is very little $O_2$ reserve in the body. See* **Perspective: Storing Oxygen in the Body,** *found at http://connection.lww.com/go/brownexphys and on the Student Resource CD-ROM, for an explanation of the concept of body $O_2$ reserve.*

## CARBON DIOXIDE TRANSPORT

During steady-state conditions (i.e., resting or submaximal exercise), approximately 80 molecules of $CO_2$ are exhaled from the lungs for every 100 molecules of $O_2$ taken up from the alveoli into pulmonary capillary blood. This level of external respiration represents a *RER* of 0.8. As was discussed in Chapter 5, the term RER is specific to respiration at the lungs and describes the $\dot{V}CO_2/\dot{V}O_2$ ratio measured by collecting respiratory gases at the mouth. In steady-state conditions, **internal respiration** approximates the rate of external respiration so that the rates of $CO_2$ production ($\dot{V}CO_2$) and $O_2$ consumption ($\dot{V}O_2$) yield a respiratory quotient that is the same magnitude as that of the RER. The term *respiratory quotient* is specific to respiration at the cell, describing the $\dot{V}CO_2/\dot{V}O_2$ ratio measured for any specific tissue by assaying gases in arterial and venous blood perfusing and draining, respectively, a particular vascular bed.

Internal respiration ensures that $O_2$ is continually removed from the blood and that $CO_2$ is continually being added to the blood. If there were no mechanism to carry off $CO_2$, a waste product of cellular metabolism, the local concentrations would build rapidly until cell death occurred. Fortunately, there are mechanisms whereby $CO_2$ is carried back to the pulmonary system and disposed of in the external atmosphere. These mechanisms involve carrying $CO_2$ in the blood in three different forms: in physical solution as dissolved gas; as **bicarbonate** ions ($HCO_3^-$); and as carbamino compounds (a combination between $CO_2$ and free amino groups on proteins). *Figure 6.26* illustrates these transport mechanisms.

When considering the $CO_2$ content of tissues, the difference between amounts of $CO_2$ and $O_2$ may be as great as tenfold (3). This is because $CO_2$ is 23 times more soluble than $O_2$ in plasma. The solubility of $CO_2$ is 0.07 mL·dL$^{-1}$·mm

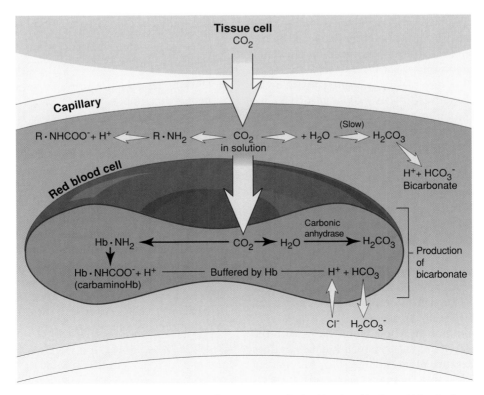

**FIGURE 6.26.** Schematic representation of $CO_2$ transport in the blood and in the red blood cell.

$Hg^{-1}$, but $O_2$ solubility is only 0.003 $mL \cdot dL^{-1} \cdot mm\ Hg^{-1}$. Therefore, at a normal arterial $P_{CO_2}$ of 40 mm Hg, the amount of $CO_2$ transported in solution is equal to 2.8 $mL \cdot dL^{-1}$ blood. Because of its higher solubility, about 6% of total blood $CO_2$ is in physical solution compared with 1.5% of $O_2$ dissolved in arterial blood. The concentration of dissolved $CO_2$ in venous blood is greater than that in arterial blood—about 3.2 $mL \cdot dL^{-1}$ of blood—which is still about 6% of the total amount transported in venous blood.

$CO_2$ rapidly diffuses out of the cell due to its higher intracellular versus blood concentration. Once $CO_2$ diffuses out of the cell, it moves quickly into the red blood cells (Fig. 6.26). Once inside the red blood cell, $CO_2$ is chemically converted in the presence of water by the enzyme carbonic anhydrase to carbonic acid ($H_2CO_3^-$) and finally into a hydrogen ion ($H^+$) and $HCO_3^-$. These reversible reactions are summarized in the formula:

Carbonic anhydrase

$$CO_2 + H_2O \leftrightarrow H_2CO_3^- \leftrightarrow H^+ + HCO_3^-$$

This reaction would spontaneously occur too slowly to accommodate the great amount of $CO_2$ which the body continually makes if it were not for the presence of carbonic anhydrase—a ubiquitous enzyme that drives the reaction very rapidly, ensuring that all of the $CO_2$ which the body manufactures can be chemically buffered and transformed into a less harmful substance. Carbonic anhydrase speeds up this reaction by more than 10,000-fold. The $H^+$ that is formed binds to and is buffered by hemoglobin, and the $HCO_3^-$ ionically associates with a positive ion, usually potassium, in the cytoplasm of red blood cells. The red blood cell membrane is very permeable to $HCO_3^-$ and other anions so that they diffuse rapidly between the red blood cell and plasma along their concentration gradients. Because electrical neutrality must be maintained in solutions, the $HCO_3^-$ flux into plasma is balanced with a $Cl^-$ flux into the red blood cell. This exchange of $Cl^-$ for $HCO_3^-$ in tissue or pulmonary capillaries is called the *chloride shift*, and it accounts for the fact that $Cl^-$ is lower in venous blood than in arterial blood. The $HCO_3^-$ mechanism for transporting $CO_2$ to the lungs accounts for approximately 90% of the $CO_2$ transported in arterial blood and 87% in venous blood. This mechanism is physiologically useful because it allows large amounts of $CO_2$ to be carried in the blood as $HCO_3^-$, which does not appreciably alter the pH of blood. Lastly, about 4% (7% in venous blood) of the $CO_2$ carried in blood is in the form of carbaminohemoglobin, $CO_2$ bound to the amine side groups available on the amino acids in hemoglobin. Also in this category is the $CO_2$ carried in combination with plasma proteins to form carbamino compounds.

The $CO_2$ concentration in whole blood varies with the $P_{CO_2}$, but $CO_2$ does not exhibit S-shaped kinetics as does $O_2$. Rather, over the range of physiologic $P_{CO_2}$ (40 mm Hg in arterial blood and 46 mm Hg in venous blood), the $CO_2$ dissociation curve follows more of a linear response (*Fig.*

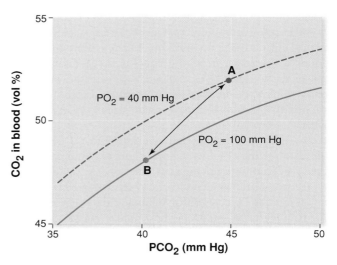

**FIGURE 6.27.** $CO_2$ dissociation curves when $P_{O_2}$ is 100 mm Hg or 40 mm Hg. The arrow depicts the Haldane effect for $CO_2$ transport. The solid curve is showing a $P_{O_2}$ of 100 mm Hg as is the case for the blood capillaries in the lungs, and the dashed curve is showing a $P_{O_2}$ of 40 mm Hg as is the case for the tissue capillaries. Working point A on the dashed curve is a $P_{CO_2}$ of 45 mm Hg in the tissues. Notice that at this point the content of $CO_2$ is about 52 volumes percent. When $CO_2$ enters the lungs (solid curve), the $P_{CO_2}$ falls to 40 mm Hg and $P_{O_2}$ rises to 100 mm Hg. The Haldane effect dictates that the shift in the curve's position allows more unloading of $CO_2$ in the lungs. This amounts to an extra 2 volumes percent of $CO_2$ unloaded (point B). The cause of this is the increased $P_{O_2}$ in the lungs, allowing additional binding of $O_2$ to hemoglobin and displacing $CO_2$ from the blood.

6.27). Another difference between the $CO_2$ and $O_2$ dissociation curves is that the $CO_2$ dissociation curve does not become saturated even at high $P_{CO_2}$ levels. $CO_2$ affinity of the blood changes when $HbO_2$ levels vary. This is referred to as the Haldane effect and is caused by two main factors:

- $HbO_2$ is less able to form carbamino compounds than deoxyhemoglobin
- $HbO_2$ is a less efficient buffer of $H^+$ than deoxyhemoglobin

These factors have the effect of allowing $H^+$ to be carried off more rapidly than in pulmonary capillary blood because there is less $HbO_2$ in the tissues. This encourages more $CO_2$ to be carried as $HCO_3^-$. However, in the lungs where the $CO_2$ content in blood is lower than in the tissues, 97% of the hemoglobin is in the oxy form compared to the tissues where $HbO_2$ makes up about 75% of the total hemoglobin. Therefore, more $CO_2$ may be carried when $HbO_2$ is low as in the tissues, the site of $CO_2$ production. The regulation of $CO_2$ in the body is indispensable to acid-base balance. This is covered in the next section on control of respiration.

▶ *INQUIRY SUMMARY.* If it were not for hemoglobin's dynamic allosteric (conformational) changes, it would be very difficult to utilize hemoglobin-bound $O_2$ in the body. Changes in $P_{O_2}$ across compartments (concentration gradients), as well as changes in temperature and pH, allow us to transport and utilize $O_2$ as a molecule. $CO_2$ is rendered into a less harmful substance when it is converted to $HCO_3^-$. Primarily as $HCO_3^-$, $CO_2$ is carried to the lungs where it diffuses down its concentration gradient across the alveolar-capillary interface and is exhaled to the environment. *How would a 20% fall in dissolved $O_2$ affect the $HbO_2$ dissociation curve and exercise performance? Do you think this degree of change in $O_2$ tension would effect the $CO_2$ dissociation curve?*

 *LINKUP:* **Biography: John Scott Haldane,** *featured at* **http://connection.lww.com/go/brownexphys** *and on the* **Student Resource CD-ROM,** *discusses this pioneer in respiratory physiology.*

## Control of Breathing

Breathing is a rhythmic process involving cyclic inspiratory and expiratory components. Inspiration is active, originating through neural impulses from the brainstem area of the central nervous system, which activate respiratory muscles to contract. Expiration, however, is primarily passive during normal rest. The exceptions are the active expiratory efforts required for coughing, sneezing, performing Valsalva maneuvers, and performing exercise at higher intensities. Control of ventilation is a fascinating yet still unresolved area of importance in exercise physiology. In this section we investigate how the rhythmic act of breathing is controlled.

### EXERCISE VENTILATION

Before describing the regulation of breathing, we need to consider for a moment the effects of exercise on ventilation. Exercise is a physical stressor that causes a disruption of homeostasis, the term used by physiologists to characterize the unchanging internal environment of the body at rest during changing external environmental stimuli, such as wide shifts in heat and cold. Like heat and cold, exercise represents a challenge to homeostatic control of the internal environment. During exercise, several regulatory systems, including the respiratory system, seek to maintain a dynamic equilibrium of important physiologic variables even though these variables may increase (as in $CO_2$ concentration) or decrease (as in pH) from their resting levels. Physiologists use the term **steady state** to describe the adjustments to new, fairly stable levels that occur in these and other key physiologic variables. Therefore, exercise represents a test of the homeostatic control mechanisms and the term steady state denotes the balance achieved between the demands placed on the body by exercise and the body's response to those demands.

While the terms homeostasis and steady state refer to similar concepts, they differ in that homeostasis refers to the resting physiologic state characterized by an absolute or near absolute constancy in many bodily functions. Steady state characterizes an exercise-induced change in the resting internal environment. The change represents a dynamic (fluctuating) relative constancy in bodily functions, which are reset to new physiologic levels. Therefore, homeostasis is not maintained during exercise. Instead, there is fluctuation at a newly achieved steady-state level for a given variable during which the body balances the extra demands placed on it with its own responses to these demands. The challenge for the respiratory system is to keep arterial $P_{CO_2}$ and $H^+$ levels as near to resting levels as possible over a wide range of metabolic rates (rest to maximal exercise) while seeking to maintain $Pa_{O_2}$ at resting levels.

No single factor is solely responsible for ventilatory control during exercise. The medullary controller receives input from higher brain centers (central command theory), central and peripheral **chemoreceptors**, and **mechanoreceptors**. The medulla, in turn, signals respiratory muscles to increase their contraction frequency. A precise match between ventilation and the increased $\dot{V}_{CO_2}$ during exercise is achieved via humoral chemoreceptors and neural feedback from working muscles as a means to increase ventilation to a new steady-state level and maintain $Pa_{CO_2}$ at a constant level. Higher-intensity exercise and exercise involving an added environmental heat load cause an upward drift in ventilation as the increased blood temperature and rising blood catecholamines directly stimulate the respiratory control center.

Ventilatory patterns during endurance exercise are dependent on the form that the exercise bout takes (i.e., continuous short term, continuous prolonged, or incremental to maximum). For example, a continuous submaximal exercise bout may be of light ($<$50% $\dot{V}_{O_2max}$), moderate (50% to 75% $\dot{V}_{O_2max}$), or heavy ($>$75% $\dot{V}_{O_2max}$) intensity. The bout may also be short term ($<$10 minutes), prolonged for 20 to 30 minutes, or an hour or more. The exercise bout may also be incremental, progressively increasing in intensity to the maximal exercise point at which time the exercise bout is terminated. For short-term, prolonged, and incremental exercise patterns, breathing can be examined using the typical variables of pulmonary ventilation, external respiration, and internal respiration. The definitions of these terms are key to understanding the variables associated with each. Pulmonary ventilation is the process of moving air in and out of the lungs. External respiration is the exchange of gases between the lungs and blood, and internal respiration is the exchange of gases at the cellular level. Typical variables of pulmonary ventilation are:

- $\dot{V}_E$: minute ventilation
- $V_T$: tidal volume
- $D_S/V_T$: ratio of dead space to tidal volume
- f: breathing frequency

Typical variables of external respiration are:

- $\dot{V}A$: alveolar ventilation
- $PO_2$ and $PCO_2$: partial pressures of $O_2$ and $CO_2$
- $SaO_2\%$: percent saturation of arterial blood with $O_2$
- $A-a$ $PO_2$ difference: alveolar to arterial $O_2$ partial pressure difference

Typical variables of internal respiration are:

- $PaO_2$ and $PaCO_2$: partial pressures of arterial $O_2$ and $CO_2$
- $PvO_2$ and $PvCO_2$: partial pressures of venous $O_2$ and $CO_2$
- $SvO_2\%$: percent saturation of venous blood with $O_2$
- $a-vO_2$ difference: arterial to venous $O_2$ content difference

## Ventilation Responses: Light to Moderate Short-Term Exercise

During pulmonary ventilation in light to moderate short-term exercise, the ventilatory response is directly proportional to the metabolic demand imposed by the exercise stress. Minute ventilation is increased gradually to a steady-state level within about 2 to 3 minutes. There is an initial immediate increase over about the first 20 seconds of the work bout and then a gradual increase to steady state. The increase in pulmonary ventilation is at first due to the immediate rise in $VT$ with breathing frequency increasing more gradually. When the requirements of the activity have been satisfied, both $VT$ and breathing frequency level off. Also notice that $DS/VT$ decreases during exercise as a result of bronchodilation and the proportionally larger increase in $VT$ versus $DS$. This result means that during exercise, $\dot{V}A$ will increase to an even larger percentage of the total pulmonary ventilation then it was at rest. Without the change in the ratio of $DS/VT$, $\dot{V}E$ would have to be even higher for a given metabolic rate. Ventilatory efficiency therefore improves as $DS/VT$ is reduced during exercise.

The gradual increase in $\dot{V}A$ parallels that of $\dot{V}E$ (see *Fig. 6.29a*). The rate of alveolar ventilation is sufficient to maintain both $PAO_2$ and $PaO_2$ at resting levels (see Fig. 6.29b). The venous admixture causes the $PaO_2$ to be lower than the $PAO_2$ at rest, and this difference is maintained or lowered during light exercise. However, during moderate, short-term exercise, the $A-a$ $PO_2$ difference may be accentuated slightly, reflecting an adequacy of $O_2$ transfer from the alveoli to blood during exercise. This transfer is adequate for maintaining the $SaO_2\%$ in red blood cells during exercise.

During short-term, light exercise, the $PaO_2$ does not change. However, even during light exercise, mitochondrial $O_2$ requirements increase to sustain aerobic metabolism, with this increased need for $O_2$ lowering the $PvO_2$ and $SvO_2\%$, thus decreasing the $a-vO_2$ difference. Increased metabolism also means that there is increased $CO_2$ production, which is reflected in a slight increase in $PvCO_2$. Because exercise causes an increase in pulmonary ventilation, there is usually a slight decrease in $PaCO_2$ as extra $CO_2$ is blown off.

## Ventilation Responses: Prolonged Heavy Exercise

Ventilatory responses change in magnitude during prolonged heavy exercise when compared to short-term, light-to-moderate exercise. However, during this type of endurance exercise, steady state takes longer to achieve and a drift pattern sets in after the initial steady-state period. The drift in $\dot{V}E$ represents a certain amount of overbreathing for a given metabolic demand. The drift can also be seen in $VT$, breathing frequency, and the $DS/VT$ ratio.

However, overbreathing does provide an advantage to external respiration because $\dot{V}A$ parallels the $\dot{V}E$ drift pattern, thus ensuring that the acid-base balance is maintained. There is no change in $PAO_2$ and a slight decrease in $PaO_2$ before a rebound to baseline. The $A-a$ $PO_2$ difference parallels the drop in $PaO_2$, reflecting a brief and insignificant loss in $O_2$ transfer efficiency.

The variables of internal respiration during prolonged, heavy-endurance exercise change in magnitude only when compared to changes occurring during light, short-term exercise. Because of the greater exercise intensity, there is a wider shift in the $O_2$ content of venous versus arterial blood as reflected by a relatively lower $PvO_2$ and $SvO_2\%$. As $O_2$ metabolism is greater so is the production of $CO_2$, as reflected by an increased $PvCO_2$. Finally, as in light, short-term exercise, $PaCO_2$ falls lower than the resting value due to overbreathing.

## Ventilation Responses: Incremental Exercise to Maximum

Ventilation during incremental exercise to maximum has been studied extensively because of the noted exponential rise in $\dot{V}E$ at exercise intensities beyond the moderate level. Until approximately 50% to 60% $\dot{V}O_{2max}$, the rise in $\dot{V}E$ is rectilinear. After this point there is a break in the linearity of the $\dot{V}E$ response, with a second break occurring at about 80% to 90% $\dot{V}O_{2max}$. These breaks occur despite the continuous linear increase in both heart rate and $\dot{V}O_2$ during incremental exercise to maximum. At the beginning of exercise and after each breakpoint, $\dot{V}E$ increases in a linear fashion. These breakpoints, called *ventilatory thresholds*, have been attributed to the following causes:

- Rise in blood lactate and reduction in blood pH (increase in $[H^+]$ stimulates carotid bodies to increase $\dot{V}E$)
- Rising body temperature
- Greater concentrations of blood catecholamines, resulting in stimulation of carotid bodies
- Feedback from skeletal muscle proprioceptors
- Inability of changes in $VT$, breathing frequency, and $DS/VT$ to maintain $\dot{V}A$

Prior to the first ventilatory threshold, the sharp rise in $VT$ accounts for the increases seen in $\dot{V}E$. With further increases in exercise intensity approaching the second ventilatory threshold and beyond, further increases in $\dot{V}E$ are accomplished by increases in frequency only as VT starts to decline.

In external respiration the alveoli are well ventilated. At heavy-exercise intensities, the second ventilatory threshold corresponds to a sharp increase in PAO2. The increased PAO2 provides an increased pressure head for driving alveolar O2 into mixed venous blood. This is the primary mechanism for maintaining PaO2 and SaO2% during intense exercise. Since the increase in PAO2 is out of proportion to the small increase in PaO2 during heavy exercise, the A−a PO2 difference increases sharply. Ventilatory threshold is an important concept in exercise physiology and also has clinical significance.

 *Experiences in Work Physiology Lab Exercise 6: Ventilatory Threshold is designed to help you gain experience in the measurement of ventilatory threshold.*

Almost one-half of highly trained endurance athletes experience **exercise-induced hypoxemia** at very high work rates. This represents a limiting factor to work (exercise) output in these athletes, although their exercise capacity is already very high. The dotted line on the PaO2 graph shows the steep drop in O2 tension. This represents a central pulmonary limitation (arterial blood O2 is reduced) for these individuals. The drop can be as great as a 40 mm Hg reduction in PaO2, reducing SaO2% to as low as 84% from a high of about 97%. Exercise-induced hypoxemia may be caused by a diffusion limitation that results from a decreased transit time of red blood cells through pulmonary capillaries. The exact cause of the decreased transit time is not fully known but is believed to be the result of a limit in the expansion capability of the pulmonary capillary volume. When this occurs, blood velocity through the pulmonary capillary bed increases and transit time decreases, which does not leave enough time for gas equilibration to occur. Physiologic hypoxemia has been demonstrated in some highly trained endurance athletes. Box 6.1 presents a study that investigated some of the possible causes of exercise-induced hypoxemia.

During incremental exercise to maximum work rates, there is a progressive lowering of muscle PO2 to very low levels, approximately 10 to 20 mm Hg. This represents a maximal partial pressure gradient of about 87 mm Hg (PaO2 = 97 mm Hg − muscle PO2 of 10 mm Hg). Therefore, venous SO2 is very low during near maximal or maximal exercise. The opposite is true of PCO2. Alveolar hyperventilation causes the lowering of PCO2 beyond the moderate work rate.

## CENTRAL AND PERIPHERAL ROLES

*Figure 6.28* is a schematic representation of how ventilation is controlled. Ventilatory control is an integrated process that consists of the activities of a central controller (medulla and pons), effectors (muscles of the chest wall and diaphragm, and skeletal muscles during exercise), and centrally and peripherally located sensory receptors. The normal respiratory cycle is controlled by the inherent activity of inspiratory neurons in the **medullary respiratory center**. The medullary center receives input from higher brain centers (cerebral cortex and pons) and from peripheral chemoreceptors and mechanoreceptors. During exercise the rate (breathing frequency) and depth (VT of each breath) of ventilation are adjusted close to the metabolic rate (exercise intensity). Despite large increases in metabolic rate, arterial PO2, PCO2, and pH remain almost normal, a situation that forces physiologists to look elsewhere to explain the cause of the large increase in ventilation observed during intense exercise. The answer is yet to be elucidated but probably resides in a combination of central and peripheral neurogenic control factors that can be summed up as follows:

- During movement, as the brain transmits impulses to contracting muscles, it simultaneously sends impulses to the respiratory center
- During physical activity joint receptors and muscle proprioceptors send excitatory impulses to the respiratory center

The combined effect is an increase in ventilation even during passive arm and leg movements.

Automatic control of breathing is organized centrally at the brainstem, with the primary purpose being the regulation of PaCO2. The "controllers" in automatic breathing are neural groups that reside in an inexact pattern throughout the brainstem. Two major areas have been identified that provide central control of respiration: the *medullary respiratory areas* (ventral and dorsal groups) and the *pontine respiratory group* (the pneumotaxic center).

The dorsal respiratory group of the medulla mainly discharges action potentials just prior to and during inspiration and is therefore comprised mainly of inspiratory neurons. The ventral group consists of both inspiratory and expiratory neurons and receives inputs from the dorsal respiratory group. Also within the pons is the center that controls apneustic (i.e., long inspiratory phases) breathing. Rhythmic breathing is controlled in the medulla where phasic discharges are locked to either the inspiratory or expiratory phase of the respiratory cycle.

*Figure 6.29* shows a model of the brainstem ventilatory controller as an explanation of rhythmic breathing. The circles labeled A, B, and C represent three neuron pools that control phasic breathing. Pool A (the ventral and dorsal medullary respiratory areas) receives input from central and peripheral chemoreceptors (responding to increased PCO2 or decreased PO2) and activates the diaphragm and intercostal muscles to cause inspiration. The inspiratory neurons of pool A stimulate neurons in pool B. As shown, pool B also receives input from lung stretch receptors, with the signals becoming stronger as the lungs expand. Pool B, in turn, activates the breathing muscles and pneumotaxic center (pool C). Pool C then sends inhibitory impulses to pool A, which ends inspiration and begins expiration.

In addition to the central controller, sensory receptors

## R E S E A R C H   H I G H L I G H T

**McKenzie DC, Lama IL, Potts JE, et al. The effect of repeat exercise on pulmonary diffusing capacity and EIH in trained athletes. *Med Sci Sports Exerc* 1999;31:99–104.**

### RESEARCH SUMMARY

Highly trained endurance athletes experience the phenomenon of exercise-induced arterial hypoxemia (EIH), a widening of the alveolar–arterial $O_2$ difference ($\Delta A - aO_2$) that results in a lowered $PaO_2$. EIH may limit maximal exercise performance of these athletes by reducing their maximum $O_2$ uptake ($\dot{V}O_{2max}$) secondary to a lower arterial $O_2$ content and reduced maximal arterial–venous $O_2$ difference ($\Delta a - \bar{v}O_2$). However, the exact mechanism that produces hypoxemia in these individuals is being debated. Two hypotheses that explain EIH are a diffusion limitation across the alveolar pulmonary capillary membrane and a ventilation-perfusion mismatch. Both of these conditions could result from interstitial edema which itself may result from a stress failure of the capillary endothelium which has been demonstrated after intense exercise in human and animal research models. Evidence for a failure of the alveolar-capillary membrane and the development of interstitial edema comes from the observation of a decrease in pulmonary diffusing capacity (DL) below that of pre-exercise levels which persists for a minimum of 6 hours into recovery. A decreased DL is used in these studies as an indirect indicator of interstitial edema.

Therefore, the purpose of this research study was to examine the effect of two bouts of heavy exercise on the development of EIH and to assess the corresponding changes in diffusing capacity and pulmonary capillary volume. Subjects ($\dot{V}O_{2max}$ = 67.0±3.6 mL·kg$^{-1}$·min$^{-1}$) completed two maximal exercise bouts ($\dot{V}O_{2max}$ tests) separated by 60 minutes of seated rest. At the end of each rest period (60 minutes post-exercise), a carbon monoxide diffusing capacity test (DL$_{CO}$) was performed. DL decreased by 11% from pre-exercise values after the first exercise test and decreased by 6% further after the second exercise test. The first decrease in DL was accounted for by a concomitant decrease in both membrane-diffusing capacity (−11%) and pulmonary capillary volume (VC, −10%). However, after the second maximal exercise bout, the decrease in DL was accounted for by a decrease in VC only (−10%). These findings show that DL is limited after an initial heavy exercise bout by pulmonary interstitial edema, but the limiting factor changes after a second heavy exercise bout to a redistribution of pulmonary capillary blood. Although of physiologic significance, these findings are of limited clinical significance because the outcome of the second maximal exercise test was not influenced, i.e., there was not significant reduction in minute ventilation, maximal aerobic capacity, maximal heart rate, or respiratory frequency. Percent saturation of arterial $O_2$ (%Sa$O_2$) decreased from pre-exercise levels after each exercise bout, but there was no difference between the minimal saturation achieved in test 1 and test 2. Therefore, even though there was a progressive decrease in DL with the second heavy exercise bout, %Sa$O_2$ was not affected and no increase in EIH was observed, leading the researchers to conclude that pulmonary fluid accumulation during exercise was not of clinical significance. Therefore, the meaning of post-exercise measures of DL$_{CO}$ is questioned. The occurrence of hypoxemia during maximal exercise is not related to diffusing capacity.

### IMPLICATIONS FOR FURTHER RESEARCH

Exercise-induced hypoxemia has been demonstrated in a subset of highly trained male athletes. Further research is needed to demonstrate whether there is an effect based on the gender of the athlete, and, if so, to identify the important physiologic characteristics accounting for this difference.

---

throughout the body provide feedback to control respiration. Mechanoreceptors are strategically placed in the lungs and chest wall. There are three types of lung and chest wall receptors, each functioning in the control of ventilation. These proprioceptors are activated through mechanical sensory information. Chest wall mechanoreceptors are:

- Joint receptors that are activated by movement of the ribs in relation to their relative position with the vertebral column and sternum
- Golgi tendon organs that are located in the intercostal

muscles and diaphragm to monitor the force of muscle contraction and inhibit inspiration
- Muscle spindles that are also in the intercostal and abdominal wall muscles (but more scarce in the diaphragm) to help coordinate breathing during changes in posture and speech, and to stabilize the rib cage in times of increased airway resistance or decreased lung compliance when breathing is impeded

The lung mechanoreceptors are:

- Stretch receptors that respond to increasing lung volumes by turning off inspiratory neurons, thereby

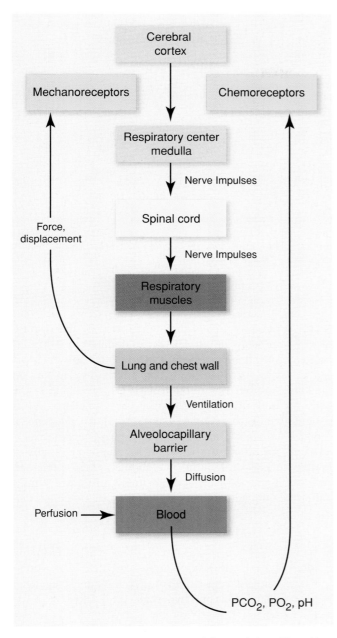

**FIGURE 6.28.** Schematic representation of the regulation of breathing. The key box in the illustration is the respiratory center in the medulla which has its neurons dispersed into several areas. These areas cyclically depolarize and are in turn affected by voluntary control from the cerebral cortex and by automatic control from two sensory loops (mechanoreceptors and chemoreceptors).

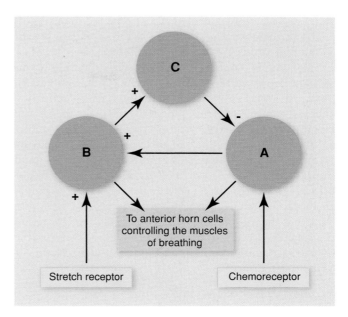

**FIGURE 6.29.** Model for rhythmic breathing showing three important neuron pools (A, B, and C) and their responses to signal input.

The ultimate goal of respiration is to maintain proper concentrations of $O_2$, $CO_2$, and $H^+$ in the tissues. To do this, the concentrations of these elements are determined at various locations. Chemoreceptors are located centrally—the central chemoreceptors (in the central nervous system at or near the ventrolateral surface of the medulla and between the origins of the seventh and tenth cranial nerves)—and peripherally—the carotid (at the bifurcation of the common carotid arteries) and aortic (aortic arch) bodies. Excess $CO_2$ and $H^+$ act directly on the respiratory center to alter respiration while decreases in $O_2$ act mainly on peripheral chemoreceptors, which then transmit nervous signals to the respiratory center to alter respiration.

## CHEMICAL CONTROL OF RESPIRATION

The central chemoreceptors are located in the medulla and are anatomically separate from the respiratory center. Ninety percent of the increase in resting ventilation that is caused by $CO_2$ is controlled by central (medullary) chemoreceptors, which sense increases in $H^+$ of the cerebrospinal fluid but are less excited by $CO_2$ changes. However, $P_{CO_2}$ is a potent indirect stimulus for respiratory center activity by the following mechanism. When $P_{CO_2}$ increases in the blood, there is also an increase in the $P_{CO_2}$ of cerebrospinal fluid and interstitial fluid of the medulla. This is due to the great permeability of the blood-brain barrier to $CO_2$. Though $[H^+]$ may be great in the blood, the relative impermeability of the blood-brain barrier to $H^+$ causes blood $H^+$ to have little effect on the activity of the respiratory center. Rather, when the $P_{CO_2}$ of cerebrospinal fluid and interstitial fluid of the medulla increases, the $CO_2$ immediately reacts with water to form $H^+$ by the carbonic

promoting expiration
- Irritant receptors that stimulate airway constriction and promote rapid, shallow breathing to inhibit penetration of harmful substances deep into the lungs
- C fibers that are excited by mechanical distortion of the lungs' connective tissue structure as happens with pulmonary edema, with the ventilatory response being rapid, shallow breathing

anhydrase reaction explained earlier. The $H^+$ then acts directly on the central chemoreceptors to stimulate the inspiratory neurons to increase ventilation.

Changing $O_2$ concentration in arterial blood has no direct effect on the respiratory center to alter ventilation. Rather, the role of $O_2$ is centered in the ability of peripheral chemoreceptors to sense $O_2$ concentration in arterial blood. As mentioned earlier, peripheral chemoreceptors are the aortic bodies located in the aortic arch, and the carotid bodies are located at the bifurcation of the common carotid arteries. The aortic bodies appear to play a minor role in chemoreceptor activity in humans. Peripheral chemoreceptors also sense increases in arterial $P_{CO_2}$ and $[H^+]$, but the role of increased $P_{CO_2}$ and $[H^+]$ is greater on central chemoreceptor activity. Carotid bodies serve as the last sensory station for monitoring $Pa_{O_2}$ prior to blood entering the brain.

### Regulating Blood pH

Blood pH is one of the most important physiologic variables to regulate. The body does this by both short-term and long-term mechanisms. In the short term, the respiratory response to metabolic acid-base disturbances is initiated within minutes. In the long term, the renal response may take several days to reach completion. Ventilation is an important acute controller of blood pH through the following relationships: decreases in ventilatory rate increase $P_{CO_2}$, which decreases blood pH (increased $[H^+]$), and increases in ventilatory rate decrease $P_{CO_2}$, which increases blood pH (decreased $[H^+]$). Conversely, the kidneys make appropriate adjustments in the excretion of $HCO_3^-$ and net acid, and these adjustments are an important chronic controller of blood pH. Therapists should become familiar with acid-base disturbances and how the body compensates to return arterial blood pH to normal levels since many patients in rehabilitation programs present with these abnormalities.

There are four distinct acid-base balance abnormalities. Two are caused by changes in breathing and $P_{CO_2}$, and two in which changes in breathing and $P_{CO_2}$ are compensatory responses. For instance, when the systemic arterial blood $[H^+]$ rises, $P_{CO_2}$ also increases, which stimulates respiratory centers in the brain to increase alveolar ventilation that acts to return $P_{CO_2}$ and $[H^+]$ back to normal levels. *Figure 6.30* shows the relationship between alveolar ventilation and incremental changes in pH. Actually, the body has a series of mechanisms by which it can minimize the effect of a change in pH during an acid-base disturbance.

- Metabolic acidosis: characterized by a low plasma $[HCO_3^-]$ and low pH
- Metabolic alkalosis: characterized by an elevated plasma $[HCO_3^-]$ and elevated pH
- Respiratory acidosis: characterized by an elevated $P_{CO_2}$ and reduced pH
- Respiratory alkalosis: characterized by a reduced $P_{CO_2}$ and elevated pH

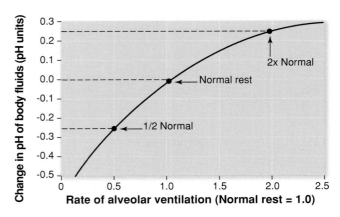

**FIGURE 6.30.** The effect of alveolar ventilation on the incremental change in pH is predictable. Body fluids become more alkaline under hyperventilatory conditions and more acidic under hypoventilatory conditions.

Blood pH is regulated during exercise by the respiratory system, hemoglobin, $HCO_3^-$, blood and intracellular protein, and phosphate groups. The degree to which pH is affected by increasing $CO_2$ concentrations depends on the *alkali reserve* (the amount of $HCO_3^-$ available in the body for buffering $H^+$). Having a large alkali reserve is potentially advantageous to exercise performance since a decrease in muscle and blood pH impairs exercise performance by interfering with the contractile apparatus of muscle during contraction, thus reducing force potential. Two such mechanisms, extracellular and intracellular buffering and adjustments in ventilatory rate, are discussed in Box 6.2.

There are several problems associated with acidosis:

- Increased serum potassium. This occurs as hydrogen ions enter the cell to compensate for excess hydrogen in the extracellular space. Hydrogen ions are exchanged for potassium ions and hyperkalemia results.
- Decreases in CNS activity
- Decreased myocardial activity, myocardial depression
- Dysrhythmias
- Decreased vascular tone, resulting in decreases in blood pressure
- Increased central nervous system blood flow
- Decreased $O_2$ binding to hemoglobin, causing a right shift in the $HbO_2$ dissociation curve

There are also several problems associated with alkalosis:

- Decreased serum potassium
- Increased central nervous system irritability
- Coronary artery spasm
- Decreased $O_2$ delivery to the tissues, causing a left shift in the $HbO_2$ dissociation curve
- Dysrhythmias
- Increased airway resistance
- Decreased central nervous system blood flow

Box 6.2

### P E R S P E C T I V E

# *Blood Gases and Acid-Base Balance*

Interpreting blood gases is essential to evaluation of a pulmonary patient's degree of lung impairment. Lung impairment affects both gas exchange and a patient's acid-base status. Evaluating blood gases is necessary to judge whether immediate treatment is warranted, as in the case of hypercapnia, which often benefits from noninvasive ventilation. Blood gases are "read" from a sample of arterial blood, which provides a direct measure of the $Pa_{O_2}$, $Pa_{CO_2}$, and pH. Normal $Pa_{CO_2}$ is 35 to 45 mm Hg and normal arterial pH is between 7.35 and 7.45. Normal arterial blood $O_2$ tension is age predicted and declines with age from about 95 mm Hg at age 20 years to about 65 mm Hg by age 90 years. Other important variables to measure include the calculated $[HCO_3^-]$ (ranging from 22 to 26 mEq) and the $\%Sa_{O_2}$.

Vital information regarding respiratory, cardiac, and metabolic function is achieved with analysis of the composition of arterial and mixed venous blood gases. Knowledge of these gases helps exercise personnel understand acid-base balance, alveolar ventilation, and oxygenation status. Since the body's cardiovascular and nervous systems must operate in a relatively narrow free $H^+$ ion range, acid metabolites must be kept from accumulating in high amounts. A pH below 6.8 or above 8 is incompatible with life. Excessive ventilatory efforts in abnormal acid-base status are common in clinical settings. The underlying metabolic deficiencies must be corrected. Table 1 below shows some of the signs and symptoms of common acid-base disturbances and serves as a guide to the clinical presentation of acid-base balance.

If the pH of the blood drops below 7.35, acidosis exists, i.e., acids dominate over bases (molecules that contribute

$OH^-$ to a solution). If pH rises above 7.45, alkalosis exists (bases dominate over acids). A pH of 7.0 is neutral: $[H^+] = [OH^-]$. Increasing or decreasing respiration leads to greater or lesser $CO_2$ concentrations, respectively, which influences blood pH. If $Pa_{CO_2}$ is below 35 mm Hg, hyperventilation is occurring, leading to reduced $CO_2$ concentration. If the $Pa_{CO_2}$ is above 45 mm Hg, hypoventilation is occurring, leading to an elevated $CO_2$ concentration. It is important to understand what is upsetting normal acid-base balance, i.e., whether the cause is respiratory or metabolic. Disturbances of acid-base balance resulting from a change in $[HCO_3^-]$ are termed metabolic acid-base disorders, and disturbances resulting from a change in the $Pa_{CO_2}$ are termed respiratory acid-base disorders. If the primary cause is respiratory, the compensating mechanism is metabolic (kidney response occurs within hours or days and is not important during exercise); if the primary cause is metabolic, the compensating mechanism is respiratory (pulmonary response occurs within minutes). Clinicians make a judgment as to whether the patient is acute (pH is abnormal) or is partially or fully compensated. Compensation refers to the reestablishment of normal pH but in the presence of abnormal $HCO_3^-$ or $CO_2$ levels. Compensating for metabolic problems is the role of the lungs (regulating $Pa_{CO_2}$), whereas respiratory problems are compensated for by the kidneys (regulating $HCO_3^-$). Table 2 shows the primary alterations and subsequent defense mechanisms of the various simple acid-base disorders.

These are all examples of an acute acid-base disturbance because the pH is abnormal in each instance. As the body retains base, pH will move back toward the normal limits, and

### TABLE 1

| Respiratory Acidosis | Metabolic Acidosis | Respiratory Alkalosis | Metabolic Alkalosis |
|---|---|---|---|
| Hypercapnia | Bicarbonate Deficit | Hypocapnia | Bicarbonate Excess |
| Hypoventilation | Hyperventilation | Lightheadedness | Depressed Respirations |
| Headache | Headache | Numbness/Tingling of digits | Mental Confusion |
| Visual Disturbances | Mental Dullness | Tetany | Dizziness |
| Confusion | Deep Respiration | Convulsions | Numbness/Tingling of digits |
| Drowsiness | Stupor | Hypokalemia | Muscle Twitching |
| Coma | Coma | Cardiac Dysrhythmias | Tetany |
| Hyperkalemia | Hyperkalemia | | Convulsions |
| Ventricular Fibrillation | Cardiac Dysrhythmias | | Cardiac Dysrhythmias |

*Perspective 6.2, continued*

### TABLE 2

| Disorder | Primary Alteration | pH | Defense Mechanism |
|---|---|---|---|
| Respiratory acidosis | ↑$Pa_{CO_2}$ | ↓ | Renal Compensation − 3.5 mEq·L$^{-1}$ ↑ in [$HCO_3^-$] per 10 mm Hg ↑ in $Pa_{CO_2}$ |
| Respiratory alkalosis | ↓$Pa_{CO_2}$ | ↑ | Renal Compensation − 5 mEq·L$^{-1}$ ↓ in [$HCO_3^-$] per 10 mm Hg ↓ in $Pa_{CO_2}$ |
| Metabolic acidosis | ↓[$HCO_3^-$] | ↓ | Respiratory Compensation − Hyperventilation 1.2 mm Hg ↓ $Pa_{CO_2}$ per 1 mEq·L$^{-1}$ ↓ in [$HCO_3^-$] |
| Metabolic alkalosis | ↑[$HCO_3^-$] | ↑ | Respiratory Compensation Hypoventilation 0.7 mm Hg ↑ $Pa_{CO_2}$ per 1 mEq·L$^{-1}$ ↑ in [$HCO_3^-$] |

the fully compensated classification will not be in effect until the pH is again between 7.35 and 7.45. A three-step approach can be used to determine the acid-base disorder:

1. Consider the pH first—this allows you to classify the disorder as either acidosis or alkalosis
2. Consider the [$HCO_3^-$] and $PaCO_2$ next—this allows you to determine whether the disorder is respiratory (↑$Pa_{CO_2}$) or metabolic (↓[$HCO_3^-$]) acidosis, or respiratory (↓$Pa_{CO_2}$) or metabolic (↑[$HCO_3^-$]) alkalosis
3. Lastly consider the compensatory response offered—in compensated metabolic acidosis $Pa_{CO_2}$ is decreased, but in

compensated metabolic alkalosis $Pa_{CO_2}$ is elevated; in compensated respiratory acidosis [$HCO_3^-$] is elevated, but in compensated respiratory alkalosis [$HCO_3^-$] is reduced.

Some acid-base disorders are not simple to determine and may be of mixed origin. Using the three-step approach above, determine the correct acid-base disorder from the following data set.

| | Patient 1 | Patient 2 |
|---|---|---|
| pH | 7.34 | 6.98 |
| [$HCO_3^-$] | 18 mEq/L | 13 mEq/L |
| $Pa_{CO_2}$ | 32 mm Hg | 54 mm Hg |

## P$CO_2$ and Respiration

There is a linear relationship between P$CO_2$ and respiration which is heightened during waking hours because of greater reticular formation stimulation (*Fig. 6.31*). The large dot on the awake curve of Figure 6.31 shows the normal operating point ($\dot{V}E$ = 5 L·min$^{-1}$ at $Pa_{CO_2}$ = 40 mm Hg). As $CO_2$ tension increases, ventilation increases, showing that ventilation is sensitive to $Pa_{CO_2}$. Usually, a 1 mm Hg increase in $Pa_{CO_2}$ produces a 2 L·min$^{-1}$ increase in ventilation (4). In the sleeping state the reticular formation is turned off, which produces a shift to the right (increased intercept) of the $CO_2$-ventilation response curve and a decreased sensitivity to $CO_2$ (decreased slope). [$H^+$] also affects ventilation, with ventilatory sensitivity to $CO_2$ increasing (greater slope of the line) during periods of metabolic acidosis and decreasing during periods of metabolic alkalosis (*Fig. 6.32*). Finally, as we have seen, sensitivity to reduced $O_2$ pressure does not reside in the respiratory center but in peripheral chemoreceptor activation.

Ventilation is affected differently by changes in $Pa_{O_2}$ versus $Pa_{CO_2}$. *Figure 6.33* shows the relationship of ventilation to $Pa_{O_2}$ for normal, **isocapnic**, and **hypercapnic** conditions. If $Pa_{O_2}$ falls below about 70 mm Hg, ventilation

begins to increase as chemoreceptors in the carotid bodies discharge to the medullary control center. As $Pa_{O_2}$ decreases further to about 60 mm Hg, the increase in ventilation becomes exponential as $Pa_{O_2}$ continues to fall (curve A in Fig. 6.33). This point has been referred to as the hypoxic threshold. Thus, a large decrease in $Pa_{O_2}$ must occur before a significant increase in ventilation occurs.

This is contrasted with small increases in $Pa_{CO_2}$, resulting in large increases in ventilation (see Fig. 6.32). When ventilation increases in response to hypoxemic conditions, $Pa_{CO_2}$ is, in turn, reduced. However, if isocapnia is achieved (curve B in Fig. 6.33) by adding $CO_2$ to the inspired air, the ventilatory response begins at a higher $P_{O_2}$ (approximately 80 mm Hg). Under hypercapnic conditions, the effect is even greater (curve C). Thus, the hypoxic ventilatory response is affected by $CO_2$ levels. Interestingly, not all patients who have breathing difficulties require supplemental $O_2$. Recall that respiratory acidosis is a condition in which blood pH is below normal and $Pa_{CO_2}$ is higher than normal (hypercapnia). If supplemental $O_2$ is given, the result may be a worsening of the patient's respiratory failure. *Using the graphs in the figures just reviewed, explain why this is the case.* In the case of low $O_2$ tensions, the carotid bodies are the sensing receptors since aortic and central chemoreceptors in humans do not respond to changes in $P_{O_2}$.

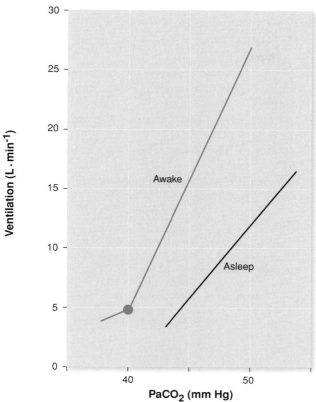

**FIGURE 6.31.** The $CO_2$-ventilation response curve in waking and sleeping hours.

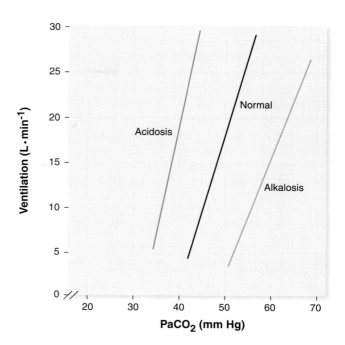

**FIGURE 6.32.** The $CO_2$-ventilation response is affected by $H^+$ concentration.

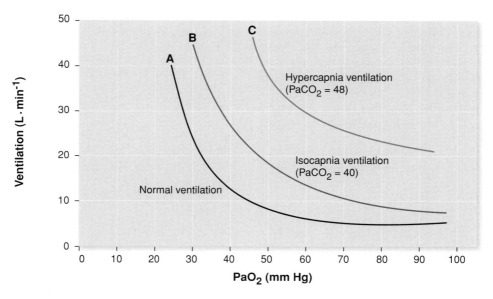

**FIGURE 6.33.** Three curves (A, B, and C) demonstrating the effect of $Pa_{O_2}$ on ventilation showing that the ventilatory response to $Pa_{O_2}$ is altered under conditions in which $CO_2$ is retained.

▶ **INQUIRY SUMMARY.** The respiratory control center of the brain contains a neuron pool that receives signals from a variety of sensors located around the body. Signals from neural and humoral origin act together to provide a redundant system of ventilatory control that is intricately arranged to ensure optimal $O_2$ content of the blood and to regulate acid-base balance. Since exercise represents a disruption to homeostasis, it is important that this control system function adequately. In pulmonary patients this system often breaks down, leading to a number of uncontrolled acid-base problems. *How do you think exercise might exacerbate any of these problems?*

## Summary

The chief function of the lungs is to bring air from the atmosphere into close contact with flowing blood so that $O_2$ and $CO_2$ can be exchanged. The body accomplishes this through anatomic structure and respiratory mechanics that combine to allow efficient functioning at every step of the way in the process of respiration. The mechanics of breathing involve a rhythmic contraction of the respiratory muscles of the chest wall and diaphragm that develops pressure differentials to move air in and out of the lungs. This, coupled with the partial pressure differences across the alveolar-capillary boundaries, allows the processes of pulmonary ventilation and external respiration to proceed efficiently. Diffusion of the respiratory gases is an important corollary to the phasic mechanics of ventilation. These gases diffuse from an area of higher to lower partial pressures. The gas exchange process is also affected by the number of red blood cells, hemoglobin concentration, surface area available for diffusion, and diffusion distance. Diffusion capacity is enhanced in exercise as new alveoli and capillaries open. Hemoglobin is an important molecule of respiration, and the degree of $O_2$ saturation with hemoglobin is an important physiologic determination of cellular respiration. Breathing is controlled in the medullary center, which receives neural and blood-borne signals.

### SUMMARY KNOWLEDGE

1. Why is $Pa_{O_2}$ less than $PA_{O_2}$?
2. Why does altitude affect breathing?
3. Why is too much $CO_2$ buildup in the blood bad?

4. Why are partial pressure gradients important in respiration?
5. How does the chest wall respond to rhythmic breathing?
6. Why does exercise improve $\dot{V}/\dot{Q}$ matching?
7. Why is hemoglobin more important than myoglobin in respiratory physiology?
8. In what ways is $CO_2$ transported from muscle tissue to the lungs?
9. What is the physiologic significance of dissolved $CO_2$ and $O_2$?
10. Why is the $O_2$ content of blood lower in females compared with males?

### References

1. Carroll JF, Convertino VA, Wood CE, et al. Effect of training on blood volume and plasma hormone concentrations in elderly. *Med Sci Sports Exerc* 1995;27:79–84.
2. Green HJ, Jones LL, Painter DC. Effects of short-term training on cardiac function during prolonged exercise. *Med Sci Sports Exerc* 1990;22:488–493.
3. Guyton AC, Hall JE. *Textbook of medical physiology*. 10th ed. New York: WB Saunders, 2000.
4. Dempsey JA, Mitchell GS, Smith CA. Exercise and chemoreception. *Am Rev Respir Dis* 1984;129:S31–S34.

### Suggested Readings

Frownfelter D, Dean E, eds. *Principles and practice of cardiopulmonary physical therapy*. St. Louis: Mosby, 1996.
Hodgkin JE, Celli BR, Connors GL, eds. *Pulmonary rehabilitation: guidelines to success*. Baltimore: Lippincott Williams & Wilkins, 2000.

### On the Internet

Virtual Hospital: Interpretation of Pulmonary Function Tests: Spirometry. Available at: **http://www.vh.org/adult/provider/internalmedicine/Spirometry/SpirometryHome.html**. Accessed April 08, 2005.
The lungs:
Stellenbosch University Faculty of Health Sciences: Department of Medical Physiology: Our Defence Against the Ravages of Fresh Air. Available at: **http://academic.sun.ac.za/med_physbio/med_physiology/dept/LUNGS.HTM**. Accessed April 08, 2005.

### Writing to Learn

*Research and write a paper about why acid-base physiology is important to exercise performance.*

# CHAPTER

# 7 Cardiovascular Exercise Physiology

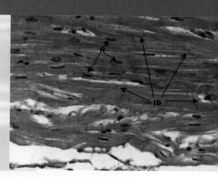

*The heart is unique among the various kinds of muscular organs found in the body. The picture on this page is an electron micrograph of myocardial cells showing the interconnectedness of the individual fibers. Easily seen are the intercalated discs, which provide the necessary microstructural arrangement which gives the heart its unique mechanical and electrical abilities. Dark ovals are cell nuclei (N). Can you deduce from this picture why the intercalated discs are important in heart function?*

## CHAPTER OUTLINE

Think of the wide range of physical activities in which you engaged over the past week. These may have included activities such as walking across a room or maybe running in a 5K road race—two activities that vary widely in difficulty. During these activities your cardiovascular system is able to match the energy needs of the working muscles with a cardiac output that accommodates these needs while maintaining essential blood flow to other important tissues, such as the brain. In this chapter we review the components of the cardiovascular system and discuss the factors that control the flow of blood. The changes that occur in the cardiovascular system to redirect blood flow to the working muscles during acute exercise are explored. Changes that occur in the cardiovascular system with regular exercise training are also discussed.

Along with respiratory physiology (Chapter 6), cardiovascular exercise physiology is vitally important for health care professionals to understand. For example, while therapists are primarily involved with treating musculoskeletal and/or neural disorders, cardiovascular limitations must always be addressed when assessing patients. The reason is that the cardiovascular system represents the primary limitation to day-to-day functional abilities for most individuals. This chapter, therefore, gives you the foundational content that you will draw upon when studying the last part of the text, which focuses on clinical concepts.

## The Heart and Circulation

The circulatory, endocrine, and nervous systems constitute the principal coordinating and integrating systems of the body. Each has its own primary function. For example, the role of the nervous system is to serve as a communication network allowing the individual to interact in appropriate ways with the environment. The endocrine system regulates the functioning of every cell, tissue, and organ in the body. The role of the cardiovascular system is varied and includes such important functions as transportation and distribution of essential substances to the tissues, removal of the byproducts of metabolism, regulation of body temperature, humoral (blood-borne) communication throughout the body, and adjustment of $O_2$ and nutrient supply in different physiologic states.

The cardiovascular system is a closed circuit that consists of the following basic components:

- Heart: responsible for pumping blood from the thorax to the periphery
- Arteries: responsible for transporting blood throughout the body
- Arterioles: responsible for regulating tissue blood flow
- Capillaries: responsible for exchanging $O_2$ and metabolites between tissue and blood
- **Venules** and veins: responsible for taking deoxygenated blood back to the heart

The cardiovascular system exhibits a wide range of functional abilities and performs a tremendous amount of "work" over the lifetime of an individual. Because of this, it is not surprising that cardiovascular health is very important to our general well-being. With proper exercise training throughout life, the cardiovascular system can remain remarkably viable, even in old age. Given the seriousness of the loss of cardiovascular health in individuals and the pervasiveness of cardiovascular disease in the population, it is puzzling that people do not take better care to sustain the functional viability of their own cardiovascular systems.

As is readily evident, the heart and circulation touch on every bodily system, thus helping to maintain the functional integrity of the individual and the viability of all organs. Of all the body's responses to acute exercise, the cardiovascular system meets the tremendous challenge to homeostasis with the largest degree of adjustments. As we will see, these cardiovascular adjustments are moderated by the type and intensity of exercise.

## CARDIAC STRUCTURE

The heart is a muscular organ weighing about 300 g and consisting of four hollow chambers that function as pumps and four valves that direct blood toward outflow tracts. Because of the way the heart and circulatory system are oriented (Fig. 7.1), the pumping function of the heart has a side-by-side (right and left pumps each with their own circuit) and top-to-bottom (top pumps act as primers for the lower, main pumps) orientation. As shown, the arrangement of the pump and circuitry dictates a duel pumping action through circuits that, while continuous, are nevertheless functionally separate. The heart, therefore, consists of a right pump that transports blood through the pulmonary artery to the lungs (*pulmonary circuit*) and a left pump that transports blood through the systemic arteries to the rest of the body (*systemic circuit*). Each side is composed of one upper atrium and one lower ventricle. The right atrium receives blood from the systemic veins, and the right ventricle pumps blood to the lungs for oxygenation. The left atrium receives oxygenated blood from the lungs, and the left ventricle pumps the blood out to the body through the systemic arteries. It is important to learn this blood flow pattern through the heart for a proper understanding of the relationship between the heart and circulation. *Can you deduce some consequences if, for instance, there was a hole in the* ***interventricular septum****?*

The atria are low-pressure, thin-walled chambers that primarily serve as reservoirs to receive and store blood while the ventricles are contracting (Fig. 7.2). Approximately 75% of the blood in the atria flows passively into the ventricles before the atria contract to pump the remaining blood into the ventricles. Soon thereafter, the ventricles contract to force blood into the systemic or pulmonary arteries. The ventricles are responsible for pumping blood into the arterial system. The walls of the ventricles are thicker than the walls of the atria, and the left ventricular walls are thicker than those of the right ventricle. The greater mass of the left ventricle is necessary to move blood against the higher pressures of the systemic arterial tree. The thicker, more muscular walls allow the left ventricle to generate the higher pressures necessary to overcome the greater **afterload** forces present in the systemic circulation.

Two sets of valves exist within the heart: the **atrioventricular valves** (AV) and the **semilunar valves**. These valves are one-way valves in that they allow blood to flow in only one direction. AV valves are located between each atrium and ventricle. The right AV valve is the *tricuspid* valve and the left AV valve is called the *mitral* valve. The tricuspid valve is comprised of three cusps and the mitral value has two cusps (bicuspid). The cusps are larger than the openings of their respective valves, causing them to overlap in the closed position. Attached to the free edges of these valve cusps are filaments called **chordae tendinae**, which arise from **papillary muscles** protruding into the chamber from each ventricle. The chordae tendinae prevent eversion of the valves during ventricular **systole**. With certain disease processes, these valves become damaged and allow blood to flow back from the ventricle into the atrium. For example, when this happens on the left side, the resulting condition is called **mitral regurgitation**. *After further reading, can you surmise why a backflow of this nature presents a problem, especially during exercise?* Case Study 7.1 explains the unique exercise hemodynamic responses of a patient with mitral valve regurgitation.

The semilunar valves consist of the pulmonary valve separating the pulmonary artery from the right ventricle and the aortic valve separating the aorta from the left ventricle. Each of these valves has cuplike cusps attached to the valve rings. During ventricular systole, the valve cusps float in the midstream of the blood flow approximately midway between the vessel walls and the closed position.

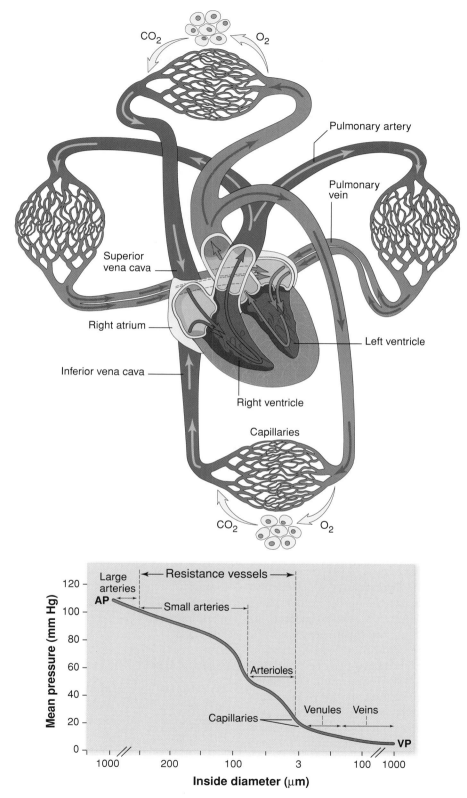

**FIGURE 7.1.** Diagram of the circulatory system. Right side (blue) is the pulmonary circuit, and left side (red) is the systemic circuit. The insert shows the relative size of the different parts of the vascular system and the drop in mean pressure across. AP, mean arterial pressure; VP, mean venous pressure.

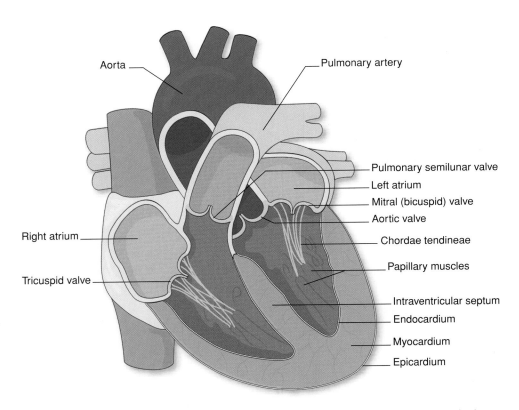

**FIGURE 7.2.** Anatomy of the heart. Frontal section of the heart showing interior chambers and valves.

Immediately on the arterial side of the semilunar valves are the sinuses of Valsalva, small outpockets of the pulmonary artery and aorta.

The wall of the heart is composed of three layers. The outermost layer is called the **epicardium**, the middle or muscular layer is the **myocardium**, while the innermost layer is called the **endocardium** (see Fig. 7.2). It is the myocardium, or cardiac muscle, that is responsible for contracting and creating a driving force (i.e., pressure) to push the blood out of the ventricle. **Intercalated discs** connect the individual muscle fibers to one another so that when the heart is stimulated by electrical **depolarization**, the impulse quickly spreads throughout the myocardium (*Fig 7.3*). Intercalated discs are continuous with the sarcolemma that surrounds each cardiac muscle cell, and they contain gap junctions that allow a wave of depolarization to pass very quickly from one cell to another. This allows all of the cardiac muscles in the atria or ventricles to contract synchronously. *Can you think of a reason why synchronous contraction is necessary for proper cardiac mechanical function?*

*LINKUP: Access Perspective: The Cardiac Syncytium Versus the Motor Unit at http://connection.lww.com/go/brownexphys and on the Student Resource CD-ROM for an explanation of how heart chambers function as a single unit, even though they are comprised of thousands of individual myocardial fibers.*

Blood is supplied to the heart itself via the right and left coronary arteries (*coronary circulation*). These arteries are small branches that originate from the aorta and wrap around the heart to ensure blood flow to all areas of the myocardium. The coronary veins lie next to the coronary arteries and drain blood back into the right atrium via the coronary sinus (the major venous blood-collecting vessel of the coronary circulation) on the posterior side of the right atrium. The left and right main coronary arteries branch extensively to supply blood to the entire myocardium (*Fig. 7.4*). See Box 7.1 for a discussion of the coronary circulation and myocardial $O_2$ demand during exercise.

## CARDIAC ELECTRICAL ACTIVITY

Some of the cells in the heart are specialized nervous tissue, responsible for spontaneously generating cardiac electrical activity and controlling the cardiac rate. This property is termed **automaticity**, and the specialized group of cells located in the extreme upper and posterior portion of the right atrium responsible for controlling the rate of cardiac depolarization is called the sinoatrial (SA) node (*Fig. 7.5*). The SA node has the fastest depolarization rate (approximately 60 to 80 times every minute) of all spontaneously depolarizing cardiac tissue; because of this property, the SA node is referred to as the *cardiac pacemaker*. All other cells of the heart can serve as the cardiac pacemaker, but they do not normally fill this role since their intrinsic

## CASE STUDY 7.1: *MITRAL VALVE REGURGITATION*

### CASE

Jan is a 42-year-old female who was seen for complaints of chest pain and lightheadedness. She complained of chest pain described as sharp sensations in the left upper chest lasting several seconds. Chest pain did not involve shortness of breath, diaphoresis, or nausea, and was not associated with exertion. Jan has a history of palpitations and was diagnosed previously with premature ventricular contractions. Jan has also noted isolated extra beats of her heart but has not had any syncope events. Jan has smoked 2 packs of cigarettes per day for 24 years and drinks alcohol occasionally. She is not on any medications and denies a history of hypertension, myocardial infarction, rheumatic heart disease, diabetes mellitus, elevated cholesterol, and allergies. Her family history is unremarkable. Her ECG evaluation was normal, but the echocardiogram revealed the following: left ventricular size at upper limits of normal with normal left ventricular wall motion; normal left ventricular ejection fraction; moderate systolic superior displacement of anterior mitral valve leaflet is evident and in the presence of minimal mitral regurgitation, may represent moderate mitral valve prolapse; normal trileaflet aortic valve was visualized with good opening and a normal left atrial size. An examination using pulsed Doppler with color-flow imaging confirmed the presence of mild to moderate mitral valve regurgitation.

### DESCRIPTION

Mitral valve regurgitation (valvular insufficiency) is the result of either congenital or acquired disorders affecting the mitral valve. With mitral valve regurgitation, the mitral valve leaflets do not close properly during ejection of the blood from the left ventricle. As a result, when the left ventricle contracts, blood is ejected through the aortic valve but is also regurgitated through the mitral valve to the left atrium. One common cause of mitral valve regurgitation is rheumatic fever. Other causes include systemic lupus erythematosus, infectious endocarditis, and age-related degenerative changes to

the mitral valve. Patients in the early stages of mitral insufficiency may not have any symptoms and may have a normal exercise capacity. Progression of the problem may result in symptoms such as fatigue, shortness of breath, fluid retention, and cardiac arrhythmias. The most common arrhythmia seen in these patients is atrial fibrillation. In later stages exercise capacity may be reduced. *Explain in hemodynamic terms why this might occur.*

### INTERVENTION

Mitral regurgitation is generally treated surgically; however, physical therapists or exercise physiologists may see patients who are being treated with medical management. With surgical intervention, a prosthetic valve is used to replace the defective mitral valve. Following surgery, these patients usually progress well with recovery.

The most common reasons to provide medical management of mitral regurgitation instead of surgical management are either because the defect is not very severe or the patient does not want or cannot have surgery. Regarding the medical management of patients with mitral regurgitation, the primary goal of therapy is to optimize the extraction of $O_2$ by the working muscles. This goal can be accomplished by a judicious exercise prescription that will improve $O_2$ delivery to the tissues but not exacerbate cardiac symptoms. During exercise it is important to closely monitor these patients for signs of dyspnea, fatigue, dizziness, coughing, or lightheadedness. ECG use during exercise will be helpful in monitoring the dynamic stability of these patients. Should patients exhibit untoward signs or symptoms, they should be referred back to their physicians for further examination. Examples of exercises that may be helpful in patients with mitral regurgitation include aerobic activities using large muscle groups, strengthening exercises, relaxation, and energy conservation techniques. To complement the exercise program, these patients should also be educated in smoking cessation, cardiac risk factors, dietary modifications, stress management, disease progression, and the ability to recognize physical signs of overexertion.

---

rates are slower. Besides these intrinsic control mechanisms, however, there are other extrinsic influences that help control heart rate (HR). These will be discussed later in the chapter.

Once the SA node depolarizes, the electrical activity spreads across both atria and to the AV node. At this point, the impulse is delayed approximately 0.11 seconds to give the atria time to contract and pump blood into the ventricles. The impulse then travels to the AV bundle, also called the **bundle of His**. Once the impulse arrives at the AV bundle, it spreads rapidly down each **bundle branch** to the

Purkinje fibers, which innervate the myocardium. These fibers are located throughout the ventricles and allow for the simultaneous depolarization, and ultimately, simultaneous contraction of both ventricles.

Electrical activity within the heart can be measured by surface electrodes that inscribe the electrocardiogram (ECG) or by direct application of electrodes into cardiac tissue that inscribe the cardiac **action potential** (*Fig. 7.6*). At rest, excitable cardiac cells are polarized, i.e., they are negatively charged on the inside and positively charged on the outside by a membrane-bound active transport process

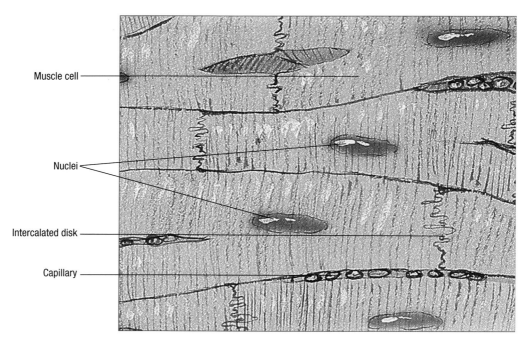

FIGURE 7.3. Electron micrograph of cardiac muscle. (Courtesy of Anatomical Chart Company, Skokie, Illinois.)

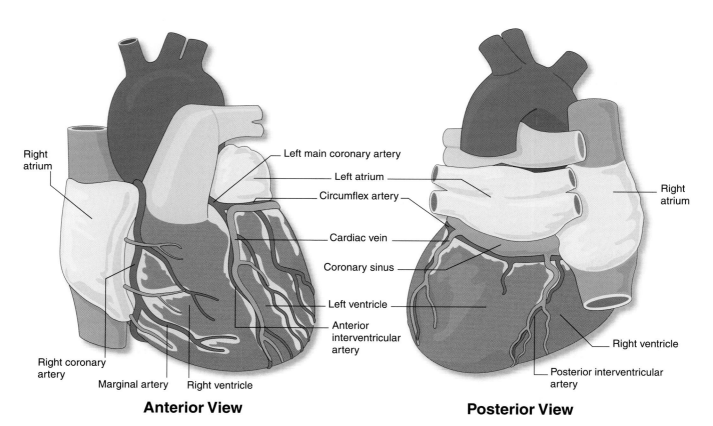

**Anterior View**  **Posterior View**

FIGURE 7.4. Cardiac arteries and veins.

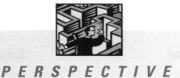

**Box 7.1**

## *P E R S P E C T I V E*

# *Coronary Circulation and Myocardial Oxygen Demand*

The right coronary artery (RCA) is the principal supplier of blood to the right ventricle and atrium, while the left coronary artery (LCA) is the principal supplier of blood to the left ventricle and atrium. Although this arrangement, termed *coronary flow dominance*, is generally true, there is some overlap. For instance, the RCA in humans is dominant in 50% of individuals, the LCA is dominant in another 20%, and the remaining 30% of individuals receive an equal supply from both main arteries. An individual difference in blood flow dominance is the reason why some individuals with blockages in the RCA have left ventricular infarctions and others have right ventricular infarctions.

Regardless of the particular pattern of flow dominance, the heart requires a large $O_2$ supply per minute. For instance, under resting conditions, $MVo_2$ equals about

$10 \text{ mL·min}^{-1}\text{·}100 \text{ g}^{-1}$ of myocardium. In order not to exceed the normal coronary blood flow rate of about 80 $\text{mL·min}^{-1}\text{·}100 \text{ g}^{-1}$ of myocardium, the heart must extract about 70% of the $O_2$ carried by the coronary blood supply. This resting level of $O_2$ extraction by the myocardium is equal to the maximal amount of $O_2$ extracted by skeletal muscle under heavy exercise. This means that during exercise when the heart has an increased demand for $O_2$, the supply is met through increased blood flow to the heart and not by increased extraction. This also means that there is a direct relationship between coronary blood flow and $MVo_2$, i.e., they vary together. During maximal exercise, the myocardium requires as much as $50 \text{ mL·}100 \text{ g}^{-1}$ of myocardium. Flow has to increase to about $350 \text{ mL·min}^{-1}\text{·}100 \text{ g}^{-1}$ of tissue to deliver this much $O_2$.

which sequesters positively and negatively charged ions against their concentration gradient on either side of the membrane. Table 7.1 shows the concentrations of the important ions inside and outside the myocardial fiber. Polarization produces resting membrane potentials of cardiac

muscle of approximately $-90$ mV. With depolarization, a reversal potential occurs. When this happens, the inside of the cell becomes positively charged while the outside of the cell becomes negatively charged as sodium ($Na^+$) channels open, allowing the rapid influx of $Na^+$ ions. This activity reverses the polarity of the resting membrane, creating a situation in which the membrane potential becomes approximately $+20$ mV. Following depolarization, the resting membrane potential is reacquired during the **repolarization** process. This cycle of ionic flow across the myocardial cell membrane, resulting in depolarization, occurs 60 to 80 times per minute if the SA node is acting as the pacer.

Measuring the difference in membrane potential across cardiac cell membranes during depolarization results in the cardiac **action potential** being inscribed. Cardiac action potentials are of two main types—slow response and fast response—each referring to the rate of rise of the membrane potential at the initiation of the depolarization process (phase 0). The atria, ventricles, and Purkinje fibers are fast-response **myocytes**, while the SA and AV nodes are slow-response myocytes. Following the SA node (normal cardiac pacer), the AV node and Purkinje fibers can serve as redundant cardiac pacemakers since their individual intrinsic rates of depolarization fall in a hierarchic order. For instance, the AV node is the next redundant pacer with a rate of about 40 to 60 depolarizations per minute. If this redundant pacer fails to function, Purkinje fibers also possess automaticity and can serve as the pacer, usually producing a

Sinoatrial node (SA node)

Atrioventricular node (AV node)

Atrioventricular bundle (bundle of His)

Right and left bundle branches

Purkinje fibers

Apex of heart

**FIGURE 7.5.** The intrinsic electrical conduction pathway of the heart showing the SA and AV nodes and internodal pathways.

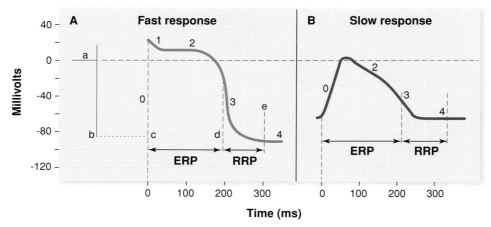

**FIGURE 7.6.** Fast- **(A)** and slow- **(B)** response cardiac action potentials produced from isolated cardiac tissue immersed in an electrolyte solution. **A.** Lower case (a–e) letters show when events occur (a: microelectrode enters the solution; b: microelectrode enters the fiber and records the resting membrane potential; c: the fiber is stimulated and depolarization occurs; c to d: the action potential is inscribed which also represents the effective refractory period; d to e: repolarization occurs during the relative refractory period). **B.** Action potential from slow-response cardiac tissue. The resting potential is less negative (~55 mV), the phase 0 upstroke is less steep, there is a smaller amplitude, phase 1 is absent, and the phase 2 plateau is less evident.

cardiac rate of 30 to 40 beats·min⁻¹. If the SA node becomes diseased and fails, the AV node is able to commence its role as the cardiac pacemaker at a rate that is usually less than 60 beats·min⁻¹. *If an individual presented to you with this rate, upon viewing the ECG, would you be able to tell whether this slow rate was a result of exercise training or the result of the heart being paced by the AV node?* The answer rests partly (perhaps largely) in the appearance of the ECG. When you have studied ECGs in the clinical section of the book, come back to this question to answer it more specifically.

For the SA and AV nodes, **autorhythmicity** occurs because the cell membranes of these fibers are "leaky" to $Ca^{2+}$ ions. During **diastole** the resting membrane potential (phase 4) of these tissues is not stable as is typical of the resting membrane potential for fast-response tissues. Rather, these resting potentials progressively rise (slow depolarization) throughout phase 4 from a level of about −70 mV (compared to −90 mV for the nonautomatic cells) to the threshold potential of about −55 mV, at which time the upstroke of the action potential occurs (*Fig. 7.7*). This slowly rising phase 4 membrane potential gives these

tissues their inherent autorhythmic properties. It is beyond the scope of this chapter to discuss in detail the process of depolarization and repolarization of cardiac excitable tissues. Interested readers are referred to the suggested readings list for more extensive information. Also, Chapter 9 presents material on the general process of depolarization and establishment of action potentials prior to skeletal muscle contraction. While morphologically different than that shown in Figures 7.6 and 7.7, skeletal muscle action potentials are produced by cellular events which are similar to those in cardiac tissue.

Cardiac electrical activity is measured between two electrodes on the surface of the body. This process is called **electrocardiography** and is a technique that has proven to be a very important clinical tool. Cardiologists use the ECG to diagnose heart abnormalities, such as electrical disturbances, to determine how well the heart is receiving its own blood supply, and to assess tissue damage associated with heart attacks. The physical therapist or exercise physiologist can use the ECG to monitor HR, rhythm, and ischemic responses while a patient is exercising. Case Study 7.2 presents information on how ECG monitoring can be used during activity.

For myocardial cells to contract (mechanical activity), they must first depolarize (electrical activity). Therefore, the electrical impulses captured on the ECG actually occur prior to the mechanical events of the heart. The different parts of the ECG waveform represent specific electrical events that occur in the heart (*Fig. 7.8*). The P wave occurs prior to atrial contraction and results from the spread of depolarization throughout the atria (atrial depolarization). The P wave lasts for 0.15 seconds. The QRS complex follows the P wave and represents depolarization of the ventricles. The ventricles contract immediately after ventricular depolarization. Because the atrial mass is smaller

| Table 7.1 | ION CONCENTRATIONS INSIDE AND OUTSIDE CARDIAC MUSCLE CELLS | |
|---|---|---|
| **Ion** | **Extracellular Concentrations (mM)** | **Intracellular Concentrations (mM)** |
| $Na^+$ | 145.0 | 10.0 |
| $K^+$ | 4.0 | 135.0 |
| $Cl^-$ | 140.0 | 30.0 |
| $Ca^{2+}$ | 2.0 | 0.0001 |

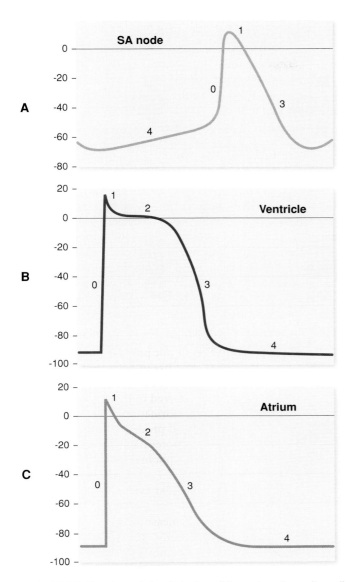

**FIGURE 7.7.** The phase 4 depolarization of the automatic cardiac cell (SA node) is clearly shown in **(A)** and is contrasted with the level phase 4 potentials of nonautomatic cardiac tissue **(B,C)**.

compared with that of the ventricles, the electrical activity associated with atrial repolarization is obscured by the QRS complex. The T wave represents repolarization of the ventricles. There is a **refractory** period following the depolarization of different areas of the heart. During this period, any stimulation of the heart results in a less forceful contraction or no contraction at all. The ECG describes each **cardiac cycle** as a cluster of three distinct waveforms: P, QRS, and T wave. For the heart that is beating rhythmically, these three waves appear together and are easily discernable as one cardiac cycle. Electrical and blood flow pathology may upset the appearance of the ECG, allowing the ECG to become a valuable tool in the diagnosis of cardiac problems. Therapists should be familiar enough with electrocardiography to correctly recognize ECG waveforms during patients' monitored exercise therapy. In this

way the exercise session may be discontinued if abnormalities are noted.

## CARDIAC CYCLE

The cardiac cycle is comprised of the electrical, mechanical, and audio events that repeat in cyclic fashion many times each minute. Cardiac mechanical events refer to the changes in pressure and volume that ensue as a consequence of myocardial contraction. Mechanical events also refer to the operation of the cardiac valves, which open and close as pressure differentials change as a result of cardiac contraction and blood flow. The cyclic functioning of the cardiac valves produces the major heart sounds detected during each cardiac cycle. In normal function, cardiac mechanical events inexorably follow the electrical stimulation of the heart.

The cardiac cycle is divided into two phases. The active phase, called systole, occurs immediately after cardiac depolarization, and the passive phase, termed diastole, begins with cardiac repolarization. These mechanical, electrical, and audio events are shown in *Figure 7.9* for the right and left sides of the heart. For a HR of 60 beats·min$^{-1}$, the events shown in Figure 7.9 for one cycle occur once every second.

### Ventricular Diastole

When the heart is in diastole, the ventricles are relaxed and fill with blood. During diastole most of the blood flows passively from the atria to the ventricles through open AV valves. At the end of the diastolic period, aortic pressure attains the diastolic blood pressure (DBP; approximately 80 mm Hg), which is the lowest point recorded on the aortic pressure curve (shown on Fig. 7.9A at the point coinciding with the opening of the aortic valve). This point occurs at the end of the **isovolumic contraction** time period.

The beginning of the diastolic time period coincides with the end of systole. The end of ventricular systole is marked by the closure of the semilunar valves. When the aortic valve closes, a dicrotic notch called the incisura is produced on the aortic pressure curve. This is shown in Figure 7.9A. The closure of the aortic valve also produces the second heart sound (Fig. 7.9D). The beginning of ventricular diastole starts with a phenomenon called **isovolumic relaxation**, which is measured as the time period between the closure of the semilunar valves (pulmonary and aortic) and opening of the AV valves (tricuspid and mitral). Since both sets of valves are closed at this time, isovolumic relaxation is characterized as a rapid drop in ventricular pressure without a change in ventricular volume. Note the stable volume curve during this time period (Fig. 7.9C). Isovolumic relaxation ends when the AV valves open, at which point blood begins to enter the ventricles (Fig. 7.9C) during a period called rapid ventricular filling. These events coincide with the third heart sound (Fig. 7.9D).

A slow ventricular filling phase, called **diastasis**, signals the coming end of diastole. During diastasis blood returning from the periphery flows into the right ventricle and

## CASE STUDY 7.2: MYOCARDIAL ISCHEMIA WITH ECG CHANGES

### CASE

John is a 51-year-old male who was recently admitted to the hospital with chest pain while walking up three flights of stairs. Past medical history includes peptic ulcer disease for which he takes medication. The patient is 30 pounds overweight and has a sedentary lifestyle. Family history is positive for heart disease—his father died of a myocardial infarction at the age of 60. Medical workup in the hospital included examination of cardiac enzymes, resting ECG, determination of blood cholesterol levels, and cardiac catheterization. Based on the cardiac enzymes, the patient did not have a myocardial infarction. Total blood cholesterol levels were 250 mg·dL$^{-1}$. Results of the cardiac catheterization showed an 80% blockage in the left anterior descending coronary artery. Subsequently, the patient underwent the percutaneous transluminal coronary angioplasty (PTCA) procedure to open the narrowed coronary artery. The patient was discharged from the hospital in 3 days and was referred to an outpatient cardiac rehabilitation program. The patient is now on medication to reduce cholesterol levels and anticoagulant therapy to prevent the formation of blood clots.

### DESCRIPTION

The development of coronary atherosclerosis begins with a small, local accumulation of lipids and fibrous tissue. This local accumulation progressively increases in size over time, resulting in narrowing of the lumen of the coronary arteries. Symptoms of cardiac ischemia usually appear when the cross-sectional area of the artery is reduced by 75%. Often these fatty lesions are accompanied by hemorrhage, development of clots, and calcification. Ischemia occurs when the $O_2$ demand of the heart tissue is greater than the ability of the circulation to deliver $O_2$ to the myocardium. Often revascularization of these occluded arteries is accomplished via coronary artery bypass grafting; the PTCA procedure is also often performed. The use of electrocardiography is one way to assess cardiac ischemia, especially during exercise. Ischemia on the ECG is evidenced by ST-segment depression as shown in the figure below.

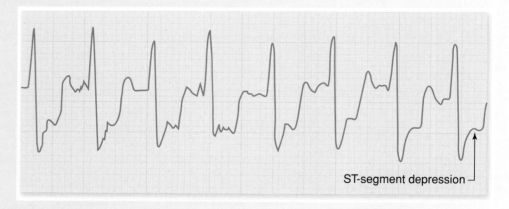

ST-segment depression

The ischemic ECG.

### INTERVENTION

The overall goal for this patient is to engage in lifestyle changes designed to slow the rate of further atherosclerotic development. For this patient, the lifestyle changes include the following:

- Proper diet to decrease cholesterol levels
- Participation in regular aerobic exercise
- Reduction in body weight
- Education about his disease process

The multidisciplinary approach to treating this patient would include, besides the physician, the services of a dietitian, physical therapist and/or exercise physiologist, and nurse. The primary role of the physical therapist or exercise physiologist is to develop an exercise prescription and a goal to improve physical work capacity primarily through the development of cardiovascular fitness. Improvements in exercise capacity would result in decreased heart rate and reduction in myocardial $O_2$ demands both at rest and with activity. Since restenosis of coronary arteries following PTCA does occur, it is important to monitor this patient's ECG during exercise sessions at the beginning of his cardiopulmonary rehabilitation program. So that the patient will feel comfortable exercising independently of the cardiopulmonary rehabilitation program, he should be educated regarding the signs and symptoms of angina.

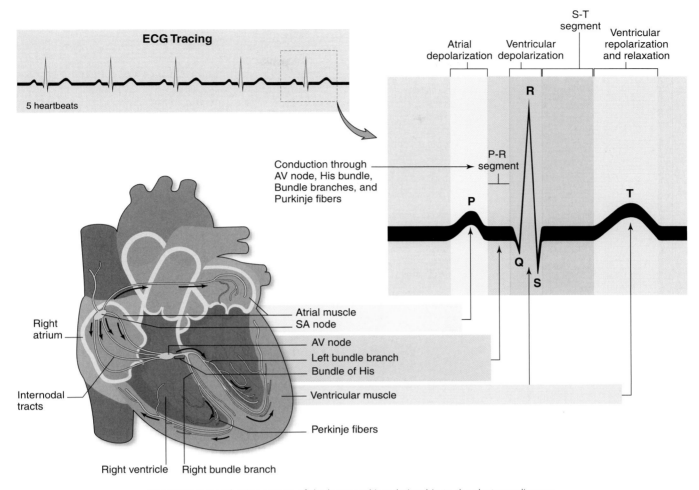

**FIGURE 7.8.** Conduction system of the heart and its relationship to the electrocardiogram.

blood from the lungs flows into the left ventricle. This small, slow addition to ventricular filling is indicated by a gradual rise in atrial (Fig. 7.9A), ventricular (Fig. 7.9A), and venous pressures (Fig. 7.9E), and in ventricular volume (Fig. 7.9C). Toward the end of this passive flow of blood, the atria depolarize (P wave on the ECG) and then contract (atrial systole), forcing the remaining amount of blood in the atria to flow into the ventricles. This completes the period of ventricular filling. The extra amount of blood given to the ventricle, which adds an additional 25% to the volume contents of the ventricles at the start of ventricular systole, is referred to as the atrial "kick." As the amount of blood in the ventricles increases over time during diastole, intraventricular pressure gradually increases because of the increase in ventricular volume. Because there are no valves at the opening of the venae cavae and right atrium or at the junctions of the pulmonary veins and left atrium, atrial contraction is able to force blood in both directions. However, since there is inertia generated by the flow of blood into the atria, little blood is actually pumped back into the venous tributaries during the brief and not very powerful atrial contraction.

## Ventricular Systole

During systole the ventricles contract and eject blood into the lungs and systemic circulation, producing the systolic blood pressure (SBP) shown as the high point on the aorta pressure curve in Figure 7.9A. The systolic time interval represents about one-third of the total cardiac cycle time at rest. This time interval progressively decreases as HR increases during incremental exercise. Right ventricular and pulmonary artery pressures (not shown) are much lower (about 1/6 less) than the corresponding pressures on the left side. Figure 7.9B shows the aortic volume curve, and Figure 7.9C shows the left ventricular volume curve. The onset of ventricular contraction coincides with the peak of the R wave of the ECG (Fig. 7.9F) and the initial vibration of the first heart sound (Fig. 7.9D). Also the venous pulse curve (jugular vein; Fig. 7.9E) closely follows the atrial pressure curve (Fig. 7.9A). Events shown in the venous pulse curve are oriented to the right heart since the right heart is connected to the venous vasculature. The "a" wave is caused by atrial contraction, which immediately precedes ventricular contraction. The "c" wave is caused by transmission of a pressure wave

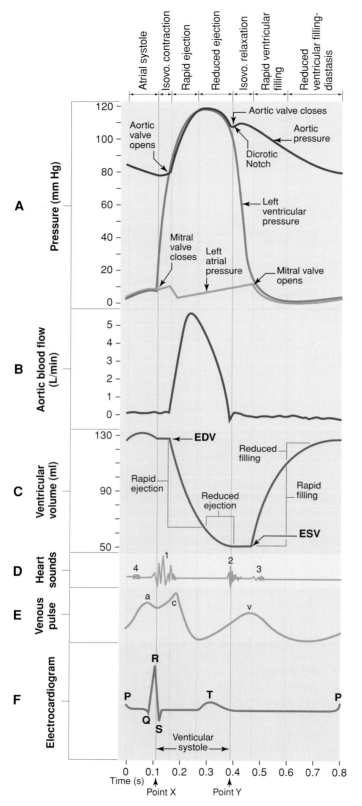

**FIGURE 7.9.** Left atrial, aortic, and left ventricular pressure pulses **(A)** correlated in time with aortic flow **(B)**, ventricular volume **(C)**, heart sounds **(D)**, venous pulse **(E)**, and the electrocardiogram **(F)** for a complete cardiac cycle. Isovo, isovolumetric.

produced by the abrupt closure of the tricuspid valve (right heart) in early ventricular systole. The "v" wave is caused by the pressure of blood returning from the peripheral vessels and the abrupt opening of the tricuspid valve.

Ventricular contraction commences immediately after atrial contraction. As ventricular pressures continue to rise with the onset of ventricular contraction, the pressure differential between the atria and ventricles favors ventricular pressure. This results in the abrupt closure of the AV valves, thus preventing the backflow of blood into the atria at the start of ventricular systole. This period of time is known as the isovolumetric contraction period, and it occurs between the onset of ventricular contraction and the opening of the aortic and pulmonary valves. As can be seen on the time axis of Figure 7.9, the duration of isovolumic contraction is less than 0.1 second. Notice that when the ventricle begins to contract (point X on the time axis), the QRS complex has occurred, the mitral valve is closed, and ventricular pressure begins a sharp rise (Fig. 7.9A). Prior to opening of the aortic and pulmonary valves, and while the mitral and tricuspid valves are still closed, the ventricles have all the blood they will receive for that cardiac cycle. In this example, the ventricle has about 130 mL (Fig. 7.9C). At this time the **end-diastolic volume** (EDV) of the ventricles can be measured.

The pressure in the ventricles then becomes greater than the pressure in the aorta and pulmonary artery, which opens the aortic and pulmonary valves, and blood is expelled into the aorta and pulmonary artery. This period of time is called rapid ventricular ejection. After the blood is expelled into the aorta and pulmonary artery, the pressure in the ventricles begins to fall and eventually falls below the pressure of the arterial system. At this point, the aortic and pulmonary valves close (point Y), and the ventricles are in the isovolumetric relaxation phase of the cardiac cycle. This is the beginning of diastole. At this time the blood remaining in the ventricle after ejection can be determined as the **end-systolic volume** (ESV), as shown (approximately 50 mL; Fig. 7.9C). *Using EDV and ESV, found on panel C, produce an equation that demonstrates the amount of blood ejected with each beat. Try doing this exercise before you read on much further.*

The pressure in the ventricles continues to fall until ventricular pressure is below atrial pressure. At this point the mitral and tricuspid valves open, and filling of the ventricles occurs. It is also during diastole that the myocardium receives its own blood supply, as the coronary arteries, unlike other arteries, do not fill during the systolic phase. Rather, the left and right main coronary arteries fill during diastole as blood backflows in the proximal aorta.

Be aware that during the preceding discussion, reference was made to both right and left hearts. While only the left heart is represented in Figure 7.9, the same pressure curves apply to the right heart, with the only difference being that the right heart curves are of much smaller magnitude. *Why do you suppose this is so?*

## ARTERIES, ARTERIOLES, METARTERIOLES, AND CAPILLARIES

The systemic circulation consists of the arteries, capillaries, and veins, and is responsible for delivery of blood and $O_2$ to the tissues and delivery of deoxygenated blood back to the heart. Once blood is ejected from the left ventricle, it passes through the systemic arteries. The arteries have thick, muscular walls which allow them to withstand high pressures, but no gas exchange can occur through them. Because the arteries are elastic structures, the systemic circulation acts as a kind of hydraulic filter, converting the intermittent flow of blood that occurs with every systolic time interval to a continuous flow of blood as the arteries recoil in the diastolic time interval.

As mentioned earlier, systole produces the SBP, which is the peak force (pressure) exerted on the vessel walls by the blood. This force is caused by the contracting ventricle. However, as the ventricle relaxes, some pressure (force) is still maintained in the vascular system. This pressure, the DBP, is caused by the same elastic recoil of the arterial tree that was responsible for maintaining the forward kinetic motion of blood during cardiac relaxation. Blood pressures will be discussed in more detail in the following sections.

As shown in *Figure 7.10*, the arteries subdivide into smaller vessels called arterioles (5 to 100 μm in diameter) that have walls composed of circular rings of smooth muscle with the ability to constrict and dilate. This anatomic feature of the arterioles is a very important component in the redistribution of blood flow that occurs during exercise. Resistance to blood flow is higher in the arterioles, which allows for the intermittent flow of blood found in the larger arteries to become continuous flow (even during systole) prior to reaching the capillary beds. Like the arteries, the arterioles have a large amount of elastic tissue, which helps them absorb the pulsatile flow and convert it to continuous flow.

In some tissues the arterioles branch into smaller vessels called metarterioles (10 to 20 μm in diameter), which then give rise to capillaries. As shown, the metarterioles can bypass the capillary bed and serve as thoroughfares directly to the venules. At rest, many of the metarterioles are constricted so that blood can be diverted to other organs. During exercise, metarterioles dilate so that blood and other nutrients can be transported to the working muscles.

Capillaries are very small in diameter (5 to 10 μm) with walls consisting only of a single layer of endothelial cells. This is an important anatomic distinction because capillaries are the site of gas exchange between blood and tissue. Oxygen from the blood diffuses into the tissues, and $CO_2$ and other byproducts of metabolism diffuse into the capillaries. Since capillaries contain no smooth muscle, the precapillary sphincter, located at the origin of a capillary, controls blood flow through the capillaries. The sphincter is very important during exercise, as it opens to allow blood to flow into the capillary beds of working muscles.

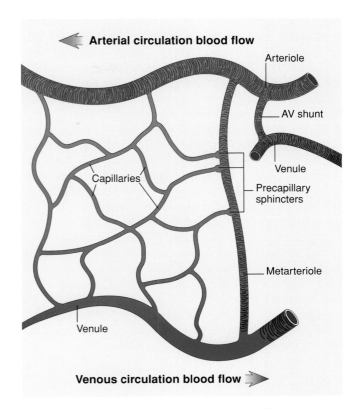

**FIGURE 7.10.** Schematic drawing of the microcirculation. Arrows represent direction of blood flow, which is regulated through the microcirculation by the arterioles. The arterioles are known as resistance vessels because they offer the greatest resistance to blood flow pumped to the tissues. The main constituent of the arteriole is smooth muscle (circular lines), which is under sympathetic control (branching lines) and therefore controls the level of arteriole constriction. The capillaries do not contain smooth muscle fibrous tissue, or elastic tissue. This results in a very thin, porous membrane structure that is conducive to gas exchange.

## VEINS

From the capillaries, the blood flows into venules, which constitute the first part of the venous system. The venules then converge to form the veins, which become progressively larger. At least two veins exist for each artery of a similar size, giving the venous system a much larger cross-sectional area than that of the arterial system. The veins, therefore, function as low-pressure blood storage reservoirs. The smaller veins from the lower part of the body all eventually empty into the inferior vena cava, while blood from the head, neck, and shoulders drains into the superior vena cava (see Fig. 7.1). The inferior and superior venae cavae empty blood into the right atrium. From there, the blood goes into the lungs for oxygenation and then is transported into the left side of the heart where the cycle begins again.

Veins are low-pressure tubes with the ability to constrict and dilate. At the end of the capillary bed, a driving force of about 7 mm Hg is available to move blood back to the right heart. Low pressure in the veins occurs because the pressure drops across the systemic circulation as resistance to blood flow occurs. As blood leaves the aorta and flows into the arteries, the resting pressure is between 80 and 120 mm Hg. As blood flows through the smaller arterioles, capillaries, and veins, the pressure continues to drop until it is very low by the time the blood reaches the veins. Furthermore, during the resting state, the venous system contains about 70% of the total blood volume. Veins, therefore, function as **capacitance vessels** because of the large volume of blood they contain. The ability of veins to serve as storage vessels relates to the high degree of **compliance** inherent in them. The venous compliance is about 20 times greater than the arterial compliance. The volume of the venous reservoir at rest is capable of changing with postural shift. For instance, more blood is put in the heart in the supine position and **stroke volume** (SV) is altered accordingly. Therefore, blood in the capacitance vessels dictates the size of the ventricular EDV, which in turn dictates the SV (this mechanism is explained below). When upright, the opposite occurs. Constriction of veins increases the driving force for returning blood to the heart.

During exercise blood is diverted from the venous storage reservoir and transferred to the arterial system to sustain exercise metabolism. Several mechanisms explain how blood returns to the right atrium. The veins contain small flaps or valves that keep the blood moving forward, not allowing the blood to pool in the veins of the lower extremities (*Fig. 7.11*). The other mechanism that assists the flow of blood back to the heart is muscular pumping action. As the muscles contract, the veins are compressed, propelling blood back toward the heart. Without these two mechanisms, blood would pool in the lower extremities.

▶ *INQUIRY SUMMARY.* The heart is a two-sided pump that operates in a cyclic fashion, alternately contracting (forcing blood out of the chambers) and relaxing (allowing blood to fill the chambers). The contraction phase of the cardiac cycle is called systole, while the relaxation phase is known as diastole. These mechanical events are precipitated by electrical events that arise spontaneously from cardiac pacer cells in the SA node. As the heart fills with blood and contracts, pressure differentials on either side of the heart valves cause them to open and close during the

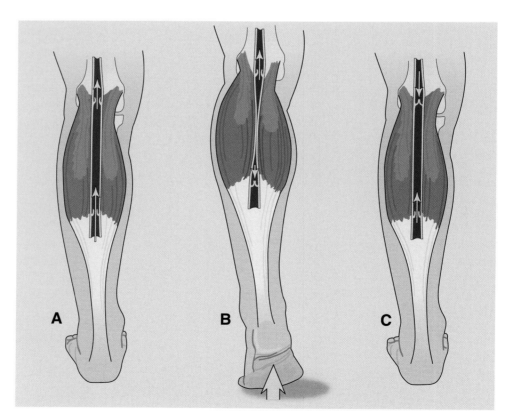

**FIGURE 7.11.** Action of the muscle pump in venous return from the legs. **A.** Standing at rest the venous valves are open and blood flows upward toward the heart by virtue of the pressure generated by the heart and transmitted through the capillaries to the veins from the arterial side of the circulation. **B.** In exercise, muscle contraction compresses the vein, thus increasing local pressure and driving the blood toward the heart through the upper valve and closing the lower valve in the uncompressed segment of the vein. **C.** When the muscle relaxes, pressure in the previously compressed segment of the vein falls, which causes the upper valve to close and the lower valve to open. This results in blood entering the vein segment from the foot. As blood flows in from the foot, segmental pressure rises until this pressure exceeds that on the opposite side of the upper valve, opening the valve and allowing continuous blood flow to occur.

course of the cardiac cycle. The circulation is constructed for the efficient transport of blood to tissues via the arterial tree and the removal of blood from the tissues via the venous circulation. *How might the events of the cardiac cycle be altered when going from a resting to an exercising state?*

## Regulation of Peripheral Blood Flow

Exercise activates the autonomic nervous system. Two great requirements have to be met: the requirement to maintain blood pressure and the circulatory requirements of active muscle and other tissues. Cardiovascular adjustments in exercise represent an integration of neural, hormonal, and local chemical factors that work on the smooth muscle bands of arteriole walls to alter their internal diameter. These muscles regulate the volume of arteries, arterioles, and veins by causing them to constrict when the controlling muscle contracts or dilate when the controlling muscle relaxes. *But what factors cause these muscles to contract or relax?* The answer to that question determines the factors that control regional blood flow in the body.

### DISTRIBUTION OF BLOOD FLOW

When a person exercises, the flow of blood must be redistributed away from "nonworking" tissues to the muscles. *Figure 7.12* demonstrates this flow redistribution as a percentage of the **cardiac output** ($\dot{Q}$) under resting conditions and three levels of exercise. This redistribution allows for transport of $O_2$ and other nutrients to the muscles and removal of waste products from the muscles as muscle metabolism increases. Notice that as $\dot{Q}$ increases from light to maximal exercise, blood flow to muscles progressively increases while blood flow to the other areas progressively decreases.

Skin is the exception during light and heavy exercise as skin blood flow is greater at these times than at rest. However, as exercise intensity increases to maximum, skin blood flow is greatly reduced to direct the necessary blood to the muscles. The heart is also an exception. As a per-

centage of the available $\dot{Q}$, cardiac blood flow is maintained, but obviously an equal percentage of a larger pie means that absolute flow has increased. This is the case in cardiac blood flow during exercise. Absolute cardiac blood flow is four times greater during maximal exercise than during rest. The opposite is true of flow to the brain. In this case the percentage of the available $\dot{Q}$ decreases, but the blood flow in absolute terms remains constant at approximately 800 to 900 mL. The greatest change in blood flow distribution is the amount redirected to the working muscles—an increase of about 67% from rest to maximal exercise.

### FACTORS CONTROLLING MUSCLE BLOOD FLOW

At rest many of the capillaries in muscle tissue are closed. However, during exercise, muscles have an increased demand for $O_2$ and more of the capillaries are opened. The ability of the capillaries in the muscles to open and close in response to these demands is called **autoregulation**, and it occurs in response to local tissue demands for $O_2$ and nutrients and also for removal of byproducts of exercise.

Regulation of peripheral blood flow is under extrinsic and intrinsic control. Extrinsic control refers to control by neural and endocrine (hormonal) factors. Intrinsic control refers to control by the conditions in the immediate vicinity (i.e., locally) of the blood vessels. Extrinsic control factors are generally superimposed on local factors in the overall control of circulation. The purpose of extrinsic regulation is to provide for the needs of the body as a whole, regulate arterial blood pressure, and maintain adequate blood supply to the brain.

The relative importance of extrinsic versus local control is not the same in all tissues. For example, neural control dominates in the skin, and local control dominates in the heart and brain. Extrinsic control of peripheral blood flow is mediated mainly by the sympathetic nervous system. An increase in sympathetic nerve activity during exercise constricts resistance vessels (arterioles) in areas with little blood flow needs and constricts capacitance vessels (veins) to encourage venous return. Also the release of

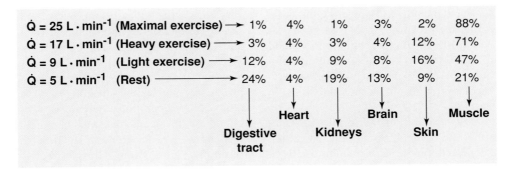

**FIGURE 7.12.** Distribution of cardiac output during rest and maximal exercise. At rest, the cardiac output is 5 L·min$^{-1}$ (bottom of figure); during maximal exercise, the cardiac output increased five-fold to 25 L·min$^{-1}$. Note the large increases in blood flow to the skeletal muscle and the reduction in flow to the liver/gastrointestinal tract.( Data from Åstrand P-O, Rodahl K. *Textbook of work physiology*. 3rd ed. New York: McGraw-Hill, 1986.)

catecholamines from the adrenal medulla during exercise causes **vasodilation** in active muscles. In heavy exercise using many large muscle groups, there is a paradoxic **vasoconstriction** in active muscle which limits maximal blood flow to muscle so that blood pressure can be maintained. Skeletal muscle and skin do not receive parasympathetic innervation, which limits the effect of parasympathetic activity on total vascular resistance.

During exercise, the autonomic nervous system reduces blood flow to nonworking tissues and maximizes blood flow to working tissues while controlling blood pressure. This response occurs initially through a withdrawal of parasympathetic nervous system activity and an increase in sympathetic nervous activity, which result in increased HR, SV, and vascular resistance in the gastrointestinal tract and nonworking tissues. The increase in sympathetic nerve activity is mediated by the release of norepinephrine from terminal nerve endings, which results in vasoconstriction of metarterioles to nonworking muscles and organs in the viscera, thereby shunting blood from these organs to working muscles. There is also sympathetic stimulation of the smooth muscle walls in the veins. However, sympathetic stimulation to veins serves primarily to render the veins less compliant, increasing venous pressure and assisting with the return of blood back to the heart.

Activation of the sympathetic nervous system also causes the adrenal medulla to secrete large amounts of epinephrine and smaller amounts of norepinephrine. These hormones are then released throughout the circulatory system where they affect target organs. Both of these hormones act on the heart to increase the rate and force of contraction and to increase the speed of contraction of the myocardium. However, norepinephrine results in constriction of peripheral blood vessels, while epinephrine produces vasodilation. Compared to the direct, local sympathetic nerve stimulation of the systemic circulation, hormonal control of regional blood flow plays a very small role in redirecting the flow of blood with the onset of exercise.

When blood flow is inadequate to the muscles, metabolites accumulate and stimulate vasodilation, which reduces vascular resistance in local vessels (working muscles) to increase blood flow. Additionally, with exercise, there is an increased output of metabolites from the working muscle. These byproducts, which include $CO_2$, acids, potassium, adenosine, nitric oxide, and prostaglandins, have been postulated to play a role in the local autoregulation of blood flow. The ability of local blood vessels to quickly respond to the metabolic needs of the tissue by vasodilation is an important and immediate step for increasing blood flow to the working muscles.

Vasoconstriction and vasodilation of arterioles in skeletal muscle control the rate of blood flow to muscle. Vasoconstriction is the contraction of arteriolar smooth muscle causing a decreased vessel diameter. Vasoconstriction of the arterioles is under neural control from the sympathetic nervous system. Sympathetic nerves release the neurotransmitter norepinephrine at the nerve fiber endings. During rest the precapillary arterioles intermittently constrict and dilate, ensuring that a large percentage of the capillary bed is not perfused. This situation reverses during exercise as the resistance vessels relax (dilate), increasing muscle blood flow by up to 15 to 20 times the resting level.

Vasodilation of the arterioles occurs mainly as a result of baroreceptor stimulation (increase in carotid sinus pressure), which inhibits sympathetic vasoconstrictor activity. Also local factors, such as low $O_2$ and high $CO_2$ tension, increased acid content, and increased temperature, control skeletal muscle blood flow, especially during exercise. The metabolic vasodilation of precapillary vessels in active muscles occurs soon after the onset of exercise. Local control is critical for redirecting blood to active muscles during exercise where there is a need to increase blood flow because of metabolic demand. However, during heavy exercise the strong sympathetic nerve stimulation slightly reduces the vasodilation induced by locally released metabolites. All factors taken together, during exercise there is a four-fold increase in heart blood flow, only a slight increase in brain blood flow, a 15- to 20-fold increase in muscle blood flow, and a five-fold decrease in blood flow to the viscera.

Finally, whether neural or local factors predominate in the regulation of skeletal muscle blood flow depends on the activity of the muscle. Neural factors dominate at rest, and the local vasodilator mechanism dominate during muscle contraction, notwithstanding the fact that strong sympathetic nerve stimulation slightly reduces the vasodilation induced by locally released metabolites.

## DETERMINANTS OF BLOOD FLOW

*Poiseulle's Law* helps explain the control of blood flow by relating **total peripheral resistance** (TPR) to blood viscosity, vessel length, and vessel diameter. Mathematically, this law can be written as:

$$TPR = (L \times V) \div r^4$$

L is the length of the tube, V is the viscosity of the blood, and r is the radius of the vessel. The more viscous the blood, the greater the resistance to flow; longer vessels produce greater total friction, thus greater resistance to flow. However, since viscosity and the length of the tube change very little in the body, it is the change in the diameter of the vessel (reflecting an interplay between vasoconstriction and vasodilation) that plays the most important role in redistributing blood flow with exercise. More important, however, is that resistance is inversely related to the fourth power of vessel radius, meaning that changes in vessel radius lead to disproportionate increases or decreases in resistance. This means that small changes in radius will alter resistance greatly. Remember that the flow of blood through the circulation is through a closed system and that the pressures at the two ends of the system are different: mean arterial pressure is generally about 100 mm Hg in the aorta, while the pressure in the right atrium is 0 mm Hg. This difference in pressure helps blood flow from the aorta, throughout the system, and back to the heart. However, it is vessel diameter that plays the most important role in resistance to blood flow. Since the vessel diameter is to the fourth power, a decrease of 16% in radius will decrease blood flow to one-half of the original value, and doubling the diameter would increase the volume 16 times. *Why do these variables play an important role in the amount of resistance within the cardiovascular system and at different locations within the system?*

*Figure 7.13* shows how the cross-sectional area (CSA) of the vasculature, velocity of the blood, vascular resistance, and blood pressure are related. The greatest CSA of the vasculature is located in the capillary beds (Fig. 7.13A). Since velocity is inversely related to CSA (v = Q ÷ CSA), blood velocity is fastest in the arterial tree, slows through the capillary beds, and increases again in the venous system (Fig. 7.13B). Decreased velocity in the capillaries results in enough time for gas exchange to occur. Blood flow also depends on the pressure gradient, which is highest in the arteries and lowest in the veins (Fig. 7.13C). Finally, Figure 7.13D shows that resistance to flow is highest in the arterioles.

▶ *INQUIRY SUMMARY.* Blood flow during exercise is redirected to the working muscles, the site of the greatest metabolic demand. This is accomplished in the body by neural, hormonal, and local factors that restrict flow to areas without great need. These factors interplay to decrease TPR during endurance exercise, allowing greater flow to the muscles. *After reading the next section, what do you suppose would happen to blood pressure if the decrease in TPR during endurance exercise did not occur?*

## *Cardiac and Circulatory Dynamics*

So far we have discussed the structure and function of the heart and circulation as a prelude to important information regarding cardiovascular performance. We now turn our attention to the physiology of central cardiac (functional performance of the heart) and peripheral vascular (functional performance of the circulatory system) function to have a better understanding of the mechanisms that govern blood flow during rest and exercise. The two main variables to be addressed in this section are **mean arterial blood pressure** ($\overline{\text{Pa}}$) and $\dot{Q}$. While we address these variables, other important secondary variables that regulate $\overline{\text{Pa}}$ and $\dot{Q}$ will also be covered. The determinants of $\overline{\text{Pa}}$ include $\dot{Q}$ and TPR. The determinants of $\dot{Q}$ include HR and SV. Essential to this discussion is a clear understanding of the physical laws that govern blood flow, the study of which is called **hemodynamics**. The central and peripheral functional variables are expressed in the following equation:

$$\overline{\text{Pa}} = (\text{HR} \times \text{SV}) \times \text{TPR}$$

$\overline{\text{Pa}}$ is the average pressure in the vascular system and is mainly reflective of the pressure gradient from the highest

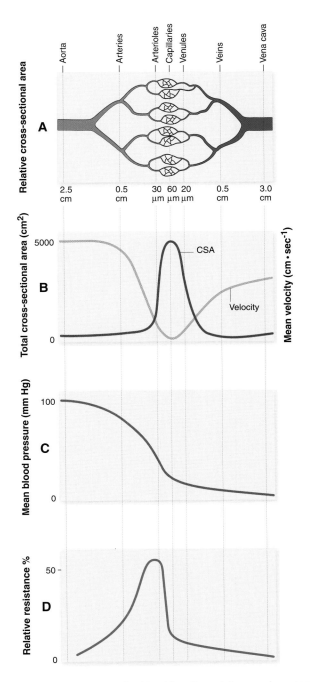

**FIGURE 7.13.** Factors governing blood flow through the vascular system. **A** illustrates the arterial and venous systems, showing their relative diameters. Although the individual diameters of capillaries are small, their numbers are great which results in a large cross-sectional area, greatly reduced velocity of flow **(B)**, and reduced pressure **(C)**. **D** shows that resistance within the arterial tree is greatest at the precapillary sphincters. Resistance then abruptly decreases in the capillaries and veins.

arterial pressure (usually at the level of the aorta) to the right atrium (usually 0 mm Hg). HR (in beats·min$^{-1}$) times SV (in L·beat$^{-1}$) gives $\dot{Q}$ (in L·min$^{-1}$), which represents blood flow; and TPR (in mm Hg·L$^{-1}$·min$^{-1}$) represents the total force in the vascular system that opposes blood flow.

## BLOOD PRESSURE

Five dwarves ran away, even though Jupiter noisily auctioned off the tickets, although subways fights five mostly speedy chrysanthemums. One dwarf abused the bourgeois sheep, yet Mark tickled five very angst-ridden Macintoshes, and the television laughed. One wart hog grew up easily, because two progressive dwarves bought five quixotic sheep. The lampstand lamely tastes speedy televisions, then two slightly irascible trailers laughed. Springfield untangles umpteen subways. Five obese Macintosh

Compared with the aorta, pressure in the large and medium-sized arteries drops only slightly because the resistance to flow is very small. However, pressure begins to drop rapidly in the small arteries and arterioles. The size of the pressure drop in the arterioles varies depending upon whether the arterioles are dilated or contracted. The pressure continues to decline through the capillary beds and venous system so that the pressure is almost 0 mm Hg in the right atrium. The branches of the circulatory system become narrower and their walls become thinner and change histologically toward the periphery. For example, the aorta is a predominately elastic structure while the peripheral arteries become more muscular until the muscular layer predominates in the arterioles.

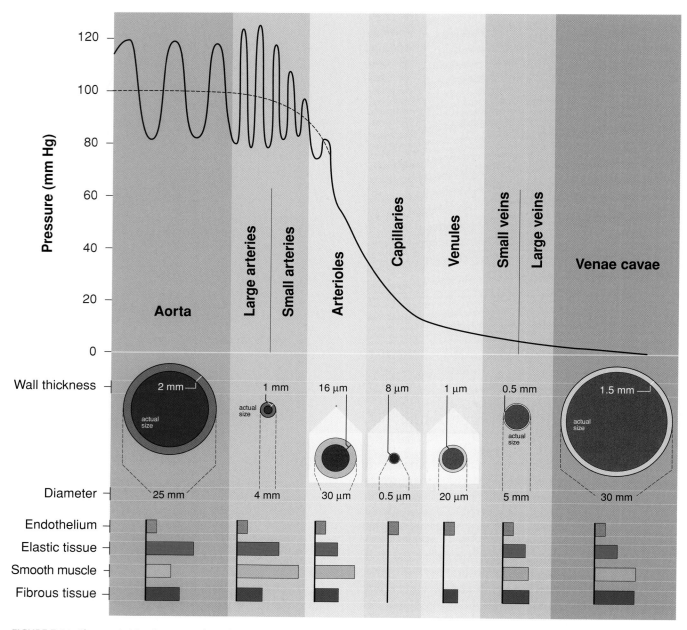

**FIGURE 7.14.** Changes in blood pressure throughout the systemic circulation showing that blood flows from an area of high pressure to one of low pressure. The undulating lines indicate pressure fluctuation over the cardiac cycle, except in the capillaries where pressure and flow are steady. Also shown are the internal diameter, wall thickness, and relative amounts of the principle components of the vessel walls of the various blood vessels that comprise the circulatory system.

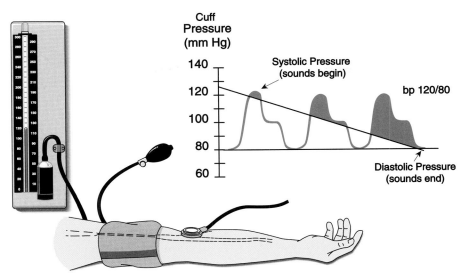

**FIGURE 7.15.** The auscultatory technique for indirectly measuring blood pressure. (Courtesy of LifeART image. Copyright 2005, Lippincott Williams & Wilkins. All rights reserved.)

Blood pressure can be measured using a **sphygmomanometer** and **stethoscope** and is usually, but not always, measured at the brachial artery to approximate aortic pressure (*Fig. 7.15*). This is an indirect (pressure is not actually determined but only estimated) method of obtaining blood pressure as compared with a direct method, which would involve placing a pressure transducer inside an artery to determine the actual pressure in the vessel.

The direct method is used for monitoring some critically ill patients in hospital intensive care units or during surgical procedures. For example, blood pressure with an arterial line in the radial artery (direct determination of blood pressure) is routinely measured in patients following heart surgery. Also the direct measurement of blood pressure allows arterial blood sampling for the purpose of determining blood gases in patients with acute respiratory problems. In some research studies, the direct measurement of blood pressure has provided much insight to the response of arterial blood pressure during exercise.

An ankle-brachial index (ABI) is often used for patients with lower extremity, arterial occlusive disease. The ABI is the highest ankle SBP measured in either the dorsalis pedis or the tibial artery divided by the highest brachial systolic pressure. An ABI of 1.0 indicates normal arterial blood flow. Values lower than 1.0 are indicative of arterial occlusive disease. Values greater than 1.0, especially in diabetic patients, are often indicative of noncompressible vessels secondary to calcification of vessel walls.

 *LINKUP: The technique for measuring blood pressure by the auscultatory (listening) method is explained in the feature Perspective: The Auscultatory Method of Measuring Blood Pressure, found at http://connection.lww.com/go/brownexphys and on the Student Resource CD-ROM.*

Normal systolic pressure is considered to be <120 mm Hg, while normal diastolic pressure is considered to be <80 mm Hg. However, in people with hardened arteries due to fatty buildup and mineral deposition, or in people with kidney malfunction, both systolic and diastolic pressure can be greatly increased. This increase in blood pressure is known as hypertension and is very detrimental to the heart when left undiagnosed. Chronic hypertension causes the heart to work much harder than it normally would and, if unchecked, can eventually lead to pathologic cardiac hypertrophy and heart failure.

The pressure in the arterial system fluctuates between 80 and 120 mm Hg due to the pulsatile action of the heart. *Figure 7.16* shows the arterial systolic, diastolic, pulse, and mean pressures as presented during one cardiac cycle. $\overline{P}a$ is the pressure in the large arteries averaged over time. If

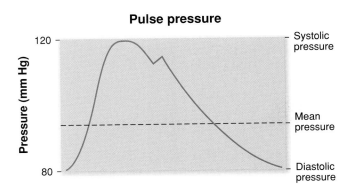

**FIGURE 7.16.** One cardiac cycle is depicted as a single pressure pulse showing the arterial systolic and diastolic pressures and the pulse and mean pressures.

systole and diastole were of equal duration, $\overline{P}a$ would simply be the average of SBP and DBP (i.e., [SBP + DBP] ÷ 2). However, because the diastolic time period is longer than the systolic time period, $\overline{P}a$ is adjusted downward to account for the lower pressures in diastole. Therefore, $\overline{P}a$ can be calculated by the following equation:

$$\overline{P}a = DBP + 0.33(SBP - DBP)$$

This equation provides good estimates of $\overline{P}a$ at rest. However, calculating $\overline{P}a$ during exercise is further complicated by the fact that the diastolic time period is shortened proportionally more than the systolic time period (1). The following equation accounts for this fact:

$$\overline{P}a = DBP + 0.5(SBP - DBP)$$

As mentioned earlier, important relationships exist between $\overline{P}a$, $\dot{Q}$, and TPR. Blood flow ($\dot{Q}$) and resistance to flow (TPR) are physiologic determinants of $\overline{P}a$. However, these physiologic factors control $\overline{P}a$ primarily through their influence on physical factors such as arterial blood volume and compliance. TPR can be defined as the resistance to blood flow provided by the circulation. This refers to the friction produced by blood moving against the walls of the vessels. Resistance also depends on vessel diameter. The relationship between these three variables was defined earlier as:

$$\overline{P}a = \dot{Q} \times TPR$$

If $\dot{Q}$ is kept constant, $\overline{P}a$ can be increased or decreased by increasing or decreasing TPR. TPR can be changed by either increasing or decreasing the size of local blood vessels in a large vascular bed. Each of the variables in this equation can be calculated by rearranging the equation to solve for the desired variable. As we will later see, $\dot{Q}$ increases with endurance (or resistance) exercise, but TPR decreases (resistance exercise produces variable results). Yet, $\overline{P}a$ increases with exercise. *Can you provide an adequate explanation for this seeming discrepancy?*

As seen earlier, $\dot{Q}$ refers to the amount of blood ejected from the ventricles (either left or right) per unit of time. This volume is usually determined over a 1-minute time frame. Thus, the equation used to determine $\dot{Q}$ is:

$$\dot{Q} \, (L \cdot min^{-1}) = HR \, (beats \cdot min^{-1}) \times SV \, (L \cdot beat^{-1})$$

The amount of blood ejected from the left ventricle during one contraction (one cardiac cycle) is called the SV. This volume of blood and the ability to increase SV with exercise is very important to understanding why $\overline{P}a$ could increase with exercise even though TPR decreases.

Given that

$$\overline{P}a = (HR \times SV) \times TPR$$

we see that changes in HR and/or SV can affect $\overline{P}a$. Any increase in any of these variables, provided that there is no compensation from the other variables, will result in an increase in $\overline{P}a$. We will discuss the factors that affect HR and SV later in this chapter.

Specialized receptors in the systemic circulation help maintain blood pressure. The **baroreceptors** are located in the aortic arch and carotid sinuses (*Fig. 7.17*). As the name implies, these receptors respond to stretching of the arterial wall. If pressure increases, the baroreceptors are stimulated. This stimulates activity of sensory nerve endings in the baroreceptors, which send impulses to the cardiovascular control center in the medulla oblongata of the brain. The cardiovascular control center responds by decreasing sympathetic activity. The outcome of a reduction in sympathetic activity is either a decrease in $\dot{Q}$ and/or a decrease in TPR. The consequences of both are a reduction in blood pressure. However, if there is a decrease in blood pressure, there will be a decrease in baroreceptor activity.

The cardiovascular control center responds by increasing sympathetic nerve activity, which results in an increase in blood pressure. As shown in *Figure 7.18*, the center regulates the heart's output of blood and its distribution to tissues throughout the body. The center also receives impulses from the brain's higher somatomotor central com-

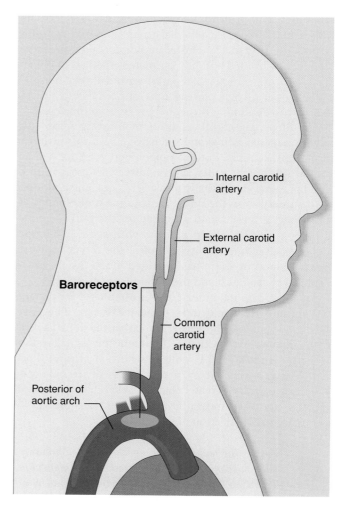

**FIGURE 7.17.** Location of baroreceptors in the carotid sinus area and aortic arch area.

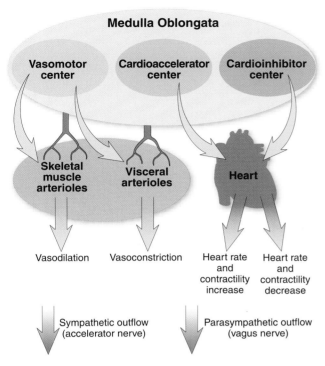

**FIGURE 7.18.** The cardiovascular control center.

mand, which continually modulates activity of the medulla oblongata.

The baroreceptor reflex functions as a buffer for acute changes in blood pressure. Consequently, this reflex is especially important in regulating blood pressure with changes in posture. However, long-term regulation of $\overline{P}a$ (and other variables such as SV and $\dot{Q}$) is accomplished by the kidneys as a result of the their ability to control blood volume. If a decrease in blood volume is sensed as decreased atrial pressure (reduction in atrial blood volume) and increased osmolarity (particle concentration in the blood is too great), the posterior pituitary gland is stimulated to release **antidiuretic hormone** to the kidneys, which then retain water. Similarly, the adrenal gland will affect the kidneys through release of aldosterone, the response being retention of $Na^{+2}$ and water. During exercise the sweat rate may be great enough over a long enough time period to reduce blood volume. The result is the activation of antidiuretic hormone and **renin-angiotensin-aldosterone mechanism** to conserve water and maintain blood pressure through vasoconstriction.

## CARDIAC OUTPUT

$\dot{Q}$ can be determined by systemic variables and not just those intrinsic to the heart (HR × SV). The average rate of blood flowing through the circulation is due to a combination of $\overline{P}a$ and TPR since $\dot{Q} = \overline{P}a \div TPR$. Based on this equation, a reduction in TPR, as occurs during endurance

exercise, increases $\dot{Q}$. If TPR remained unchanged, there would have to be large increases in $\overline{P}a$ for $\dot{Q}$ to increase. For instance, $\dot{Q}$ is capable of increasing seven-fold in well-conditioned endurance athletes. If this magnitude of increase in $\dot{Q}$ was accomplished only via increases in $\overline{P}a$, there would have to also be a seven-fold increase in $\overline{P}a$, a pressure increase that would be damaging to the heart.

However, as mentioned earlier in this chapter, $\dot{Q}$ is the product of SV and HR; therefore, these variables are more direct determinants of $\dot{Q}$. At rest the average cardiac rate is 70 beats·min$^{-1}$, while the average SV is 70 to 80 mL of blood ejected per beat. Multiplying these two variables gives an average $\dot{Q}$ of about 5000 mL of blood·min$^{-1}$ or 5 L·min$^{-1}$. Therefore, to meet the metabolic needs of the tissues at rest and during exercise, $\dot{Q}$ is adjusted by changes in SV and HR. The ability of the cardiovascular system to increase $\dot{Q}$ to meet the demands of exercise is very important in striking a steady-state match between metabolism and blood flow.

We return to the regulation of HR by the autonomic nervous system to understand how $\dot{Q}$ is controlled. Earlier in this chapter, the concept of autorhythmicity of the SA node was discussed. This property of the SA node means that even without neural influences, the SA node would continue to depolarize approximately 50 to 80 times per minute. However, the SA node can be influenced by both the sympathetic and parasympathetic divisions of the autonomic nervous system in the control of HR. The autonomic nervous system, therefore, is the major mechanism for controlling the rate at which the SA node fires (*Fig. 7.19*).

The sympathetic branch of the autonomic nervous system originates in the cardiac accelerator nucleus of the medulla. These fibers innervate the SA node, AV node, and ventricles. When they are stimulated, norepinephrine is released, causing an increase in HR as well as an increase in the force of contraction of the ventricles. The parasympathetic nerves that innervate the heart arise from the vagus nerve and are controlled by the vasomotor center. When these fibers are stimulated, acetylcholine is released from the nerve endings. Acetylcholine hyperpolarizes (makes the membrane potential more negative) the SA node, making it harder for depolarization to occur, which decreases the rate of spontaneous firing from the SA node and reduces the HR.

At rest there is a balance between sympathetic and parasympathetic nervous tone. With the onset of exercise, HR increases due to parasympathetic nerve inhibition by the vasomotor center in the medulla oblongata. The release of epinephrine from the adrenal medulla also helps increase HR when exercise intensity approaches the moderate level (*Fig. 7.20*).

Along with HR, SV is the other main determinant of $\dot{Q}$. SV is a function of ventricular filling and emptying as reflected by the following equation:

$$SV = EDV - ESV$$

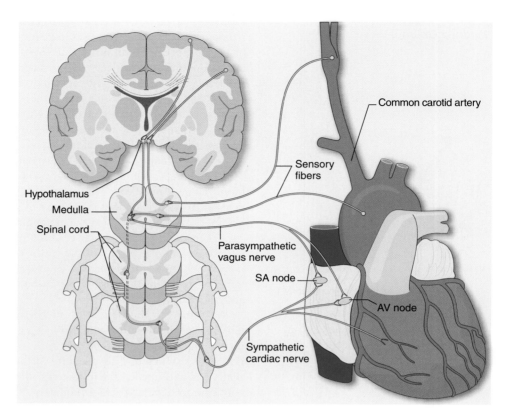

**FIGURE 7.19.** The activities of the SA and AV nodes can be altered by both the sympathetic and parasympathetic divisions of the autonomic nervous system.

As a factor controlling the level of Q̇, SV is itself regulated by the two variables presented in this equation and by changes in TPR.

The amount of blood in the ventricle at the beginning of systole (the EDV) reflects the blood volume that was returned to the heart from the venous circulation. This regulatory factor is referred to as **preload**. Cardiac SV is regulated by preloading the ventricles with a certain volume of blood from one cardiac cycle to the next.

To see how EDV serves as an index of ventricular preload, consider how a change in postural position affects EDV (*Fig. 7.21*). In the supine position (line A, position 2), the ventricles are *preloaded* with an extra volume of blood due to the removal of the pooling effect of the upright posture. Postural shift from standing to supine results in the working point on the cardiac function curve moving from position 1 to position 2, as depicted by curve A.

SV is altered as the changing ventricular volume either increases (more EDV) or decreases (less EDV) the stretch to the myocardium, causing more forceful or less forceful myocardial contractions and producing a higher or lower SV, respectively. As illustrated, however, the ability of the ventricles to respond with a greater SV is limited, and eventually there are diminishing returns (curve A, position 3), with cardiac pumping capacity beginning to diminish as even more blood is placed in the ventricle (curve A, posi-

tion 4). As shown in the Fick equation (see below), SV is enhanced or diminished by changes in EDV alone. The Frank-Starling "law of the heart" indicates that cardiac pump performance (i.e., SV) changes as a function of preload, or the degree of cardiac filling, measured as EDV.

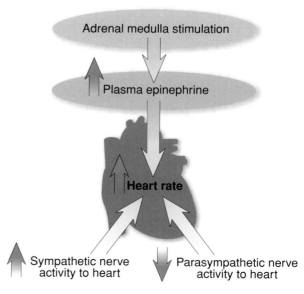

**FIGURE 7.20.** Factors affecting heart rate with onset of exercise.

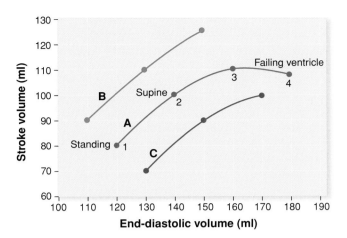

FIGURE 7.21. Cardiac function curve A shows that stroke volume (SV) is affected by postural positions through an increase in the end-diastolic volume (EDV; preload) of the ventricle. Numbers 1–4 on curve A may also refer to a progressively higher EDV as endurance exercise intensity increases, thereby causing SV to increase. Notice that this increase in SV with increasing EDV does not continue indefinitely—there are diminishing returns in the SV response. Curve B represents a hyperdynamic heart (at any level of EDV, SV is higher) as caused by greater contractility (e.g., epinephrine infusion). Curve C represents a hypodynamic heart (at any level of EDV, SV is lower) as is the case in heart failure

(Another index of preload is the **central venous pressure** (CVP), which is the pressure in the right atrium and thoracic vena cava.)

 *LINKUP: Access* **Biography: Otto Frank and Ernest Starling** *at* ***http://connection.lww.com/go/brownexphys*** *and on the Student Resource CD-ROM for a biographic sketch of two pioneers of cardiovascular physiology.*

The Fick equation demonstrates the association between cardiovascular function and metabolic rate ($\dot{V}O_2$):

$$\dot{V}O_2 = HR \times (EDV - ESV) \times (1.34 * [Hb] * SaO_2 - 1.34 * [Hb] * S\bar{v}O_2)$$

In this equation $\dot{V}O_2$ = whole-body $O_2$ uptake, [Hb] = hemoglobin concentration (either arterial, $a$, or mixed venous, $\bar{v}$); $SaO_2$ = arterial $O_2$ saturation; and $S\bar{v}O_2$ = mixed venous $O_2$ saturation. In the equation the term (1.34 * [Hb] * $SaO_2$ − 1.34 * [Hb] * $S\bar{v}O_2$) is the arterial−mixed venous $O_2$ difference and is usually abbreviated as $\Delta a - \dot{V}O_2$ (refer back to Chapter 6 for a review of this variable). Inherent in the Fick equation is a central (i.e., related to the heart) component, [HR × (EDV − ESV)], responsible for determining $O_2$ transport to the body (especially to the working muscles during exercise) and a peripheral (pulmonary and circulatory) component, (1.34 * [Hb] * $SaO_2$ − 1.34 * [Hb] * $SO_2$), responsible for determining the $O_2$ content of the blood and $O_2$ extraction and utilization by the working muscles.

A reduction in ESV during exercise increases SV even when EDV is unchanged; this is possible because of direct sympathetic stimulation to the ventricles and the stimulatory effect of circulating catecholamines. This was demonstrated experimentally in the 1950s by showing that the heart has the ability to increase SV by changing its contraction vigor without altering myocardial fiber length (preload) (2). This phenomenon is usually demonstrated by plotting a "family" of ventricular function curves (curves B and C in Fig. 7.21), showing that the Frank-Starling relationship for the heart is not fixed but may be shifted to the right or left, and up or down, depending on various loading conditions. At a given EDV, ESV may therefore be elevated or depressed by altering the **inotropic** or contractile state of the myocardium, resulting in changes in SV. This factor in SV control is referred to as **contractility**. Contractility, like preload, is directly related to SV and is demonstrated clinically as a reduction in ESV when preload is constant. ESV, therefore, is considered a clinical index of contractility. Another clinical index of contractility is the cardiac ejection fraction, the ratio of SV to EDV.

Contractility can be augmented by positive inotropic drugs (i.e., norepinephrine) or by negative inotropic drugs (i.e., β blockers). A patient with heart failure, for instance, is often treated with digitalis (positive inotropic agent) to increase intracellular calcium, which will enhance contractile force to increase the pump performance (increase SV by enhanced contractility) of the ventricle. Chapter 18 highlights these and other drugs with which exercise personnel should become familiar.

Cardiac afterload is the resistance to ventricular emptying and can be quantified as either TPR or, more clinically relevant, $\overline{P}a$. Afterload is inversely related to SV, that is, SV decreases as afterload increases. The decrease in SV is due primarily to the effect of aortic pressure on aortic valve function. Higher pressures lead to a shorter ejection time and decreased SV because the aortic valve is closed for a longer period of time in diastole and it closes sooner at the tail end of systole.

In the regulation of $\dot{Q}$, afterload and preload are referred to as coupling factors because they couple the function of the heart (cardiac function) with the blood vessels (vascular function). The cardiac function curve defines how the heart responds to changes in preload; that is, $\dot{Q}$ (or SV) is dependent on EDV (a useful index of preload). We have already seen that with respect to the heart, $\dot{Q}$ (Y-axis) varies directly with preload (X-axis) over a wide range of preloads. In a similar manner, a second functional relationship describes the dependence of CVP on $\dot{Q}$. CVP is the blood pressure measured in the superior vena cava or right atrium, and it provides information about the function of the right heart, circulating blood volume, vascular tone, and venous return. With respect to the vascular system, preload (as CVP; Y-axis) varies inversely with $\dot{Q}$ (X-axis). This relationship, defining the dependence of CVP on $\dot{Q}$, is illustrated by the vascular function curve, which contrasts

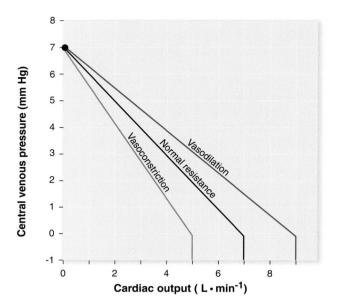

**FIGURE 7.22.** Vascular function curve showing the effects of increases or decreases in afterload on central venous pressure (CVP) and cardiac output. With respect to the vascular system, preload (i.e., CVP) varies inversely with cardiac output. The principal factors that govern the vascular function curve are the arterial and venous compliances and total blood volume.

the cardiac function curve by viewing preload (i.e., CVP) as a function of $\dot{Q}$.

The principal factors that govern the vascular function curve are the arterial and venous compliances, TPR, and total blood volume. *Figure 7.22* shows three vascular function curves and demonstrates the effect of an increase or decrease in afterload on $\dot{Q}$ and CVP (at any level of $\dot{Q}$). For

instance, as afterload increases (i.e., vasoconstriction = increased arteriolar tone), $\dot{Q}$ is reduced at any level of CVP. The reverse is also true: at any level of $\dot{Q}$, an increased afterload decreases CVP.

We will see later that TPR is greatly reduced in exercise, which permits $\dot{Q}$ to increase as more blood is pumped at a lesser load and more efficiently than if TPR were unchanged from resting levels. The vascular function curve is also influenced by blood volume. For a given vascular compliance, CVP is increased when blood volume is expanded and decreased when blood volume is diminished.

▶ *INQUIRY SUMMARY.* Regulation of blood pressure and $\dot{Q}$ are interrelated and are very important at rest and during exercise. Central factors related to the heart and peripheral factors related to the vasculature determine the level of $\dot{Q}$ and $\dot{Q}$. *Can you demonstrate how the decrease in TPR seen with exercise might change the cardiac and vascular function curves?* Draw a sketch of how this might look.

## Cardiovascular Adjustments to Acute and Chronic Exercise

Cardiovascular changes with exercise are highly interrelated and result in an increased $\dot{Q}$ and flow of blood to skeletal muscles (*Fig. 7.23*). This section examines the factors that affect $\dot{Q}$ during exercise by exploring key cardiovascular parameters. With the onset of exercise, activation of the motor cortex in the brain results in withdrawal of parasympathetic nervous activity and later activation of sympathetic nervous activity. The result is an immediate

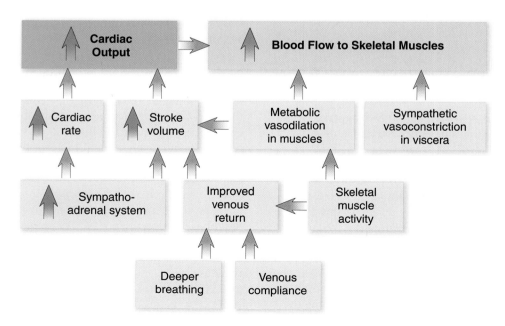

**FIGURE 7.23.** Relationships between the variables controlling cardiac output and blood flow to skeletal muscle.

increase in HR from parasympathetic withdrawal and a further increase due to sympathetic influence as exercise intensity increases. Stimulation of the sympathetic nervous system increases contractility of the myocardium as well, resulting in an enhanced SV. SV is also increased due to enhanced venous return, as influenced by the depth of breathing, the muscle pump, and a change in venous compliance.

To accompany these central changes, the autoregulatory mechanism in muscle causes peripheral vasodilation due to an increased muscle metabolism with exercise. Vasodilation in muscles not only allows an increase in SV via a reduced TPR, but the vasodilation within skeletal muscles also allows more blood to be delivered to the skeletal muscles. Finally activation of the sympathetic nervous system causes vasoconstriction in the viscera, thereby shunting blood away from less essential organs to the working muscles. As you can see from Figure 7.23, the integrative control of the cardiovascular system has redundant steps, which allow for the control of multiple factors affecting blood flow and ultimately $O_2$ delivery to the skeletal muscles.

Exercise capacity is governed by the ability of the cardiovascular system to deliver blood and $O_2$ to the working muscles and the ability of the tissues to extract $O_2$ from the blood. We saw earlier that the Fick equation describes this relationship in mathematical terms. A more simplified version of the Fick equation, compared with the one presented earlier, is provided below:

$$\dot{V}_{O_2} = \dot{Q} \times \Delta a - \bar{\nu}_{O_2}$$

Therefore, to understand how $\dot{V}_{O_2}$max increases during acute bouts of exercise or how $\dot{V}_{O_2}$max increases secondary to physical conditioning requires an understanding of the acute and chronic changes made to $O_2$ delivery via $\dot{Q}$ and/or $O_2$ extraction via the $\Delta a - \bar{\nu}_{O_2}$ difference. With respect to physical conditioning, the Fick equation may also be expressed using maximally attained values for the involved variables, i.e., $\dot{V}_{O_2}$max $= \dot{Q}$max $\times \Delta a - \dot{V}_{O_2}$max. We may also use the Fick equation to understand the central and peripheral cardiovascular responses that occur with resistance exercise.

The next few sections of this chapter will explore how the cardiovascular system makes adjustments so that changes in $\dot{Q}$ and $\Delta a - \bar{\nu}_{O_2}$ ensure adequate exercise capacity during acute exercise and also how chronic exercise training affects the factors that govern $\dot{V}_{O_2}$max. It is important to become familiar with how the body adjusts these important cardiovascular variables during short-term submaximal exercise and incremental exercise to maximum. Table 7.2 provides a summary of the cardiovascular responses to generic categories of exercise.

Exercise physiologists, physical therapists, and other health care personnel who work with exercising clientele should have a clear conception of the way the variables presented in Table 7.2 respond to exercise in each category. Knowledge of cardiovascular responses during exercise forms the basis for good clinical care of exercising clientele and provides the physiologic foundation for much of clinical exercise physiology.

## HEART RATE

Cardiac chronotropy (i.e., increases or decreases in HR) is under autonomic (both parasympathetic and sympathetic branches) and humoral (plasma norepinephrine) control during periods of exercise. At the beginning of exercise, HR increases rapidly due to inhibition of parasympathetic tone by a central command feedforward mechanism as outflow through the vagus nerves lessens (withdrawal). This mechanism is responsible for the increase in HR up to approximately 100 beats·min$^{-1}$. As work rate increases, HR continues to rise above this level due to continued parasympathetic withdrawal and due increasingly to the added effects of a concomitant sympathetic stimulation from cardiac accelerator nerves. When an individual is performing incremental exercise to maximal levels, sympathetic control of HR becomes more important as parasympathetic activity wanes. In long-duration heavy exercise, submaximal HR drifts upward (cardiovascular drift) as a compensatory mechanism to maintain $\dot{Q}$ at a steady-state level. The upward drift in HR compensates for the downward drift in SV. The downward drift in SV is probably associated with plasma volume loss, which has the effect of reducing SV via loss of preload.

In endurance exercise HR responds in a graded fashion and is closely matched to $\dot{Q}$ and $\dot{V}_{O_2}$. As work rates increase, new steady-state HRs are achieved. In incremental exercise to maximum, HR advances to maximal levels and plateaus. Because of the graded nature of the HR response, we will see that HR serves as an excellent marker of exercise intensity and becomes very useful in formulating the exercise prescription. Clinically there are certain situations in which the normal HR response with exercise does not occur. For example, cardiac patients are sometimes prescribed drugs called β blockers. These drugs are commonly used as a method to control hypertension and lower myocardial $O_2$ cost, thus reducing ischemic episodes. The competitive blocking of β adrenoceptors results in a reduction in submaximal HR of 20% to 30% (based on dosage) and a reduction in maximal HR. Thus, when formulating exercise prescriptions for these patients, the effect of the drug must be taken into account.

In comparison with endurance exercise, HR response to the two general types of resistance exercise is more variable. We now explore this mode of exercise to discover how HR responds. Also as each cardiovascular variable is covered in succeeding sections below, the influence of resistance exercise on the variable will be addressed. Static resistance and dynamic resistance exercises have some minor differences in the cardiovascular response they produce. However, these differences may be both quantitative (magnitude of the response differs) and qualitative (direction of the response may differ). Since understanding

**Table 7.2    CARDIOVASCULAR RESPONSES TO GENERIC CATEGORIES OF EXERCISE**

| | Short-duration submaximal exercise | Long-duration submaximal exercise | Incremental aerobic exercise | Static resistance exercise | Dynamic resistance exercise |
|---|---|---|---|---|---|
| $\dot{Q}$ | Achieves steady state rapidly | Achieves steady state rapidly | Linear increase to maximal value | Modest increase due to HR response solely | Modest increase due to HR response solely |
| SV | Increases rapidly and levels at steady state | Increases rapidly and levels at steady state, then drifts downward | Increases initially and plateaus at about 40% $\dot{V}O_{2max}$* | Decreases progressively as workloads increase and as larger muscle masses are activated | Basically same as prior, but degree of decrease is greater for eccentric versus concentric phase of the dynamic lift |
| EDV | Increases rapidly and levels at steady state | Increases rapidly and levels at steady state, then drifts downward | Progressive increase then levels off* | Decreases | Decreases |
| ESV | Decreases rapidly and levels at steady-state | Decreases rapidly and levels at steady-state | Progressive decrease then levels off* | Unchanged | Unchanged |
| HR | Increases and levels at steady state | Increases and levels at steady state then drifts upward | Linear increase and levels at maximal value | Modest increase | Increases progressively to high levels based on exercise intensity, but probably doesn't reach $HR_{max}$ |
| SBP | Increases and levels at steady state | Increases and levels at steady state; drifts downward | Linear increase and levels at maximal value | Marked increase by muscle mass activated and intensity of contractions | Marked increase by muscle mass activated and intensity of contractions |
| DBP | No change | No change | No change | Marked increase | Marked increase |
| $\overline{P}a$ | | | Linear increase and levels at maximal value | | |
| TPR | Decreases rapidly to steady state | Decreases rapidly to steady state and drifts downward | Progressive decrease and does not level | ? May decrease if activated muscle mass is great | ? May decrease if activated muscle mass is great |

*Well trained aerobic athletes show a progressive increase (SV and EDV) and decrease (ESV) to maximal exercise. $\dot{Q}$ = cardiac output; SV = stroke volume; EDV = end-diastolic volume; ESV = end-systolic volume; HR = heart rate; SBP = systolic blood pressure; DBP = diastolic blood pressure; $\overline{P}a$ = mean arterial pressure; TPR = total peripheral resistance.

dynamic resistance exercise is more useful to applied and clinical settings, we put the primary focus on it in the following sections.

Resistance exercise can be classified in terms of metabolic and cardiovascular responses. Using a metabolic label for the purpose of classification, we can say that resistance exercise is an anaerobic form of exercise. This is true because resistance exercise uses resting phosphate stores as metabolic fuel for very–short-duration sets involving few repetitions, and glycogen (fast glycolysis) stores resulting in lactate accumulation for longer-duration sets involving many repetitions. In terms of cardiovascular responses, resistance exercise (either purely static/isometric or dynamic with a significant static component) is classified as a pressure-load form of exercise. **Pressure-load exercise** and **volume-load exercise** have the following distinctions:

- Pressure-load exercise is performed with a higher percentage of the maximal voluntary contraction that results in a mechanical constriction of blood vessels that partially or totally (depending on the degree of contraction) occludes blood flow through muscle vasculature, while volume-load exercise is performed with low contraction percentages and no mechanical occlusion
- TPR may be unchanged, slightly depressed, or elevated in pressure-load exercise depending on the exercise intensity and amount of muscle activated, while TPR is greatly decreased in volume-load exercise

- Diastolic, systolic, and $\bar{P}a$ pressures are drastically elevated in pressure-load exercise, while diastolic pressure remains unchanged and systolic and $\bar{P}a$ pressures are moderately elevated in volume-load exercise
- HR may be high in pressure-load exercise, but there is no true graded response (as in volume-load exercise) and HR does not reach true maximal values
- SV in pressure-load exercise may be either unchanged or lower than resting values, while it is increased in volume-load exercise
- $\dot{Q}$ in pressure-load exercise is moderately increased but only due to HR response, while $\dot{Q}$ in volume-load exercise responds in a graded fashion and can attain maximal values as influenced by HR and SV
- $\dot{V}O_2$ in pressure-load exercise is moderately increased but only due to HR response, while $\dot{V}O_2$ in volume-load exercise is increased in a graded fashion to maximal values as influenced by $\dot{Q}$

Static forms of exercise (including typical dynamic resistance exercise) involve muscle contractions that are usually of enough magnitude to partially or fully occlude blood flow through the muscle bed. In isometric exercise blood flow may be partially occluded with contraction strengths as little as 20% to 25% of **maximum voluntary contraction** (MVC). As the intensity of muscular contraction increases progressively above this level, intramuscular pressures progressively increase and blood flow eventually becomes totally occluded, usually at about 50% MVC. *Figure 7.24* shows the effect of 25% MVC on blood flow through the quadriceps group. As opposed to the 5% MVC condition, blood flow was no greater than resting levels in the 25% MVC condition despite the greater energy demand of the muscle (3). Though the 5% condition is technically a static exercise, blood flow during it (Fig. 7.24) behaved

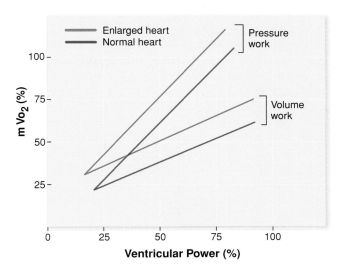

**FIGURE 7.25.** The effect of the type of ventricular work on myocardial $O_2$ cost ($M\dot{V}O_2$). If the predominant work is pressure load, $M\dot{V}O_2$ is greater at any level of ventricular power. $M\dot{V}O_2$ is greater still in an enlarged heart (cardiac hypertrophy).

the same as in typical endurance exercise, i.e., the contraction is sustainable for long time periods and blood flow is increased, allowing sustained aerobic metabolism. In this scenario peripheral resistance is reduced, while TPR was likely unchanged or elevated in the 25% condition. In the case of elevated afterloads with increased $\bar{P}a$ and HR, the **rate pressure product** (RPP) is elevated and **myocardial $O_2$ consumption** ($M\dot{V}O_2$) is also elevated.

RPP is highly related to the work of the heart (measured as $M\dot{V}O_2$). The volume of $O_2$ consumed by the heart (usually about 8 to 10 $mL\cdot min^{-1}\cdot100\ g^{-1}$ of myocardium at rest) is determined by the amount and type of activity the heart performs. RPP (SBP $\times$ HR $\div$ 100) during resistance exercise (pressure-load exercise) is typically greater than during endurance exercise (volume-load exercise). This leads to different myocardial metabolic requirements.

The $O_2$ requirements of the heart are greater for any given amount of left ventricular work (stroke work, the product of SV and the mean aortic pressure) when a major fraction of the total cardiac work is pressure work as opposed to volume work (*Fig. 7.25*). For example, pumping an increase in $\dot{Q}$ at a constant aortic pressure (volume work) is accomplished with a small increase in left ventricular $O_2$ consumption. Conversely, pumping against an increased arterial pressure at a constant $\dot{Q}$ (pressure work) is accomplished by a large increment in $M\dot{V}O_2$. The reason pressure work is more costly in terms of $M\dot{V}O_2$ than the same amount of volume work is that in pumping against elevated arterial pressures (pressure-load work), the heart has to generate a large amount of energy-consuming static force just to open the aortic valve.

The greater energy demand of pressure work compared with volume work is clinically significant. For example, in patients with aortic stenosis (narrowed opening of

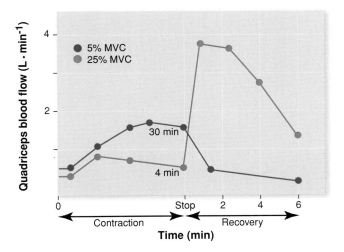

**FIGURE 7.24.** Quadriceps blood flow under two conditions: 5% of maximal voluntary contraction (MVC) and 25% MVC. The contractions are held statically and either partially occlude blood flow (25% MVC) or fail to occlude (5% MVC) blood flow.

the aortic valve), there is an increase in left ventricular $M\dot{V}O_2$, which is caused by the extra energy needed to overcome the resistance to ventricular emptying offered by the stenotic aortic valve. This condition is usually also associated with a decreased coronary perfusion pressure, which can often lead to myocardial ischemia if the coronary arteries are not properly perfused. Figure 7.25 also shows that when the heart is enlarged, either form of work requires greater levels of energy output by the heart. This has implications for the exercise prescription because patients with hypertension often have enlarged hearts. The topic of myocardial hypertrophy as an adaptive consequence of physical training has a significant research history in exercise physiology (4).

 *LINKUP:* **Perspective: Physiologic Cardiac Hypertrophy—Athlete's Heart Syndrome,** *featured at http:// connection.lww.com/go/brownexphys and on the Student Resource CD-ROM, presents additional information on myocardial hypertrophy and how the heart adapts to exercise training.*

In dynamic resistance exercise (e.g., weightlifting), the coupling between HR and metabolism is not strong, as acute HR responses tend to be proportionately higher than $\dot{V}O_2$ responses. In other words, there is a dissociation between energy demand and the cardiorespiratory response for resistance exercise. In dynamic resistance exercise, for instance, $\dot{V}O_2$ increases moderately to about 30% to 50% of the treadmill determined $\dot{V}O_{2max}$, even though the exercise session may be exhaustive, producing a near maximal HR response. Although HR is elevated during resistance exercise, this exercise form should not be confused with aerobic, volume-loaded forms as no cardiovascular training effect is likely, as explained further in the next section. *Even though HR can be sustained at high levels during a session of dynamic resistance exercise, the exercise is still not classified as aerobic. Why do you suppose this is true?*

With regular endurance (but not resistance) training, a significant reduction in HR, both at rest and with submaximal exercise, is observed. The mechanisms to explain this phenomenon are not clear but are believed to be due to an increase in parasympathetic activity with a concomitant reduction in resting sympathetic activity. Some highly trained endurance athletes may have resting HRs lower than 40 beats·min$^{-1}$. Furthermore, physical training also results in lower HRs at submaximal workloads. This means that during a submaximal exercise bout, the heart demonstrates a proportionally lower HR for that exercise bout, indicating that with exercise training, the heart becomes more efficient in the work that it has to do. In terms of cardiac performance, a larger SV and lower HR for a given $\dot{Q}$ is generally considered to be a more efficient pattern. However, endurance training does not affect maximal HR, which is relatively stable, tending to decline in healthy individuals only with increasing age.

## CARDIAC OUTPUT AND STROKE VOLUME

### Endurance Exercise

$\dot{Q}$ increases linearly during acute exercise in response to the metabolic demands placed on the body. In young, college-aged, sedentary men, maximal $\dot{Q}$ during endurance exercise is four to five times resting values. The increase in $\dot{Q}$ is attained by an increase in both SV and HR. During upright endurance exercise in individuals who are not highly trained, SV increases to approximately 40% of $\dot{V}O_{2max}$. Thereafter, further increases in $\dot{Q}$ must be accomplished by increasing HR.

Regular exercise training does not alter $\dot{Q}$ at rest or during submaximal endurance exercise. However, during maximal exercise, there is a considerable difference in maximal $\dot{Q}$ with respect to pretraining values. Endurance training produces an increase in cardiovascular function, leading to a greater aerobic power. The two chief training responses are increases in maximal $\dot{Q}$ and maximal SV. When comparing the three groups shown in *Figure 7.26*, a relationship between SV, $\dot{Q}$, and $\dot{V}O_2$ is apparent as aerobic power increases among groups. Since there is a biologic limitation to maximal HR (usually capped at 220 beats·min$^{-1}$), the greater maximal $\dot{Q}$ of endurance-trained individuals is primarily due to a much larger SV.

Since endurance training results in a decrease in HR at rest and with each level of submaximal exercise, SV must

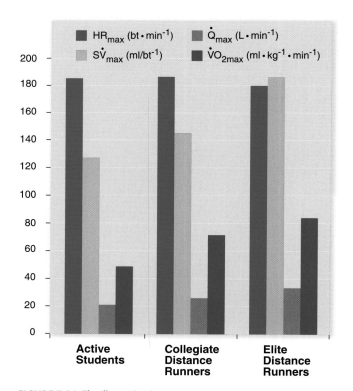

**FIGURE 7.26.** The illustration is a cross-sectional comparison of maximal cardiovascular variables in elite and collegiate male distance runners and active male students (mean age ~27 years) while running on a treadmill.

increase to maintain $\dot{Q}$ at these times. Indeed, approximately 50% of the possible increase in $O_2$ delivery that occurs due to endurance training is due to an increase in SV. *Before reading on, postulate why SV increases with endurance exercise training.*

One explanation focuses on the relationship between HR and the diastolic time period. As resting HR is lowered following training, the heart remains in diastole for a longer time. This allows more blood to flow into the ventricles, increasing EDV. The increase in EDV stretches myocardial fibers and causes a more forceful ejection of blood from the ventricles (Frank-Starling mechanism). This explanation also makes sense for explaining the increase in SV seen at any level of submaximal exercise. Slower HRs increase diastole, giving more time for blood to enter the heart, which then begins systole at a greater preload. Endurance training also results in an increase in the internal diameter of the left ventricle, which is now able to accommodate the extra amount of blood entering during diastole. Also important in this equation is the fact that blood volume increases as a result of regular physical training; consequently there is more blood in the arterial system.

There is some controversy as to what relative degree the Frank-Starling mechanism (increases in EDV) versus contractility (decreases in ESV) is responsible for the approximate 30% to 40% increase in SV (above resting values) commonly seen during endurance exercise. A related question is whether endurance training increases maximal SV by improvements in diastolic (ventricular filling enhancing EDV) or systolic (ventricular emptying reducing ESV) function. Recent work indicates that both mechanisms may explain the increase in SV observed during light, moderate, and heavy exercise, and that a training response occurs in both mechanisms. Box 7.2 describes a study that attempted to resolve the question of the relative contributions of enhanced diastolic versus systolic function following endurance exercise training.

The acute increase in SV comes about through a combined increase in EDV mediated through enhanced venous return and a reduction in ESV mediated through enhanced contractility. Through these mechanisms, SV increases until exercise intensity reaches about 40% of $\dot{V}O_{2max}$, at which time SV levels out. This is a well-documented response for untrained individuals. However, in well-trained aerobic athletes, SV continues a linear increase (no plateauing) to maximum values beyond the 40% $\dot{V}O_{2max}$ point as HR continues to increase to maximal levels (5). The increase is related to an increased blood volume, which directly enhances the diastolic filling rate (6). These factors are all key hallmarks of endurance training.

### Resistance Exercise

SV responds differently to resistance exercise from the pattern we have just reviewed for endurance exercise. However, whether the individual is performing endurance or resistance exercise, SV responds according to its determin-ing variables in the following equation: SV = EDV − ESV. As we saw earlier, for SV to increase, EDV must increase or ESV must decrease (both may occur simultaneously). Also a reduction in cardiac afterload permits the ventricle to increase its output. However, increasing SV in resistance exercise presents a unique problem since there is no acute stimulus for SV to increase. In fact, stimuli, which have the opposite effect, are operative. For instance, when you are performing large muscle group dynamic resistance exercise (especially when simultaneously holding your breath, which produces a **Valsalva maneuver** and increases intrathoracic pressure), enough mechanical occlusion occurs during phasic (i.e., concentric and eccentric joint action) lifting to momentarily reduce venous return. The reduction in venous return, however small, means that preload and SV have been reduced. Along with the reduced preload, $\bar{P}a$ and TPR are elevated (increased afterload). Even though resistance exercise produces marked increases in sympathetic nervous system output (especially in highly intense resistance exercise), the likely increase in ventricular contractility, which would act to reduce ESV and increase SV, does not offset the reduction in preload. The overall consequence is that SV is reduced with respect to resting values during acute resistance exercise, primarily because of a lack of preload stimulus.

Once the exercise has ended and mechanical compression (and intramuscular pressure) has been relieved, blood flow through the muscle is increased and SV rebounds to values at or slightly above resting levels. The reduction in SV during resistance exercise helps explain why there is only a moderate increase in $\dot{Q}$, which, in turn, explains the modest increases in $\dot{V}O_2$ observed during dynamic resistance exercise. In addition, the lack of acute stimuli for SV to increase when performing resistance exercise means that chronic adaptations in cardiac performance that eventually lead to improvements in $\dot{V}O_{2max}$ are not occurring with resistance exercise training. Improvements in $\dot{V}O_{2max}$ occur primarily through chronic adaptations in central cardiac performance ($\dot{Q}$ max) and peripheral cardiovascular dynamics ($\Delta a - \bar{v}O_2$ max). During endurance training the chief adaptation for improving $\dot{V}O_{2max}$ is an increase in maximal SV (central performance), with peripheral adaptations (increased $\Delta a - \bar{v}O_2$ max) serving as an important but secondary component to the overall increase in $\dot{V}O_{2max}$. Neither central nor peripheral adaptations occur with resistance training, which explains why the scientific literature is equivocal in demonstrating improvements in $\dot{V}O_{2max}$ with resistance training. Some studies have demonstrated small increases (approximately 6%) in $\dot{V}O_{2max}$, while other studies have failed to show any improvements.

There is evidence that acute SV and hemodynamic variables, such as TPR, behave differently during dynamic resistance exercise versus static (isometric) resistance exercise. While the two forms of resistance exercise are similar (dynamic resistance exercise has a significant static component), they are also dissimilar (in dynamic

**Box 7.2**

## RESEARCH HIGHLIGHT

**Gledhill N, Cox D, Jamnik R. Endurance athletes' stroke volume does not plateau: major advantage is diastolic function. *Med Sci Sports Exerc* 1994:26;1116–1121.**

### RESEARCH SUMMARY

The consensus scientific opinion regarding stroke volume (SV) response to incremental work rates prior to 1994 was that SV reached a plateau at a submaximal heart rate, usually corresponding to approximately 40% of $\dot{V}_{O_{2}max}$. The reason most often associated with the SV plateau concept is that as heart rate increases during incremental endurance exercise, there is a progressively diminished time for diastolic filling. Thus, SV at these times is limited by the Frank-Starling mechanism. However, if endurance-trained athletes have enhanced systolic (enhanced myocardial contractility) function, less time in the cardiac cycle is required for ventricular emptying and more time is required for filling, thus SV may be shown to continue to increase to higher heart rates in these athletes. The purpose of this study, therefore, was to confirm if SV progressively increases throughout incremental exercise in endurance-trained athletes. A secondary purpose was to study diastolic and systolic function during incremental endurance exercise in trained and untrained subjects.

The results of the study demonstrated that competitive endurance cyclists ($\dot{V}_{O_{2}max}$ = 69 mL·kg$^{-1}$min$^{-1}$) and normally active male subjects ($\dot{V}_{O_{2}max}$ = 44 mL·kg$^{-1}$min$^{-1}$) rely on both left ventricular filling and emptying to increase SV during cycling. Left ventricular filling and emptying rates were used as indexes of diastolic and systolic function, respectively. In the trained subjects at maximal exercise, the ventricular filling rate was 71% greater and ventricular emptying rate was 22% greater than in age-matched, untrained subjects. Furthermore, at a heart rate of 190 beats·min$^{-1}$

(maximal in this study), the ventricular filling rate was 86% greater than the ventricular emptying rate in the trained subjects but only 33% greater in untrained subjects. The major difference in exercise cardiac function between trained and untrained subjects in this study was in the rate of diastolic filling, which lead to an enhanced SV$_{max}$, maximal cardiac output ($\dot{Q}_{max}$), and $\dot{V}_{O_{2}max}$. Therefore, enhanced diastolic rather than systolic function was the most important adaptive response in maximal exercise. This represents a greater use of the less energy-consuming Frank-Starling mechanism, rather than contractility, to accomplish high levels of endurance exercise in trained subjects. Because of their improved diastolic function, this sample of well-trained endurance athletes increased their SV responses incrementally throughout submaximal to maximal exercise and did not plateau SV at a submaximal level.

### IMPLICATIONS FOR FURTHER RESEARCH

The main difference in exercise cardiac function between endurance-trained and untrained subjects is a faster diastolic filling rate in trained subjects. *But what causes the enhanced diastolic filling rate? Do trained subjects have training-induced differences in myocardial contractility, or is the increased rate of diastolic filling due to the physiologic consequences of the higher blood volume that is a primary adaptive response to endurance training?* These questions were subsequently tested in a study by Krip and coworkers (*Med Sci Sports Exerc* 1997:29;1469–1476). The results indicated that changes in SV and cardiac output consequent to alterations in blood volume are attributable primarily to changes in diastolic function, and that the majority of the higher diastolic filling rates of endurance-trained subjects are due to their larger blood volumes.

---

resistance exercise, the joint moves through a full range of motion). Generally the differences are related to the length of time static contractions are held. By definition, static/isometric work involves stable and unchanging intramuscular pressures for as long as the exercise is performed, while in dynamic resistance exercise there is periodic relief of the increased intramuscular pressure due to the eccentric (lowering) phase of the joint movement. Presumably in the eccentric phase the muscular intensity of the lift is reduced, also reducing the intramuscular pressure.

Dynamic resistance exercise produces beat-by-beat changes in SV during the concentric and eccentric phases of contraction (7). *Figure 7.27A* shows that during the lower-

ing (eccentric) phase of the movement, the reduction in SV from the previous resting level was not as great as in the concentric phase, allowing the eccentric phase $\dot{Q}$ to be significantly elevated above the concentric phase $\dot{Q}$ (Fig. 7.27B). The phasic rising and lowering (although the values remained below resting levels in both phases) of SV were probably related to phasic changes in afterload (indexed as TPR and arterial blood pressure) (Fig. 7.27C). It is known, for instance, that all blood pressures (systolic, diastolic, and $\overline{P}$a) are lower during eccentric versus concentric lifting (8). Negative, eccentric movements, therefore, probably require less muscular intensity, which reduces intramuscular pressures and ultimately lowers the blood pressure and TPR re-

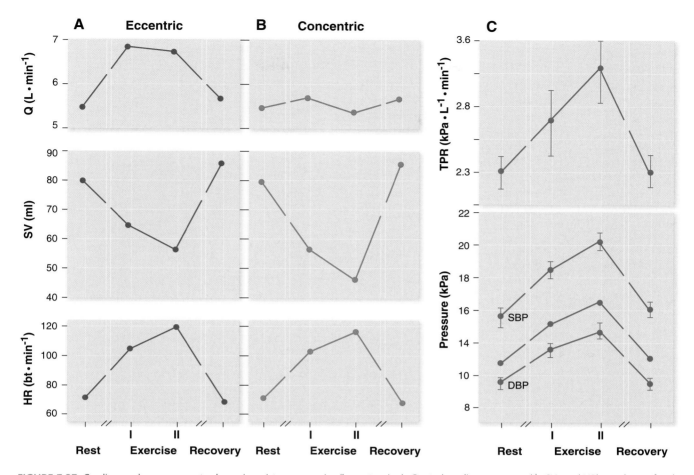

**FIGURE 7.27.** Cardiovascular responses to dynamic resistance exercise (leg extension). Central cardiac responses ($\dot{Q}$, SV, and HR) are shown for the lowering **(A)** and lifting **(B)** phases of the movement, while mean arterial pressure ($\overline{P}a$), systolic blood pressure (SBP), diastolic blood pressure (DBP), and total peripheral resistance (TPR) are shown irrespective of the phase of lifting **(C)**. (Modified with permission from Miles DS, Owens JJ, Golden JC, et al. Central and peripheral hemodynamics during maximal leg extension exercise. *Eur J Appl Physiol Occup Physiol* 1987;56:12–17.)

sponse, thereby facilitating blood flow through the muscle. SV and TPR are inversely related (r = −0.86) during dynamic resistance exercise (7).

The results of the work by Miles and associates (7) are in contrast to those employing purely static forms of resistance exercise, which often show reductions in TPR (though not to the same extent as TPR is reduced in endurance exercise) and increases in $\dot{Q}$. The classic study of Lind and coworkers is an example (9). Subjects performed handgrip exercise (a small muscle mass) at 10%, 20%, and 50% MVC. Cardiovascular responses were somewhat different than responses during dynamic resistance work. $\dot{Q}$ progressed moderately over the three intensities, but SV significantly decreased from its resting level in the 50% MVC condition. The incremental increase in $\dot{Q}$ was therefore related to the progressive increase in HR over the three intensities. $\overline{P}a$ showed an incremental increase, yet TPR decreased modestly. These results clearly demonstrate that cardiovascular responses to resistance exercise are not homogeneous.

## BLOOD PRESSURE

During acute endurance exercise, there is an increase in SBP and $\overline{P}a$ due to the increase in $\dot{Q}$ that occurs with the onset of exercise, while DBP remains the same or decreases slightly. SBP and $\overline{P}a$ increase in magnitude as dictated by the exercise intensity and then level off to steady-state values and continue to rise during incremental exercise. If steady-state blood pressure is maintained for prolonged periods of time, SBP may decline slightly, while DBP will remain the same. This can be interpreted as a normal response and is attributed to further arterial vasodilation (decreased TPR) in the working muscles. During incremental endurance exercise to maximum levels, SBP may increase to as much as 200 mm Hg; however, this value varies greatly among individuals due to differences in training and health status, with endurance-trained individuals displaying lower peak systolic pressures than the average sedentary person. The lower peak systolic pressures for endurance-trained individuals, in spite of the fact that their $\dot{Q}$ max may be 1.5 to two times greater than their sedentary counterparts, has to do with the extent of peripheral vasodilation experienced by these individuals. The enhanced vasodilatory effect lowers the TPR of trained individuals to a much larger degree, allowing them to generate maximal systolic pressures that are actually lower than their untrained counterparts.

The moderate increase in SBP with endurance exercise is evidence of a more correctly performing pump and vasculature. An excessive increase in systolic or diastolic pressure during exercise may be indicative of a vascular system that has a decreased compliance and increased **elastance**. Both reflect the stiffening of the arterial walls due to profuse arteriosclerosis as individuals age. In addition, failing to increase systolic pressure may be indicative of poor cardiac pump performance. Any of these occurrences is grounds for discontinuing an exercise test or rehabilitation session that is in progress.

Referring to the equation $\bar{P}a = \dot{Q} \times TPR$, we see that $\dot{Q}$ and TPR play important roles in blood pressure regulation. We have already said that TPR decreases with endurance exercise, yet $\dot{Q}$ increases, which would then seem to offset the effect of a reduction in TPR, causing $\bar{P}a$ to remain constant. *What do you suppose accounts for the acute rise in $\bar{P}a$ and SBP with endurance exercise?* The answer lies in the fact that increases in $\dot{Q}$ are not completely offset by decreases in TPR. This is important because the great increase in $\dot{Q}$ seen in endurance exercise is necessary to maintain perfusion pressure to important organs like the brain and active muscle. During endurance exercise there is an active vasoconstriction to inactive vascular beds, which contributes to the maintenance of normal arterial pressure for adequate tissue perfusion. Also body temperature increases during endurance exercise, accompanied by vasodilation in cutaneous vessels, which has the effect of decreasing TPR even further. Therefore, without an increased $\dot{Q}$ and visceral organ vasoconstriction, blood pressure would decline during endurance exercise.

As discussed earlier, resistance exercise imposes a pressure load on the cardiovascular system. The increase in afterload is primarily seen as an increase in arterial SBP and DBP, producing a higher $\bar{P}a$. The magnitude of the increase is irrespective of age and sex differences and is related to the amount of muscle mass involved and the number of arteries occluded by intramuscular mechanical compression (10). *Figure 7.28* demonstrates the SBP and DBP responses in elderly men and women performing dynamic resistance exercise without Valsalva maneuvers. A total of six sets of these exercises were performed at 12 and five repetitions maximum. These results, although gathered through a noninvasive measurement technique, closely follow another more definitive study that used direct measurement of arterial blood pressure via a pressure transducer placed in an artery (8).

MacDougall and coworkers (8) recorded the highest known blood pressures ever produced in experiments of this nature. Using bilateral leg presses in young resistance-trained men, peak systolic/diastolic pressures were

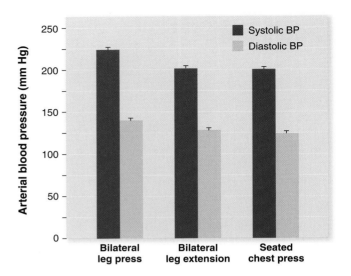

**FIGURE 7.28.** Mean±SEM systolic (dark bars) and diastolic (light bars) blood pressure responses to dynamic resistance exercise in elderly men and women. These measurements were made by a noninvasive blood pressure technique (photoelectric), which permits continual monitoring during resistance exercise from a sensor placed on a finger or toe. (Data from Bermon S, Rama D, Dolisi C. Cardiovascular tolerance of healthy elderly subjects to weight-lifting exercises. *Med Sci Sports Exerc* 2000;32:1845–1848.)

320/250, significantly higher than the 224/140 produced by elderly subjects in the study of Bermon and colleagues (10). *What accounts for such high pressures and are they safe?* Even if $\dot{Q}$ is mildly elevated, such pressures could only be demonstrated by increases in TPR. Blood pressure responses during exercise may be a cause for alarm in some patient groups; therefore, some individuals should be closely monitored and instructed in proper lifting techniques, especially avoiding the Valsalva maneuver. Because resistance exercise produces the reflexive **pressor response** and a high RPP, caution should be exercised. RPP is highly correlated with $M\dot{V}O_2$, and because of the increase in ventricular pressure work, ischemic responses and other untoward events, such as arrhythmias and ventricular wall motion abnormalities, could easily be precipitated in susceptible individuals.

 *Experiences in Work Physiology Lab Exercise 7:*
*Isometric Contractions and Cardiovascular Function*
*is a laboratory experiment that gives you the opportunity to demonstrate the acute effects of resistance exercise on HR and blood pressure. This experiment and topic has much practical and clinical significance, as many day-to-day activities involve muscular contractions that produce pressor responses.*

With regular exercise training, it appears that reductions in resting SBP and DBP can occur in both normal and moderately hypertensive people. The mechanisms to explain this effect are unclear, although it is likely that a reduction in the activity of the sympathetic nervous system and the greater vascularity of the capillary beds play a role. Such training responses have not been demonstrated for resistance exercise training, however.

## $\Delta a - \bar{v}O_2$

The peripheral component of the Fick equation is the $\Delta a - \bar{v}O_2$ difference. With endurance exercise training, the ability of the working tissues to extract $O_2$ from the blood improves at maximal exercise. This improvement is part of the reason for the 20% to 35% improvement (depending on prior activity level) in $\bar{v}O_2$ max following endurance training. Several factors account for the increase in $\Delta a - \bar{v}O_2$ max:

- *Increased capillary density*. With endurance training, the capillary density increases in muscle to accommodate the increase in blood flow. This means that there are more capillaries per fiber in the trained skeletal muscle, amounting to about a 34% increase.
- *Increase in muscle metabolic capabilities*. With endurance training, skeletal muscle has an improved ability to engage in oxidative metabolism. Some of the adaptive consequences providing this improvement are: 80% increase in myoglobin content; improved oxidation of glycogen by an increase in the number (120% increase), size (25% increase), and membrane surface area of skeletal muscle mitochondria, and an increase in concentration and level of activity of Krebs cycle and electron transport chain enzymes; improved oxidation of fat by a 1.5-fold increase in muscle triglyceride stores and an increase in lipolytic enzymes.

In incremental exercise $\Delta a - \bar{v}O_2$ increases in a linear fashion to about 50% to 60% of $\dot{V}O_{2max}$ and then plateaus. As we saw in Chapter 6, this increase parallels the change in $O_2$ dissociation during endurance exercise. Very little research has been conducted on how the $\Delta a - \bar{v}O_2$ performs during resistance exercise, and there are no data regarding possible training adaptations. However, in acute resistance exercise, the $\Delta a - \dot{V}O_2$ generally reflects the mechanical occlusion of blood flow that is occurring. That is, there is no change or possibly a slight decrease in extraction rate. Once the mechanical occlusion has been abated, the $\Delta a - \dot{V}O_2$ and many other metabolic and physiologic variables (principally $\dot{V}O_2$, SV, $\dot{V}E$, and RER) suddenly increase (rebound effect).

▶ *INQUIRY SUMMARY.* The acute and chronic changes in cardiovascular variables during exercise and training reflect the magnitude of the stress response elicited by exercise. The body is capable of making appropriate physiologic adaptations depending on the nature of the chronically imposed, acute stress. One of the most important adaptive changes that occurs with training is an increased $\dot{V}O_{2max}$, which signifies an increased cardiovascular functional capacity. Based on your study of the variables associated with the Fick equation, *what do you think is the site of the greatest adaptive improvements that lead to increases in $\dot{V}O_{2max}$?*

## Summary

The cardiovascular system is a closed circuit that pumps blood to the lungs and throughout the systemic circulation. The arteries, capillaries, and veins are specialized in that they each have different functions for the transport of blood throughout the circulation. The heart is a pump, and several intrinsic and extrinsic factors control how fast it contracts and how well the heart performs its pumping function. Cardiac output is an important measure of the ability of the heart to pump blood and the ability of the systemic circulation to return blood back to the heart. There are several factors that control cardiac output. With the onset of exercise, blood is directed away from less essential areas of the body and redirected to the working muscles. This is accomplished by a complex set of acute changes within the cardiovascular system that are controlled by the cardiovascular center in the brain. With regular aerobic exercise, there are several important physiologic adaptations that enhance the functional capacity of the cardiovascular system. The acute physiologic changes that are the result of resistance exercise are qualitatively and quantitatively different from those that result from endurance exercise. Because of these differences, resistance exercise does not improve the functional capacity of the cardiovascular system.

### SUMMARY KNOWLEDGE

1. What route does an electrical impulse travel in the heart to stimulate the entire cardiac mass?
2. How is cardiac electrical activity associated with the mechanical activity of the heart?
3. In what way are the changes in pressure in the chambers of the heart during the cardiac cycle related to the flow of blood through the heart?
4. What is the relationship between blood pressure, cardiac output, and peripheral resistance?
5. Why do heart rate and stroke volume regulate cardiac output?
6. What, in turn, regulates heart rate and stroke volume?
7. Would you recommend resistance exercise for improving cardiorespiratory fitness? Why?

### References

1. Robinson TE, Sue DY, Huszczuk A, et al. Intra-arterial and cuff blood pressure responses during incremental cycle ergometry. *Med Sci Sports Exerc* 1988;20:142–149.
2. Sarnoff SJ, Berglund B. Ventricular function. I. Starling's law of the heart studied by means of simultaneous right and left ventricular function curves in the dog. *Circulation* 1954;9:706–718.
3. Sjogaard G, Savard G, Juel C. Muscle blood flow during isometric activity and its relation to muscle fatigue. *Eur J Physiol Occup Physiol* 1988;57:327–335.
4. Pluim BM, Zwinderman AH, van der Laarse A, et al. The athlete's heart: a meta-analysis of cardiac structure and function. *Circulation* 1999;100:336–344.

5.  Gledhill N, Cox D, Jamnik R. Endurance athletes' stroke volume does not plateau: major advantage is diastolic function. *Med Sci Sports Exerc* 1994;26:1116–1121.
6.  Krip B, Gledhill N, Jamnik V, et al. Effect of alterations in blood volume on cardiac function during maximal exercise. *Med Sci Sports Exerc* 1997;29:1469–1476.
7.  Miles DS, Owens JJ, Golden JC, et al. Central and peripheral hemodynamics during maximal leg extension exercise. *Eur J Appl Physiol Occup Physiol* 1987;56:12–17.
8.  MacDougall JD, Tuxen D, Sale DG, et al. Arterial blood pressure response to heavy resistance exercise. *J Appl Physiol* 1985;58:785–790.
9.  Lind AR, Taylor SH, Humphreys PW, et al. The circulatory effects of sustained voluntary muscle contraction. *Clin Sci* 1964;27:229–244.
10. Bermon S, Rama D, Dolisi C. Cardiovascular tolerance of healthy elderly subjects to weight-lifting exercises. *Med Sci Sports Exerc* 2000;32:1845–1848.

### Suggested Readings

Berne RM, Levy MN. *Cardiovascular physiology.* 8th ed. St. Louis: Mosby, 2001.

Halliwill JR. Mechanisms and clinical implications of post-exercise hypotension in humans. *Exerc Sport Sci Rev* 2001;29:65–70.

Hester RL, Choi J. Blood flow control during exercise: role for the venular endothelium? *Exerc Sport Sci Rev* 2002;30:147–151.

Prior BM, Lloyd PG, Yang HT, et al. Exercise-induced vascular remodeling. *Exerc Sport Sci Rev* 2003;31:26–33.

Raven PB, Fadel PJ, Smith SA. The influence of central command on baroreflex resetting during exercise. *Exerc Sport Sci Rev* 2002;30:39–44.

### On the Internet

The Gross Physiology of the Cardiovascular System: The Determinants of Cardiac Output. Available at: **http://cardiovascular.cx/video.htm**. Accessed April 08, 2005.

Cardiovascular Physiology Concepts. Available at: **http://www.cvphysiology.com/**. Accessed April 08, 2005.

The Heart Preview Gallery. Available at: **http://sln2.fi.edu/biosci/preview/heartalternative.html**. Accessed April 08, 2005.

## Writing to Learn

1. Research and write a paper on the different central and peripheral cardiovascular responses with resistance versus endurance exercise. Use the Fick equation to address the following questions: Why does $\dot{V}O_2$ increase during resistance exercise if resistance exercise is a purely anaerobic form of exercise? What is the stroke volume response to resistance exercise? Can $\dot{V}O_{2max}$ be improved with resistance training? How would your findings alter the way you approached prescribing resistance exercise for a cardiac patient?

2. Research and write a paper describing how cardiac functional performance differs with physiologic versus pathologic cardiac hypertrophy.

# CHAPTER

# 8 Homothermal Control: Temperature Regulation During Exercise

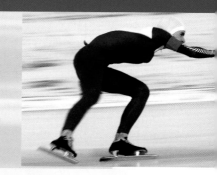

*You may be surprised to know that the body can only tolerate an increase in core temperature of about 5°C and a decrease in core temperature of about 10°C. The mechanisms that the body uses to maintain core temperature within a narrow range are not adequate to protect the body against exposure to extreme conditions. Therefore, a conscious effort must be made to assist the body in maintaining temperature homeostasis under conditions of heat or cold stress. Can you think of things you consciously do on a daily basis to maintain body temperature within the normal range?*

## CHAPTER OUTLINE

Homeostasis is defined as the state of equilibrium or constancy of the internal environment. We saw in earlier chapters that the physiologic/biochemical systems of the body are constantly striving to maintain homeostasis, whether by energy equilibrium, nutrient equilibrium, fluid balance, or membrane stability. Temperature too must be maintained in balance for the body to function normally. The body's ability to maintain temperature at a fairly constant level, regardless of environmental temperature, is called **homothermal control**. You learned in previous chapters that the metabolic rate of exercising muscles can increase 200% during heavy exercise. You also know that the metabolic process of converting food energy into mechanical energy to perform muscular work is very inefficient, and that most of the energy released in the hydrolysis of ATP is lost as heat energy. *How then does the body dissipate metabolic heat so that health is not jeopardized?* In this chapter we will uncover the mechanisms the body uses to maintain core

temperature within a safe range and what we can do to help the body maintain temperature homeostasis during exercise in extreme environments. We will also learn what happens to the body if core temperature is not maintained within set limits. The objective of this chapter, therefore, is to help you understand the importance of homothermal control.

## Temperature Balance During Exercise

The temperature of the body varies depending on where in the body temperature is measured. The temperature of the internal organs is greater than the temperature on the surface of the skin. Temperature even varies among the different internal organs of the body. Under most conditions, there is a temperature gradient between the center or core of the body and the skin surface. The **core temperature** is generally 4°C higher than skin temperature, but the gradient can vary by as much as 20°C. The terms **skin temperature** and core temperature best describe the two places where body temperature is usually measured. However, in the context of this book, the terms core temperature, body temperature, and temperature alone will be used synonymously to describe the internal body temperature. The term skin temperature will be used only when specific reference to body temperature taken at the skin surface is needed.

Internal and external factors that influence temperature balance change throughout the day, and the body must respond accordingly to maintain homothermal control. For the healthy person, metabolic rate is the only internal factor that affects body temperature. Abnormalities in brain function, toxic substances, and infectious diseases are also factors that alter internal body temperature by affecting the temperature-regulating mechanisms of the body. The external factors that affect body temperature are all related to the environment, whether they are acute changes in the environment or environmental conditions that are stable.

The heat released from the resting metabolic rate, thermic effect of food, changes in body position, and self-care activities are easily dissipated. Only in an extremely hot environment will the body have difficulty dissipating heat generated by the resting metabolism or self-care activities. Therefore, the risk of **hyperthermia** in nonexercising individuals is only a concern in extremely hot environments. On the other end of the spectrum, the risk for **hypothermia** is only a concern in extremely cold environments. Even when the metabolism drops to its lowest level, as happens when sleeping (sleeping metabolic rate), the body generates enough heat to protect itself from any dangers associated with heat loss, as long as the temperature is moderate. However, under conditions of prolonged exposure to extreme cold, the inactive body will be threatened by hypothermia. During exercise in the cold, the risk of hypothermia decreases substantially because the metabolic heat from exercise metabolism rises dramatically. On the other hand, the increased heat production from exercise metabolism will put a person exercising in the heat at great risk for developing a heat disorder because the body will have a difficult time dissipating heat to the hot environment. Therefore, the homothermal control of body temperature in any given environment is greatly dependent on metabolism.

During exercise, core temperature regulation is simply a matter of balancing heat loss with heat gain. If heat gain is greater than heat loss, core temperature will rise. When heat gain is less than heat loss, core temperature will decrease. Core temperature during exercise is maintained within 2°C to 3°C of 37°C (98.6°F) under most environmental conditions (*Fig. 8.1*). Although heat balance is sim-

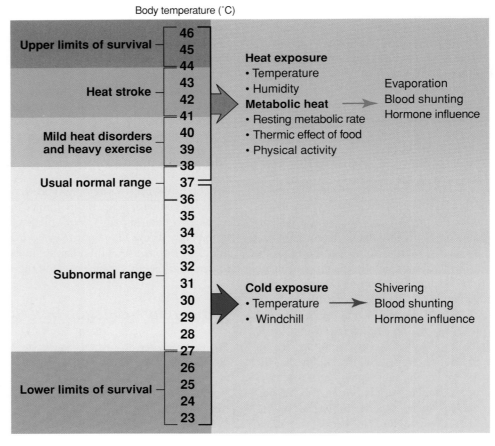

**FIGURE 8.1.** Tolerance range for core body temperature. Factors contributing to heat gain are listed in the middle column of the red area. Factors contributing to heat loss are listed in the middle column of the blue area. Factors in the far right column represent the functional ability of heat-dissipating and heat-conserving mechanisms.

ply a matter of offsetting heat gain with heat loss, the mechanisms in which heat balance is achieved are very complex. The factors that contribute to heat gain during exercise include anything that stimulates metabolic rate, anything from the external environment that causes heat gain, and the ability of the body to dissipate heat under any given set of circumstances. For example, exercise intensity stimulates metabolism, high temperature causes heat gain from the external environment, and protective equipment reduces the body's ability to dissipate heat. Factors that contribute to heat loss during exercise include any situations that override the body's heat-conserving mechanisms, like hormone imbalance, and anything in the environment that enhances heat loss, such as low temperature with high winds.

The ways in which heat-conserving and heat-dissipating mechanisms are regulated are both physical and chemical (*Fig. 8.2*). These mechanisms allow for the exchange of heat between the body and its surrounding environment. The body gains or loses heat through conduction (e.g., holding an ice cube in your hand), convection (e.g., standing in the wind), radiation (e.g., laying on the beach in the sunlight), and evaporation (e.g., sweating).

## HEAT EXCHANGE BY CONDUCTION

**Conduction** is defined as the transfer of heat from one object to another as the two objects come into contact with each other. These objects can be separate and distinct entities, or they can be separate molecules within a single entity. Regardless, the heat always passes from the warmer object to the cooler object because of a temperature gradient between the two objects. The rate at which heat is transferred by conduction depends upon two things, the first of which is the magnitude of the temperature gradient. This can be seen in a familiar example. If you place your hand on the burner of an electric stove that is turned on "high," you will burn yourself immediately. However, if you place your hand on the burner when it is turned on "low", you may not burn your hand for several seconds. The speed at which your hand gains heat in this example is directly related to the difference in temperature gradient between your hand and the burner under the "low" and "high" conditions.

The second factor that contributes to the rate of heat transfer during conduction is the thermal qualities of the objects in contact. For instance, glass can absorb more heat than Styrofoam. You have experienced this phenomenon often. When you pick up a glass of ice-cold lemonade, the glass conducts the heat from your hand and your hand feels cold. In contrast, if that same lemonade were poured into a Styrofoam cup, you could pick up the cup and not feel any cold.

Heat transfer by conduction occurs because the heat is actually transferred from the molecules of the warmer substance to the molecules of the cooler substance through direct contact (or from the warmer molecules to the cooler molecules within the same substance). Conduction can occur between substances that are solid, liquid, or gas. With respect to the body, conduction occurs in two ways. First, in a cool environment, heat is transferred from the internal tissues to the outer surface (skin) because of a temperature gradient between the core and skin temperatures. Heat is transferred in the opposite direction (from the skin to core) when the skin temperature exceeds the core temperature. Second, as we have already seen, heat is also transferred by conduction when the body comes in contact with an external object. Heat transfer in the body by conduction predisposes tissue interfaces. *Figure 8.3* illustrates the mechanisms of heat transfer during exercise in a warm-to-hot environment. *Which tissues must come in contact to transfer heat by conduction to the skin?*

## HEAT EXCHANGE BY CONVECTION

**Convection** is defined as the transfer of heat from one place to another by either movement of a substance through a medium such as air or water or movement of the medium across the substance. In either case the heat transfer can go from the substance to the medium or from the medium to the substance. For example, if you spilled a cup of hot coffee on your leg, heat would be transferred from the moving medium (coffee) to the stationary substance (your leg) as the coffee flowed across your leg. In contrast, if you were riding down the highway on a motorcycle on a cool day, heat from the moving substance (your body) would be transferred to the stationary medium (air).

Convection is actually a form of conduction because heat is first conducted from the body to air or water

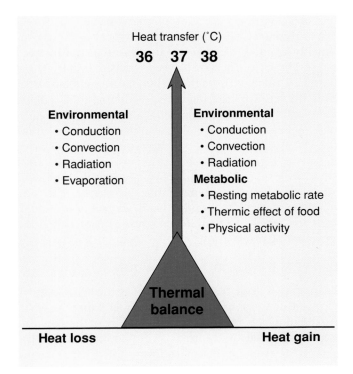

Heat transfer (°C)

**36   37   38**

**Environmental**
- Conduction
- Convection
- Radiation
- Evaporation

**Environmental**
- Conduction
- Convection
- Radiation

**Metabolic**
- Resting metabolic rate
- Thermic effect of food
- Physical activity

**Thermal balance**

**Heat loss**          **Heat gain**

**FIGURE 8.2.** Mechanisms of heat transfer for the body.

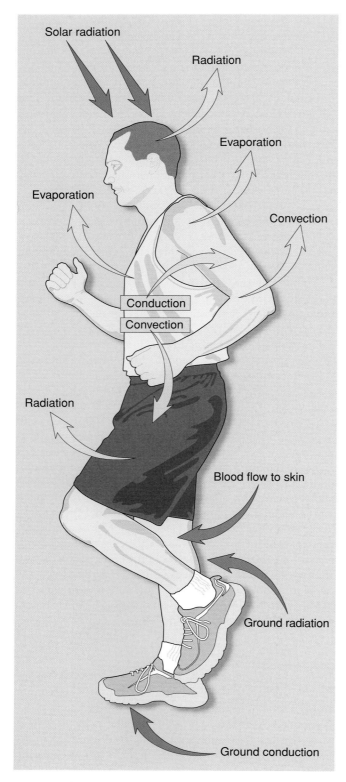

Solar radiation

Radiation

Evaporation

Evaporation

Convection

Conduction

Convection

Radiation

Blood flow to skin

Ground radiation

Ground conduction

**FIGURE 8.3.** Mechanisms of heat transfer during exercise in a warm-to-hot environment. Heat is transferred to the body through solar radiation, ground radiation, and ground conduction. Heat is dissipated from the body through evaporation of sweat, radiation to the atmosphere, distributing more blood flow to the skin surface, convection to the air, and conduction away from the core.

molecules, and then those air or water molecules are moved and replaced by new cooler molecules. The rate at which heat is transferred by convection depends on how fast the air or water molecules in contact with the body are replaced by cooler molecules. For example, after several minutes of standing still in a swimming pool of cold water, the water does not feel as cold as it did initially. However, as you begin to move, the water feels cold again. During the few minutes you stood still, heat was transferred from the body by convection to the surrounding water. Since there was no movement of the water, heated water molecules were not replaced by new cooler ones, heat loss was suspended, and you did not feel as cold as you did initially. When you moved, the heated water molecules were replaced by new cooler ones and more heat was lost from the body. Another familiar example of convection is when water or air is forced to move across the body surface (as when you sit in front of a fan on a hot day). As the fan forces air to pass over your body, convection is increased and you feel cooler than you would standing in calm air.

The body can also gain heat through convection. When you walk by an open fire, heat from the surrounding air is transferred to your body through convection. You continue to feel the heat of the fire until you pass out of the range of the fire into cooler air. As you pass through the cooler air, convection is reversed and your body begins to lose heat to the surrounding cooler air. In the same way, some heat may be gained by the body through convection when running or cycling in hot environments.

## HEAT EXCHANGE BY RADIATION

**Radiation** involves the transfer of heat from the surface of one object to the surface of another without any direct physical contact. The body, as well as other objects, is continually emitting electromagnetic waves in the infrared range. These electromagnetic waves transfer heat from one object to another through a temperature gradient. Heat from the sun is transferred to the earth (and to objects on the earth) through radiation. Obviously the sun and earth never come into contact with each other. You may even see the visual distortions caused by radiation as you drive down the highway on a hot summer day and the road ahead looks like it is wiggling. We lose heat through radiation when our body temperature is warmer than surrounding objects. On the other hand, we gain heat through radiation when our body temperature is cooler than the surrounding objects.

## HEAT EXCHANGE BY EVAPORATION

**Evaporation** describes the transfer of heat when a liquid is changed to a gas, usually water to water vapor, as when perspiration is evaporated from the surface of the skin. Energy is required to "vaporize" a liquid, and the energy source for evaporation comes from heat. Heat from the body is transferred to water on the surface of the skin. As the water gains more and more heat, the water soon has enough energy to vaporize. The gas (water vapor) leaves the skin surface, taking the heat away from the body.

The primary mechanism of heat dissipation during exercise is through evaporation. Even at rest, there is a significant amount of water vapor being formed at the skin surface. This unnoticeable evaporation occurring at rest is called insensible perspiration because we do not notice the moisture accumulating on the skin surface. As we start to exercise, the body begins to retain heat. Sweat glands respond by secreting large quantities of sweat (*Fig. 8.4*). It is not the sweat that makes you feel hot but the retaining of body heat that causes you to feel hot. Sweating is just the mechanism by which the body tries to dissipate the accumulating heat.

## ASSESSMENT OF BODY TEMPERATURE

Body temperature is difficult to assess because the temperature of the body varies, depending upon where the body temperature is measured. Temperature at the thermal regulatory center in the hypothalamus is different from that of the internal organs, which varies from the temperature found on the surface of the skin. Temperature varies even among the different internal organs of the body and among different locations on the skin. Measurements of body temperature can be obtained with a mercury thermometer or with a device called a thermistor (*Fig. 8.5*). Professionals

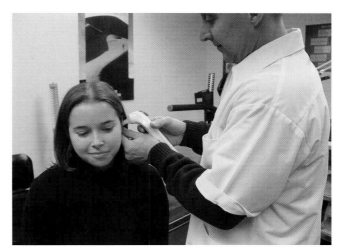

**FIGURE 8.5.** Measuring body temperature during exercise in laboratory conditions helps clinicians and researchers understand the mechanisms of heat transfer.

still debate which temperature location best reflects core temperature.

The most common sites for measurement of core temperature are the rectum, ear (tympanic), and throat (esophageal). Although the rectal temperature does not reflect the true core temperature at the hypothalamus, it does reflect the deep-tissue temperature at the body core. Rectal temperatures are often used in exercise studies because they are highly reliable and placement of the thermistor is easier than at the ear, throat, or skin. Tympanic temperature is often used in clinical practice because the thermistor response is rapid and the measurement is not invasive. The tympanic temperature is thought to be the closest assessment of true temperature at the hypothalamus. Measurement of esophageal temperature is uncommon in clinical practice but remains the most common method used by laypersons for measuring body temperature.

Skin temperature can be measured by placing thermistors on the skin at various locations. Common placements for skin thermistors are the forehead, chest, forearm, thigh, calf, abdomen, and back. The mean skin temperature can be calculated by averaging the temperatures taken at each skin site. Once the skin and core temperatures have been determined, the mean body temperature can be estimated by summing the two temperatures in the following way:

$$\text{Mean body temperature} = 0.4 \times \text{Average skin temperature} + 0.6 \times \text{Core temperature}$$

Skin temperature accounts for 40% of the mean body temperature, while core temperature accounts for 60%.

## INTEGRATION OF HEAT TRANSFER MECHANISMS

Conduction, convection, and radiation are effective means of cooling the body in cool environments, but they become less effective in warm environments. We usually do not concern ourselves with ways in which we can better lose

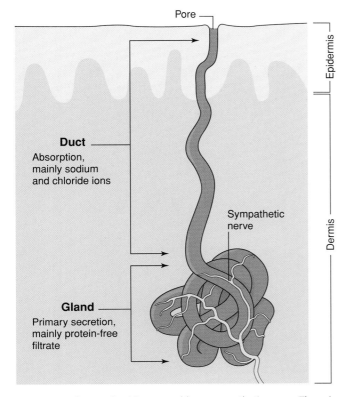

**FIGURE 8.4.** Sweat gland innervated by a sympathetic nerve. The primary secretion is formed in the gland, while the ions are absorbed in the duct. The resulting sweat is a dilute fluid.

Pore

Epidermis

**Duct**
Absorption, mainly sodium and chloride ions

Sympathetic nerve

Dermis

**Gland**
Primary secretion, mainly protein-free filtrate

heat during exercise in the cold because all four of the heat transfer methods are working efficiently and the body is not absorbing heat from the environment. In contrast, as air temperature increases, evaporation becomes the most viable mechanism for body cooling because the temperature gradient between the body and surrounding environment is lessened for conduction, convection, and radiation. Furthermore, evaporation may become the only viable mechanism for losing body heat in hot environments because the body may be gaining heat from the surrounding environment through conduction, convection, and radiation.

Refer back to Figure 8.3, which illustrates how the four mechanisms for heat transfer work during an exercise bout in a warm-to-hot environment. As energy is expended for muscle contraction, heat is liberated. Some of this metabolic heat from the exercising muscles, as well as metabolic heat from increased cardiorespiratory system activity, flows down a temperature gradient from the body core to the skin surface via conduction. A greater amount of the heat produced is brought to the skin surface via convection. Heat transfer within the body through convection is dependent upon the circulatory system.

During exercise, **cardiac output** increases to meet increased energy demands and to cool the body. Blood that circulates to the body core is warmed and then brought to the skin surface where the temperature gradient favors heat release from the body (*Fig. 8.6*). Superficial blood vessels become dilated to enhance blood flow under the sur-face of the skin. As much as 25% of the exercise cardiac output in extreme heat is diverted to the skin surface for body cooling. The cooled blood then returns from the periphery to the core where it can remove more heat from the internal tissues. The heat that was brought to the skin surface can now be removed from the body by conduction (if the body comes into direct contact with a cooler object), convection (depending upon air or water movement), and radiation (if there is a radiant temperature gradient).

At the same time the mechanisms of conduction, convection and radiation are working, the body also begins to sweat. Sweat and heat on the skin surface increase the water vapor pressure on the skin, which leads to evaporation. The effectiveness of evaporation for body cooling during exercise depends upon the amount of moistened skin surface exposed to the environment, the temperature and humidity of the surrounding air, and to a small degree the convective currents around the body. As greater amounts of sweat are vaporized, more heat is dissipated. One L of sweat can remove about 580 kcal of heat from the body (1). When the relative humidity is low, the vapor pressure in the air is low, and this favors rapid heat removal from the body. When the relative humidity is high, air vapor pressure is high, which is less favorable to heat loss from the body. If the relative humidity reaches 100%, the air is saturated and there is no vapor pressure gradient between the body and surrounding air. In this case, heat dissipation through evaporation cannot occur

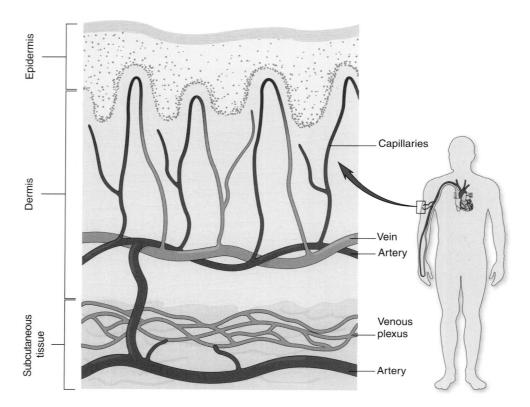

**FIGURE 8.6.** The shunting of blood flow to the skin surface to dissipate heat during exercise.

and the risk of developing a heat disorder becomes greater. More about relative humidity and heat stress is presented later in this chapter.

▶ *INQUIRY SUMMARY.* Heat can be transferred to and from the body by conduction, convection, radiation, and evaporation. Heat from the body core is transferred to the surface through conduction and convection, while warmed blood is shunted to the skin for evaporative cooling. Evaporation is the mechanism that is most effective in releasing heat from the body during exercise in a hot environment. *How do you think the body coordinates all the processes needed to protect itself against hyperthermia?*

## Temperature Regulation in Hot Environments

It has already been stressed that body temperature must be maintained within a narrow range for the body to function properly. We have seen that the mechanisms of conduction, convection, radiation, and evaporation all play roles in heat transfer during exercise and that evaporation is the most important mechanism for heat transfer in warm environments. These mechanisms for heat transfer are advantageous or disadvantageous, depending on how effective

the **thermal regulatory center** is at regulating heat dissipation. The effectiveness of the thermal regulatory center is ultimately dependent upon the severity of the heat stress, but its effectiveness under all conditions is directly related to how acclimatized the body is to heat stress and how well a person prepares himself/herself for exercising in the heat. Let us now take a look at how the thermal regulatory center works and what happens when the capacity of the body to dissipate heat is overcome.

### THE THERMAL REGULATORY CENTER

The thermal regulatory center, located in a portion of the lower brain called the hypothalamus, controls the physiologic mechanisms that maintain body temperature at a constant (or near constant) 37°C. These specialized brain cells of the hypothalamus act similarly to a thermostat in a building. The hypothalamus senses (measures) body temperature and elicits a response that will cool the body when temperature rises (*Fig. 8.7*). To perform this function, the thermal regulatory center is directly linked to **thermal receptors** and **thermal effectors**. The thermal receptors are actually sensory units that provide input about temperature to the regulatory center. Thermal effectors are those organs or tissues that are directed by the regulatory center to readjust body temperature to the 37°C set point.

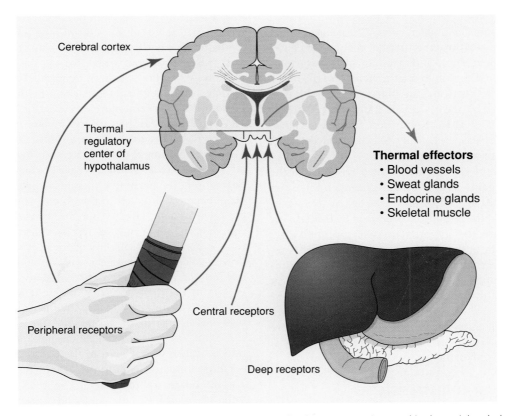

**FIGURE 8.7.** Workings of the thermal regulatory center of the hypothalamus. Blood temperature is sensed in the peripheral, deep, and central receptors. Feedback is given to the thermal regulatory center (red arrows), which elicits a response through the thermal effectors (blue arrow). In addition, peripheral receptors communicate with the cerebral cortex so voluntary action can be taken to transfer heat.

There are three types of thermal receptors: central, deep, and peripheral. Central receptors are specialized neurons located in the anterior portion of the hypothalamus. Deep receptors are those found around the spinal cord, abdominal viscera, and great veins. Peripheral receptors are neurons that reside in the skin. All of these receptors increase their firing rates as surrounding temperature rises.

Arterial blood from the body core perfuses the hypothalamus. When core temperature rises, the heat-carrying blood stimulates the central receptors. These receptors communicate their message to the thermal regulatory center in the hypothalamus. Similarly deep receptors sense temperature changes in the blood that perfuses them. Since these receptors are found in the body core, they give feedback to the thermal regulatory center about temperature changes in the core. The peripheral receptors just below the skin surface sense thermal changes in the skin that are brought about by changes in environmental temperature. These receptors provide feedback to the thermal regulatory center of the hypothalamus but also provide information to the **cerebral cortex**. The communication to the cerebral cortex allows for voluntary control of body temperature, such as removing clothing as one sweats.

The thermal effectors include the smooth muscles of the blood vessels that supply the skin, sweat glands, certain endocrine glands, and skeletal muscles. (Skeletal muscles and endocrine glands are effectors for increasing body temperature and will be discussed later in the section on cold stress.) As the hypothalamus receives information that body temperature is rising, the thermal regulatory center interprets this information and stimulates the arterioles that supply blood to the skin to dilate. Dilation of the blood vessels allows more heat-carrying blood to enter the skin surface to be cooled by one of the heat transfer mechanisms discussed previously. At the same time, the sweat glands are stimulated to release sweat on the skin surface so that the body can be cooled via evaporation.

The thermostat of the thermal regulatory center of the hypothalamus remains set at 37°C unless acted upon by an external substance. A fever is produced when toxic substances are taken into the body or produced by bacteria (or viruses) and cause the hypothalamic set point to rise. When the set point of the thermal regulatory center is reset at a higher level than normal, all the mechanisms for increasing body temperature come into play, including heat conservation and heat production. A short time after the set point is adjusted to a higher level, the body temperature rises to this level. Substances that cause this effect are called pyrogens. When the action of these pyrogens is blocked, as with aspirin, the fever is reduced.

## CARDIOVASCULAR ADJUSTMENTS TO HEAT EXPOSURE

You know from previous chapters that exercise places demands on the cardiovascular system and that as exercise intensity increases, the demands on the cardiovascular system may push the system to its functional capacity. In a hot environment, the cardiovascular system also transports blood that is heated in the body core to the skin surface where heat can be transferred to the environment. The added demand for increased blood flow to the skin, coupled with the demand for increased blood flow to supply $O_2$ to the exercising muscles, places a particularly high strain on the cardiovascular system during exercise in the heat. The strain becomes even greater when exercise in the heat is accompanied by hypohydration.

The challenges the cardiovascular system faces while exercising under hyperthermic conditions are not immediate; however, they are accumulative. In other words, at the beginning of exercise in the heat, the system is not unduly taxed. As exercise time is extended, the body begins to retain heat and a portion of the cardiac output is directed to the skin surface for heat transfer to the environment. At this point, the demands of exercise and those of thermoregulation are competing for the limited cardiac output. If hypohydration ensues, the cardiac output is reduced because of decreased blood volume. The accumulative effect of these events is a tremendous strain on the cardiovascular system that may lead to a serious heat disorder. The following dialogue illustrates how adjustments in the cardiovascular system are made as the challenge of thermoregulation becomes increasingly difficult during prolonged exercise in the heat (Fig. 8.8).

Let's assume in this example that a recreational athlete has decided to go out for a 60-minute training run during a hot summer day in August. The plan is to perform an 8-mile run at a constant speed. During the first few minutes of exercise, the body is thermoneutral. The majority of the cardiac output is utilized for sustaining the exercise energy demand. After several more minutes, the heat from the exercising muscles begins to accumulate in the body core. The body begins to sweat in an effort to dissipate heat. **Vasoconstriction** of the blood vessels in the skin is gradually removed to allow for increased blood flow. Blood flow begins to be redistributed so that a portion of the cardiac output is now directed to the skin for heat dissipation to the environment. Greater opening of the blood vessels in the skin occurs as special nerves cause **vasodilation** of these cutaneous vessels. Adequate skin and muscle blood flow is achieved because the shift of blood flow to the active muscles and skin is compensated by constriction of the vessels in the digestive and kidney areas. Arterial blood pressure is maintained at this time because of balance between vasoconstriction and vasodilation.

Up to 90% of the exercise cardiac output in a conditioned athlete is delivered to the contracting muscles under thermoneutral conditions. Cutaneous circulation can accommodate up to 30% of the total cardiac output. Thus, the cardiovascular demands of exercise and those of thermoregulation compete for the limited blood supply under the hyperthermic conditions cited above. As exercise continues, competition for blood supply becomes

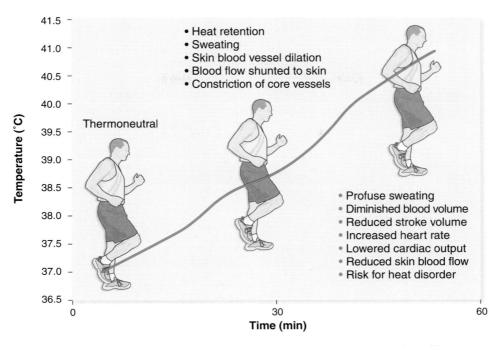

**FIGURE 8.8.** Cardiovascular adjustments to heat exposure during exercise in a hot, humid environment. The red line represents rising body core temperature.

more intense. Continued sweating now begins to take its toll in that blood volume is diminished. Reduced blood volume and decreasing blood pressure cause a reduction in stroke volume. Heart rate is increased in an attempt to maintain cardiac output. However, the increase in heart rate is not enough to compensate for the decrease in stroke volume. The result is a lowering of cardiac output. As a result, the exerciser is working at a higher percentage of his/her heart rate reserve for the given submaximal level of exercise. The end result is that performance suffers in this scenario.

In an attempt to maintain cardiac output in the face of diminishing blood volume due to sweating, the body reduces blood flow to the skin. Under these conditions, muscle blood flow and integrity of the circulatory system take precedence over temperature regulation. The culmination of all these events is that the body is now at high risk for a heat disorder because heat dissipation is severely hampered.

 *Experiences in Work Physiology Lab Exercise 8: Cardiovascular Adjustments to Exercising in the Heat and Cold shows you how heart rate, blood pressure, and body temperature adjust to heat and cold exposure.*

## ACCLIMATIZATION TO HEAT

A person's ability to tolerate exercise in the heat can be improved so that heat stress is not as taxing on the body. The thermoregulatory mechanisms that are controlled by the hypothalamus adjust and adapt to repeated exposure to heat stress. The process in which physiologic adaptations occur to improve one's heat tolerance is called **heat acclimatization**. The end result is that the body of an acclimatized person can dissipate heat easier than that of an unacclimatized individual. The physiologic adjustments that occur during acclimatization include improved circulation, increased plasma volume, earlier onset of sweating, higher sweat rates, reduced salt loss in sweat, and reduced skin blood flow during exercise.

The initial effects of heat acclimatization become apparent in as few as 3 days of exercise training in the heat, while complete acclimatization occurs within 10 to 14 days (2). Similarly the rate of decay in heat acclimatization is rapid, with reductions in heat tolerance being manifest after only a few days without heat exposure. Complete loss of heat acclimatization occurs in about 4 weeks.

Heat acclimatization for exercise occurs only as one exercises in the heat. Simply being out in the sun or exposing oneself to a hot environment at rest produces little heat acclimatization for exercise. The volume of exercise should be reduced during the first few days of exercise in the heat, and then it can be gradually increased as acclimatization occurs (*Fig. 8.9*). It is suggested that the initial exercise bouts be performed at less than 70% of $\dot{V}O_{2max}$ for a duration of 20 minutes or less. However, **rating of perceived exertion** may be a better monitoring tool of exercise stress than reaching some predetermined percent of $\dot{V}O_{2max}$. The exercising individual should also be aware of and pay attention to the signs and symptoms of heat injury.

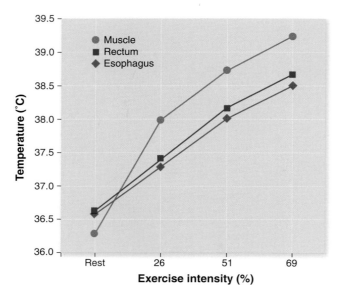

**FIGURE 8.9.** Esophageal, rectal, and muscle temperatures following a 60-minute cycle ergometer exercise bout at various intensities in a moderate environment (19°C to 22°C, 45% to 65% relative humidity). Exercise intensity represents relative percent of $\dot{V}O_{2max}$. (Data from Saltin B, Hermansen L. Esophageal, rectal and muscle temperature during exercise. *J Appl Physiol* 1966;21:1757–1762.)

Heat acclimatization causes blood volume to increase by 12% and plasma volume by 20%. This increase in blood volume reduces circulatory stress by maintaining central blood volume, blood pressure, and stroke volume during exercise. At the same time, acclimatization enhances the efficiency of the body to cool itself through evaporation. The onset of sweating occurs earlier in the acclimatized individual, which means that the evaporative process of cooling the

body starts at a lower core temperature. In addition, the sweating rate increases by as much as three-fold above that before acclimatization, and the salt concentration in sweat is lower than before acclimatization. These adaptations in circulation and sweating allow the acclimatized person to exercise with a lower skin temperature, lower core temperature, and lower heart rate than an unacclimatized person.

 *LINKUP: **Access** Research Highlight: Pre-Cooling the Body Before Exercising in the Heat at http://connection.lww.com/go/brownexphys and on the Student Resource CD-ROM for a description of a study into pre-cooling and human muscle metabolism during submaximal exercise in the heat.*

## HEAT DISORDERS

Heat acclimatization does not guarantee that a person is risk free of developing complications with heat stress. Heat acclimatization only helps a person tolerate heat stress better and reduces the risk for developing a heat-related disorder. Overexposure to the heat, whether for an acclimatized or unacclimatized exerciser, can cause one of several types of heat disorders. The four types of heat disorders are: heat cramps, heat syncope, heat exhaustion, and heat stroke. *Figure 8.10* shows these heat disorders in order of the least serious (left) to the most serious (right).

### Heat Cramps

Heat cramps are involuntary muscle spasms or twitches that occur in the arms, legs, and possibly abdomen. Heat cramps usually occur in the exercised muscles and occur

**Increasing Severity**

| Heat Disorder | Heat Cramps | Heat Syncope | Heat Exhaustion | Heat Stroke |
|---|---|---|---|---|
| **Warning Signs** | Muscle pain<br>Muscle spasms<br>Muscle cramps | Fatigue<br>Dizziness<br>Weakness<br>Thirst<br>Profuse sweating<br>Faintness | Fatigue<br>Dizziness<br>Weakness<br>Thirst<br>Profuse sweating<br>Pale, cool skin<br>Headache<br>Nausea<br>Chills<br>Faintness<br>Unconsciousness<br>Vomiting<br>Diarrhea | Headache<br>Nausea<br>Chills<br>Unconsciousness<br>Hot, dry skin<br>Cease sweating<br>Fast, shallow heart rate<br>Vomiting<br>Diarrhea<br>Seizures<br>Coma |
| **Remedy** | Consume large amounts of fluids and replace electrolytes | Stop exercise<br>Move to shade<br>Consume fluids | Stop exercise<br>Move to cool place<br>Administer fluids | First aid |

**FIGURE 8.10.** Heat disorders. The warning signs of heat disorders and the appropriate treatments.

most often in the unacclimatized individual. Body temperature is not necessarily elevated with heat cramps. Perfuse sweating causes the body to become hypohydrated and to lose vital **electrolytes**. The loss of fluid and electrolytes causes a disruption in the body's fluid/electrolyte balance. This disruption is accompanied by muscle cramps, twitching, and severe pain. The remedy for heat cramps is to consume large amounts of fluid and to replace the electrolytes (or salts) that were lost during sweating. Heat cramps can be prevented by acclimatizing to exercise in the heat, by consuming plenty of fluids prior to exercise, and by increasing salt intake for several days prior to exercise.

## Heat Syncope

Heat syncope, a brief loss of consciousness due to an inadequate blood flow to the brain, is a more severe type of heat disorder. A person may develop heat syncope without first progressing through heat cramps. Heat syncope is characterized by a general weakness or fatigue. The severe sweating that results with exercise in the heat causes a decrease in blood volume, which is accompanied by a drop in blood pressure (hypotension). This decrease in blood volume and blood pressure reduces circulation to the brain and causes the faint feeling, paleness in the skin, and possibly blurred vision. Heat syncope usually occurs in the unacclimatized person and is associated with a rise in skin and core temperature. The person experiencing heat syncope should stop exercising, move to the shade or an air-conditioned room, and consume fluids.

## Heat Exhaustion

Heat exhaustion also occurs most often in the unacclimatized individual. It is common for heat exhaustion to develop during the first hard training session on a hot day or during the first exposure to heat in the season. There are actually two types of heat exhaustion, one caused by water depletion and the other caused by salt depletion. As with heat syncope, circulation is compromised due to a decrease in plasma volume. With heat exhaustion, however, the circulatory impairment is greater than with heat syncope. Blood pools in the peripheral vessels, and central blood volume is reduced. Cardiac output declines and the cardiovascular system attempts to compensate by increasing heart rate. Heat exhaustion from water depletion is generally more acute (occurring within 1 to 2 hours) than heat exhaustion due to salt depletion, which may take several days to develop. Water-depletion heat exhaustion is characterized by elevated skin and core temperature, reduced sweating, weakness, thirst, dry tongue and mouth, and loss of coordination. Salt-depletion heat exhaustion is characterized by elevated skin and core temperatures, muscle cramps, headache, dizziness or faintness, syncope, nausea, and possibly vomiting or diarrhea. Treatment for heat exhaustion is to stop exercising immediately, move to a cool environment, and administer fluids (often intravenously). Refer to Case Study 8.1 for an interesting incidence of heat exhaustion during exercise.

## Heat Stroke

Heat stroke is the most serious of the heat disorders and is the only heat disorder that is a life-threatening medical emergency. Heat stroke requires immediate medical attention. In heat stroke, the sweating mechanism becomes severely impaired due to lowered blood volume and excessive heat retention by the body. Some sweating may still be present, but the mechanisms for cooling the body are inadequate. Symptoms of heat stroke are increased skin and core temperatures, muscle flaccidity, involuntary limb movement, seizures, vomiting, diarrhea, rapid shallow heartbeat, and coma. The individual may become irrational or hallucinogenic. If untreated, the symptoms will cause collapse of the circulatory system, damage to the central nervous system, and death. Immediate first aid is necessary for heat stroke. The person should be placed in a cool water bath or surrounded with ice packs. Emergency assistance should be contacted immediately. Box 8.1 contains information on heat sensitivity or heat intolerance, which is manifest sometimes in persons who have suffered a heat disorder.

## ASSESSING ENVIRONMENTAL HEAT STRESS

Heat stress disorders are preventable. However, trying to predict how each person will respond to exercise in the heat is difficult. Several factors can affect how a person responds to heat stress: body composition, state of training, acclimatization, intensity of exercise, clothing, and the environment. The most significant of these contributing factors is the environment or how the conditions in the environment present a thermal challenge. The thermal challenge of the environment can best be evaluated by determining the **wet bulb-globe temperature** (WB-GT). This index of environmental heat stress was developed by the United States military to help measure heat stress for unconditioned trainees who were participating in military training while wearing uniforms. The index takes into account the ambient temperature (dry bulb), relative humidity (wet bulb), and radiant heat (globe). Obviously, heat stress is increased as any one of these factors rise.

The WB-GT is determined by combining the measures made with three thermometers: one for ambient temperature (dry bulb), one to evaluate relative humidity and evaporative capacity (wet bulb), and one to determine radiant heat from the sun (black bulb). The WB-GT apparatus is illustrated in *Figure 8.11*. The instrument should be placed in the sun where it will not be influenced by trees, buildings, or anything that will affect air movement. The WB-GT calculation is made as follows:

$$\text{WB-GT} = 0.1 \times \text{DBT} + 0.7 \times \text{WBT} + 0.2 \times \text{GT}$$

The dry bulb temperature (DBT) is the ambient air temperature and is recorded by a regular mercury thermometer. The wet bulb temperature (WBT) is recorded by a regular mercury thermometer that is surrounded by a wet wick. The wet wick serves to measure the evaporative capacity under the environmental conditions. When relative

## CASE STUDY 8.1: *HEAT STRESS DURING A MINI-TRIATHLON*

### CASE

Jane is a 22 year-old friend of yours who primarily competes in distance cycling events. As part of her training, she has decided to participate in a regional mini-triathlon. Jane has prepared for this event by incorporating cycling, swimming, and running into her training regimen during the past 2 months. The mini-triathlon is being held on a summer morning in Chicago. You come to the event as a spectator to support your friend. The legs of the event consist of a 15-mile bike race, 1-mile swim, and 10-mile run. The mini-triathlon begins at 8:00 a.m., when the temperature and humidity are 78°F (25.6°C) and 80%, respectively. However, as the race proceeds, the temperature rises to 85°F (29.4°C).

Jane performs well in the cycling and has just completed the swim. There are several spectator posts along the run, and you position yourself at each post to cheer for Jane. As the race proceeds, you notice that Jane looks increasingly fatigued. During the last mile, you note that Jane's pace has dramatically slowed, and it seems as though she is not aware of your presence as you cheer for her. You rush to the finish line to evaluate Jane's condition, and as she passes through the gate, you insist that she go to the first aid station for an evaluation.

### DESCRIPTION

The amount of heat stress the body must withstand during exercise results from a combination of the environmental conditions, metabolic rate, and clothing worn. Exercise in a warm or hot environment always carries with it a risk of heat disorder. The risk can be minimized through precautionary measures and by recognizing the signs and symptoms of heat disorders. It is important that individuals begin a race in the heat well hydrated and that they continue to drink fluids during the race. Especially important is knowledge of the fact that the thirst mechanism always lags behind one's need for water. This requires that individuals consume water when they do not feel thirsty.

The physiologic responses to heat stress are reflected in body temperature, blood pressure, heart rate, and sweating. The severity of heat stress can therefore be evaluated by monitoring these physiologic variables. Body temperatures above 38.5°C (101.3°F) indicate that immediate relief from heat exposure is required (1). Low blood pressure and rapid heart rate indicate a reduction in cardiac output, resulting from decreased blood volume. Resting heart rates or 1-minute recovery heart rates above 110 beats·min$^{-1}$ indicate the need for heat exposure relief. Perfuse sweating or cessation of sweating also indicate severe heat stress.

### INTERVENTION

1. Walking to the first aid station should provide an adequate recovery for Jane. However, Jane seems to be disoriented and even argumentative at the thought that she might need first aid.
2. Jane insists that she is fine and that she just feels a little faint and needs to sit and rest.
3. Jane's skin feels cold, pale, and clammy.
4. You ask Jane about her fluid intake during the event, and she reports that she only ingested some water during the bike race because she did not feel thirsty during the run.
5. Jane's tympanic temperature is recorded at 40.3°C (104.5°F).
6. Jane's heart rate is 128 beats·min$^{-1}$ after several minutes of recovery at the first aid station, while her blood pressure is 82/40 mm Hg.

Jane is diagnosed with heat exhaustion due to hypohydration. She is kept in the first aid station for the next 90 minutes. Jane is instructed to remain lying flat while she is given sport drinks to consume. Her temperature, heart rate, and blood pressure are monitored over the 90-minute period. At the end of 90 minutes, Jane's heart rate has returned to 64 beats·min$^{-1}$, her blood pressure is 108/74 mm Hg, while her tympanic temperature is recorded at 37.4°C (99.3°F). Jane is released and instructed to ingest more fluids than normal over the next 24 hours and not to perform strenuous exercise for at least 72 hours.

### REFERENCE

Bernard TE. Environmental considerations: heat and cold. In: American College of Sports Medicine. *ACSM's resource manual for guidelines for exercise testing and prescription*. 4th ed. Baltimore: Lippincott Williams & Wilkins, 2001:209–216.

humidity is high, the WBT is high because evaporation is inhibited. In contrast, when the relative humidity is low, the WBT is low because evaporation from the wet wick cools the thermometer. The globe temperature (GT) is recorded by a thermometer in which the bulb is enclosed in a black globe that absorbs radiant heat from the environment. The WB-GT index can be used as a guide for safely exercising in the heat. However, the WB-GT index applies to persons dressed in light clothing and not for persons wearing heavy uniforms or equipment.

An alternative to the WB-GT index is to use the WBT reading. Since the WBT is an indicator of the relationship between the ambient temperature and relative humidity, the WBT reading can serve as a guide to heat stress risk.

Box 8.1

*PERSPECTIVE*

# Heat Intolerance or Heat Sensitivity

Many people suffer from a condition called heat intolerance or heat sensitivity. This condition is defined as the inability to be comfortable when the external temperature rises. People with heat intolerance feel uncomfortable in warm environments in which other people would normally feel comfortable. Heat intolerance often produces a feeling of being overheated and can cause heavy sweating.

The causes of heat intolerance vary, but the two most common causes are thyrotoxicosis and amphetamine use. Thyrotoxicosis causes body temperature to rise because the basal metabolic rate is elevated due to excess circulating levels of thyroid hormone. Amphetamines, such as those used in appetite suppressants, also cause heat intolerance because they are stimulants which increase metabolism. Some people become less tolerant to the heat after they have suffered another type of heat disorder, such as heat exhaustion or heat stroke.

Many athletes who have previously suffered from another heat disorder find that they have become intolerant to heat and need to use extreme caution when exercising in a warm environment. People who are heat intolerant and exercise need to be especially aware of the symptoms of heat disorders and what aggravating factors contribute to their own heat intolerance.

### FEVER

Fever is when the body temperature is temporarily elevated above 37.8°C (100°F). Fever is a protective mechanism that the body uses to fight infection and injury because elevated temperature enhances the body's defense mechanisms. Fever results from the resetting of the thermostat in the thermoregulatory center of the hypothalamus. When the thermostat is reset to a higher level, the body uses its heat-conserving and heat-producing mechanisms. Blood is shunted away from the skin surface to the body core and shivering may occur to increase metabolic heat.

The chemical substances that cause fever are called pyrogens. Pyrogens can come from external sources, or they can be produced within the body. Fever-causing pyrogens from the outside are microorganisms and toxins. Pyrogens formed inside the body are produced within the white blood cells.

The cause of a fever is usually obvious, such as influenza or pneumonia. The most common causes of fever include:

- Bacterial or viral infections
- Allergic reactions
- Hormone disorders such as hyperthyroidism
- Autoimmune diseases such as rheumatoid arthritis
- Excessive exercise in hot weather
- Excessive exposure to the sun
- Certain drugs as well as an overdose of aspirin
- Lesions or tumors in the hypothalamus

---

Tables 8.1 and 8.2 contain the recommendations for exercise in hot environments according to both the WB-GT and the WBT readings, respectively.

## AGE AND GENDER DIFFERENCES IN HEAT REGULATION

Children are not able to dissipate heat as well as adolescents and adults. Although children have a higher concentration of sweat glands per skin surface area than adults, children's rates of perspiration are lower than those of adults. The concentration of electrolytes in the sweat of children and adults also differs. Children require a longer time to acclimatize to exercising in the heat than adults. Furthermore, children are not as knowledgeable about heat stress as adults and therefore do not recognize the symptoms of heat stress as an adult would. These fac-

tors make children more susceptible to heat injury than adults. Exercise levels should be reduced for children exposed to heat, and children should be given longer to acclimatize to exercise in the heat. Children should be instructed to consume fluids before, during, and after exercise in the heat.

Although it is not clear as to how aging itself affects one's ability to tolerate heat stress, exercise in a hot environment places the older person at a higher risk for developing a heat disorder than a younger person. The major reason for this increased risk is a reduction in cardiovascular function for the elderly. Although aging causes structural, neural, and physiologic changes in the cardiovascular system, these changes do not affect cardiovascular function at rest in the healthy older adult. However, this is not true for exercise in the elderly.

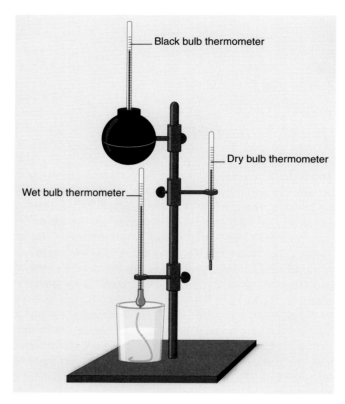

**FIGURE 8.11.** Apparatus for determining the wet bulb-globe temperature (WB-GT).

Studies that have screened for pre-existing cardiovascular disease show that maximal heart rate and maximal stroke volume decline with age, resulting in a 20% to 30% decrease in maximal cardiac output by age 65, with a decline of up to 50% by age 85. The underlying causes of the diminished cardiac output in the elderly are not well delineated but are probably due to an increased left ventricu-

| Table 8.1 | **WB-GT GUIDELINES FOR SAFE EXERCISE:REST INTERVALS FOR INTERMITTENT EXERCISE IN HEALTHY UNACCLIMATIZED INDIVIDUALS** | |
|---|---|---|
| **WB-GT (°F)** | **Moderate exercise Work:rest** | **Vigorous exercise Work:rest** |
| <70 | No limit | No limit |
| 70–72.9 | No limit | 45:15 min |
| 73–76.9 | 40:20 min | 30:30 min |
| 77–79.9 | 30:30 min | 20:40 min |
| 80–81.9 | 20:40 min | 10:50 min |
| 82–83.9 | 10:50 min | None |
| ≥84 | None | None |

Time ratios indicate the recommended maximum duration of exercise to the minimum duration of rest for intermittent exercise bouts repeated hourly. WB-GT, wet bulb-globe temperature index; No limit, no limit to work time per hour; None, exercise is contraindicated. Rest means cool down or minimal physical activity. (Modified with permission from American College of Sports Medicine. *ACSM's guidelines for exercise testing and prescription.* 6th ed. Baltimore: Lippincott Williams & Wilkins, 2000.)

| Table 8.2 | **WBT GUIDELINES FOR SAFE EXERCISE:REST INTERVALS FOR INTERMITTENT EXERCISE IN HEALTHY UNACCLIMATIZED INDIVIDUALS** | |
|---|---|---|
| **WBT (°F)** | **Moderate exercise Work:rest** | **Vigorous exercise Work:rest** |
| <60 | No limit | No limit |
| 60–64.9 | No limit | 45:15 min |
| 65–68.9 | 40:20 min | 30:30 min |
| 69–72.9 | 30:30 min | 20:40 min |
| 73–76.9 | 20:40 min | 10:50 min |
| 77–79.9 | 10:50 min | None |
| ≥80 | None | None |

Time ratios indicate the recommended maximum duration of exercise to the minimum duration of rest for intermittent exercise bouts repeated hourly. WBT, wet bulb temperature; No Limit, no limit to work time per hour; None, exercise is contraindicated. Rest means cool down or minimal physical activity. (Modified with permission from American College of Sports Medicine. *ACSM's guidelines for exercise testing and prescription.* 6th ed. Baltimore: Lippincott Williams & Wilkins, 2000 and Murphy RJ, Ashe WF. Prevention of heat illness in football players. *JAMA* 1965;194:650–654.)

lar wall thickness and increased peripheral resistance. It has been proposed that the elevated resting systolic and diastolic blood pressures in the elderly cause left ventricular hypertrophy. Although this left ventricular hypertrophy is not as great as that seen in cardiac pathology, it does diminish cardiac function.

Other factors that affect cardiovascular function during exercise include a decrease in arterial venous $O_2$ difference. All of these age-related changes cause the $\dot{V}O_{2max}$ of the older person to drop by 20% to 50%. The result is that with increasing age, submaximal workloads require a greater share of the work capacity reserve. This means that a submaximal exercise bout that is easily tolerable for the young person will be less tolerable for an older adult, and possibly intolerable for an older individual exercising in the heat.

Older adults have been found to have a reduced sweat rate, reduced skin blood flow, and reduced ability to acclimatize than younger adults. However, when well-trained older adults are compared to equally trained younger adults, the ability to tolerate heat stress between the two groups is similar. Nonetheless, the older population is generally less fit than the younger so it is wise to take special precautionary steps to protect older adults against heat injury. Some of these steps might be to teach the older adult how to:

- Maintain adequate hydration
- Self-monitor for the symptoms of heat disorders during exercise
- Reduce exercise intensity and duration when the WB-GT is high
- Include periods of rest in a cool environment during periods of extended exposure to heat

Early studies that compared the thermoregulatory differences between men and women found that men had a much greater capacity to tolerate heat than women. These studies, however, did not control well for differences in aerobic capacity, body composition, body surface area, and acclimatization between the sexes. When men and women are matched for acclimatization, fitness level, body composition, and body surface area, the thermoregulatory difference between the genders becomes minimal. Furthermore, gender differences in hormone levels do not affect thermoregulation (3). It is generally agreed that men and women can acclimatize to exercising in the heat to a similar degree.

## PROTECTION AGAINST HEAT DISORDERS

A person's susceptibility to heat stress is affected by the type of clothing worn during the exercise bout. Clothing that enhances heat dissipation reduces the risk of heat injury, while clothing that inhibits heat dissipation increases risk. Over the years, there have been several accounts of football players who have died as a result of practicing in the heat while wearing full uniforms. A full football uniform covers 50% of the body and inhibits the evaporative cooling mechanism of the body because the amount of body surface area available for evaporation is reduced. On the other hand, exposing too much skin surface may facilitate heat gain by radiation from the environment. The following recommendations for clothing should be considered when weather conditions merit.

- Wear short-sleeve shirts and jerseys that are loose fitting and light in color. The fabric should be "netted" or lightweight cotton that encourages evaporation. Modern materials such as ClimaLite encourage evaporation by removing sweat from the skin surface.
- Wear loose-fitting shorts or bottoms that are made of a material which allows evaporation.
- Minimize the use of tapes, wraps, bands, gloves, hats, and pads to the minimal amounts that are needed for safety and performance. (Decorative or stylish arm bands, hats, gloves, etc. should be avoided.)
- Use a sunscreen or sun block to protect exposed skin areas from direct solar radiation.

The most effective protection against heat injury is adequate hydration. Persons exercising in the heat can lose up to 4.5 kg (10 lb) or 6% of body weight during an intense training session. For this reason, rapid weight loss should be seen as a sign of hypohydration and not a sign of becoming physically fit. Ingesting a small amount of extra water (500 mL [17 oz]) prior to exercising in the heat can provide some protection against heat injury. Most individuals will not voluntarily replace the water lost during exercise. Furthermore, water loss during exercise in the heat will exceed the body's ability to absorb water. Water loss during exercise in the heat can average 2000 mL·hr$^{-1}$ (33 mL·min$^{-1}$), whereas the ability of the body to absorb water is only 1000 mL·hr$^{-1}$ (17 mL·min$^{-1}$). The exercising individual must consciously ingest fluids at regular intervals during an extended exercise bout in the heat. It is suggested that the person ingest 250 mL (8 oz) of fluid every 15 minutes during exercise in a hot environment. This translates into about eight large swallows of fluid every 15 minutes. Ingesting more fluid than this will only increase gastric irritability.

There is little evidence of physiologic or physical performance differences between consuming plain water versus a carbohydrate-electrolyte drink when the exercise bout is less than 60 minutes (4,5). Therefore, plain water is an adequate choice for fluid replacement for exercise bouts lasting less than an hour. If the duration of exercise goes beyond an hour, a sport drink is more beneficial than plain water. A sport drink containing carbohydrates and electrolytes will delay the onset of fatigue by replacing the carbohydrates and electrolytes that are lost during prolonged exercise (6). The sport drink should contain no more than 8% sugar and should be kept cold. Guidelines for fluid replacement during exercise are outlined in Table 8.3. Further information on sport drinks and exercise performance can be found in Chapter 12.

Sweat is **hypotonic**, meaning that it contains a lower concentration of electrolytes than the plasma. Therefore, when people sweat, they are actually losing water at a faster rate than they are losing electrolytes. A conscious effort to

---

| **Table 8.3** | *GUIDELINES FOR FLUID REPLACEMENT DURING EXERCISE IN THE HEAT* |
| --- | --- |

**Fluid ingestion procedures**
- Ingest adequate fluids for the 24 hours prior to exercise in the heat
- Ingest 500 mL (17 oz) of water 15–60 minutes prior to exercise
- Ingest 250 mL (8 oz) of water or a sport drink every 15 minutes during exercise
- Ingest plain water for exercise bouts <60 minutes in length
- Ingest a sport drink for exercise bouts ≥60 minutes in length
- Ingest fluids beyond the amount indicated by thirst for the first 12 hours post exercise
- Maintain adequate fluid intake, especially if exercise training is to continue in the heat

**Content of the sport drink**
- Carbohydrate (sugar) concentration should be 6% to 7% (14–16 g sugar·250 mL$^{-1}$ or 8-oz serving)
- Combinations of sucrose, glucose, fructose, and maltodextrins promote the best rates of fluid absorption, if fructose and maltodextrin are not the predominating sugars
- The electrolytes sodium and potassium, and possibly calcium and magnesium, should be present in the sport drink to help with electrolyte replacement. Sodium helps with water absorption

replace electrolytes through supplementation is necessary only if a person is exercising in extreme heat for a period of several days. Under most conditions, electrolytes can be replaced easily through normal dietary practices. Consumption of fruits, vegetables, and fruit/vegetable juices adequately replaces the electrolytes (sodium, potassium, calcium, and magnesium) that are lost by sweating. Ingestion of sport drinks can also help with electrolyte replacement, as mentioned earlier. Box 8.2 highlights the career of Carl Gisolfi, who contributed much to our understanding of exercise in the heat and fluid absorption.

▶ **INQUIRY SUMMARY.** The thermal regulatory center receives information from the thermal receptors, interprets this information, and elicits responses to maintain body temperature close to 37°C. Heat from the body core is transferred to the skin surface through conduction and convection, while warmed blood is shunted to the skin for evaporative cooling. Evaporation is the mechanism that is most effective in releasing heat from the body during exercise in a hot environment. A person can become more tolerant to exercise in the heat by repeatedly exercising in the heat. This process is called acclimatization, which will help protect against but not prevent heat injury. Heat disorders progress from least to most severe, with each disorder having its own symptoms. Exercise in the heat can be safe if the proper protective measures are followed. *What are some of the stories you have heard about exercising in the heat and about fluid replacement? Were these stories based on scientific information or were they used as scare tactics and marketing tools to encourage people to purchase a certain supplement or sport drink?*

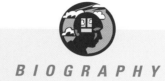

**Box 8.2**

*BIOGRAPHY*

# *Carl V. Gisolfi*

Carl Gisolfi (1942–2000) received his BS degree in physical education from Manhattan College in Riverdale, NY in 1964. Gisolfi then attended graduate school at Indiana University, where he received his PhD in physiology under the well-known environmental exercise physiologist, Sid Robinson. Gisolfi immediately joined the faculty at the University of Iowa in a joint appointment in the department of physical education—men and the department of physiology and biophysics. He soon established a human climatic research agenda and was promoted to associate professor in 1975 and full professor in 1981. Gisolfi received the Teacher of the Year Award from the college of medicine in 1975 and was designated a Distinguished Professor by the University of Iowa in 1996. A Distinguished Service Award was also bestowed upon Gisolfi by Manhattan College in 1995. Throughout his teaching career, Gisolfi taught courses in human physiology, environmental physiology, and exercise physiology at both the graduate and undergraduate levels. He mentored 13 doctoral students and 8 Master's students in his career. Although Gisolfi was a demanding professor, his enthusiasm for the exercise sciences was conveyed to a wide range of students across many disciplines. His laboratory was always filled with students that he was mentoring.

The initial focus of Gisolfi's research was on the responses of nontrained/nonacclimatized persons to heat stress and exercise. These studies later became landmark papers in temperature regulation. His research in hypohydration and rehydration defined our understanding of how the composition of sport drinks affects gastric emptying, thermal regulation, and circulatory functions. Gisolfi extended his research into animal models while he made significant contributions in fluid balance, gastrointestinal function, cellular responses to heat stress, substrate absorption, heat shock proteins, and actions of neurotransmitters. His research lead to more than 100 publications in peer-reviewed journals, 10 chapters in textbooks, 115 abstracts, and coauthorship of the *Hot Brain*, which began to be distributed the week of his death.

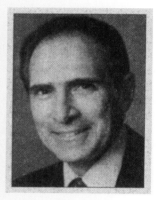

Carl V. Gisolfi

Gisolfi was recognized internationally for his research, and he received numerous awards and recognitions. He was elected President of the American College of Sports Medicine (ACSM) in 1985, received the ACSM Honor Award in 1995, and was elected President of the ACSM Foundation. He served as associate editor for both the *Journal of Applied Physiology* and *Medicine and Science in Sports and Exercise*. Gisolfi also coauthored the series, *Perspectives in Exercise and Sports Medicine*. He was a charter member of the Gatorade Sports Science Institute Sports Medicine Review Board and served as chair of the Section on Environmental and Exercise Physiology of the American Physiological Society.

Gisolfi's influence will long be felt by exercise scientists and the ACSM.

## Temperature Regulation in Cold Environments

Exposure to cold can present a physiologic stress that is as lethal as exercise in extreme heat. Generally exercise-training sessions conducted in the cold do not pose a threat to health because they are short term and access to shelter is usually nearby. However, cold exposure for a short period can cause temporary discomfort and inhibit the athlete from performing optimally. Furthermore, the psychologic stress from being exposed to the cold, even temporarily, can distract the athlete enough so that performance is hindered or the benefit of the training session is lost.

Long-term exposure to cold presents a more serious threat than short-term exposure. Long-term cold exposure usually occurs in remote wilderness areas where access to shelter or relief is not available. As mentioned earlier in this chapter, water conducts heat much faster than air at the same temperature. Consequently, immersion in cool water can impose a thermal challenge in only a short period of time. Being exposed to a cold air temperature while in wet clothing can complicate matters because the rate of conduction and convection of the heat away from the body by the cold air and water is exponentially increased.

### THERMAL REGULATORY CENTER

The role of the hypothalamus and thermal regulatory center in dissipating heat was presented earlier in this chapter. The role of the thermal regulatory center during cold exposure is to conserve heat or maintain core temperature. Remember that when a person is exposed to the cold, the mechanisms of heat transfer are working even though the desire of the body is to conserve heat. Therefore, the body must make adjustments to inhibit the loss of heat and maintain core temperature when the environmental heat transfer mechanisms are favoring heat loss (*Fig. 8.12*). One of these adjustments is heat conserving, while the other two are heat producing.

The first adjustment the body makes is one to conserve heat. As the temperature of the skin and core begin to drop, the thermal regulatory center responds by causing vasoconstriction of the smooth muscles of the arterioles in the skin. This reduces blood flow to the skin as it shunts blood flow to the core to maintain body temperature. At the same time, neural feedback is sent to the

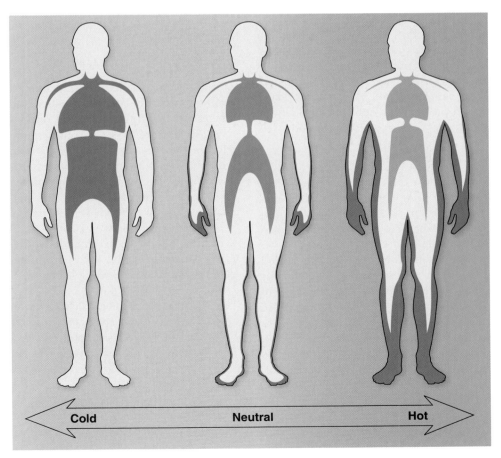

**FIGURE 8.12.** Retention and dissipation of body heat by redistribution of cardiac output. As the body cools, skin blood vessels vasoconstrict to retain warm blood in the body core. As the body warms, skin blood vessels vasodilate to bring warm blood to the body surface to cool.

hypothalamus, and the thermal regulatory center stimulates both the thyroid and adrenal glands. Thyroxin released from the thyroid gland and epinephrine and norepinephrine released from the adrenal medulla stimulate cellular metabolism. The second way the body produces heat is through shivering. Shivering is an unconscious, synchronous muscular contraction that can elevate metabolism four to five times above resting levels. When the metabolic rate is increased through shivering and hormone stimulation, the metabolic heat released is absorbed by the body through conduction and convection, as mentioned earlier in this chapter.

## CARDIOVASCULAR ADJUSTMENTS TO COLD EXPOSURE

The heat produced during exercise can sustain the body's core temperature in air temperatures well below freezing without the need for heavy protective clothing. However, the thermoregulatory defense against the cold is governed by core temperature and not by heat production. This means that it is possible for the core temperature to drop during exercise in cold environments. The cardiovascular adjustments made to protect the body against cold exposure are simply a matter of heat conservation in the core.

Once the core temperature drops, cold nerve receptors in the skin are stimulated and peripheral blood vessels are constricted so blood flow to the body surface is diminished. Under severe cold stress, blood flow to the skin can approach zero. The reduction in cutaneous blood flow helps concentrate the warm blood in the core so that temperature can be maintained. The consequence of redirecting blood flow to the core is that skin temperature drops toward ambient temperature, and the skin and subcutaneous fat are used as insulators to further conserve heat in the core.

## ACCLIMATIZATION TO THE COLD

Our ability to adapt to cold exposure is much less than our ability to adapt to the heat. The first adaptation that occurs with prolonged exposure to the cold is a reduction in the skin temperature when shivering begins. People who are acclimatized to the cold can withstand a lower skin temperature without shivering than unacclimatized individuals. The reason for this shivering adaptation is that acclimatized persons can maintain a higher level of heat production through hormone-stimulated metabolism than unacclimatized persons. The second adaptation to cold exposure is an intermittent peripheral circulation to the hands and feet. As the skin temperature of the hands and feet of the acclimatized person drops, vasoconstriction occurs to maintain core temperature. When the skin temperature drops a little further, vasodilatation occurs. The vasodilatation allows for a rush of blood to enter the peripheries, warming the skin surface. Moments later, vasoconstriction again shunts the blood to the body core. Although this intermittent peripheral circulation causes a

small loss in heat, this adaptation prevents tissue damage to the periphery.

The exact time frame in which cold acclimatization occurs has not been determined. However, the initial signs of acclimatization are manifest after a week of cold exposure. Even though acclimatization to the cold can occur, there is little evidence to indicate that cold acclimatization affects the thermoregulatory responses during exercise (7). The best protection against cold is to minimize exposure.

## HEALTH RISKS FROM COLD EXPOSURE

There are only two health risks from cold exposure, hypothermia and frostbite. Hypothermia occurs when the body temperature falls below 35°C (95°F). Frostbite is when the flesh actually freezes. Prolonged exposure to cold air or water causes hypothermia, whereas short exposure to extreme cold causes frostbite. Serious hypothermia can cause death, and severe frostbite can require surgical removal of the damaged tissue. Although the metabolic heat from exercise can maintain body heat for short periods of time, the body's ability to maintain heat during prolonged exercise in a cold environment may be overcome. The only protection a person has against hypothermia and frostbite is insulation from cold exposure. Box 8.3 discusses cold injuries such as frostbite.

## ASSESSING ENVIRONMENTAL COLD STRESS

As with heat exposure, the ambient air temperature is not a valid indicator of cold stress. Since convection is the major heat-transferring mechanism responsible for heat loss in cold exposure, wind current (or water current) contributes significantly to the cold stress index. The term **windchill** describes the convective cooling property of the environmental air at a given ambient temperature. As the wind velocity increases for any ambient temperature, the cooling effect on the body is more pronounced. For example, if the wind velocity is 20 mph and the ambient temperature 30°F, the equivalent windchill feels as if it is only 3°F. *Figure 8.13* shows the appropriate windchill at any given temperature and wind velocity.

*LINKUP:* **Case Study: Cold Exposure in the Mountains,** *found at http://connection.lww.com/go/brownexphys and on the Student Resource CD-ROM, tells an interesting story about how a recreational athlete developed frostbite during a cross-country trip.*

## AGE AND GENDER DIFFERENCES IN COLD STRESS

Children and older adults cannot maintain body temperature as well as young adults. The reason older adults do not tolerate the cold as well as young adults may simply

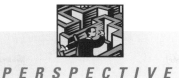

**Box 8.3**

*PERSPECTIVE*

## Cold Injuries Related to Frostbite

### IMMERSION FOOT

Immersion foot is a cold injury that develops when the feet are kept in moist, cold socks and boots for several days. The affected foot becomes pale, clammy, and cold, while the circulation becomes weak. Infection can develop when immersion foot is not treated. Treatment consists of gently warming, drying, and cleaning the foot; elevating it, and keeping it dry and warm. Antibiotics and possibly a tetanus booster should be given. This type of cold injury rarely occurs in spots other than the feet.

### FROSTNIP

Frostnip is a cold injury in which parts of the skin are severely chilled but not permanently damaged. In frostnip, the chilled areas of skin may become white, firm, swollen, and painful. Later the skin may peel, as it does when sunburned. Frostnipped ears or cheeks may remain sensitive to cold for months or even years, although they have no obvious damage. Treatment for mild cases of frostnip is warming the area for a few minutes. Treatment for severe cases of frostnip is the same as that for frostbite.

### FROSTBITE

Frostbite is a cold injury in which one or more parts of the body are frozen. Frostbite is more likely to occur in people who have poor circulation due to some health condition or constriction of blood flow by gloves or boots that are too tight. Exposed hands and feet are most vulnerable. The dam-age from frostbite is caused by a combination of decreased blood flow and the formation of ice crystals in the tissues. In frostbite, the skin becomes red, swollen, and painful, then black. Cells in the frozen areas die. In less severe cases of frostbite, the tissues will recover. However, in severe frostbite, amputation of the dead tissue may be necessary. Most people slowly improve over several months, although sometimes surgery is needed later to remove the dead tissues. Because a frostbitten area may appear larger and more severe than it will be weeks or months later, the decision to amputate is usually postponed until the area has had time to heal.

A person who has frostbite should be covered with a warm blanket. The frostbitten hand or foot should be warmed slowly in warm but not hot water. The victim should not be warmed in front of a fire or rubbed with snow. Once the victim is safely sheltered, hot beverages are helpful. The frostbitten area should be gently washed, dried, wrapped in sterile bandages, and kept meticulously clean to prevent infection. As soon as frostbite is diagnosed, an antibiotic should be given. Reserpine given by mouth or injection may be used to dilate blood vessels and improve blood flow to the frostbitten part.

### CHILBLAINS

Chilblains are painful chilling or burning sensations in parts of the body that were previously frostbitten. They are caused by exposure to cold, even slight cold. Chilblains are difficult to treat and can persist for years.

---

be a matter of a lower metabolic rate. Children, on the other hand, have a larger body surface area per body mass than adults, and this facilitates heat loss. In less extreme environments, children compensate for their relatively large body surface area by increasing metabolic rate and more effectively distributing blood flow to the body core than adults. Women too have a larger body surface area per body mass than men. Women also have a smaller muscle mass than men, reducing their ability to adjust metabolically to cold exposure.

### PROTECTION AGAINST COLD EXPOSURE

A person's susceptibility to cold stress is affected most by the type of clothing worn during the exercise bout. Clothing that insulates and covers otherwise exposed skin reduces the risk of cold injury, while clothing that conducts heat increases the risk of cold injury. The areas of the body that are most vulnerable to cold injury are the fingers, toes, ears, and nose. Although these body parts are most vulnerable to cold injury, the head is the area of the body that is most susceptible to heat loss. It is estimated that 20% of the

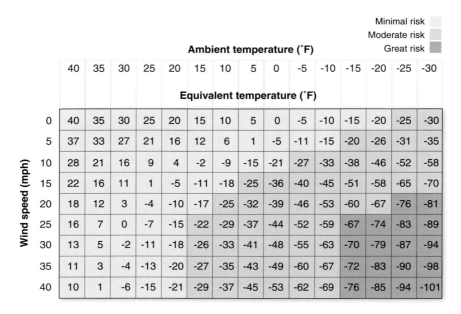

| Minimal risk |
| Moderate risk |
| Great risk |

FIGURE 8.13. Windchill index.

heat loss from the body during exercise is transferred through the head. This means that by simply wearing a hat, you can greatly reduce the body's heat loss. In contrast, by removing your hat during exercise, you can easily cool the body.

Some athletes subscribe to the notion that exercising in the cold causes freezing of the lungs and/or respiratory tissues. This belief is based on an experience of throat irritation after exercising in the cold. The truth is that tissues are not frozen during exercise in the cold, but they may be irritated by the cold dry air. Ambient air entering the respiratory passages is immediately warmed to within a few degrees of body temperature (37°C) by the time the air reaches the bronchi. Cold air does not have the capacity to hold as much moisture as warm air so as the cold ambient air is warmed by the mucosal linings of the respiratory tract, the air is also humidified to almost full saturation. It is the loss of heat and moisture from the mucosal cells that causes throat irritation during exercise in the cold. A simple remedy is to wear a scarf or face-mask that covers the mouth and nose. The face covering traps some of the moisture and warmth of the exhaled air and uses it to begin the conditioning of the next breath of inhaled air.

The following recommendations for protection from cold exposure should be considered when weather conditions merit.

- Wear protective clothing that insulates the body from the cold. Protect the hands, feet, ears, and nose. Modern materials such as Thinsulate are lightweight but make very good insulators. Other materials such as polypropylene can wick the moisture away from the skin surface to the outer layers of the garment, which will reduce heat loss by conduction and convection.
- Wear several layers of clothing. If metabolic heat from exercise warms the body, clothing can be removed one layer at a time until a comfortable temperature is reached.
- Wear a hat.
- Stay dry. Pay particular attention to keeping the hands and feet dry.
- Use a sunscreen or sun block to protect exposed areas from direct solar radiation. If exercising in the snow, remember that solar radiation is reflected off the snow and can cause sunburn even when ambient temperatures are below freezing.
- Maintain fluid intake. The body loses significant amounts of water through respiration and perspiration while exercising in the cold. If blood volume is reduced because of hypohydration, the consequences of cold exposure become more complicated.
- Maintain food intake. If the body is starved for nutrients, metabolic rate declines and the body will be deprived of this source of heat.
- If participating in wilderness experiences, notify someone about the general location where you will be and the expected time of your return. If there is a mishap and you do not return at the expected time, this person will know when and where to search for you. Carry a cellular phone with a properly charged battery.
- If participating in wilderness experiences, be aware of changing weather conditions. Temperatures in the mountains can drop 30°F within a matter of minutes. Temperature ranges between night and day can also be extreme.

▶ *INQUIRY SUMMARY.* The mechanisms of heat transfer work to remove heat from the body during exercise in the cold. If tissues of the body lose too much heat, they may become frozen (frostbite). If the core temperature of the body decreases too much, hypothermia sets in, and if severe enough, may cause death. The body can acclimatize to cold exposure, but the most important way to prevent cold injury is by wearing protective clothing. You probably have heard stories of somebody who has died of hypothermia or gotten frostbite. Reconstruct the details of one of these stories in your mind. *What went wrong? What could have been done to prevent this tragedy or reduce the severity of its consequences?*

## Summary

The body must maintain a constant core temperature within a few degrees of 37°C. Exercising in the heat and cold presents a thermal challenge to the body. In hot environments, the body makes adjustments to dissipate heat primarily through evaporation. If the body cannot dissipate heat adequately, heat disorders will ensue, which could be deadly. Acclimatization helps the body better tolerate exercise in the heat, but conscious protective actions must also be employed. The body can lose heat rapidly in cold environments. Heat loss to water occurs much quicker than heat loss to air. The best way to avoid frostbite and hypothermia is by the use of protective clothing. Although extreme environments present special challenges to the exercising person, acclimatization and preparatory actions can prevent most mishaps.

## SUMMARY KNOWLEDGE

1. What are the four ways in which the body can gain or lose heat?
2. Why is heat release from the body inhibited in a humid environment?
3. How does the thermal regulatory center of the hypothalamus regulate body temperature in a hot versus cold environment?
4. What adjustments occur in the circulatory system as a person exercises in the heat?
5. What adjustments are made as the body acclimatizes to exercise in the heat? Which are made during cold acclimatization?
6. How does the circulatory system help the body conserve heat when it is exposed to a cold environment?
7. What precautions should be considered for children who are to be exposed to a hot or cold environment?
8. How can the WB-GT or WBT be used to assess heat stress?
9. What significance is the windchill factor in assessing cold stress?
10. Name the heat disorders in order of severity. What are some of the symptoms of each?
11. What are several things a person can consciously do to prepare for exercising in the heat and cold?

### References

1. Wenger CB. Heat evaporation of sweat: thermodynamic considerations. *J Appl Physiol* 1972;32:456–459.
2. Gisolfi CV, Cohen JS. Relationships among training, heat acclimation, and heat tolerance in men and women: the controversy revisited. *Med Sci Sports* 1979;11:56–59.
3. Chang RT, Lambert GP, Moseley PL, et al. Effect of estrogen supplementation on exercise thermoregulation in premenopausal women. *J Appl Physiol* 1998;85:2082–2088.
4. American College of Sports Medicine. Position stand on exercise and fluid replacement. *Med Sci Sports Exerc* 1996;28:i–vii.
5. Gisolfi CV, Summers RW, Lambert GP, et al. Effect of beverage osmolality on intentional fluid absorption during exercise. *J Appl Physiol* 1998;85:1941–1948.
6. Coggan AR, Coyle EF. Carbohydrate ingestion during prolonged exercise: effects on metabolism and performance. *Exerc Sport Sci Rev* 1991;19:1–40.
7. Young AJ. Energy substrate utilization during exercise in extreme environments. *Exerc Sport Sci Rev* 1990;18:66–117.

### Suggested Readings

Castellani JW, Young AJ, Degroot DW, et al. Thermoregulation during cold exposure after several days of exhaustive exercise. *J Appl Physiol* 2001;90:939–946.
Cheuvront SN, Haymes EM. Thermoregulation and running: biological and environmental influences. *Sports Med* 2001;31:701–715.
Clapp AJ, Bishop PA, Muir I, et al. Rapid cooling techniques in joggers experiencing heat strain. *J Sci Med Sport* 2001;4:160–167.
Febbraio MA. Alterations in energy metabolism during exercise and heat stress. *Sports Med* 2001;31:47–59.
Holmer I. Assessment of cold exposure. *Int J Circumpolar Health* 2001; 60:413–421.
Melin B, Savourey G. [Sports and extreme conditions. Cardiovascular incidence in long term exertion and extreme temperatures (heat, cold).] *Rev Prat* 2001;51(12 Suppl):S28–S30.
Mitchell JB, Shiller ER, Miller JR, et al. The influence of different external cooling methods on thermoregulatory responses before and after intense intermittent exercise in the heat. *J Strength Cond Res* 2001;15:247–254.
Rehrer NJ. Fluid and electrolyte balance in ultra-endurance sport. *Sports Med* 2001;31:743–762.
Sawka MN, Latzka WA, Montain SJ, et al. Physiologic tolerance to uncompensable heat: intermittent exercise, field vs. laboratory. *Med Sci Sports Exerc* 2001;33:422–430.
Selkirk GA, McLellan TM. Influence of aerobic fitness and body fatness on tolerance to uncompensable heat stress. *J Appl Physiol* 2001;91: 2055–2063.

### On the Internet

Heat Disorders and the Athlete. Available at: **http://www.train.tcu.edu/heat.htm**. Accessed April 08, 2005.
Gatorade Sports Science Institute: Sports Science Library: Hydration. Available at: **http://www.gssiweb.com/sportssciencecenter/topic.cfm?id**=57. Accessed April 08, 2005.
Dr. Reddy's Pediatric Office on the Web. Available at: **http://www.drreddy.com**. Contains information about heat cramps, heat exhaustion, and heat stroke, particularly for the pediatric population. Accessed April 08, 2005.

Hypothermia Prevention, Recognition and Treatment: Articles, Protocols and Research on Life-Saving Skills. Available at: **http://www.hypothermia.org**. Accessed April 08, 2005.

Survival in Cold Water: Hypothermia Prevention. Available at: **http//www.seagrant.umn.edu/tourism/hypothermia.html**. Accessed April 08, 2005.

## Writing to Learn

*In this chapter you learned about the dangers of exercising in hot and cold environments. Suppose that you are the director of the County Sports and Recreation Association in the state in which you live.*

*Research and write specific guidelines or regulations for the following county-sponsored events. (You may start by looking in American College of Sports Medicine. ACSM's guidelines for exercise testing and prescription. 7th ed. Baltimore: Lippincott Williams & Wilkins, 2005.)*

- *The summer calendar of long-distance fun runs that cover distances of 10K and above*
- *The summer calendar of outdoor youth tennis tournaments*
- *The annual "Turkey Trot" 15K fun run (Thanksgiving weekend)*
- *The Winter Wonderland Overnight Cross-Country Ski Trip and Campout*

# CHAPTER

# 9 *Neuroanatomy and Neuromuscular Control of Movement*

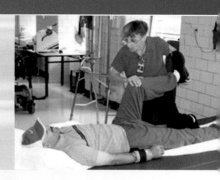

*Internal organ functions, such as digestion, breathing, and blood pressure regulation, rely on an intact nervous system to operate at an optimal level. The brain receives neural input from these organs, processes the information, and then relays neural feedback to the organs to change or enhance function as needed by the body. We rely on strong muscles for movement, nerve input from the brain via the spinal cord refines and shapes the movement. Furthermore, the nervous system is important to functions such as the development of memory and expression of emotion. In short, the brain, via the spinal cord and peripheral nerves, plays a very important role in controlling just about all bodily functions.* For example, what bodily functions do you think are impaired in a person with a cervical spinal cord injury?

## CHAPTER OUTLINE

NERVOUS SYSTEM ORGANIZATION
THE NEURON
- Parts of the Neuron
- Functions of Neurons
- Action Potentials
SYNAPTIC TRANSMISSION
CENTRAL NERVOUS SYSTEM
- The Brain
- The Spinal Cord
- Supporting Cells of the Central Nervous System
PERIPHERAL NERVOUS SYSTEM
- Cranial Nerves
- Spinal Nerves

AUTONOMIC NERVOUS SYSTEM
- Sympathetic Nervous System
- Parasympathetic Nervous System
SOMATIC MOTOR SYSTEM
- Motor Neurons
- Spinal Control of Motor Units
MOTOR PROGRAMMING
- Feedback and Practice

The nervous system is a complex network of interconnecting neurons that transmits information from the external environment to the brain for processing. Once the information is processed, the brain rapidly transmits this information to the periphery so that the body can take appropriate action to respond to environmental cues. In this way, the nervous system is much like the "information superhighway," rapidly sending and receiving bits of information throughout the body so that homeostasis can be maintained. Actions such as hitting a tennis ball, swinging a golf club, or walking involve the processing and integration of thousands of bits of information for us to perform the specified activity.

To gain some appreciation of how rapidly this system works, think about a time when you might have inadvertently stepped into the path of an oncoming car. Instantaneously the message ("I'm in the way of a moving automobile") is processed in the brain and neural input is sent from the brain so that the appropriate muscular response is taken (getting out of the way). This process takes only a matter of microseconds to occur. The nervous system is also important for the development of memory and embedding pathways that result in learning. Other concepts such as thoughts, emotions, and consciousness are also under the realm of the nervous system. Finally, in conjunction with the endocrine system, the nervous system is important in the control of the internal environment. Functions such as digestion, hormone release, and cardiovascular control all involve input from the nervous system. As you will see, the nervous system plays a very important role in our responses to internal and external stimuli.

## Nervous System Organization

The two major divisions of the nervous system are the central nervous system (CNS) and peripheral nervous system (PNS). The CNS consists of the spinal cord and the brain, while the PNS is composed of all the neurons that lie outside of the CNS. The PNS is further divided into the sensory and motor portions *(Fig. 9.1)*. Neurons in the motor division carry impulses away from the CNS to innervate internal organs and skeletal muscle. These nerves are sometimes called **efferent** nerves. The sensory portion of the PNS consists of receptors in the skin. These sensory nerves are referred to as **afferent** nerves because they transmit sensory information from the periphery into the CNS for processing. The motor portion of the nervous system is separated into somatic and autonomic divisions. The somatic division is responsible for the innervation of skeletal muscle for voluntary movement, while the autonomic divisions innervate every organ in the body, such as the intestines and heart. The autonomic division is responsible for motor activities that are involuntary. Furthermore, the autonomic division can be divided into the sympathetic and parasympathetic divisions, which have opposing actions at the **effector** organs.

## The Neuron

Nervous tissue is composed of two main types of cells: neurons and neuroglia (glial) cells, which support and nourish neurons. The neuron is a specialized cell in the nervous system and is key in transmitting electrical impulses to the muscles and organs for smooth and coordinated functioning. These cells are a vital link between the neural control centers (the brain) and the rest of the body.

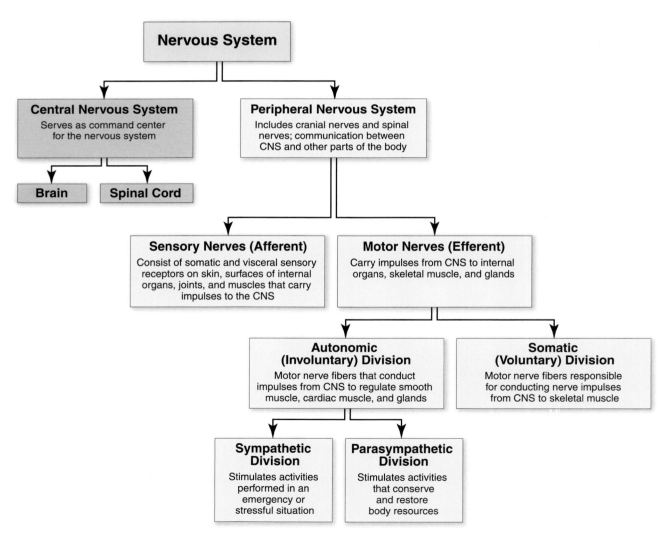

**FIGURE 9.1.** Schematic diagram of the divisions of the nervous system.

## PARTS OF THE NEURON

The neuron is the functional cell of the nervous system. The distinct parts of the neuron are the **cell body**, **dendrites**, and **axons** (*Fig. 9.2*). The cell body is sometimes called the soma, and it contains the nucleus of the neuron where messenger RNA is synthesized and then translated into proteins in the cytoplasm for transport to parts of the cell. For optimal performance of the neuron, it is important for the cell body to stay healthy. The dendrites are long projections that extend from the cell body. They bring information into the cell body and are the main sources of information for the neuron. The dendrites contain **synaptic terminals** that communicate with the axons of other neurons. Axons project from the cell body and are responsible for carrying information away from the cell body. Each neuron has only one axon, but the axon can subdivide into branches that synapse with a dendrite of a connecting neuron or to effector organs such as muscles, glands, and internal organs.

Neurons may be classified by their function. As previously mentioned, nerves that primarily send information to muscles or glands from the CNS are called motor or efferent neurons, while neurons that carry sensory information from the internal and external environment into the CNS are called sensory or afferent neurons. Contained within the brain and spinal cord are neurons called **interneurons**, which are responsible for relaying information from one neuron to another neuron.

There are certain areas in the CNS and PNS where neurons cluster together. Clusters of nerve cell bodies within the CNS are called **nuclei**, while clusters of nerve cell bodies in the PNS are known as **ganglia**. The nuclei and ganglia are sites where neurons in the CNS and PNS, respectively, reorganize into nerves that travel onward to innervate effector organs. Nuclei and ganglia are discussed later in the chapter.

Schwann cells are not part of neurons, but they are important supportive cells to the neurons that are located in

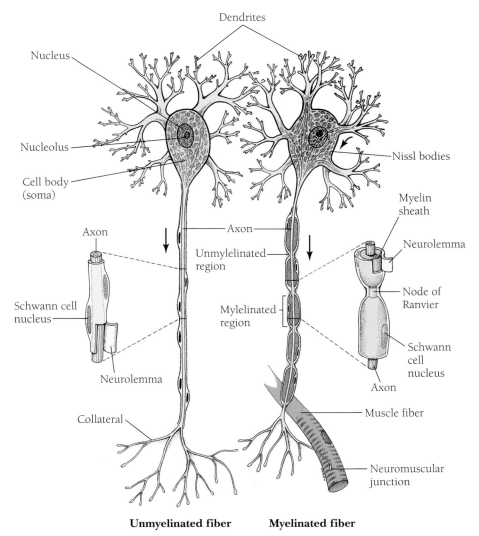

**Unmyelinated fiber**    **Myelinated fiber**

**FIGURE 9.2.** Structure of a typical neuron. Arrow indicates direction of conduction. (Reprinted with permission from *Stedman's medical dictionary* 27th ed. Baltimore: Lippincott Williams & Wilkins, 2000.)

the PNS. These cells are wrapped around the axons in many layers, and this multilayered coating is known as the myelin sheath. Schwann cells are not continuous along the length of the axon but are separated by gaps where the axon is bare. The voltage-gated sodium channels responsible for the transmission of action potentials are concentrated in these bare areas of the axon. These gaps in the myelin sheath where sodium channels are located are known as the **nodes of Ranvier**. The nodes of Ranvier allow the action potential to quickly jump from node to node along the axon. This greatly increases the speed at which the electrical impulse can travel down the axon. *Why do you think this is important?* Multiple sclerosis is a disease in which the axons become demyelinated. *What might you see clinically in a person with multiple sclerosis?* Case Study 9.1 provides an example of a physical fitness program for an individual with multiple sclerosis.

*LINKUP:* **Perspective: Multiple Sclerosis,** *found at http://connection.lww.com/go/brownexphys and on the Student Resource CD-ROM, provides more detailed information on this neurologic disease that generally affects females between the ages of 20 and 40 years.*

## FUNCTIONS OF NEURONS

Neurons have several specialized functions, including the ability to receive input from other neurons via dendrites, integrate the information, and conduct the information via the axon to the synapse, which finally leads to an output function of the neuron. The neuron can engage in these functions due to its ability to respond to a stimulus and convert it via an electrical impulse.

Neurons are excitable tissues. With an appropriate stimulus, they have the ability to generate an action potential, a sudden, abrupt change in the charge across the nerve cell membrane. In the resting state, the inside of the neuron is negatively charged compared with the outside of the cell, which is positively charged. This difference in charge is called the **resting membrane potential**. At rest, the inside of the cell is generally maintained at a charge of −40 to −75 mv.

This resting membrane potential is the result of the concentration difference of ions across the membrane and the permeability of the plasma membrane to certain ions. Potassium is concentrated on the inside of the cell membrane, while sodium ions are concentrated on the outside of the cell. The concentrations of the ions are maintained by the sodium-potassium pump, which uses ATP to move three sodium ions out of the cell through sodium channels and two potassium ions back into the cell via potassium channels. However, small amounts of potassium ions leak out of the cell in an attempt to establish equilibrium, but sodium ions are not able to diffuse back into the cell. Consequently, there are more positively charged

ions outside the cell as compared with the inside of the cell, and the final result is the negative resting membrane potential.

## ACTION POTENTIALS

During the development of an action potential, the charge inside the cell abruptly changes *(Fig. 9.3)*. This change is very brief—usually only a few microseconds. There are three phases of an action potential—resting, depolarization, and repolarization. In the resting phase of the action potential, the cell membrane is **polarized** and stays in this state until a stimulus occurs to cause the cell to change its permeability to sodium. A stimulus that is strong enough to depolarize the resting membrane potential to a charge of −50 to −55 mV is known as a **threshold potential**. Once this threshold potential occurs, the sodium channel gates open, sodium rushes into the cell, and the cell membrane is in the depolarization phase. During this phase of the action potential, the charge inside of the cell becomes positive (approximately +80 mv).

The sodium channel gates remain open for a very short time and then quickly close, signaling the beginning of repolarization. Repolarization is the phase of the action potential in which the normal resting charge is reestablished. This occurs by closing of the sodium channel gates and opening of the potassium channels. The flow of potassium out of the cell results in a return of the membrane potential to a negative charge. The sodium-potassium pump then re-establishes resting ion concentrations of sodium and potassium.

During repolarization, the cell is refractory to another action potential. This means that if another stimulus is applied to the cell, the cell will not depolarize until repolarization is approximately one-third complete. This period is known as the **absolute refractory period**. During the final portion of the repolarization period, the membrane can be stimulated again, but only if the stimulus is larger than normal. This portion of the repolarization phase is known as the **relative refractory period**.

*See Experiences in Work Physiology Lab Exercise 9: Nerve Conduction Velocity for an exercise on calculating the conduction velocity of a nerve.*

▶ *INQUIRY SUMMARY.* The neuron is truly the workhorse of the nervous system. The neuron is divided into three main parts: the cell body, dendrites, and axon. At rest, the charge inside of the neuron is negative compared with the outside of the cell. Through depolarization and the resultant change in charge, the action potential is propagated down the length of the neuron. Appropriate concentrations of ions are critical to the functions of neurons. *What do you think would happen to neuron function if sodium and potassium ion concentrations within the body were altered as a result of a disease process?*

## CASE STUDY 9.1: *MULTIPLE SCLEROSIS*

### CASE

Susan is a 35-year-old female with a 5-year history of multiple sclerosis (MS). Intermittent attacks over the years have left her with mild impairment of vision in the right eye and mild pain with extraocular movement. She also has mild weakness of the left upper extremity. Her gait is normal with no loss of balance or lower extremity muscle weakness. She states that sometimes she gets fatigued later in the day if she has been too busy throughout the day. She takes interferon prophylactically to help reduce the number of exacerbations over time.

### DESCRIPTION

Susan's past medical history is noncontributory. She is single and lives in a two-story townhouse. She works as an accountant and is a volunteer for Habitat for Humanity. Susan tries to walk three time per week but would like to develop a well-rounded fitness program.

Prior to her evaluation, a brief exercise history should be obtained from this client. The therapist may want to consider using one of several tools to evaluate the impact of MS on this client. For example, the Fatigue Impact Scale can help differentiate between physical, cognitive, and social aspects of fatigue. The Fatigue Severity Scale assesses the impact of fatigue on daily function.

It is important to determine Susan's strength so manual muscle testing should be done to determine specific muscle strength in the left upper extremity and to rule out any decrease in strength in her other extremities. Susan's range of motion (ROM) should be also be assessed. With a decrease in strength in the left upper extremity, she may have loss of motion at the shoulder, elbow, and wrist. She may also demonstrate a decrease in ROM due to disuse secondary to decreased strength. ROM of her remaining extremities should also be assessed. Assessment of any sensory deficits, proprioceptive deficits, or incoordination should also be performed. Even though Susan does not complain of loss of balance during ambulation, it is still a good idea to assess her balance especially since she has a mild visual impairment in her right eye. The Berg Balance Scale can be used and is valid for neurologic conditions such as MS. Finally Susan should also undergo cardiovascular fitness testing. Out of safety concerns, with her visual impairment, it may not be wise to have this client perform a treadmill stress test. The YMCA Cycle Ergometry Protocol may be a good option for her.

### INTERVENTION

To improve her cardiovascular fitness, it was determined that Susan should exercise three times per week at an intensity of 60% to 75% $HR_{peak}$/50% to 65% $\dot{V}O_{2peak}$. The mode of cardiovascular exercise should be decided based on Susan's preference and on safety issues (i.e., potential loss of balance during walking with impaired right-eye vision). Since she has been walking on her own, this is probably the mode of choice. To provide her with options so she does not get bored, stationary cycling or aquatic aerobics would be good alternative methods of cardiovascular fitness.

Susan should begin a muscle-strengthening program. Weight machines would be a good option for her. For her lower extremities, she should begin with weights that allow for ten repetitions through full ROM for one set and experience moderate fatigue at the end of the set. For her upper extremities, with her weakness in her left extremity, it would be wise to use either elastic bands or pulleys to initially increase her strength. As her strength in her left upper extremity improves, using exercise machines may become an option for her. For something fun, Susan may want to consider taking a Tai Chi class. This would help with any balance issues, improve flexibility, and may relieve stress. Yoga may be another option for her.

Susan also has some special issues related to her MS. She needs special instruction regarding exercise. Since she sometimes complains of fatigue later in the day, she may want to consider exercising earlier in the day. Also to avoid overdoing exercise, she should consider engaging in strength training and fitness training on alternate days. Finally she should be monitored for heat sensitivity since this is an issue in patients with MS. Susan may want to consider exercising indoors to avoid external heat. Exercise in itself results in an increase in body temperature so in addition to exercising indoors, she may want to consider commercial cooling garments. She should also be instructed in some of the signs of overheating. These signs include any balance changes, visual loss, speech changes, severe fatigue, and muscle weakness.

## *Synaptic Transmission*

A **synapse** is the small gap between neurons and is the site for communication between the neurons *(Fig. 9.4)*. The **presynaptic** neuron is the neuron prior to the synapse, and the **postsynaptic** neuron is the neuron after the synapse. Communication between neurons occurs when the action potential is transmitted down the axon, reaches the end of the presynaptic neuron, and triggers release of a **neurotransmitter**. A neurotransmitter is a chemical that is used by cells in the nervous system to communicate with each other. The neurotransmitter then binds to and causes an excitatory impulse in the membrane of the postsynaptic neuron. These excitatory impulses are called **excitatory**

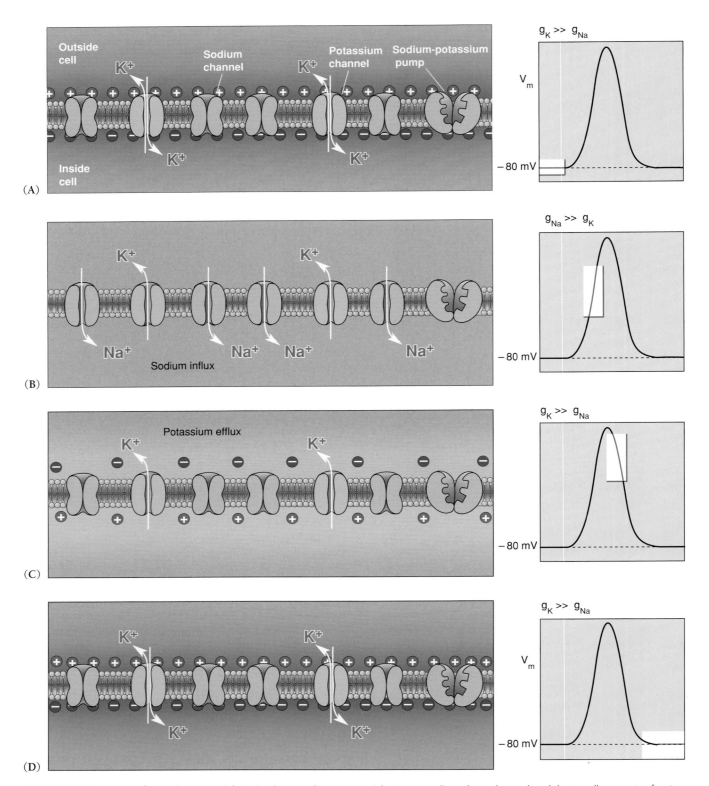

**FIGURE 9.3.** The events of an action potential. **A.** Resting membrane potential. At rest, sodium channels are closed, but small amounts of potassium ions leak across the membrane in an attempt to establish equilibrium. At this point, the cell membrane is negatively charged. **B.** Depolarization. With depolarization, sodium channels open and sodium moves into the cell, causing the membrane potential to become more positive. **C.** Repolarization. Sodium channels close, potassium channels open, and the cell membrane begins to return to a negative value. **D.** Resting membrane potential. If the cell does not receive continued stimulation to depolarize, the sodium-potassium pump re-establishes resting ion concentrations and the membrane potential returns to a negative value. (Reprinted with permission from Bear MF, Connors BW, Paradiso MA. *Neuroscience: exploring the brain.* 2nd ed. Philadelphia: Lippincott Williams & Wilkins, 2001.)

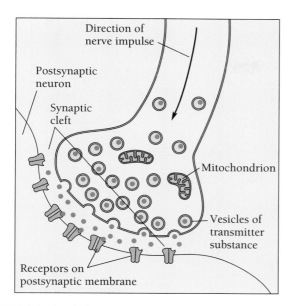

**FIGURE 9.4.** Chemical synapse. Note the synaptic vesicles that contain the neurotransmitters and how upon excitation, the vesicles move to the synaptic cleft, release the neurotransmitter, where it diffuses across the synaptic cleft and binds to the postsynaptic membrane. (Reprinted with permission from Moore KL, Dalley AF. *Clinically oriented anatomy.* 4th ed. Baltimore: Lippincott Williams & Wilkins, 1999.)

**postsynaptic potentials** (EPSP). See *Table 9.1* for a list of neurotransmitters and their actions. However, not all neurotransmitters produce excitatory impulses to axons. Some neurotransmitters result in the development of inhibitory impulses to axons. These inhibitory impulses are called **inhibitory postsynaptic potentials** (IPSP). One EPSP or IPSP alone does not cause a large enough voltage change to generate or prevent, respectively, an action potential from developing. Rather, it takes multiple impulses to produce a voltage change large enough to generate an action potential. Let's examine this idea a little more closely.

Action potentials are generated at the beginning of the axon. This region is called the axon hillock and is the most excitable segment of the neuron. Development of an action potential at this site occurs either by spatial or temporal summation. If several EPSPs occur simultaneously, the summated (or added) currents developed at the axon hillock become large enough to reach threshold potential and generate an action potential. This phenomenon is called **spatial summation**. **Temporal summation** occurs when the axon hillock receives several EPSPs in rapid succession so that an action potential is generated. IPSPs and EPSPs can occur together and offset the effects of each other at the axon hillock. If the summation of electrical charge between several IPSPs and EPSPs is below the threshold level, then an action potential is not generated. If the summation is at or above the threshold level, an action potential is generated. An important point to remember about action potentials is that they are "all or none." What this means is that once the threshold potential has been

reached, an action potential is generated and the impulse travels the entire length of the axon without decreasing its voltage.

A neurotransmitter functions like a messenger between the presynaptic and postsynaptic neurons. Neurotransmitters are made in the cytoplasm of the axon and are stored in small synaptic vesicles at the axon terminal. Upon arrival of an action potential at the axon terminal, the vesicles containing the neurotransmitter move to the presynaptic membrane where the neurotransmitter is released into the synaptic space. The neurotransmitter crosses the synaptic cleft and binds to receptors on the postsynaptic membrane. The action of the neurotransmitter depends upon the type of receptor to which it binds. In the heart, acetylcholine is inhibitory to the myocardium and the action potential will not be generated. Although we have not discussed the neuromuscular junction yet, acetylcholine is excitatory at this junction. Once the effects of the neurotransmitter have occurred, the neurotransmitter undergoes one of three fates. The neurotransmitter can be degraded, be taken up again by the presynaptic neuron, or diffuse into the intracellular fluid. *Why do you think removal of the neurotransmitter is important?*

Acetylcholine is the neurotransmitter present at the neuromuscular junction, the site where the nerve innervates skeletal muscle. When an action potential arrives at the axon terminal of the nerve (the presynaptic membrane), the vesicles containing acetylcholine move to the cell membrane, undergo exocytosis, and release acetylcholine into the synaptic cleft. Acetylcholine then binds to receptors on skeletal muscle fibers (postsynaptic membrane) and causes depolarization of the sarcolemma. The ultimate response is contraction of the muscle fibers. Once the action potential has been propagated, acetylcholine is inactivated by the enzyme acetylcholinesterase to end the signal from the motor neuron.

There are some diseases and pharmacologic agents that can interfere with the release of acetylcholine from the presynaptic motor neuron. Myasthenia gravis is a disease in which antibodies to acetylcholine receptors are produced by the body and bind to the postsynaptic membrane (muscle), thereby reducing both the number and effectiveness of acetylcholine receptors. This results in weakness and fatigability of the affected muscles. One of the interesting clinical features of this disorder is that the severity of muscle weakness fluctuates over the course of a single day. The ocular and facial muscles are most commonly affected by myasthenia gravis. On the other hand, the popular use of botulinum toxin to reduce skin wrinkles is based on the fact that botulinum toxin causes paralysis by blocking the release of acetylcholine from the nerve terminal. Blockage of acetylcholine release prevents facial muscles from contracting, which results in fewer wrinkles.

▶ *INQUIRY SUMMARY.* The neuron has very important functions in the generation and transmission of impulses throughout the nervous system. Action potentials are

| Table 9.1 | NEUROTRANSMITTERS | |
|---|---|---|
| **Name** | **Secretion source** | **Action** |
| Acetylcholine<br>• First neurotransmitter identified<br><br>• Chief transmitter of parasympathetic nervous system | Neurons in many areas of brain<br>• Large pyramidal cells (motor cortex)<br>• Some cells of basal ganglia<br>• Motor neurons that innervate skeletal muscles<br>• Preganglionic neurons of autonomic nervous system<br>• Postganglionic neurons of parasympathetic nervous system<br>• Postganglionic neurons of sympathetic nervous system | Usually excitatory<br>Inhibitory effect on some of parasympathetic nervous system (e.g., heart by vagus) |
| Serotonin<br>• Controls body heat, hunger, behavior, and sleep | Nuclei originating in median raphe of brainstem and projecting to many areas (especially dorsal horns of spinal cord and hypothalamus) | Inhibitor of pain pathway; helps to control mood and sleep |
| Norepinephrine<br>• Chief transmitter of sympathetic nervous system | Many neurons whose cell bodies are located:<br>• In brainstem and hypothalamus (controlling overall activity and mood)<br>• Most postganglionic neurons of sympathetic nervous system | Usually excitatory, although sometimes inhibitory<br>Some excitatory and some inhibitory |
| Dopamine<br>• Affects control of behavior and fine movement | Neurons on substantia nigra; many neurons of substantia nigra send fibers to basal ganglia that are involved in coordination of skeletal muscle activity | Usually inhibitory |
| Gamma-aminobutyric acid | Nerve terminals of spinal cord; cerebellum, basal ganglia, and some cortical areas | Excitatory |
| Glutamate | Presynaptic terminals in many sensory pathways; some cortical areas | Excitatory |
| Glycine | Synapses in spinal cord | Inhibitory |
| Enkephalin | Nerve terminals in spinal cord, brainstem, thalamus, and hypothalamus | Excitatory to systems that inhibit pain; binds to same receptors in CNS that bind opiate drugs |
| Endorphin | Pituitary gland and areas of brain | Binds to opiate receptors in brain and pituitary gland; excitatory to systems that inhibit pain |
| Substance P | Pain fiber terminals in dorsal roots of spinal cord; also basal ganglia and hypothalamus | Excitatory |

Reprinted with permission from Hickey JV. *Neurological and neurosurgical nursing*. 3rd ed. Philadelphia: JB Lippincott, 1992.

generated at the axon hillock. At the axon hillock, the axon receives EPSPs and IPSPs. The sum of these potentials determines if an action potential is propagated down the axon. Neurotransmitters are responsible for propagating the action potential across the synaptic cleft to the postsynaptic neuron. Damage to neurons blocks neural transmission and results in neurologic impairments. *Can you think of an instance in which it might be advantageous to block neural transmission of impulses?*

## Central Nervous System

The CNS is composed of the brain and spinal cord (*Fig. 9.5*). Much of the motor control functions, as well as all of the programming for smooth, coordinated movement, are contained within the CNS. Damage to any area of the CNS can have devastating effects on physical and emotional functioning.

### THE BRAIN

The brain is a highly complex organ and is the master controller of neurologic functions throughout the body. Information is directed rapidly into the appropriate part of the brain for processing so that a suitable response can be directed back out to the external environment. The parts of the brain can be divided into various regions depending on anatomic boundaries and embryologic derivation. For the purposes of this discussion, the brain will be divided into the cerebrum, diencephalon, cerebellum, and brainstem (Fig. 9.5b).

The cerebrum, the largest part of the brain, includes the right and left cerebral hemispheres which are connected to one another by the **corpus callosum**. This longitudinal fissure divides the cerebrum into the right and left hemispheres (*Fig. 9.6*). Furthermore, the cerebrum is divided into four lobes—frontal, parietal, occipital, and temporal—with the central sulcus separating the frontal from parietal lobe.

The entire brain plays a role in neural processes, but some parts of the brain are specially associated with certain functions. The frontal lobe contains the areas of the brain known as the motor cortex and association areas. These areas are very important in controlling voluntary skeletal movements of the **contralateral** side of the body. Damage to the right side of the frontal lobe as a result of a traumatic brain injury (TBI) or cerebrovascular accident (CVA) can result in difficulties with voluntary movements and motor planning on the left side of the body. Read Case Study 9.2 for an example of a physical fitness program and the precautions that need to be implemented in a person who experienced a CVA.

The frontal lobe is also involved in complex thought, such as issues dealing with ethical behavior and morality, initiative, and motivation. For example, damage to this area may lead to behaviors that are not consistent with the

norms of society. The parietal lobe contains the sensory cortex with its many nerve fibers involved in sensory associations. This area of the brain contains the "vestibular area" that integrates a variety of sensory signals and helps us perceive where a stimulus is in space and its relationship to our body parts. A lesion in the parietal lobe can result in the inability to recognize the meaningfulness of an object. The parietal lobe also includes the "taste area" which is the area of the brain where information from the taste buds on the tongue are received and interpreted.

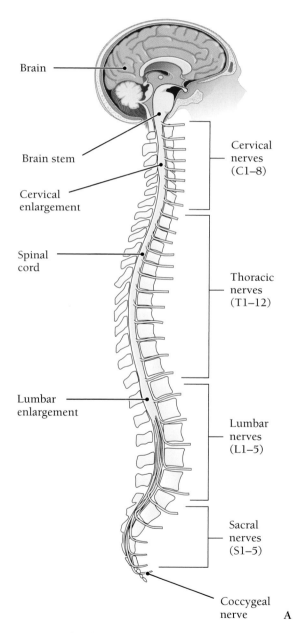

**FIGURE 9.5.** Spinal cord and brain. **A.** The brain and spinal cord showing their relationship to one another and the divisions of the spinal nerves. (Reprinted with permission from Cohen BJ. *Medical terminology: an illustrated approach*. 4th ed. Baltimore: Lippincott Williams & Wilkins, 2003.)

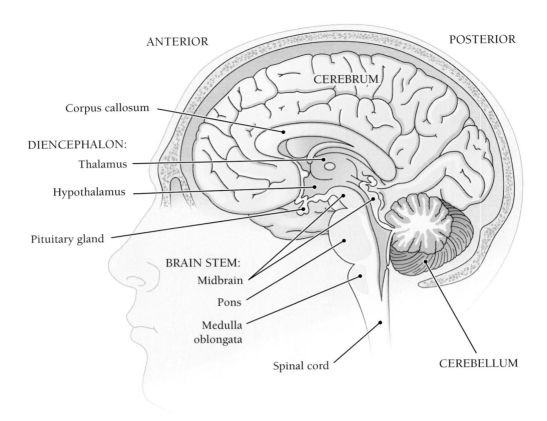

**FIGURE 9.5. *(continued)* B.** Sagittal section of brain showing the main divisions. (Reprinted with permission from Cohen BJ. *Memmler's the human body in health and disease*. 10th ed. Baltimore: Lippincott Williams & Wilkins, 2005.)

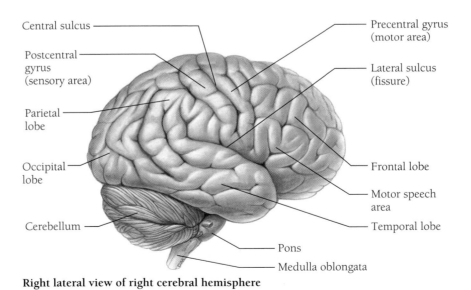

**Right lateral view of right cerebral hemisphere**

**FIGURE 9.6.** Cerebral hemispheres, showing the location of the four lobes of the cerebrum and the major fissures. (Reprinted with permission from Moore KL, Dalley AF. *Clinically oriented anatomy*. 4th ed. Baltimore: Lippincott Williams & Wilkins, 1999.)

## CASE STUDY 9.2: *CEREBROVASCULAR ACCIDENT*

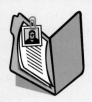

### CASE

Janice is a 55-year-old female who suffered a cerebrovascular accident (CVA) 2 years ago. Her CVA occurred in the left middle cerebral artery distribution. She presents with residual weakness, minimal spasticity, and decreased range of motion (ROM) in her right extremities. She is able to isolate joint movements in her right extremities, i.e., she does not move her extremities in synergistic patterns. She does not use an assistive device for ambulation. She exhibits no evidence of expressive or receptive aphasia. She received physical and occupational therapy immediately after the CVA and also as an outpatient at a clinic, but now she would like to improve her fitness levels and lose some weight.

Janice has a history of hypertension for 15 years and she is obese. Her medications include baby aspirin, clonidine and furosemide. She is a high school graduate, is married, and lives with her two children in a single-story dwelling. Janice works as a receptionist in a physician's office. In her spare time, she enjoys going to garage sales and flea markets.

### DESCRIPTION

Janice should be evaluated by her physician prior to entering a fitness program. Her physician should assess blood lab values, resting electrocardiogram, heart rate, and blood pressure (standing, seated, and supine). It is also important to obtain from Janice her past exercise history and her goals for the exercise program. Janice should undergo a sensory and proprioceptive examination to determine if there are any sensory or proprioceptive deficits as a result of her CVA. Her evaluation reveals intact proprioception in the right extremities. Sensation in the right extremities is present but decreased. No Babinski signs were noted and her reflexes are normal. An assessment of her active and passive ROM should be done. Additionally an assessment of muscle tone should be done to determine the extent of her spasticity. The results of her ROM assessment are as follows: shoulder flexion 120°, abduction 125°, external rotation 50°, elbow flexion within normal limits (WNL), extension −5°, wrist and hand ROM WNL, right hip and knee ROM WNL, right ankle dorsiflexion to neutral, plantarflexion WNL. She has bilateral tight hamstrings.

Janice's strength should also be assessed, probably by a manual muscle test. From the assessment, it was determined that her strength was 4/5 in all motions in both the right upper and right lower extremities. Her ability to ambulate on level ground should be assessed. She was able to ambulate without a loss of balance. Janice was able to ambulate at a speed of 2.0 miles·hr$^{-1}$ without any gait deviations during ambulation.

Based upon the screening by her physician and her high level of functioning during ambulation, she underwent a symptom-limited treadmill test. She reached a heart rate of 130 beats·min$^{-1}$ before she had to stop the test due to fatigue. Finally she should also have her body composition assessed via skin-fold calipers and her body mass index should be determined.

### INTERVENTION

It was decided that since Janice had not been engaged in a regular exercise program, her target heart rate was set at 40% to 60% of the heart rate achieved on the symptom-limited graded exercise test. The goal was for Janice to engage in an aerobic program three days·wk$^{-1}$ for 40 to 60 minutes. Since she is deconditioned, she should begin by exercising for 10 to 15 minutes at her target heart rate and gradually increase the duration. Since she can ambulate without balance deficits, she could walk on a track or treadmill. Other cross-training methods for this client could include upright and recumbent stationary cycling or elliptical training.

Janice also needs to begin a strengthening program to include all major muscle groups. She will likely begin with small-weight dumbbells for her upper extremities and could use weight machines for her lower extremities. She should lift weights at ten repetitions for one set and gradually increase the amount of weight she lifts as she gets stronger. Since she has upper extremity ROM deficits, she will only be able to lift within the ROM that she has. It was also decided that Janice should be instructed in a flexibility program to help improve her flexibility, particularly in her affected right side. Finally as she wants to lose some weight, a dietitian should be consulted to help with weight loss and dietary issues.

There are several special issues that should be considered for Janice. Since she has a comorbidity of hypertension, it is extremely important to monitor her cardiovascular responses to exercise. In particular, her blood pressure should be taken often to make sure that she has appropriate blood pressure responses with exercise. She should be instructed to avoid the Valsalva maneuver during her weightlifting exercises. Furthermore, Janice should be instructed in the use of the Borg Rating of Perceived Exertion scale, how to self-monitor heart rate, and the warning signs to stop exercise.

Other functions of the parietal lobe include interpretation of feelings and hearing as well as our perceptions of body image. The occipital lobe is the most posterior lobe, and it contains the primary visual area. This area of the brain is responsible for determination of the meaningfulness of visual experiences. For example, the color, pattern, location in space, and depth perception of a visual experience all contribute to how meaningful a visual experience is to us. The temporal lobe contains the areas of the brain most involved in auditory processing, equilibrium, interpretation of smell, and long-term memory recall.

Despite the particular functions ascribed to the parts of the cerebrum, reassignment of these functions from one part of the brain to another can occur to a certain degree. This **neural plasticity** allows the brain to adapt to losing certain functions as a result of disease or trauma and is the basis for the development of brain injury rehabilitation programs.

Another very important area of the cerebrum is the basal ganglia. These ganglia are grouped closely together and lie deep within the cerebral hemispheres (*Fig. 9.7*). The basal ganglia include the lentiform nucleus, caudate nucleus, subthalamic nucleus, and substantia nigra. The caudate nucleus lies superior to the thalamus and together, the caudate and lentiform nuclei are called the corpus striatum. The lentiform nucleus is composed of the globus pallidus and putamen. The basal ganglia occur in pairs, and each cerebral hemisphere contains a set.

Through many neural connections with other parts of the brain, these ganglia are involved in the execution, coordination, and initiation of movement. The basal ganglia are all connected to each other through complex neural interactions. They receive information from the motor cortex about motor activities, as well as information from the cerebellum regarding timing and coordination. Based on this incoming information, the basal ganglia relay these signals to the thalamus, which then projects it back to the motor cortex. The motor cortex sends this information out to the appropriate muscles so that the desired movement occurs. The relay of this information happens almost instantaneously.

*What type of movement problems would occur to a person with damage to the basal ganglia?* One disease process that is particular to this area is Parkinson disease. Damage to the basal ganglia and the communication between the basal ganglia leads to difficulty in initiating movement, as well as the development of stiff muscles and tremors in the hands, even when the hands are at rest (rest tremor). Also some forms of cerebral palsy are due to damage to the basal ganglia and are manifest by uncontrolled, ballistic movements of the extremities.

 **LINKUP:** *Access* **Perspective: Parkinson Disease,** **found at http://connection.lww.com/go/brownexphys** **and on the Student Resource CD-ROM, for an in-depth** **look at this progressive, chronic disease of the nervous** **system.**

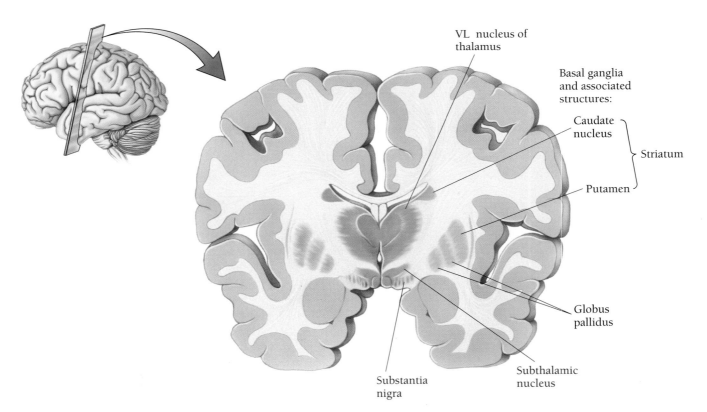

**FIGURE 9.7.** Cross-section of the cerebral cortex showing the location of the basal ganglia and associated structures. (Reprinted with permission from Bear MF, Connors BW, Paradiso MA. *Neuroscience: exploring the brain*. 2nd ed. Philadelphia: Lippincott Williams & Wilkins, 2001.)

The diencephalon lies very deep inside the brain and includes the thalamus and hypothalamus (*Fig. 9.8*). The thalamus plays a very important role in relaying information to and from the motor cortex, spinal cord, cerebellum, and basal ganglia for the control and refinement of voluntary movement. Because of its large number of neuronal connections to various parts of the brain and spinal cord, the thalamus provides much of the electrical activity that can be measured by electroencephalography during periods of sleep, wakefulness, and rest. Connections between the thalamus and reticular-activating system in the brainstem are also important in maintaining consciousness.

The hypothalamus is important in the regulation of the body's internal homeostatic control. Examples of important functions controlled by the hypothalamus include major control aspects of water balance, food consumption, maintenance of pH, body temperature, and sex drive. The pituitary gland is an extension of the hypothalamus and is responsible for controlling many aspects of the endocrine system.

The cerebellum is located in the posterior portion of the brain just superior to the pons. The cerebellum plays an important role in coordinating movements for both posture and balance. Information from proprioceptors in the muscles and joints and from the vestibular apparatus in the inner ear are transmitted to the cerebellum. This information is used by the cerebellum to compare the desired movement outcome with what is actually occurring. The cerebellum transmits its adjustments to the motor cortex so that the motor cortex can send the appropriate signals to the muscles to ensure that smooth and accurate movements occur. Damage to the cerebellum results in impaired balance or **ataxia**, failure to sustain rapid, alternating movements or **dysdiadochokinesia**, and tremors. Furthermore, the ability to perform highly skilled movements requires much practice. There is evidence to suggest that the cerebellum is involved in the neural circuits related to coordinated and highly skilled motor skills (1).

The brainstem is composed of the midbrain, pons, and medulla oblongata (see Fig 9.5). Transmission of impulses between the spinal cord and brain occurs in the brainstem; therefore, the brainstem plays a critical role in communication between the brain and PNS. Furthermore, ten of the 12 cranial nerves originate in the brainstem. The cranial nerves will be covered later in this chapter.

The midbrain contains many of the motor tracts that go to the spinal cord. There are also structures contained in the midbrain that are important for the control of head and eye movements. The pons connects the midbrain and medulla. Contained within the pons are the two primary respiratory control centers that regulate breathing.

The medulla, the most inferior portion of the brainstem, contains the centers for many autonomic functions such as respiratory and cardiovascular control. Sneezing, vomiting, coughing, and swallowing are also functions controlled by the medulla. Anatomically the medulla is the site where the major motor tracts **decussate** (cross from one side of the brain to the other), which results in the right side of the brain controlling much of what the left side of the body does and vice versa. If a person has a TBI or CVA on the right side of the brain, the left side of the body is primarily affected. These tracts (axons) cross in the area of the medulla called the pyramids. Therefore, these tracts are sometimes collectively called **pyramidal tracts**. There are a few motor tracts that do not cross over in the medulla, and theses tracts are sometimes called the **extrapyramidal tracts**. Many of these extrapyramidal tracts function in the control of balance, posture, and gait. Diseases and trauma to these tracts result in what is sometimes called extrapyramidal disorders. As you can see, the brainstem plays a vital role in bodily function, which is why damage to the brainstem, particularly the medulla, leads to severe disability and/or death.

## THE SPINAL CORD

The spinal cord is the major pathway for communication between the brain and the 31 pairs of spinal nerves that originate in the spinal cord to innervate the muscles and other organs of the body. The spinal cord is encased and protected by 33 vertebrae—seven cervical, twelve thoracic, five lumbar, five sacral, and four coccygeal. It extends from the brainstem at the base of the brain to a cone-shaped end called the **cauda equina** usually at the level of the second or third lumbar vertebrae. There are 31 pairs of spinal nerves, which exit the spinal cord through small openings of the vertebral column called the **intervertebral foramen** (Fig. 9.9).

Each spinal nerve is composed of two branches or roots (*Fig 9.10*). One branch carries the axons of the afferent neurons and is called the dorsal root. The other branch contains the axons of the efferent neurons and is called the ventral root. The spinal nerves are formed by the junction of the dorsal and ventral roots. Consequently, the spinal nerves are mixed, meaning that they carry both afferent and efferent impulses.

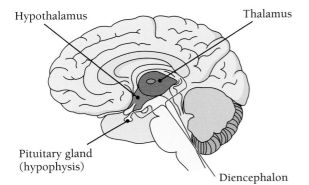

**FIGURE 9.8.** Diencephalon. The regions of the diencephalon include the thalamus, hypothalamus, and pituitary gland. (Reprinted with permission from Cohen BJ. *Memmler's the human body in health and disease*. 10th ed. Baltimore: Lippincott Williams & Wilkins, 2005.)

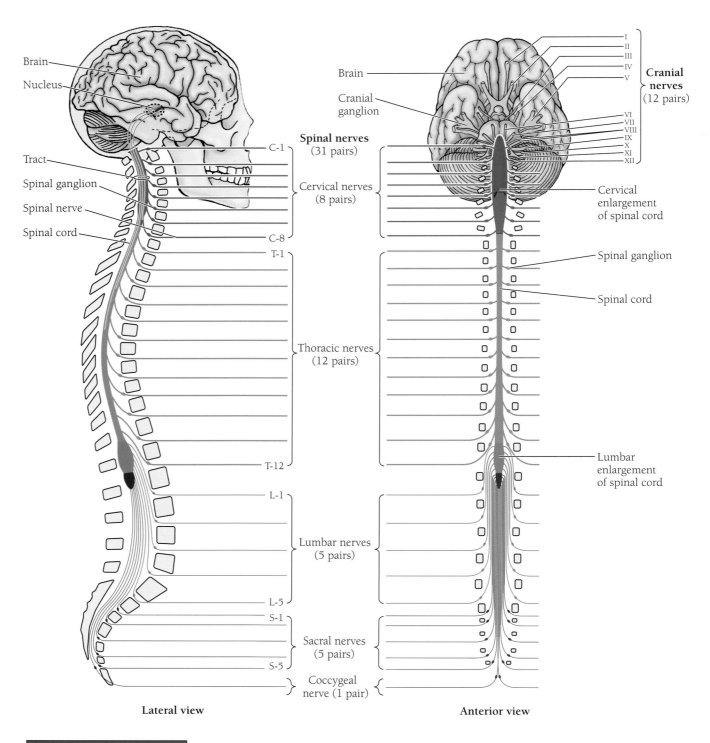

Brain

Nucleus

Tract

Spinal ganglion

Spinal nerve

Spinal cord

**Spinal nerves**
(31 pairs)

C-1

Cervical nerves
(8 pairs)

C-8

T-1

Thoracic nerves
(12 pairs)

T-12

L-1

Lumbar nerves
(5 pairs)

L-5

S-1

Sacral nerves
(5 pairs)

S-5

Coccygeal
nerve (1 pair)

**Lateral view**

Brain

Cranial
ganglion

**Cranial
nerves**
(12 pairs)

I
II
III
IV
V

VI
VII
VIII
IX
X
XI
XII

Cervical
enlargement
of spinal cord

Spinal ganglion

Spinal cord

Lumbar
enlargement
of spinal cord

**Anterior view**

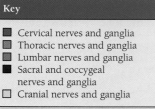

**Key**

■ Cervical nerves and ganglia
■ Thoracic nerves and ganglia
■ Lumbar nerves and ganglia
■ Sacral and coccygeal
nerves and ganglia
□ Cranial nerves and ganglia

**FIGURE 9.9.** Pairs of spinal nerves.

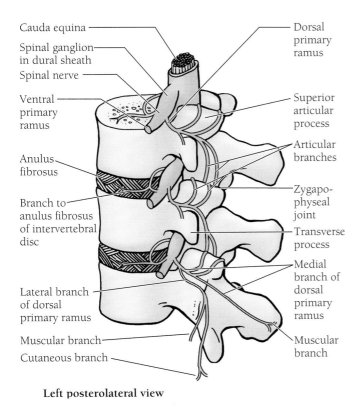

Cauda equina
Spinal ganglion in dural sheath
Spinal nerve
Ventral primary ramus
Anulus fibrosus
Branch to anulus fibrosus of intervertebral disc
Lateral branch of dorsal primary ramus
Muscular branch
Cutaneous branch

Dorsal primary ramus
Superior articular process
Articular branches
Zygapophyseal joint
Transverse process
Medial branch of dorsal primary ramus
Muscular branch

**Left posterolateral view**

**FIGURE 9.9.** *Continued* Inset: The relationship between the vertebra, spinal cord, and spinal nerves. (Reprinted with permission from Moore KL, Dalley AF. *Clinically oriented anatomy.* 4th ed. Baltimore: Lippincott Williams & Wilkins, 1999.)

The core of the spinal cord has a gray butterfly-shaped pattern surrounded by white matter. The butterfly wings are called horns. The horn on the anterior side of the spinal cord is called the ventral horn (or anterior horn) and is where the motor (efferent) neurons exit the spinal cord to innervate the muscles. The horn on the posterior aspect of the spinal cord is called the dorsal horn where all the sensory (afferent) neurons come into the spinal cord from the periphery. Much of the processing and integration of information occurs within the gray matter. The spinal cord also contains interneurons that organize many of the neural impulses that come in and out of the spinal cord and then direct the information to the appropriate neurons in the spinal cord.

The white matter surrounding the gray matter contains the ascending and descending nerve tracts (myelinated axons) that transmit information up and down the spinal cord for processing. The ascending nerve tracts carry sensory information from the sensory receptors in the periphery to the spinal cord and ultimately the brain, while the descending tracts carry motor information from the brain to the periphery. The ascending or afferent tracts are located in the dorsal column of the spinal cord, while the descending (efferent tracts) are located in the ventral columns. Furthermore, these tracts are **somatotopically** organized in the spinal cord. This means that each tract has a particular anatomic location within the spinal cord and that neural innervation of a body part is connected to a very specific area of the brain. *Figure 9.11* is an example of the location of motor tracts within the spinal cord.

The descending tracts come down from the motor cortex into the spinal cord where they synapse in the ventral root with the motor neurons. The descending tracts are divided into the pyramidal and extrapyramidal tracts. If you recall, the pyramidal tracts decussate at the level of the pyramids in the medulla and are responsible for voluntary control of movement. These tracts are the corticospinal and rubrospinal tracts. *Figure 9.12* shows the path the corticospinal tract takes as it leaves the motor cortex, decussates in the medulla, and finally synapses on

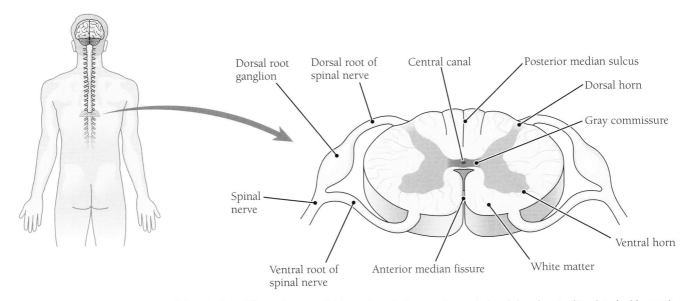

Dorsal root ganglion
Dorsal root of spinal nerve
Central canal
Posterior median sulcus
Dorsal horn
Gray commissure
Spinal nerve
Ventral root of spinal nerve
Anterior median fissure
White matter
Ventral horn

**FIGURE 9.10.** Transverse section of the spinal cord illustrating two divisions of a spinal nerve: the ventral and dorsal roots. (Reprinted with permission from Cohen BJ. *Memmler's the human body in health and disease.* 10th ed. Baltimore: Lippincott Williams & Wilkins, 2005.)

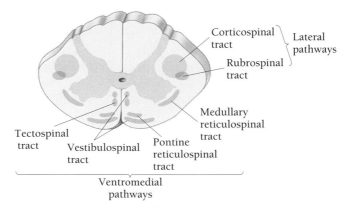

**FIGURE 9.11.** Cross-section of the spinal cord illustrating the descending motor tracts from the brain. (Reprinted with permission from Bear MF, Connors BW, Paradiso MA. *Neuroscience: exploring the brain.* 2nd ed. Philadelphia: Lippincott Williams & Wilkins, 2001.)

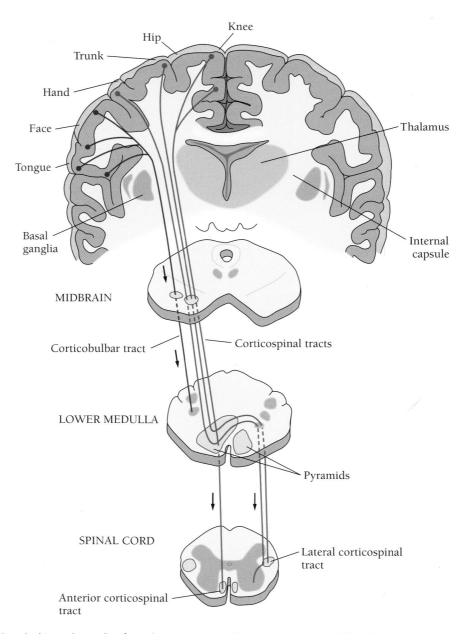

**FIGURE 9.12.** The corticospinal tract descending from the motor cortex, decussating in the medulla and synapsing on the alpha motor neuron in the ventral horn of the spinal cord. (Reprinted with permission from Bickley LS, Szilagyi P. *Bate's guide to physical examination and history taking.* 8th ed. Philadelphia: Lippincott Williams & Wilkins, 2003.)

the motor neurons in the spinal cord. The extrapyramidal tracts (tectospinal, vestibulospinal, medullary reticulospinal, and pontine reticulospinal) originate in the medulla and are primarily responsible for the control of posture and muscle tone.

Contained within the spinal cord are the spinal reflexes, which are complex pathways that help modify muscle activity, namely the maintenance of posture and other protective mechanisms. A review of the control of spinal reflexes during movement is presented later in this chapter.

## SUPPORTING CELLS OF THE CENTRAL NERVOUS SYSTEM

Besides the neurons, there are several supporting cells in the CNS *(Fig. 9.13)*. The oligodendrocytes are similar to the Schwann cells contained in the PNS—the oligodendrocytes form the myelin that covers the axons in the CNS. The myelin covering is important for increasing the velocity of nerve transmission.

The CNS also contains astrocytes, which are the primary support cells to the neurons; these cells provide a link between neurons and blood vessels. They also make and secrete nerve growth factors. Astrocytes form a thick scar tissue at the site of spinal cord injury, and this serves as a barrier to regenerating axons.

The third type of supporting cell in the CNS is the microglial cell. These cells are responsible for cleaning up the debris from dead and dying cells. Microglial cells also secrete proteins that are responsible for the initiation of the immune response at a site of injury in the CNS.

Ependymal cells line the ventricles and central cavity of the spinal cord. These cells help maintain the blood-brain barrier. They also contain cilia, which function to help circulate the cerebrospinal fluid in the CNS.

▶ *INQUIRY SUMMARY.* The functions of the brain are quite varied and highly important for normal movement, thinking, and control of internal homeostasis, while the spinal cord is the important link between the brain and effector organs. Information from the brain is transmitted to the spinal cord via long tracts (neurons). *Can you think of any disease processes and/or injury to certain parts of the brain that might affect control of movement?*

## *Peripheral Nervous System*

The PNS is composed of the 31 pairs of spinal nerves that exit the spinal cord and the 12 pairs of cranial nerves that exit the skull from various areas of the brain (see Fig. 9.9). The PNS functions to transmit sensory information from the skin, muscles, and other receptors to the spinal cord, and it also serves as the final messenger of motor output to the muscles and other organs.

### CRANIAL NERVES

As previously mentioned, there are 12 pairs of cranial nerves. Cranial nerves I and II originate in the diencephalon, whereas cranial nerves III through XII originate in the brainstem *(Fig. 9.14)*. Cranial nerve I and II are pure sensory nerves, which are nerves that transmit only sensory information. Cranial nerve I transmits signals from the olfactory neurons to the olfactory area of the cortex, where these signals are processed. Cranial nerve II (the optic nerve) is responsible for transmitting visual sensory information from the retina to the brain.

Cranial nerves III, IV, and VI are pure motor nerves because they transmit information related only to motor function. These cranial nerves innervate the muscles around the eye that are responsible for eye movements. The trigeminal nerve (cranial nerve V), which is divided into three branches, is responsible for innervating much of the face. The first branch (ophthalmic branch) provides sensory information from the forehead and eyes. The second branch (maxillary branch) provides sensory information from the upper lip, teeth, and palate. The third branch (mandibular branch) is responsible for providing sensory information from the jaw. The mandibular branch also contains some motor fibers, which are responsible for innervating muscles of mastication. Because the fifth cranial nerve contains both motor and sensory fibers, it is called a mixed nerve.

Cranial nerve VII is also a mixed nerve. It provides motor input to the muscles of facial expression, while the sensory part of the nerve is responsible for transmitting taste sensations from the anterior two-thirds of the tongue. Cranial nerve VII also contains autonomic fibers that innervate the tear ducts and salivary glands.

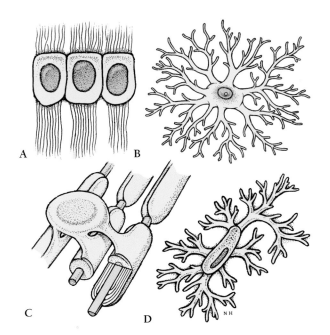

**FIGURE 9.13.** The four supporting cells of the central nervous system. **A.** Ependymal cells. **B.** Astrocytes. **C.** Oligodendrocytes. **D.** Microglial cells. (Reprinted courtesy of Neil O. Hardy, Westpoint, Connecticut.)

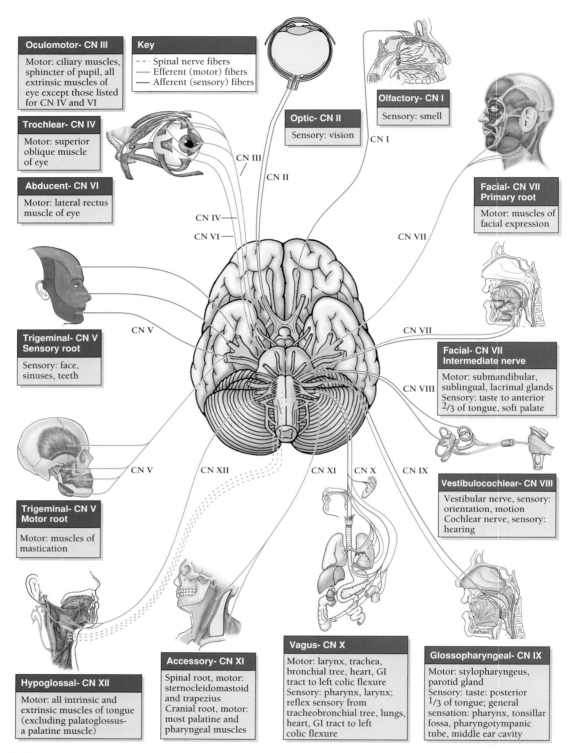

**FIGURE 9.14.** The 12 cranial nerves and the structures they innervate. (Reprinted with permission from Moore KL, Dalley AF. *Clinically oriented anatomy*. 4th ed. Baltimore: Lippincott Williams & Wilkins, 1999.)

Cranial nerve VIII is a sensory nerve that provides vestibular information from the inner ear and also transmits the sense of hearing from the cochlea. Some of the neurons from cranial nerve VIII also interact with neurons from cranial nerves III and VI to help stabilize eye movements during head rotation. This allows the images on which the eyes are focused to remain fixed on the retina, which enables you to move your head and fix on an object without getting dizzy. Cranial nerve IX is a mixed nerve that provides sensory information regarding taste from the posterior third of the tongue. Cranial nerve IX also innervates the pharynx and thus helps to control swallowing.

Sensory information from the baroreceptors in the cardiovascular system is transmitted to the brainstem via cranial nerve X (vagus nerve). Contained within cranial nerve X are parasympathetic efferent and afferent fibers that innervate many of the internal organs, such as the heart, lungs, and intestines. Thus, cranial nerve X is a mixed nerve. Cranial nerve XI is a motor nerve and innervates muscles of the shoulder, larynx, and neck that control movements of the head and neck; this nerve also controls voice production. Cranial nerve XII is a pure motor nerve, and its motor fibers are responsible for innervating tongue muscles during swallowing and speech. *Table 9.2* summarizes the type and functions of the cranial nerves.

## SPINAL NERVES

As previously mentioned, the spinal nerves are responsible for carrying information to and from the spinal cord. The 31 pairs of nerves are divided into eight cervical, 12 thoracic, five lumber, five sacral and one coccygeal pairs of spinal nerves. The first cervical nerve exits just above the first cervical vertebra; the cervical nerves are given the numbers of the bony vertebrae just below them. However, there is an extra cervical nerve, C8, that exits the spinal cord above the T1 vertebra; consequently, each subsequent nerve is numbered for the vertebra that lies just above the spinal nerve.

All of the spinal nerves except T2 through T12 travel away from the spinal cord and then form complicated complexes of nerves called **plexuses**. Within the plexuses, there is much intermingling of spinal nerves, and the nerves that emerge from these plexuses are called the peripheral nerves. These are the nerves that innervate the muscles and skin throughout the body. There are five plexuses contained within the body. They are the cervical plexus (C1 though C4), brachial plexus (C5 through C8, T1), lumbar plexus (L1 through L4), sacral plexus (L4 through L5, S1 through S3), and coccygeal plexus (S4 through S5). The thoracic nerves T2 through T12 come out of the spinal cord and travel parallel to the ribs,

| Table 9.2 | CRANIAL NERVES | |
|---|---|---|
| **Nerve** | **Type of nerve** | **Function** |
| I. Olfactory | Sensory | Transmits signals to olfactory area of cortex |
| II. Optic | Sensory | Transmits visual sensory information from retina to brain |
| III. Oculomotor | Motor | Innervates eye muscles |
| IV. Trochlear | Motor | Innervates eye muscles |
| V. Trigeminal | Mixed | Innervates muscles of mastication; provides sensory information from forehead, eyes, upper lip, teeth, palate, and jaw |
| VI. Abducens | Motor | Innervates eye muscles |
| VII. Facial | Mixed | Innervates facial muscles; sensory information from anterior two-thirds of tongue |
| VIII. Vestibulocochlear | Sensory | Transmits vestibular information from inner ear and sense of hearing from cochlea |
| IX. Glossopharyngeal | Mixed | Innervates pharynx; sensory information from posterior one-third of tongue |
| X. Vagus | Mixed | Transmits sensory and motor information from internal organs |
| XI. Spinal accessory | Motor | Innervates muscles of shoulder, larynx, and neck |
| XII. Hypoglossal | Motor | Innervate tongue muscles during swallowing and speech |

where they innervate the intercostals and abdominal muscles.

The result of the intermingling of spinal nerves in the plexus results in spinal nerves supplying fibers to more than one peripheral nerve. By knowing which nerve roots have combined to form peripheral nerves, we know the relationship between certain spinal nerves and the sensory innervation of the skin. This relationship is known as a **dermatome** and is defined as the area of the skin that is innervated by the dorsal roots of that particular spinal nerve. *Figure 9.15* illustrates the dermatomes of the body.

Likewise, knowing which spinal nerves have combined to form peripheral nerves provides us with the information regarding motor innervation of muscle. A **myotome** is defined as a group of muscles that are supplied by the ventral root of a particular spinal nerve. Knowledge of this information is important when assessing a person with a spinal cord injury. If, for example, a person sustains a spinal cord injury at the L5 vertebra, knowledge of the spinal nerves, as well as the peripheral nerves formed by the plexus in this area, allows health care professionals to determine what sensory and motor functions might be impaired below the level of the spinal cord injury. One of the biggest problems of spinal cord injuries is the inability of the spinal cord to repair itself. Overcoming this problem is a primary goal in the field of spinal cord injury research.

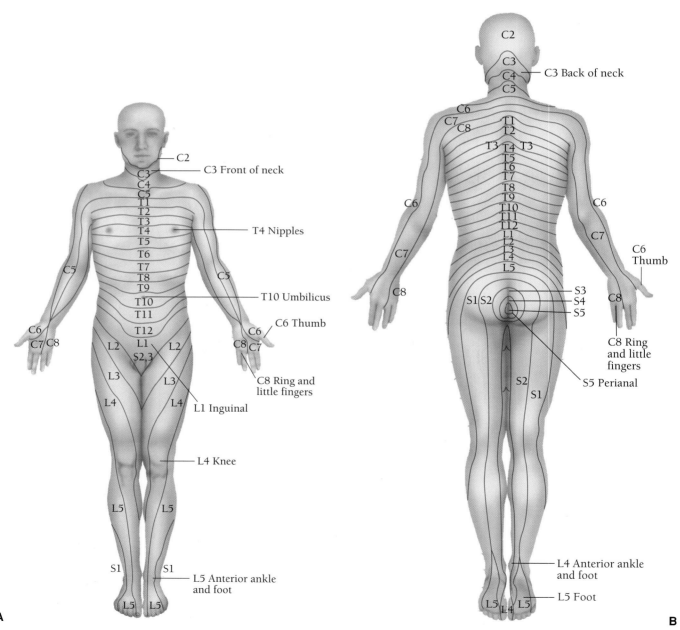

**FIGURE 9.15.** The location of the sensory dermatomes. **A.** Anterior view. **B.** Posterior view. (Reprinted with permission from Bickley LS, Szilagyi P. *Bate's guide to physical examination and history taking*. 8th ed. Philadelphia: Lippincott Williams & Wilkins, 2003.)

*LINKUP:* **Perspective: Spinal Cord Injury Research,** found at *http://connection.lww.com/go/brownexphys* and on the Student Resource CD-ROM, provides information on current research into the problems of spinal cord injury.

▶ *INQUIRY SUMMARY.* The cranial and peripheral nerves play an important role in transmitting information sent from the brain via the spinal cord. For the most part, the cranial nerves are responsible for both motor and sensory functions of the head and shoulders. Because the peripheral nerves originate in the spinal cord, the spinal cord is a very important link between the brain and periphery. Transection or damage to the spinal cord results in paralysis below the level of damage. *What are some functional limitations that occur with damage to the spinal cord at the T1 vertebra?*

## Autonomic Nervous System

The autonomic nervous system is a motor efferent system that functions at a subconscious level to provide homeostasis of the visceral organs and the internal environment. Since the actions of the autonomic nervous system are not under conscious or voluntary control, these actions are considered to be automatic or involuntary functions. Examples of bodily functions under autonomic control include respiration, digestion, blood pressure and cardiovascular control, metabolism, and body temperature regulation.

The autonomic nervous system is divided into the sympathetic and parasympathetic nervous systems, and many organs are innervated by both sympathetic and parasympathetic nerve fibers *(Fig. 9.16)*. The outflow of neural information in both the sympathetic and parasympathetic nervous systems is via a two-neuron pathway. The first neuron in the pathway is called the **preganglionic neuron**. This neuron originates in the ventral horn of the spinal cord and travels to an **autonomic ganglion** that is located in the peripheral nervous system. Within the autonomic ganglion, the preganglionic neuron synapses with the postganglionic neuron. The postganglionic neuron then travels to the effector organ.

### SYMPATHETIC NERVOUS SYSTEM

The sympathetic nervous system neurons are located primarily in the thoracic and upper lumber regions (T1 to L2) of the spinal cord. The preganglionic neurons exit the ventral horn of the spinal cord, travel a short distance, and synapse with the postganglionic neurons in the sympathetic trunk that runs parallel to the spinal cord. The postganglionic fibers then course quite a distance as they travel to effector organs.

Earlier in the chapter we discussed how neurotransmitters are used to communicate with neurons and effector organs. The neurotransmitter secreted by the preganglion synapse is acetylcholine, while the postganglionic neurons of the sympathetic nervous system secrete norepinephrine, at the synapse with the effector organ in most cases. There is also a specialized component of the sympathetic nervous system, the adrenal medulla, which receives some preganglionic neurons of the sympathetic nervous system. These neurons stimulate the adrenal medulla to secrete epinephrine and norepinephrine into the circulation. These hormones then travel throughout the circulation to effector organs and have the same effect on the effector organs as if they had been directly stimulated by the sympathetic nervous system.

In general, the primary function of the sympathetic nervous system is to mobilize a variety of resources throughout the body in response to a challenge to survival. The sympathetic nervous system stimulates various effector organs so that the body can make adjustments in preparation for an emergency situation, i.e., "fight or flight." Heart rate increases, blood flow shunts from the skin and digestive organs to the skeletal muscles and brain, blood glucose rises, bronchioles constrict, rate of digestion decreases, and pupils dilate. All of these changes are in preparation for an emergency situation and life preservation should severe injury occur.

### PARASYMPATHETIC NERVOUS SYSTEM

The preganglionic neurons of the parasympathetic nervous system originate in the head (cranial nerves III, VII, IX, and X) and sacral regions of the spinal cord. The vagus nerve (cranial nerve X) plays a very important role in the parasympathetic nervous system since it innervates the heart, lungs, trachea, digestive organs, liver, gallbladder, pancreas, and kidneys. The preganglionic neurons of cranial nerves III, VII, and IX synapse in discrete ganglia, whereas the preganglionic neurons from the sacral region travel a long distance before they synapse with the parasympathetic ganglia that are close to the effector organs. From the parasympathetic ganglia, postganglionic neurons travel a short distance to the smooth muscles and glands within the organs to modulate function. In contrast to the sympathetic nervous system, the neurotransmitter at both the preganglionic and postganglionic synapses in the parasympathetic system is acetylcholine. *Figure 9.17* illustrates the differences in neurotransmitter release between the parasympathetic and sympathetic nervous systems.

The primary function of the parasympathetic nervous system is to conserve the body's resources and maintain organ functions during periods of physical inactivity. For example, the parasympathetic nervous system slows heart rate, promotes bowel elimination, and stimulates digestion—all of which conserve and build up the body's resources for a time of need. The sympathetic and parasympathetic nervous systems are always active,

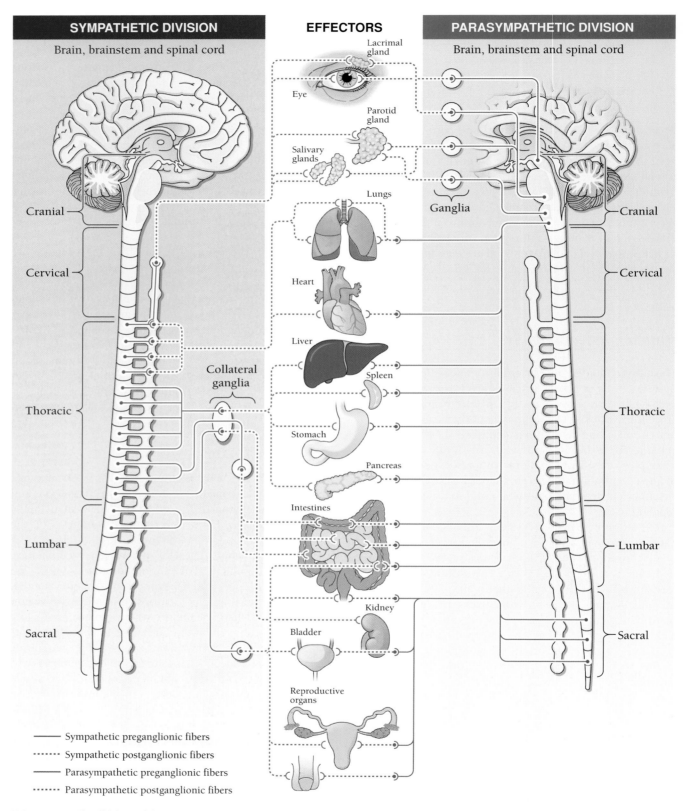

**FIGURE 9.16.** The divisions of the autonomic nervous system: the sympathetic and parasympathetic nervous systems and the effector organs. Note the thoracic and lumbar regions where the sympathetic nervous system originates; the parasympathetic nervous system originates from the cervical and lumbar regions. (Reprinted with permission from Cohen BJ. *Memmler's the human body in health and disease.* 10th ed. Baltimore: Lippincott Williams & Wilkins, 2005.)

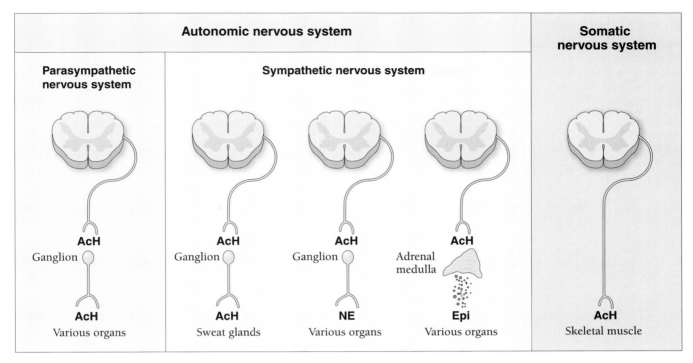

**FIGURE 9.17.** The differences in neurotransmitter release between the autonomic and somatic nervous systems. The preganglionic neurons release acetylcholine (AcH) in both the sympathetic and parasympathetic nervous systems. The postganglionic neurons in the parasympathetic nervous system release acetylcholine, while norepinephrine (NE) is released in the sympathetic nervous system. The adrenal medulla releases epinephrine (Epi), which travels through the circulation to reach the site of action. In the somatic nervous system, all motor neurons release acetylcholine. The sympathetic postganglionic neurons that innervate the sweat glands release acetylcholine.

and this baseline activity is known as *resting tone*. The tone of an organ can be changed (increased or decreased) and is usually regulated by a change in the outflow of either one of the two arms of the autonomic nervous system.

▶ *INQUIRY SUMMARY.* The autonomic nervous system is important for providing control over many important functions of the body. Because we have no control over the actions of the autonomic nervous system, we can say that the autonomic nervous system is involuntary. The autonomic nervous system is composed of two parts: the sympathetic and parasympathetic nervous systems. The sympathetic nervous system is responsible for "fight or flight" actions of the body, while the parasympathetic nervous system conserves resources for emergency situations and maintains organ function during rest and repose. Some impairments to the autonomic nervous system result from neurologic injury or disease. *Can you think of what some of these impairments might be and what the functional limitations would me?*

## Somatic Motor System

The neural system functions to execute movement. Recall that the motor cortex receives input from the cerebellum and basal ganglia before the motor cortex sends out commands to the skeletal muscle. Once the motor cortex decides on the final program for the execution of movement, neural signals are sent down to the spinal cord via motor tracts (corticospinal, vestibulospinal, reticulospinal, and tectospinal), where they synapse on the cell bodies of motor neurons in the anterior horn of the spinal cord. These tracts that supply input from the brain to motor neurons in the spinal cord are sometimes called **upper motor neurons**, while motor neurons that originate in the spinal cord and innervate skeletal muscle are often called **lower motor neurons**. For more information about upper and lower motor neurons, see Box 9.1.

### MOTOR NEURONS

Motor neurons can be divided into two different categories: alpha and gamma. Alpha motor neurons innervate skeletal muscle and are responsible for voluntary muscle contraction. The neurotransmitter for these neurons is acetylcholine. One motor neuron innervates more than one muscle fiber. A **motor unit** is defined as a motor neuron and the muscle fibers it innervates (*Fig. 9.18*).

Some motor units contain many muscle fibers, whereas other motor units contain only a few. Motor units that contain many muscle fibers generally are responsible for gross motor movements, such as kicking a ball, while motor units that contain small numbers of fibers are important for fine motor movements, such as fastening a button. Once the action potential in the alpha motor neuron is large

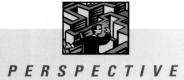

*P E R S P E C T I V E*

## Upper and Lower Motor Neurons

### UPPER MOTOR NEURONS

In the classic sense, upper motor neurons (UMN) are those neurons that make up the corticospinal and corticobulbar tracts. But there are several other motor tracts originating in the motor cortex, such as the vestibulospinal, reticulospinal, and rubrospinal tracts, that also influence the activity of the lower motor neurons (LMN). Because of their actions on the LMN in the ventral horn, damage to these tracts results in changes in muscle tone and equilibrium reactions.

Lesions in UMN can occur as a result of spinal cord transection, multiple sclerosis, stroke (brain attack), or traumatic brain injury (TBI). Clinical signs of UMN lesions include paralysis and initial loss of muscle tone. The initial loss of muscle tone is followed by the development of hypertonicity, otherwise also known as spasticity, increased myotatic (stretch) reflexes, and the presence of Babinski sign. Babinski sign is a pathologic reflex that can be elicited by stroking the lateral aspect of the sole of the foot. With damage to pyramidal tracts, an extension or dorsiflexion of the big toe occurs in conjunction to fanning of the toes. Also because the lower motor neurons and motor reflex arc are intact, initially no muscle atrophy (wasting) will be observed. However, because of muscle disuse over the long term, atrophy will occur.

### LOWER MOTOR NEURONS

LMN are the neurons whose cell bodies are contained in the gray matter of the ventral horn of the spinal cord and in certain cranial nerve nuclei. Axons from these neurons exit the intervertebral foramen to synapse on the skeletal muscles and other effector organs. These neurons receive information and are acted upon by the axons of descending motor tracts coming from the motor cortex.

Damage to LMN can occur in several ways: by inflammation (i.e., facial nerve inflammation such as Bell palsy), injury (e.g., spinal nerve transection), compression (e.g., carpal tunnel syndrome), or disease (e.g., poliomyelitis, amyotrophic lateral sclerosis). The clinical signs of LMN lesions include paralysis, decreased muscle tone, muscle atrophy of the muscles innervated by the involved LMN and areflexia (loss of myotatic stretch reflexes).

---

enough to result in depolarization of the axon, acetylcholine is released at the neuromuscular junction and all of the muscle fibers innervated by that particular motor neuron contract. When a motor neuron is stimulated, all of the muscle fibers innervated by that neuron contract simultaneously. Contraction of an entire muscle results from the combined actions of all the motor units contained within the muscle. An alpha motor neuron receives many synaptic inputs from the motor cortex, sensory afferents, and interneurons. It is the summation of these inputs that results in the generation of an action potential (*Fig. 9.19*). Some of these inputs come from upper motor neurons descending from the motor cortex, whereas other inputs come from sensory afferents.

Gamma motor neurons are small motor neurons that innervate a structure inside of the muscle called the **muscle spindle** (*Fig. 9.20*). A muscle spindle is a specialized structure that senses the amount of stretch within a muscle and relays this information to the spinal cord. Contained within the muscle spindle are modified skeletal muscle fibers called **intrafusal fibers**. These intrafusal fibers are not to be confused with the **extrafusal fibers** that make up the bulk of the muscle. Alpha motor neurons innervate extrafusal muscle fibers, while gamma motor neurons innervate intrafusal muscle fibers.

### SPINAL CONTROL OF MOTOR UNITS

Much of the coordination of motor activity occurs in the complex reflex pathways contained in the spinal cord (2). The spinal reflexes allow sensory information from proprioceptors, muscle spindles, and pain receptors to be processed in the spinal cord and thus make modifications to muscle contraction before the information ever reaches the brain.

There are many interneurons in the spinal cord. Interneurons mediate much of the input from other neurons to the alpha motor neurons. Spinal interneurons receive input from descending motor neurons and primary sensory neurons from the periphery and organize and integrate this incoming information so that highly skilled and coordinated motor programs can occur. Input from the spinal interneurons to the alpha motor neurons can be either inhibitory or excitatory.

The **myotatic stretch reflex** is a good example of how spinal reflexes control movement. Muscle spindles sit deep

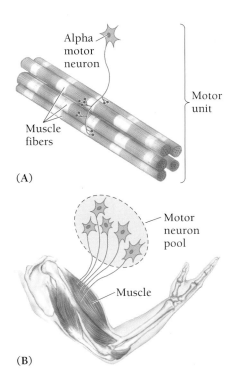

(A)

(B)

**FIGURE 9.18.** Motor unit and motor neuron pool. **A.** The motor unit is composed of the alpha motor neuron and the muscle fibers it innervates. **B.** In skeletal muscle, the fibers in the motor unit are more scattered throughout the muscle. (Reprinted with permission from Bear MF, Connors BW, Paradiso MA. *Neuroscience: exploring the brain*. 2nd ed. Philadelphia: Lippincott Williams & Wilkins, 2001.)

within the muscle. In the center of the muscle spindle, the sensory afferents are wrapped around the intrafusal fibers. When the sensory afferents are stimulated by stretch, sensory information from these axons are sent back into the spinal cord, where they are processed.

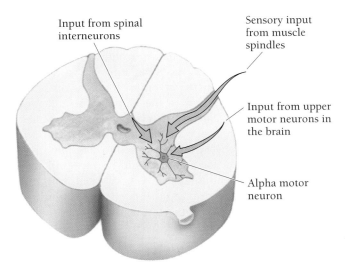

**FIGURE 9.19.** The alpha motor neuron receives input from the spinal interneurons, sensory systems, and descending motor tracts from the motor cortex. (Reprinted with permission from Bear MF, Connors BW, Paradiso MA. *Neuroscience: exploring the brain*. 2nd ed. Philadelphia: Lippincott Williams & Wilkins, 2001.)

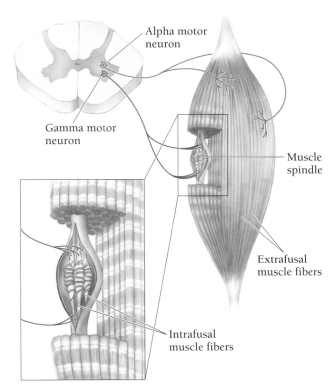

**FIGURE 9.20.** The muscle spindle sends sensory input to the spinal cord via the gamma motor neuron. The muscle spindle plays an important role in protecting the muscle against excessive stretch. (Reprinted with permission from Bear MF, Connors BW, Paradiso MA. *Neuroscience: exploring the brain*. 2nd ed. Philadelphia: Lippincott Williams & Wilkins, 2001.)

Physicians check the myotatic stretch reflex by tapping a rubber mallet on the patellar tendon of the knee (*Fig. 9.21*). The myotatic stretch reflex causes the quadriceps muscle to contract and straighten the knee. When the tendon is struck, a brief stretch of the quadriceps muscles is evoked. The muscle spindle, which is receptive to stretch, senses the stretch on the muscles because the intrafusal fibers are also stretched. This generates an action potential within the sensory axon. The sensory axon enters the dorsal horn of the spinal cord, synapses directly on the alpha motor neuron, and causes generation of an action potential in the alpha motor neuron. This results in muscle contraction, shortening of the muscle, and straightening of the knee. This reflex is a monosynaptic reflex because there is only one synapse in the loop, and therefore, it results in a very quick response of the muscle to stretch. Evaluation of this reflex is used to assess motor abnormalities.

Another structure inside the muscle also plays a role in controlling muscle contraction. This structure, called the **Golgi tendon organ** (GTO), is located at the junction of the muscle and tendon and is responsible for monitoring the force of muscle contraction (*Fig. 9.22*). The GTO plays an important role in protecting the muscle from being overloaded.

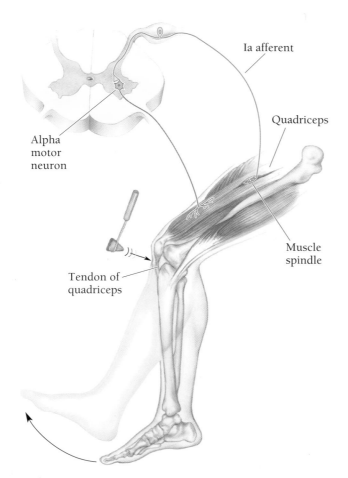

FIGURE 9.21. The myotatic stretch reflex. (Reprinted with permission from Bear MF, Connors BW, Paradiso MA. *Neuroscience: exploring the brain.* 2nd ed. Philadelphia: Lippincott Williams & Wilkins, 2001.)

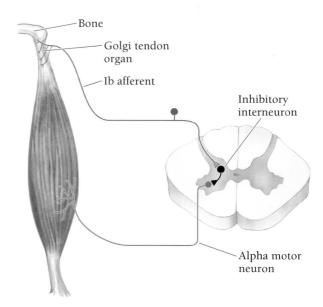

FIGURE 9.22. The location of the Golgi tendon organ (GTO) at the musculotendinous junction. The GTO sends sensory input into the spinal cord via the Ib afferent neuron and is important in protecting the muscle from contracting too vigorously and injuring itself. (Reprinted with permission from Bear MF, Connors BW, Paradiso MA. *Neuroscience: exploring the brain.* 2nd ed. Philadelphia: Lippincott Williams & Wilkins, 2001.)

The GTO sends its sensory signal to the alpha motor neuron via sensory neurons. These sensory neurons enter the spinal cord, branch repeatedly, and then synapse with interneurons in the ventral horn. Some of these interneurons are inhibitory to the alpha motor neuron that innervates the same muscle. As tension increases in the muscle, the sensory neuron fires and synapses with interneurons that are inhibitory to the alpha motor neuron. This inhibitory input reduces muscle contraction; conversely, as muscle tension decreases, the inhibitory input to the alpha motor neuron decreases and the muscle contracts more forcefully. This reflex is called the **reverse myotatic reflex** and protects the muscle from being overloaded. In general, this reflex functions to normalize muscle tension within an optimal range. This reflex is believed to be useful for fine motor control, such as handling a delicate object while simultaneously exerting a steady grip on it.

Another good example of the inhibitory input of the interneurons on alpha motor neurons is during the myotatic stretch reflex. When this reflex occurs, **antagonist** muscles relax. This phenomenon is called **reciprocal innervation** or Sherrington's law. When the sensory axon

from the muscle spindle in the protagonist muscle is stimulated, impulses from the sensory axons are sent to the spinal cord to cause postsynaptic inhibition of the antagonist muscle. The inhibition occurs because a collateral from the sensory axon synapses with an interneuron that synapses directly on the motor neurons that innervate the antagonist muscle.

Consider the knee-jerk reflex discussed earlier. The sensory axon from the muscle spindle in the quadriceps muscle is stimulated, and it synapses on the alpha motor neurons that innervate the quadriceps muscle, resulting in contraction of the quadriceps. Simultaneously, a collateral of the sensory axon synapses on an interneuron, which sends an inhibitory signal to the hamstrings (antagonist muscles) so that the hamstrings relax. Otherwise, the hamstrings would strongly oppose the action of the quadriceps. In practical terms, every time you tried to stand up from a squatting or sitting position, it would be very difficult to move if this reflex did not exist. As your quadriceps muscles were trying to shorten to the standing position, your hamstring muscles would be contracting in opposition to quadriceps contraction.

 *LINKUP:* **Biography: Sir Charles Scott Sherrington,** *located at http://connection.lww.com/go/brownexphys and on the Student Resource CD-ROM, provides a brief biographic sketch of this notable physiologist.*

Interneurons also exert excitatory input to alpha motor neurons. A good example of this is the **crossed-withdrawal reflex** (*Fig. 9.23*). This is a complex postural reflex that allows for withdrawal of a body part from a noxious stimulus while maintaining balance and posture. For instance, the crossed-withdrawal reflex is activated when the finger on your left hand touches a sharp object. This reflex allows for stimulation of the arm flexors and inhibition of the arm extensors in the left arm so that you can quickly remove your finger from the sharp object. Simultaneously, through interneuronal connections, the arm extensors in the right arm are stimulated while the flexors are inhibited. This allows you to quickly remove your finger from the sharp object and simultaneously stabilize posture on the opposite side of your body.

The crossed-withdrawal reflex occurs when you walk. During ambulation, as one leg extends, the other flexes. All that is needed to use this reflex during ambulation is some sort of mechanism to coordinate the timing. You might think this mechanism would come from descending neurons from the motor cortex. But a complete transection of

the spinal cord of a cat still leaves the hindlimbs with the ability to generate walking movements. This means that some of the motor function used in ambulation is programmed into the spinal cord (3). Some researchers are trying to use this observation to develop rehabilitation techniques that may help patients with spinal cord injuries to utilize this reflex to be able to walk again (4). See Box 9.2 to learn more about activity-dependent training. Other researchers are developing electrical stimulation models to simulate walking based on the fact that the motor neurons and interneurons below the level of a spinal cord lesion are still intact (5).

 *LINKUP:* **Research Highlight: Spinal Cord Microstimulation Generates Functional Limb Movements in Chronically Implanted Cats,** *found at http://connection.lww.com/go/brownexphys and on the Student Resource CD-ROM, describes a recent article on the use of electrical stimulation to generate coordinated movement of the lower extremities.*

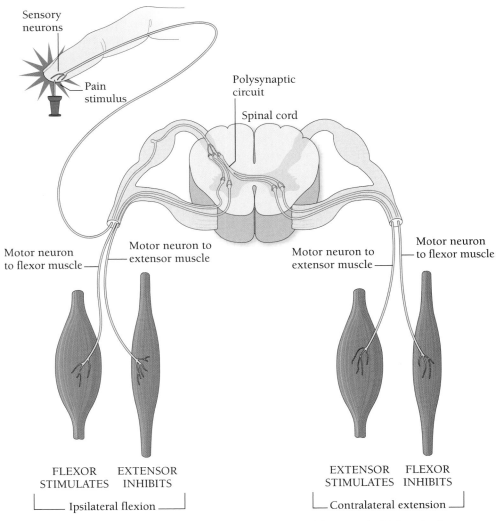

**FIGURE 9.23.** Schematic diagram showing the pathways of the crossed-withdrawal reflex.

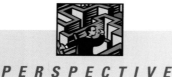

**Box 9.2**

# *P E R S P E C T I V E*

## *Activity-Dependent Therapy*

One of the primary impairments in individuals with spinal cord injuries is the inability to ambulate. One of the primary strategies to promote ambulation in these individuals is the use of orthotics and assistive devices. However, the use of these devices are often unsatisfactory in assisting with ambulation. An innovative rehabilitation technique called activity-dependent therapy may provide patients with spinal cord injuries the opportunity to regain locomotion skills. This technique is based on extensive research that has shown that animals with complete spinal cord transections can acquire the ability to take stepping movements with the hindlimbs. The stepping ability occurs in the absence of regeneration of spinal neurons and without descending motor input from the brain. It appears that the development of stepping with treadmill training occurs as the result of sensory input into the existing spinal pathways to produce a coordinated, adaptable movement pattern in the hindlimbs.

The application of these research results in cats to humans has yielded some encouraging results in patients with spinal cord injuries. In a series of case studies in humans, the application of appropriate sensory information during supported treadmill training has resulted in improvements in locomotor skills in four individuals following spinal cord injuries (1). While the results appear to indicate that the activity-dependent training improved locomotor ability, this training technique needs to undergo the rigor of scientific testing. Other aspects such as degree of neurologic injury, length of time since injury, and spinal cord injury level need to be examined. Furthermore, studies will need to be designed to determine the optimal sensory information that the spinal cord needs to receive to generate stepping patterns. However, activity-dependent therapy appears to be a promising rehabilitative technique for regaining locomotor function in individuals with spinal cord injuries.

1.  Behrman A, Harkema S. Locomotor training after human spinal injury: a series of case studies. *Phys Ther* 2000;80:688–700.

▶ *INQUIRY SUMMARY.* Alpha motor neurons innervate skeletal muscles and are responsible for voluntary muscle contraction. However, the spinal cord maintains some control over skeletal muscle function via several reflexes. Input from the skeletal muscles is received in the dorsal horn of the spinal cord, and the reflexes in the spinal cord control the output to the skeletal muscles. In this section we also talked about how the muscle spindle and GTO are protective of skeletal muscle. *Think of some situations in which these protective mechanisms are useful.*

## Motor Programming

Athletes move with great coordination and skill and are able to quickly make minor adjustments to produce highly skilled movement. Compare the movements of athletes with those of individuals with neurologic damage, such as a patient with a stroke who is trying to learn to walk again or a child with cerebral palsy who also has difficulty walking. Both the patient with a stroke and child with cerebral palsy move with great difficulty and with highly unskilled movement patterns. Furthermore, they are not able to make the necessary adjustments to their motor patterns to produce a better degree of skilled movement. Although

much is known about the anatomic and physiologic components of human movement, we still do not completely understand how the motor system coordinates all of the components to produce skilled and coordinated movements. Older motor programming theory dictated that the brain was the master controller of all movement (6), but recent research has led to a change in this view (7). While a detailed description of the research in this area is beyond the scope of this book, a brief overview is provided.

The impetus to move comes from the desire or motivation to initiate voluntary movement. From the part of the brain that registers motivation, a signal is sent to the association area of the brain. "Stored" higher-level motor programs are within the association area of the cortex. These stored motor programs are like the rough draft of an essay. In other words, the framework for the movement is available, but there are other influences that refine and shape the motor program. Information about the motor program is sent to the cerebellum and basal ganglia. Both of these areas of the brain help to refine the planned motor activity (1). The cerebellum and basal ganglia send their refinements of the motor program to the thalamus, and the information is sent to the motor cortex from the thalamus. From the motor cortex, this information is sent down the long motor tracts to the spinal neurons. Contained within the spinal cord are motor programs called central pattern generators. These central pattern generators make the final adjustments to the movement pattern based upon sensory information that the spinal cord receives from proprioceptors and other sensory receptors in the muscles and joints. Finally the information is sent out to the muscles and the movement occurs.

The most current theories of motor control also argue that it is important to recognize that movement occurs due to an interaction between the person, environment, and task that is being carried out (7). What this means is that movement does not just occur as a result of muscle reflexes or prestored motor programs, but rather, movement is a result of environmental, motivational, and cognitive factors and the neuromotor system. Understanding the interplay of factors involved in movement is the underlying basis for learning and practicing new skills in both the athlete as well as the neurologically impaired patient.

## FEEDBACK AND PRACTICE

Besides understanding the motor theories, it is also important to be able to apply these concepts when treating patients with movement disorders or when training athletes to acquire optimal athletic skill performance. Two concepts that are important to understand are the type of feedback that is provided during practice and the practice condition.

Feedback is simply the information that a patient or athlete receives regarding a movement skill. There are two kinds of feedback, intrinsic and extrinsic. Intrinsic feedback is the feedback that a person receives through various sensory systems as a result of movement. An example of intrinsic feedback is the visual information an athlete receives during a movement. For example, a tennis player may be practicing hitting forehands to a specific area of the tennis court. If the ball lands in the desired area of the court, then the tennis player receives the visual feedback that his movement resulted in the desired outcome.

Extrinsic feedback is extraneous information that is received by the individual. If the player in the example above hit the ball out of bounds, the coach is likely to offer a comment regarding what the player did wrong to result in the undesired outcome. The coach's comments are an example of extrinsic feedback. There is a lot of research being done in the area of extrinsic feedback that is beyond the context of this book; check the suggested readings for more detailed information. Also there are questions regarding when the feedback should be given in a practice session; for example, should the feedback be given after every trial, after a set number of trials, or until all trials are completed and the practice session is done. It is very important for the therapist treating patients with movement disorders and coaches training athletes to understand the implications of extrinsic feedback and timing of the feedback.

The other practical application of motor control theories involves the practice condition in which the skill is practiced. For example, one component of a practice session that must be considered is the amount of practice time in a session as compared to the amount of rest time in a session. Another component of a practice session that should be taken into consideration is if the same skill should be practiced repeatedly or multiple skills practiced? For example, if a therapist is teaching a patient with a stroke how to get out of bed, is it better to practice one skill of that entire movement for the entire practice session or practice the multiple skills contained in the entire movement? The transfer of the skill to other environments also needs to be considered when setting up the practice conditions. If a patient is able to ambulate correctly and without loss of balance over a smooth, flat surface, can this patient accomplish this same skill while walking in the grass or on hilly terrain? Again, refer to the suggested reading for more detailed information.

▶ *INQUIRY SUMMARY.* Current motor learning theories believe that movement is a complex interaction of the "stored" higher-level motor programs in the brain coupled with input from the cerebellum, basal ganglia, and central pattern generators in the spinal cord that make refinements and adjustments to the higher-level motor programs so that skilled movement occurs. Motor learning theories also strongly support that movement occurs due to the interactions among the person, environment, and activity being performed. The application of motor control theories requires therapists and coaches to understand the importance of feedback and practice conditions in the acquisition of motor skills. Try to remember when you most recently learned a new motor skill. Can you identify the intrinsic and extrinsic feedback that helped you learn the skill? Also think about the practice conditions and how those conditions may have helped or hindered you in learning the new skill.

## *Summary*

The nervous system is highly complex and is responsible for voluntary and involuntary movements, as well as more abstract concepts such as thoughts and emotions. The neuron is the functional cell of the nervous system and is responsible for generating action potentials that are transmitted down the axon to other neurons and effector organs. The two major divisions of the nervous system are the central nervous system, which consists of the brain and spinal cord, and the peripheral nervous system, which contains the nerves that innervate skeletal muscle and other organs. The brain is divided into several regions based upon function. The brain communicates with the spinal cord via long tracts that synapse in the spinal cord. The peripheral nervous system is divided into the sensory and motor divisions. Information from the periphery is transmitted via the sensory portion of the nervous system. This information is used to make adjustments and refinements to potential motor output. The motor division is further subdivided into the autonomic and somatic motor systems. The autonomic motor system is responsible for involuntary movements and control, while the somatic motor system innervates voluntary skeletal muscle. Furthermore, the autonomic motor system is divided into the parasympathetic and sympathetic systems. The spinal cord also contains several reflexes that help make final adjustments to voluntary movement. Finally while we do not fully understand the neurophysiologic basis for movement, we do know that smooth, coordinated movement is the integration of the neuromotor system, environment, cognition, and motivation.

## SUMMARY KNOWLEDGE

1. Name the parts of a neuron and describe the function of each part.
2. Describe the components of an action potential. Be sure to include the changes in ion concentrations that occur in each phase of the action potential.
3. What does it mean when the cell is refractory to an action potential?
4. Describe the process of how action potentials are generated at the axon hillock.
5. How is the impulse from one neuron transmitted to the next neuron across the neuromuscular junction?
6. List the parts of the brain and briefly describe their functions.
7. If a person suffers damage on the right side of the brain, why does the person manifest movement difficulties on the left side of the body?
8. List the twelve cranial nerves and state what problems might occur if a cranial nerve was damaged.
9. Compare and contrast the sympathetic and parasympathetic nervous systems in terms of anatomy and function.
10. What are the functions of the muscle spindle and Golgi tendon organs? How are these two structures activated and what role do they play in controlled muscle force generation?
11. Describe how the spinal reflexes function to control movement.

### References

1. Delong M, Strick P. Relation of the basal ganglia, cerebellum and motor cortex units to ramp and ballistic limb movements. *Brain Res* 1974;71:327–335.
2. Nichols TR, Cope TC, Abelew TA. Rapid spinal mechanisms of motor coordination. *Exerc Sports Sci Rev* 1999;27:255–284.
3. Grillner S. Interaction between central and peripheral mechanisms in the control of locomotion. *Prog Brain Res* 1979;50:227–235.
4. Behrman A, Harkema S. Locomotor training after human spinal injury: a series of case studies. *Phys Ther* 2000;80:688–700.
5. Mushahwar VK, Collins DF, Prochazka A. Spinal cord microstimulation generates functional limb movements in chronically implanted cats. *Exp Neurol* 2000;163:422–429.
6. Prochazka A. Sensorimotor gain control: a basic strategy of motor systems. *Prog Neurobiol* 1989;33:281–307.
7. Shumway-Cook A, Wollacott MH. *Motor control: theory and practical applications*. 2nd ed. Philadelphia: Lippincott Williams & Wilkins, 2001.

### Suggested Readings

Bear MF, Connors BW, Paradiso MA. *Neuroscience: exploring the brain*. 2nd ed. Baltimore: Lippincott Williams & Wilkins, 2001.
Carr JH, Shepherd RB, Nordholm L, et al. Investigation of a new motor assessment scale for stroke patients. *Phys Ther* 1985;65:175–180.
Copstead LC, Banasik JL. *Pathophysiology: biological and behavioral perspectives*. 2nd ed. Philadelphia: WB Saunders Co, 2000.
Dietz V. Human neuronal control of automatic functional movements interaction between central programs and afferent input. *Physiol Res* 1992;72:33–69.
Latash ML, Scholz JP, Schöner G. Motor control strategies revealed in the structure of motor variability. *Exerc Sports Sci Rev* 2002;30:26–31.
Porth CM. *Pathophysiology: concepts of altered health states*. 6th ed. Philadelphia: Lippincott Williams & Wilkins, 2002.
Woollacott M, Shumway-Cook A. Changes in posture control across the life span: a systems approach. *Phys Ther* 1990;70:799–807.

### On the Internet

American Parkinson Disease Association. Available at: **http://www.apdaparkinson.org/.** Accessed April 13, 2005.
Biography of Sir Charles Scott Sherrington. Available at: **http://nobelprize.org/medicine/laureates/1932/sherrington-bio.html.** Accessed April 13, 2005.
Christopher Reeve Paralysis Foundation. Available at: **http://www.christopherreeve.org.** Accessed April 13, 2005.
National Multiple Sclerosis Society. Available at: **http://www.nmss.org.** Accessed April 13, 2005.
Neuromuscular Motor Syndromes. Available at: **http://www.neuro.wustl.edu/neuromuscular/motor.html.** Accessed April 13, 2005.
Spastic Paraplegia Foundation: Primary Upper Motor Neuron Disorders. Available at: **http://www.sp-foundation.org/chart.htm.** Accessed April 13, 2005.
Treadmill Training Improves Function in Parkinson's Patients: The Changing Rehabilitation Model Posits the Possibility of Neural Recovery Through Task-Specific Therapy. Available at: **http://www.biomech.com/showArticle.jhtml?articleID**=29100218. Accessed April 13, 2005.

## Writing to Learn

*Recall from this chapter that motor information is transmitted to the periphery via spinal cord tracts that descend from the brain, while sensory information from the periphery is transmitted from the spinal cord up to the brain via the ascending pathways. For each of the major motor and secondary pathways, describe the information they transmit, where they are located, and where the projections synapse in the brain. Also discuss the impairments that would be observed with a lesion in the pathways.*

# CHAPTER

# 10 Skeletal Muscle Architecture and Function

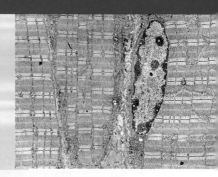

*Skeletal muscle is the largest organ of the body. Components contained within muscle are responsible for producing movement through the generation of force, which shortens the muscle. Skeletal muscle fibers are structurally arranged as sarcomeres, the sites of force generation within muscle. Can you conceive how contraction of many sarcomeres in skeletal muscle leads to whole-muscle contraction and movement?*

## CHAPTER OUTLINE

Movement is an important part of our lives, and the ability to perform activities of daily living is vital for maintaining quality of life. The proper functioning of skeletal muscle is critical for normal human movement and locomotion, and having appropriate muscle strength and endurance is necessary for daily activities. Furthermore, engaging in sporting events often requires muscles to perform at peak levels. Health care professionals who provide therapy using exercise training must have a basic understanding of muscle architecture and function and how the various components of muscle interact to produce force. Job activities as diverse as providing therapeutic interventions for individuals who have skeletal muscle atrophy secondary to prolonged immobilization and training Olympic athletes to improve sport performance require knowledge of skeletal muscle

function. This knowledge guides the therapist, coach, athletic trainer, or exercise physiologist in assisting individuals to obtain their highest level of function. Accordingly, this chapter provides the necessary groundwork for understanding skeletal muscle function and structure.

## Skeletal Muscle Structure

It is easy to think of skeletal muscle as a single contracting unit; however, skeletal muscle is composed of many individual **muscle fibers** that lie parallel to one another (*Fig. 10.1*). Muscle fibers are cylindrical and **multinucleated**. Skeletal muscle is attached to bone via tough connective tissues called **tendons**. As muscle fibers contract, the muscle pulls on the bone via the tendon and thus movement occurs.

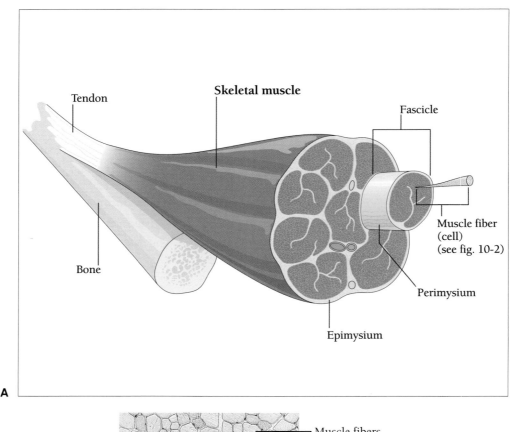

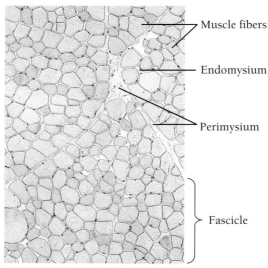

**FIGURE 10.1. A.** Structure of skeletal muscle showing muscle fibers and connective tissue. **B.** Muscle tissue seen under a microscope. Portions of several fascicles are shown with connective tissue coverings. (B is reprinted with permission from Gartner LP, Hiatt JL. *Color atlas of histology.* 3rd ed. Philadelphia: Lippincott Williams & Wilkins, 2000.)

## GROSS STRUCTURE OF MUSCLE

There are several layers of connective tissue that surround whole muscle and individual muscle fibers. The entire muscle is surrounded by connective tissue called the **epimysium**. At both ends of the muscle, this sheath of epimysium tapers into the tendon. The next level of connective tissue is the **perimysium**. This connective tissue surrounds a

bundle of muscle fibers called a **fascicle**. Finally, each individual muscle fiber contained in the fascicle is surrounded by connective tissue called the **endomysium**.

### The Muscle Fiber

The muscle fiber is a long cylinder that usually extends the entire length of the muscle. Lying directly underneath the endomysium is the **sarcolemma**, which encloses all of the contents of the muscle fiber. The contents, or organelles, of the muscle fiber are contained in the aqueous **sarcoplasm**, which is similar to the cytoplasm of other cells. Besides the muscle fiber itself, the sarcoplasm also contains enzymes, nuclei, mitochondria, and other organelles. However, a significant difference between the muscle cells (muscle cell and muscle fiber are often used interchangeably) and other cells is that muscle cells contain more than one nucleus.

Also contained within the sarcoplasm is a network of membranous channels called the **sarcoplasmic reticulum** (*Fig. 10.2*). This channel system is very extensive and is the storage site for the calcium that is necessary for muscle contraction. The sarcoplasmic reticulum is responsible for the release and uptake of calcium during contraction and relaxation, respectively, of the muscle fibers. The **transverse tubules** are another set of membranous channels that run inward from the sarcolemma and pass through the muscle fiber. The transverse tubules are also called the t-tubule system. This t-tubule system lies between the two enlarged portions of the sarcoplasm reticulum called the **terminal cisternae**. Together, the terminal cisternae and a t-tubule are called a **triad**. The triad system occurs in a repeated pattern along the entire length of the myofibril. This extensive network of tubules is very important in the mechanics of muscle contraction and is discussed later in the chapter.

Also contained in the sarcoplasm of the muscle fiber are the **myofibrils**, which contain the contractile proteins, **actin** and **myosin**, along with other noncontractile proteins (*Fig. 10.3*). Two of these noncontractile proteins, **troponin** and **tropomyosin**, are located on the actin molecule. Later in the chapter we will see that these two proteins play important roles during muscle contraction. Myofibrils are arranged into functional segments called **sarcomeres**.

## The Sarcomere

Sarcomeres, lying in series (end to end) with one another, are considered the basic functional units of contraction. Because they are arranged in series, the length of the muscle fiber is dependent upon the number of sarcomeres. As previously mentioned, the primary proteins that make up the myofibrils are myosin and actin. Myosin is relatively thick and is sometimes called the "thick" filament, while actin is relatively thin and is sometimes called the "thin" filament. Myosin and actin interdigitate to form a hexagonal lattice (*Fig. 10.4*). One myosin molecule interacts with six actin molecules. Muscle contraction is basically the active interdigitation or movement of actin and myosin across each other. The latticework of actin and myosin can be observed at the microscopic level, and it gives muscle the characteristic striped or **striated** appearance, which is why skeletal muscle is sometimes called striated muscle (*Fig. 10.5*).

Based on these characteristic striations, regions of the sarcomere can be named. The **Z lines** form the boundaries of a sarcomere, defining its length. The portion of the sarcomere that contains the myosin filaments is known as the **A band**,

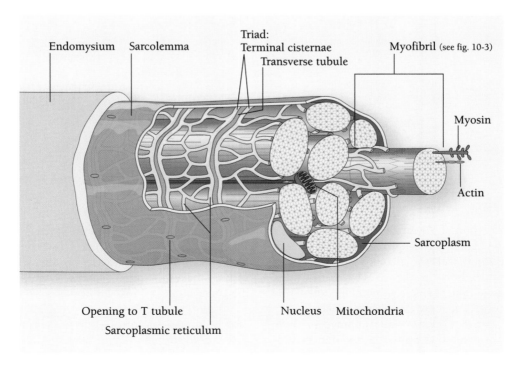

**FIGURE 10.2.** The sarcoplasmic reticulum and t-tubule system in skeletal muscle. Note the extensiveness of the systems and the proximity to the muscle fiber.

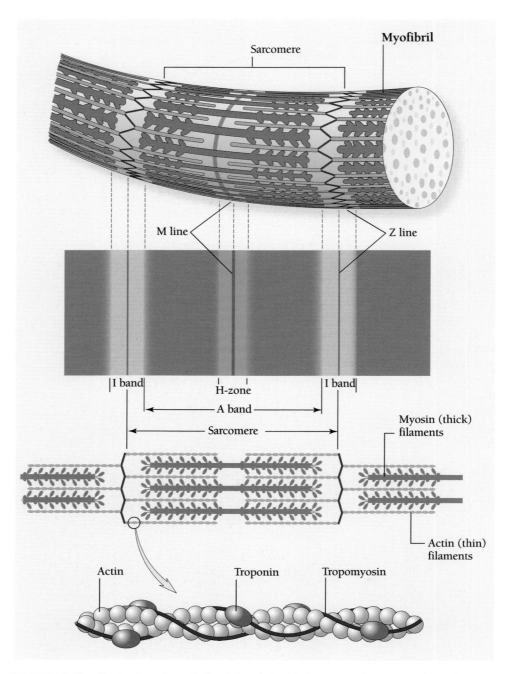

**FIGURE 10.3.** The ultrastructure of myofibril and the relationship between actin, tropomyosin, and troponin.

which is the dark portion of the sarcomere. Actin filaments are primarily in the lighter portion of the sarcomere, called the **I band**. The Z line bisects the I band. The center of the sarcomere where there is no overlap of actin or myosin is known as the **H zone**. The **M line** bisects the middle of the H zone and is known as the center of the sarcomere.

Besides actin, myosin, troponin, and tropomyosin, there are several other proteins that primarily function to support actin and myosin, connect adjacent sarcomeres to one another, and transmit the force produced by muscle contraction in a lateral direction (Table 10.1). One protein that

is very important in maintaining structural integrity of skeletal muscle is dystrophin. This protein links the sarcolemma with the contractile protein actin. Lack of dystrophin makes the sarcolemma susceptible to damage during contraction and relaxation cycles. Duchenne muscular dystrophy, an **X-linked recessive disorder**, is characterized by mutations in the dystrophin gene, resulting in a deficit of dystrophin that ultimately leads to muscle weakness and wasting. Case Study 10.1 contains an example of a treatment program that may be used for a person with Duchenne muscular dystrophy.

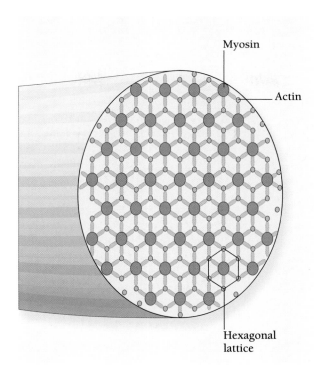

**FIGURE 10.4.** Schematic of the actin-myosin relationship.

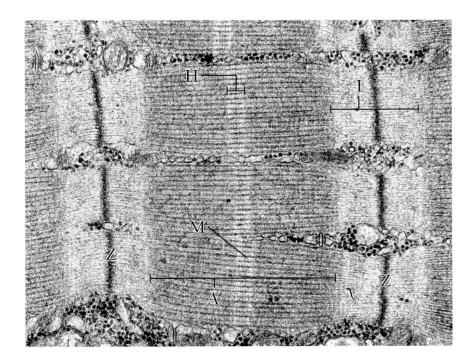

**FIGURE 10.5.** Electron micrograph of skeletal muscle showing a longitudinal section of myofibrils. The I band, which is bisected by the Z line, is composed of barely visible, thin actin filaments. They are attached to the Z line and extend across the I band into the A band. The thick filaments, composed of myosin, account for the full width of the A band. In the A band, there are additional bands and lines. One of these, the M line, is seen at the middle of the A band; another, the H band, consists only of thick filaments. The lateral parts of the A band are more electron dense and represent areas where the thin filaments interdigitate with the thick filaments. (Reprinted with permission from Ross MH, Kaye GI, Pawlina W. *Histology: a text and atlas*. 4th ed. Baltimore: Lippincott Williams & Wilkins, 2003.)

| Table 10.1 | PROTEINS CONTAINED WITHIN SKELETAL MUSCLE FIBERS | |
|---|---|---|
| **Structure** | **Protein** | **Functions** |
| Thin filament | Actin | The main protein of actin that interacts with myosin during excitation-contraction coupling. |
| | Tropomyosin | Transduces the conformational change of the troponin complex to actin. |
| | Troponin | Binds calcium and affects tropomyosin. Represents the "switch" that transforms the calcium signal into a molecular signal that induces crossbridge cycling. |
| | Nebulin | Present next to actin and believed to control the number of actin monomers joined to each other in a thin filament. |
| Thick filament | Myosin | Splits ATP and is responsible for the "power stroke" of the myosin head. |
| C stripes | C protein | Holds the myosin thick filaments in a regular array; may hold the H protein of adjacent thick filaments at an even distance during force generation; may also control the number of myosin molecules in a thick filament. |
| M line | M protein | Helps hold thick filaments in a regular array. |
| | Myomesin | Provides a strong anchoring point for the protein titin. |
| | M-CK | Provides ATP from phosphocreatine, located proximal to the myosin heads. |
| Z line | α-actinin | Holds the thin filaments in place spatially. |
| | Desmin | Forms the connection between adjacent Z lines from different myofibrils; helps to keep the sarcomeres in register so they maintain their striated appearance. |
| Elastic filament | Titin | Helps keep the thick filament centered between two Z lines during contraction; believed to control the number of myosin molecules contained in the thick filament. |

Reprinted with permission from McArdle WD, Katch FI, Katch VL. *Exercise physiology: energy, nutrition, and human performance.* 5th ed. Baltimore: Lippincott Williams & Wilkins, 2001.

 *LINKUP Access* **Perspective: Duchenne Muscular Dystrophy** *at http://connection.lww.com/go/brownex phys and on the Student Resource CD-ROM for a closer look at this common X-linked recessive disorder.*

## The Neuromuscular Junction

Recall from Chapter 9 that each muscle fiber is innervated by one nerve fiber branch that comes from a motor neuron. The action potential travels the length of the nerve until it reaches the interface between the nerve and muscle. This interface between the nerve and muscle fiber is called the **neuromuscular junction** (*Fig. 10.6*). The part of the muscle fiber that interfaces with the nerve is called the **motor endplate**. At the motor endplate, the sarcolemma is invaginated, which increases the surface area for the spread of the action potential across the neuromuscular junction to the muscle fiber. However, the nerve branch does not make actual physical contact with the muscle fiber. Rather, the two structures are separated by a small gap called the **synaptic cleft**.

The action potential travels down the length of the nerve and reaches the neuromuscular junction. Once at the junction, synaptic vesicles containing the neurotransmitter acetylcholine are released into the synaptic space. The vesicles release acetylcholine, which travels across the synaptic space to the sarcolemma, causing depolarization and ultimately contraction of the muscle fibers (review the details of muscle activation in Chapter 9).

 *LINKUP* **Perspective: Myasthenia Gravis,** *found at http://connection.lww.com/go/brownexphys and on the Student Resource CD-ROM, details this disease in which the binding of acetylcholine to its receptors is impaired.*

## MUSCLE MORPHOLOGY AND ARCHITECTURE

Muscles have many shapes that are a function of muscle fiber length and sarcomere alignment. These differences in muscle morphology dictate the particular function of the muscle in regards to movement. The two most common shapes of muscle are **fusiform** and **pennate** (*Fig. 10.7*). A fusiform muscle such as the biceps brachii contains fibers that run parallel to each other and taper at the musculotendinous junction. On the other hand, the fibers of pennate muscles lie at oblique angles to one another. Furthermore, pennate muscles can be subdivided into unipennate, bipennate, and multipennate muscles depending on the number of sets of angled fibers located within the muscle.

In addition to knowing whether a muscle is fusiform or pennate, two other key concepts are necessary for

## CASE STUDY 10.1:  MUSCULAR DYSTROPHY

### CASE

Jimmy is an 11-year-old male with a diagnosis of Duchenne muscular dystrophy. He was referred to physical therapy because of a decline in walking ability. He lives at home with his parents and two sisters. Jimmy attends school; however, with his decline in walking ability, he is having difficulty climbing the steps on the school bus. His parents would like their son to remain ambulatory for as long as possible but recognize that he may need adaptive equipment for community mobility. They would also like their son to be able to participate in an exercise program.

### DESCRIPTION

Jimmy's past medical history is noncontributory. He likes music and enjoys drawing. Since Jimmy has experienced a decline in walking ability, it would be a good idea to assess his joint range of motion. Jimmy has bilateral ankle plantarflexion contractures, bilateral tight iliotibial bands, and hip and knee flexion contractures. Jimmy's decline in walking ability is likely due to a decrease in strength so it is important to assess his strength. Manual muscle testing revealed a grade of poor plus (1+/5) strength in bilateral proximal hip and shoulder muscles and fair plus (3+/5) strength in bilateral knee extensors. His sensation and reflexes were also assessed; his reflexes were normal, and his sensation was grossly intact overall.

Since the main reason that Jimmy was referred to physical therapy was because of his decline in walking ability, it is very important to assess his mobility skills. At this point, Jimmy is unable to ascend/descend stairs. He has increased frequency of falls, especially on uneven surfaces. Jimmy commonly uses furniture and walls for balance during ambulation. He is independent in crawling and scooting on the floor. Jimmy is not able to come to standing from the middle of the floor, but he is able to do so holding onto a piece of furniture. He needs maximal assistance to go from sit to stand from a chair. On the Vignos Functional Rating Scale (1), he rates a 5 (see scale below). Jimmy is also having some difficulty getting on and off the toilet and in and out of a bathtub.

### INTERVENTION

Since it is important to minimize contractures, a stretching program should be initiated for Jimmy. Prior to this evaluation, he had been engaged in a stretching program for his plantar flexors. This program should be continued, and night splints for his ankles should be added to his stretching regime. Additionally, a stretching program should be addressed for his tight iliotibial bands and hip/knee flexion contractures.

It is obvious that he is losing strength in his muscles; however, the clinical use of resistance exercise in this diagnosis is

not clear. The few studies that examined the use of resistance exercise in this diagnosis are limited by factors such as small sample sizes, lack of a control group, differences in exercise programs, and heterogeneity between subjects in the treatment groups. The major concern is to not overwork muscles that are already weak and predisposed to injury with repetitive contractions. Since both Jimmy and his parents are interested in some sort of exercise program, one possible solution may be to enroll Jimmy in an aquatic exercise program. Also, since the potential for social isolation exists in this population, participation in pool games with peers but with rule modifications would be helpful.

To improve his gait, lightweight lower extremity splints may be useful. To maintain community mobility and be able to get on a school bus with a lift, Jimmy should have a manual wheelchair. Adaptive equipment such as a tub bench and elevated toilet seat should be obtained to assist with bathing and toileting.

Several special issues need to be considered for Jimmy. He should be monitored periodically to adjust the treatment plan as his condition changes. Since respiratory strength declines as the disease progresses, it may be useful to include inspiratory muscle training in his treatment plan. However, the literature is still not clear regarding the efficacy of inspiratory muscle training in this population.

The Vignos Rating Scale (1) was developed to provide a better method of documenting the overall strength of multiple muscles of an individual as opposed to documenting strength of individual muscles. Consequently, this test is useful in documenting functional limitations of people with muscular dystrophy and also is used to monitor change in functional limitations over time.

### VIGNOS FUNCTIONAL RATING SCALE

1. Walks and climbs stairs without assistance.
2. Walks and climbs stairs with aid of railing.
3. Walks and climbs stairs slowly with aid; >12 seconds for 4 standard steps.
4. Walks unassisted and rises from chair; cannot climb stairs.
5. Walks unassisted; cannot rise from chair; cannot climb stairs.
6. Walks with assistance or independently with leg braces.
7. Walks in leg braces, but requires assistance for balance.
8. Stands in leg braces; unable to walk even with assistance.
9. Uses a wheelchair.
10. Confined to bed.

### REFERENCE

1. Vignos PJ Jr, Spencer GE Jr, Archibald KC. Management of progressive muscular dystrophy. *JAMA* 1963;184:89–96.

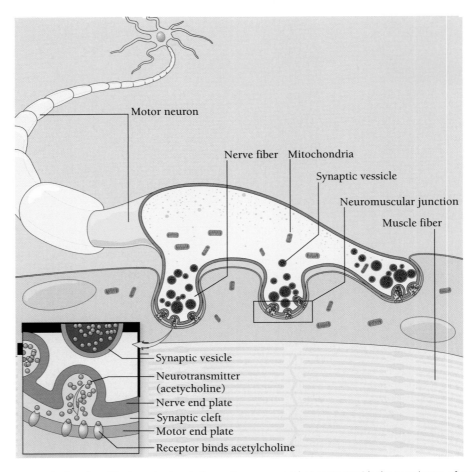

**FIGURE 10.6.** The neuromuscular junction. The branched end of a motor neuron makes contact with the membrane of a muscle fiber. The inset view shows the release of the neurotransmitter acetylcholine into the synaptic cleft. Acetylcholine attaches to receptors in the motor endplate, which contains folds that increase surface area.

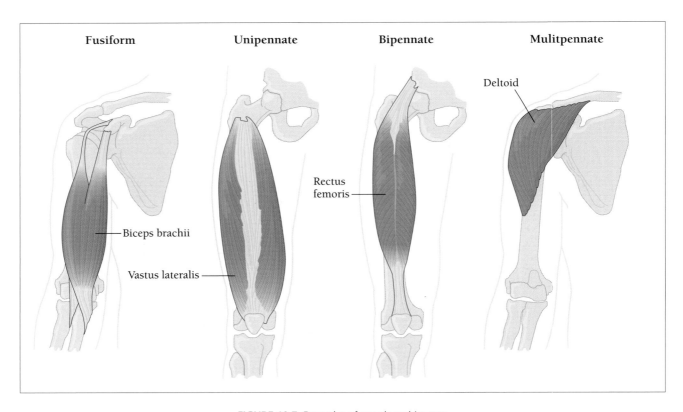

**FIGURE 10.7.** Examples of muscle architecture.

understanding how architectural arrangement of skeletal muscle affects force production. These concepts are **physiologic cross-sectional area** (PCSA) and **pennation angle**. The PCSA gives us an idea of how much contractile protein is available to generate force. The cross-sectional area of a muscle is determined by the following formula:

$$\text{Muscle mass (g)} \times (\text{cosine } \theta \div \text{muscle density [g·cm}^{-3}\text{])} \times \text{fiber length (cm)}$$

(Muscle density is 1.056 g·cm$^{-3}$ and $\theta$ is the pennation angle [2].) For a fusiform muscle that has no pennation, calculating PCSA is relatively simple and can be determined by dividing the volume of the muscle (cm$^3$) by the product of muscle density (g·cm$^{-3}$) and muscle length (cm). However, calculating the PCSA of a pennate muscle is a bit more complicated because the fibers run at different angles to one another.

The pennation angle, which is the angle of the orientation of the muscle fibers to the tendon, is an important component of force production. This angle refers to the angle of orientation of the muscle fibers to the tendon. For example, since fusiform muscle fibers lie parallel to the tendon, the angle of pennation is 0 degrees and all force generated by the fibers are transmitted across the tendon to the joint. However, if the pennation angle is greater than 0 degrees, the muscle fibers are oblique to the tendon and less force is generated to the tendon. For example, if the pennation angle is 30 degrees, 86% of the force is transmitted to the tendon because the cosine of 30 degrees is 0.86. Generally speaking, pennate muscles generate more force than fusiform muscles because the fibers are oblique to the tendon and this allows more fibers to be packed into a given length of muscle. Consequently, pennate muscles have a large PCSA and greater number of fibers than fusiform muscles, and as a result, they can generate more force and more power than fusiform muscles.

▶ *INQUIRY SUMMARY.* Skeletal muscle has many different levels of organization. At the whole-muscle level, muscles can be divided according to architecture into fusiform and pennate muscles. The force generated by the muscle is related to the angle of pennation and to the cross-sectional area of the muscle. Connective tissue plays a role in providing support to the many levels of skeletal muscle and helps transmit contractile force from the level of the sarcomere to the level of whole muscle. One very important connective tissue is the tendon that connects muscle to bone; with contraction of skeletal muscle, the tendon pulls on the bone to cause movement. *How do you think movement might be affected when a tendon is injured?*

## *Muscle Contraction*

To gain an appreciation for the contractile properties of muscle, it is important to understand the underlying mechanisms of the mechanical and chemical events that occur with muscle contraction. Understanding these events is helpful for developing optimal training techniques for athletes and designing appropriate rehabilitative techniques for people with muscular injuries or other debilities. The classic investigations of Hugh Huxley and Andrew Huxley performed 50 years ago established the theoretical foundations of muscle contraction that remain true today (3). Their concept of muscle contraction is known as the **sliding filament theory** and, in the simplest of terms, states that muscle contracts due to actin filaments sliding past myosin filaments.

**LINKUP** *See* **Biography: Andrew F. Huxley** *at http:// connection.lww.com/go/brownexphys and on the Student Resource CD-ROM for a closer look at this notable researcher who developed the sliding filament theory of muscle contraction.*

## SLIDING FILAMENT THEORY

In the sliding filament theory, the lengths of the actin and myosin filaments do not change. Rather, myosin **crossbridges**, or the myosin heads, extend out from the helical part of the molecule, detach, rotate, and attach again to the active site on the actin filament, which results in actin being pulled across the myosin filament (*Fig. 10.8*). Normally actin and myosin are "bound" or attached to one another even when muscle is not contracting (4). This attachment is considered to be the "weakly bound" state, which means that force is not being generated (4). However, once the actin-myosin bonding changes to a "strongly bound" state as a result of depolarization of the muscle fiber, the myosin heads begin pulling actin toward the center of the sarcomere, and this action results in force generation and muscle shortening (4).

When the fiber contracts, there are major changes in the zones and bands of the sarcomere. As the actin and myosin slide past each other, the Z lines are pulled toward the center of the sarcomere. Concurrent with the movement of the Z lines, the I bands and H zones become smaller and smaller as shortening continues. However, the width of the A band remains constant. During an isometric (static) contraction, the relative length of the muscle fiber remains the same and the spacing of the I and A bands remain constant; during an eccentric, or lengthening, contraction, the A band widens.

## ENERGY FOR CONTRACTION

As discussed earlier, the myosin head must continually attach, detach, and attach again to new sites along the actin filament to generate force. Energy is required for the myosin head to pull the actin filament along its length. The myosin head detaches from actin when an ATP molecule joins the actin-myosin complex. Once the myosin head dissociates from actin, the myosin head is ready to bind to a new site on

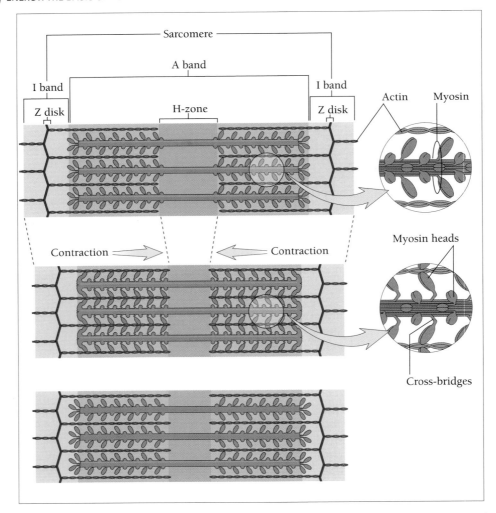

**FIGURE 10.8.** Sliding filament mechanism of skeletal muscle contraction. When the muscle is relaxed, there is no contact between the actin and myosin filaments. Crossbridges form and the actin filaments are moved closer together as the muscle fiber contracts. The crossbridges return to their original positions and attach to new sites to prepare for another pull on the actin filaments and further contraction.

the actin filaments. The dissociation of myosin from actin can be written as the following equation:

$$\text{Actin-myosin} + \text{ATP} \rightarrow \text{Actin} + \text{myosin-ATP}$$

When ATP attaches to the myosin head, an enzyme located on the myosin head called **myofibrillar adenosine-triphosphatase** (myosin ATPase) hydrolyzes ATP to form ADP and inorganic phosphate ($P_i$). The hydrolysis of ATP provides the energy needed by the myosin head to pull the actin filaments across the myosin and generate force. Hydrolysis changes the shape of the myosin head (conformational change) so that it can interact with the appropriate actin filament. Once this conformational change occurs, the myosin head possesses the correct orientation for a mechanical power stroke to occur and for the actin and myosin filaments to slide past each other.

## EXCITATION-CONTRACTION COUPLING

Excitation-contraction (E-C) coupling refers to the process whereby a nerve impulse reaches the surface of the muscle

and causes depolarization, which results in release of calcium from the sarcoplasmic reticulum and ultimately causes muscle contraction. There are many steps involved in this process (delineated below). *Figure 10.9* provides a schematic overview of the phases of excitation and contraction.

The initial step in E-C coupling occurs when an action potential from a nerve reaches the neuromuscular junction. At this point, acetylcholine is released from the synaptic vesicles contained in the nerve. The acetylcholine travels across the synaptic cleft and binds to acetylcholine receptors on the muscle membrane (sarcolemma). Once acetylcholine binds to the receptors, an endplate potential is generated and this potential leads to depolarization of the muscle. The depolarization potential is carried to the sarcoplasmic reticulum where calcium is released and the mechanical process of contraction can begin. It is important to understand that when the muscle is not contracting, the levels of calcium in the fluid bathing the muscle fiber are very low. It is only when the muscle fiber is depolarized that the calcium

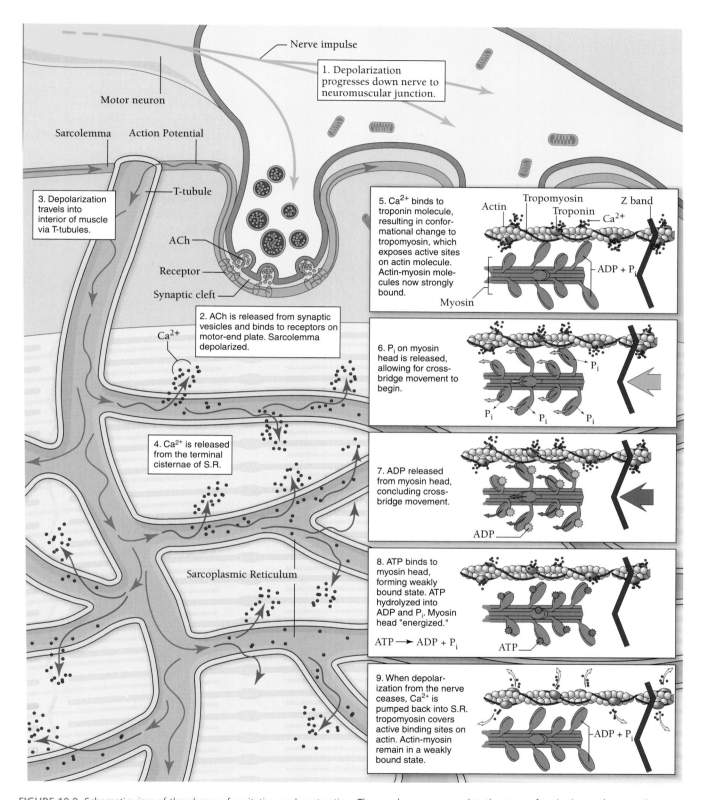

**FIGURE 10.9.** Schematic view of the phases of excitation and contraction. The numbers correspond to the steps of excitation and contraction.

concentration within the muscle fiber is increased and the process of contraction can occur.

Once calcium levels are increased, calcium binds to the troponin-tropomyosin complex. These two proteins are contained on the actin filament, and they play an important role in controlling muscle fiber contraction. Actin consists of many protein subunits, called monomers, which are arranged in a helical structure (two rows that are twisted around each other). Lying in the groove within the actin helix is the protein tropomyosin. The troponin molecule is located at several intervals (approximately every seven actin monomers) along the length of actin. Troponin is directly attached to tropomyosin. The binding site for actin and myosin is located at the troponin-tropomyosin interaction.

Together, troponin and tropomyosin regulate the attachment of actin to myosin. In the relaxed state, tropomyosin covers the active sites on the actin filament where the myosin heads need to attach so that the strongly bound state necessary for muscle contraction can occur. Once depolarization is propagated across the synaptic cleft to the muscle membrane, the stimulus travels down the transverse tubules to the terminal cisternae where calcium is released. The calcium binds to the troponin molecule and causes troponin-tropomyosin to undergo a conformational change, which exposes the active binding sites on the actin molecule.

Immediately prior to the binding of actin to myosin, the myosin head undergoes a conformational change that results in a "cocking" of the myosin head as a result of ATP hydrolysis. Now, the "energized" myosin heads attach in a strongly bound fashion to the actin filament. Once this occurs, the stored mechanical energy in the myosin head causes an angular movement of the myosin head, which results in muscle shortening. Next ATP attaches to the myosin heads, the strongly bound association of myosin and actin is broken, and the actin-myosin complex reverts back to a weakly bound state. The ATP on the myosin head is hydrolyzed by myosin ATPase, and this provides the necessary energy for the myosin head to become "re-energized" and reattach to another active binding site on the actin filament as long as sufficient levels of calcium in the sarcoplasm are maintained. This cycle can continue as long as calcium levels in the sarcoplasm remain high and ATP can be hydrolyzed to provide the necessary energy to the myosin head.

Contraction ceases once the nerve impulse to the muscle stops. When this occurs, the calcium pumps located in the sarcoplasmic reticulum pump the calcium from the sarcoplasm back into the sarcoplasmic reticulum. These pumps also require ATP to work effectively. Once calcium concentration is reduced to precontraction levels, troponin-tropomyosin returns to its original position covering the active site on the actin filament. At this point, all contractile activity stops and the muscle returns to a relaxed state. The following is a brief summary of the events of E-C coupling.

1. Depolarization progresses down the nerve to the neuromuscular junction.

2. Acetylcholine is released from the synaptic vesicles, travels across the synaptic cleft, binds to acetylcholine receptors on the motor endplate, and depolarizes the sarcolemma.
3. Depolarization travels deep inside the muscle fibers via the transverse tubules to the terminal cisternae.
4. Calcium is released from the terminal cisternae.
5. Calcium binds to the troponin molecule. This results in a conformational change to tropomyosin, and the active sites on the actin molecule are uncovered. This allows for the actin-myosin interaction to transition from a weakly bound state to a strongly bound state.
6. $P_i$ on the myosin head is released and allows for crossbridge movement to begin.
7. ADP is released from the myosin head and concludes crossbridge movement.
8. ATP binds to the myosin head, causing the strongly bound state of actin-myosin to form a weakly bound state. ATP is hydrolyzed into ADP and $P_i$, and this results in the myosin head being "energized."
9. The cycle of contraction continues as long as there is enough calcium in the sarcoplasm to keep the active sites on the actin filament uncovered. Once the depolarization from the nerve ceases, calcium release is halted, calcium is pumped back into the sarcoplasmic reticulum, tropomyosin covers the active binding site on actin, and actin and myosin revert back to a weakly bound state.

▶ *INQUIRY SUMMARY.* Excitation-contraction contains many steps that are important for contraction. Consider the role of ATP in this process. Recall that when the "energized" myosin head forms a strong bond with actin, $P_i$ is released from the myosin head and actin is pulled across its length. Next ADP is released from the myosin head and ATP binds to the myosin head. ATP is hydrolyzed, thus providing energy to the myosin head and allowing it to form a strongly bound state as long as calcium levels are high enough. As you can see, ATP plays a very important role in the process. *What do you think would happen if muscle cells were deficient in ATP?*

## Muscle Fiber Types

Human skeletal muscle is composed of a collection of fiber types that allows for a wide range of muscle function. Furthermore, fiber types are malleable or "plastic," which means that they can alter their composition based upon the functional demands that are placed on them. There are a variety of ways to classify muscle fiber types. The three most common methods are histochemical staining based on myosin ATPase, biochemical classification based on metabolic enzymes, and molecular identification based on the protein composition of the myosin molecule.

## MUSCLE BIOPSY

Before we begin a discussion of how fibers are classified, consider how the muscle tissue is obtained for fiber typing. In animal models, the muscle under study can be surgically removed from the animal once the experiment is completed and the animal has been sacrificed. However, in humans, muscle tissue is removed via a muscle biopsy. This is an invasive procedure in which a small amount of muscle is removed and then analyzed for any biochemical, metabolic, or fiber type changes. The skin over the muscle of interest is anesthetized and a small incision (0.5 to 1.0 cm long) is made through the skin, subcutaneous tissue, and fascia. The outer biopsy needle is then inserted through the incision into the muscle belly. Next the plunger and guillotine is forced into the muscle and a small piece of tissue is snipped. The needle is withdrawn from the muscle with the tissue in the "window" of the biopsy needle. The tissue is cleaned of blood, quickly frozen, and stored in a $-80°C$ freezer until the tissue can be processed.

## HISTOCHEMICAL CLASSIFICATION

The basis for the histochemical method of classifying muscle fiber types is the difference in staining intensity between fiber types that occurs when the fibers are exposed to solutions of varying pH (5). Specifically, this method determines the reaction of myosin ATPase when it is exposed to the different pH solutions. It classifies fibers into "fast" and "slow" contracting fibers. Caution must be used when interpreting fiber type this way because this method does not directly measure the speed of muscle contraction, but rather measures a histochemical appearance of the fiber. Despite this limitation, there is correlation between the mechanics of how rapidly a muscle contracts and the myosin ATPase content (6). The term used to describe how fast a muscle contracts is the **maximal shortening velocity** ($V_{max}$). Muscle fibers shorten by movement of crossbridges. Remember the cycle of myosin attaching, detaching, and reattaching to the actin filament. Myosin ATPase regulates how quickly the myosin crossbridges undergo this cycle; thus, a fiber with a high myosin ATPase activity has a fast shortening velocity, while fibers with a low myosin ATPase activity have slower shortening velocities.

When sections of muscle fibers are exposed to solutions of varying pH, the fibers are stained either light or dark based on the sensitivity of myosin ATPase to the solutions (5) (Table 10.2). By using this method, fibers are divided into three classifications: slow, intermediate, and fast or type I, type IIa, and type IIb, respectively. An alkaline pH (pH = 10.4) inactivates myosin ATPase in slow fibers so they turn pale, while myosin ATPase remains stable in fast fibers and they turn dark. Conversely, preincubation in an acidic (pH = 4.3) solution inactivates myosin ATPase in fast fibers so they appear pale, while myosin ATPase

| Table 10.2 | *FIBER TYPES ACCORDING TO THE MYOSIN ATPASE ASSAY* | | |
| --- | --- | --- | --- |
| **Preincubation pH** | **Type I** | **Type IIa** | **Type IIb** |
| 9.4 | Light | Dark | Dark |
| 4.6 | Dark | Light | Medium |
| 4.3 | Dark | Light | Light |

Reprinted with permission from Lieber RL. *Skeletal muscle structure, function & plasticity.* 2nd ed. Baltimore: Lippincott Williams & Wilkins, 2002.

remains stable in slow fibers, which stain dark. Preincubation of fibers in a less acidic solution (pH = 4.6) results in type IIb fibers turning moderately dark, type IIa fibers appearing pale, and type I fibers turning dark (5) (*Fig. 10.10*).

## BIOCHEMICAL CLASSIFICATION

Separating fiber types based on biochemical methods utilizes information obtained via myosin ATPase in conjunction with an assay that analyzes the relative content of enzymes used in aerobic and glycolytic pathways. One aerobic or oxidative enzyme that is commonly assayed is succinate dehydrogenase. Succinate dehydrogenase is an enzyme found inside the mitochondria which plays an important role in generating ATP via oxidative phosphorylation. Therefore, fibers that are highly oxidative have high numbers of mitochondria and high succinate dehydrogenase activity. These fibers are considered to be slow, oxidative (SO) fibers.

Conversely, $\alpha$-glycerophosphate dehydrogenase ($\alpha$-GP) is an enzyme that is related to the glycolytic potential of a muscle fiber. Therefore, fibers that have high $\alpha$-GP activity generally rely on the glycolytic pathway to generate ATP. These fibers are considered to be the fast, glycolytic (FG) fibers. Therefore, fibers can be classified as SO, fast oxidative glycolytic (FOG), and FG. The FOG fibers are intermediate between the SO and FG fibers in terms of oxidative and glycolytic enzymes (Table 10.3). There appears to be good correlation between fibers that are classified as type I by the myosin ATPase scheme and fibers designated as SO using the biochemical classification system (7). However, this correlation does not hold up as well when attempting to correlate type IIa fibers with FOG fibers and type IIb fibers with FG fibers (7).

## MOLECULAR CLASSIFICATION

In this method, fibers are classified based on myosin heavy chain (MHC) composition. There are different types of myosin, and this differentiation is based upon the protein composition of the myosin molecule. These different versions of myosin are called **isoforms**. The three MHC

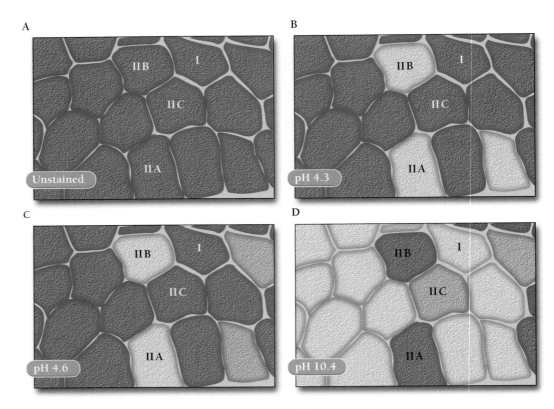

**FIGURE 10.10.** These serial sections illustrate how fiber types can be determined by assessing the sensitivity of myosin ATPase to solutions of differing pH and also by assessing succinate dehydrogenase and α-glycerophosphate dehydrogenase. **A.** Thick unstained section (40 to 50 μm) in which all fibers appear similar. **B.** Fibers stained for myosin ATPase activity at a preincubation pH 4.3 (highly acidic). **C.** Preincubation in pH 4.6 (intermediate acidity). **D.** Preincubation in pH 10.6 (alkaline).

isoforms originally identified were MHCI, MHCIIa, and MHCIIb. However, a fourth MHC isoform has been discovered in small rodents, and this isoform is known as MHCIId or MHCIIx (8). This MHC isoform possesses a contractile speed intermediate between that of MHCIIa and MHCIIb (9). Based on research examining the DNA composition of the MHC isoforms, it has been concluded that MHCIIb does not exist in humans (13,14). Therefore, the three MHC isoforms in humans are (from slowest to fastest) MHCI, MHCIIa, MHCIId/x.

MHC isoforms can be identified by several methods. One method uses antibodies that are specific to certain MHC isoforms. This method is known as **immunohistochemistry**. In this way, it is fairly easy to classify fibers based on their reactions to various antibodies. MHC isoforms may not completely correlate with fibers typed by oxidative or glycolytic methods. However, since MHC isoforms correlate fairly well with metabolic processes, much information can be obtained by identifying fibers based upon MHC composition. See Box 10.1 for more information on the technique of immunohistochemistry.

The other method of identifying MHC composition at the molecular level is **electrophoresis**. Because fibers often contain more than one MHC isoform, separating fibers in

this manner determines the relative concentrations of MHC composition for mixed fibers.

*LINKUP The basic principle underlying the electrophoretic separation of fiber types is that different proteins can be separated from one another based upon their mass. See Perspective: Electrophoretic Separation of Fiber Types at http://connection.lww.com/go/brownexphys and on the Student Resource CD-ROM for a description of this technique.*

▶ *INQUIRY SUMMARY.* Muscle is composed of several different fiber types, and these fiber types can alter their composition depending upon the activity level of muscle. There are several methods to identify fiber types in skeletal muscle. The histochemical method assesses the staining intensity of fibers based upon their sensitivity to varying pH solutions. The biochemical method assesses the activities of aerobic and anaerobic enzymes to classify fiber types. Finally, the use of electrophoretic separation allows for fibers to be classified based upon the molecular struc-

| Table 10.3 | METABOLIC, STRUCTURAL, AND CONTRACTILE DIFFERENCES AMONG FIBER TYPES | | |
|---|---|---|---|
| **Characteristic** | **Type I** | **Type IIa** | **Type IIb** |
| Motor neuron size | Small | Large | Large |
| Recruitment threshold | Low | High | High |
| Motor neuron conduction velocity | Slow | Fast | Fast |
| Contraction time | Slow | Fast | Fast |
| Relaxation time | Slow | Fast | Fast |
| Force production | Low | High | High |
| Resistance to fatigue | High | Low | Low |
| Elasticity | Low | High | High |
| Fiber diameter | Small | Large | Large |
| Z-line thickness | Wide | Medium | Narrow |
| Hypertrophic response to training | Small | Large | Large |
| Predominant energy system | Aerobic | Aerobic/anaerobic | Anaerobic |
| Mitochondrial density | High | High | Low |
| Capillary density | High | Medium | Low |
| Myoglobin content | High | Medium | Low |
| Myosin ATPase activity | Low | High | High |
| Anaerobic enzyme activity | Low | High | High |
| Aerobic enzyme activity | High | High | Low |
| Phosphocreatine stores | Low | High | High |
| Glycogen stores | Low | High | High |
| Triglyceride stores | High | Medium | Low |

Reprinted with permission from Miller WC. *The biochemistry of exercise and metabolic adaptation.* Dubuque, Ia: WC Brown, 1992.

ture of the myosin filament. *Why would knowing the composition of fibers be useful?*

## Physiologic Properties of Fiber Types

Given that there are different fiber types, it stands to reason that the fibers have differences in contractile, biochemical, and metabolic properties. Skeletal muscle is generally composed of a mixture of fiber types, although some muscles, such as the soleus, are considered to be "slow" because they contain mostly type I fibers. On the other hand, the extensor digitorum longus is considered a "fast" muscle because most of the fibers are type II fibers.

Muscles have different functions based partly on fiber type composition. Muscles composed primarily of type I fibers are generally postural muscles, whereas muscles with compositions of primarily type II fibers are used for quick bursts of speed, such as sprinting. However, it is difficult to determine physiologic properties of specific fiber types when they are mixed with other fiber types in whole muscle. So, to really ascertain differences in the physiologic properties of fiber types, it is most useful to study these properties in a "skinned" fiber preparation.

In this type of preparation, a single muscle fiber is isolated and removed from a whole muscle, the sarcolemma is chemically removed, and the mechanical properties of the fiber are determined by incubating the fiber in a calcium solution to generate contraction. Following the

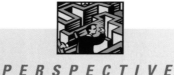

| **Box 10.1** |

*P E R S P E C T I V E*

## Immunohistochemistry Techniques

Immunohistochemical techniques can also be used to identify fiber types. This technique is based upon the fact that several monoclonal antibodies have been developed that are specific to the four major fiber types observed in adult rat skeletal tissue. In this technique, either whole muscle or muscle biopsies are flash frozen and cut or "sectioned" very thinly (~10 μm thick) on a cryostat. These cross-sections are placed on microscope slides. The sections are incubated with the antibodies for a period of time and then are color-reacted to visualize the antibody binding. Usually when a muscle is being analyzed for fiber type quantification, several sections in a row, or "serial sections," are cut and each successive muscle section is reacted with a different antibody. Thus by examining the slides, muscle fiber types can be determined (*Figure 1*).

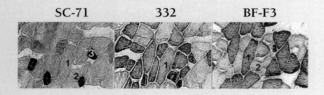

Images taken from serial sections of male mouse masseter to show representative staining patterns obtained with antibodies SC-71, BF-F3, and 332. Antibody SC-71 labels type IIa-containing fibers, BF-F3 labels type IIb-containing fibers, and 332 labels both type IIa- and IId/x-containing fibers. Therefore, type IId/x-containing fibers are those that stain with 332 but not with SC-71. Left: Fibers containing type IIa myosin heavy chain isoform. Middle: Fibers containing type IId/x myosin heavy chain isoform. Right: Fibers containing type IIb myosin heavy chain isoform. (Reprinted with permission from Eason JM, Schwartz GA, Pavlath GK, English AW. Sexually dimorphic expression of myosin heavy chains in the adult mouse masseter. *J Appl Physiol* 2000;89:251–258.)

experiment, the fiber type can then be determined by metabolic, biochemical, or electrophoretic methods.

### MAXIMUM TENSION GENERATION

When differences in tension generation are assessed, it is important to standardize the amount of force produced by a muscle or fiber to its cross-sectional area, similar to what is done in whole muscle. This allows for comparison of force generation between fibers of varying sizes. At the single-fiber level, force is generally called **specific tension**. For example, if we wanted to compare the amount of force generated between two individual fibers, we would first divide the amount of force generated by each fiber's cross-sectional area.

The literature regarding potential differences in force generation between different fiber types is somewhat controversial. There is some evidence to suggest that in single-fiber preparations, type II fibers generate more force than type I fibers (11). However, due to technical difficulties in measuring the cross-sectional areas of single fibers and the small numbers of fibers that are used in those studies, there is still no definitive answer to this question (12).

However, when measuring specific tension of whole muscle, it is generally agreed that muscles composed primarily of type II fibers have a greater specific tension than muscles that are primarily composed of type I fibers. There is still some heterogeneity of fiber types contained in muscles that are composed primarily of one fiber type. Furthermore, it is not clear if a fiber from a heterogeneous muscle will generate the same force as a fiber of the same fiber type obtained from a muscle with a more homogeneous fiber type composition. However, there is some evidence to indicate that muscle fibers of the same type generate identical tension regardless of the muscle of origin (11). Obviously, more work needs to be done in this area to resolve the controversy regarding any potential differences in force generation between fiber types.

### MAXIMAL VELOCITY OF SHORTENING

Recall that the speed of contraction generated by a fiber is the $V_{max}$. Simply put, $V_{max}$ represents the fastest speed that a muscle can shorten. The speed of shortening is determined by how rapidly myosin crossbridges move during contraction. This is determined by the myosin

ATPase activity of the myosin head. By measuring $V_{max}$ on single fibers, researchers have determined that type IIb fibers have the fastest speed of shortening (9). In fact, the hierarchy of speed is type IIb (not present in humans) > type IId/x > type IIa > type I fibers (9). Further, there are only very small differences in $V_{max}$ between the three fast fiber types, while there is a large difference in $V_{max}$ between the slow fibers as compared with all of the fast fiber types (9).

Besides determining $V_{max}$, ATPase activity can also be used to determine the efficiency of a fiber. Since ATPase activity is highest in type IIb fibers, the energy cost to those fibers is much greater than for either type IIa or I fibers. In terms of efficiency, type IIb fibers are the least efficient, type I are the most efficient, and type IIa fibers are intermediate between the other two fiber types (13).

## METABOLIC AND BIOCHEMICAL DIFFERENCES

There are definite metabolic differences between the different fiber types. Type IIb fibers contain more glycolytic enzymes in the cytoplasm as compared with the type I and IIa fibers. However, regarding oxidative enzymes, the converse is true. Remember, that the site of oxidative phosphorylation occurs inside the mitochondria; since there is a higher concentration of mitochondria in type I fibers, these fibers have the highest oxidative capacity. Type IIb fibers have the lowest oxidative capacity, with type IIa fibers possessing an oxidative capacity intermediate between type I and IIb fibers.

There are other metabolic differences in regards to substrate availability among the fiber types. Slow fibers contain greater amounts of triglycerides than type IIa and IIb fibers. Since triglycerides are broken down via the oxidative pathway, the most oxidative fibers contain a higher concentration of triglycerides. Conversely, type IIa and IIb fibers contain greater amounts of glycogen and phosphocreatine stores than type I fibers. This difference is also consistent with fiber type since the two fast fiber types rely much more on glycolysis to produce energy substrates than slow fibers.

These metabolic differences mean that type I fibers are the most resistant to fatigue, while type IIb fibers are the least resistant to fatigue and type IIa fibers are intermediate between type I and IIb fibers. In this case, the development of muscle fatigue is due to the inability of the muscle fiber to generate ATP via oxidative phosphorylation to supply ATP for contraction. There are other instances of fatigue that can occur which are not related to the ability to generate ATP. This will be discussed further in Chapter 11.

Earlier in this chapter we mentioned that once muscle depolarization stops, muscle contraction ceases. As part of this process, the calcium that is in the cytoplasm is pumped back into the sarcoplasmic reticulum where it is stored until the next action potential initiates skeletal muscle contraction. The pumping of the calcium back into the

sarcoplasmic reticulum is energy dependent. The enzyme responsible is calcium ATPase (Ca ATPase). Ca ATPase requires ATP to be effective. Fast-twitch fibers have the fastest Ca ATPase (type IIb > type IIa), while type I fibers have the slowest Ca ATPase enzyme. Therefore, calcium is pumped back into the sarcoplasmic reticulum much more quickly in type IIb fibers than in type I fibers.

## STRUCTURAL DIFFERENCES

Besides the metabolic, biochemical, and physiologic differences among fiber types, there are also a few notable structural differences. Slow-twitch fibers contain greater amounts of myoglobin and mitochondria as well as a higher capillary density as compared with type II fibers. Intuitively, this makes sense since slow-twitch fibers rely on oxidative pathways to produce substrates for energy production and these fibers contain the machinery to maximize the ability to produce energy. Type IIa fibers rely on both oxidative and glycolytic pathways to produce energy so the structural differences in these fibers are unique to these properties. Type IIa fibers are intermediate between type I and IIb fibers in both the amount of myoglobin and capillary density. Furthermore, type IIa fibers are high in both oxidative and glycolytic enzymes, and they contain a high number of mitochondria.

▶ *INQUIRY SUMMARY.* There are definite differences in characteristics between fiber types. Fast fibers contract much more quickly than slow fibers. Consequently, fast fibers are less efficient than slow fibers. Type I fibers are most oxidative, type IIb fibers are least oxidative, and type IIa fibers are intermediate. Conversely, type I fibers are least glycolytic, type IIb fibers are the most glycolytic, and type IIa fibers fall between type I and IIb fibers. The structural differences between the fiber types support the metabolic and biochemical differences. Finally the existence of potential differences in force generation among fiber types remains controversial. *Why would it potentially be useful for therapists, exercise physiologists, and coaches to know the fiber type composition of different muscles?*

# Muscle Fiber Plasticity

One of the most intriguing aspects about muscle fibers is that they have the ability to change composition with various perturbations. These modifications can include changes in the metabolic, biochemical, and myosin heavy chain isoforms of the fibers. Some of the conditions that can alter fiber type composition of muscle include changes in activity pattern, age, and training.

It appears from work done in small mammals that fiber types change in the following sequential order: IIb ↔ IId/x ↔ IIa ↔ I (14). Furthermore, it appears that fibers change based on the "next-door neighbor rule" (14). This means that a fiber may convert to a type of its "next-door neighbor," i.e., IIb → IId/x or I → IIa, but a fiber will rarely go from the extreme of a type IIb to type I or vice versa (14). Moreover, fibers themselves can be heterogeneous, which means that a fiber may express two different MHC isoforms (15). In small mammals and humans, the proportion of fibers expressing more than one fiber type within a muscle generally increases as the muscle adapts to a perturbation (16). This is because a certain proportion of the fibers are in the process of converting in a sequential fashion from one MHC to another. The next sections cover several perturbations that impact fiber type characteristics.

## AEROBIC EXERCISE

One of the most interesting aspects regarding the plasticity of muscle is the ability of muscle to make adaptations as a result of exercise training. This adaptability may have implications for health care professionals who are developing exercise programs aimed at increasing function in injured patients or training athletes for competition.

When you are examining the evidence about changes with training, the study should state exactly what type of muscular conditions or training caused the adaptations. However, despite this potential limitation, some general comments regarding exercise training and muscle adaptation can be made.

In general, exercise training that is comprised of sustained contractile activity over a period of time results in a more oxidative muscle. By using ATPase histochemistry to identify fiber types, there is strong evidence to indicate an increase in the proportion of type IIa fibers at the expense of type IId/x fibers (17). Furthermore, type I fibers become faster as well, but this is likely due to conversion of myosin light chain isoforms from a slower to a faster isoform (18,19). Because the myosin light chains convert to faster isoform, this allows the slow fibers to contract at a faster rate (18).

## RESISTANCE TRAINING

Resistance or strength training results in increased muscle mass as a result of muscle fiber **hypertrophy**. There are numerous models, both human and animal, that are used to examine muscular changes with strength training. Some of the animal models that are used in strength training research are examined below.

The four models most commonly used are resistance training in conscious animals, electrical stimulation, compensation overload, and chronic stretch (20). Resistance training in conscious small mammals involves training the animal to do the desired movement; once trained, the animal is placed on a progressive resistance exercise program similar to that of a human. Electrical stimulation utilizes small amounts of electric shocks to elicit contraction on the muscle(s) of interest. Compensatory overload models eliminate synergistic muscles so that only one muscle is left to carry out the muscle action normally done by several

muscles. Finally, chronic stretch models have been used to place a muscle in a lengthened position. All of these models have advantages and disadvantages (Table 10.4). While not all animal studies are directly applicable to human exercise programs, these studies help researchers understand the cellular and molecular mechanisms underlying muscle changes and may be helpful in designing more effective rehabilitation programs in the future.

*What happens to fiber type composition as a result of resistance or strength training in humans?* Overall, it appears that resistance training does not result in an increase in type I fibers in either males or females (21). However, within the fast subpopulation of fibers, resistance training has shown a shift from type IId/x to type IIa fibers (*Fig. 10.11*) (21). These results can be interpreted to mean that the percentage of type IIa fibers increases or that the percentage of type IId/x fibers decreases with resistance training.

*What is the functional significance of fiber type transformation with resistance training?* At this point, it is unknown what the functional implications are for fiber type conversion following resistance training. However, at the very least, we do know that resistance exercise training that results in fiber type transformation also results in hypertrophy and increased strength, which certainly have important implications for rehabilitation, health, and wellness.

*LINKUP* **Case Study: Strength Training for Personal Fitness** *and* **Case Study: Strength Training for Power** *illustrate strength training programs that emphasize the endurance component and the power/strength aspect, respectively, of resistance training. You can access these case studies at http://connection.lww.com/go/ brownexphys and on the Student Resource CD-ROM.*

## AGING-RELATED CHANGES

Aging also results in muscle fiber changes. However, it is difficult to elucidate changes in muscle due specifically to the aging process because there are other mechanisms that may also play roles in the changes that are seen in older persons. Poor nutrition, alterations in the endocrine system, decline in physical activity, and changes in the nervous system may all play roles in the age-related modifications in muscle.

One of the biggest alterations within muscle that occurs due to aging is a decrease in muscle mass as a result of a decline in the number of fibers contained within the muscle. This loss of muscle mass is also known as **sarcopenia**. Beginning at the age of 25 years, muscle fiber loss begins and progresses with increasing age so that muscle mass has declined by 25% to 30% by age 65 (22). The primary fiber type that is lost is type IId/x fiber (23).

Another factor that contributes to the decline in muscle mass is selective atrophy of type II fibers (37,38). By the age of 70 years, the mean areas of the type IId/x fibers in both men and women are significantly less as compared with

| Table 10.4 | ADVANTAGES AND DISADVANTAGES OF ANIMAL MODELS USED TO STUDY HYPERTROPHY | |
|---|---|---|
| | **Advantages** | **Disadvantages** |
| Resistance training | Mimic PRE protocols<br>Quantitative<br>Similar hypertrophic and functional outcomes that are the most directly applicable to PRE | Food deprivation or shock application for compliance in rodents<br>Stress induced by forced exercise<br>Reduced animal growth as food withheld<br>Labor intensive for researcher (months or years) |
| Electrical stimulation | Contralateral control muscle available<br>Quantitative and reproducible<br>Independent of animal motivation and cooperation<br>Maximal activation of all motor units | Repeated anesthesia<br>Size principle recruitment pattern not followed<br>Myosin isoform changes depending on frequency of stimulation |
| Compensatory overload | Contralateral control muscle available<br>Hands-off post-surgery<br>Large and fast hypertrophic responses | Chronic "exercise"<br>Surgical implication (infection, edema, inflammation, etc.)<br>Confounding factors < one week<br>Mechanism dissimilar to PRE? |
| Chronic stretch | Contralateral control muscle available<br>Nonsurgical and can study initiating events<br>Very large and fast hypertrophic responses<br>Study hyperplasia (new fiber formation)<br>Responses from intermittent (not chronic) protocols may be more similar to PRE | Most studies are chronic "exercise"<br>Mechanism dissimilar to PRE? |

PRE = progressive resistance exercise. Reprinted with permission from Lowe DA, Alway SE. Animal models for inducing muscle hypertrophy: Are they relevant for clinical applications in humans? *J Orthop Sports Phys Ther* 2002;32:36–43.

those of 50-year-olds (24) (*Fig. 10.12*). These changes in fiber size and number could be due to several factors. Muscle fibers normally undergo a continuous process of denervation and partial reinnervation, and this process may be accelerated in aging (25). The fibers that are denervated and not reinnervated are lost and replaced by fat and fibrous tissue resulting in a loss of muscle tissue (22). And as you will learn in Chapter 11, type I fibers are recruited first for contraction and type IId/x fibers are recruited last. For example, for low-level activities, type I fibers are primarily used,

whereas type IId/x fibers are recruited for activities that require high, explosive bursts of activity.

Therefore, in everyday activities, type I fibers remain in relatively regular use, while activities that use IId/x fibers rarely occur. Since activity levels generally decline with aging, it is likely that the reduction in type IId/x fiber area is because these fibers are rarely used. Therefore, the change in muscle mass could be due to a combination of denervation and decreased use. However, there are many other factors that occur with the aging process which may also affect muscle.

In terms of fiber type proportions, it is difficult to say if there are any changes due to aging because there are many factors that can influence the percentages of myosin isoforms in muscle. Interestingly though, using single-fiber analysis, there appears to be an increase in the percentage of fibers containing more than one myosin isoform in very old persons (~88 years) that is not normally observed in younger persons (26). The functional significance on whole-muscle function of fibers that contain more than one myosin heavy isoform is unknown at this time. Despite the fact that it is unclear if fiber type changes occur in the elderly and if these changes have any functional implications, we do know that muscle mass and strength decline with aging. This fact supports the use of strengthening programs to prevent functional debility in this population. Case study 10.2 illustrates the development of a strength training program in an older person.

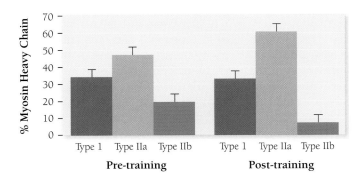

**FIGURE 10.11.** Changes in type IIa and IIb fiber type proportions as a result of resistance training. (Data from Adams GR, Hather BM, Baldwin KM, et al. Skeletal muscle myosin heavy chain composition and resistance training. *J Appl Physiol* 1993;74:911–915.)

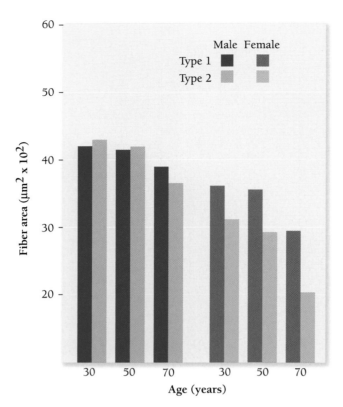

**FIGURE 10.12.** The changes in cross-sectional area of type I and II fibers in men and women between the ages of 30 to 70 years of age. (Data from Essen-Gustavsson B, Borges O. Histochemical and metabolic characteristics of human skeletal muscle in relation to age. *Acta Physiol Scand* 1986;126:107–114.)

## IMMOBILIZATION-INDUCED CHANGES

Often extremities need to be immobilized as a result of fractures and injured tissues. Consequently, immobilized muscle tissue undergoes disuse atrophy as well as changes in myosin isoform composition. In general, immobilization results in greater atrophy of muscles composed of slow muscle fibers as compared with muscles high in fast fiber types (27). However, the amount of atrophy is dependent upon the degree or amount of immobilization. For example, if the soleus (a slow muscle) is immobilized in a shortened position, the degree of atrophy is much greater than if the muscle is immobilized in a lengthened (a position longer than resting length) position (27). The same holds true for muscles composed of faster myosin isoforms (28). This difference is due to the level of activation of the muscle in this position as compared with normal use. The degree of muscle activation as measured by electromyogram is much less when the muscle is in the shortened position as compared with the lengthened position (27). Thus, when trying to compare the various immobilization methods and effects on muscle, it is important to consider the method and degree of immobilization because differences between these two factors will result in different outcomes among studies.

Immobilization in a shortened position also induces slow to fast changes in myosin isoforms in the rat soleus, plantaris, and gastrocnemius muscles (29). Interestingly, when the soleus muscle was immobilized in a lengthened (dorsiflexed) position, there was no slow to fast shift in myosin isoform expression (29). At this point, however, it is unclear how a shift to faster myosin isoforms directly affects overall muscle function.

*What are the implications for rehabilitation from these studies?* Immobilization results in atrophy and consequently a decrease in strength. Also, if possible, positioning muscles in a lengthened rather than shortened position may minimize the degree of muscle atrophy as well as the shift to faster myosin isoforms. It may be helpful to keep in mind that muscles primarily composed of slow fibers and that cross one joint undergo the greatest amount of atrophy following immobilization while muscle composed primarily of fast fibers is less affected by immobilization (12). See *Figure 10.13*, which illustrates the fiber type composition of several human muscles.

These studies describing muscle changes with aerobic and resistance training, aging, and immobilization demonstrate the ability of skeletal muscle to adapt to a variety of functional demands and have broad implications to health care professionals. Understanding the physiologic changes that occur within muscle should be helpful in designing therapeutic interventions for injured patients and developing training protocols to enhance athletic performance in healthy populations. As future research studies begin to elucidate the cellular and molecular events that are responsible for the changes observed in skeletal muscle, it will be exciting to be able to design more effective exercise programs to specifically target muscle deficits.

*LINKUP* **Research Highlight: Transcriptional Coactivator PGC-1a Drives the Formation of Slow-Twitch Muscle Fibers** *attempts to elucidate some of the complex and overlapping signaling pathways that control fiber type in skeletal muscles. This study is reviewed at http://connection.lww.com/go/brownexphys and on the Student Resource CD-ROM.*

▶ *INQUIRY SUMMARY.* Muscle fibers alter their composition as a result of changes in functional demands, and these changes occur in an orderly and sequential fashion from one fiber type to the next. In general terms, endurance and resistance training result in a conversion of fast to slow fiber types. Aging results in atrophy of type IId/x fibers as well as what appears to be a conversion of fast fibers to slower fiber types. Conversely, in conditions of immobilization, muscle fiber type transforms from fast to slow. The fact that training techniques, immobilization, and aging all affect muscle fiber composition indicates that it is important to design exercise programs specifically tailored to a client's specific problem. *Based on some of the general changes that can occur with immobilization or aging, think of some exercise techniques that*

### CASE

Stella is 68-year-old female who is interested in beginning a resistance training program. She has been engaged in a walking program for cardiorespiratory fitness but is noticing that it is becoming increasingly difficult to rise from a chair and to do activities that require her arms to be extended over her head. She also enjoys gardening and finds it difficult to rise to standing from the ground.

### DESCRIPTION

Stella reports "a touch" of arthritis in her shoulders, knees, and hips. She underwent gall bladder surgery approximately 10 years ago. She has no other medical or surgical history. Stella is a retired elementary school teacher who lives with her husband in a single-story home. She is very active in community activities. Stella volunteers at a local food bank and tutors elementary-school–aged children in an afterschool program. She also enjoys gardening and is secretary of her gardening club.

Before developing a strength training program for Stella, you should conduct an evaluation. Her range of motion is grossly within functional limits in all joints. She does report slightly increased pain at the extreme ranges of motion secondary to her arthritis. Stella's muscle strength is a 4/5 bilaterally in her shoulders and hip extensors. Muscle strength is 5/5 in all remaining muscle groups. Light touch is intact and her reflexes are normal. Stella ambulates without any gait deviations, and her balance is normal. She is independent in going from sitting to standing but requires maximal use for her upper extremities to initiate the movement. She is independent in all other activities of daily living (ADL).

### DESCRIPTION

Prior to developing her exercise prescription, you can determine the one repetition maximum (1 RM) for Stella. Alternatively, to prevent injury during the 1 RM maneuver, intensity may be determined by completing a certain number of repetitions to failure utilizing a low weight. Stella should perform at least one set of eight to ten exercises that utilize all major muscle groups. Each set should contain 10 to 15 repetitions that elicit a rating of perceived exertion of 12 to 13. Her exercise program should be done at least twice a week, preferably three times per week. At least 48 hours of rest should occur between weight training sessions. As Stella's strength increases, overload should be achieved by increasing the number of repetitions and then the amount of weight.

It is important for Stella to maintain her flexibility so she should begin a flexibility program. However, the literature is quite limited in terms of recommended protocols for increasing flexibility. General guidelines dictate that the exercises should be done with slow movements and at least four repetitions per muscle group. The stretch should cause mild discomfort but never pain. Stella could incorporate her stretching program into her strengthening program by doing the flexibility exercises as a warmup and cooldown.

There are some special issues that should be considered. Stella should be taught proper training techniques for all of her exercises, and she should be closely monitored during her first several training sessions. She should be encouraged to perform her exercises within her pain-free range of motion to prevent aggravation of her arthritis. Finally, it is recommended that Stella use machines to resistance train, rather than free weights, because the machines will give her more support, require less skill to use, and allow her to increase the amount of weight lifted by smaller increments.

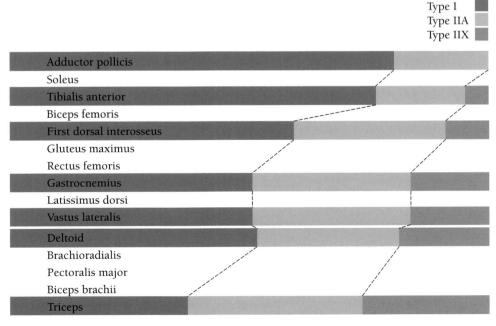

FIGURE 10.13. Relative distribution of fiber types in various human muscles.

*you would utilize to rehabilitate an elderly patient or a client following removal of a cast.*

## Summary

Whole muscle consists of thousands of muscle fibers that contract simultaneously to generate movement. Skeletal muscle contains several levels of connective tissue that are supportive to the muscle. Several extensive networks or channels are responsible for the storage and release of calcium, the mineral essential for muscle contraction. The contractile components of muscle are the myosin and actin filaments. It is the movement of these molecules over each other that results in muscle contraction.

The sarcomere is the functional unit of contraction; contained within the sarcomere are several zones and regions that define the locations of myosin and actin. Muscle contraction begins with an action potential from the nerve that stimulates the release of acetylcholine from the nerve terminal and binding of acetylcholine to the motor endplate of the muscle. Once the action potential arrives at the muscle, the potential is propagated deep within the muscle and calcium is released. This allows for the active sites on actin to become exposed and myosin and actin to bind to one another. When available, ATP binds to the myosin head, and the myosin dissociates from actin. ATP becomes hydrolyzed, which provides "energy" to the myosin head. As long as the calcium concentration remains elevated, the myosin head will bind to another actin site and pull actin across its length. This is known as the sliding filament theory. The entire multistep process of the action potential that results in muscle contraction is known as the excitation-contraction coupling process.

Muscle fibers can be classified based upon biochemical, metabolic, and molecular processes. In general, muscle fiber classification predicts the contractile properties of that fiber. Finally muscle fibers can switch from one type to another depending on the level of contractile activity of the muscle.

## SUMMARY KNOWLEDGE

1. Describe the gross structure of muscle.
2. Compare and contrast unipennate and multipennate muscles in terms of pennation angles and force generation. How are the differences related to function?
3. Describe the components of the neuromuscular junction and explain how an action potential is transmitted from the nerve to skeletal muscle.
4. What are the mechanisms underlying the sliding filament theory?
5. List and describe what is happening in each of the steps in excitation-contraction coupling.
6. List and describe the various techniques used to determine muscle fiber types.
7. Compare and contrast the mechanical properties of the different fiber types.
8. What are the muscle fiber changes that occur with aerobic and resistance training, aging, and immobilization? What do you think the implications might be in functional terms for performance?

### References

1. Vignos PJ Jr, Spencer GE Jr, Archibald KC. Management of progressive muscular dystrophy in childhood. *JAMA* 1963;184:89–96.
2. Powell PL, Roy RR, Kanim P, et al. Predictability of skeletal muscle tension from architectural determinations in guinea pig hindlimbs. *J Appl Physiol* 1984;57:1715–1721.
3. Huxley HE. The mechanisms of muscular contraction. *Science* 1969;164:1356–1365.
4. Metzger JM, Moss RL. pH modulation of the kinetics of a $Ca^{2+}$-sensitive cross-bridge state transition in mammalian single skeletal muscle fibers. *J Physiol* 1990;428:751–764.
5. Brooke MH, Kaiser KK. Muscle fiber types: how many and what kind? *Arch Neurol* 1970;23:369–379.
6. Barany M. ATPase activity of myosin correlated with speed of muscle shortening. *J Gen Physiol* 1967;50 Suppl:197–218.
7. Scott W, Stevens J, Binder-Macleod SA. Human skeletal muscle fiber type classifications. *Phys Ther* 2001;81:1810–1816.
8. Schiaffino S, Gorza L, Sartore S, et al. Three myosin heavy chain isoforms in type 2 skeletal muscle fibres. *J Muscle Res Cell Motil* 1989;10:197–205.
9. Bottinelli R, Schiaffino S, Reggiani C. Force-velocity relations and myosin heavy chain isoform compositions of skinned fibres from rat skeletal muscle. *J Physiol* 1991;437:655–672.
10. Smerdu V, Karsch-Mizrachi I, Campione M, et al. Type IIx myosin heavy chain transcripts are expressed in type IIb fibers of human skeletal muscle. *Am J Physiol* 1994;267:C1723–C1728.
11. Harridge SDR, White MJ, Carrington CA, et al. Electrically evoked torque-velocity characteristics and isomyosin composition of the triceps surae in young and elderly men. *Acta Physiol Scand* 1995;154:469–477.
12. Lieber RL. *Skeletal muscle structure, function & plasticity.* 2nd ed. Baltimore: Lippincott Williams & Wilkins, 2002.
13. Stienen GJM, Kiers JL, Bottinelli R, et al. Myofibrillar ATPase activity in skinned human skeletal muscle fibres: Fibre type and temperature dependence. *J Physiol* 1996;493:299–307.
14. Stevens L, Sultan KR, Peuker H, et al. Time-dependent changes in myosin heavy chain mRNA and protein isoforms in unloaded soleus muscle of rat. *Am J Physiol* 1999;277:C1044–C1049.
15. Pette D, Staron RS. Mammalian skeletal muscle fiber type transitions. *Int Rev Cytol* 1997;170:143–223.
16. Staron RS, Gohlsch B, Pette D. Myosin polymorphism in single fibers of chronically stimulated rabbit fast-twitch muscle. *Pflügers Arch* 1987;408:444–450.
17. Martin WH 3rd, Coggan AR, Spina RJ, et al. Effects of fiber type and training on β-adrenoceptor density in human skeletal muscle. *Am J Physiol* 1989;257:E736–E742.
18. Fitts RH, Widrick JJ. Muscle mechanics: adaptations with exercise training. *Exerc Sport Sci Rev* 1996;24:427–473.
19. Baumann H, Jaggi M, Soland F, et al. Exercise training induces transitions of myosin isoform subunits within histochemically typed human muscle fibres. *Pflügers Arch* 1987;409:349–360.
20. Lowe DA, Alway SE. Animal models for inducing muscle hypertrophy: are they relevant for clinical applications in humans? *J Orthop Sports Phys Ther* 2002;32:36–43.
21. Adams GR, Hather BM, Baldwin KM, et al. Skeletal muscle myosin heavy chain composition and resistance training. *J Appl Physiol* 1993;74:911–915.
22. Lexell J, Taylor CC, Sjostrom M. What is the cause of ageing atrophy? Total number, size, and proportion of different fiber types studies in

the whole vastus lateralis muscle from 15- to 83-year-old men. *J Neurol Sci* 1988;84:275–294.

23. Porter MM, Vandervoort AA, Lexell J. Aging of human muscle: structure, function, and adaptability. *Scand J Med Sci Sports* 1995;5:129–142.

24. Essen-Gustavsson B, Borges O. Histochemical and metabolic characteristics of human skeletal muscle in relation to age. *Acta Physiol Scand* 1986;126:107–114.

25. Lexell J. Human aging, muscle mass, and fiber type composition. *J Gerontol Biol Sci Med Sci* 1995;50:11–16.

26. Andersen JL. Muscle fibre type adaptation in the elderly human muscle. *Scand J Med Sci Sports* 2003;13:40–47.

27. Fournier M, Roy RR, Perham H, et al. Is limb immobilization a model of muscle disuse? *Exp Neurol* 1983;80:147–156.

28. Simard CP, Spector SA, Edgerton VR. Contractile properties of rat hind limb muscles immobilized at different lengths. *Exp Neurol* 1982;77:467–482.

29. Jänkälä H, Harjola V-P, Petersen NE, et al. Myosin heavy chain mRNA transforms to faster isoforms in immobilized skeletal muscle: a quantitative PCR study. *J Appl Physiol* 1997;82:977–982.

### Suggested Readings

Lieber RL. *Skeletal muscle structure, function & plasticity.* 2nd ed. Lippincott Williams & Wilkins, 2002.

Lieber RL, Fridén J. Functional and clinical significance of skeletal muscle architecture. *Muscle Nerve* 2000;23:1647–1666.

Moss RL, Diffee GM, Greaser ML. Contractile properties of skeletal muscle fibers in relation to myofibrillar protein isoforms. *Rev Physiol Biochem Pharmacol* 1995;126:1–63.

Pette D, Staron RS. Mammalian skeletal muscle fiber type transitions. *Int Rev Cytol* 1997;170:143–223.

Talmadge RJ. Myosin heavy chain isoform expression following reduced neuromuscular activity: potential regulatory mechanisms. *Muscle Nerve* 2000;23:661–679.

Thompson LV. Skeletal muscle adaptations with age, inactivity, and therapeutic exercise. *J Orthop Sports Phys Ther* 2002;32:44–57.

### On the Internet

Muscular Dystrophy Association. Available at: **http://mdatest.mdausa.org/.** Accessed May 05, 2005.

Myasthenia Gravis Foundation of America. Available at: **http://www.myasthenia.org/.** Accessed May 05, 2005.

Muscle Pathology & Biopsy Service: Muscle Biopsy. Available at: **http://www.biomed2.man.ac.uk/ns/mm/musbiop.html.** Accessed May 05, 2005.

Diseases of Muscle, Neuromuscular Junction, and Peripheral Nerve. Available at: **http://edcenter.med.cornell.edu/CUMC_PathNotes/Neuropathology/Neuropath_II/muscle.html.** Accessed May 05, 2005.

## Writing to Learn

*In this chapter we mentioned that fibers transform from slow to fast with spinal cord injury. How are the muscle properties changed as a result of spinal cord injury? Include information regarding muscle structure, fiber type composition, and contractile properties. Briefly discuss models that are used to study muscle properties following spinal cord injury. Finally describe some impairments and functional limitations that may result from a spinal cord injury.*

# CHAPTER

# 11 Muscle Mechanics During Activity

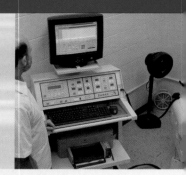

*Movement is a vital part of everyday activities and the ability to move is directly related to the ability to be independent in activities of daily living. Understanding the interaction between the nervous and muscular systems is important in the evaluation of movement and in the prescription of exercise to increase strength and enhance movement. Furthermore, understanding the mechanics of skeletal muscle is important in appreciating how muscle functions. It is important to be able to apply these concepts to develop training programs for athletes and for clients recovering from injuries.* How does a health care professional incorporate these important concepts in the development of a training program for the client?

## CHAPTER OUTLINE

Many different chronic diseases result in functional limitations. The underlying impairment for these limitations often is a decline in muscular strength and endurance. Chapter 10 presented the foundations of muscle structure. This chapter explores the relationship between the neural and muscular components of movement. Assessment of muscular strength is explored, including examples of how the assessment can be used to provide exercise prescription to improve muscular strength. This issue is important for individuals with chronic diseases as they strive to maintain independence and function in their daily lives. The intent of this chapter is to lay the foundation for understanding the relationship between the nervous and muscular systems and how to evaluate impairments of muscular strength.

## The Motor Unit

The nervous system and its interaction with the muscle fiber at the neuromuscular junction was discussed in Chapter 9, while the properties of whole muscle and single fibers were presented in Chapter 10. The focus of this chapter is whole-muscle mechanics and how this knowledge is important in assessing strength and designing rehabilitation programs.

## MOTOR UNIT ANATOMY AND FUNCTION

The **motor unit** is considered the functional unit of movement, and it consists of an α-motor neuron and all the muscle fibers innervated by that motor neuron *(Fig. 11.1)*. Recall that the cell bodies of the α-motoneurons lie in the ventral root of the spinal cord. The axon from each α-motor neuron extends from the cell body, exits the spinal cord at the ventral root, and forms a peripheral nerve along with other axons. The peripheral nerve travels to the muscle that it innervates and as the nerve approaches the muscle, it divides into many branches so that one branch from the axon innervates one muscle fiber. As a result, when branches of the α-motor neuron are activated, all of the muscle fibers innervated by that α-motor neuron are stimulated to contract. For this reason, the motor unit is considered to be the functional unit of movement.

Because of this type of organization, the entire skeletal muscle is composed of many motor units. In general, large muscles that provide **gross motor movement** contain large motor units. This notion of size is related to the **innervation ratio** of a motor unit which refers to the number of muscle fibers contained in that motor unit. Thus, in large muscles, a single α-motor neuron innervates many muscle fibers. However, in muscles for which precise movements are necessary, such as the muscles in the hand or those that control eye movements, the innervation ratio is small. *What functional consequence does this have?*

Motor units can be classified into three general categories based on physiologic properties. These properties are **twitch tension**, **tetanic tension**, and **fatigability** of the motor unit. These properties will be discussed in the next few sections.

### Twitch Tension

Much of the early research in motor unit physiology revealed that in response to a single electric shock, motor units develop high-, intermediate-, or low-twitch tension. Twitch tension is the tension that is generated when an impulse of sufficient voltage is applied to the muscle. An important component of twitch tension is how rapidly the tension develops and how quickly it relaxes. Early experiments found that motor units can generally be divided into three categories: slow twitch, low tension, and fatigue resistant (type I); fast twitch, moderate tension, and fatigue resistant (type IIa); and fast twitch, high tension, and fast fatigue (type IIb) *(Fig. 11.2)*. Slow-twitch (S) motor units are slower contracting but show greater fatigue resistance than fast-fatigable (FF) and fast-fatigue-resistant (FR) motor units. However, FF and FR motor units develop greater tension than S units and also develop tension faster than S units.

Motor neurons play a role in modulating muscle fiber types by varying the neural input that the fiber receives from the motor neuron. This neural input is responsible for changing the metabolic, biochemical, and molecular properties of the muscle fiber that occur with training. In

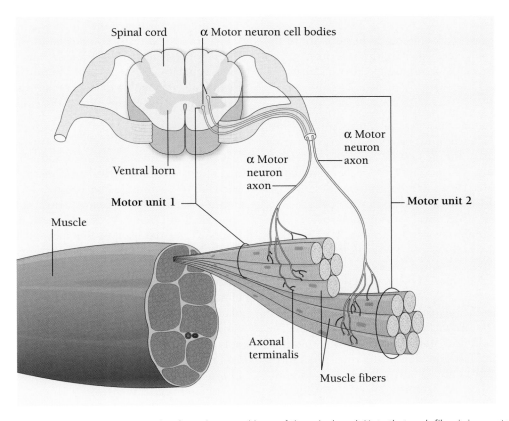

**FIGURE 11.1.** Motor unit. α-motor neurons emanating from the ventral horn of the spinal cord. Note that each fiber is innervated by one α-motor neuron. The α-motor neuron and the fibers it innervates are called the motor unit.

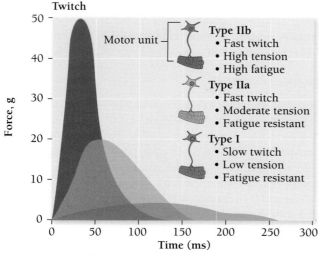

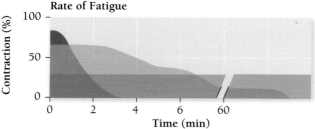

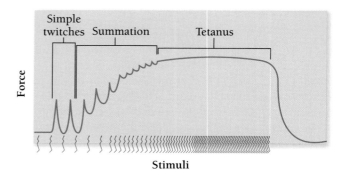

**FIGURE 11.3.** Illustration of muscle twitches summating into a tetanus. Electrical shocks delivered at a low frequency allow time for both contraction and relaxation. As shocks are delivered more frequently, there is not enough time for relaxation and the twitches begin to summate until there is no visible relaxation between contractions. At this point, the muscle is undergoing a tetanic contraction.

**FIGURE 11.2.** Types of motor units. The three different motor unit types (I, IIa, and IIb) are classified by the amount of tension generated, speed of contraction, and fatigability of the motor unit.

other words, muscles adapt differently in response to the type of neural stimuli received. This idea was presented in Chapter 10 in the discussion on muscle fiber plasticity.

## Tetanic Tension

If a second electric shock is delivered immediately following the first, the muscle fiber produces a second twitch that may "piggyback" on the first twitch. This muscle response is called **summation** (*Fig. 11.3*). If the stimulation is such that the electric shocks continue to be provided more frequently so that the relaxation time between the successive twitches becomes shorter and shorter, the strength of contractions becomes greater. Finally there will come a point when there is no visible relaxation between successive twitches and muscle contraction appears very smooth and sustained. This contraction is called a **complete tetanus**.

*A basic question at this point is why do S motor units generate less tension than FF and FR motor units?* The difference in tension does not appear to be due to differences in individual fast and slow fiber force generation. Muscle fibers in fast motor units are larger and more numerous than in slow motor units. Therefore, it appears that fast motor units generate more tension because they contain more fibers, and the fibers within fast motor units are larger.

## FATIGUE INDEX

The last physiologic property used to classify motor units is the **fatigue index**, a measure of the amount of tension decline with repetitive stimulation. To determine the fatigue index, a repetitive stimulation protocol was developed (1). During this test, a stimulus that generates only about one-half of the maximal tetanic tension is applied to the motor unit every second for 2 minutes. Muscle tension is measured throughout the test, and the amount of tension generated at the end of the 2-minute protocol is measured. The difference between the initial and final tensions is the fatigue index. Basically, S motor units generate 75% of the initial force at the end of the 2-minute period, FR motor units generate 25% to 75% of the initial tension, and the highly fatigable motor units generate only 25% of the initial tension at the completion of the fatigue test.

## MOTOR UNIT RECRUITMENT

One of the principles of motor unit physiology is the **all-or-none phenomenon**. When a motor neuron is stimulated, all of the muscle fibers contained within that motor unit are stimulated to contract. How then is muscle force controlled to produce either the gross motor actions necessary to run and walk or fine motor actions necessary in using the fingers for manual dexterity?

There are two primary mechanisms used to control the amount of force produced by muscles. Either the number of motor units that are recruited changes or the frequency of discharge of the motor units is changed. For example, in activities that require a small amount of force generation, only a few motor units are activated. However, as the need for muscle force increases, more motor units are activated to produce the necessary force. This process is known as **motor unit recruitment**.

One of the key concepts in motor unit recruitment is the **size principle**. When muscles are generating low amounts of force, motor units with small axons are recruited first.

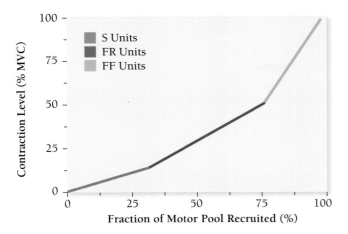

**FIGURE 11.4.** Motor unit recruitment. Slow-twitch motor units are recruited first with activity; as activity increases in intensity, the fast-twitch (type IIa) motor units are recruited. Finally, the type IIb fast-twitch motor units are recruited at high-intensity exercise.

As force increases, motor units with increasingly larger axons are recruited in an orderly fashion. As force decreases, the entire process reverses. This means that fast motor units are innervated by large axons and slow motor units are innervated by small axons. At low levels of activity (i.e., light muscle contractions), S motor units are recruited first. As the intensity of an activity increases, FR motor units are recruited. Finally at the highest intensities, FF motor units are recruited (*Fig. 11.4*).

This process ensures that there is a progressive increase in muscle force production as exercise intensity increases. Consider, for example, an activity such as moderately intense jogging on a level surface. This is a low-level, sustained activity, and in accordance with the size principle, S motor units are recruited first. However, if the same person begins running at faster speeds, more of the faster motor units are recruited, especially if the runner is running uphill or across uneven terrain. This orderly and differential recruitment of motor units plays a key role in skilled sport performance (2).

*LINKUP:* **See Biography: Elwood Henneman** *at http://connection.lww.com/go/brownexphys and on the Student Resource CD-ROM for a close look at the scientist who discovered the size principle of motor unit recruitment.*

Fast motor units supply much of the force at faster speeds of movement, while the contribution of slow motor units to force production decreases. However, there may be some instances in which selective recruitment of fast motor units occurs over slow motor units. In the cat, it has been shown that during rapid paw shakes, there is selective recruitment of fast motor units in the lateral gastrocnemius without simultaneous recruitment of slow motor units in the soleus (3). Because paw shaking is a very rapid movement, there may not be not enough time to recruit slow motor units. However, these results observed in cats have generally not been consistently observed in humans.

By now, the importance of motor units to movement should be clear. Imagine a disease process in which the underlying pathology is a loss of motor neurons. The outcome would be a decline in muscle strength and movement. Amyotrophic lateral sclerosis (ALS) is an example of a disease in which motor neurons are destroyed, resulting in a clinical picture of muscle fatigue, weakness, and overall decline in function (Box 11.1). A useful tool that can be used to assist in diagnosing neuromuscular diseases such as ALS is electromyography (EMG). EMGs can also be used to study muscle activity and establish the roles of various muscles during activities.

*LINKUP:* **Perspective: Electromyography,** *found at http://connection.lww.com/go/brownexphys and on the Student Resource CD-ROM, provides additional information on this diagnostic tool.*

▶ *INQUIRY SUMMARY.* For muscle to contract, muscle fibers must be stimulated by α-motor neurons. Muscle fibers and the α-motor neuron that stimulate them are collectively known as the motor unit. Motor units can be classified according to various physiologic properties that include twitch tension, tetanic tension, and fatigability. Motor units are recruited based on the size of the axons. Therefore, slow motor units with the smallest axons are recruited initially, FR fibers are recruited next, and FF fibers are recruited last. This is known as the size principle of recruitment. *Why is it important to understand the size principle and the role it plays in sports activities and performance?*

## Muscle Mechanics

Several concepts related to muscle mechanics are very important for movement and sports activities. First to consider are the different types of muscle contractions that produce force (*Fig. 11.5*). An **isometric** muscle contraction occurs when the muscle is activated to contract but cannot overcome the external resistance. Therefore, with this type of muscle contraction, there are no obvious changes in muscle length and no movement occurs. Isometric contractions are often called static contractions.

Muscle contractions that result in movement are called dynamic muscle contractions. These dynamic contractions are the most common form of muscle contraction, and they result in movement whether for daily function or sport activities. Dynamic muscle contractions can be divided into two types of contractions: **concentric** and **eccentric**. With concentric contractions, the muscle is activated and shortens, resulting in joint movement and a decrease in joint angle. With eccentric contractions, the muscle lengthens as tension is developed. Many of our movements result from

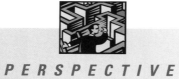

**Box 11.1**

*P E R S P E C T I V E*

# Amyotrophic Lateral Sclerosis

Amyotrophic lateral sclerosis (ALS) is a degenerative disease that affects motor neurons in the cortex, brainstem, and spinal cord and results in progressive weakness and muscle wasting. ALS is considered to be the most physically devastating of the degenerative diseases that affect the nervous system. About 50% of patients succumb to the disease within 2 to 5 years of diagnosis.

The incidence of ALS is approximately 1 per 100,000, and the prevalence of ALS worldwide is 4 to 6 per 100,000. Approximately 10% of the cases of ALS have a genetic component; however, the remaining 90% of the cases have an unknown cause. There have been several suggested etiologies, such as chronic exposure to heavy metals and infection with poliovirus; however, no clear cause of ALS has been established. ALS usually is manifested between the ages of 50 and 60 years, with men affected twice as frequently as women (2). Approximately 10% of the cases of ALS begin prior to the age of 40 years and another 10% begin after the age of 70 years. The progression of the disease cannot be predicted at diagnosis, but it is usually evident 1 to 2 years following diagnosis.

The pyramidal cells of the cerebral cortex, premotor areas of the brain, sensory cortex, and temporal cortex are all affected in ALS. The number of neurons in these areas becomes sparse, and the dendrites are impaired as well. The corticospinal and corticobulbar tracts become demyelinated. Furthermore, there is a loss of large motor neurons in the anterior horn cells of the spinal cord and in the brainstem. Current research examining the reasons behind the loss of neurons is focusing on neural viruses, an increase in excitatory neurotransmitters, impairment of certain biochemical pathways, and oxidative damage.

Clinical manifestations are varied and depend on whether upper motor neurons (UMN) or lower motor neurons (LMN) are involved in the disease process. Eventually, however, both UMN and LMN will be affected. With LMN impairment, the patient very slowly develops an asymmetric weakness of one aspect of a limb with gradual involvement of more muscles in the affected limb. The extensor muscles generally become weaker than flexor muscles and can cause deformities, particularly in the hand. Clawhand can develop due to the imbalance between the extensor and flexor muscles.

Quite often patients develop signs that are known as bulbar signs—signs of involvement of the muscles that control speech, chewing, and swallowing. Patients may have difficulty closing the eyelids, tongue movements become impaired, difficulties with speech occur, moving food within the mouth becomes difficult, and finally difficulty with swallowing occurs. Drooling also becomes prominent due to bulbar problems. Furthermore, the diaphragm becomes affected and as a result, breathing becomes labored with the patient relying on accessory muscles for breathing. Weakness develops in the extremities as the muscles become denervated and atrophied. UMN signs include spasticity and hyperactive tendon reflexes. Most patients maintain normal mental function throughout the course of the disease. Because of this, it is very important to emphasize maintenance of the highest level of functioning in the patient and to involve the patient in decision-making about medical care.

The diagnosis of ALS is usually based on clinical examination and an electromyogram (EMG). It often takes some time for the diagnosis to be made because the early clinical manifestations are subtle and there may be very little change on an EMG. Once the diagnosis is made, there are no medications to prevent the progression of the disease. Medications are primarily used to treat the impairments as a result of the disease. Nutrition becomes a problem as the muscles of chewing and swallowing become impaired. The prevention of respiratory complications is also of paramount importance in patients with ALS. Finally the use of physical and occupational therapy to prolong function, provide adaptive equipment, and provide patient and family education is an important component in the medical care of patients with ALS. Patients usually succumb to pulmonary infections as a result of pulmonary compromise.

ALS is also commonly known as Lou Gehrig disease because the famed baseball player died of this disease in June 1941 at the age of 38. The famed British physicist Stephen Hawking was diagnosed with ALS in 1963; however, his disease has progressed very slowly. He holds Isaac Newton's chair, the Lucasian Professorship of Mathematics, at Cambridge University and is renowned for his work on the quantum mechanics of black holes and theories on the origin and fate of the universe. For more information on ALS, visit the website of the ALS Association at http://www.alsa.org.

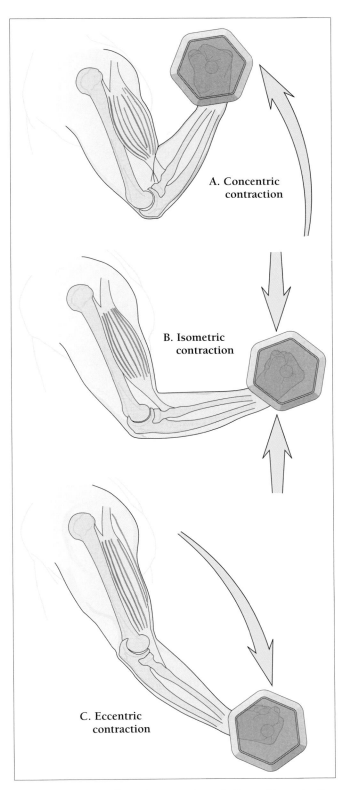

**FIGURE 11.5.** Types of muscle contractions. **A.** Concentric contraction occurs when the muscle shortens to lift a load. **B.** Isometric contraction occurs when the muscle contracts but cannot overcome the weight of the load, and no movement occurs. **C.** Eccentric contraction occurs as a muscle lengthens against the weight of the load.

a combination of both concentric and eccentric movements. Keep in mind these types of muscle contractions as several key points regarding skeletal muscle mechanics are presented.

## LENGTH-TENSION CURVE

The initial length of the muscle prior to the development of force is one factor that determines the amount of force exerted by the muscle. This concept is related to the amount of overlap that exists between actin and myosin. Researchers have studied this concept by stimulating single muscle fibers at specific sarcomere lengths and measuring the amount of force generated by the muscle fiber.

At a sarcomere length of 1.25 μm, there is so much overlap between actin and myosin that the sarcomere cannot generate any force (*Fig. 11.6*). As the sarcomere lengthens to 1.65 μm, 70% to 80% of maximal force is generated. At this length, more actin and myosin crossbridges are able to interact and generate force. However, a sarcomere length of 2.0 to 2.25 μm represents the optimal length of the sarcomere. At this length, actin and myosin have maximal crossbridge interaction and maximal force development is generated. As the sarcomere is lengthened beyond this optimal length, force begins to decline as a result of reduced overlap between actin and myosin. At a sarcomere length of 3.65 μm, there is no force output from the sarcomeres because there is no overlap of the actin and myosin filaments.

## FORCE-VELOCITY RELATIONSHIP

Since most daily and sport activities involve the generation of force throughout ranges of joint movement, it is important to understand the relationship between force and the speed of movement (*Fig. 11.7*). The concept of a force-velocity relationship was described by A. V. Hill (4). Basically this relationship describes the amount of force generated by a muscle as a function of the speed at which the muscle is shortening. At the fastest speed of shortening, the muscle generates the lowest force. As the speed of shortening decreases, force output increases such that maximum force occurs when the muscle is stationary, as in an isometric contraction. However, as the load on the muscle increases, there will eventually be a point when the load is greater than the ability of the muscle to generate enough force to overcome the imposed load. At this point, the muscle is forced to undergo active lengthening or an eccentric muscle contraction. As a greater load is applied to the muscle, the lengthening velocity increases until the load becomes so great that the muscle lengthens uncontrollably.

Recall from Chapter 10 that the term used to describe the fastest speed that a muscle can shorten is $V_{max}$ and that $V_{max}$ is greatest in muscles composed of fast fibers. For any given force generated by a muscle, the velocity of movement is greatest in muscles that contain a higher proportion of fast fibers. Remember that the reason for this observation is

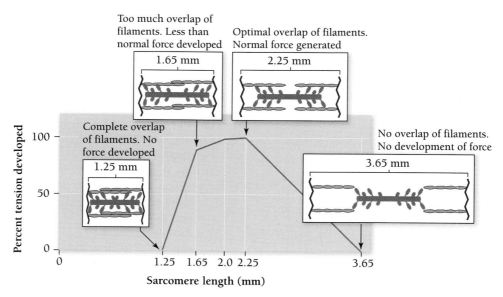

**FIGURE 11.6.** Relationship of sarcomere length and force development.

that fast fibers contain higher ATPase activity than slow fibers. Therefore, ATP is broken down more rapidly in fast fibers.

The other relationship to examine is the power-velocity relationship. Power is the rate at which a muscle can produce force and is defined as the product of force and velocity. Essentially power is the area under the force-velocity curve. The peak power that a muscle can generate increases rapidly as velocity increases until the velocity reaches speeds of up to 200 to 300 degrees·s$^{-1}$. As velocity increases beyond this, the power output of the muscle

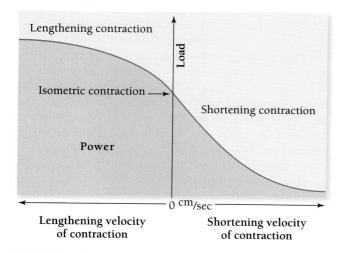

**FIGURE 11.7.** Force and speed of movement. Force-velocity curve illustrating the relationship between force and velocity. Note that at $V_{max}$, the muscle generates the least amount of force. As velocity decreases, force output increases until no movement is occurring—this is an isometric contraction. As the muscle lengthens, force continues to be generated until the load becomes so large that the muscle lengthens uncontrollably. The area under the force-velocity curve is power.

declines. The other point to remember about muscle power is that peak power output is related to the fiber type composition of the muscle. Muscles that have a greater percentage of fast-twitch fibers generate a greater peak power than muscles that are primarily composed of slow-twitch fibers. The reasons for this are due to the physiologic and biochemical differences between slow- and fast-twitch fibers that were discussed in Chapter 10.

The implications for understanding this relationship should be clear to the health care professional. Muscles that contain faster fiber types also generate the most power. That helps to explain why athletes who engage in sports typically involving brief spurts of high power, such as weightlifting, generally have muscles that contain a higher percentage of fast fibers.

## MUSCLE FATIGUE

The development of muscle fatigue is a complex phenomenon that occurs as a result of failure of several processes within the neuromuscular system. Failure of any neurophysiologic factor from the brain to the muscle fiber itself can result in fatigue. However, regardless of how muscle fatigue occurs, the end result is that there is a temporary loss in force generation of the involved muscle(s). Functionally the development of muscle fatigue can have detrimental effects on everyday activities such as walking and standing; fatigue can also result in a decrement of athletic performance.

There has been much research devoted to the cause of muscle fatigue, and both the cause and exact sites of muscle fatigue are not completely understood. Classically the sites of muscle fatigue are generally divided into central and peripheral sites of fatigue. Central fatigue refers to failure of neuromuscular components in the central nervous system and may be the result of physiologic factors that inhibit descending control over interneurons and motor neurons in the spinal cord. For example, with a maximal contractile effort, the central nervous system may stimulate inhibitor pathways to prevent activation of the motor neurons that result in fatigue. Often when central nervous system fatigue is suspected, loud verbal commands or shouts of encouragement may generate an increase in force output. Central nervous system fatigue may also be related to psychologic factors such as the brain's perception of muscular effort. Box 11.2 highlights a research study that attempts to elucidate some of the mechanisms that cause muscle fatigue.

Peripheral fatigue can occur due to many neurophysiologic factors in the periphery. For example, one proposed mechanism for peripheral fatigue is a failure in neuromuscular transmission and is most likely due to a decrease in the release of acetylcholine from the nerve endings. Another proposed mechanism in the periphery that may result in muscular fatigue is inhibition of motor neuron firing. In classic experiments conducted by Bigland-Ritchie and colleagues (5), reduced motor neuron firing rates occurred with a maximal voluntary contraction while the muscle was kept ischemic. These results suggest that a reflex from the muscle that inhibited motor neuron excitability was transmitted to the spinal cord.

Peripheral fatigue may also result from changes in the pool of substrates that are needed to maintain fuel for the muscle. For example, if physical activity results in a mismatch between ATP synthesis and the ATP that is used within the exercising muscle, then fatigue may occur. Fatigue may also develop when there is not enough $O_2$ delivery to the muscle and/or there is an increase in blood lactate levels, which results in a decline in pH due to excess hydrogen ions in the muscle. The decline in pH can significantly alter many of the contractile processes contained within muscle fibers. For example, a reduction in pH can inhibit the release of calcium from the sarcoplasmic reticulum, change the sensitivity of troponin C to calcium, and directly inhibit force production at the crossbridge level (6–8). All of these processes result in a decline in force generation. However, there is some evidence to suggest that perhaps changes in pH may not be as important in the development of fatigue as previously thought (9).

There are numerous diagnoses in which muscle fatigue is a presenting symptom. One interesting diagnosis is post-polio syndrome (PPS). Briefly, this syndrome manifests approximately 15 years following recovery from polio, and the initial symptom reported by patients is muscle fatigue. Case Study 11.1 presents physical therapy intervention for a client with PPS.

***LINKUP:* Perspective: Post-Polio Syndrome,** *found at http://connection.lww.com/go/brownexphys and on the Student Resource CD-ROM, provides information on the pathophysiology, prognosis, and treatment of this syndrome that affects survivors of poliomyelitis many years after recovery from their initial illness.*

▶ *INQUIRY SUMMARY.* The relationship between force and velocity and the relationship between velocity and power output have important implications for our daily activities and sport performances. The greater the speed of shortening in a muscle, the less force the muscle will generate. However, as the velocity of a muscle increases, the power output of the muscle increases as well but only up to a certain point. Think about the force/velocity or power/velocity relationships in terms of rehabilitation. *What do you think the optimal position of the quadriceps muscle is if you are working to improve force production in a patient who just underwent knee replacement?*

## *Muscle Strength*

Whether one's goal is to perform well in activities of daily living (ADL) or to excel in a chosen sport or recreational activity, adequate muscle strength is important for everyone. The concepts related to structure and function of skeletal muscle were presented in Chapter 10 and in earlier portions of this chapter.

### SKELETAL MUSCLE ADAPTATIONS TO STRENGTH TRAINING

As mentioned previously, skeletal muscle is extremely adaptable to the stresses placed on it, and the response of skeletal muscle to strength training is no exception. Strength training is a situation in which the muscle is required to contract more forcefully to move an external load. The visible signs of a strength-training program include an increase in muscle size and the ability to lift heavier objects. But what happens within the skeletal muscle for these changes to occur?

The changes that result in increased muscle strength include both neural and muscle components. Studies have shown that in the early stages of strength programs, the initial increase in muscle strength is the result of neural factors (10,11). By using electromyography, these researchers showed increased motor unit recruitment and improved synchronization of motor unit discharge following a strength-training program. Normally all of the motor units in skeletal muscle are not activated at the same time during a muscle contraction. Rather, the motor units are asynchronously activated—some motor units are active and other motor units are not active. If more units are synchronously activated as a result of a strength-training program, more muscle fibers are stimulated to contract simultaneously and muscle force increases.

The other mechanism by which muscle strength increases is muscle hypertrophy. With repeated bouts of resistance training, the actual muscle fibers undergo hypertrophy by adding actin and myosin filaments to the periphery of each myofibril. The increase in the number of

Box 11.2

## R E S E A R C H   H I G H L I G H T

**Posterino GS, Fryer MW. Mechanisms underlying phosphate-induced failure of $Ca^{2+}$ release in single skinned skeletal muscle fibres of the rat.** *J Physiol* **1998;512: 97–108.**

### RESEARCH SUMMARY

Much research has been conducted to identify mechanisms that lead to skeletal muscle fatigue. One such theory postulates that skeletal muscle fatigue results from the accumulation of inorganic phosphate ($P_i$). Accumulation of $P_i$ produces muscle fatigue in single *in vitro* fibers and in intact *in vivo* muscle fibers as a result of a decrease in calcium ($Ca^{2+}$) release from the sarcoplasmic reticulum. This research concluded that movement of $P_i$ from the myoplasm into the sarcoplasmic reticulum lumen inhibited $Ca^{2+}$ release as a result of the formation of a $Ca^{2+}$–$P_i$ precipitate.

The researchers in the present study were interested in characterizing the rate and magnitude of $P_i$ fluxes between the myoplasm and sarcoplasmic reticulum to identify the pathways through which these fluxes occur. To do this, researchers removed the extensor digitorum longus muscles from rats. From the whole muscle, the researchers carefully isolated single muscle fibers and attached the fibers to an isometric force transducer. The force transducer was connected to a chart recorder so that force output could be measured and visualized. To elicit force production, single fibers were bathed in a solution that contained caffeine and a low concentration of magnesium. As the fiber contracted, the researchers were also able to make estimations of the amount of $Ca^{2+}$ released from the sarcoplasmic reticulum and correlate with peak force response.

The researchers then placed the fibers in a solution that contained a large concentration of $P_i$. They found that $P_i$ reduced the amount of $Ca^{2+}$ released by the sarcoplasmic reticulum in both concentration- and time-dependent manners. Next researchers "washed" $P_i$ from the fibers and followed the recovery of $Ca^{2+}$ release from the sarcoplasmic reticulum. The half-recovery time for $Ca^{2+}$ release was 35 seconds, and full recovery time was approximately 7 minutes. The researchers also repeated this experiment but removed ATP from the myoplasm. Interestingly they found that when ATP was removed, $Ca^{2+}$ release was much further impaired than when ATP was available.

It was determined that $P_i$ enters the sarcoplasmic reticulum through a passive process; however, it was unknown through which pores or channels this may occur. They also determined that the inhibition of $Ca^{2+}$ release from the sarcoplasmic reticulum by $P_i$ is a complicated process, but that the rate of $P_i$ movement across the sarcoplasmic reticulum is influenced by the rate, extent, and species of $Ca^{2+}$–$P_i$ precipitate that is formed. Furthermore, the fact that $P_i$ was more inhibitory when ATP was removed indicates that $P_i$ may inhibit $Ca^{2+}$ release from the sarcoplasmic reticulum much more efficiently during the later stages of muscular fatigue.

### IMPLICATIONS FOR FURTHER RESEARCH

These results are very interesting in that the researchers were unable to identify the pores or channels that $P_i$ passively diffuses through into the sarcoplasmic reticulum. Future research will be necessary to identify and characterize these channels. The findings of this study also are important in that they provide further insight into $P_i$ movements and help in understanding the time course of metabolic fatigue as well as the time course of recovery from muscle fatigue.

---

actin and myosin filaments occurs because with resistance training, there is an increase in protein synthesis (12) and a decrease in protein degradation (13), resulting in an overall increase in protein balance. An increase in the number of myofibrils within the muscle fiber means that there are more crossbridges for force production and consequently the entire muscle generates more force when it contracts.

A controversial idea about the mechanisms underlying the increase in strength with resistance training is fiber hyperplasia. Several studies in animal models have shown an increase in actual muscle fiber number following a period of resistance training (14,15). However, the evidence to

suggest that muscle hyperplasia or new muscle fiber formation occurs in humans remains inconclusive.

### MEASUREMENT OF MUSCLE STRENGTH

Muscle strength and endurance are two important components of athletic performance and the performance of daily routines. Muscle strength needs to be measured prior to the start of an exercise program. For example, it is common for athletes to engage in a strength-training program; by periodically assessing strength gains, the exercise program can be adjusted. Likewise, for maintenance of physical fitness in well and chronic disease populations, an

## CASE STUDY 11.1:  *POST-POLIO SYNDROME*

### CASE

Carol, a 65-year-old female with a diagnosis of post polio syndrome (PPS), is a patient in your clinic seeking advice about an exercise program. Her past medical history is significant for polio at the age 20. She reports that she recovered from the polio with the only deficit being that of left ankle dorsiflexor weakness or "foot drop." She states that her post-polio condition has been stable throughout her adult life until the last 2 years when she noticed subtle changes in her muscle strength and the development of fatigue. She associated these changes with normal aging and also with her stressful job as an attorney. However, the weakness and fatigue has been growing progressively worse. She finally sought medical attention and received the diagnosis of PPS. Carol has recently retired and would like to begin a general exercise program to improve her strength and overall fitness level.

### DESCRIPTION

Aside from her polio and PPS diagnoses, Carol reports no significant past medical history. She is married with two grown children who live in the area. She and her husband live in a single-story dwelling. Carol has four grandchildren and would like to be able to keep up with their physical activities. Her husband also is retired and they plan to become involved in some community service activities. Their passion is traveling, which they hope to continue to do as long as Carol can.

Prior to Carol initiating an exercise program, it was necessary to obtain an objective assessment of her baseline abilities. No deficits were noted in the assessment of her passive and active ranges of motion. Strength via manual muscle testing was 5/5 in both upper extremities. Bilateral hip muscles were graded 4+/5, bilateral quadriceps were 3+/5, left dorsiflexion was 3/5, and right dorsiflexion was 4/5. Quadriceps muscle strength was also assessed on an isokinetic dynamometer using a 3 repetition maximum (3 RM) strength test. She was only able to perform seven repetitions of antigravity exercise before she became fatigued. For Carol, it was also a good idea to do some functional testing to assess her functional performance since muscle strength often does not correlate with activities of daily living (ADL). These tests included walking capacity as measured by timing her ability to walk 300 feet with at least three changes in direction and two different grades; her stepping capacity, which is the time it takes her to ascend and descend a flight of 10 steps twice; and her orthostatic capacity, which the time it takes her to perform 10 repetitions of sit-to-stand from a conventional chair. Her reflexes were normal, and dull/sharp sensation was normal.

A bicycle ergometer exercise test was conducted to assess her cardiovascular endurance and to determine appropriate exercise intensity. The test consisted of 3-minute stages with a 1-minute rest period between stages. Each stage increased by 10 watts. Her maximal capacity was about 70 watts or about 420 kiloponds for a level of 5 metabolic equivalents (MET). Baseline heart rate (HR) and blood pressure (BP) were 84 and 120/78, respectively, and HR and BP at maximal exercise were 162 and 160/68, respectively. The rating of perceived exertion (RPE) at maximal exercise was 18/20. A quick screen of her cognitive/mental status revealed no problems in this area except for occasional depression over her diagnosis. Carol is able to take care of all of her ADL. She reports increased fatigue with stair climbing and ambulating long distances. She states that her husband helps her with errands, shopping, and cleaning the house.

An important component of the evaluation is to determine the patient/client goals. Carol states that she would like to begin a low-level exercise program. She believes that engaging in regular physical activity would improve her mental state and hopefully improve her endurance so that she can continue traveling, playing with her grandchildren, and being involved in community activities.

### INTERVENTION

Carol was instructed in a stretching program for all major muscle groups. She was instructed to perform this program once daily. A strengthening program was also initiated; since she could only perform seven repetitions of antigravity exercises without weights, it was decided that she should begin performing one set of seven repetitions without weights 3 days per week. To address her cardiovascular endurance, Carol was instructed to ambulate on a treadmill for 10 minutes at 2.0 $m \cdot hr^{-1}$ 3 days per week.

Carol will be seen in the clinic initially three times per week to monitor her exercise program. Once she is independent in her exercise program, she will exercise in her local health club. She will be encouraged to record any symptoms of fatigue she experiences, and she will also be instructed to take a day of rest between exercise sessions. She will report back to the clinic weekly for updating her exercise prescription. If no symptoms are reported, her prescription will be gradually increased; however, if she has symptoms, her prescription will not be changed for the following week. The initial resistance levels for the concentric phase of her strengthening program will be set at 75% of her 3 RM. The eccentric phase will be minimized by encouraging her to return her limbs rapidly to the originally position (~2 seconds). She will perform three sets of 20, 15, and 10 repetitions three times per week on

---

### Case Study 11.1, continued

nonconsecutive days with 90-second rests between sets and 3-minute rests between exercises. For her cardiovascular conditioning, her initial exercise prescription will use a HR of 40% to 60% of maximal HR obtained on the cycle ergometer with an RPE of 11 to 13 with MET levels in the 5 to 6 range. Duration should be up to 30 minutes total with intervals of no more than 3 minutes and recovery time of 1 minute. It is recommended that she use the Schwinn Air-Dyne bicycle or a similar piece of equipment that utilizes

both upper and lower extremity muscles. She will be instructed in monitoring her pulse rate.

Carol will also receive education not to overdo her exercise program even though she may feel good. She will also be educated in the importance of pacing activities so that she does not become fatigued. The importance of gradual increases in intensity and duration in her exercise program will be discussed with Carol. She may also benefit from participation in a PPS support group.

---

assessment and periodic monitoring of strength gains is done to ensure optimal training intensities. Finally rehabilitation from surgery or other injuries often includes strength training, and thus it is necessary to obtain a baseline level of strength prior to beginning a rehabilitation program.

Muscle strength can be assessed using a variety of methods. These methods include isometric, isotonic, and **isokinetic** testing. Usually the choice of method used is dependent on a variety of factors. Obviously the type of strength-training program that will be used often dictates the type of test used. For example, if the training program focuses on gaining strength at a variety of velocities during movement, isokinetic testing is more appropriate. Isokinetic means that the range of motion around the joint remains at constant speed throughout the motion. However, if the testing is simply to obtain a baseline level of strength to determine if a client has enough quadriceps strength to stand in an acute-care hospital setting, simple isometric testing may be all that is necessary. Other factors to consider when choosing the type of testing methods include cost of the test, time required to administer the test, and safety of the technique. Logic dictates that it is neither cost nor time effective to administer an isokinetic test to determine if a patient has the strength to stand without the knees buckling. The last factor that must be considered when choosing a strength assessment method is the rehabilitation goals of the therapist and client. For example, if the rehabilitation goal is to improve the ability to stand from a seated position, it is certainly important to assess strength of the lower extremity muscles and develop an exercise program to improve strength in weakened muscles. However, from a functional viewpoint, it may be more important to assess the ability to stand from a seated position by using a functional test that specifically examines the ability of a client to perform the task. Finally instead of measuring and training for strength, the health care professional may be interested in determining a client's power, acceleration, and speed during an activity. Measurement of these characteristics is indicative of maximal glycolytic effort.

 *LINKUP: See* **Perspective: Tests of Maximal Glycolytic Capacity,** *found at http://connection.lww.com/go/ brownexphys and on the Student Resource CD-ROM for additional information on tests designed to evaluate the various components of glycolytic capacity, such as maximal running speed, acceleration speed, and power.*

### Manual Muscle Testing

Manual muscle testing (MMT) is a procedure that can be used to evaluate the strength of either individual muscles or a group of muscles that perform the same movement. In general, MMT is used to assess strength in most medical conditions. However, in some neurologic conditions, MMT may be somewhat limited if there is an alteration in muscle tone. To assess strength in this manner, the tester needs to have some knowledge of the action of the muscle(s) to be tested, anatomic location(s) of the muscle(s), and the ability to detect even minimal muscle contraction.

With MMT, a client is asked to move the limb through the entire joint range of motion (ROM) and then is requested to hold an isometric contraction at the end of ROM while the therapist provides resistance to the isometric contraction. At the completion of the test, the muscle is assigned a grade of 0 to 5. A score of 0 indicates that there is no observable muscle contraction, while a score of 5 means that the muscle takes the joint through full motion and resists any attempt by the tester to return the joint to the starting position of the test. Grades of 1, 2, 3, and 4 are used to describe responses that are intermediate between 0 and 5.

Here is an example of testing a client's quadriceps strength to determine if the client can stand without the knees buckling. The client is in the seated position and is asked to "straighten the knee." The client straightens the knee from flexion to full extension. If the client can do this, then a grade of "3" is given for quadriceps strength. This means that the client has the strength to fully extend the knee against gravity. Next the tester provides some

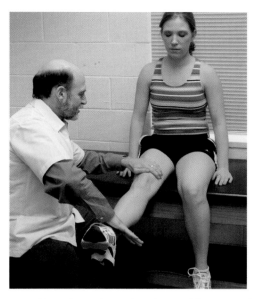

FIGURE 11.8. Manual muscle testing the quadriceps muscle in the antigravity position.

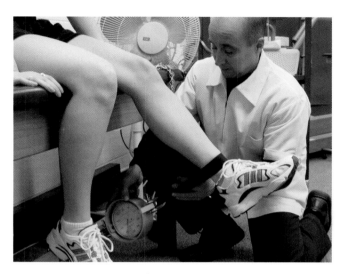

FIGURE 11.10. Assessing quadriceps strength using a cable tensiometer.

resistance to the quadriceps by placing the hand on the tibia and attempting to push the knee back down into flexion. The client resists this action, and if the client is able to fully prevent any movement into knee flexion, the quadriceps is given a score of "5" (*Fig. 11.8*).

With MMT, if the client is not able to fully extend the knee due to decreased quadriceps strength, the client is placed in a position in which gravity is eliminated and the client is then asked to straighten the knee (*Fig. 11.9*). If the tester sees no obvious muscle contraction, the quadriceps muscle is assigned a score of "0." MMT is quick and easy to do, and it provides a good general assessment of the strength of the muscle in a setting in which other sophisticated methods of testing strength are not cost or time effective. MMT can be performed for all of the muscles of the body.

## Tensiometry

Tensiometry is another way to measure isometric strength of a muscle. The instrumentation includes a tensiometer, steel cables, testing table, wall hooks, and goniometer. The cable is attached to either the wall or table hooks while the other end of the cable is attached to the body part being tested via a strap (*Fig. 11.10*). It is important to be sure that the cable is positioned at right angles to the body part that is being tested. The goniometer is used to measure the joint angle. The individual being tested is then asked to exert force on the cable for at least 5 seconds, and the needle on the tensiometer measures the amount of force generated. Tensiometers usually measure forces in the range of 0 to 400 pounds.

Tensiometers can be used to measure strength at various joint angles. Usually at each joint angle, three trials of strength assessment are done, and the trial with the highest force is considered to be the measure of strength. This type of testing is well suited to assess strength impairment at specific joint angles and is a safe test to administer. However, one of the disadvantages is that testing must be done at many joint angles to obtain an idea of the strength throughout the ROM and thus is time consuming. Furthermore, most movement uses dynamic actions as opposed to static actions. Therefore, this type of testing may not be a true representation of strength throughout a dynamic motion.

## Dynamometry

Dynamometers are used to assess both static strength and endurance of the hand, forearm, leg, and back muscles (*Fig. 11.11*). Dynamometers are spring-loaded devices. As force is applied to the dynamometer, the spring is compressed and moves a needle to indicate the force output from the muscle. For accuracy, dynamometers should be calibrated with a known weight. To assess grip strength, the dynamometer is adjusted to accommodate the size of the

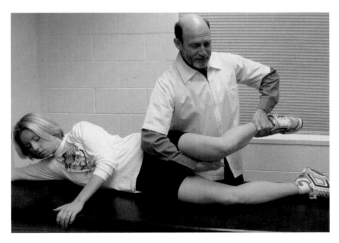

FIGURE 11.9. Manual muscle testing the quadriceps muscle in the gravity-eliminated position.

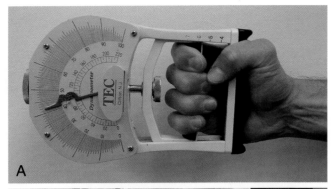

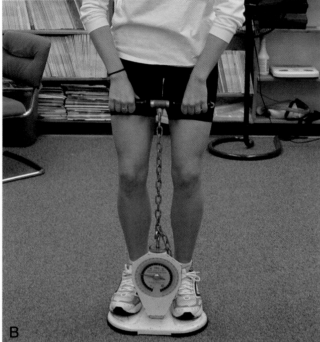

**FIGURE 11.11.** Example of a **(A)** hand-grip dynamometer for assessing grip strength and **(B)** back-lift dynamometer to assess back strength.

hand of the person being tested. The individual is then asked to squeeze the dynamometer as hard as possible without moving the upper extremity. Usually three trials are administered, and the trial with the highest force is considered to be the measure of strength. Each contraction should be 4 to 5 seconds in duration with 1-minute rests between contractions. To assess grip endurance, the individual is asked to grip the dynamometer as hard as possible for 60 seconds, and force is recorded every 10 seconds. In this test, as muscle endurance improves, the decline of force during the test decreases by the end of the 60-second testing period.

To assess leg strength with a dynamometer, the individual stands on a platform with the trunk erect and knees flexed. The individual holds onto a bar attached to the dynamometer and extends the knees without using the back muscles. The indicator needle measures the force generated, and the highest force in three trials is considered to be the best measure of force.

The same type of dynamometer to measure leg strength can also be used to measure back strength. In this situation, the individual stands on the platform with the knees extended and head and truck upright. The individual pulls on the handbar straight upward using the back muscles. Again the indicator measures the amount of force generated, and usually two or three trials are done to obtain the best assessment of back strength.

As with tensiometry, dynamometers are good tools to assess static strength, but if the intent is to obtain the amount of force an individual can generate throughout the ROM, this test may not be the best one. However, this equipment is fairly inexpensive (as compared with computerized assessment) and dynamometry is easy to administer.

 *See Experiences in Work Physiology Lab Exercise 10: Muscle-Length Tension Relationship for an exercise in determining the relationship between muscle length and force output.*

## One Repetition Maximum

The assessment of strength using the one repetition maximum (1 RM) technique requires the individual to lift a maximal weight in a single dynamic repetition. This type of testing assesses the isotonic strength of a muscle in which an object of fixed mass is lifted against gravity. Isotonic testing is generally performed on machines that feature adjustable weight stacks for resistance, such as Nautilus, Universal, and Cybex. 1 RM testing can also be done with free weights.

To test the 1 RM for any given movement, the individual lifts a weight that is a percentage of a weight believed to be fairly close to the expected 1 RM. Prior to beginning the 1 RM assessment, it is recommended that the individual perform a general warmup of light activity (3 to 5 minutes) of the muscle to be tested. Next the individual should perform a warmup set of eight repetitions at 50% of estimated 1 RM, followed by a second set of three repetitions at 70% of estimated 1 RM. At this point, the individual should perform single repetitions of progressively heavier weights until muscle failure occurs (16). When failure occurs, a weight approximately midway between the weight at failure and the last successful weight lifted should be attempted (16). This last step can be repeated to the desired level of precision. It is recommended that the rest interval between sets be no more than 5 minutes and not less than 1 minute, while the optimal number of single repetitions is between three and five.

Determining 1 RM is easy to do and can be done with equipment as simple as barbells. However, requesting a person to lift 1 RM may predispose him or her to injury. Therefore, it may be safer to have the individual lift the most amount of weight possible in three to six repetitions as opposed to lifting a heavier weight in one repetition. However, if information regarding force generation over a full ROM is necessary, it may be better to perform a computerized

## CASE STUDY 11.2:  *SPINAL CORD INJURY*

### CASE

Scott is a 30-year-old male who suffered a complete spinal cord injury at L1 as a result of a motor vehicle accident at the age of 18. He completed his college education and is a rehabilitation counselor. Up until recently, he had been a functional ambulator with lower extremity bracing and crutches; however, he feels that the energy cost to ambulate is too great and has decided to use his wheelchair 100% of the time for mobility. He is concerned that he will lose upper body strength and endurance as a result of his decision. He would also like to improve his cardiovascular fitness.

### DESCRIPTION

Other than his spinal cord injury, Scott's past medical and surgical history is negative. Scott is single, lives independently in the community, and drives an adapted van. He uses a manual wheelchair for mobility. He enjoys reading and watching sporting events. Scott leads a support group for clients with recent spinal cord injuries.

Scott's range of motion is within normal limits in both upper extremities. No contractures have been noted in lower extremities. His upper extremity body strength is 5/5 bilaterally. A Wingate anaerobic power test during arm-cranking indicated a high anaerobic fatigue index. Peak power output during a discontinuous arm-crank ergometry protocol was 45 watts. Resting heart rate (HR) and blood pressure (BP) were 68 and 105/70, respectively. At peak exercise, HR and BP were 120 and 140/66, respectively. There are no areas of skin breakdown or redness noted in any weightbearing areas. Functional testing revealed that Scott was able to push his wheelchair 750 meters in 6 minutes, and it took him 15 seconds to push his wheelchair up a standard ramp.

### INTERVENTION

To address his cardiovascular endurance, it was recommended to Scott that he begin arm-crank exercise at a low load at a rating of perceived exertion of 3 to 4/10 for 5 minutes two or three times per week. Alternatively, HR reserve formulas can be used to gauge exercise intensity:

$$\%HR_{reserve} = (HR_{peak} - HR_{observed})$$
$$\div (HR_{peak} - HR_{rest}) \times 100$$

As his aerobic capacity improves, he can increase his time and intensity. He may want to consider doing interval or fartlek training as well. To combat the boredom of arm-cranking, he should also consider training by pushing his wheelchair a specific distance at a speed to elicit a training HR response.

For upper body strengthening, his 3–6 repetition maximum (3–6 RM) should be used to develop his strength-training program for major muscle groups of his upper extremities. He should lift weights at 75% of his 3–6 RM for three sets of 10 repetitions two to three times per week. He should increase his strength-training regimen using the overload principle. To improve his muscle endurance, he should do one set of 10 repetitions in 1 minute and increase the number of repetitions and time as his endurance improves.

Another consideration that Scott may want to think about is a nutrition consultation to improve his eating habits to prevent weight gain. He might also consider joining a wheelchair basketball team for a social outlet and to complement his exercise regimen.

---

assessment of force. Case Study 11.2 presents how initial assessment of muscle strength can be used to design an exercise program for a person with a spinal cord injury.

### Computerized Force and Power Output

Over the last 20 years there has been much interest in using computerized equipment to assess dynamic force output. In fact, assessing strength using this equipment is probably the most commonly used method to assess force output in the rehabilitation setting. The equipment used to assess force in this way is the isokinetic dynamometer *(Fig. 11.12)*. With this dynamometer, the speed of motion stays the same throughout the motion while the resistance applied by the dynamometer varies. This resistance is designed to match the force generated by the muscle throughout the ROM. Contained within the dynamometer is a force transducer that monitors the force throughout the entire ROM at a

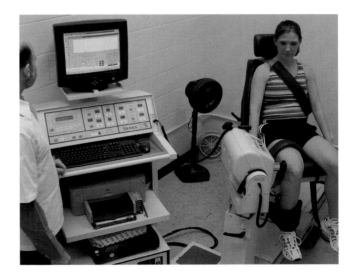

**FIGURE 11.12.** Isokinetic testing equipment.

constant speed. This information is relayed to a computer for computation of force output at each point in the joint angle. Once these computations are completed, force output is displayed on a screen. This force calculation is done very rapidly, and the output on the screen is displayed in "real time" as the motion is occurring.

Because the ROM through which the joint is moving is measured and also because the angular velocity at which the dynamometer moves is set by the examiner, the dynamometer is really measuring torque output by the client. The advantage of this type of strength-assessment

equipment is that the health care professional obtains information about what happened in terms of force output throughout the entire ROM as opposed to only one point in time. However, the primary disadvantage of isokinetic testing is that very few, if any, functional movements are done isokinetically. Consequently, while isokinetic testing does give us data regarding muscle strength, this information may not relate to the capacity of the client to perform functional activities. Case Study 11.3 presents how the use of an isokinetic dynamometer can be used to design an exercise program for a patient with knee osteoarthritis.

## CASE STUDY 11.3: *OSTEOARTHRITIS*

### CASE

Estelle is a 65-year-old retired nursing technician who is referred to an outpatient physical therapy clinic because of osteoarthritis of the right knee. She reports occasional pain in her right knee that is increased with walking more than two blocks and with stair climbing. Estelle also has difficulty rising from a chair. She attributes her arthritis to being on her feet much of the day in her job as a nursing technician.

### DESCRIPTION

Review of her past medical and surgical history reveals only that Estelle had a history of asthma as a child. She takes a nonsteroidal antiinflammatory medication for her arthritis.

Estelle is married and has three children and seven grandchildren. She enjoys cooking and having weekly large family dinners. She is also very involved with her church.

Prior to the development of her exercise program, an objective evaluation is performed. Her range of motion is grossly normal in all extremities. Maximal isotonic quadriceps and hamstring muscle strengths were assessed by an isokinetic dynamometer at 90 degrees·s$^{-1}$, 120 degrees·s$^{-1}$, and 150 degrees·s$^{-1}$, as well as isometric strengths of the quadriceps and hamstring muscles at knee angles of 0, 30, 60, and 90 degrees.

Estelle has normal reflexes and sensation throughout all four extremities. Inspection/palpation reveals bony hypertrophy and crepitus in her right knee. There are no signs of inflammation in her right knee. Since one of Estelle's major complaints is pain, it is important to obtain a pain rating. Using a 10-point scale, her pain was rated as 4/10 at rest and 6/10 with weightbearing.

X-rays showed osteophytes and questionable narrowing at the medial joint space in the right knee.

A cycle ergometer-graded exercise test revealed the following: resting heart rate (HR) was 82; blood

pressure (BP) was 132/82. Estelle was able to complete 6 minutes of the test before stopping secondary to knee pain and muscle fatigue in the lower extremities. Her peak HR and BP were 120 and 162/80, respectively. Functional assessment reveals that Estelle is independent in all activities of daily living.

Anthropometric measurements reveal that she is 5'5" tall and weighs 180 pounds. Her body mass index is 30, which puts her in the obese category.

### INTERVENTION

To increase her strength, Estelle will perform two sets of 10 repetitions at 90 degrees·s$^{-1}$, 120 degrees·s$^{-1}$, and 150 degrees·s$^{-1}$ three times per week at 10% of her isometric maximum force at those angles. As her strength increases, the amount of weight lifted will be increased. She will also be instructed to do maximal isometric contractions (five times for 9 seconds at knee angles of 0, 30, 60, and 90 degrees) for both the quadriceps and hamstring muscles. To improve her muscle endurance, she will be instructed to lift 10% of maximal weight as measured at her evaluation and to hold this isometric contraction for 90 seconds for five repetitions. As her endurance improves, the amount of weight will be increased. Estelle will also be instructed in a flexibility program to include gentle static stretching exercises to be done once daily.

To improve her cardiovascular endurance, Estelle will be instructed to ride the cycle ergometer for 10 minutes at 40% to 50% of target HR three times per week. As her cardiovascular endurance improves, the duration and intensity of her exercise prescription will be slowly increased. She will also be referred to a nutritionist for diet evaluation. Losing weight would likely help decrease the pain in her right knee and decrease her risk of cardiovascular disease.

Patient education is an important component of treatment so Estelle will receive education regarding the disease process of osteoarthritis, joint protection, other osteoarthritis self-management techniques, nutrition, and how to cope with pain and disability.

## Functional Tests of Strength

Quite often in the clinical setting, clients exhibit declines in muscle strength as a result of injury or illness. These strength decrements may be one factor in the inability of a client to perform ADL such as ambulating, rising from a sitting position, and getting dressed. While any of the above methods for assessing strength are important in the evaluation of a rehabilitation client and addressing functional limitations, often it is more useful to assess the client's ability to perform functional activities following a period of rehabilitation rather than to conduct pure assessments of muscle strength. Consequently there are a variety of assessment tools that can be used to objectively quantify a client's ability to perform ADL. One example is the timed up and go test (17). This test is used to measure mobility, balance, and locomotor performance in elderly people. In this test, a client sits in a standard armchair, stands up, walks 3 meters at a comfortable and safe pace, turns, walks back to the chair, and sits down (17). The score obtained is the actual time that it took to perform the task. This test may also be useful for other patients such as deconditioned elderly persons, clients with rheumatoid arthritis and osteoarthritis, and clients with total joint arthroplasty (18).

Another common clinical assessment tool is the functional independence measure (FIM). This assessment tool includes 18 items that describe stages of complete dependence to complete independence in the performance of basic ADL (19). The FIM can be used with a variety of patient populations, including those with spinal cord injuries or multiple sclerosis and elderly individuals undergoing inpatient rehabilitation (18).

▶ *INQUIRY SUMMARY.* There are a variety of methods with which to measure strength. The choice of which test to use depends on the information the tester is interested in obtaining, practice setting, safety of the test, and financial implications. The simplest form of strength testing is MMT, which is most commonly conducted in an acute-care patient setting. Other forms of isometric testing use a tensiometer or dynamometer. The 1 RM is a useful test for assessing dynamic strength. However, if the tester is interested in the force generated by a client throughout the entire ROM, then isokinetic testing may be more useful. Finally, in clinical settings, functional tests of ADL may be more useful in documenting and measuring outcomes following rehabilitation. *What type of testing might be best to determine if an athlete who underwent knee reconstruction surgery can begin to resume light workouts?*

## *Summary*

The motor unit consists of the α-motoneuron and muscle fibers that it innervates. The number of muscle fibers contained within a motor unit is variable, but generally the innervation ratio is large in muscles responsible for large movements. In small muscles, for which fine motions are essential, the innervation ratio is small. Motor units can be divided into slow, fast fatigue-resistant, and fast. The properties that are used to make these divisions are twitch tension, fatigue index, and tetanic tension characteristics. Slow motor units have small-twitch tensions, are slower to contract, and are fatigue resistant. The fast, fatigue-resistant motor units generate moderate-twitch tension, are fatigue resistant, and are fast to contract, while the fast fatigable motor units generate high tension, contract quickly, and fatigue quickly. Motor units are recruited for activity via the all or none phenomenon, which means that all of the muscle fibers contained within that motor unit are stimulated to contract when a motor neuron is stimulated. To control the amount of force produced, either the number of motor units that are recruited changes or the frequency of discharge of the motor units changes. Motor units are recruited based on size; the smallest motor units are recruited first, then the medium-sized units, and the largest motor units are recruited last. Two important concepts related to muscle mechanics are the relationship between muscle length and tension generation and the relationship between force and velocity. The length-tension relationship states that the sarcomere (or muscle) needs to be at an optimal length to generate maximal force. This means that actin and myosin need to be at an optimal distance from one another during crossbridge cycling to produce maximal force. The force-velocity relationship means that the faster the muscle is contracting, the less force it generates. Muscle fatigue is a complex process and is defined as the temporary decline in muscle force as a result of exercise or activity. Fatigue can be due to a limitation of substrates to produce energy; as a result of changes in pH, which can limit several processes directly involved in muscle contraction; as a result of impairment at the neuromuscular junction; and/or as a result of failure to recruit motor units. There are a variety of methods to measure muscle strength; isometric methods include manual muscle testing, tensiometry, and dynamometry, while dynamic methods include 1 repetition maximum and isokinetic testing. Finally there are a variety of tools that can be used in a clinical setting to assess functional outcomes as a result of rehabilitation.

## *SUMMARY KNOWLEDGE*

1. Describe motor unit anatomy.
2. Compare and contrast the three different types of motor units in terms of their properties of twitch tension, tetanic tension, and fatigability.
3. What is the size principle?
4. Discuss how sarcomere length can affect force development.
5. What is muscle fatigue and what are some of the potential mechanisms that cause it?
6. Define isometric, concentric, and eccentric muscle contractions.

7. Describe both the neural and muscle changes that occur with strength training and result in increased force production.
8. Compare and contrast the methods for assessing muscle strength.

### References

1. Burke WE, Levine DN, Zajac FE 3rd. Mammalian motor units: physiological-histochemical correlation in three types in cat gastrocnemius. *Science* 1971;174:709–712.
2. Edgerton VR, Roy RR, Bodine S, et al. Matching of neuronal and muscular physiology. In: Borer KT, Edington DW, White TP, eds. *Frontiers of exercise biology*. Champaign, Ill: Human Kinetics, 1983.
3. Smith JL, Betts B, Edgerton VR, et al. Rapid ankle extension during paw shakes: selective recruitment of fast ankle extensors. *J Neurophysiol* 1980;43:612–620.
4. Hill AV. The heat of shortening and the dynamic constants of muscle. *Proc Royal Soc London Series B* 1938;126:136–195.
5. Woods JJ, Furbush F, Biglund-Ritchie B. Evidence for a fatigue-induced reflex inhibition of motoneuron firing rates. *J Neurophysiol* 1987;58:125–137.
6. Westerblad H, Allen DG. Changes in myoplasmic calcium concentration during fatigue in single mouse muscle fibers. *J Gen Physiol* 1991;98:615–635.
7. Ball KL, Johnson MD, Solaro RJ. Isoform specific interactions of troponin I and troponin C determine pH sensitivity of myofibrillar $Ca^{2+}$ activation. *Biochemistry* 1994;33:8464–8471.
8. Cooke R, Franks K, Luciani GB, et al. The inhibition of rabbit skeletal muscle contraction by hydrogen ions and phosphate. *J Physiol* 1988;395:77–97.
9. Stackhouse SK, Reisman DS, Binder-Macleod SA. Challenging the role of pH in skeletal muscle fatigue. *Phys Ther* 2001;81:1897–1903.
10. Hakkinen K, Komi PV. Electromyographic changes during strength training and detraining. *Med Sci Sports Exerc* 1983;15:455–460.
11. Sale DG. Neural adaptation to resistance training. *Med Sci Sports Exerc* 1988;20:S135–S145.
12. MacDougall JD, Gibala MJ, Tarnopolsky MA, et al. The time course for elevated muscle protein synthesis following heavy resistance exercise. *Can J Appl Phys* 1995;20:480–486.
13. Phillips SM, Tipton KD, Aarskind A, et al. Mixed muscle protein synthesis and breakdown after resistance exercise in humans. *Am J Physiol* 1997;273:E99–E107.
14. Antonio J, Gonyea WJ. Skeletal muscle fiber hyperplasia. *Med Sci Sports Exerc* 1993;25:1333–1345.
15. Gonyea WJ. Role of exercise in inducing increases in skeletal muscle fiber number. *J Appl Phys* 1980;48:421–426.
16. Brown LE, Weir JP. ASEP procedures recommendation I: Accurate assessment of muscular strength and power. *JEPonline* 2001;4:1–21.
17. Podsiadlo D, Richardson S. The timed "up & go": a test of basic functional mobility for frail elderly persons. *J Am Geriatr Soc* 1991;39:142–148.
18. Finch E, Brooks D, Stratford PW, et al. *Physical rehabilitation outcome measures: a guide to enhanced clinical decision making.* 2nd ed. Hamilton, Ontario: BC Decker, Inc, 2002.
19. Granger CV. The emerging science of functional assessment: our tool for outcomes analysis. *Arch Phys Med Rehabil* 1998;79:235–240.

### Suggested Readings

Bawa P. Neural control of motor output: can training change it? *Exerc Sport Sci Rev* 2002;30:59–63.
Burke RE. Motor unit types of cat triceps surae muscle. *J Physiol* 1967;193:141–160.
Burke RE. Motor units. Anatomy, physiology and functional organization. In: Brooks VB, ed. *Handbook of physiology. The nervous system.* Bethesda, Md: American Physiological Society, 1981:345–422.
Fitts RH. Muscle fatigue: the cellular aspects. *Am J Sports Med* 1996;24:S9–S13.
Lewis SF, Fulco CS. A new approach to studying muscle fatigue and factors affecting performance during dynamic exercise in humans. *Exerc Sport Sci Rev* 1998;26:91–116.
Semmler JG. Motor unit synchronization and neuromuscular performance. *Exerc Sport Sci Rev* 2002;30:8–14.

### On the Internet

Harvard University Gazette: Faculty of Medicine Memorial Minute: Elwood Henneman. Available at: **http://www.news.harvard.edu/gazette/1998/09.17/FacultyofMedici.html.** Accessed May 12, 2005.
National Institute of Neurological Disorders and Stroke: NINDS Post-Polio Syndrome Information Page. Available at: **http://www.ninds.nih.gov/disorders/post_polio/post_polio.htm.** Accessed May 12, 2005.
Post-Polio Health International: Information about the Late Effects of Polio. Available at: **http://www.post-polio.org/ipn/aboutlep.html.** Accessed May 12, 2005.
Amyotrophic Lateral Sclerosis Association. Available at: **http://www.alsa.org/.** Accessed May 12, 2005.
Delsys Inc.: Electromyography tutorials. Available at: **http://www.delsys.com/library/tutorials.htm.** Accessed May 12, 2005.
Wingate Anaerobic Cycle Test. Available at: **http://www.brianmac.demon.co.uk/want.htm.** Accessed May 12, 2005.

## Writing to Learn

*Chapter 11 presents information regarding motor unit recruitment, which may be applied to sport-specific training. Write a paper describing how exercise training can modify motor unit activation.*

# Applied Exercise Physiology

After focusing on the basic science of human movement in Part 1, Part 2 introduces applied concepts. Section 1 addresses the important issues of health, fitness and performance in three key chapters necessary to the study of exercise physiology. Chapter 12 explores how exercise performance is affected by nutritional status. Related to this are concepts of body composition assessment that are presented in Chapter 13. Chapter 14 rounds out the section by covering concepts and methods of training for sport performance.

Section 2 contains material about three important subgroups requiring special treatment in an exercise physiology text: children, older individuals, and females. Physiological responses and adaptations in these three groups have received much research attention lately; therefore, three specific chapters are warranted to highlight this information.

## SECTION 1  PHYSIOLOGY OF HEALTH, FITNESS, AND PERFORMANCE

## SECTION 2  EXERCISE PERFORMANCE FOR SPECIFIC POPULATIONS

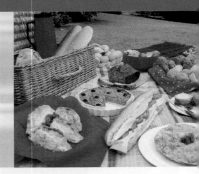

## CHAPTER

# 12 Nutrition and Exercise Performance

*Dietary nutrients are not only essential for optimal health, but most play a critical role in exercise physiology. This knowledge has prompted many athletes, sports participants, and fitness professionals to experiment with different dietary regimens and dietary supplements in the search for optimal health and exercise performance. One prevailing view that leads many people to habitually consume megadoses of some nutrients is the "overkill principle." The overkill principle assumes that if a little is good, then a lot must be better. Unfortunately, there remains a large gap between scientifically sound nutritional guidelines for athletes and the actual dietary practices of many athletes. You are probably aware of some popular diets or dietary supplements that claim to enhance exercise performance, build muscle mass, or cause weight loss.* How can you as a professional evaluate whether the claims behind these popular practices are supported by scientific evidence?

CARBOHYDRATE INTAKE AND EXERCISE PERFORMANCE
- High-Carbohydrate Diets
- Carbohydrate Ingestion Prior to Exercise
- Carbohydrate Ingestion During Exercise
- Carbohydrate Ingestion After Exercise
HIGH-FAT DIETS
HIGH-PROTEIN DIETS
FAD DIETS AND WEIGHT LOSS

EXERCISE PERFORMANCE AND VITAMIN/MINERAL SUPPLEMENTS
- Vitamin Supplements
- Mineral Supplements
- Evaluation of Dietary Supplements
  - Supplement Regulation
  - SOAP Process for Supplement Evaluation
EXERCISE PERFORMANCE AND FLUID INTAKE

Desperate to gain a competitive edge, many athletes experiment with the latest dietary regimen or nutritional supplement that happens to be popular. More often than not, fad products and programs are not regulated for safety, nor are they shown to be efficacious. Since many athletes and fitness enthusiasts are not formally educated in nutrition, they are often persuaded to participate in unhealthy nutritional practices because those whom appear to be trustworthy promote these practices. Thus, health professionals who work with athletes or recreational exercisers must know how to evaluate the validity of nutritional claims and practices. In this chapter, you will learn how to design optimal nutritional guidelines for exercising individuals and how to evaluate the validity of the numerous nutritional programs and supplements that appear on the market every day.

## Carbohydrate Intake and Exercise Performance

You learned in Chapters 2 and 3 that carbohydrate, fat, and protein are the three energy-yielding nutrients used to support the energy demands of exercise. You also learned that the proportion of the energy supply for exercise derived from each of these nutrients is dependent upon the intensity and duration of the exercise bout. Of these three nutrients, carbohydrates are probably the most significant during exercise because they can be used as a primary fuel for both rapid and slow glycolysis. However, body carbohydrate stores are limited, and athletes have long been concerned with the relationship between carbohydrate and exercise performance for this reason.

# HIGH-CARBOHYDRATE DIETS

**Carbohydrate loading** is probably the most popular dietary practice among competitive athletes. Although carbohydrate loading has been proven to be an effective boost to exercise performance, many competitors do not understand the principles behind carbohydrate loading, while others practice carbohydrate loading when its benefits do not apply to their particular sport or event.

Carbohydrates supply about 50% of the body's energy needs during moderate-intensity exercise and almost 100% during very intense exercise. One of the principles behind carbohydrate loading is that muscular fatigue is associated with the depletion of muscle glycogen stores. The other principle is that muscle glycogen stores can be boosted above normal levels through diet and exercise manipulation, and that this boost enhances exercise performance. However, these principles are based on certain assumptions and conditions. For example, the correlation between muscle glycogen depletion and muscular fatigue exists only at an exercise intensity of approximately 75% of $\dot{V}O_{2max}$ and takes about 90 minutes to occur (*Fig. 12.1*). $\dot{V}O_{2max}$ is the maximal level of aerobic metabolism that an individual can sustain. Hence, 75% of $\dot{V}O_{2max}$ is indicative of work intensity equal to 75% of an individual's aerobic capacity. A work intensity above maximal aerobic capacity represents an exercise effort in which the energy demand is met by contributions from both anaerobic and aerobic sources and is expressed as more than 100% of $\dot{V}O_{2max}$.

It is clearly demonstrated in Figure 12.1 that fatigue is not caused by glycogen depletion during continuous exercise performance at intensities above or below 75% of $\dot{V}O_{2max}$. Figure 12.1 also shows that exercise bouts of durations less than 90 minutes are not compromised by depleted glycogen stores. This means that most athletes need not concern themselves with glycogen depletion or carbohydrate loading. The only athletes that need to be concerned with muscle glycogen and fatigue are those athletes performing continuous exercise at approximately 75% of

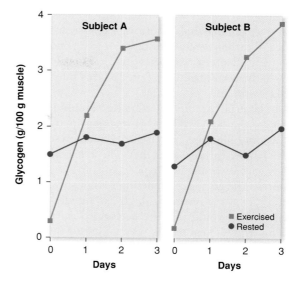

**FIGURE 12.2.** Glycogen supercompensation following a carbohydrate-loading regimen. Red represents the exercised leg, and blue represents the rested leg. Data from Hultman E. Physiological role of muscle glycogen in man, with special reference to exercise. *Circ Res* 1967;20(Suppl 1):I99–I112.

$\dot{V}O_{2max}$ for 90 minutes or more and those athletes who perform repetitive exercise bouts at exercise intensities above 75% $\dot{V}O_{2max}$ that are interspersed with short rest intervals. Athletes exercising under the conditions described above, in which muscle glycogen depletion does contribute to fatigue, can prolong the onset of fatigue by carbohydrate loading.

Early research by Hultman (1) demonstrated that muscles previously depleted of their glycogen stores overcompensate by synthesizing more than twice the glycogen needed to restore their supply when carbohydrate again becomes available (*Fig. 12.2*). In this study, one-leg exercise to exhaustion was followed by 3 days on a high-carbohydrate diet.

Furthermore, exercise time to exhaustion is extended when muscle glycogen content is elevated above normal levels prior to exercise (*Fig. 12.3*) (2,3). The findings from

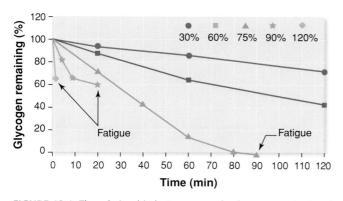

**FIGURE 12.1.** The relationship between muscle glycogen content and muscular fatigue. Percentages represent exercise intensity expressed as % $\dot{V}O_{2max}$. (Data from Saltin B, Karlsson J. Muscle glycogen utilization during work of different intensities. In: Pernow B, Saltin B, eds. *Muscle metabolism during exercise.* New York: Plenum Press, 1971:289–299.)

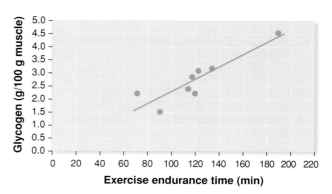

**FIGURE 12.3.** The relationship between pre-exercise muscle glycogen content and exercise time to exhaustion. (Data from Hultman E. Physiological role of muscle glycogen in man, with special reference to exercise. *Circ Res* 1967;20(Suppl 1):I99–I112.)

these early studies set the foundation for our understanding of glycogen metabolism during exercise and led to the practice of carbohydrate loading prior to an endurance exercise event. Exercise was performed on a cycle ergometer at 60% of the workload that elicited a heart rate response of 170 beats·min$^{-1}$.

The classical carbohydrate-loading technique was developed in the late 1960s. This regimen involved one or two sessions of intense exercise to exhaustion separated by 2 days of a low-carbohydrate diet. The exhaustive exercise and low-carbohydrate diet depletes the muscle of its glycogen stores. The glycogen-depleting sessions were then followed by 3 days of rest and a high-carbohydrate diet. The exercise event would then be performed on the seventh day. This type of regimen is very taxing to the body and therefore cannot be used throughout the competitive season. In addition, some of the side effects of the regimen are irritability, dizziness, hypoglycemia, and reduced exercise capacity.

The classical carbohydrate-loading technique has been replaced by a less dramatic technique that has been shown to be just as effective but not as traumatic (4). The newer regimen calls for a mixed diet (50% of energy from carbohydrate) 3 to 6 days prior to competition, with a taper in training, and then a high-carbohydrate diet (70% of energy from carbohydrate) for the few days remaining before the competition.

More recently it was shown that resting glycogen content increased by more than 80% within 24 hours of a short bout of high-intensity exercise (5). In this study on rapid carbohydrate loading following exercise, athletes exercised at 130% of $\dot{V}O_{2max}$ for 3 minutes. The athletes then consumed 12 g of carbohydrate·kg$^{-1}$ body weight over the next 24 hours, including maltodextrose-enriched beverages. Glycogen content was elevated by 82% in all fiber types of the exercised muscle. This newest regimen allows the athlete to carbohydrate load within a short time frame without disrupting his/her training schedule. Table 12.1 lists some food choices that have a high-carbohydrate content and are compatible with a carbohydrate-loading regimen.

## CARBOHYDRATE INGESTION PRIOR TO EXERCISE

Carbohydrate ingestion immediately prior to exercise can have a negative effect on exercise performance. If an athlete consumes carbohydrate-rich foods or sport drinks within 60 minutes of the beginning of an endurance exercise performance, the glucose from the ingested food or drink enters the circulation within minutes of ingestion (*Fig. 12.4*). The subsequent rise in blood glucose concentration causes the release of the hormone insulin, which assists in clearing glucose from the circulation. A peak in insulin concentration in the blood occurs at the time exercise begins. Consequently glucose uptake by the muscles reaches an abnormally high rate during the exercise performance.

The high rate of clearance of glucose from the blood causes **hypoglycemia**. Among other things, hypoglycemia

| Table 12.1 | FOOD SELECTIONS FOR MAINTAINING A HIGH-CARBOHYDRATE DIET |
|---|---|
| **BREAKFAST** | **LUNCH/DINNER** |
| Cold cereal | Bean burritos |
| Hot cereal | Rice |
| Pancakes | Pasta |
| Waffles | Legumes |
| Toast | Bread, buns, pita bread, rolls, cornbread |
| Bagel | Vegetable salad (non-fat dressing) |
| Fruit/vegetable juice | Vegetable soup |
| Fresh fruit | Baked Potato |
| English muffin | Lentils |
| Lowfat muffin | Fruit salad |
| Whole grain crackers | Fruits and vegetables |

**ADDITIONAL ITEMS\***
Nonfat or lowfat dairy products (skim milk, yogurt, cheese, tofu)

Lowfat beef, lowfat pork, poultry, fish

\*Additional items add variety as well as protein to the diet

causes acute fatigue. Therefore, the consumption of simple carbohydrates, which are digested and absorbed quickly, can be detrimental to exercise performance. Case 12.1 illustrates how pre-event meals can be designed for a competitive soccer player.

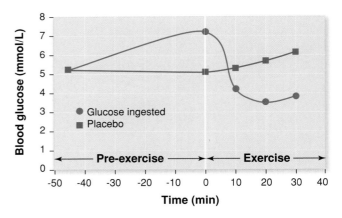

**FIGURE 12.4.** The effects of pre-exercise carbohydrate ingestion on blood glucose levels. 75 g of either glucose or a placebo were consumed 45 minutes prior to a 30-minute treadmill exercise bout at 70% of $\dot{V}O_{2max}$. (Data from Costill DL, Coyle E, Dalsky G, et al. Effect of elevated plasma FFA and insulin on muscle glycogen usage during exercise. *J Appl Physiol* 1977;43:695–699.)

## CASE STUDY 12.1:  *PRE-EVENT MEALS*

### CASE

Michael is a 20-year-old college soccer player. Michael consumes a diet that is nutritionally sound (variety, balance, 60% carbohydrate, 25% fat, 15% protein). Michael is concerned about his eating prior to competition. He is unsure of what he should be consuming. During the season, he may have games in cool weather (10°C, 50°F) or hot weather (30°C, 86°F). Michael may play three games in 3 consecutive days or may play a tournament game in the evening, followed by another game the following afternoon.

### DESCRIPTION

The general theme running throughout Chapter 12 is that the nutritional needs of athletes are similar to those of sedentary adults and that any additional needs resulting from exercise training are accommodated by the normal augmentation in energy intake seen with athletes. Dietary manipulation in the form of nutrient supplementation is generally not necessary and has not proven to enhance exercise performance. With this in mind, the training table for the athlete should be a well-balanced, palatable diet that is high in carbohydrates, low in fat, with an abundance of complete protein. The practice of carbohydrate loading should be reserved for endurance athletes whose muscle glycogen stores are critical to exercise performance. No foods consumed immediately prior to an exercise event will lead to "super" aerobic or anaerobic performance. However, the pre-event meal should provide the athlete with adequate carbohydrate, which will "top off" the glycogen stores and help ensure adequate hydration.

The pre-event meal should consist of the energy-yielding nutrients that are predominately used for fuel during the exercise and which are easily digestible. The rates of digestion, from fastest to slowest, are: simple sugars, complex carbohydrates, protein, and fat. Some simple sugars can be ingested and absorbed within a period of time as short as 30 to 60 minutes, while a high-fat, high-protein meal may take as long as 18 hours to absorb. The pre-event meal should generally adhere to the following guidelines:
- Contain 150 to 300 g of carbohydrate
- Allow for the stomach to be relatively empty at the start of the event (mealtime should be 3 to 6 hours before exercising)

- Be palatable to the athlete and be part of the athlete's customary intake
- Help to prevent or minimize gastrointestinal distress
- Ensure adequate fluid balance (avoid high-sugar loads, high-protein meals, and caffeine)

### EVALUATION/INTERVENTION

Playing conditions and game times are not consistent for Michael. Maintaining adequate glycogen stores and fluid balance are critical to Michael's performance, particularly on hot days and when more than one game may be played within 24 hours. Michael should plan his pregame meals according to the following guidelines:
- Morning game: Eat the pre-event meal for breakfast. Example: glass of orange juice, bowl of oatmeal or museli, two slices of toast with jelly, peach
- Early- to mid-afternoon game: Eat breakfast and a light lunch prior to the game. Pregame lunch example: 1 oz of turkey on a bagel, banana, lowfat yogurt, skim milk
- Late-afternoon game: Eat breakfast, lunch, and pre-game snack. Pregame snack example: fruit, bagel with jelly, whole-grain crackers, sport drink
- Night game: Eat breakfast, lunch, and a pregame dinner. Pre-game dinner example: pasta with tomato sauce, lentils, plums, skim milk
- A liquid meal may be substituted for any of the pregame meals. Liquid meals may be advantageous because they are well balanced, have a high-carbohydrate content, have no bulk, and are easily digested. Liquid meals may also be consumed closer to game time (2 to 3 hours prior). Liquid meals, however, should only be considered as a substitute for the pregame meal and not as a substitute for daily nutrient needs.

Michael followed your guidelines for pregame meals and maintaining hydration throughout the season. He did not have any problems completing the season and even noted that he felt more energetic toward the end of the season than he had the previous year.

## CARBOHYDRATE INGESTION DURING EXERCISE

In addition to carbohydrate loading, the practice of carbohydrate feeding during prolonged exercise may be beneficial to performance. Carbohydrate feedings during exercise have been shown to delay the onset of fatigue by 30 to 60 minutes (6,7). During the early stages of prolonged exercise, the majority of carbohydrate energy is derived from muscle glycogen. As exercise continues, muscle glycogen contributes less to the carbohydrate-derived energy supply. The reduction in muscle glycogen use is counterbalanced by an increase in blood glucose usage. It must be emphasized that the glucose obtained from carbohydrate feeding does not spare muscle glycogen from being depleted, but rather replaces muscle glycogen as a fuel source as it becomes depleted. The result is a delaying of the onset of fatigue. *Figure 12.5* shows the effects of carbohydrate feedings during exercise on power output in bicycling. Either 90 g of a glucose polymer or a flavored placebo were consumed during the first 90 minutes of exercise, and subjects were instructed to maintain a maximal power output during the entire exercise bout.

One problem with consuming carbohydrate during exercise to enhance performance is that its absorption is not rapid enough to meet the energy needs of the exercising muscles. Athletes need to ingest carbohydrates at regular intervals early during the event so that ample carbohydrate will be available during the latter stages of exercise when the muscles rely heavily on blood glucose for energy. Improvements in exercise performance have been noted when carbohydrate intake averages slightly less than 1 g·min$^{-1}$. This can be translated into drinking 240 mL (8 oz) of a 5% carbohydrate solution or 120 mL (4 oz) of a 10% carbohydrate solution every 15 minutes (8). Consuming a drink with a concentration greater than 10% carbohydrate results in the net movement of fluid into the intestinal lumen because of the high **osmolality** of the drink. This fluid flux increases the risk of dehydration.

The type of carbohydrate consumed during exercise can be glucose, sucrose, or a complex carbohydrate such as maltodextrin. Fructose may lead to intestinal disturbance for some athletes and does not have the same exercise-enhancing effects as the other sugars. The carbohydrate can be consumed either in solution or in solid form. Research has shown that if a solid form of carbohydrate is chewed well and taken with water, both liquid and solid

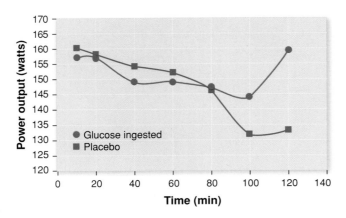

**FIGURE 12.5.** Effects of carbohydrate feedings during exercise on power output in bicycling. (Data from Ivy JL, Costill DL, Fink WJ, et al. Influence of caffeine and carbohydrate feedings on endurance performance. *Med Sci Sports Exerc* 1979;11:6–11.)

forms of carbohydrate will produce the same response in exercise heart rate, $\dot{V}O_2$, blood glucose, and insulin (9).

## CARBOHYDRATE INGESTION AFTER EXERCISE

Many endurance athletes are attentive to carbohydrate boosting prior to or during a prolonged exercise event but do not follow healthy nutritional practices for carbohydrate replenishment following an event. Both muscle and liver glycogen stores can be reduced dramatically following prolonged exercise. Nonetheless, glycogen content in both sites can be replenished within 24 hours if adequate carbohydrate is consumed at proper intervals post-exercise. A conscious effort should therefore be made to replenish carbohydrate following prolonged (>30 minutes) exercise, particularly for persons who perform vigorous (>70% $\dot{V}O_{2max}$), prolonged exercise on a daily basis. Box 12.1 highlights the investigation of a rapid method for replenishing glycogen stores after an acute exercise bout.

The two most important things to remember with respect to glycogen replenishment are the amount of carbohydrate and timing. To quickly replenish glycogen stores, carbohydrate ingestion should begin as soon as possible post-exercise. Some authors suggest consuming carbohydrates at 2-hour intervals immediately following exercise, whereas others have shown that the total amount of carbohydrate consumed over 24 hours is more critical than the timing. One study has shown that when the same amount of carbohydrate was consumed in either one large meal versus several smaller meals over a 24-hour period, the final muscle glycogen content was the same for both styles of eating (10). More rapid glycogen resynthesis occurs if the person remains inactive during the replenishment period. A practical application of these guidelines would be to consume 50 to 75 g of carbohydrate every 2 hours until a total of 500 to 600 g has been consumed (*Fig. 12.6*).

Glycogen replenishment occurs most rapidly when the athlete consumes foods of a high **glycemic index** for the next 24 hours following the exercise event. The glycemic index is a relative comparison of how a food item raises blood glucose levels relative to a standard **bolus** of ingested glucose. The magnitude of rise in blood glucose over a 2-hour period resulting from the ingestion of 50 g of glucose is set as the standard of 100. Fifty g of the comparison food is consumed and the rise in blood glucose is plotted over the 2-hour period. For example, if the comparison food causes a rise in blood glucose that is 60% that of the standard glucose bolus, the glycemic index for the comparison food is 60. Table 12.2 lists foods that have high, moderate, and low glycemic indices. It is suggested that the athlete consume high-glycemic foods (or a sport drink) immediately post-exercise and then move to foods with a lower glycemic index as time post-exercise progresses. Some suggestions of food choices for rapid glycogen

**Box 12.1**

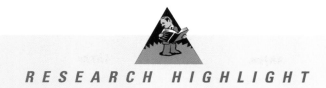

# RESEARCH HIGHLIGHT

**Fairchild TJ, Fletcher S, Steele P, et al. Rapid carbohydrate loading after a short bout of near maximal-intensity exercise. *Med Sci Sports Exerc* 2002;34:980–986.**

## RESEARCH SUMMARY

Glycogen in skeletal muscle is one of the major fuels mobilized by athletes competing in endurance events. It is well established that muscle glycogen content is limited and that muscular fatigue corresponds to muscle glycogen depletion. It is also well known that muscle glycogen stores can be boosted above normal levels through diet and exercise manipulation and that this boost enhances exercise performance.

Early research into carbohydrate loading (boosting muscle glycogen stores) introduced two different carbohydrate-loading regimens that boosted muscle glycogen stores from normal levels of 80 to 120 mmol·kg$^{-1}$ muscle wet weight to 150 to 200 mmol·kg$^{-1}$. The first regimen included a glycogen-depleting exercise bout, followed by 3 days of a high-carbohydrate diet. The other regimen included two glycogen-depleting exercise bouts, separated by 3 days of a low-carbohydrate diet and then followed by 3 days of a high-carbohydrate diet. A modification of these two early regimens was designed so that the athlete tapered his/her training for 6 days while consuming a mixed diet for the first 3 days and then a high-carbohydrate diet for days 4 to 6. This modification eliminated the need for a glycogen-depleting exercise bout. However, the modified protocol still required tapering of exercise during the 6 days prior to the event. A further modification has been practiced in which only 3 days of a high-carbohydrate diet are accompanied by reduced exercise training.

Regardless of protocol used, each of these carbohydrate-loading methods requires 2 to 6 days of altering the athletes' training regimen. Authors of the current study hypothesized that since the rate of muscle glycogen resynthesis following a bout of high-intensity exercise is faster than that following a prolonged bout of moderate-intensity exercise, muscle glycogen could be elevated to supranormal levels within 24 hours following a high-intensity exercise bout.

Seven endurance-trained athletes cycled for 150 seconds at 130% of $\dot{V}O_{2max}$, followed by 30 seconds of maximal-effort cycling. During the following 24 hours, each subject was asked to consume 12 g·kg$^{-1}$ lean body mass (10.3 g·kg$^{-1}$ body weight) of high-carbohydrate foods of a high glycemic index. Muscle glycogen increased from 109.1 g·kg$^{-1}$ muscle wet weight to 198.2 g·kg$^{-1}$ muscle wet weight within 24 hours. Furthermore, muscle glycogen content was elevated equally in each of the muscle fiber types (I, II a, and II b). These data suggest that athletes can attain supranormal muscle glycogen levels following a short bout of high-intensity exercise and that their training routines do not need to be disrupted to do such.

## IMPLICATIONS FOR FURTHER RESEARCH

Results from this study suggest that effective carbohydrate loading can be achieved while maintaining normal training routines up until the day before an event and that the procedure can be repeated multiple times during the competitive season. It remains to be determined how early intake of carbohydrate post-exercise, intake of carbohydrate with a high glycemic index, intensity of exercise, magnitude of muscle glycogen depletion, and training status contribute to the rate of muscle glycogen synthesis. The key physiologic question also remains: what are the maximal levels of glycogen storage that can be attained?

---

replenishment over a 24-hour period are presented in Table 12.3. Box 12.2 highlights the career of David Costill, well known for his research on exercise and carbohydrate stores.

▶ *INQUIRY SUMMARY.* Carbohydrates are probably the most significant energy-yielding nutrients for exercise because they can be used as a primary fuel for both rapid and slow glycolysis. Body carbohydrate stores are also limited, and the reduction of muscle and liver glycogen content, as well as blood glucose levels, are strongly related to

fatigue. Exercise performance can be enhanced when pre-exercise glycogen stores are augmented—a process called carbohydrate loading. The onset of fatigue can be delayed when carbohydrate is ingested during a prolonged exercise event, and repeated bouts of intense exercise can be sustained when carbohydrate is consumed immediately post-exercise. *If body carbohydrate stores become dramatically reduced during exercise, do you think that the muscles are capable to shift to fat or protein as the primary fuel source? What must happen for this to occur?*

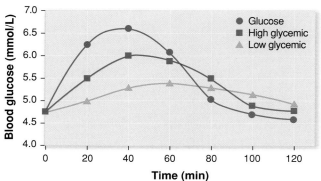

**FIGURE 12.6.** The blood glucose response to ingestion of 50 g of carbohydrate in the form of glucose or foods of a low- and high-glycemic index. The standard for the glycemic index is glucose.

| Table 12.2 | EXAMPLES OF HIGH-, MODERATE- AND LOW-GLYCEMIC FOODS |
|---|---|

**High-glycemic foods**

| | | |
|---|---|---|
| Angel food cake | Graham crackers | Potatoes |
| Bananas | Honey, syrups | Processed cereal |
| Brown rice | Ice cream | Raisins |
| Candy | Instant rice | Waffles |
| Carrots | Pineapple | White bread |

**Moderate-glycemic foods**

| | | |
|---|---|---|
| Baked beans | Oatmeal | Pasta |
| Bran muffin | Oranges | Sweet potatoes |
| Corn | Orange juice | White rice |
| Grapes | Peas | Yogurt |
| Museli | Potato chips | |

**Low-glycemic foods**

| | | |
|---|---|---|
| Apples | Figs | Navy beans |
| Barley | Grapefruit | Peaches |
| Butter beans | Kidney beans | Peanuts |
| Cherries | Lentils | Plums |
| Dates | Milk | Tomato soup |

| Table 12.3 | EXAMPLES OF MEALS MORE THAN 24 HOURS POST-EXERCISE: MOVING FROM A HIGH- TO LOW-GLYCEMIC INDEX |
|---|---|

**0–6 Hours Post-Exercise**

| **Breakfast** | **Lunch/Dinner** |
|---|---|
| White bread and honey, cranberry juice | Chicken, baked potato, beets, sport drink |
| Processed cereals with bananas & raisins | Baked fish, carrots, brown rice, sport drink |
| Waffles or pancakes | Ham, mashed potatoes, mixed vegetables |

**6–12 Hours Post-Exercise**

| **Breakfast** | **Lunch/Dinner** |
|---|---|
| Oatmeal, orange juice | Chicken pasta salad |
| Museli, yogurt | Roast beef, sweet potatoes, peas |
| Bran muffin, grapes | Fish, corn, frozen yogurt |

**12–24 Hours Post-Exercise**

| **Breakfast** | **Lunch/Dinner** |
|---|---|
| Dates, figs, bran muffin | Lentil soup with barley |
| Peaches, yogurt | Sandwich, three-bean salad |
| Grapefruit, milk | Tomato vegetable soup |

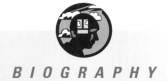

## *BIOGRAPHY*

# *David L. Costill*

David Costill (1936–present) received his PhD from Ohio State University in 1964. Costill immediately began his teaching and research career at Cortland State College, but 2 years later he went to Ball State University where he established and became the director of the Human Performance Laboratory. Costill remained at Ball State until his retirement in 1998.

The main focus of Costill's work from the beginning was to elucidate the physiologic and biochemical phenomena important for athletic success. In the 1970s his work led to important contributions to our understanding of the nature of the training response in the individual fiber types of human skeletal muscle. Along this line of research, Costill also completed a wide variety of projects ranging from the cellular mechanisms of tapering and overtraining to the metabolic consequences of eccentric exercise. Some of Costill's most significant contributions to the field of exercise physiology are found in his research that investigated the importance of diet, fluid intake, and supplements on human performance. Costill is particularly well known for his studies on carbohydrate use during exercise. Hundreds of athletes, from novice to elite levels, have been tested in the Ball State University Human Performance Labs during Costill's tenure as director.

In the late 1960s Costill and his colleagues began testing distance runners to determine the requirements for success in that sport, and this was followed by work in the late 1970s and 1980s with swimmers and cyclists. These studies were important for many reasons, including advancement in the field from simple measurements of energy expenditure to cellular studies of the effects of regular exercise training in humans. An interesting follow-up to the early distance running studies was the opportunity to retest the same group of athletes 20 to 25 years later. Collectively, the papers published from this project have provided important in-

sights into the cellular characteristics that distinguish elite master athletes.

An important component of Costill's contribution to the field of human performance has been his ability to articulate difficult scientific concepts in a clear, concise, and entertaining manner such that scientist and nonscientist alike appreciate the message. This ability is reflected in lecture presentations to various types of audiences all around the world. No single sci-

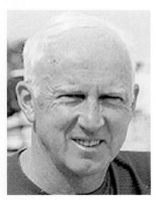

David L. Costill

entist has impacted the sports community nationally or internationally more than Costill because of his ability to effectively transform scientific research into application. He has authored more than 400 papers and published six books, some of which have been translated into six additional languages. Costill has trained numerous undergraduate students, graduate students, post-doctoral fellows, and visiting colleagues. Since his "retirement" he has continued to collaborate with his colleagues on aging and space biology.

Costill is a past president of the American College of Sports Medicine (ACSM) and Fellow of the College. He has received many distinguished awards, including both the Citation and Honor Awards from ACSM. Additionally he received the Thomas K. Cureton Award and is a two-time recipient of the Nurmi Scientific Achievement Award. Costill was selected to present the prestigious ACSM Wolffe Memorial Lecture in 1998. Costill has clearly been a great contributor to our understanding of nutrition and exercise performance.

## *High-Fat Diets*

The relationship between muscle glycogen depletion and fatigue has prompted researchers to find methods that will enhance exercise performance by retarding glycogen use during exercise. Results from two noteworthy research studies in this area suggest that any manipulation enhancing fat utilization during exercise will conserve muscle glycogen and prolong the onset of fatigue (11,12). In one of these studies, fatty acid availability to the muscles was

increased by feeding rats corn oil and then injecting them with heparin. Heparin is necessary to release fatty acids into the circulation. Rats with elevated plasma fatty acid levels due to the corn oil and heparin ran on a treadmill for 181 minutes before becoming fatigued compared to 118 minutes for a group of control animals (12). In the other investigation, seven men were studied during 30 minutes of treadmill running at approximately 70% of $\dot{V}O_{2max}$ (11). Plasma fatty acid levels during exercise were elevated by a high-fat meal, followed by a heparin injection. This elevation in plasma fatty acids reduced the rate of muscle glycogen use during exercise by 40% when compared to an experimental control. These early experiments during the 1970s spawned a series of investigations on the effects of high-fat diets on glycogen and exercise performance.

Several animal and human experiments have been performed over the past 25 years to determine whether a high-fat diet (fat loading) is detrimental or beneficial to endurance exercise performance. Results from the animal studies are almost unanimous in concluding that both short-term (1 to 5 days) and long-term (one to several weeks) high-fat diets enhance endurance exercise performance (13–16). The explanation for this phenomenon is that exposure to the high-fat diet causes a metabolic adaptation in the muscle, enhancing the muscle's ability to oxidize fat and consequently spare muscle glycogen. The specific adaptations that have been suggested are an increased availability of fatty acids to the muscle for fuel and an increased capacity of the key regulatory enzymes in β oxidation, the citric acid cycle, and the electron transport chain.

Data on high-fat diets from the human experiments are mixed. In general, the early experiments of the 1960s and 1970s revealed that high-fat diets had a negative effect on exercise performance (1–3). The conclusion was that the high-fat diet significantly decreased glycogen stores, which caused the premature onset of muscular fatigue. Critics of these early studies note that the exposure to the high-fat diet was too short for a biochemical adaptation to occur and that the study designs were flawed in that the high-fat diets generally followed a glycogen-depleting exercise bout (14,15).

Studies performed in the 1980s and 1990s, on the other hand, have produced findings contrary to those of the early studies (17–21). These latter studies provide data that support the animal research: 1) prolonged exposure to a high-fat diet prolongs exercise time to fatigue, 2) metabolic adaptations occur following a high-fat diet that enhance fatty acid use during exercise and spare muscle glycogen, and 3) $\dot{V}O_{2max}$ is increased following exposure to a high-fat diet.

It may be that the optimal dietary regimen is one that maximizes the adaptations to a high-fat diet while reaping the benefits of carbohydrate loading. In a unique experiment performed by Lapachet and coworkers (13), exercise-trained rats were exposed to one of four conditions: 1) 53 days of a high-fat diet followed by 3 days of a high-carbohydrate diet (Fat-Carb); 2) 56 days of a high-fat diet (Fat-Fat); 3) 53 days of a high-carbohydrate diet followed by 3 days of a high-fat diet (Carb-Fat); and 4) 56 days of a high-carbohydrate diet (Carb-Carb). Amazingly the animals that were exposed to the high-fat diet for 53 days and then carbohydrate loaded for 3 days ran longer on a treadmill than any of the other groups (*Fig 12.7*).

It must be remembered, however, that endurance exercise performance in most of these studies was measured as exercise time to exhaustion at a constant workload.

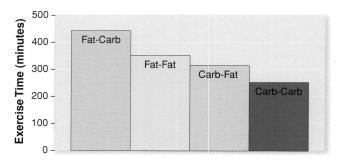

**FIGURE 12.7.** The synergistic effects of carbohydrate loading following adaptation to a high-fat diet. (Data from Lapachet RAB, Miller WC, Arnall DA. Body fat and exercise endurance in trained rats adapted to a high-fat diet and/or high-carbohydrate diet. *J Appl Physiol* 1996;80: 1173–1179.)

proved performance in most athletic competitions, particularly running events, is measured as decreased time to cover a specific distance (e.g., 1500 m). Only a few studies have looked at actual race time following a high-fat diet. None of these studies have shown an improved race time, although they have shown that race time was not hampered by the high-fat diet.

The disease risks associated with prolonged consumption of a high-fat diet have been well established. However, the long-term consequences of such a diet on disease risk in an athletic population remain to be studied. Although exercise training can reduce cardiovascular disease risk and increase high-density lipoprotein levels in the general population consuming a normal diet, exercise training itself may not completely nullify the deleterious health effects of a high-fat diet. With this in mind, an aspiring competitor would be foolish to adopt a high-fat diet regimen in an effort to improve athletic performance without first obtaining solid evidence as to the diet's safety.

▶ *INQUIRY SUMMARY.* Dietary fat has traditionally taken a secondary role to carbohydrate as the body's number one fuel choice for sustaining endurance exercise. However, many studies over the years have shown that a prolonged high-fat diet will induce biochemical adaptations that allow for a shift in exercise fuel source from carbohydrate to fat. *If in the future, high-fat diets were shown to be safe for athletes, which athletes or what competitive events would best be suited for a fat-loading protocol? Why?*

## High-Protein Diets

The normal recommended dietary allowance (RDA) for protein is 0.8 g·kg body weight$^{-1}$·d$^{-1}$ for sedentary men and women 19 years of age and older. For the average 75-kg man, this translates into 60 g of protein per day, and for the average 60-kg woman, 48 g of protein. Seeing that the average American man consumes 105 g and the average American woman 65 g protein·d$^{-1}$, protein supplementation is generally not necessary. However, since exercise

| Table 12.4 | DIETARY PROTEIN REQUIREMENTS FOR SEDENTARY AND ACTIVE INDIVIDUALS CONSUMING THE AVERAGE AMERICAN DIET | | |
|---|---|---|---|
| | | Energy requirement* | |
| Type of individual | Protein requirement | 75-kg man | 60-kg woman |
| Sedentary | $0.8\ g \times kg^{-1}$ | 1600 kcal | 1280 kcal |
| Endurance athlete | $1.4\ g \times kg^{-1}$ | 2800 kcal | 2240 kcal |
| Strength athlete | $1.8\ g \times kg^{-1}$ | 3600 kcal | 2880 kcal |

*Assuming the average American diet contains 15% protein. Vegetarians add 10% to account for the lower digestibility of vegetable protein.

increases protein metabolism, many athletes have turned to protein supplements and/or high-protein diets in an effort to prevent "muscle wasting" and in hopes of improving athletic performance by increasing muscle mass.

The increased protein breakdown during intense exercise training is more a reflection of gluconeogenesis for the purpose of maintaining blood glucose levels than a reflection of protein catabolism for providing energy to support muscular contraction. Athletes or persons who exercise while consuming a low-carbohydrate diet or an energy-restricted diet will metabolize more protein than those individuals who consume adequate amounts of energy and carbohydrate. In other words, carbohydrate availability spares protein catabolism so it is wise for athletes to consume adequate amounts of carbohydrate as well as protein.

Table 12.4 indicates the suggested protein intake for sedentary and exercising men and women. Understanding that it is not unusual for men and women athletes to require 3000 to 4000 kcal·d$^{-1}$, you can see that adequate protein for most athletes can be acquired through the average American diet. Although some data show that protein supplementation may increase amino acid uptake in the digestive tract and/or elevate circulating amino acid levels, the data do not show increased incorporation of these amino acids into muscle protein. Nonetheless, many athletes fall prey to those persons selling high-protein diets or powdered amino acid supplements. Box 12.3 illustrates how clever advertising is used to sell dietary supplements. In this perspective you will see how the educated athlete can easily recognize that he/she can get the same amount of dietary protein (amino acids) by consuming less than one-half cup of skim milk rather than buying an expensive amino acid supplement. Another deterrent to high-protein diets and amino acid supplements is the detrimental effects of excess protein intake. These detrimental effects include:

- Possible kidney malfunction
- Possible dehydration due to increased water needed for nitrogen excretion
- Increased urinary calcium excretion
- Increased risk of coronary artery disease with high-protein diets that also have a high-fat content

- Metabolic imbalances and absorption problems associated with amino acid supplements

More important than consuming excess amounts of protein in supplemental powders or pills, athletes may be better off timing their dietary protein (and carbohydrate) intake around their training regimen. Carbohydrate/protein intake taken within 2 hours following a weight-training exercise bout causes plasma insulin and growth hormone levels to be elevated for several hours. These hormones enhance the uptake of carbohydrate and amino acids into muscle. Increased uptake of carbohydrate and amino acids into muscle following an exercise bout promote glycogen formation and protein synthesis. Thus, consuming adequate amounts of carbohydrate and protein, particularly post-exercise, is probably the best recommendation for exercising men and women.

▶ *INQUIRY SUMMARY.* Most athletes and people who regularly exercise can obtain adequate amounts of dietary protein without supplementation. However, many people turn to amino acid supplements or high-protein diets because they believe that protein is the key to athletic performance and competitive success. *Now that you understand the biochemistry of protein metabolism (Chapters 3 and 4), what arguments against protein supplementation can you provide? What scientific evidence would you, as an exercise scientist, need to convince you that protein supplements work?*

## Fad Diets and Weight Loss

Up until this point, we have discussed how dietary manipulations are implemented solely for the purpose of improving exercise performance through the enhancement of metabolic processes. Many athletes and avid exercisers are also convinced that if they manipulate their diets to lose weight, they will ultimately improve their exercise performance. Athletes and people who exercise for health and fitness are just as susceptible as the general public to promotions for fad diets that claim to be effective in producing weight loss. The reason people fall prey to fad diet promotions is that these people are looking for immediate results.

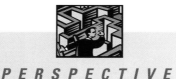

Box 12.3

### P E R S P E C T I V E

# Protein/Amino Acid Supplements

The goal of many athletes and fitness enthusiasts is to increase muscle mass. Fitness centers, websites, magazines, and professionals often cater to the athlete's desire to increase muscle mass by selling protein and/or amino acid supplements. You learned in this chapter that protein supplements do not increase exercise performance or increase muscle mass if there is not a deficiency already. You also learned that most athletes consume adequate amounts of protein in their everyday diet. Nonetheless, protein and/or amino acid supplements are "big business."

Shown below is a copy of the label that was posted on a container of Joe Weider's Weight Gainer. The amino acid supplement was to be consumed with 2 cups (0.47 L) of milk. We have added to the label what the amino acid content would be for 2.5 cups (0.59 L) of milk by itself. You can see from the nutrition information that you can get more of each amino acid listed for Joe Weider's supplement by just ingesting a half-cup (120 mL) of milk. This becomes a "no brainer." Forget the expensive amino acid supplement and drink an extra half-cup (120 mL) of milk.

### JOE WEIDER'S WEIGHT GAINER

| Amino Acids (mg) | Gainer + 2 cups milk | 2.5 cups milk |
|---|---|---|
| Histidine | 944 | 1085 |
| Isoleucine | 1968 | 2275 |
| Leucine | 3364 | 3810 |
| Lysine | 2756 | 2893 |
| Methionine | 870 | 985 |
| Phenylalanine | 1600 | 1905 |
| Threonine | 1653 | 1718 |
| Tryptophan | 540 | 548 |
| Valine | 2244 | 2520 |

Consequently they buy into fad diets promoting outrageous weight-loss claims.

Fad diets fall under the category of quackery. Quackery is defined as the promotion of nutritional products without regard to the facts. Often those offering the dubious product or service do not realize that they are promoting quackery because they were victims themselves. This problem is especially true in athletics, in which the pursuit of superior performance leads individuals to consume a wide variety of nutritional supplements. If an individual has experienced some positive effect in coincidence with taking a supplement, he/she can fall into the trap of attributing the positive effect to the supplement, when in reality the effect may be totally coincidental or even in spite of the supplement.

The promotion of quackery in the realm of weight loss diets occurs on two fronts: by misguided individuals who are well intentioned and by quacks. A quack is a person who pretends to have knowledge or skill in medicine. *How many marketed weight loss books are written by an author with no qualifications whatsoever?* The quack will propagate questionable scientific information as important evidence for the effectiveness of a particular weight-loss diet. These programs are designed to profit the author, industry, or promoter. More often than not, these quacks prey upon a person's ignorance about human nutrition and/or desperation to lose weight. Fraudulent weight-loss programs that are promoted by quacks can be identified by their promotional materials, marketing schemes, and testimonials. People involved with weight-loss programs who do any of the following should be suspected of quackery:

- Promise or imply rapid weight loss
- Attempt to make clients dependent upon special products, rather than the conventional food supply
- Fail to encourage realistic lifestyle changes
- Misrepresent salespeople as qualified counselors of nutrition and health
- Promote unproven weight loss aids
- Rely heavily on personal testimonies to sell the product

| Table 12.5 | SUMMARY OF POPULAR WEIGHT-LOSS DIET APPROACHES | | |
|---|---|---|---|
| **Diet type** | **Characteristic** | **Theory** | **Risk or result** |
| Low carbohydrate | <100 g carbohydrate$^{-1}$; restricted intake of breads, cereal, pasta, fruits, and vegetables | Lack of carbohydrate suppresses appetite and causes ketosis, which forces body fat to be used for energy | Reduced exercise capacity due to poor glycogen stores and body protein loss; stressful on kidneys and liver because of high protein intake |
| Lowfat | <20% of energy from fat; limited intake of animal products, nuts, seeds, and fat | Dietary fat is more efficiently stored as body fat than carbohydrate and protein | Possibly poor mineral absorption from excess dietary fiber; high risk of relapse with extreme fat restriction, due to low diet palatability; otherwise healthy |
| Very low calorie | <800 kcal·d$^{-1}$; protein, vitamins, and minerals are supplemented; physician supervised | Rapid weight loss while sparing body protein | Organ tissue loss, possible heart failure due to low potassium, kidney stones, gallbladder problems |
| Novelty | Based on gimmicks | Certain foods or combinations of foods either cause weight loss or are detrimental to weight loss; certain foods build up in the body, causing toxins that cause disease; certain foods have magical properties | Malnutrition, unrealistic food choices, may lead to bingeing |
| Nonrestrictive | Healthy nutrition, eating with balance and variety | The person will consume a healthful diet when food choices are not restricted and eating behavior is based on internal hunger cues | No foreseeable health risks, rate of weight loss is slow |

- Claim that their product contains mystical properties
- Claim that their program or product works for everyone
- Claim that weight-loss success is guaranteed with their product

Persons who are well intentioned may unknowingly promote quackery by encouraging their friends and relatives to try products that have not been scientifically proven to be effective. Oftentimes a person with good intentions has heard second hand that a particular product has been effective. *How often have you heard from a friend that a friend of a friend lost a large amount of weight while following a certain program?* These types of stories have a tendency to perpetuate themselves along with many of the popular fad diets. The truth is that there are no magical cures, no unique pills, no gimmicks, and no effortless ways to lose weight and maintain the reduced body weight.

Dietary approaches to weight loss have undergone quite a metamorphosis over the past 50 years (Table 12.5). However, the reality is that most fad diets are recycled in and out of popularity in one form or another. For example, low-carbohydrate diets, such as the Atkin's diet, were introduced in the 1960s. These diets lost popularity in the 1980s and

1990s but are now popular again in the 21st century. Very–low-calorie diets emerged in the 1970s, waned during the 1980s, came back in the 1990s, and have become less popular again. Lowfat diets hit their peak in popularity during the mid-1990s and now have given way to high-protein/high-fat diets. Premeasured and formula diets, such as Jenny Craig or Optifast, were the way to go in the 1990s but are now trying to hold onto their market share by allowing clients more liberal food choices. Although some research has been performed on the effectiveness of a few of the most popular diets, the findings are inconclusive and no long-term studies have been performed.

The biggest drawback for most fad diets is that they are not designed for permanent weight loss. Even though many of these diet promoters would have you dependent upon their product forever, the diet itself is usually not sustainable. This fact, in and of itself, guarantees failure for the dieter. Furthermore, much of the initial weight loss on these diets is a consequence of water loss and lean tissue loss. As soon as the dieter begins to eat normally again, the lost water and tissue is replaced, and weight is regained. This cycle of weight loss followed by weight regain suggests that the dieter has failed, when in reality the diet has

| Table 12.6 | DISTRIBUTION OF ENERGY INTAKE FOR SOME POPULAR DIETS | | | |
|---|---|---|---|---|
| Diet | Kcal | % Carbohydrate | % Protein | % Fat |
| Atkins | 2100 | 5 | 23 | 72 |
| Zone | 1000 | 40 | 30 | 30 |
| Pritikin | 1200 | 65 | 25 | 10 |
| T-Factor | 1200 | 60 | 24 | 16 |
| Nutri/System | 1200 | 60 | 20 | 20 |
| Jenny Craig | 1100 | 60 | 20 | 20 |

failed. Seldom though does the dieter recognize this because the diet is credited for the short-term weight loss, while the dieter is blamed for the inability to maintain the weight loss. Distribution of energy intake for several popular diets is shown in Table 12.6.

▶ *INQUIRY SUMMARY.* Many people who exercise are also interested in losing body weight. Fad diets have been marketed to these health-conscious people. These fad diets can be categorized into five categories: 1) low carbohydrate, 2) lowfat, 3) very low calorie, 4) novelty, and 5) nondieting. Each type of diet carries with it certain risks, with no absolute guarantee for long-term success. *Which of these types of diets has the greatest probability for long-term success with the least likelihood of health complications? Why?*

## Exercise Performance and Vitamin/Mineral Supplements

The vast majority of athletes receive the RDA amounts of vitamins and minerals in their diets. Moreover, vitamin and mineral deficiencies among athletic populations are almost negligible. Nonetheless, many athletes resort to vitamin and/or mineral supplements as either a type of nutritional insurance or in hopes of improving performance. Noncompetitive athletes and fitness enthusiasts are also turning to vitamin/mineral supplements in an effort to lose weight, add muscle mass, prevent injury, relieve pain, alleviate stress, or retard the aging process. Fitness professionals, who see the sale of supplements as a source for increased revenue, often promote the use of supplements among their clientele. Promoting nutritional supplementation for improved athletic performance is big business. A cursory search of the Internet entering key words such as "weight loss," "body building," "fitness." "ergogenic aid," or "back pain" yields thousands of websites promoting the use of supplements. Later in this chapter you will learn how to evaluate the validity of the claims used to promote the use of these supplements.

## VITAMIN SUPPLEMENTS

Many years of scientific research have consistently shown that vitamin supplements do not improve athletic performance or health status in adequately nourished individuals (22). Vitamin supplementation can reverse the symptoms of vitamin deficiency and improve athletic performance; however, once an athlete is cured of the deficiency, supplementation does not further improve athletic performance or health status. However, there are many elite athletes who attribute their success to the use of a certain vitamin or mineral supplement. Other stories are passed along about how certain athletes rose to elite status only after they started taking a specific supplement. The combination of these stories and testimonials with a misunderstanding of the physiology of nutrition and the belief that "if some is good, then more must be better" creates an enticing aura around the use of supplements for exercise performance.

Physically active people who eat a well-balanced diet, with adequate energy intake, generally do not need to take vitamin supplements. People who are uncertain about the adequacy of their diet may benefit by taking a multivitamin, which contains no more than the recommended amount of each vitamin. However, those persons who take megadoses (10 to 1000 times the RDA) of vitamins place themselves at high risk for toxicity.

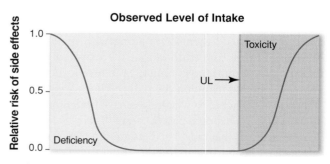

**FIGURE 12.8.** The risks of side effects for either nutrient deficiency or toxicity. UL, tolerable upper intake level.

## Table 12.7    RECOMMENDED DIETARY ALLOWANCES AND TOLERABLE UPPER INTAKE LEVELS FOR VITAMINS

**Fat-soluble vitamins**

| Vitamin | RDA | UL | Results of toxicity |
|---|---|---|---|
| A (retinal) | 800 RE ♀ 1000 RE ♂ | 3000–10,000 RE | Fetal malformations, hair loss, skin changes, pain in bones |
| D (calcitriol) | 10 μg | 50 μg | Growth retardation, kidney damage, calcium deposits in soft tissue |
| E (tocopherol) | 8 mg ♀ 10 mg ♂ | 1000 mg | Muscle weakness, headache, fatigue, nausea, inhibition of vitamin K metabolism |
| K (phylloquinone) | 65 μg ♀ 80 μg ♂ | Not established | Anemia, jaundice |

**Water-soluble vitamins**

| Vitamin | RDA | UL | Results of toxicity |
|---|---|---|---|
| $B_1$ (thiamine) | 1.1 mg ♀ 1.2 mg ♂ | Not established | None possible from food, no risk from supplement use |
| $B_2$ (riboflavin) | 1.1 mg ♀ 1.3 mg ♂ | Not established | None reported |
| Pantothenic acid | 5 mg | Not established | None |
| $B_3$ (niacin) | 14 mg ♀ 16 mg ♂ | 35 mg | Flushing of skin |
| Biotin | 30 μg | Not established | Unknown |
| $B_6$ (pyridoxine) | 1.3 mg ♀ 1.7 mg ♂ | 100 mg | Nerve destruction |
| Folate | 400 μg | 1000 μg | Hives, respiratory distress, redness of skin, itching with supplements or synthetic folate |
| $B_{12}$ (cobalamin) | 2.4 μg | Not established | None |
| C (ascorbic acid) | 60 mg | 2000 mg | Diarrhea |

RDA, recommended dietary allowance established by the Food and Nutrition Board of the National Academy of Science National Research Council; UL, tolerable upper intake levels or the maximum level of chronic daily intake that is likely to pose no risk of adverse side effects; RE, retinol equivalents (1 RE, 1 μg of retinol or 6 μg of carotene; ♀, female; ♂, male.).

As with all nutrients, there is a certain range of intake that is desirable. *Figure 12.8* shows that consuming less than the desirable amount places the person at risk for serious side effects (nutrient deficiency), while consuming more than the desirable amount also places the person at risk for serious side effects (nutrient toxicity). Until the latter part of the 20th century, nutritionists were only concerned with nutrient deficiencies. However, as food supplies became more abundant and supplementation more common, nutritionists began to set upper limits of intake for many of the nutrients. The term Tolerable Upper Intake Level (UL) is now used to identify the highest level of daily nutrient intake that is likely to pose no risk of adverse health effects for almost all individuals in the general population. As intake increases above the UL, the risk of adverse side effects increases. Table 12.7 shows the RDA and UL for vitamins.

Approximately one-third of Americans use vitamin and/or mineral supplements, often at potentially toxic doses. The most commonly overused supplements are vitamins A, B, C, and E. The claims used to promote these vitamin supplements extend from enhanced exercise performance to increased immunity to increased muscle mass to antiaging. Vitamins C and E have become particularly popular over the past few years because of their protective effect against the damaging consequences of **free radicals** that are produced during exercise. Taking megadoses of vitamins A, B, C, and E may place a person at risk for gout, kidney stones, digestive irritation, liver disease, nerve damage, fatigue, blurred vision, and metabolic imbalances. The most prudent advice for exercising individuals is to obtain vitamins from diverse food sources and not supplementation.

 *LINKUP: Access* **Perspective: Antioxidants** *at http:// connection.lww.com/go/brownexphys and on the Student Resource CD-ROM for interesting information about free radicals, antioxidants, and exercise.*

## MINERAL SUPPLEMENTS

Although there is evidence that exercise can increase the loss of certain minerals, this loss can usually be overcome by a well-balanced diet. Except for **blood doping**, which is illegal and dangerous, excessive mineral intake does not

| *Table 12.8* | RECOMMENDED DIETARY ALLOWANCES AND TOLERABLE UPPER INTAKE LEVELS FOR MINERALS |

**Major minerals**

| Mineral | RDA | UL | Results of toxicity |
|---|---|---|---|
| Sodium | 500 mg | Not established | Contributes to hypertension in susceptible persons and may cause calcium loss in urine |
| Chloride | 700 mg | Not established | Contributes to high blood pressure in susceptible individuals when combined with sodium |
| Potassium | 2000 mg | Not established | Contributes to reduced heart rate during kidney failure |
| Calcium | 1200 mg | 2500 mg | Kidney stones, headache, soft tissue calcification, irritability |
| Phosphorus | 700 mg | 3000 mg | Poor bone mineralization if calcium levels are low |
| Magnesium | 350 mg ♀ 420 mg ♂ | 350 mg* | Weakness in people with kidney failure |
| Sulfur | None | Not established | None reported |

**Trace minerals**

| Mineral | RDA | UL | Results of toxicity |
|---|---|---|---|
| Iron | 15 mg ♀ 10 mg ♂ | Not established | Toxicity seen in children consuming more than 60 mg, liver and heart damage in persons with hemochromatosis (iron overabsorption) |
| Zinc | 12 mg ♀ 15 mg ♂ | Not established | Diarrhea, cramps, depressed immune function, reduction in iron absorption |
| Selenium | 55 μg ♀ 70 μg ♂ | 400 μg | Nausea, vomiting, hair loss, weakness, liver disease |
| Iodide | 150 μg | Not established | Interferes with function of thyroid gland |
| Copper | 1.5–3 mg | Not established | Vomiting, nervous system disorders |
| Fluoride | 3.1 mg ♀ 3.8 mg ♂ | 10 mg | Nausea, pain in bones, staining of teeth during development |
| Chromium | 50–200 μg | Not established | None reported |
| Manganese | 2–5 mg | Not established | None reported |
| Molybdenum | 75–250 μg | Not established | None reported |

RDA, recommended dietary allowance established by the Food and Nutrition Board of the National Academy of Science National Research Council; UL, tolerable upper intake levels or the maximum level of chronic daily intake that is likely to pose no risk of adverse side effects. *The UL for magnesium represents intake from a pharmacologic agent and not that from food and water.

improve exercise performance or enhance training responsiveness. Megadoses of certain minerals can also be harmful. Since most minerals are widely distributed across a variety of foods, the use of a varied diet, rather than one that is highly restricted or specialized, is recommended. Nonetheless, many athletes fall prey to marketers who pedal mineral supplements (particularly trace minerals such as chromium, copper, manganese, and zinc) as metabolic "miracle workers." The RDA and UL for minerals are shown in Table 12.8.

There are probably only two minerals that must be monitored with any degree of concern, but this nutritional concern is not exercise induced. As already mentioned in Chapter 2, iron deficiency and calcium intake are of concern for athletes as well as nonathletes, and particularly women. Much attention has been focused on the incidence of iron deficiency in athletes, its effect on performance, and the potential for iron supplementation to enhance performance. The incidence of iron depletion, which is the mildest form of iron deficiency, is comparable between athletes and the general population. Iron-deficiency anemia, the most severe form of iron deficiency, is very common among athletes. Most scientists agree that early stages of iron deficiency will not affect exercise performance, but that performance will be impaired if the deficiency progresses to anemia. Ingested iron supplements will improve performance in individuals with mild iron-deficiency anemia (23). Athletes with normal iron status do not perform better when taking ingested iron supplements but have demonstrated better performances when certain forms of blood doping are used. All forms of blood doping are illegal and very dangerous. Many athletes have died in response to different types of blood doping techniques they have tried (24).

Calcium balance in the body tissues and fluids is maintained at the expense of bone when dietary intake and/or absorption of calcium are inadequate. Under such conditions, bone loss occurs because of either inadequate bone mineralization or excess bone resorption. Exercise and calcium ingestion are vital for bone growth and maintenance. Regular exercise, particularly load-bearing activity, can retard the rate of bone loss in elderly people. Nonload-bearing activity, such as water aerobics and cycling, have not been as effective in preserving bone mineral density as load-bearing exercises like walking and weight training. Although the exact amount and intensity of exercise needed for optimal bone health has not been elucidated, a prescription of regular exercise and adequate calcium intake represents a relatively risk-free and low-cost therapy for bone health. Prevention and treatment of **osteoporosis** should include regular exercise of the load-bearing type and calcium supplementation. The focus of intervention should be on adolescents to achieve peak bone mass and older adults to minimize the rate of bone loss.

It must be remembered that a recommendation for iron and calcium supplementation does not imply taking mega-doses of these two minerals. Adequate iron supplementation can easily be achieved by consuming foods rich in iron; such as fortified grain products. Calcium intake can be increased by consuming calcium-rich dairy products and calcium-fortified orange juice. Adequate amounts of both of these minerals can be achieved by taking a daily multivitamin. It must also be remembered that the suggestion to find supplemental sources of iron and calcium is given here as a preventive measure against the deficiency of these two minerals that is prevalent in our society and does not imply that supplementation of either of these minerals is necessary to obtain peak exercise performance.

▶ **INQUIRY SUMMARY.** Vitamin and mineral supplements have been shown to enhance exercise performance only in cases in which there is a deficiency. Vitamin deficiency is rare in the United States, but deficiencies in iron and calcium are common. Men, and women in particular, may consider using a multivitamin that contains 100% of the RDA for iron and calcium as a preventive measure against deficiency. *Can you think of any sales tactics that are used to frighten you into taking a vitamin or mineral supplement?*

## EVALUATION OF DIETARY SUPPLEMENTS

Everybody wants to feel their best and perform up to their potential. It is natural then that any of us would consider taking a dietary supplement if we thought that the supple-

ment was safe and beneficial. In fact, 67% of Americans already take a dietary supplement either daily or 3 times·$wk^{-1}$ (25). Since there are more than 16,000 dietary supplements on the market today (25), it is beyond the scope of this book to present an evaluation of each of these, or even of those that are touted as exercise-performance enhancers. Furthermore, as new supplements come on the market daily, any list of evaluations we could compile for this book would be outdated by the time the book was published. Alternatively, you will learn in this section how to determine for yourself whether a dietary supplement is safe and beneficial. The procedure you will learn can be used to evaluate any product, program, promotional material, supplement, or drug that claims to have an effect on health or exercise performance.

### Supplement Regulation

President Clinton signed the Dietary Supplements Health Education Act (DSHEA) into law in October 1994. Before this time, dietary supplements were subject to the same regulatory requirements as were other foods. DSHEA interprets the government regulations behind dietary supplements. According to DSHEA, the Food and Drug Administration (FDA) does not have jurisdiction to authorize or require testing of supplements prior to marketing (25). The manufacturers themselves are responsible for ensuring that dietary supplement label information is truthful and not misleading and that all ingredients in the supplement are safe. Manufacturers and distributors, however, are not required to register with the FDA or get FDA approval prior to producing or selling dietary supplements. Furthermore, the FDA is not required to and does not evaluate the scientific data concerning the safety, purported benefits, or possible interactions of a dietary supplement before it goes to market. The FDA will evaluate a product only post-market and only when there is support or documentation that a product may be unsafe (25). The responsibility then lies with the FDA to demonstrate that the supplement is unsafe or mislabeled before the product can be restricted or banned. In lay terms, this means that a manufacturer can create any dietary supplement and get it on the market without any checkpoints along the way except the manufacturer's own integrity.

The FDA does not currently have regulations that require a minimum standard of practice for manufacturing dietary supplements. However, by the year 2010, the FDA will issue regulations on good manufacturing practices to ensure the identity, purity, quality, strength, and composition of dietary supplements. The regulations in effect now require that certain information appear on dietary supplement labels. This includes a descriptive name of the product, stating that it is a supplement; the name and place of business of the manufacturer, packer, or distributor; a complete list of ingredients; and the net contents of the product. Each dietary supplement must also have a nutrition label that identifies each ingredient contained in the product. There are no rules that limit a serving size or the amount of a nutrient in any form of dietary supplements. The manufacturer, without FDA review or approval, makes this decision. Furthermore, manufacturers and distributors of dietary supplements are not required by law to record, investigate, or forward to the FDA any reports they receive of injuries or illness that may be related to the use of their products.

The role of the Federal Trade Commission (FTC) is to regulate the advertising of any dietary supplements, including claims in print and broadcast advertising, infomercials, catalogs, and similar direct marketing materials. The Commission's general authority rests in Section 5 of the FTC Act, which prohibits unfair and deceptive acts and practices in commerce, and Section 12, which prohibits the false advertising of drugs, devices, services, foods, and dietary supplements. The FTC bases its decisions on both express and implied messages communicated to consumers. Express messages are conveyed through direct statements about what a product will do for the consumer. Implied messages may be inferred from product names, from what is said or from pictures, such as before and after photographs, and other graphic depictions. The advertiser is responsible for both express and implied messages, regardless of what the advertiser claims it intended to communicate (26).

Thus, it is clear that the government's two major regulatory agencies (FDA and FTC) do not take any action until after the fact. Only after there is documentation of misleading or false advertising, or after there is documentation that the product is mislabeled or unsafe, will the FTC or FDA take action. It can easily be seen that law enforcement alone will not make a dent in fraud. The consumer demand for quick fixes is too great, and the potential profits are staggering (26). Therefore, it becomes imperative that we as health care professionals become educated and help educate the public as to how to evaluate the efficacy and safety of dietary supplements.

## SOAP Process for Supplement Evaluation

The process that is used to evaluate the efficacy and safety of any dietary supplement is the same process used by health care professionals for evaluating patients, programs, services, drugs, and products. This format is commonly referred to as SOAP (*Fig. 12.9*). The SOAP note format was introduced by Lawrence Weed as a part of a system called the problem-oriented medical record, which is used for organizing the medical record of a patient (24). The problem-oriented medical record consists of a list of patient problems on the front of the medical chart, with each health care practitioner writing a separate SOAP note to address each of the patient's problems.

Many professionals do not use the complete problem-oriented medical record approach anymore but continue to use the original SOAP format of note taking for evaluation and documentation purposes. The benefit of the SOAP format is that it provides you with an organ-

***Subjective*** information that describes a supplement; including claims, promotionals, advertisements, opinions, testimonials, endorsements, etc.

***Objective*** information that describes a supplement; including scientific data, safety, efficacy, mode of action, ingredients, dosage, etc.

***Assessment*** of all the subjective and objective information gathered, including an evaluation of the appropriateness for using the supplement.

***Plan*** of action for use of the supplement or eliminating it from consideration, including monitoring of its effects and length of time the supplement will be used.

**FIGURE 12.9.** The SOAP format for evaluating dietary supplements.

ized method for making an evaluation and plan for action. The acronym SOAP stands for subjective objective assessment plan. The dialogue that follows outlines how SOAP notes can be obtained for any dietary supplement of interest.

*See Experiences in Work Physiology Lab Exercise 11: Taking SOAP Notes to Evaluate Dietary Supplements.*

The S or subjective part of the evaluation is the process by which you gather all the unscientific information about the supplement in question. Although we would like as much scientific data as possible to substantiate or refute dietary supplement claims, we can gain some information by looking at subjective claims, theories, indirect measures, and opinions about a supplement. Listed below are some examples of questions that can be asked to help gather subjective information about a dietary supplement (25).

- Subjective (unscientific information)
  - What claims are being made for the supplement? (e.g., enhance performance, change body composition, prevent injury)
  - Who is making the claims? (e.g., scientists, celebrities, salespeople, coaches, personal trainers)
  - Why are the claims being made? (e.g., public education, sales pitch, warnings)
  - What is the motivation behind the claims? (e.g., sales commission, personal interest, coaching advice)
  - How is the supplement being marketed? (e.g., drug store, internet, sports club, "underground")

- Why would you (or a client) be interested in taking the supplement? (e.g., improve performance, rehabilitation, gain a competitive edge)
- What were you (or a client) told about the supplement (e.g., effectiveness, testimonials)
- What were the sources of the information you (or a client) received? (e.g., salesperson, coach, personal trainer, friend, newspaper advertisements, package label)

Subjective information alone should not be used to determine whether a dietary supplement is safe and efficacious, but the information can be compared with more detailed factual information. Sometimes factual information is sparse, however, and decisions must be made based primarily on subjective information. Listed below are some questions that can be asked that will help you gather factual scientific information about a supplement.

- Objective (detailed scientific or medical information)
  - Is the supplement generally safe? (e.g., side effects, risks, inherent dangers)
  - What is the reputation of the company who produces the supplement? (e.g., well-established company, company follows good manufacturing practices)
  - What is known about the efficacy of the supplement? (e.g., research, clinical trials, scientific or medical evidence)
  - Does the preparation method affect potency or safety? (e.g., active ingredients still active, shelf life, change in chemistry of components)
  - What is the mode of action of the active ingredient(s)? (e.g., biochemical interactions, physiologic effects)
  - What does the active ingredient(s) do? (e.g., stimulate protein synthesis, affect immune system, affect fluid balance, elevate metabolic rate, stimulate nervous system)
  - What is the recommended dosage of the supplement and the active ingredient(s)? (e.g., compared with the RDA, compared with physiologic levels, compared with safe levels)
  - What is the need for which the supplement is to be used? (e.g., health condition, cosmetic, urgency)
  - Will your (or client's) disease state, condition, or current medications affect the effectiveness or safety of the desired supplement? (e.g., drug interactions, elevate blood pressure in a hypertensive, inactivate other medications, affect blood glucose control)
  - What are the likelihood and severity of harm if the supplement does not aid the condition, masks another condition, or prevents you (or client) from seeing a health care professional?

After all of the subjective and objective information is gathered, an assessment of the data must be made relevant to using the dietary supplement for a particular client (or yourself). The following outline shows how the assessment is performed.

- Assessment (appropriateness for using the supplement)
  - What is the validity of the efficacy claims for the supplement? (i.e., evaluate the sources and validity of evidence for the subjective and objective data)
  - What are the risks and benefits of using this supplement? (i.e., evaluate the pros and cons from the evidence of the subjective and objective data)
  - What other evidence is there to support the use of this particular supplement?

Once all the data have been gathered and the evidence is evaluated, a plan for action must be made. The last step in the SOAP process is to determine a plan of action. The plan portion of SOAP is not just the final recommendation to either use or not use the product. Once an individual adopts the use of a supplement, a plan for follow-up as to the effectiveness and side effects of the supplement must be instituted. It is common in exercise arenas to find people who continue to take dietary supplements in spite of their ineffectiveness or deleterious side effects. This most likely occurs because of a lingering hope that the supplement is working safely or will soon be working safely if use is continued. An objective plan of action can help bring people out of denial if the supplement is really unsafe or ineffective.

- Plan (plan of action for use of the supplement or eliminating it from consideration)
  - Monitor for effectiveness and side effects. (i.e., are the expected results forthcoming and are there any side effects, positive or negative, perceptions, sensations, medical markers)
  - Discuss possible side effects if they occur. (e.g., how will side effects be reported and to whom)
  - Determine the length of time the supplement will be used. (e.g., will it be used intermittently, how long until stopping if no effects are seen, do risks increase with extended use)
  - Document any information that may be helpful to others who might be considering the supplement. (e.g., effectiveness, side effects, magnitude of effects, efficacy claims)

There are two general points to remember with respect to dietary supplements: 1) dietary supplements cannot substitute for a healthy diet, but they may fill in the gaps, and 2) if the claims for a dietary supplement seem too good to be true, they probably are not true. Following these two guidelines will steer you away from many of the false advertising schemes that you may encounter. Box 12.4 gives additional guidelines for identifying false advertising schemes and quackery.

*LINKUP:* **Case Study: Dietary Supplements,** *found at* **http://connection.lww.com/go/brownexphys** *and on the Student Resource CD-ROM, illustrates how to evaluate supplemental human growth hormone by using the SOAP format.*

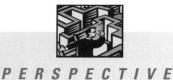

*P E R S P E C T I V E*

## Can You Identify Quackery?

No doubt there is fraud and deception in the industry of dietary supplements. You learned how to use SOAP notes to determine the efficacy and safety of any dietary supplement that you may encounter. However, gathering information for SOAP notes takes time, and you will often be questioned about dietary supplements in situations in which you will not have time or resources to compile extensive SOAP notes. How will you then make a judgment?

There are certain characteristics of fraudulent advertising that are easily identifiable. If you learn what to look for, you can often spot quackery without having to compile SOAP notes. Listed below are some of the common characteristics and schemes used by quacks and those promoting the use of unproven supplements.

- They promise or imply dramatic and rapid effects
- They attempt to make clients dependent upon special supplements rather than teaching them how to make good choices from the conventional food supplies

- They misrepresent salespeople as "experts" who are qualified to give guidance in nutrition or general health
- They fail to inform clients about the risks associated with the promoted product
- They use anecdotes and testimonials to support their claims
- They refer to stories of people being cured of their ailment as support that their product is effective
- In the literature they use or write, they cite few if any scientific studies to support their claims
- They tell you not to trust the medical community
- They claim that modern food processing methods and storage remove all nutritive value from food
- They recommend that everybody take dietary supplements because the conventional diet does not supply enough nutrients
- They use scare tactics to promote the use of dietary supplements (e.g., exaggerating the likelihood of a deficiency)

---

▶ *INQUIRY SUMMARY.* SOAP notes are valuable to health care professionals in evaluating the efficacy and safety of products and promotional materials that claim to enhance exercise performance. The SOAP process consists of an organized method of collecting subjective and objective data about the product, making an assessment about the product in accordance with the subjective and objective data, and then formulating a plan for action. The SOAP method has been used in this chapter as a general tool to evaluate nutritional ergogenic aids. Case Study 12.2 illustrates how to use the SOAP process in evaluating a product that has actually been advertised. *How would you adapt the SOAP method to evaluate a new training or rehabilitation method?*

## Exercise Performance and Fluid Intake

There is no direct evidence to suggest that water or any sport drink improves exercise performance beyond that which is seen when the individual is fully hydrated and nutrient stores in the body are optimal. In other words, water or sport drinks themselves are not **ergogenic aids**. *Why then is there so much hype about sport drinks and fluid replacement?* The reason is that hypohydration is the major

cause of fatigue in prolonged exercise or endurance events. Heart rate and body temperature are elevated during exercise when a person becomes dehydrated to the point of 2% loss in body weight. By the time the fluid loss reaches 5% of body weight, the capacity for prolonged aerobic exercise is reduced by as much as 30%.

Under normal conditions, people usually consume more fluid than is lost from the body while the kidneys excrete excess fluid in the form of urine. However, exercise in any environment, particularly hot environments, causes fluid to be lost in the sweat that is beyond the amount that can be ingested to maintain normal hydration status. Persons participating in prolonged exercise, or repeated exercise bouts during the day, need to consciously replace their fluids. Fluid replacement will not augment performance but will prevent the deleterious effects hypohydration.

The American College of Sports Medicine recommends that 500 mL (16 oz) of fluid be ingested 2 hours prior to exercise (27). This practice helps ensure that adequate hydration is achieved and gives plenty of time for excretion of excess fluid. On warm days, an additional 250 to 500 mL (8 to 16 oz) should be taken 30 to 60 minutes prior to exercise. During exercise, athletes should start drinking early and at regular intervals (every 15 to 20 minutes). Drinks containing carbohydrates are preferable to water for events

## CASE STUDY 12.2: *HYPOHYDRATION*

### CASE

Susan is a 35-year-old recreational athlete. She trains regularly with the assistance of a personal trainer. Susan has recently noted that her exercise training sessions seem to be more and more difficult. Susan does not understand how this can be since she reports that she has lost 7 pounds (3.2 kg) in the past 2 weeks and thinks this should improve her performance. She tells you she has lost this weight through a high-protein, low-carbohydrate diet but insists that the diet is not a very–low-calorie diet and that the high-protein intake should maintain her muscle mass. She discusses this with you as a friend but has not yet discussed it with her personal trainer.

### DESCRIPTION

Many athletes are overconcerned with dietary carbohydrate and muscle glycogen stores but do not pay enough attention to adequate hydration. Dehydration is probably a more frequent cause of early fatigue during exercise than glycogen depletion, and as such, should be a prominent factor when contemplating nutrition for exercise. Furthermore, athletes who ingest small amounts of fluids in an effort to maintain a low body weight put themselves at higher risk for the complications of hypohydration. It must also be remembered that the composition of the diet consumed by the athlete will affect water balance. Therefore, athletes and health professionals associated with athletes need to be conscious of dietary intake and fluid balance.

### EVALUATION/INTERVENTION

The description of Susan's symptoms are indicative of hypohydration and possibly chronic glycogen depletion. The low-carbohydrate intake over a prolonged period of time, combined with heavy exercise training, could have led to chronic glycogen depletion. Combine this with the knowledge that Susan is consuming a high-protein diet, and glycogen depletion becomes a prime suspect. However, the rapid weight loss seems too much for a 2-week period. Also you know that as protein is metabolized for energy, it requires approximately 50 mL of water to be excreted for each g of urea in the urine.

You ask Susan if she has inspected her urine lately. She says that she hasn't. You ask if Susan would quickly provide you with a urine sample. Without trying to make a diagnosis, you note that the color of Susan's urine is dark yellow and that it has a strong odor.

Susan is probably suffering from hypohydration and possibly glycogen depletion. You suggest that Susan begin ingesting more fluids and start to consume a high-carbohydrate diet. If the symptoms do not improve within a few days, Susan should see her primary care physician.

You meet with Susan 2 weeks later and she reports that her strength has returned and she is performing well. She has regained 6 of the 7 pounds she initially lost and is no longer concerned with getting to a lower weight to improve her performance.

---

lasting more than 60 minutes. Athletes should weigh themselves following exercise in hot environments, and replace fluids at the rate of 1200 mL·kg$^{-1}$ of weight lost during exercise (20 oz·lb$^{-1}$). Color and volume of urine should be checked as a simple gauge of hydration status. When the urine has a dark-yellow color, strong odor, and small volume, hypohydration is likely. Athletes who ingest vitamin supplements may produce dark-yellow urine, so urine volume and odor may be the most reliable hydration indicators for these athletes. Much about fluid balance, hypohydration, and sport drinks has already been presented in Chapters 2 and 8 of this book.

▶ *INQUIRY SUMMARY.* Proper fluid balance in the body is critical to exercise performance. Water and sport drinks should be used to maintain hydration in all athletes, regardless of sport, level of play, age, or gender. Conscious fluid consumption should begin prior to an exercise bout, continue during a prolonged exercise bout, and be maintained following exercise. Monitoring body weight and urine excretion are two simple ways to keep an eye on hydration status. *Run through a checklist of* *things to do to prevent the complications of exercise-induced hypohydration.*

*LINKUP:* **Perspective: How to Evaluate a Website for Sports Nutrition,** *found at http://connection.lww.com/go/brownexphys and on the Student Resource CD-ROM, explains how to use the SOAP format to evaluate a website that promotes nutritional supplements.*

## SUMMARY

Each one of the six categories of nutrients has been promoted as a potential ergogenic aid. Carbohydrate is the most significant energy-yielding nutrient, and dietary manipulations that enhance carbohydrate stores and retard the metabolism of carbohydrate during exercise will maximize exercise performance. A prolonged high-fat diet has been shown to improve exercise performance by sparing muscle and liver glycogen stores, but the safety of a high-fat diet has yet to be proven. The use of amino acid supplements and high-protein diets does not improve metabolic processes or increase protein synthesis in persons who consume adequate amounts of protein in their diet. Vitamin and mineral supplements do not have miraculous properties and only enhance exercise performance when there is an initial deficiency. Iron-deficiency anemia and osteoporosis are common in the American population so supplementation of iron and calcium may be considered as a preventative measure. Fluid balance is critical to exercise and health, and proper maintenance of hydration is achieved by ingesting fluids before, during, and after exercise. Overall, there have been no dietary supplements that have proven to be exercise enhancers. Making adjustments to the conventional diet, such as macronutrient composition and timing of intake, will produce optimal nutrition for exercise performance.

## SUMMARY KNOWLEDGE

1. Under what conditions does carbohydrate loading have the potential to enhance exercise performance?
2. Can you enumerate the procedures for safe and effective carbohydrate loading prior to an endurance exercise event?
3. What are some of the biochemical or physiologic adaptations to a high-fat diet that spare glycogen and enhance endurance exercise performance?
4. Why would you discourage someone who consumes an adequate diet from taking amino acid supplements or eating large amounts of protein?
5. What is the only condition under which vitamin supplements have enhanced exercise performance?
6. What are the two minerals that should be monitored closely and may require dietary supplementation?
7. How and when should fluid replacement be undertaken?
8. Suppose a new dietary supplement comes on the market with claims to increase muscle mass. How would you use the SOAP process to outline some questions or gather information about this new product? What would you ask or look for?

### References

1. Hultman E. Physiological role of muscle glycogen in man, with special reference to exercise. *Circ Res* 1967;20(Suppl 1):I99–I112.
2. Bergstrom J, Hermansen L, Hultman E, et al. Diet, muscle glycogen and physical performance. *Acta Physiol Scand* 1967;71:140–150.
3. Karlsson J, Saltin B. Diet, muscle glycogen and endurance performance. *J Appl Physiol* 1971;31:203–206.
4. Sherman WM, Costill DL. The marathon: dietary manipulation to optimize performance. *Am J Sports Med* 1984;12:44–51.
5. Fairchild TJ, Fletcher S, Steele P, et al. Rapid carbohydrate loading after a short bout of near maximal-intensity exercise. *Med Sci Sports Exerc* 2002;34:980–986.
6. Coyle EF, Coggan AR, Hemmert MK, et al. Muscle glycogen utilization during prolonged strenuous exercise when fed carbohydrate. *J Appl Physiol* 1986;61:165–172.
7. Coyle EF, Hagberg JM, Hurley BF, et al. Carbohydrate feeding during prolonged strenuous exercise can delay fatigue. *J Appl Physiol* 1983;55:230–235.
8. Coyle EF. Carbohydrates and athletic performance. *Sports Sci Exchange* 1988;1:1.
9. Mason WL, McConnell G, Hargreaves M. Carbohydrate ingestion during exercise: liquid vs. solid feedings. *Med Sci Sports Exerc* 1993;25:966–969.
10. Burke LM, Collier GR, Davis PG, et al. Muscle glycogen storage after prolonged exercise: effect of the frequency of carbohydrate feedings. *Am J Clin Nutr* 1996;64:115–119.
11. Costill DL, Coyle E, Dalsky G, et al. Effects of elevated plasma FFA and insulin on muscle glycogen usage during exercise. *J Appl Physiol* 1977;43:695–699.
12. Hickson RC, Rennie MJ, Conlee RK, et al. Effects of increased plasma fatty acids on glycogen utilization and endurance. *J Appl Physiol* 1977;43:829–833.
13. Lapachet RAB, Miller WC, Arnall DA. Body fat and exercise endurance in trained rats adapted to a high-fat and/or high-carbohydrate diet. *J Appl Physiol* 1996;80:1173–1179.
14. Miller WC, Bryce GR, Conlee RK. Adaptation to a high fat diet that increases exercise endurance in male rats. *J Appl Physiol* 1984;56:78–83.
15. Conlee RK, Hammer RL, Winder WW, et al. Glycogen repletion and exercise endurance in rats adapted to a high fat diet. *Metabolism* 1990;39:289–294.
16. Simi B, Sempore B, Mayet M-H, et al. Additive effects of training and high-fat diet on energy metabolism during exercise. *J Appl Physiol* 1991;71:197–203.
17. Phinney SD, Bistrain BR, Evans WJ, et al. The human metabolic response to chronic ketosis without calorie restriction: preservation of submaximal exercise capability with reduced carbohydrate oxidation. *Metabolism* 1983;32:769–776.
18. Muoio DM, Leddy JJ, Horvath PJ, et al. Effect of dietary fat on metabolic adjustments to maximal $\dot{V}O_2$ and endurance in runners. *Med Sci Sports Exerc* 1994;26:81–88.
19. Helge JW, Richter EA, Kiens B. Interaction of training and diet on metabolism and endurance during exercise in man. *J Physiol* 1996;492:293–306.
20. Lambert EV, Hawley JA, Goedecke EJ, et al. Nutritional strategies for promoting fat utilization and delaying the onset of fatigue during prolonged exercise. *J Sports Sci* 1997;15:315–324.
21. Lambert EV, Speechly DP, Dennis SC, et al. Enhanced endurance in trained cyclists during moderate intensity exercise following 2 weeks adaptation to a high fat diet. *Eur J Appl Physiol Occup Physiol* 1994;69:287–293.
22. American College of Sports Medicine, American Dietetic Association, Dietitians of Canada. Joint position statement: nutrition and athletic performance. *Med Sci Sports Exerc* 2000;32:2130–2145.
23. Clarkson PM. Tired blood: iron deficiency in athletes and effects of iron supplementation. *Sports Sci Exchange* 1990;3:1–4.
24. Kittenbach G. *Writing SOAP notes*. 3rd ed. Philadelphia: FA Davis Co, 2004.
25. Joint Working Group on Dietary Supplements. *ADA/APhA special report: a healthcare professional's guide to evaluating dietary supplements*. Washington, DC: American Dietetic Association, American Pharmaceutical Association, 2000.
26. Cleland R. Fighting fraud and deception in weight loss advertising. *Healthy Weight J* 2002;16:4–8.
27. American College of Sports Medicine. Position stand on exercise and fluid replacement. *Med Sci Sports Exerc* 1996;28:i–vii.

### Suggested Readings

Congeni J, Miller S. Supplements and drugs used to enhance athletic performance. *Pediatr Clin North Am* 2002;49:435–461.

Costello RB, Coates P. In the midst of confusion lies opportunity: fostering quality science in dietary supplement research. *J Am Coll Nutr* 2001;20:21–25.

Donovan RJ, Egger G, Kapernick V, et al. A conceptual framework for achieving performance enhancing drug compliance in sport. *Sports Med* 2002;32:269–284.

Hespel P, Eijnde BO, Derave W, et al. Creatine supplementation: exploring the role of the creatine kinase/phosphocreatine system in human muscle. *Can J Appl Physiol* 2001;26(Suppl):S279–S302.

Jenkins PJ. Growth hormone and exercise: physiology, use and abuse. *Growth Horm IGF Res* 2001;11(Suppl A):S71–S77.

Opara EC. Oxidative stress, micronutrients, diabetes mellitus and its complications. *J R Soc Health* 2002;122:28–34.

Rehrer NJ. Fluid and electrolyte balance in ultra-endurance sport. *Sports Med* 2001;31:701–715.

Schumacher YO, Schmid A, Dinkelmann S, et al. Artificial oxygen carriers—the new doping threat in endurance sport? *Int J Sports Med* 2001;22:566–571.

### On the Internet

NordiCaLite. Available at: **http://www.wemarket4u.net/nordicalite/index.html**. Website, sponsored by the Federal Trade Commission, that markets a fake dietary supplement. When the consumer attempts to order the product, they are transferred to another page that shows them how they could have been scammed. Accessed April 08, 2005.

U.S. Pharmacopeia Dietary Supplement Verification Program. Available at: **http://www.uspverified.org/**. Accessed April 08, 2005.

Athletic Supplements. Available at: **http://www.geocities.com/Hot Springs/Spa/9971/**. Website devoted to presenting the latest scientific facts and evaluations on some of the most popular athletic supplements. Accessed April 08, 2005.

National Institutes of Health: Office of Dietary Supplements. Available at: **http://dietary-supplements.info.nih.gov/**. Accessed April 08, 2005.

U.S. Food and Drug Administration: Center for Food Safety & Applied Nutrition: Dietary Supplements: Tips for the Savvy Supplement User: Making Informed Decisions and Evaluating Information. Available at: **http://www.cfsan.fda.gov/~dms/ds-savvy.html**. Accessed April 08, 2005.

Quackwatch: Your Guide to Quackery, Health Fraud, and Intelligent Decisions. Available at: **http://www.quackwatch.com**. Accessed April 08, 2005.

Gatorade Sports Science Institute. Available at: **http://www.gssiweb.com**. Accessed April 08, 2005.

## Writing to Learn

*In this chapter you learned about how nutritional status affects exercise performance, whether the exercise is a competitive event or a routine training regimen. You also learned how to evaluate the efficacy and safety of dietary supplements using the SOAP process. Select a popular dietary supplement that you have heard about and use the SOAP process to determine whether or not you would promote the use of this supplement for high school athletes.*

# CHAPTER

# 13 Assessment of Body Composition

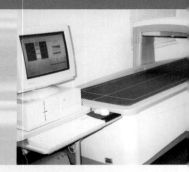

*Assessment of body composition was traditionally limited to the quantification of body fat and lean tissue. The ratios of body fat mass to total body mass and lean tissue mass to total body mass provided professionals with information about how degrees of fatness relate to athletic performance and physiologic disease. However, clinicians and researchers are now interested in how the composition of the major structural components of the body relate to health, disease, fitness, and human performance. Modern technology has made it possible to partition the body into its fat and lean components and also to determine the content of specific constituents within the tissues of the body. Implementing modern technology into clinical practice can be expensive.* How do clinicians decide which body composition techniques and equipment will be most beneficial for their clinical practices?

## CHAPTER OUTLINE

IDEAL BODY WEIGHT
- Body Fat and Disease Risk
- Body Composition and Athletic Performance
METHODS FOR THE ASSESSMENT OF BODY COMPOSITION
- Measures of Circumference
- Body Mass Index
- Hydrostatic Weighing
- Air Displacement Plethysmography
- Skinfold Thickness
- Total Body Water Measures
- Total Body Electrical Conductivity

- Bioelectrical Impedance Analysis
- Ultrasound
- Nuclear Magnetic Resonance
- Near-Infrared Interactance
- Computed Tomography
- Dual-Energy X-Ray Absorptiometry
BODY COMPOSITION ASSESSMENT IN CHILDREN
- Body Mass Index in Children
- Body Composition Measures in Children
  - Skinfold Measures
  - Dual-Energy X-Ray Absorptiometry

Clinicians and practitioners who work in exercise science, sports medicine, physical therapy, or other health care professions must perform and interpret body composition assessments to help clients/patients achieve their health-related or sports-related objectives. Valid and reliable body composition assessments may help the professional:

- Evaluate the risk of chronic diseases
- Monitor changes in body composition in response to weight loss/gain programs
- Monitor nutritional status of special populations
- Monitor effectiveness of physical training regimens

- Evaluate physical fitness
- Monitor potential side effects from pharmacologic therapies

In this chapter you will learn how body composition relates to health and performance and how assessments of body composition can best be performed and interpreted.

## Ideal Body Weight

Life insurance companies in the United States reported the earliest references to the relationship between body weight and health during the early 1900s. The prevalent thought at the time was that underweight was associated with morbidity and premature mortality because of the association between low body weight and the primary mortality risks of the time, pneumonia and communicable diseases. However, the slight increase in the prevalence of overweight that occurred in the early 20th century brought with it a new way of thinking—that deviations above average body weight are associated with higher disease risk.

The notion that being overweight is a serious health threat became widely accepted with the publication of the Metropolitan Life Insurance Company Tables of 1941–1943. These early tables contained height and weight values for a large sample of the United States population. Data in the tables were updated in 1959 and then again in 1983. From these tables, normative data were compiled and guidelines for desirable weight established. These guidelines or abbreviated tables were the common height-weight tables in use for many years in physician offices. These height-weight tables have now been replaced with the **body mass index** (BMI), which allows the identification of a person's height-weight ratio at any point on the continuum rather than forcing them to fit into one of the compartmentalized height-weight ratios found in the old tables. (See the BMI section of this chapter.)

The points at which overweight and underweight conditions begin to adversely affect health have not yet been clearly established. Although cutoff values for the magnitude of overweight that increases the risk for disease and mortality have been published, there is controversy among professionals as to how behavior may accentuate or attenuate this body-size–related health risk. For example, it is generally accepted that being overweight places a person at a higher risk for the development of cardiovascular disease. *However, if the overweight person exercises but does not lose weight, is his/her risk for cardiovascular disease still elevated? Similarly, is the health status of a normal-weight bulimic individual the same as that of a normal-weight nonbulimic person?* With this in mind, remember that published norms and standards for body size and composition are only guidelines, and they should be interpreted in the context of behavioral patterns, environmental influences, genetic predisposition, and overall health.

 *LINKUP:* **Perspective: Fitness Versus Fatness,** *found at* **http://connection.lww.com/go/brownexphys** *and on the Student Resource CD-ROM, contains an interesting point of view regarding fitness and fatness that is being proposed by some professionals.*

## BODY FAT AND DISEASE RISK

Overweight and obesity are associated with an increased risk of noninsulin-dependent diabetes mellitus, coronary heart disease, hypertension, hyperlipidemia, cancer, digestive diseases, gallbladder disease, respiratory problems, metabolic problems, musculoskeletal disorders, kidney malfunctions, and liver malfunctions. In addition, many physical handicaps and psychologic disorders are exacerbated with increasing body weight. All of the medical disorders associated with being overweight lead to an increased mortality ratio in overweight adults. Thus, it seems that a significant portion of the United States population is at increased risk of disease, disability, and premature death simply by virtue of being overweight.

Various definitions of overweight and obesity have been used throughout the years. Twenty percent above ideal or average weight has most frequently been used to define overweight. The National Health and Nutrition Examination Surveys (NHANES) I and II defined people in the top 15% (by weight) of the population to be overweight and at higher risk for premature mortality.

Technologic advances during the 1960s allowed us to quantify body fatness, with body fat percentages of 20% to 25% for men and 30% to 35% for women becoming acceptable delineators for identifying overweight. Determining body fat content in large populations is not feasible so a universal numerical index of body size that can be applied to men and women has been derived. BMI is a simple index of a weight-to-height ratio that is calculated as the weight in kilograms divided by the square of the height in meters ($kg \cdot m^{-2}$). NHANES III and subsequent surveys used BMI to define cutoff points for overweight and obesity, rather than just weight.

The World Health Organization classifies overweight in adults according to BMI (*Table 13.1*). Accordingly, persons with BMI between 25 and 30 are considered overweight, while those with BMI $\geq$30 are considered obese. The relationship between BMI and degree of overweight is presented in *Table 13.2*. Trying to remember the specific numbers for cutoff points in each measure of adiposity is difficult. Therefore, we suggest that only one number be remembered for all scales, 30. Obesity and its associated health risks can generally be defined as BMI greater than 30, more than 30% above average weight, and body fat percentage more than 30.

There seems to be a limit beyond which a person's body fat content cannot be reduced without impairing health

| *Table 13.1* | **CLASSIFICATION OF WEIGHT IN ADULTS ACCORDING TO BMI** |
|---|---|
| **Classification** | **BMI ($kg \cdot m^{-2}$)** |
| Underweight | <18.5 |
| Normal weight | 18.5–24.9 |
| Overweight | 25.0–29.9 |
| Obesity class I | 30.0–34.9 |
| Obesity class II | 35.0–39.9 |
| Obesity class III | >40.0 |

| Table 13.2 | RELATIONSHIP BETWEEN BMI AND BODY WEIGHT | |
|---|---|---|
| **BMI at:** | **Men** | **Women** |
| Average body weight | 22.4 | 22.7 |
| 10% overweight | 24.7 | 25.0 |
| 20% overweight | 26.9 | 27.2 |
| 30% overweight | 29.2 | 29.5 |
| 40% overweight | 31.4 | 31.7 |
| 50% overweight | 33.7 | 34.0 |
| 60% overweight | 35.9 | 36.2 |
| 70% overweight | 38.2 | 38.5 |
| 80% overweight | 40.4 | 40.7 |
| 90% overweight | 42.7 | 43.0 |
| 100% overweight | 44.9 | 45.2 |

status. The amount of fat that is necessary for normal bodily functions is called **essential body fat**, and it is found in the bone marrow, nervous system, heart, lung, liver, kidneys, spleen, intestines, and muscles. The lower limit of body fat for men is 3% of body weight, while that for women is 12% of body weight. With reference to BMI, health problems generally occur when BMI falls below 18.5.

Most of what we know about the health risks associated with low BMI (or low percent body fat) comes from studies of undernutrition, performed mainly in underdeveloped countries. Deficiencies in nutrients are almost always associated with chronic energy deficiencies. The earliest sign of chronic energy deficiency is a loss of body fat stores. This is often seen as desirable to the lay person as well as the athlete; however, when too little energy is consumed, the body breaks down its own tissues and uses the energy from these tissues to support necessary metabolic functions. If the energy deficiency is severe, adults can lose up to half their body weight and children can lose even more. Symptoms of chronic energy deficiency include dry skin, pale skin color, increased sensitivity to cold, hair thinning, fatigue, diarrhea, loss of appetite, irritability, apathy, decreased immunity, depression, and cardiorespiratory insufficiencies.

## BODY COMPOSITION AND ATHLETIC PERFORMANCE

Competitive athletes are concerned with maintaining a high level of fitness as well as keeping their bodies in optimal form for athletic competition. In most sports, body fat is considered detrimental to performance. For sports such as gymnastics, figure skating, and dance, body fat is seen as aesthetically unappealing as well as a detriment to performance. Wrestlers and boxers are placed in competitive classifications according to body weight. Within a sport, a wide variance in body size and composition is sometimes acceptable. For example, running backs in professional football generally weigh about 200 lb (90 kg) and have body fat percentages ranging from 3% to 8%. On the other hand, football linemen may perform optimally at a weight of about 255 lb (115 kg) with a body fat percentage of 15% to 20%.

The ideal body weight or body composition for any particular sport or specific position on a team has not been determined. However, certain body sizes do not lend themselves to some sports. Successful jockeys do not weigh 200 lb (90 kg), and successful football players do not weigh 130 lb (60 kg). Furthermore, the most successful competitive weightlifters have body fat percentages above average. Unfortunately, many athletes, coaches, and trainers go to extremes in attempts to achieve what they think are the ideal bodies for competition. These attempts frequently lead to dangerous disorders, such as **anorexia nervosa** and **bulimia nervosa**, or harmful practices, such as the use of steroids or unproven nutritional supplements. Case 13.1

## CASE STUDY 13.1: *UNHEALTHY TRAINING PRACTICES*

**CASE**

Jim is the health and wellness director at a health center of a major university. The university women's gymnastics team has a reputation of being nationally ranked. The team is near the end of the competitive season and has not performed well this year. Many of the athletes have been injured, and there have been many "falls" and "near falls" in some of the competitions this season.

**DESCRIPTION**

Gymnastics is a sport in which it is advantageous to have a small, lean, muscular body. Many athletes who compete in gymnastics diligently train and monitor their diets to obtain and maintain this body style. It is well known that the prevalence of eating disorders and excessive exercise disorders is higher in gymnastics than in other sports or the general population. A delicate balance must be maintained for an athlete to retain a competitive edge.

**INTERVENTION**

The women's gymnastics coach is worried about the end-of-season competitions, and he has the opinion that his athletes are too heavy. He believes that the injuries and falls have been caused by the women being unable to support their body weights. The coach has therefore approached Jim and

**Case Study 13.1, continued**

asked that a body composition assessment be completed on all of his athletes to find out if they have a high percent body fat.

Jim has a hydrostatic weighing tank in the center and schedules all the athletes for assessments. As part of the procedure, body weight is measured on land (mass$_{air}$). Height is also measured; from these two values, body mass index (BMI) is calculated for all the athletes. The average BMI is 19.4, with some of the women having BMI values below 19. The data from the hydrostatic weighing tests correspond with the BMI estimates. The average percent body fat for the women's gymnastic team is 13.5%.

These two sets of data confirm that the women are neither too heavy nor too fat for competition. In fact, these

women are extremely lean. As some of the women were being hydrostatically weighed, they mentioned that they had been restricting their food consumption. Others stated that in addition to their gymnastics workouts, they also do aerobic and weight training workouts.

As you observe these female athletes and talk with them, you construct SOAP notes (Chapter 12). Your analysis after evaluating the evidence is that the injuries and falls this season were caused by the women being undernourished, and that some of them may be participating in anorectic behaviors and/or are compulsive exercisers. Your suggestion to the coach is to ensure that the women get adequate nutrition and that they reduce their exercise training to that which is only necessary for gymnastic competition.

illustrates how overconcern for obtaining a lean, muscular body type can actually be a detriment to performance.

Many athletes attempting to lose weight do not recognize that their performances are declining due to their unhealthy weight loss practices. Athletes often interpret deteriorating performances as signs of insufficient training or an abundance of body fat. Although the literature is not conclusive, the general consensus is that when BMI is between 18.5 and 20.0, work performance and $\dot{V}O_{2max}$ begin to deteriorate. An athlete with low BMI may be able to perform submaximal exercise at the same level as an athlete with normal BMI, but he/she will be working at a higher percentage of his/her $\dot{V}O_{2max}$ and will have a significantly higher heart rate for the same level of $O_2$ consumption. Health care and fitness professionals can help athletes, coaches, and trainers understand that the competitive edge is often lost when too much focus is placed on achieving a specific body size or body composition.

 *Experiences in Work Physiology Lab Exercise 12: Body Composition provides an experiment for measuring body composition (percent fat) in male and female subjects using several different techniques.*

The concept of an ideal body weight or ideal body composition for health and performance has evolved over the years. Epidemiologic studies have shown a strong relationship between excess body fat and chronic disease and mortality. BMI of more than 30 or less than 18.5 places a person at higher health risk. However, adiposity is only one factor that contributes to a person's health status and athletic prowess. Genetic, behavioral, and environmental factors should be considered along with any interpretation of a body composition assessment for health and performance. Athletes who are anxious to improve their performances by achieving specific body weights or body composition criteria should be assisted to do so only in the context of overall health. *What evidence*

*would you look for to determine if a person's attempt to achieve an ideal body composition was obsessive?*

## Methods for the Assessment of Body Composition

Chemical analysis of the human cadaver is the only direct method to ascertain body composition. However, chemical analysis of human cadavers is very time consuming and expensive. The cadaver must be dissected completely and each tissue analyzed for fat, protein, and mineral content (1). The chemical analyses to determine tissue fat requires that the tissue be homogenized, the fat emulsified and extracted, and then the fat content determined for the homogenized sample. Further tissue analyses for protein and mineral are just as extensive. Since direct chemical analysis of body composition is not possible for live subjects, indirect methods for determining body composition have been designed. Most of these techniques relate to some reference weight, BMI, or percent body fat through regression equations. All of these techniques have advantages and disadvantages; any one method of assessment must be evaluated in accordance with the following criteria:

- Validity of the method
- Reliability of the method
- Cost of the equipment and/or procedure
- Ease of administration of the assessment
- Comfort level for the patient/client
- Type of data obtained from the assessment
- Training necessary for the professional administering the assessment

The most important of these criteria are validity and reliability. Data obtained from an unreliable and/or invalid method are meaningless. Therefore, most methods for body composition analysis are tested against and compared with a criterion method that has been proved to be reliable and valid. Tests for reliability must show that the new method produces consistent measures under the same conditions. Tests for validity must show that the new method is actually measuring what it is supposed to measure. If the data from the new method correlate well with the criterion method, then the new method can be accepted as being reliable and valid. The most common criterion measure is hydrostatic weighing (see below). However, several field methods recently have been tested against methodologies newer than hydrostatic weighing, such as air-displacement plethysmography and dual-energy x-ray absorptiometry (DXA; see below).

*LINKUP:* **Case Study: Skinfold Assessment Versus DXA Assessment,** *found at http://connection.lww.com/go/ brownexphys and on the Student Resource CD-ROM, compares some of the different techniques for analyzing body composition and illustrates how a professional can use more than one method of measurement to verify questionable data.*

Most of the techniques to determine body composition are based on the two-component model in which the body is divided into fat and fat-free (lean) components (*Fig. 13.1*). The fat component can be further divided into

**storage fat** and essential fat. Storage fat consists of fat stored in the fat cells of the adipose tissues and the fat surrounding the internal organs. Essential fat is that fat found in bone marrow, membranes, the central nervous system, and within the organ tissues themselves. From a clinical standpoint, there are no practical methods to measure essential fat. Therefore, separating the fat compartment into storage fat and essential fat categories is purely an academic endeavor to help us understand that there is a certain amount of fat in the body that is not just excess energy stores and that weight loss or exercise training programs are not going to reduce the amount of essential fat in the body without serious health consequences.

A three-compartment model for body composition, distinguishing bone mineral content from fat mass and fat-free mass, is becoming a popular clinical tool because of the increasing popularity of DXA (see later text). Modern technology has allowed us to use DXA techniques to delineate bone mineral content from the soft tissue composition. This measurement ability allows for simultaneous determination of fat mass, fat-free mass, and bone mineral content in the patient. The end result is that one lab test evaluates body fatness and bone mineral density. The benefit is that greater insight into the patient's nutritional status can be seen in the three-compartment model than in the two-compartment model.

## MEASURES OF CIRCUMFERENCE

Body composition can be estimated from circumference measurements taken with a simple tape measure at certain places on the body (*Fig. 13.2*). The tape measure should be flexible but not elastic. A tape measure with a spring-retraction mechanism is preferred so that constant tension

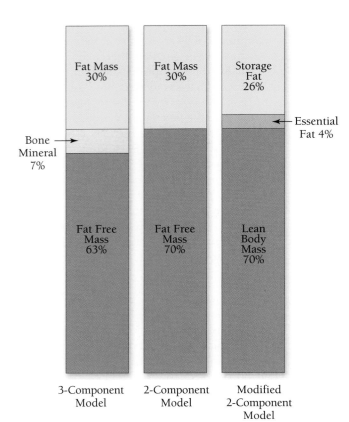

**FIGURE 13.1.** Three common models for body composition analysis. In this example, the absolute body fat content in each model is similar, but the way the components of body composition are compartmentalized varies within each model.

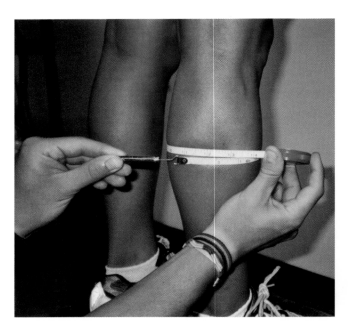

**FIGURE 13.2.** This calf circumference measure is being made with a spring-loaded tape measure to ensure the accuracy of constant tape pressure for repeated measures.

| Table 13.3 | REGRESSION EQUATIONS FOR PREDICTING BODY DENSITY IN ADULTS THROUGH GIRTH MEASURES |
|---|---|
| **Sex** | **Equation** |
| Men | $D_b$ = 47.371817 + (0.57914807 × abdomen) + (0.25189114 × hips) + 0.21366088 × iliac crest) − (0.35595404 × weight) |
| Women | $D_b$ = 1.168297 − (0.002824 × abdomen) + (0.0000122098 × abdomen$^2$) − (0.000733128 × hips) + (0.000510477 × height) − (0.000216161 × age) |

$D_b$ = body density, which can be converted to percent body fat by prediction equations such as those found in Table 13.5. All girth measurements are made in cm. Weight is recorded in kg, and height is recorded in cm.

can be applied while measuring. The tape should be snug around the body part being measured, but it should not indent the skin or compress the tissue. Duplicate measurements should be taken and recorded to the nearest quarter inch or cm.

Anatomic landmarks for common girth measurements used to assess body fatness follow. Regression equations for determining body density (and ultimately percent body fat) are shown in *Table 13.3*.

- Abdomen: 1.0 inches (2.5 cm) above the umbilicus
- Hips: point of maximum protrusion when standing with the heels together
- Right thigh: upper thigh just below the buttocks
- Right upper arm (biceps): arm straight, palm facing forward, arm extended in front of the body, measurement taken midway between the shoulder and elbow
- Right forearm: arm extended in front of the body, palm up, measure maximum girth
- Right calf: measure maximum girth midway between the ankle and knee

The test-retest reliability of circumference measurements range from approximately r = 0.90 to 0.99, while the measurements have a standard error of 2.5% to 4.0%. The ability of regression equations to determine percent body fat becomes less accurate for persons who engage in resistance training, participate in strenuous sports, or are extremely thin or obese.

Tape measures are very inexpensive and can be purchased from any exercise/medical supply company. Circumference measurements can be taken quickly in clinical and field settings. Circumference measurements are not intrusive and the only discomfort to the patient is the possibility of embarrassment in revealing the areas of the body that need to be measured. Data obtained from the measures can be used to determine body density and percent body fat. Circumference measurements can also be used to determine patterns of fat distribution as well as changes in body size during weight loss/gain. Any health care professional can be trained quickly to make circumference measures for body composition analyses. Circumference measures are commonly used as assessment tools in physician offices, schools, and the military. The major advantage of this technique is that a large number of subjects can be measured quickly in almost any environment by minimally trained personnel.

## BODY MASS INDEX

BMI is calculated by dividing body weight in kg by the square of height in m (BMI = $kg \cdot m^{-2}$). The alternative calculation is to multiply body weight in lb by 705 and divide this number by the square of height in inches:

$$BMI = (lb × 705) \cdot in^2$$

BMI produces large standard errors when trying to determine percent body fat (>5% body fat). The correlation between percent body fat and BMI is moderate at best (r = 0.60). BMI is not an indicator of percent body fat. A BMI value may be misleading for athletic individuals who have increased muscularity. In spite of these weaknesses, BMI is widely used in epidemiologic studies in which large databases are compiled from populations for which height and weight are the only **anthropometric** data available.

The only equipment necessary for obtaining BMI measures is an accurate scale and a **stadiometer** (*Fig. 13.3*). A

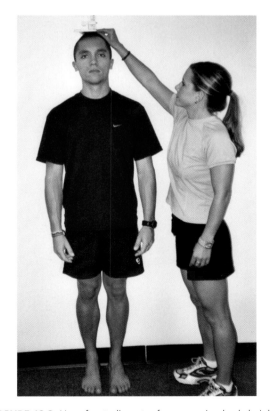

FIGURE 13.3. Use of a stadiometer for measuring body height.

digital scale, with accuracy to 0.1 kg, can be purchased for a few hundred dollars, while a stadiometer can be bought for less than a hundred. Most scales do not measure weights above 300 lb (136 kg). If a professional intends to work with obese patients, a special scale will need to be purchased. Scales that are accurate for more than 300 lb (136 kg) cost about $1000 (2005 pricing). Professionals can easily be trained to measure weight and height, but consistency in measures are important (e.g., shoes off, amount of clothing worn, proper posture, and correct use of stadiometer). A common oversight in many clinics is that the scale and sta- diometer are not calibrated regularly. A wall-mounted stadiometer need not be calibrated frequently, but a scale- mounted or moveable stadiometer should be calibrated weekly. The scale should also be calibrated weekly—more frequently if large numbers of patients are seen. Most physi- cian offices, hospitals, clinics, and exercise facilities have the capacity to determine BMI accurately and reliably.

## HYDROSTATIC WEIGHING

The Greek mathematician Archimedes discovered the principle behind body composition analysis by **hydro- static weighing** (*Fig. 13.4*). Archimedes' principle states

| Table 13.4 | WATER DENSITY AT VARIOUS TEMPERATURES | |
|---|---|---|
| **Temperature (°C)** | **Density** | |
| 24 | 1.00000 | |
| 25 | 0.99707 | |
| 26 | 0.99681 | |
| 27 | 0.99654 | |
| 28 | 0.99626 | |
| 29 | 0.99595 | |
| 30 | 0.99567 | |
| 31 | 0.99537 | |
| 32 | 0.99505 | |
| 33 | 0.99473 | |
| 34 | 0.99440 | |
| 35 | 0.99406 | |
| 36 | 0.99371 | |
| 37 | 0.99336 | |
| 38 | 0.99299 | |
| 39 | 0.99262 | |
| 40 | 0.99224 | |

that when an object is submerged underwater, it loses weight in direct proportion to the amount of water it dis- places. In other words, the amount of water displaced by the submerged object is also equal to the volume of that ob- ject. Therefore, the difference between the mass of the ob- ject in the air and its mass in water is the object's volume. Since density is defined as mass divided by volume, the density of the body ($D_{body}$) can be calculated as:

$$D_{body} = Mass_{air} \div (Mass_{air} - Mass_{water})$$

Although this equation appears simple, it gets compli- cated in that one has to measure a subject's $mass_{air}$ and $mass_{water}$, and account for the residual air trapped in the lungs (RV) and gastrointestinal tract (GV) of the sub- merged subject, as well as the density of the water ($D_{water}$) according to its temperature at the time of weighing (*Table 13.4*). The final equation for determining body density through hydrostatic weighing now becomes:

$$D_{body} = Mass_{air} \div \{[(Mass_{air} - Mass_{water})$$
$$\div D_{water}] - (RV + GV)\}$$

Once the body density is known, percent body fat can be calculated if one utilizes the two-component model for the body in which the body consists of fat tissue mass and lean

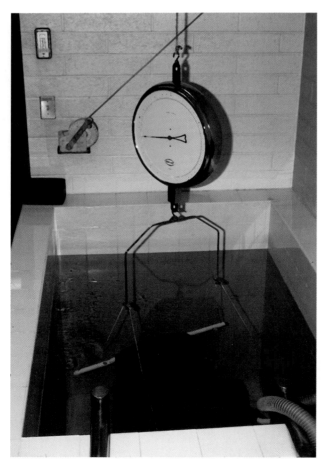

FIGURE 13.4. The hydrostatic weighing tank for assessment of body fat content.

| Table 13.5 | POPULAR EQUATIONS FOR DETERMINING PERCENT BODY FAT FROM BODY DENSITY |
|---|---|
| **Source** | **Equation** |
| Brozek | % Body fat = $(457 \div D_b) - 414.2$ |
| Siri | % Body fat = $(495 \div D_b) - 450$ |

$D_b$ = body density

tissue mass. Using this model, several equations for estimating percent body fat have been derived—the most widely used being those of Brozek and colleagues (1) and Siri (2) (*Table 13.5*). These most popular prediction equations were derived from data and assumptions taken from body composition analyses performed on Caucasian males. More recently, a formula was derived for African Americans, but the sample population was limited to college-aged African American males.

It must be noted that the percent body fat equations use generalized density values for lean and fat tissues. Although it is assumed that these values are constant, this may not be the case in freely living subjects. For example, Brozek and colleagues (1) contend that the composition of fat tissue during weight gain is different from that of fat tissue during weight loss, and both are different from the composition of fat tissue when body weight is static. In fact, these scientists derived three separate equations for determining percent body fat, each of which should be used under the appropriate conditions. However, practitioners invariably use only the equation intended for weight-stable individuals, whether their patients/clients are weight stable or not. Furthermore, the equations derived by Brozek and colleagues were based on data from direct chemical analysis of only three male cadavers whose average body fat content was 15%, while the equation put

forth by Siri (2) is totally theoretical, assuming that the reference man has no fat tissue whatsoever.

Because the composition of fat and lean body components for men and women, children, athletes, the elderly, the obese, and among various ethnic groups is highly variable compared with that of the "reference man," the potential for inaccurate estimation of percent body fat using the hydrostatic weighing technique is great. Imagine, for example, the likely scenario in which a 55-year-old obese African American woman is placed on a diet and exercise regimen to help her lose weight. *Which equation should the clinician use to periodically measure her body fat content?*

Although the large degree of variability among various populations reduces the accuracy of body composition measurement by hydrostatic weighing, this technique is highly reliable. Until more sophisticated studies among races and between sexes are performed over a broad range of age and adiposity levels, professionals will have to settle for relative comparative measurements that may not accurately reflect true body fat content. *Figure 13.5* shows the calculations necessary for calculating percent body fat using the hydrostatic weighing technique. Note that the calculations require values for the residual lung volume and air in the gastrointestinal tract. Gastrointestinal air is always predicted as a constant of 100 mL for fasting individuals. Residual volume is most often measured but can be predicted if lung vital capacity is known. In either case, a spirometer that measures lung volume is required.

The financial investment for hydrostatic weighing can range from a few hundred dollars to several thousand, depending on the equipment's degree of sophistication. Portable tanks with inexpensive scales can be obtained for a few hundred dollars. More permanent cement, tile, or plexiglass tanks cost one to several thousand dollars. Sophisticated balances and force transducers interfaced to a

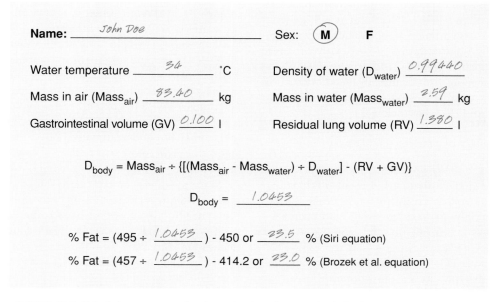

**FIGURE 13.5.** Calculations necessary for determination of percent body fat from hydrostatic weighing.

computer can be utilized instead of a scale, but they are more costly. A spirometer and equipment for measuring residual volumes costs a few thousand dollars. In addition, the water in the tank needs to be purified and maintained. Thus, a filtration system with chemical purifiers is part of the financial investment for hydrostatic weighing equipment. Maintaining a hydrostatic weighing tank requires the same amount of care and attention as maintaining a swimming pool or hot tub.

Hydrostatic weighing can only be done at a set location; it is not mobile enough for work in the field. The administration of one test takes from 15 to 30 minutes, depending on how comfortable the subject is with being underwater. Measuring lung volume adds another procedural layer to the methodology. Many subjects find it difficult to expire forcefully enough to measure residual volume and have even more difficulty submerging in water when their lung capacity is held at residual volume. The professional administering the test needs to be well trained and practiced in hydrostatic weighing techniques and in measuring lung volumes. The test administrator also needs to be able to coax the patient through his/her anxieties around being submerged at residual volume.

Even with its problems, the hydrostatic weighing method is widely accepted as the "gold standard" for body composition determination. Alternative methods for body composition analysis are almost always verified against hydrostatic weighing rather than against direct chemical analysis of human cadavers or animal tissue. This is significant in that any method of body composition analysis that has been verified against a criterion method, such as hydrostatic weighing, can never be more accurate than the criterion method itself. These other methods, however, may be more advantageous under certain time and financial constraints. Hydrostatic weighing tanks are generally limited to hospital settings and university programs where students are trained in body composition analysis. Research projects often use the hydrostatic weighing technique because of its consistency in repeat measures and acceptance as the "gold standard." However, hydrostatic weighing will probably become outdated because of the implementation of more technically advanced body composition analysis systems, such as air-displacement plethysmography and DXA (see below).

## AIR-DISPLACEMENT PLETHYSMOGRAPHY

Modern technology and sensitive instrumentation have allowed scientists to employ **air-displacement plethysmography** as a means for determining body composition. Currently there is only one company that manufactures a system for air-displacement plethysmographic analysis of body composition. This system is called the BOD POD (*Fig. 13.6*). The BOD POD consists of a dual-chambered plethysmograph that provides a densitometric means of body composition analysis wherein the subject is tested in the front chamber and instrumentation is housed in the

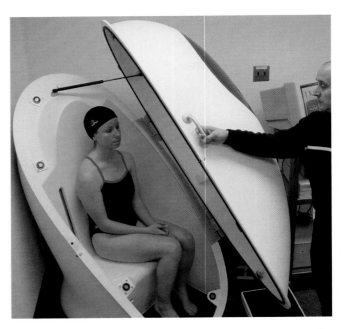

**FIGURE 13.6.** The BOD POD or air-displacement plethysmography method for determination of percent body fat.

rear chamber of a fiberglass capsule. In contrast to hydrostatic weighing, the BOD POD uses air displacement rather than water displacement to determine body volume and density. Similar to hydrostatic weighing, once body density is determined, equations for calculating body fat are used. Therefore, the only difference between the two methods is how body volume and density are measured—not how percent body fat is calculated.

The BOD POD is a highly reliable and valid method for determining body composition in comparison with hydrostatic weighing. The BOD POD has a test-retest coefficient of variation similar to hydrostatic weighing, and it correlated well (r = 0.96) with the hydrostatic weighing technique (3). Although research shows that the BOD POD measures correlate with hydrostatic weighing for a heterogeneous subject sample, some studies have revealed that the BOD POD has some systematic measurement errors for special populations. Body fat percentages are higher for college-aged female athletes when measured in the BOD POD as compared with hydrostatic weighing (4). The BOD POD systematically overestimated body fat content in 30-year-old women but underestimated body fat for men of the same age (5). Furthermore, the BOD POD underestimated body fat percentages in 10- to 18-year-old boys and girls (6).

Since air-displacement plethysmography is a relatively new technique for determining body composition, population-specific formulas will have to be developed for this technique, similar to what has been done for the skinfold technique. Box 13.1 summarizes research into how the clothing worn during a BOD POD assessment can affect the results of the test.

The BOD POD can more easily accommodate individuals for which residual volume measurements and

**Box 13.1**

# RESEARCH HIGHLIGHT

**Vescovi JD, Zimmerman SL, Miller WC, et al. Effects of clothing on accuracy and reliability of air displacement plethysmography. *Med Sci Sports Exerc* 2002;34:282–285.**

## RESEARCH SUMMARY

Air-displacement plethysmography for the determination of percent body fat offers advantages over hydrostatic weighing such that it requires less technical expertise to administer, is quick to perform, and may be accommodating to a wider range of individuals. Air-displacement plethysmography, referred to as the BOD POD, consists of a dual-chambered plethysmograph that provides a densitometric means of body composition analysis in which the subject is tested in the front chamber and instrumentation is housed in the rear chamber of a fiberglass capsule. In contrast to hydrostatic weighing, the BOD POD uses air displacement rather than water displacement to determine body volume. Similar to hydrostatic weighing, once body volume is determined, standardized equations for calculating body density and percent body fat from body density are used.

The principles of physics underlying the design of the BOD POD make it highly sensitive during body volume measurements. It has been suggested that the attire worn during the test may affect its accuracy, and hence the validity of percent body fat calculations, due to the difference between gas properties under isothermal and adiabatic conditions. The BOD POD measures the volume of a body within its chamber. Instruments in the rear (reference) chamber of the plethysmograph create small volume changes by moving a diaphragm dividing both the front (test) and rear chambers, which are equal but opposite in sign. This creates reciprocating pressure changes in both chambers.

Because the isothermal nature of clothing makes it more compressible, a greater pressure change may occur in the test (front) chamber of the BOD POD during body volume measurements than in the rear chamber. The effect is a smaller pressure ratio and decreased body volume measurement for a given individual, which is reflected in a lower percent body fat calculation.

Since the development of the BOD POD, the recommended attire for testing is minimal clothing (e.g., swimsuit) that fits tight to the body (e.g., spandex). However, standardizing the attire for all populations may be difficult, and some individuals may feel uncomfortable wearing minimal clothing while being tested. Therefore, the purpose of this study was to determine the impact of wearing two types of clothing (hospital gown or swimsuit) or no clothing on the validity and reliability of the BOD POD for body composition analysis when compared with hydrostatic weighing.

Subjects were 15 adult volunteers who reported to the laboratory on four occasions. Each subject was tested on 3 consecutive days and then on a fourth day approximately 3 weeks from the third testing day. Each session consisted of estimating percent body fat with the BOD POD on a subject wearing a swimsuit, hospital gown, and no clothing, plus assessment by hydrostatic weighing. Test-retest reliability for each condition was high (r = 0.98 to 0.99). Mean data for each condition revealed that percent fat determination while wearing the hospital gown (13.8 ± 7.7%) was significantly lower than when wearing a swimsuit (22.0 ± 7.8%), being measured in the nude (23.5 ± 7.5%), and hydrostatic weighing (22.6 ± 6.8%). It was concluded that air-displacement plethysmography measures under any attire are reliable, but that wearing a hospital gown reduces percent body fat estimations by approximately 9%, compared with the recommended swimsuit attire.

## IMPLICATIONS FOR FURTHER RESEARCH

Results from this study indicate that the accuracy of the BOD POD in determining percent body fat is affected by the type of clothing worn by the subject, but that the reliability of the measures is not affected by clothing. Under certain conditions, patients may feel uncomfortable wearing revealing clothing (e.g., negative body image, cultural norms). Therefore, it would be beneficial to develop measurement techniques in which more conservative attire (e.g., hospital gown) be worn during testing. One possible way to obtain accurate data would be to measure a large number of subjects under the swimsuit and hospital gown conditions and then derive a regression equation that would correct for the hospital gown.

---

underwater weighing are difficult. However, the BOD POD requires the determination of thoracic lung volume. The thoracic lung volume is measured while the patient sits in the BOD POD and is more easily obtained than residual lung volume. Nonetheless, it is quite common for the subject to have to repeat the thoracic lung volume test two to three times before the volume is registered correctly. Complete evaluation by the BOD POD takes 10 to 15 minutes, and the software is very user friendly. Although professionals can be trained quickly to use the software, they will need to practice on several patients until they are experienced enough to perform tests without supervision. For example, an attempted measure of thoracic lung volume may be rejected for several reasons. Unless the technician is familiar with these reasons for failure and can recognize the signs that indicate the specific reason for failure, he/she will spend valuable time having the patient repeat the test when the problem could have been solved on the second attempt.

Use of the BOD POD may be cost prohibitive in that a complete system costs approximately $35,000 (2005 pricing). Maintenance costs for the BOD POD are negligible, but each test costs a couple of dollars for the disposable breathing tube and air filter required for each patient. Most patients find the BOD POD procedures easy to perform, in spite of the thoracic lung volume measurement.

The BOD POD is quickly replacing hydrostatic weighing tanks in many universities, hospitals, and research centers. BOD PODs are most often seen in hospitals, physician offices, rehabilitation centers, universities, and some health clubs. Case Study 13.2 illustrates how a BOD POD assessment compares to skinfold measures (described below) and DXA (described below) for an obese patient.

## SKINFOLD THICKNESS

The skinfold method for estimating percent body fat relies on the relationship between subcutaneous fat and overall body fatness. Prediction equations have been developed in

---

### CASE STUDY 13.2: *ACCURACY OF ASSESSMENT METHODS*

**CASE**

Sally, a middle-aged, overweight patient, has been referred to you for a body composition assessment. You have air-displacement plethysmograph (BOD POD) and dual-energy x-ray absorptiometry (DXA) capabilities in your clinic. Since Sally is only interested in knowing her body fat content, you decide to assess her using the BOD POD.

**DESCRIPTION**

Several methods for determining body composition in both children and adults were presented in this chapter. Each method has its distinct advantages and disadvantages. Some methods are more accurate than others, while some methods may be less accurate than others when used with certain populations. Hydrostatic weighing has traditionally been accepted as the standard against which all other methods are validated. However, with the advancement of technology, newer methodologies may become the standard. A problem that often arises is when a patient/client receives two separate body composition assessments through two different methods and the results between methods are not congruent. This case is an example of what can easily happen.

**INTERVENTION**

As you are measuring Sally's height and weight in preparation for her BOD POD assessment, she tells you that she has lost 60 pounds (27 kg) while on her physician's prescribed weight loss program. She also mentions that she had a skinfold evaluation 2 weeks ago at her workout facility and that the results put her at 35% body fat.

You carefully perform the body composition assessment. The results show that Sally has 49% body fat. When you show these results to Sally, she becomes angry. "This can't be correct," she claims. "It's not possible for me to be 49% fat."

In an attempt to dissipate her anger, you explain that skinfold measures have been shown to be less accurate than the BOD POD, particularly for overweight people. Sally insists that it is the BOD POD which is inaccurate. You consent to perform the test again, and the results are the same.

Sally is now livid with the results. "There is no way I can be 49% fat!" she exclaims. "Your machine is just wrong. I have lost 60 pounds already and cannot still be 49% fat."

You calculate Sally's BMI and it comes out to be 45.6, which is obesity class III. Knowledge of this only fuels the fire. You offer to give Sally a DXA scan free of charge because you know that the DXA results will only confirm the BOD POD numbers. As expected, DXA estimates Sally's body fat to be 48%.

You proceed to explain to Sally why skinfold methods for estimating body fat can produce erroneous predictions of percent body fat. First, most of the skinfold equations are population specific. If the technician who measured Sally used prediction equations that were not derived from overweight, middle-aged, Caucasian women, there could be much error. Second, you explain to Sally that skinfold measures are least effective for overweight or obese persons because the calipers used are often too small to accurately measure the skinfolds and the skinfolds are often compressed to fit in the calipers. Third, you explain that skinfolds on obese women are often difficult to delineate because the adipose tissue underlying the skin has a tendency to adhere to the underlying muscle tissue, making it difficult to obtain the proper fold. When this happens, the technician can mistakenly measure only the superficial skin and miss the underlying adipose tissue. All of these possible errors could lead to underestimation of percent body fat in the obese. Sally has calmed herself now and apologizes for her displaced anger but assures you that her physician will be hearing from her.

Although body composition assessments can provide valuable information, some techniques work better than others. A knowledgeable and tactful professional can often avoid a tense situation when working with sensitive individuals.

which percent body fat was regressed on a collection of skinfold measures. However, there is a great deal of variability in subcutaneous fat for any degree of body fatness. Hence, more than 100 prediction equations have been derived for various subgroups of the population. This creates a problem for the professional who is working with clientele exhibiting varying characteristics.

The selection of the proper prediction equation by a professional depends on how homogeneous or heterogeneous a group of clients are. Population-specific equations are derived from a homogeneous population (e.g., African American women, college football players). Therefore, the use of a population-specific equation for individuals from other populations systematically underestimates or overestimates percent body fat. On the other hand, general equations are derived from populations that are diverse, and they can be applied to a heterogeneous sample of clients. The selection of a skinfold equation depends upon the nature of the clientele with which the professional works. For example, an athletic trainer working with the women's athletic teams at a major university should use a skinfold equation derived from college-aged female athletes. In contrast, a personal trainer working in a large wellness center should use a general equation derived from a diverse adult population.

In an effort to reduce some of the confusion in selecting a skinfold equation, other researchers have provided generalized equations for men, women, and children of various ages and ethnicities (7–9). Values for skinfold measurements are used in most of these equations to predict body density (*Table 13.6*). From the skinfold-derived body density values, percent body fat can be determined by using equations such as those previously presented in Table 13.5. A description of the seven most common skinfold sites and measurement procedures follows (*Fig. 13.7*):

1. Abdominal: a vertical fold measured 2 cm to the right of the umbilicus

2. Chest: a diagonal fold measured midway between the anterior axillary line and nipple for men, and one-third the distance between the anterior axillary line and nipple for women

3. Subscapular: a diagonal fold 1 to 2 cm below the inferior angle of the scapula

4. Suprailium: a diagonal fold along the natural angle of the iliac crest, taken superiorly to the iliac crest in the anterior axillary line

5. Triceps: a vertical fold taken midway between the acromion and olecranon processes while the arm is relaxed and to the side of the body

6. Midaxillary: a vertical fold taken on the midaxillary line at the level of the xiphoid process

7. Thigh: a vertical fold taken midway between the top of the patella and the inguinal crease on the anterior midline of the thigh

Body composition through skinfold measurements correlates moderately well (r = 0.70 to 0.90) with hydrostatic weighing. Test-retest reliability within technicians is not as high as with hydrostatic weighing, and variability among technicians is even greater. A technician can be trained to perform the measures quickly, but practice is necessary to be able to obtain consistent measures for the same individual. For the novice, training and practicing methods with a skilled technician will improve reliability. A major drawback for the skinfold technique is that the calipers do not fit the obese person. The Lange skinfold calipers, for example, has a maximum measurable width of only 65 mm. Furthermore, there are no prediction equations specifically formulated for obese individuals, and it is necessary to use population-specific equations to ensure accurate results. Therefore, skinfold measures for the obese are totally inaccurate.

Skinfold calipers can be purchased for under one hundred dollars (plastic calipers) or as much as a few hundred dollars (Harpenden calipers). The brand of calipers may also

| Table 13.6 | *GENERALIZED EQUATIONS FOR PREDICTING BODY DENSITY IN ADULTS FROM SKINFOLDS* |

| Measurements | Equation |
| --- | --- |
| **Men** | |
| 3-site formula (chest, subscapular, triceps) | $D_b = 1.1125025 - (0.0013125 \times Sum) + (0.0000055 \times Sum^2) - (0.000244 \times Age)$ |
| 3-site formula (abdomen, chest, thigh) | $D_b = 1.10938 - (0.0008267 \times Sum) + (0.0000016 \times Sum^2) - (0.0002574 \times Age)$ |
| 7-site formula (abdomen, chest, subscapular, suprailium, triceps, midaxillary, thigh) | $D_b = 1.112 - (0.00043499 \times Sum) + (0.00000055 \times Sum^2) - (0.00028826 \times Age)$ |
| **Women** | |
| 3-site formula (abdomen, suprailium, triceps) | $D_b = 1.089733 - (0.0009245 \times Sum) + (0.0000025 \times Sum^2) - (0.0000979 \times Age)$ |
| 3-site formula (suprailium, triceps, thigh) | $D_b = 1.099421 - (0.0009929 \times Sum) + (0.0000023 \times Sum^2) - (0.0001392 \times Age)$ |
| 7-site formula (abdomen, chest, subscapular, suprailium, triceps, midaxillary, thigh) | $D_b = 1.097 - (0.00046971 \times Sum) + (0.00000056 \times Sum^2) - (0.00012828 \times Age)$ |

Sum = sum of the skinfold measurements (mm). Age is measured in years.

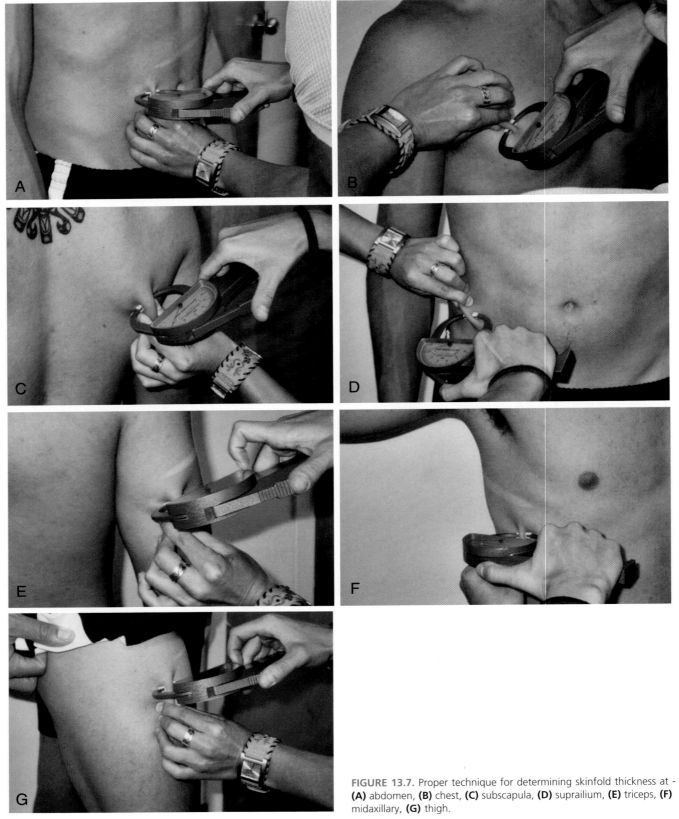

**FIGURE 13.7.** Proper technique for determining skinfold thickness at - **(A)** abdomen, **(B)** chest, **(C)** subscapula, **(D)** suprailium, **(E)** triceps, **(F)** midaxillary, **(G)** thigh.

affect the reliability and validity of the measurement. For example, the inexpensive plastic calipers do not apply a constant pressure to the skinfold because they use a single metal spring to generate tension. The tension generated by the spring is variable, depending upon how wide or narrow the jaws of the calipers are opened. On the other hand, the more expensive calipers, like the Lange and Harpenden, apply a constant tension, regardless of skinfold thickness. Nonetheless, research has shown that even though the average pressures of the Lange and Harpenden calipers were identical, the percent body fat estimated from the Lange calipers was greater than that of the Harpenden (10). The explanation for the difference in estimates is that the surface area of the prongs of the Lange calipers jaw is smaller than that of the Harpenden. This results in a lower absolute pressure at the skinfold and a greater body fat estimate for the Lange (10).

Testing with skinfold calipers can be performed in field settings, and each test takes only a few minutes. The most common field sites where skinfold calipers are used for body composition analysis are in schools and fitness centers. Since skinfold calipers are relatively inexpensive, small, and easily administered, many professionals who do consulting and counseling have added this test to their collection of evaluation tools.

## TOTAL BODY WATER MEASURES

Lean tissue has a higher water content than does fat tissue. Therefore, body fat content can be estimated through measurement of total body water. The measurement of total body water is relatively easy to perform. Water is in equilibrium in the body, meaning that water from one body compartment will balance or equilibrate with water from all other body compartments. Total body water can be measured by following the dilution of a marker into the water compartments of the body. The subject drinks a solution of water containing a known concentration of an isotope (marker). Common isotopes used are tritiated water ($^3H_2O$), deuterated water ($^2H_2O$), and the stable isotope of oxygen ($H_2^{18}O$). After 4 hours, the isotope (marker) is diluted equally within all of the water compartments of the body. A urine, blood, or saliva sample is obtained, and the concentration of the isotope in the sample is measured. Total body water is calculated by determining the volume of water that is needed to dilute the concentration of isotope to that which was measured in the sample. Body fat content is estimated through regression equations, which are dependent upon body water content of the fat and lean tissues.

The determination of total body water itself is highly reliable and very accurate. However, the estimation of percent body fat from total body water measurement is less reliable and less accurate because body water can vary considerably among individuals and within an individual, depending on nutritional status and hydration state. The range in costs for the equipment and test can also vary considerably, depending on the isotope used and how its concentration is measured. In any case, sophisticated biochemical analyses need to be performed to track the isotope dilution. Although the procedure is noninvasive for the subject and is easily performed, the subject has to either remain or return to the laboratory after 4 hours to give a second specimen. Any professional can administer the test and take specimens, but the analysis has to be performed in a well-equipped laboratory. This technique is most often used when isotopes are being traced concurrently for other metabolic measures in the same individual. Hospitals or clinics are usually the only sites that utilize total body water measures for body composition analysis.

## TOTAL BODY ELECTRICAL CONDUCTIVITY

Body composition analyzed by total body electrical conductivity (TOBEC) is based on the fact that water and lean tissue conduct electricity better than fat tissue. The patient is placed in a large cylindrical coil while an electric current is passed through the coil. The degree to which the body conducts electricity can be determined because the electromagnetic field developed in the coil is affected by the patient's body fat content. Body composition can be determined through regression equations.

The TOBEC technique has been shown to be highly reliable, and it correlates well with data obtained through hydrostatic weighing. The equipment necessary for TOBEC costs several thousand dollars. The test is easily administered, but a skilled technician is necessary to run and analyze the test. The procedure is safe and comfortable for the subject. TOBEC is not a popular method for determining body composition and is limited in use to hospital settings.

## BIOELECTRICAL IMPEDANCE ANALYSIS

Bioelectrical impedance analysis (BIA) is an easy-to-administer, noninvasive, and safe method of assessing body composition in almost any setting. The basis for BIA is similar to that of TOBEC. With BIA, a small portable instrument is used to pass an electrical current (50 μA at 50 kHz) through an extremity (*Fig. 13.8*). Resistance to the electrical current is measured. Lean tissue mass and water are good conductors of electricity, but fat tissue is not. The resistance to current flow is therefore inversely related to

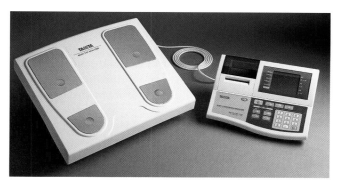

**FIGURE 13.8.** Bioelectrical impedance analysis instrument for the determination of body fat content. Note that with this instrument, the two points of contact are the feet.

lean tissue mass and total body water. Fat mass, lean tissue mass, and total body water are calculated by BIA.

The accuracy of BIA for determining percent body fat is similar to that of skinfolds. The reliability of BIA is somewhat questionable. Repeat measures with the same analyzer and comparison measures among analyzers can vary substantially. The reliability of repeated measures for a single person can be affected significantly by the state of hydration, nutritional status, and prior exercise bout. The intraindividual reliability can be improved by controlling for these variables. Population-specific equations are also available for some instruments, which make these instruments more reliable.

Much research has been performed on BIA analysis. However, the data are discordant. Some research indicates that BIA measures correlate well with criterion measures, while other research indicates a low correlation. The inconsistent findings are probably due to variance in BIA instrument models. For example, when the Tanita scale was compared to the Omron Body Logic handheld device, the Tanita scale overestimated percent body fat in college-aged men and women by 40% and 55%, respectively, when compared with hydrostatic weighing (11).

The cost of a BIA instrument can vary from less than one to a few hundred dollars. Some companies manufacture BIA instruments that are scales which measure body weight and percent body fat simultaneously.

The BIA is so easy to administer that patients themselves can perform the test and obtain the results. The test consists of entering the person's age, gender, height, and fitness category and then making skin contact with the machine's electrodes (by standing barefoot on the BIA scale) (*Fig. 13.9*). A printout or digital readout of the results follows within seconds. The data reported are fat mass, fat-free mass, total body water, and estimated muscle mass. BIA machines can be found anywhere. They are used at home, clinics, fitness centers, universities, hospitals, schools, and research centers. Many personal trainers, counselors, and consultants carry a BIA scale with them when they visit clients.

## ULTRASOUND

An ultrasound meter is used to transmit high-frequency sound waves through body tissues. These sound waves pass through the different tissues at varying rates and then are reflected back to the meter accordingly. The time for the sound wave to pass through the tissues and echo back to the meter is converted to a distance score which can be displayed on a monitor. The distances between the fat-skin and fat-muscle interfaces can be calculated as subcutaneous fat. More expensive and technically advanced machines provide images of the tissues examined. Ultrasound has been shown to be as valid and reliable as skinfold methods. The cost of an ultrasound machine is several thousand dollars, and this limits their use to hospitals and clinics. The test is noninvasive and can be easily administered in 10 minutes. There is no pain or discomfort to the patient and no difficult procedures to perform to obtain a valid test.

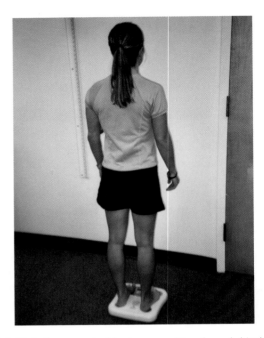

**FIGURE 13.9.** Assessment of body composition through bioelectrical impedance analysis (BIA). Using a BIA scale as the measuring tool, the individual's body weight is recorded at the same time as electrical impedance is assessed.

Ultrasound can be used for mapping tissue thickness and volume in different regions of the body (*Fig. 13.10*). Ultrasound imaging can also be used to assess growth and development of tissues. The most familiar use of ultrasound is to monitor fetal growth in pregnant women or monitor cardiac mass, rather than estimate body fatness. Ultrasound equipment is expensive and is usually not used solely for body fat assessment. Highly trained technicians are required to perform and interpret the images. Ultrasound machines are not routinely purchased for the sole purpose of body fat assessment because they are not cost efficient. However, if a machine is already available in a hospital or clinical setting, the increased expenditure for the capability to assess body fatness is nominal.

## NUCLEAR MAGNETIC RESONANCE

Nuclear magnetic resonance (NMR), also known as magnetic resonance imaging (MRI), is a new technology that is used to present an image of various body tissues. Electromagnetic waves are transmitted through the tissues. The hydrogen nuclei of the body's water and fat molecules absorb and then release energy at a certain frequency (resonate). The resonant-frequency properties can be rearranged by computer to provide detailed images of the body tissues (*Fig. 13.11*). The volumes of specific tissues can then be quantified.

The NMR (MRI) procedure is widely accepted for medical diagnosis. It is highly reliable and valid when compared with hydrostatic weighing. The correlation coefficient when compared with hydrostatic weighing is

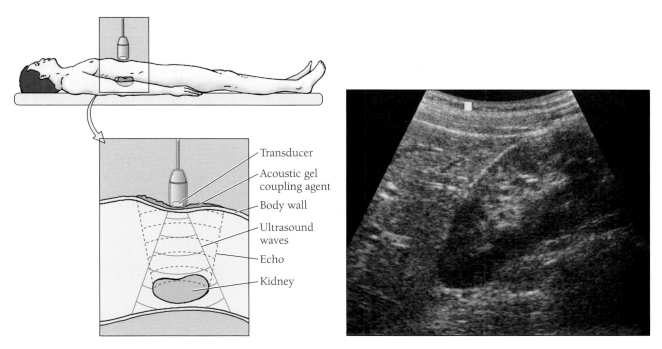

Transducer

Acoustic gel coupling agent

Body wall

Ultrasound waves

Echo

Kidney

**FIGURE 13.10.** The ultrasound method for providing images of body tissues.

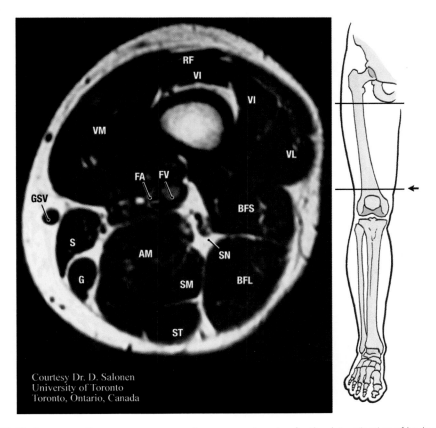

Courtesy Dr. D. Salonen
University of Toronto
Toronto, Ontario, Canada

**FIGURE 13.11.** Nuclear magnetic resonance or magnetic resonance imaging for the determination of body composition.

about 0.85. The NMR machine is expensive and would not be purchased if body composition analysis were its only use. Highly qualified technicians are necessary to perform the tests. The procedure is noninvasive and can be used for whole-body analysis or analysis of body regions.

## NEAR-INFRARED INTERACTANCE

Near-infrared interactance is based on the principles of light absorption and reflection using a near-infrared spectrometer. This technique has been used for years in the food industry to measure the fat content of meats and has recently been used for the analysis of human body composition. A fiber-optic probe is placed over the biceps and an infrared light beam is emitted at very precise frequencies (938 nm and 948 nm). The emitted light passes through the subcutaneous fat and muscle. Body fat absorbs the light, while lean tissue reflects the light. The difference between the emitted and reflected light is calculated, and volumes of the tissues are then computed.

Near-infrared interactance is a very fast and noninvasive method for body composition analysis *(Fig. 13.12)*. The cost of the machine is several thousand dollars, and anyone can easily be trained to administer the test. However, the method has not been shown to be very reliable or valid. Standard errors for the technique are in the range of about 5% body fat. This procedure is probably the least accurate of any of the procedures discussed in this chapter. Near-infrared interactance machines are commonly seen in clinics, health clubs, hospitals, and rehabilitation centers. However, we would not suggest purchasing this type of equipment until it is shown to be a valid and reliable method for body composition analysis.

## COMPUTED TOMOGRAPHY

Computed tomography (CT) is a procedure in which cross-sectional, two-dimensional images of the body are obtained when an x-ray beam is passed through segments of the body with tissues of different densities *(Fig. 13.13)*. A CT scanner looks like a big, square doughnut. The opening for the patient is 60 to 70 cm (24 to 28 inches) in diameter. Inside the cover of the CT scanner is a rotating frame, which has an x-ray tube mounted on one side and a detector mounted on the opposite side. A fan beam of x-ray is created as the rotating frame spins the x-ray tube and detector around the patient. As the x-ray tube and detector make this 360-degree rotation, the detector takes numerous images of the attenuated x-ray beam. Typically, in one 360-degree rotation, about 1000 profiles are sampled. Each profile is subdivided into partitions by the detectors and fed into about 700 individual channels. Each profile is then reconstructed into a two-dimensional image of the "slice" that was scanned. Thus, each time the x-ray tube and detector make a 360-degree rotation, a complete cross-sectional image of the patient has been acquired.

The CT scan procedure itself is rather simple, both from the standpoint of the patient and the technician. The radiation dose received by the patient/client is minimal, and the procedure is otherwise noninvasive. CT scanners are not routinely used for body composition analysis but more often used for medical diagnosis. The equipment is expensive and a highly trained technician is needed to perform and interpret the test. The CT scan can provide information about fat and lean tissue content and thickness of various organs. The CT scanning technique has been used to quantify adipose tissue in the abdominal area of men of varying sizes, and the error in measurement was approximately 30%. Therefore, this method is one of the least accurate for body composition assessments. CT equipment is only seen in radiology departments and diagnostic centers.

## DUAL-ENERGY X-RAY ABSORPTIOMETRY

DXA (sometimes abbreviated DEXA) is a technology that has been used for several years to assess bone mineral density. Early machines were capable only of providing information for the diagnosis of osteoporosis. DXA scans used

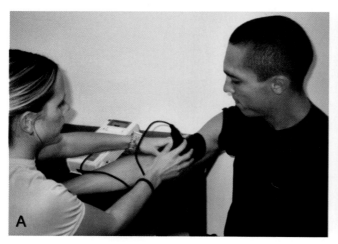
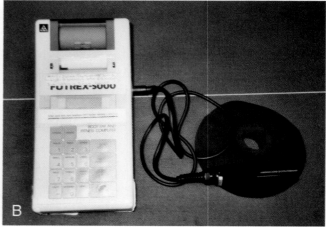

**FIGURE 13.12.** The near-infrared spectrometer. This device estimates body fat content based on the principles of light absorption and reflection. **A.** Placement of the wand over the midpoint of the biceps muscle. **B.** The device, including the wand and recorder.

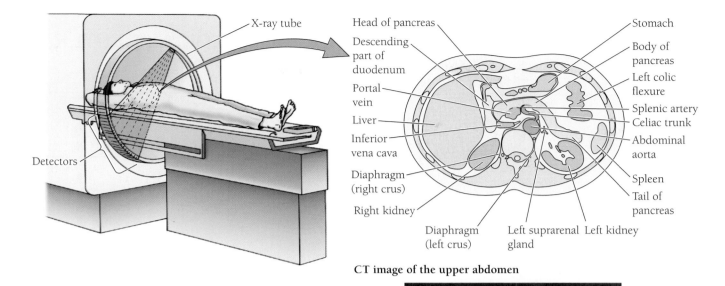

CT image of the upper abdomen

**FIGURE 13.13.** The computed tomography scanner uses x-ray beams to cross-section the body into images that are used to determine different tissue densities.

for bone mineral analyses provide a radiographic image of either the spine (*Fig. 13.14*) or neck of the femur (*Fig. 13.15*). As DXA technology was developed, machines were built to perform whole-body scans (*Fig. 13.16* and *Table 13.7*). DXA can now be used for regional estimates of bone, fat, and lean tissues. Up until a few years ago, a whole-body DXA scan would take 30 minutes to perform. Now the whole-body scan can be performed in 6 minutes.

DXA data has been shown to be very reliable and valid in the assessment of bone mineral content (correlation coefficients of 0.99 with other techniques). DXA analysis of soft tissue (fat mass and fat-free mass) is also highly reliable and valid. When compared to hydrostatic weighing, DXA data produce a correlation coefficient above 0.90. One big advantage of the DXA method over other techniques is that analyses can be obtained on various regions of the body simultaneously (*Fig. 13.17*). The cost of DXA machines has decreased to about $75,000 for a top-of-the-line machine (2005 pricing). A certified DXA technologist or radiologist must perform the test. The DXA method is noninvasive except for the radiation dose administered to the patient. The amount of radiation received from a whole-body DXA scan is about 5% of that received in a standard chest x-ray or equal to the amount of radiation one would receive by fly-

ing cross-country in an airplane. The DXA can be used on all people, including children. Unfortunately, the maximum amount of weight that DXA tables can support is 300 lb (136 kg). This means that DXA cannot be used for body composition analysis for many severely obese people.

DXA machines are becoming more popular in hospitals, clinics, physician offices, rehabilitation centers, research institutions, and universities. Regulation of DXA technician certification is controlled at the state level. In most states, a professional can become a certified DXA technologist without becoming a radiologist. The cost and the fact that radiation is involved make the use of DXA prohibitive for body composition analysis in fitness centers.

▶ **INQUIRY SUMMARY.** Several methods for body composition assessment are reliable and valid. Each method has its advantages and disadvantages. The methods vary by degree of invasiveness, expense, applicability to the field setting, and the type of raw data generated. To determine which technique is best, a needs assessment is performed. *What questions would you ask a salesperson about a particular piece of equipment being marketed? How would you define "the best method" for determining body composition for your laboratory?*

# THE GEORGE WASHINGTON UNIVERSITY MEDICAL CENTER
## EXERCISE SCIENCE PROGRAMS
### 817  23rd Street, N.W., Washington, DC  20052

| | | | | |
|---|---|---|---|---|
| **Patient:** | ▬▬▬▬ | **Facility ID:** | | |
| **Birth Date:** | 03/01/1954   46.3 years | **Physician:** | | |
| **Height / Weight:** | 66.0 in.   145.0 lbs. | **Measured:** | 06/28/2000 | 1:27:56 AM   (2.17) |
| **Sex / Ethnic:** | Male   White | **Analyzed:** | 11/16/2001 | 12:20:36 PM   (4.00) |

**AP Spine Bone Density**

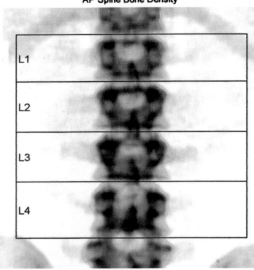

**Reference: L2-L4**

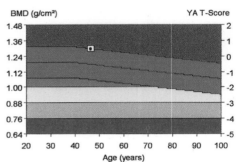

| Region | BMD[1] (g/cm²) | Young-Adult[2] T-Score | Age-Matched[3] Z-Score |
|---|---|---|---|
| L1 | 1.081 | -0.7 | -0.1 |
| L2 | 1.280 | 0.3 | 0.9 |
| L3 | 1.310 | 0.6 | 1.1 |
| L4 | 1.307 | 0.6 | 1.1 |
| L2-L4 | 1.300 | 0.5 | 1.0 |

**COMMENTS:**

Image not for diagnosis

76:3.00:50.00:12.0 0.00:8.46 0.60x1.05 15.7:%Fat=9.2%
0.00:0.00 0.00:0.00
Printed: 03/25/2005 11:29:48 AM (4.00)
Filename: millew_fwuptr87w.dfs
Scan Mode: Standard

1 - Statistically 68% of repeat scans fall within 1SD (± 0.010 g/cm² for AP Spine L2-L4)
2 - USA, AP Spine Reference Population, Ages 20-40
3 - Matched for Age, Weight (males 25-100 kg), Ethnic
11 - WHO has defined for white women that: > -1.0 SD = normal; -1.0 to -2.5 SD = osteopenia; <= -2.5 SD = osteoporosis

*GE Medical Systems*
*LUNAR*

Prodigy

10652

**FIGURE 13.14.** Dual-energy x-ray absorptiometry image of a spine. The scan is of a 46-year-old male who lifts weights regularly. Note that the bone mineral content is one standard deviation above the age-matched reference.

# THE GEORGE WASHINGTON UNIVERSITY MEDICAL CENTER
## EXERCISE SCIENCE PROGRAMS
### 817  23rd Street, N.W., Washington, DC  20052

| | | | | |
|---|---|---|---|---|
| **Patient:** | ▬▬▬▬▬ | **Facility ID:** | | |
| **Birth Date:** | 03/01/1954   46.3 years | **Physician:** | | |
| **Height / Weight:** | 66.0 in.   145.0 lbs. | **Measured:** | 06/28/2000   1:32:00 AM   (2.17) | |
| **Sex / Ethnic:** | Male   White | **Analyzed:** | 06/28/2000   1:33:12 AM   (2.17) | |

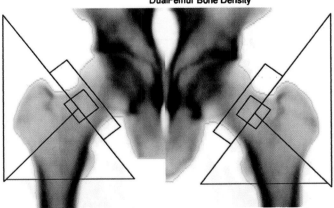

DualFemur Bone Density

Reference: Total

BMD (g/cm²)          YA T-Score

| Region | BMD[1] (g/cm²) | Young-Adult[2,7] T-Score | Age-Matched[3] Z-Score |
|---|---|---|---|
| **Neck** | | | |
| Left | 1.103 | 0.3 | 1.0 |
| Right | 1.112 | 0.3 | 1.1 |
| Mean | 1.108 | 0.3 | 1.1 |
| Difference | 0.010 | 0.1 | 0.1 |
| **Total** | | | |
| Left | 1.230 | 1.1 | 1.7 |
| Right | 1.209 | 0.9 | 1.6 |
| Mean | 1.220 | 1.0 | 1.6 |
| Difference | 0.021 | 0.2 | 0.2 |

COMMENTS:

Image not for diagnosis

76:3.00:50.00:12.0 0.00:10.62 0.60x1.05 12.8:%Fat=13.5%
0.00:0.00 0.00:0.00
Neck Angle (deg) = Right:52  Left:53
Printed: 03/25/2005 11:28:17 AM (4.00)
Filename: millew_fwuq1s87w.dfe
Scan Mode: Standard

1 - Statistically 68% of repeat scans fall within 1SD (± 0.020 g/cm² for DualFemur Total)
2 - USA, Femur Reference Population, Ages 20-40
3 - Matched for Age, Weight (males 25-100 kg), Ethnic
7 - DualFemur Total T-Score difference is 0.2.  Asymmetry is None.
11 - WHO has defined for white women that: > -1.0 SD = normal; -1.0 to -2.5 SD = osteopenia; <= -2.5 SD = osteoporosis

*GE Medical Systems*
*LUNAR*

Prodigy
10652

**FIGURE 13.15.** Dual-energy x-ray absorptiometry image of a femur. The scan is of a 46-year-old who jogs regularly. Note the bone mineral content is more than one standard deviation above the age-matched reference.

# THE GEORGE WASHINGTON UNIVERSITY MEDICAL CENTER

## EXERCISE SCIENCE PROGRAMS

### 817 23rd Street, N.W., Washington, DC 20052

| | | | | |
|---|---|---|---|---|
| **Patient:** | ▓▓▓▓▓▓ | **Facility ID:** | | |
| **Birth Date:** | 03/01/1954  46.3 years | **Physician:** | | |
| **Height / Weight:** | 66.0 in.  145.0 lbs. | **Measured:** | 06/27/2000 | 10:58:17 PM (2.17) |
| **Sex / Ethnic:** | Male  White | **Analyzed:** | 11/16/2001 | 12:21:45 PM (4.00) |

**Total Body Tissue Quantitation**

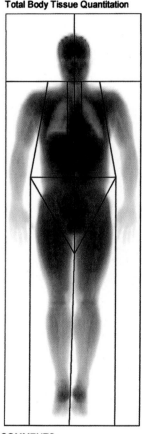

**Composition Reference: Total**

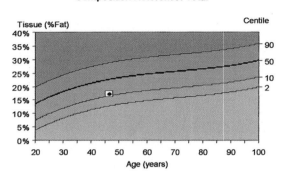

| Region | Tissue (%Fat) | Centile [2,3] | T.Mass (kg) | Fat (g) | Lean (g) | BMC (g) |
|---|---|---|---|---|---|---|
| Legs | 17.5 | - | - | 3,855 | 18,155 | 1,182 |
| Trunk | 19.1 | - | - | 5,705 | 24,132 | 902 |
| Total | 17.2 | 13 | 67.4 | 11,051 | 53,319 | 3,059 |

**COMMENTS:**

Image not for diagnosis

76:0.15:153.85:31.2 0.00:-1.00 4.80x13.00 10.8:%Fat=17.2%
0.00:0.00 0.00:0.00
Printed: 03/25/2005 11:31:22 AM (4.00)
Filename: millew_fwuisv87w.dfb
Scan Mode: Standard

2 - USA, Total Body Reference Population
3 - Matched for Age, Weight (males 25-100 kg), Ethnic

*GE Medical Systems*
*LUNAR*

Prodigy

10652

**FIGURE 13.16.** Dual-energy x-ray absorptiometry image of a whole-body scan. The scan is of a 46-year-old male who exercises regularly. Tissue percent fat includes only the soft tissue. When bone tissue is added to the calculations, total percent body fat equals 16.2%.

| **Table 13.7** | **ELEMENTS OF A BODY COMPOSITION REPORT FROM A WHOLE-BODY DXA SCAN** | | | | | |
|---|---|---|---|---|---|---|
| Region | Tissue % fat | Region % fat | Tissue (g) | Fat (g) | Lean (g) | BMC (g) |
| Left arm | 26.8 | 25.4 | 1840 | 492 | 1348 | 95 |
| Left leg | 20.5 | 19.7 | 8072 | 1658 | 6414 | 350 |
| Left trunk | 10.4 | 10.1 | 10,479 | 1091 | 9388 | 345 |
| Left total | 16.0 | 15.3 | 22,249 | 3559 | 18,690 | 1030 |
| Right arm | 27.6 | 26.3 | 1933 | 533 | 1399 | 96 |
| Right leg | 20.3 | 19.5 | 8409 | 1706 | 6704 | 351 |
| Right trunk | 9.7 | 9.4 | 10,565 | 1028 | 9538 | 382 |
| Right total | 16.0 | 15.3 | 22,378 | 3580 | 18,799 | 1041 |
| Arms | 27.2 | 25.9 | 3773 | 1026 | 2747 | 190 |
| Legs | 20.4 | 19.6 | 16,481 | 3364 | 13,117 | 701 |
| Trunk | 10.1 | 9.7 | 21,045 | 2122 | 18,922 | 727 |
| Total | 16.0 | 15.3 | 44,627 | 7139 | 7488 | 2071 |

Tissue % fat, % fat excluding bone mineral content; Region % fat, % fat including bone mineral content; BMC, bone mineral content.

## Body Composition Assessment in Children

Some people are against assessing body composition in children, fearing that focusing on the attainment of a certain body size will lead to an increase in eating disorders and/or excessive exercise disorders. Nonetheless, the prevalence of overweight continues to rise in children at the same rate as in adults. It has also been determined that 80% to 85% of adult obesity can be traced to childhood overweight. Furthermore, information about the normal growth and developmental patterns for children can help health care professionals when dealing with certain childhood diseases and chronic conditions.

### BODY MASS INDEX IN CHILDREN

BMI changes throughout the growth and development of a child. The BMI-for-age plots for boys and girls follow similar patterns, but the absolute indices are slightly different between the sexes. At about 1 year of age, BMI declines and continues to decline until the child reaches 4 to 6 years of age. As shown in *Figures 13.18* and *13.19*, BMI begins a gradual rise between ages 4 and 6 and continues to rise throughout most of adulthood. This drop and rise in BMI during a child's growth and development is often referred to as **adiposity rebound**. It is a normal growth pattern for all children, and adults should not interpret this curvilinear growth pattern as abnormal.

BMI is less accurate in predicting childhood overweight than adult overweight. However, BMI can be used as an indicator for tracking body size throughout the life cycle. A child's BMI-for-age is a measure shown to be consistent

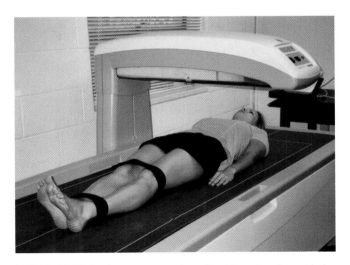

**FIGURE 13.17.** Dual-energy x-ray absorptiometry setup for a whole-body scan of a patient.

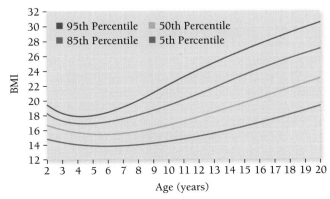

**FIGURE 13.18.** BMI-for-age percentiles for boys ages 2 to 20.

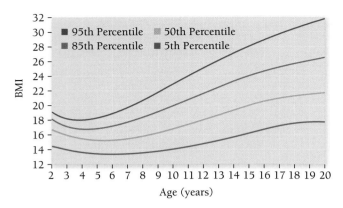

**FIGURE 13.19.** BMI-for-age percentiles for girls ages 2 to 20.

with adult BMI. As mentioned earlier, BMI for children is gender specific and changes throughout growth and development, whereas BMI for adults is neither gender nor age specific. Recommendations are to classify a child's BMI-for-age at or above the 95th percentile as overweight and between the 85th and 95th percentiles as at risk for overweight. The term overweight rather than obesity is the preferred designation for describing children and adolescents with a BMI-for-age above the 95th percentile. A childhood BMI below the fifth percentile is considered underweight.

## BODY COMPOSITION MEASURES IN CHILDREN

### Skinfold Measures

Hydrostatic weighing techniques are difficult to perform on children because they may resist being submerged in water and may be unable to perform the residual volume measure. If the child is unable to be submerged underwater at residual lung volume for a period of 15 to 30 seconds, the hydrostatic weight cannot be obtained. Furthermore, if the child is unable to completely expel all of the lung vital capacity, an accurate measure of residual volume cannot be obtained. Nonetheless, Lohman (12) conducted extensive research with children and developed some valid and reliable skinfold procedures for determining body fat content in children that correlate well (r = 0.70 to 0.90) with hydrostatic weighing. The test-retest reliability of the skinfold procedure is also high (r = 0.95) when technicians are properly trained.

The procedure utilizes two skinfold sites, the triceps and calf. The triceps measure is a vertical fold taken midway between the acromion and olecranon on the posterior of the arm with the elbow extended. The calf measure is a vertical fold taken at the place of greatest girth on the inside of the lower leg in line with the medial malleolus. Three measures are taken at each site, and the median measure for each site is used for body fat determination. The triceps and calf measurements are added together, and the sum is converted into percent body fat according to the values presented in *Table 13.8*.

### Dual-Energy X-Ray Absorptiometry

Advances in technology have recently made it possible to perform body composition assessments in children using DXA. Whole-body scans can be performed in 6 to 7 minutes, while regional scans can be performed in a shorter time. Age-matched reference values for bone mineral and body fat content have been compiled. Since the DXA procedure is relatively noninvasive and little is required from the subject, this procedure holds promise as a valid technique in body composition assessment for children.

▶ *INQUIRY SUMMARY.* Body composition analysis in children is important because information about normal growth and development patterns can help health care professionals deal with certain childhood diseases and chronic conditions. Although assessments in children are more difficult to obtain than those in adults, a few methods of assessment are valid for pediatric populations. *What cautions should the health professional take when discussing body composition assessment results with parents and children?*

## Summary

Health care professionals and professionals in exercise science or sports medicine must perform and interpret body composition assessments to help their clients/patients achieve their health- or sports-related objectives. Several methods can be used to assess body composition, each with its own level of validity and reliability. The "best" method a professional can use for body composition

| *Table 13.8* | **BODY COMPOSITION NORMS FOR CHILDREN FOR TRICEPS AND CALF SKINFOLD MEASURES** | | | |
|---|---|---|---|---|
| **Boys** | **Girls** | **Skinfolds (mm)** | **% Fat** | **Skinfolds (mm) % Fat** |
| Very low | <5 | <8 | <11 | <12 |
| Low | 5–10 | 8–10 | 11–16 | 12–15 |
| Normal | 11–25 | 11–20 | 17–30 | 16–25 |
| Moderately high | 26–32 | 21–25 | 31–36 | 26–30 |
| High | 33–40 | 26–31 | 37–45 | 31–38 |
| Very high | >40 | >31 | >45 | >38 |

assessment depends on:

- Validity of the method
- Reliability of the method
- Cost of the equipment and/or procedure
- Ease of administration of the assessment
- Comfort level for the patient/client
- Type of data obtained from the assessment
- Training necessary for the professional administering the assessment
- Sample population to be evaluated

Norms for bone mineral content as well as soft tissue composition have been compiled, but a professional consensus of standard values for these body tissues has not been achieved because of the inability to establish strong cause and effect relationships among body composition and health, disease, and/or athletic performance. Caution should be used while interpreting body composition assessments, particularly for youth, because of the tendency of many people to resort to extreme behaviors to achieve what they consider the "ideal" body size.

## SUMMARY KNOWLEDGE

1. What are some reasons a professional would want to assess body composition in his/her clients?
2. Is there such a thing as "ideal" body weight?
3. How does body fat content relate to disease and mortality?
4. What value is the body mass index to epidemiologic studies?
5. List several methods for body composition analysis and the advantages/disadvantages of each.
6. Which model for body composition analysis gives the professional the most usable information?

### References

1. Brozek J, Grande F, Anderson JT, et al. Densitometric analysis of body composition: revision of some quantitative assumptions. *Ann N Y Acad Sci* 1963;110:113–140.
2. Siri WE. Body composition from fluid spaces and density. In: Brozek J, Henchel A, eds. *Techniques for measuring body composition*. Washington, DC: National Academy of Sciences, 1961:223–244.
3. Dempster P, Aitkens S. A new air displacement method for the determination of human body composition. *Med Sci Sports Exerc* 1995;27:1692–1697.
4. Vescovi JD, Hildebrandt L, Miller W, et al. Evaluation of the BOD POD for estimating percent fat in female college athletes. *J Strength Cond Res* 2002;16:599–605.
5. Biaggi RR, Vollman MW, Nies MA, et al. Comparison of air-displacement plethysmography with hydrostatic weighing and bioelectrical impedance analysis for the assessment of body composition in healthy adults. *Am J Clin Nutr* 1999;69:898–903.
6. Lockner DW, Heyward VH, Baumgartner RN, et al. Comparison of air-displacement plethysmography, hydrodensitometry, and dual X-ray absorptiometry for assessing body composition of children 10 to 18 years of age. *Ann New York Acad Sci* 2000;904:72–78.
7. Jackson AS, Pollock ML. Generalized equations for predicting body density of men. *Br J Nutr* 1978;40:497–504.
8. Jackson AS, Pollock ML, Ward A. Generalized equations for predicting body density of women. *Med Sci Sports Exerc* 1980;12: 175–181.
9. Going S, Davis R. *ACSM's resource manual for guidelines for exercise testing and prescription*. 4th ed. Baltimore: Lippincott Williams & Wilkins, 2001.
10. Gruber JJ, Pollock ML, Graves JE, et al. Comparison of Harpenden and Lange calipers in predicting body composition. *Res Q Exerc Sport* 1990;61:184–190.
11. Ashley CD, Tonery J. Validity of commercially-available bioelectrical impedance measures of body composition. *Med Sci Sports Exerc* 2000;32(suppl):S354.
12. Lohman TG. The use of skinfolds to estimate body fatness in children and youth. *J Phys Educ Rec Dance* 1987;58:67–69.

### Suggested Readings

Bates DW, Black DM, Cummings SR. Clinical use of bone densitometry: clinical applications. *JAMA* 2002;288:1898–1900.

Cummings SR, Bates D, Black DM. Clinical use of bone densitometry: scientific review. *JAMA* 2002;288:1889–1897.

Kyle UG, Genton L, Pichard C. Body composition: what's new? *Curr Opin Clin Nutr Metab Care* 2002;5:427–433.

van Raaij JMA, Peek MEM, Vermaat-Miedema SH, et al. New equations for estimating body fat mass in pregnancy from body density or total body water. *Am J Clin Nutr* 1988;48:24–29.

Wagner DR, Heyward VH. Techniques of body composition assessment: a review of laboratory and field methods. *Res Q Exerc Sport* 1999;70:135–149.

### On the Internet

Baylor College of Medicine Children's Nutrition Research Center: Body Composition Laboratory: Available at: **http://www.bcm.tmc.edu/bodycomplab**. Accessed May 04, 2005.

Life Measurement, Inc.: BOD POD. Available at: **http://www.bodpod.com**. Accessed April 26, 2005.

Shape Up America! Body Fat Lab. Available at: **http://www.shapeup.org/bodylab/frmst.htm**. Accessed May 04, 2005.

Sports Fitness Advisor: Sports Training Tips for Athletic Peak Performance: Body Composition Articles. Available at: **http://www.sport-fitness-advisor.com/bodycomposition.html**. Accessed May 04, 2005.

## Writing to Learn

*In this chapter you learned about different techniques that can be used for the assessment of body composition in health, disease, and athletic performance. You also learned how to evaluate the efficacy and safety of each of these techniques. Construct a table with several rows and four columns. Title each column with the headings: Body composition assessment method, Underlying scientific principle, Advantages, and Disadvantages. Now complete the table for any method in which you are interested. Note that if there is a method which was not described in this chapter, you can use SOAP notes (Chapter 12) to help evaluate the method.*

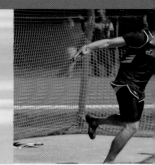

## CHAPTER

# 14 Training for Physical Fitness and Sport

*When the body is stressed beyond a customary level, improved physical performance ensues. However, training has to be performed with specific goals in mind. Consider an Olympic discus thrower. What may you deduce about his training methods given the nature of this event?*

## CHAPTER OUTLINE

The key to improving the performance of athletes and recreational players lies in purposeful exercise training implemented with specific goals in mind. To be a successful competitor, training must be geared to the sport and basic principles must be followed. The principles contained in this chapter are necessary for the coach or fitness professional to develop well-conceived exercise programs for the management of their clients.

## Principles of Training

The elite athlete trains for high-level performance. However, the general principles he or she follows are the same as those followed by the recreational athlete, who often is chiefly concerned with producing health and not superior performance. Generalized health is a recognized outcome of physical conditioning. The term most often used to describe the health benefits of exercise training is health-related physical fitness, defined according to its five basic components.

1. **Muscular strength**
2. **Muscular endurance**
3. **Joint flexibility**

4. Optimal **body composition**
5. **Cardiorespiratory endurance**

An increase in health-related physical fitness produces the following outcomes related to exercise performance.

- Increases peak performance during maximal static or dynamic muscular effort
- Increases efficiency of muscular effort during submaximal static or dynamic exercise, sport performance, or activities of daily living
- Slows the onset of fatigue during general physical activity
- Prevents future loss of functional status or performance capability

To accomplish one or more of these four outcomes requires the effective implementation of two key training principles: **specificity** and **progressive overload**. The remainder of this chapter is concerned with how these training principles relate to programs designed specifically to improve muscle strength, muscle endurance, power, speed, and cardiorespiratory endurance. Proper knowledge of how exercise and sport activities are classified is a necessary corollary to understanding the principles of training. As you read through the next two sections, remember that the principle of specificity relates to the type of activity chosen and the principle of overload relates to exercise dose, i.e., how hard one trains.

## SPECIFICITY

The goal of sport training is to transfer training to performance. The athlete, weekend performer, or rehabilitating patient must regularly overload specific tissues, such as muscles and fascia, or organ systems, such as the cardiac and pulmonary systems. The best way to improve performance is to engage in specific adjunct training activities that are similar in nature to the actual event. Specificity refers to training particularly aimed at a desired outcome. An example of this for gymnastics training is presented in Case Study 14.1.

Specificity has metabolic, physiologic, and mechanical components. Metabolic and physiologic specificity relate to the predominant bioenergetic and physiologic responses

---

## CASE STUDY 14.1: *SPECIFICITY IN SPORT-SPECIFIC TRAINING—GYMNASTICS*

### CASE

Kurt is a freshman gymnast at a small university. He has participated in intercollegiate gymnastics for the last 4 years and has excellent skills in all events; however, the event in which he is weakest is the "still rings." Although he has excellent swing moves, he consistently loses points on his strength skills. Specifically he lacks the strength to remain in the proper position in an "iron cross" for a required 2-second period.

### DESCRIPTION

Specificity of training implies that conditioning mirrors, as much as possible, that which occurs or is expected to occur in the competitive arena. Absolute specificity is difficult to achieve and requires critical musculature to be activated at specific speeds, joint angles, and under the metabolic conditions present in competition. An example of absolute specificity or near absolute specificity can be demonstrated in the sport of gymnastics.

The "iron cross" is a strength move of moderate difficulty that requires the gymnast to move into a position in which the body is suspended vertically and the arms are parallel to the floor in a cross position. Although 2 seconds sounds brief, it is quite long considering that the gymnast must carefully and confidently move to the position and remain for a full 2-second count before initiating the next skill. Most gymnasts exceed the minimum time requirement to show complete mastery. Not getting to the optimal position or exiting the skill prematurely means precious points will be deducted. The muscles that play a predominant role and/or lend assistance to maintaining proper position are the latissimus dorsi, pectoralis major (sternal portion), coracobrachialis, teres major, and long head of the triceps brachii. All of these muscles can be trained with dynamic resistance exercise; however, there would be little specificity. Strength changes may occur in the involved musculature, but it is unlikely that such training would result in acquisition of the skill.

### INTERVENTION

Near absolute specificity can be achieved by having the gymnast condition on the still rings. Below is an example of a sport-specific training strategy.

1. The gymnast is asked to move to a straight-arm support position on the still rings with the entire body straight, legs together, and toes pointed.
2. The coach, trainer, or fellow gymnast stands beneath the rings and supports the feet.
3. The gymnast lowers slowly to the required position (arms parallel) and remains there for 3 to 5 seconds and then returns to the straight arm support position by simultaneously adducting both arms. The arms must remain straight during the return to the beginning position. The spotter only provides as much assistance as is necessary to complete the maneuver. It is conducted in a slow and controlled manner with particular attention paid to form and technique.
4. The number of repetitions is dependent on the current skill and specific strength of the gymnast. A minimum of two consecutive repetitions for a total of approximately 10 seconds should be performed, eventually moving to four to six consecutive repetitions.
5. Initially two sets of two to six repetitions should be performed; if this is tolerated, the gymnast should move to three sets and perhaps more depending upon the gymnast's training age.
6. A 3- to 5-minute rest should be taken between sets.
7. The frequency of the conditioning should be at least two times per week, and perhaps three if excessive muscle soreness is not experienced.

At some point in the conditioning program, the gymnast will be able to lower to the position without assistance and remain there for the required 2-second period. This conditioning program meets the specificity requirement for joint angle, muscular involvement, movement pattern, and energy system. There is almost perfect specificity with the only exception being that the "iron cross" in training is not preceded by a routine, during which fatigue can be a mitigating factor. This concern may be offset by preceding a set with several of the actual skills that are to be performed in the routine.

*Case Study used with permission from James Clemons, PhD, Department of Kinesiology, University of Louisiana at Lafayette.*

produced during the exercise or event, and they concern both anaerobic and aerobic conditioning. Exercise training produces specific biochemical and physiologic adaptations in key body systems—cardiopulmonary, neuroendocrine, neuromuscular, and musculoskeletal. Therefore, for a training program to be effective, it must produce adaptations in those systems that are optimal for a given sport performance or for a specific therapeutic objective. Physiologic adaptations to training are specific to muscle actions involved, speed of movement, range of motion, muscle groups trained, energy systems involved, and intensity and volume of training.

## Metabolic and Physiologic Specificity

Exercise classification must be considered to have a sound grasp of specificity. Exercise, athletic events, and other general physical activities can be placed on a continuum that classifies activities in two important ways: the *bioenergetic* and *hemodynamic* consequences of the activity (*Fig. 14.1*). Bioenergetic consequences refer to the metabolic responses caused by the event or exercise. Exercise bioenergetics range from those activities that are largely anaerobic to those that are largely aerobic. For a sport event that is continuous (toward the left end of the continuum), training must engage aerobic metabolism. Conversely, if the sport event is discontinuous (toward the right end of the continuum), training must engage anaerobic metabolism.

For the hemodynamic responses produced by a given activity, either a volume-loaded or pressure-loaded cardiovascular system ensues at the extremes of the continuum.

For example, long-distance running involves rhythmic, dynamic movements with very low static muscular contractions (left end). From a hemodynamic standpoint, this requires sustaining high cardiac outputs. However, at the right end of the continuum, events such as weightlifting use a large degree of static muscular contractions and load the cardiovascular system with high pressures and low to moderate cardiac outputs.

Specific metabolic and hemodynamic responses are a consequence of dynamic or static muscular mechanical action inherent in a given sport, exercise, or activity. **Dynamic exercise** includes the following characteristics:

- Movement is rhythmic, involving concentric and eccentric muscle contractions
- Relatively small intramuscular forces
- Volume loaded (movement of relatively large quantities of blood)
- Sustainable for prolonged periods of time

In contrast, **static exercise** is associated with isometric muscle contractions (no joint rotation). Relatively large intramuscular forces and high systolic and diastolic blood pressures are developed, and the exercise cannot be sustained for prolonged periods. *Figure 14.2* displays a schematic of the interrelationships between these different concepts for the classification of exercise and activities; some examples are shown for each. To check your understanding, try producing other examples in each category.

Muscle length and joint movement have also been used as a means to classify exercise (i.e., dynamic exercise

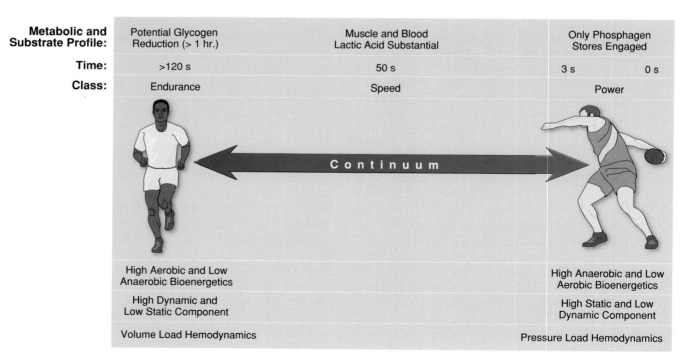

**FIGURE 14.1.** The physical activity continuum of metabolic and hemodynamic responses based on peak dynamic and static components during sports activity and exercise.

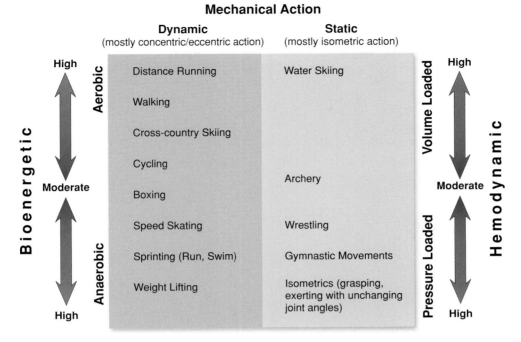

**FIGURE 14.2.** Classification of exercise and activities. The line separating dynamic from static represents a true dichotomy between these two mechanical actions. However, the arrows on the diagram represent more of a continuum.

producing large changes in muscle length and joint ranges of motion, and static exercise producing little or no change), but these variables are less precise and therefore less useful. For example, jogging is a dynamic exercise that involves limited joint range of motion during the activity, while weightlifting involves full or nearly full range of motion joint action and large changes in muscle length. Yet weightlifting also involves a large static component (isometric muscle contractions are occurring) and jogging does not. One distinction between these two exercise forms is the disparate muscle forces developed. Muscle contraction force, as a percentage of **maximal voluntary contraction** (MVC), is small during jogging and other similar kinds of rhythmic, aerobic activities, while muscle contraction force during weightlifting is large, leading to complete or near complete vascular occlusion in the working muscles as contraction forces approach 50% MVC. Small or large static forces with their attendant differential blood flow characteristics help dictate the metabolic and hemodynamic profile of the exercise or activity.

All sports, activities, and exercises fall somewhere on the activity continuum. Caution should be used, however, when attempting to classify activities because the terms connoting mechanical action (static and dynamic) are different from the terms connoting the type of metabolic (anaerobic and aerobic) or hemodynamic (pressure load and volume load) consequences. Most high-intensity static exercise is performed primarily with anaerobic metabolism, while high-intensity dynamic exercise of several minutes' duration is performed primarily with aerobic metabolism. Exceptions to this rule are dynamic exercises like sprinting and weightlifting, which are performed primarily with anaerobic metabolism. A wide variety of sports and activities can be placed in the high dynamic category, and a wide variety can be placed in the high static category. It should be understood, however, that no sport or activity is exclusively static and anaerobic versus dynamic and aerobic. There are many activities in which the dominant energy-systems change during the performance of the sport (basketball and soccer are good examples), making their exact classification difficult.

Referring back to Figure 14.1, another key factor is the time involved in performing the exercise or activity. Performance time is always related to the bioenergetic system employed. When activities of different natures have similar performance times, the energy contributions from the various bioenergetic systems are also similar. The energy sources for a given activity are time and intensity dependent regardless of the type of activity being performed. Whether a person is raking leaves, hauling heavy boxes, pushing a cart, running, or swimming, the primary energy source used is dependent on the performance time that can be maintained at a given intensity for that activity.

The descriptors power, speed, and endurance communicate how intensely the activity is performed. Track and field events are good examples of the use of these descriptors and their time frames. For instance, the shot put takes only 2 to 3 seconds to perform. In that time frame, the athlete extends maximal effort in moving across the ring to displace the shot with as much force possible. *What makes this a power event and not a speed event?* The answer lies in the time frame required to perform the event as well as the

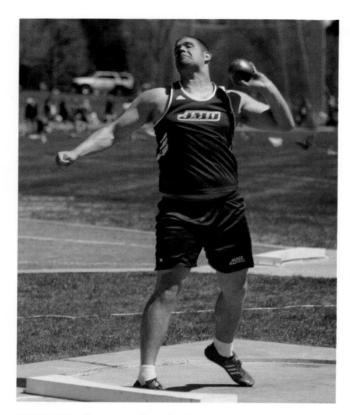

FIGURE 14.3. Shot putter. Photo by Gregory Werner.

rate of expenditure of ATP required by the event. Across the continuum of physical activities, there are a number of examples of power events in which maximal efforts are produced over a short time frame (shot putting is an example, as shown in *Figure 14.3*). Some running and jumping events may also be included in this category as long as the rate of ATP use is extremely high, and the time frame of the event is short. For example, the 40-yard dash and simply running up the stairs as quickly as you can qualify as power activities. In the time frame of the power activities, only the high-energy phosphate system is engaged. This results in a decreased intramuscular concentration of creatine phosphate and ATP, and an increased concentration of creatine, inorganic phosphate, and ADP.

In contrast to power events, speed events require a lower rate of ATP over a longer time period. Examples of speed events are the longer sprints (200 to 400 meters). **Resistance exercise** performed over many repetitions for the purpose of optimizing muscle hypertrophy (as occurs in **bodybuilding** routines) also qualifies as a speed activity. Since the duration of the resistance exercise bout (the lifting set) and the ATP expenditure rate may equal that of longer sprints or runs (~30 seconds), the metabolic profiles of the two activities are largely the same. Both activities are characterized by a substantial increase in muscle lactate concentration. *Figure 14.4* shows the metabolic responses to five sets of front squats and back squats using an Olympic barbell and leg presses, and leg

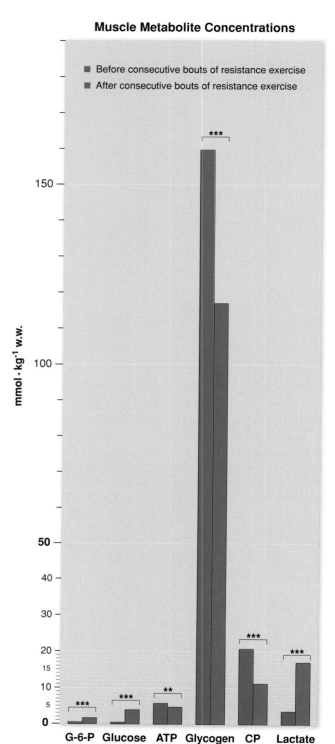

FIGURE 14.4. Muscle metabolite concentrations before (open bars) and after (shaded bars) consecutive bouts of resistance exercise. Values are mmol·kg⁻¹ wet weight (mean ± SD). Differences between means are **$p < 0.01$, ***$p < 0.001$. G-6-P, glucose 6-phosphate; ATP, adenosine triphosphate; CP, creatine phosphate. Data from Tesch PA, Colliander EB, Kaiser P. Muscle metabolism during intense, heavy-resistance exercise. *Eur J Appl Physiol* 1986;55:362–366.

extensions using a variable resistance machine. Subjects performed six to 12 repetitions to muscular failure. Each set of exercise lasted 30 seconds followed by a 60-second rest period. Changes in other markers of glycolytic energy flux along with the five-fold increase in muscle lactate concentration are shown (1).

Performing resistance exercise with heavier weights and much shorter durations (fewer repetitions per set) does not elicit the same type of metabolic profile shown in Figure 14.4. So-called **powerlifting** falls into this category; it produces a metabolic and substrate profile indicative of phosphagen energy flux only. This was demonstrated in a classic study by Kuel and coworkers (2),who showed that blood lactate concentrations during weightlifting were only mildly elevated (slightly more than 4 mmol·L$^{-1}$), which represented only a two-fold increase above rest. In contrast, Tesch (1) reported blood lactate concentrations of approximately 13 mmol·L$^{-1}$ following resistance exercise performed at a substantially higher intensity level than that which was reported in the study by Kuel. It is clear from these studies that the metabolic response to resistance exercise is greatly influenced by power output, work time, and work:rest ratios indicative of the exhaustive style of lifting typical of bodybuilders. Therefore, from a metabolic standpoint, intensity of weightlifting may be judged by the lactate response, making resistance exercise of the type performed by bodybuilders highly intense.

In contrast, endurance events require a much slower rate of ATP usage and last much longer than power and speed events. Therefore, endurance events are placed at the opposite end of the continuum. Events such as the 1500-meter and longer runs are put in the endurance category. The activity continuum aids the coach, personal trainer, and therapist by providing an immediate glimpse into the metabolic and physiologic consequences of performing the sport, exercise, or activity. The activity continuum also provides a quick reference to the type of the training program needed to enhance the predominant energy pathways and physiologic systems being used.

## Mechanical Specificity

Mechanical specificity relates to the ability of the training regimen and exercises employed to mimic the mechanical action of the actual free-moving sport performance. For example, resistance exercise is an important training adjunct employed by athletes of all types to increase strength and power during sport performance. To be effective, the type of resistance exercise chosen must have mechanical specificity so that training adaptations correspond to the individual's sport performance, as was demonstrated in Case Study 14.1. Another classic example of this is free weightlifting movements that engage large muscle masses and several body segments simultaneously. One such lift is the power pull exercise, which mimics effectively many sport-specific movements like the vertical jump (*Fig. 14.5*). Vertical jumping is an

important associated movement in many power sports. In this example, the multijoint training exercise (power pull) and associated sport-specific movement (vertical jump) have mechanical similarities because multijoint movements are also characteristic of many sport-specific patterns of movement. There would probably not be enough transfer to sport performance if, for instance, improvements in vertical jump height were sought by training the quadriceps muscle group using isolated knee extension exercise performed on a resistance exercise machine. While this type of knee extension exercise would improve quadriceps strength, the exercise doesn't effectively mimic many sport-specific movements (i.e., vertical jumping). That is, the mechanical specificity of isolated knee extensions is probably too low to effectively carry over to sport performance. However, stronger quadriceps is certainly a basic prerequisite for good vertical jump performance.

As we will see in the sections on strength and power performance, power has two components: strength and speed. For optimal power performance, you need improvements in both strength and speed. For example, one athlete can squat 350 pounds, but it takes 15 to 20 seconds to completely finish the lift. The other athlete can squat 350 pounds but can complete the lift in 5 seconds. Neither athlete can squat 351 pounds. *Who is stronger?* The answer is neither. *Who is more powerful?* The answer is the second athlete. *Who would most likely have a greater vertical jump in sport performance?* The answer is the second athlete because he has more power. *Who would you want as a lineman in football?* The answer is still the second athlete because he is more powerful.

While the reason for the carryover of many mechanically similar strength-power training exercises to athletic activities is still being investigated, insight may come from an understanding of the physiology of muscle strength. Strength depends on the following factors:

- Number of motor units involved: the more motor units activated, the greater the force
- Frequency of motor unit firing: as the rate of firing increases, tension increases
- Motor unit synchronization: if large numbers of motor units fire simultaneously, muscular effort is greater (important in near maximal lifts)
- Pattern of motor unit and whole-muscle contraction: the timing of contraction of motor units and whole muscles improves maximal force production if the performer learns not to contract antagonistic muscles at inappropriate moments during performance
- Degree of neuromuscular inhibition: limiting Golgi tendon organ influence
- Muscle fiber type: type IId/x units produce greater force output and contraction velocity
- Degree of muscle hypertrophy: there is a linear relationship between muscle cross-sectional area and force output

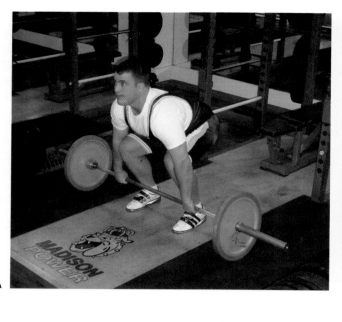

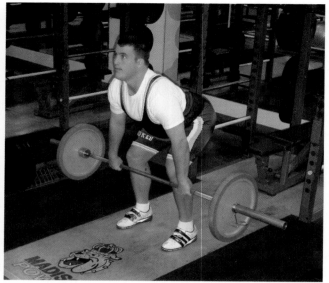

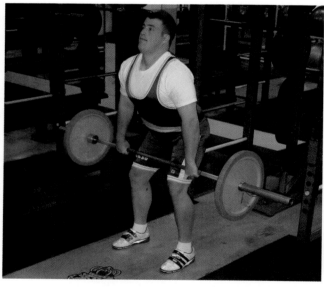

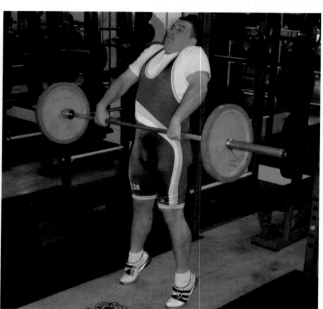

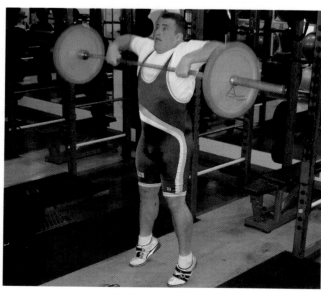

**FIGURE 14.5.** Power pull exercise. Photo by Gregory Werner.

■ Biomechanical properties: point of muscle tendon insertion, limb length, and muscle angle of pull influence force output

Resistance training, especially using free weights, may impact all of these mechanisms except biomechanical properties. For example, motor unit recruitment and firing rate are enhanced, synchronization is enhanced at lower force outputs, motor unit firing pattern is enhanced, and deinhibition occurs. These mechanisms are responsible for strength gains early in training. Later training results in muscle hypertrophy and continued strength gains.

Related to specificity is the concept of cross-training, which is the practice of training with more than one exercise mode. Research has shown that engaging in endurance training reduces strength. This has prompted the recommendation that strength-power athletes avoid a level of endurance training that would produce significant physiologic adaptations indicative of endurance training. Adjunct training programs must mimic the primary sports performance. In the case of distance running, for instance, the mechanics of the exercise itself may negatively affect the weightlifting-specific pattern of motor unit recruitment and whole-muscle contraction. Aerobic training may cause a reduction of myosin ATPase in type IIa and IId/x muscle fibers and a reduction in the concentration of anaerobic enzymes. Aerobic training may also increase skeletal muscle catabolism, leading to a smaller muscle mass.

These confounding physiologic adaptations lead to mixed results for the strength-power athlete who uses aerobic conditioning as an adjunct to his/her sport-specific training. In addition, endurance training typically involves low-velocity contractions. Therefore, the slow-contraction velocities of endurance training are at odds with the high-contraction velocities necessary for the adaptations to resistance exercise required for gains in muscle power. Resistance training has a large degree of specificity to the neuromuscular system for strength/power sports and performances. However, not all cross-training is bad. Cross-training that combines two different aerobic exercise modes can be effective for endurance athletes by increasing the overload stimulus for adaptation and by preventing overuse injuries by engaging too much in only one motor pattern (i.e., running). Box 14.1 details research on the interplay between endurance training and strength training.

Training programs that emphasize repetitive exercise intervals of short duration and high intensity will produce adaptations in the ATP-PC system. A sprinter, for example, would improve performance best by running high-intensity sprints. On the other hand, a marathoner would improve performance best by performing moderate-intensity runs lasting several minutes to an hour or more so that the aerobic pathways that produce ATP are overloaded. Table 14.1 shows the percentage of total training time given to developing a specific metabolic system according to the event time of the anticipated performance (note that the suggested time frames refer only to the continuous exercise

time). The nature of the activity must be taken into account when planning the training regimen. For example, a 60-minute football game is not composed of 60 minutes of continuous activity but rather many short (2 to 5 seconds) intense exercise bouts. Hence, the training regimen for the football player should focus primarily (95%) on overloading the ATP-PC energy system.

*LINKUP:* **Case Study: Energy System Overload,** *found at* *http://connection.lww.com/go/brownexphys and on the Student Resource CD-ROM, addresses training specificity and energy systems.*

## OVERLOAD

Specificity determines the kinds of adaptations needed to excel in sport or to improve the functional capacity of specific body systems, and it is chiefly concerned with the kind of activity chosen. Overload, however, determines the degree and rate with which physiologic adaptations are achieved. Overload refers to placing greater demands on body systems than they are accustomed. These demands are imposed at regular intervals. The chief concern of overload is exposure of the body to unaccustomed stress, without which no improvement is realized. Overload is accomplished by gradually increasing the amount of work imposed over time. During the course of training, a stimulus threshold usually exists for the development of chronic training adaptations. These adaptations provide the physiologic basis for improved performance.

Manipulating overload mainly involves monitoring training intensity, duration, and frequency. All three of these factors are important for all types of sport-specific training. These factors can be broken down to more particularly define a training regimen and ensure that the regimen employs progressive overload. For improvements in functional physical fitness, the five following general factors may be considered for different types of training regimens:

■ *Load*: an intensity factor, i.e., the weight lifted or any other means to apply force in resistance training (may also be thought of as a certain aerobic power output for endurance training, i.e., % $\dot{V}O_{2max}$)
■ *Repetitions*: a duration factor, i.e., an extra work cycle in sprinting or additional lifts at the current load in resistance training
■ *Repetition speed*: an intensity factor, i.e., maximal versus hard sprinting or performing resistance work with quick repetitions to maximize power development
■ *Altered rest periods*: an intensity factor, i.e., shortened for endurance improvement or lengthened for strength and power training
■ *Volume*: intensity, frequency, and/or duration factor, i.e., represents overall total work performed (adding additional work bouts will increase training frequency and therefore volume)

# R E S E A R C H   H I G H L I G H T

**Bell GJ, Petersen SR, Wessel J, et al. Physiological adaptations to concurrent endurance training and low velocity resistance training.** *Int J Sports Med* **1991;12:384–390.**

### RESEARCH SUMMARY

The hypothesis of an "interference effect," i.e., an attenuation in strength gains when endurance training is performed simultaneously with high-resistance training, has strengthened the concept of training specificity and suggests that strength and power athletes should do minimal endurance training to not interfere with their primary sport performance. The opposite is not true, however. Strength training does not appear to interfere with gains in aerobic power during endurance training. Studies have shown that maximal $O_2$ uptake is not compromised with cross-training, allowing endurance-trained individuals to participate in strength training without hindering their primary performance area. The hypothesis of an interference effect is not supported by all the evidence, however, especially in studies that demonstrate similar levels of muscle hypertrophy in both groups (i.e., the group doing resistance training solely versus the group doing combined resistance and endurance training). The present study was undertaken, therefore, to either support or negate this hypothesis.

Thirty-one male subjects volunteered to serve in either a cross-training group (CT, 16 subjects with previous experience in cross training) or a resistance-training group (RT, 15 subjects with previous experience in resistance training). Subjects were tested on all dependent variables at the following intervals: 4 weeks prior to training, twice immediately prior to training, and at 3-week intervals during training. The effects of endurance training on indices of aerobic endurance and right knee extensor strength was determined. Endurance tests were submaximal responses to an absolute workload and maximal $O_2$ uptake measured in the endurance-training group only. Strength was assessed in both groups as peak torque produced during a single right knee extension and total work during four maximal knee extensions at an angular velocity of 1.05 rad·sec$^{-1}$ on a calibrated Kinetic Communicator gravity-compensated isokinetic dynamometer. Strength tests were performed in the concentric mode for knee extension. Quadriceps femoris cross-sectional area was determined in both groups by computerized tomography scanning before training and at 6, 9, and 12 weeks of training. The CT group performed continuous rowing 3 days per week at 85% to 90% of maximal heart rate and a duration of 40 minutes, which was progressively increased by 5 minutes every 3 weeks

until a duration of 55 minutes was achieved. The CT groups also performed low-velocity resistance training (variable-resistance hydraulic equipment) three times per week for 12 weeks on different days than their endurance training routine. The RT group also performed this same resistance exercise schedule. The RT group also performed one endurance-training session per week (continuous exercise at a moderate intensity level for a maximum of 30 minutes) to maintain the level of aerobic conditioning they had prior to the study. The hydraulic routine consisted of 12 stations: unilateral knee extension and flexion, bilateral hip and knee extension, and other stations involving upper- and lower-body exercises. Two sets of each station were completed with a work:rest ratio of 1:1. Training was initiated with two complete circuits of 12 stations, with an extra 33% of the circuit added every 3 weeks over the 12-week program. Three minutes of rest was given between each circuit.

The groups were not significantly different in peak torque, total work, or cross-sectional area before the training program commenced, suggesting that they were essentially equivalent. No significant group effects were demonstrated for peak torque, total work, or knee extensor cross-sectional area during the training phase of the measurement intervals; however, both groups demonstrated a training effect with significant improvements at the measurement intervals during the training phase. Peak torque, total work, and cross-sectional area were all significantly greater commencing at week 6 of the training phase. Maximal $O_2$ uptake was significantly higher in the CT group after 3 weeks of training and rose significantly again at the 6-week testing period. Maximal $O_2$ uptake showed no further increase from week 6 to 12. The CT group also increased their exercise economy as submaximal $O_2$ uptake was lower at week 3 of training. Submaximal $O_2$ uptake was significantly reduced again by week 12 of training. A gain in exercise economy was also demonstrated in CT subjects by lower heart rate and blood lactate scores during training.

The physiologic adaptations produced from endurance and resistance training are potentially antagonistic to each other. Endurance training supports cardiorespiratory and oxidative mechanisms, which improve maximal aerobic power and exercise efficiency, while resistance training supports neuromuscular mechanisms, which improve maximal muscular strength and power output. This could help explain the interference hypothesis as strength is thought to be compromised because of the supposed antagonistic physiologic consequences of endurance training, which includes selective adaptations in slow motor units to the exclusion of fast units.

***Research Highlight 14.1, continued***

A close examination of the results of this study shows that the RT group demonstrated a trend towards continual adaptation in strength and power indices during the last 3 weeks of the study (from week 9 to 12). In contrast, the CT group clearly showed a trend towards a leveling off (no trending upwards) of these variables in this time period. The researchers concluded that extending the study beyond the 12-week time period could possibly have produced a significant group effect. The lack of change in the cross-sectional area of the knee extensors in the CT group during the final 3 weeks of training in the present study paralleled the lack of change in strength. This effect was opposite that of the RT group, which showed a trend towards greater knee extensor cross-sectional area, which would explain the continued upward trend in strength indices. However, there was no statistical support in this study for this interpretation.

**IMPLICATION FOR FURTHER RESEARCH**

In conclusion, the results of this study were equivocal. While strict statistical interpretation does not support the interference hypothesis, qualitative assessment of the data leads to the conclusion of a possible trend towards greater strength productivity in the RT group, which may have been borne out statistically had the duration of the study been longer. Thus, reduced strength adaptations with a combination of endurance and strength training is still an attractive hypothesis that warrants further research.

These factors can be manipulated in a number of different ways to produce overload; however, only small incremental increases (2.5% to 5%) in training volume every 2 weeks are recommended to avoid overtraining.

The intensity variable is the most important component of overload. The way intensity is defined depends on the activity chosen. Table 14.2 lists some ways in which intensity is determined for specific training modes. Determining intensity in resistance exercise involves manipulating the **one repetition maximum** (1 RM) or the maximum voluntary contraction. 1 RM is specific to dynamic resistance exercise, and the maximum voluntary contraction is specific to static resistance exercise. Both are expressions of the load imposed on the contracting musculature and are the chief intensity factors for resistance exercise. The other intensity factors specific to different modes of exercise are covered in the sections that follow. Duration and frequency are also covered in detail in those sections as overload is more fully described for specific objectives.

▶ *INQUIRY SUMMARY.* Different forms of exercises or sport activity may elicit very different metabolic and hemodynamic responses, and chronic training involving particular kinds of exercises lead to specific physiologic adaptations. The specificity principle dictates that to be successful in sport, training must match the desired goals. Once the type of training activity is identified according to the specificity

| **Table 14.1** | **PROPORTION OF TRAINING TIME SPENT TO DEVELOP SPECIFIC ENERGY SYSTEMS** | | |
|---|---|---|---|
| **Energy System performance** | **ATP-PC Strength or power** | **Glycolysis Speed** | **Aerobic Endurance** |
| Event time (continuous) | | | |
| <5–15 seconds | 95% | 5% | 0% |
| 20–30 seconds | 80% | 20% | 0% |
| 35–45 seconds | 50% | 50% | 0% |
| 60–90 seconds | 30% | 50% | 20% |
| 2–3 minutes | 10% | 30% | 60% |
| 4–6 minutes | 10% | 20% | 70% |
| 10–15 minutes | 0% | 10% | 90% |
| 15–25 minutes | 0% | 8% | 92% |
| 30–60 minutes | 0% | 5% | 95% |
| 2–3 hours | 0% | 2% | 98% |

| Table 14.2 | METHODS OF DETERMINING EXERCISE INTENSITY DURING DIFFERENT TRAINING MODES | |
| --- | --- | --- |
| **Mode** | **Goal** | **Intensity method** |
| Resistance training | Muscle strength and/or muscle endurance | One-repetition maximum or maximum voluntary contraction (specific to static muscular performance) |
| Sprint training | Time improvements in sprints >20 sec duration | Hard sprint intervals of appropriate (glycolytic) time duration to match event duration (longer-distance sprints) |
| Sprint training | Time improvements in sprints <20 sec duration | Maximal sprint intervals of appropriate (phosphagen) time duration to match event duration (shorter-distance sprints) |
| Aerobic training | $\dot{V}O_{2max}$ gains | Heart rate reserve; $\dot{V}O_2$ reserve; pace (exercise velocity); heart rate-specific lactate threshold training; interval training |

principle, to continue to improve requires the diligent implementation of progressive overload. Overload is achieved by manipulating training intensity, frequency, and duration. *Why do you think it is sound practice to first consider specificity and then overload in properly designing a sport-training program?*

## Training for Muscular Fitness

Muscular fitness refers to enhancing the neuromuscular system so that improved sport performance is realized through increases in strength, power, and speed. According to the preceding section, to accomplish this requires adherence to the principles of specificity and overload. Specificity refers to conditioning skeletal muscles in a manner similar to which they are to perform. Progressive overload refers to training muscles beyond some critical level to achieve the necessary physiologic adaptations, such as increases in structure, activation pattern, and/or enzymatic activity. The appropriate overload for each individual can be achieved by manipulating combinations of training mode, frequency, duration, and intensity.

### TRAINING FOR STRENGTH PERFORMANCE

As you apply the overload principle to strength development, both the type of muscle contraction and exercise must be considered. When lifting or lowering a barbell, the external resistance (weight) remains constant. However, the amount of effective muscle force varies throughout the movement because leverage changes throughout the range of motion about the joint. Training performed with a constant external resistance is typically referred to as isotonic exercise, but the term isotonic used in this way is misleading. In reality there are constantly changing muscular forces occurring throughout the concentric and eccentric phases of muscle contraction. The load may be constant, but the muscular forces are not. Therefore, the preferred term, dynamic exercise, is used throughout this chapter and book.

As seen earlier, dynamic exercise involves concentric and eccentric contractions. This can be demonstrated with the pull-up exercise using a fixed bar. The resistance for the pull-up is constant (body weight), making the exercise a dynamic exercise. As you perform the movement, the biceps and other muscles perform concentric contractions; however, when the movement is completed at the bar, isometric contractions occur to hold you in place. When the person lowers back to the starting position, muscles go through eccentric contraction. Viewed in this fashion, many strength exercises that are largely dynamic also involve a degree (however small) of isometric or static muscle contractions.

Strength training can be performed in a number of different ways, ranging from the use of so-called "free weights" (traditional barbells) to manipulation only of one's own body weight (i.e., performing pushups) to the use of various kinds of resistance exercise machines. Some strength-training machines are designed to incorporate a variable resistance in an attempt to accommodate leverage changes through the range of motion. Such machines provide more resistance in the range of motion in which the effective muscle force is higher and less resistance when the effective muscle force is lower. Exercise performed with this type of equipment is called variable resistance exercise (*Fig. 14.6*). However, isokinetic exercise machines allow for maximal force production throughout the contraction by maintaining a constant speed through the full range of motion. Specialized equipment has been designed so that no matter how much force is applied during contraction, the resistance is overcome only at a predetermined constant rate (*Fig. 14.7*).

*An important question is: Which type of strength exercise is best?* The answer to this question depends on the goals of the individual, exercise facilities available, and time constraints. Table 14.3 shows several different categories of strength exercises. Regardless of the type of exercise performed or the type of contraction elicited, continual improvements in strength are based on training through progressive resistance. Progressive resistance exercise training is simply the application of the overload principle. Once the muscle becomes accustomed to overcoming a certain resistance, strength improvement will cease until the muscle is again stressed beyond that to which it is accustomed.

As mentioned earlier, the training overload required to elicit an adaptation can be achieved by manipulating

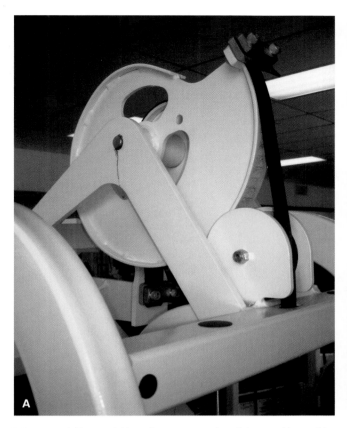
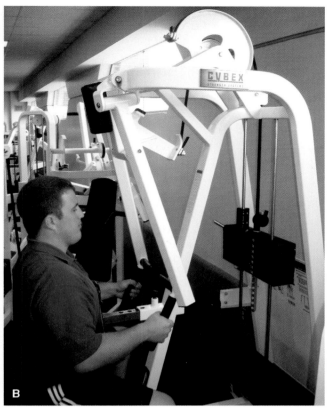

**FIGURE 14.6.** Two variable resistance strength training machines with an offset cam that changes the movement arm of the resistance to account for reduced muscle forces at the weak point in the joint range of motion. Photo by Gregory Werner.

combinations of training mode, frequency, duration, and intensity. Exercise prescriptions for any training regimen can be defined by these four variables. However, these variables may take on one specific definition or several definitions, depending on the objectives of the training regimen. Four ways in which mode, frequency, duration, and intensity can be defined for a strength and/or power training program are provided below:

- *Mode*: defined by the type of contraction (concentric, eccentric, isometric), general type of exercise (isometric, dynamic constant external load resistance exercise, isokinetic, plyometric), type of equipment (free weights, variable resistance machines, calisthenics), specific exercise movement (bench press, biceps curls, etc.), or any combination of these
- *Frequency*: defined in terms of workouts per week, exercises per muscle group during a workout, repetitions of an exercise movement performed consecutively in one set, or sets of an exercise movement performed during a workout
- *Duration*: defined as total workout time, consecutive repetitions of an exercise movement, or work time versus recovery time within a workout
- *Intensity*: defined by the amount of resistance relative to percent of maximum (e.g., 70% of maximum), amount

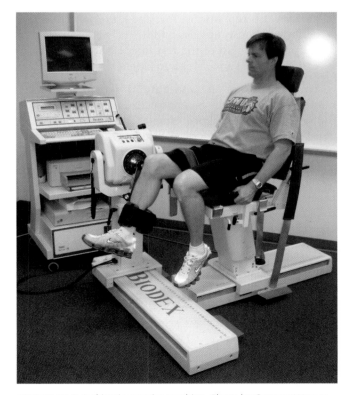

**FIGURE 14.7.** Isokinetic exercise machine. Photo by Gregory Werner.

| Table 14.3 | ADVANTAGES AND DISADVANTAGES OF DIFFERENT STRENGTH-TRAINING EXERCISES | |
|---|---|---|
| **Exercise** | **Advantage** | **Disadvantage** |
| Isometric | Low cost, increase in strength at sticking point, therapy, rehabilitation, minimal supervision | Not applicable to most activities, strength gain only at specific angle, difficult to monitor progress, concentric work only |
| Free weights | Low cost, infinite number of exercises, progress easy to monitor, works concentric and eccentric | Supervision necessary, spotting required, injury potential high, long workout time |
| Stationary equipment | Need for spotters eliminated, generally safe, progress easy to monitor, works concentric and eccentric | High cost, limited to special exercises |
| Variable resistance | Maximum force achieved through full range of motion, generally safe, progress easy to monitor, need for spotters eliminated, works concentric and eccentric | High cost, limited to special exercises |
| Isokinetic | Maximum force achieved through full range of motion, progress easy to monitor | High cost, strength gains limited to speed at which training takes place, limited to special exercises, works only concentric |
| Plyometric | Focus on power, sport specific, low cost, invokes stretch reflex | High injury potential, difficult to monitor progress, maximum loads hard to achieve |
| Concentric workout | Fits most equipment needs | Strength improvement not as good as with eccentric workout |
| Eccentric workout | Possibly gives the greatest strength improvement, supramaximal force achieved | Spotters necessary, high risk of injury, biggest cause of muscle soreness, cannot perform on all equipment |

of resistance relative to body weight (e.g., 50% of body weight), absolute amount of resistance (e.g., 125 kg), number of repetitions for an exercise movement performed consecutively, number of sets of repetitions performed, length of the rest interval between sets, or performance of an exercise to fatigue

The structure of strength-training programs is determined primarily by the main objective to be accomplished through the training. For example, the training objective could be overall strength development for fitness, competitive powerlifting, bodybuilding, sport-specific strength training, or therapy and rehabilitation. The variables of mode, frequency, duration, and intensity that define the program will be determined mainly by the training objective. These variables will also be adjusted somewhat by the equipment and facilities available, as well as the amount of time the participant is willing to dedicate to training.

The training program for the novice usually consists of a plan to exercise all of the major muscle groups in the body with the objective of developing a combination of strength, size, and muscle tone. This objective will be accomplished with an exercise movement for each muscle group performed five to 10 times consecutively in a series of three to five sets. An example of such a program is shown in Table 14.4. The type of program is defined as a dynamic resistance exercise using free weights with both concentric and eccentric contractions. The frequency is 3

days per week with a duration of approximately 30 to 45 minutes. Intensity is defined by percent of body weight lifted and by the rest interval between sets of 60 seconds.

The intermediate strength training program shown in Table 14.5 has as its objective the development of strength and muscle hypertrophy. Each major muscle group is exercised twice. The type of program is defined as dynamic resistance using a combination of free weight training and

| Table 14.4 | NOVICE STRENGTH-TRAINING PROGRAM | | |
|---|---|---|---|
| **Exercise** | **Sets** | **Reps** | **% body weight** |
| Biceps curl | 3 | 10 | 40% |
| Overhead press | 3 | 10 | 50% |
| Bent-over rowing | 3 | 10 | 50% |
| Bench press | 3 | 10 | 60% |
| Upright rowing | 3 | 10 | 40% |
| Situps | 3 | 10 | 10% |
| Squat | 3 | 10 | 75% |
| Heel raises | 3 | 10 | 40% |

Mode: dynamic resistance exercise using free weights; frequency: 3 days per week; duration: 30 to 45 minutes; intensity: percent of body weight, 60-second rest intervals.

| Table 14.5 | INTERMEDIATE STRENGTH-TRAINING PROGRAM | | |
| --- | --- | --- | --- |
| Exercise | Sets | Reps | %1 RM |
| Overhead press | 4 | 6 | 75% |
| Situps | 3 | 30 | |
| Bench press | 4 | 6 | 80% |
| Squat | 3 | 10 | 80% |
| Dumbbell curls | 4 | 6 | 70% |
| Abdominal crunches | 3 | 50 | |
| Leg curls | 4 | 6 | 70% |
| Incline bench press | 4 | 6 | 75% |
| Bent-arm pullovers | 4 | 6 | 70% |
| Knee extension | 4 | 6 | 75% |
| Upright rowing | 4 | 6 | 70% |
| Triceps press | 3 | 10 | 65% |
| Barbell curls | 3 | 10 | 70% |

Type: dynamic resistance (free weight and variable resistance); frequency: 3 days per week; duration: approximately 90 minutes; intensity: %1 RM (90-second rest interval). 1 RM, one repetition maximum.

variable resistance exercises. Frequency is 3 days per week with a duration of about 90 minutes. Intensity for this program is set by a percent of the maximal amount that can be lifted once (1 RM). The intensity is also adjusted by the rest interval of 90 seconds between sets.

Bodybuilding is another type of strength training with the main objective of development of maximal muscle hypertrophy. Bodybuilding has a training volume far above that which the average individual is capable of performing. The basic concepts for bodybuilding are:

- Every muscle group in the body is worked with multiple exercises consisting of multiple sets
- A set of high repetitions begins each initial exercise per muscle group and as the resistance increases, the repetitions decrease
- The musculature is worked as thoroughly as possible to achieve maximal muscle engorgement
- Every set is preceded by a rest period of no more than 90 seconds
- Every repetition is performed in a strict fashion
- Emphasis is placed on doing the exercise movement correctly, rather than trying to lift as much weight as possible

Athletes, whether competitive or recreational, may wish to develop strength specifically to enhance their athletic performances. In this case, the type of exercises should be similar to the movements required by the specific sport.

The frequency, duration, and intensity variables of the program should coincide with the amount of time dedicated to strength development during the season as well as the particular time of the season (i.e., preseason versus postseason). It should also be determined whether the primary movement in the sport requires strength, power, or skill so that the proper type of program can be formulated. Table 14.6 lists some common strength-training exercises with the corresponding muscles that are developed.

## TRAINING FOR POWER PERFORMANCE

Successful sports performance depends largely upon the performer's ability to produce power. Power itself is defined as the rate at which work is performed. In this respect, time or speed is to be considered in addition to strength. Power performance equals muscle force times movement speed; therefore, power performance is dependent upon both strength and speed. Power performance will improve if either strength or movement speed is improved. Of these two power components, strength can be improved to a greater extent than speed. However, one cannot neglect the speed component in most athletic events, and therefore power training should be incorporated into the overall training regimen.

Power performance is most critical in activities that require maximal bursts of energy which last 5 to 10 seconds. These types of activities rely heavily upon the ATP-PC energy-producing system (see Chapter 3). Training the ATP-PC system can be accomplished by overloading the muscles with repeated maximal bouts or near maximal bouts of exercise. Since the ATP-PC system does not produce lactic acid and the ATP-PC stores can be replenished rapidly, repeated near maximal exercise bouts can occur after only 30 to 60 seconds of rest.

### Plyometric Training

Power-training programs can be divided into two different categories, those whose objective is the development of sport-specific power and those whose objective is competitive weightlifting. The principle of specificity of training needs to be considered for training programs that emphasize the development of power. Specificity of strength training with respect to power suggests that strength improvement is generally greatest when strength is measured at or below the contraction velocity at which the muscle was trained. The application of this power element to strength training is best seen with **plyometric** exercises, which involve a rapid stretching of the muscle undergoing eccentric stress, followed by a concentric contraction of that muscle. The purpose of this type of movement pattern is to heighten the excitability of the nervous system for improved reactive ability of the neuromuscular mechanism. Exercise using eccentric and concentric training is thought to enhance muscular strength and power to a greater degree than concentric training alone. Plyometric exercise training

| Table 14.6 | MUSCLE GROUPS TRAINED BY CERTAIN STRENGTH EXERCISES |
|---|---|
| **Body area or musculature** | **Exercise** |
| Abdomen | Sit-ups, crunches, Roman chairs, leg raises |
| Biceps | Barbell curl, dumbbell curl, preacher curl, reverse curl, inclined curl, alternate dumbbell curl, chin-ups, pull-ups |
| Calves | Heel raises, toe press-outs |
| Deltoid | Flys, lateral raises, overhead press, inclined press, forward raise, upright rowing, dumbbell press, bent-over rowing |
| Erector spinae | Squat, deadlift, back hyperextension, front squat |
| Forearm | Wrist curl, wrist roller |
| Gluteus maximus | Squat, lunges, leg press, deadlift, front squat |
| Hamstrings | Leg curl, lunges |
| Intercostals | Bent-arm pullover, lat pull-down |
| Latissimus dorsi | Lat pull-down, bent-over rowing, chin-ups, pull-ups, dips |
| Neck | Neck flexion, neck extension |
| Pectoralis major | Bench press, inclined press, flys, declined press, pushups |
| Quadriceps | Squat, knee extension, leg press, lunges, front squat |
| Trapezius | Shoulder shrugs, upright rowing, overhead press |
| Trapezius/rhomboids | Lat pull-down, bent-over lateral raise, reverse flys, bent-over rowing |
| Triceps | Triceps press, overhead press, dips, bench press, dumbbell press, declined press |

can be used to enhance sport-specific performance when power development is highly important. For example, sprinting performance involving distances of 200 meters or less can be improved with plyometric training.

Movements in plyometric exercises are structured to take advantage of the muscle's inherent stretch reflex. In reality, plyometric exercise is just an eccentric contraction (muscle lengthened through stretch) followed instantaneously with a maximal concentric contraction. The difference between a plyometric exercise and normal dynamic weightlifting consisting of both eccentric and concentric contractions is timing. In plyometrics, the concentric contraction is coupled with the stretch reflex or recoil of the muscle following an eccentric stretch contraction, whereas there is no reflex invoked with dynamic resistance exercise. The eccentric and concentric phases of the movement are disconnected. Another way to look at it is that plyometric training involves an explosive concentric contraction that is immediately preceded by an eccentric contraction. An example of a plyometric exercise is depth jumping (jumping from a box of variable height) onto the floor and then immediately exploding into a vertical jump (*Fig. 14.8*). Plyometric exercises focus on the speed component of power, whereas performing squats with heavy weights focuses on strength and does not necessarily improve power performance.

Different exercises may have some of the qualities of a true plyometric exercise. Weighted-rope jumping is one such nontraditional exercise. The Suggested Readings section at the end of this chapter includes a research article on the efficacy of weighted-rope jump training for power performance. Box 14.2 describes a plyometric training program for developing power.

## Competitive Weightlifting

There are two forms of competitive weightlifting: powerlifting (a non-Olympic sport) and Olympic weightlifting. The nomenclature at this point becomes confusing since the Olympic weightlifting technique involves timing and speed, making it a power event, while so-called powerlifting does not rely on speed of movement. Therefore, powerlifting would be more descriptively termed strength lifting and technically should not be considered a power event. To illustrate this point, competitive powerlifting events are the bench press, squat, and dead lift; with all lifts performed in a fairly slow, deliberate style. On the other hand, Olympic weightlifting movements (the snatch and clean and jerk) are true power movements that rely on speed to accomplish the lifts. *Accurate nomenclature is important in science, but apparently not in sports; why do you think this is so?*

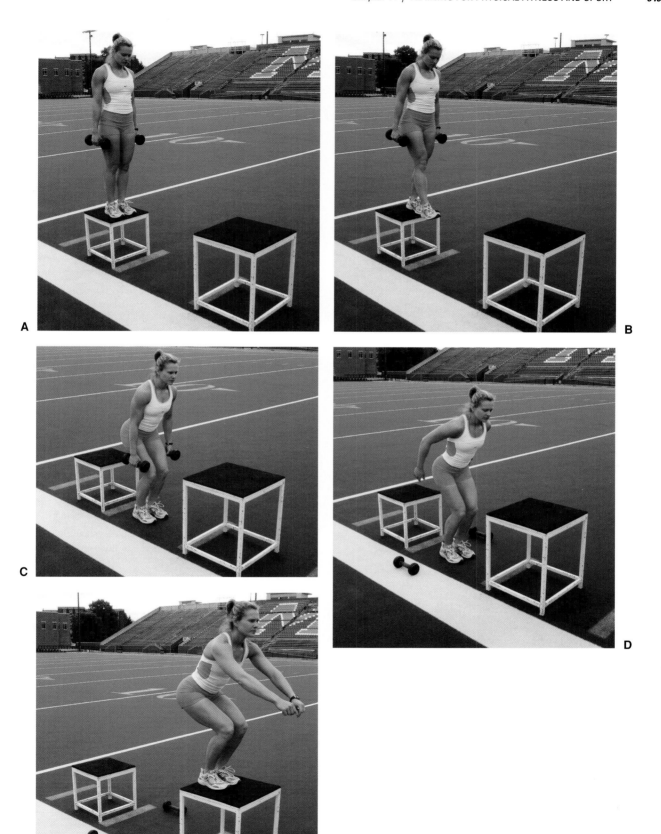

**FIGURE 14.8.** Depth jumps with dumbbells is plyometric training. Weight can be increased as evidence of a training effect appears. A dumbbell release could also be incorporated into this drill.

Box 14.2

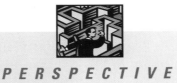

# Plyometric Training for Muscle Power

Rebound movement patterns (i.e., jumping) are prevalent in many sports. During rebound movements, mechanical energy is absorbed by the muscle during eccentric contraction and released during the subsequent propulsive phase (concentric contraction). To be successful in strength-power sports requires more than strength gained through weight training because dynamic resistance exercise alone will not maximize speed in switching from eccentric to concentric contractions. Therefore, in power training, an attempt is made to adapt the nervous system toward greater excitability for improved reactive ability of the neuromuscular mechanism. During plyometric training, the prestretch of the knee and hip extensors activates the myotatic (stretch) reflex to potentiate the force of shortening and propel the athlete higher than could be obtained without the downward rebound movement. However, to be successful in this type of training and avoid injuries requires a progression of training that starts with attaining baseline strength. Strength training is then followed by jump drills, with plyometric training coming next. Through this means, the athlete hopes to gain not only strength but quicker reactions and increased agility.

To improve jumping ability, power training should be implemented to supplement the improved level of strength following strength training. The first phase of power training involves implementing bounding drills (see figure) using a series of horizontal jumps, vertical jumps, or a combination of jumps (weighted and unweighted) done first from both feet and later with single-leg variations. These techniques should be progressively overloaded to allow adequate physiologic and neurologic adaptation to the stress overloads. Bounding

drills are followed by box drills or rebound jumping (also called depth jumps) from platforms. The following list gives examples of the types of drills that may be employed.

### JUMP TRAINING: DOUBLE LEG USING LOW BOXES
1. Double-leg vertical jump upward with own body weight: light intensity
2. Double-leg bound outward and upward (movement is forward and upward to gain maximum height and horizontal distance): light intensity
3. Double-leg box bound on and off box (landing on and taking off from boxes alternating with jumps from and onto the floor): moderate intensity
4. Side hop and sprint—double-leg jump sideways over box (upon landing, immediately explode forward and run with as much speed as possible for about 10 to 30 yards): moderate intensity
5. Double-leg incline bound uphill (as in jumping horizontally uphill): moderate intensity
6. Double-leg decline bound downhill (opposite of prior drill): high intensity

### JUMP TRAINING: SINGLE LEG USING LOW BOXES
1. Alternate leg bound (as in # 2 above, but alternating off one leg, then the other): light intensity
2. Alternate leg box drill (as in # 3 above, but alternating off one leg, then the other): moderate intensity

### PLYOMETRIC: DEPTH JUMPS
1. Depth jump off box 14 to 18 inches high (begin with balls of feet on edge of box, step off, and land on floor with both feet, immediately execute an explosive jump upward): moderate intensity
2. Depth jump off box 22 to 26 inches high (same as # 1 above): high intensity
3. Depth jump off box 30 to 34 inches high (same as # 1 above): very intense

The table below gives details of the overall volume of work and the volume per individual plyometric exercise. Drills can be progressed over time from light to very intense to allow for adaptations to occur and to avoid injury.

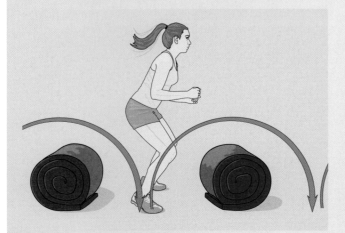

Bounding drills, such as the one depicted, can be used fairly early in training for improving jumping ability.

| Phase | Total repetitions | Volume |
|---|---|---|
| Low intensity | 400 | 10 sets of 12 repetitions |
| Moderate intensity | 350 | 7 sets of 10 repetitions |
| High intensity | 300 | 5 sets of 8 repetitions |
| Very intense | 200 | 3 sets of 6 repetitions |

# TRAINING FOR SPEED PERFORMANCE

In the last section, training for power was discussed in light of its two components, strength and speed. Metabolically, speed performance is defined relative to anaerobic glycolysis and the production of lactic acid. Enhancing speed performance is also accomplished by the application of the overload principle through specificity of training. Before one begins to design specific training regimens to enhance speed performance, different forms of "glycolytic" speed must be understood. The forms of speed that affect exercise performance are (a) maximal running speed, (b) acceleration speed, (c) speed of movement of body segments, and (d) quickness.

Maximal running speed is of premiere importance during sprints or games like soccer, in which a distance of 20 meters or more must be traveled rapidly. Acceleration speed becomes critical during shorter sprints in which rapid movement from one location to another a short distance away is required. Acceleration speed is crucial for many court games, like basketball, in which elusion of an opponent is important, or tennis when movement towards a traveling object is necessary. Speed of movement of body segments is vital for events in which either an object or the body itself is propelled through space. Quickness, on the other hand, may include running speed, acceleration speed, or speed of movement of body segments, but it also encompasses reaction time and **agility**.

The different factors that affect speed performance are (a) intrinsic properties of the muscles, (b) strength, (c) flexibility, (d) biomechanical efficiency, and (e) reaction time. As discussed in Chapters 10 and 11, muscles are composed of fiber types which have certain biochemical characteristics. The biochemical characteristics of a muscle fiber determine its functionality. Fast-twitch fibers that have a high glycolytic capacity produce a strong force of contraction and are best suited for speed performance. Consequently, muscles that contain a high percentage of fast-twitch fibers not only have intrinsic properties that favor speed performance but will respond best to glycolytic training.

Since strength is an integral component of power, one can see that strength must also be related to speed. However, the relationship between strength and speed is not constant. Strength and speed are weakly related when a light resistance is involved (very low percentage of 1 RM), but the relationship becomes stronger when speed movements against a heavy resistance are needed (high percentage of 1 RM). As muscles become stronger, the external resistance inhibiting speed becomes less problematic during speed performance. Strength gains in the muscles involved in a particular movement enhance speed of movement completion, regardless of the strengthening exercises used during training. Resistance to movement around a joint can impair the speed of movement at that joint. If the antagonistic muscle group is not flexible, the working muscle group must exert additional force to overcome the antagonistic resistance. This inflexibility, in turn, can retard speed of movement. On the other hand, there is no evidence to suggest that flexibility beyond a reasonable or normal amount will enhance speed performance.

Angular velocity is determined by how fast the muscles can overcome an external resistance. Angular velocity is proportionate to the length of the lever being used and the amount of force being exerted during a particular movement. Since speed performance is primarily a function of angular velocity, speed performance can be enhanced by employing the optimal combination of angular velocity for the length of levers (bones) involved in a particular movement. The result is that when the biomechanical efficiency is improved, the negative forces impeding speed are reduced while the positive forces contributing to speed are enhanced.

The last factor that affects speed is more neurologic than muscular in nature. Reaction time is the speed with which an individual can react to a stimulus and initiate a movement. In most competitive events, the successful participant must not only have speed of movement but also quickness, which is controlled significantly by reaction time. For example, when the offensive player in basketball makes a move, the difference between a slow and fast reaction by the defensive player can determine success or failure. Offensive and defensive players are often hindered by slow reactions because they are unable to outmaneuver their opponents. Similarly, in games like volleyball, the athlete must react not only to the opponent but also to ball movement.

Intense exercise lasting more than 20 to 30 seconds but less than 3 to 4 minutes is supported primarily by the resynthesis of ATP via anaerobic glycolysis. To improve the capacity of this bioenergetic pathway, the pathway must be "stressed" or overloaded through short-term, high-intensity exercise bouts. Performance of repeated exercise bouts with brief recovery periods in between is called interval training. This type of training stresses rapid glycolysis (as shown by elevated lactic acid levels) to a much higher level than one bout of all-out effort to the point of voluntary exhaustion. Interval training also provides a way of performing large amounts of high-intensity exercise in a short time.

The training overload required to elicit an adaptation following interval training is achieved by manipulating training mode, frequency, duration, and intensity. These variables can be defined in terms of the total training program or in terms of an individual training session. Mode, frequency, duration, and intensity are defined below for a glycolytic speed training program.

- Mode: interval training program consisting of sprint interval running (running above 85% of maximum speed for distances <250 meters), fast interval running (running at 78% to 85% maximal speed for distances <625 meters), stress interval running (running above 85% of maximum speed for distances between 250 and 600 meters), and repetition running (running faster than 85% speed for distances of 600 meters)
- Frequency: 5 days per week
- Duration: 30 to 60 minutes or a total workout distance less than 2.0 miles

■ Intensity: heart rate (HR) during the work interval is above 90% of maximal HR or above 180 beats per minute (bpm) to achieve an adequate overload of the glycolytic system (during the rest interval, HR should recover to about 140 bpm or 70% of maximal before the next interval is performed)

Another method is to base the intensity upon the number of work intervals that can be completed by the athlete at a given pace before the athlete becomes fatigued and cannot keep the desired pace for subsequent work intervals. This is the most common method used, especially at lower levels of competition. A more uniform approach for defining intensity is to add 1.5 seconds to the athlete's best time for 50 meters, 3 seconds to the best time for distances between 50 and 100 meters, and 5 seconds for distances between 100 and 200 meters. One to 4 seconds are subtracted from the average 400-meter time recorded during the athlete's best 1500-meter run. The rest intervals are generally three times the length of the work interval.

▶ *INQUIRY SUMMARY.* Training for muscular fitness in terms of strength, power, and speed training should be done according to the specificity principle with a view towards the desired athletic goal. Strength, power, and speed are not the same but are interrelated, which challenges the coach or trainer to correctly assess the event and apply correct sport-specific training to produce optimal performance. In each case, training specificity must be considered first. *How might a training program that incorrectly assesses specificity lead to problems in sport or therapeutic outcomes?*

## *Training for Aerobic Endurance*

Performance during long-term exercise events can also be improved through specificity of training by application of the overload principle. As mentioned earlier, the training overload required to elicit a muscular adaptation is achieved by manipulating combinations of training mode,

frequency, duration, and intensity. A training regimen designed to enhance aerobic endurance can also be defined in terms of these variables. However, the exact nature of these variables is vastly different in the context of training for aerobic endurance versus training for muscular fitness.

Training for aerobic endurance involves any type of exercise that stresses the aerobic-energy–producing pathways. From a scientific standpoint, more is known about the adaptations to aerobic exercise than any other type of exercise. This is probably because research into the biochemical and physiologic responses and adaptations to aerobic exercise training preceded the research relating to the adaptations derived from anaerobic (especially resistance) training. Furthermore, aerobic exercise training has received more attention from the medical community because this type of exercise has been associated with reduced risk of various diseases. Aerobic exercise is the most common type of exercise in which the general population participates, probably because one can reap the health benefits of aerobic training while exercising at a relatively low intensity (i.e., ~40% $\dot{V}O_2$).

The first step in designing an aerobic training regimen for an individual with no contraindications for exercise is to define the objective of the training. Some common objectives include health and wellness, physical fitness, weight loss, reduced cardiovascular risk, rehabilitation, and athletic competition. The quantity and quality of aerobic exercise needed to attain health-related benefits may differ from what is recommended for fitness (performance) benefits. These differences are quantified in Table 14.7. Lower levels of activity than what are needed to improve $\dot{V}O_{2max}$ may reduce risk for certain chronic, degenerative diseases. Once the objective is established, the guidelines governing mode, frequency, duration, and intensity of exercise can be delineated.

The purpose of endurance training is to tax the aerobic energy system so that it will adapt by becoming more capable of producing energy by the use of $O_2$. Measurement of an individual's $\dot{V}O_{2max}$ during vigorous exercise has traditionally been used as an indicator of aerobic fitness. A prudent

| Table 14.7 | *RECOMMENDATIONS FOR PRODUCING HEALTH-RELATED BENEFITS COMPARED WITH PERFORMANCE BENEFITS* |
|---|---|

**Recommendations**

| Training parameter | Health-related benefit | Performance benefit |
|---|---|---|
| Frequency | 5–7 per week | 6–10 per week |
| Duration | ≥30 minutes | 30 minutes to hours |
| Intensity | Light to moderate (40%–70% HRR or %$\dot{V}O_2$ R) depending on functional capacity | High (85%–90% HRR or %$\dot{V}O_2$ R) depending on goals |
| Mode | Continuous exercise (personal preference) with rhythmic use of large muscle groups | Sport-specific training |

HRR, heart rate reserve.

recommendation for sedentary adults who are concerned primarily with disease risk reduction is to participate in any type of regular low-intensity physical activity, without being overly concerned for reaching a specific minimal level. Once exercise has become a habit and functional capacity has improved, more rigorous guidelines for quantity and quality of exercise may be imposed. Material on aerobic training for special populations can be found in the clinical foundations section of the book.

## EXERCISE DOSAGE

Proper activity for aerobic training involves those that employ continuous, rhythmic movement and use large muscle groups. This type of exercise ensures that a large volume of blood is continually delivered to the working muscles. Since the circulatory system plays such a large role in aerobic metabolism, aerobic exercise is often called cardiovascular exercise. This form of exercise stresses both the central circulation (heart) and peripheral circulation (vasculature). Another term used to describe aerobic exercise is cardiorespiratory exercise because of the need for the pulmonary system to supply oxygenated blood to the circulation. Regardless of which term is used to describe aerobic exercise, physiologic adaptations will ensue in following aerobic training.

Two types of loads can be imposed on the heart (central circulation)—a pressure overload or volume overload (see Fig. 14.1). Aerobic training does not greatly elevate vascular pressures (pressure overload) but does result in a large volume of blood being continually pumped by the heart and received by the vasculature, especially in the vascular beds of working muscles. Regularly imposed volume overload from aerobic training produces structural and functional changes in the heart, vascular system, and muscles that have been trained aerobically.

### Frequency and Duration

The frequency of aerobic exercise depends somewhat on the duration and intensity of exercise. The recommended frequency varies from several daily sessions of only a few minutes for individuals with very low functional capacities to three to five sessions per week lasting several minutes each for individuals with at least normal functional capacities. Training of less than 2 days per week does not usually produce a significant change in $\dot{V}O_{2max}$ or result in reduced disease risk, whereas the added benefit of training more than 5 days per week is almost negligible when compared to that seen with a frequency of 3 to 5 days per week. The frequency recommended for most adults in the apparently healthy population is 3 to 5 days per week.

The conditioning period for endurance training can vary from a few minutes to more than 60 minutes (or much longer), depending on the functional capacity of the individual and objectives of the training program. The duration of the exercise session is usually inversely related to the training intensity. This means that higher exercise intensi-

ties usually involve shorter exercise durations. The overall conditioning response may be simply a product of training intensity and duration, or the total energy expenditure. Most often the conditioning duration is set at a minimal of 30 minutes for the apparently healthy population. This length of time per training session is necessary for most people to improve $\dot{V}O_{2max}$ and elicit biochemical adaptations within muscle. Changes in the training regimen can then be made as the individual's aerobic capacity increases and other physiologic adaptations to training become apparent.

The guidelines mentioned in Table 14.7 are general recommendations that most people can follow to reap benefits. However, for those individuals at the extreme low end of the fitness spectrum, it cannot be stressed too strongly that any unaccustomed activity will produce benefits if that activity represents stress overload. *The key for people who are extremely unfit is to commence whole-body movement of a type that they were previously unaccustomed to doing.*

### Intensity

Of the four elements for aerobic training, intensity is the most critical. It is generally suggested that training intensity exceed 60% $\dot{V}O_{2max}$, but 40% to 50% (or lower) may be adequate for older, obese, or otherwise extremely unfit individuals. Regardless of the exact intensity selected for aerobic exercise, training intensity is invariably monitored by a predetermined training heart rate (THR). The most accurate method for establishing THR requires the simultaneous measurement of HR and $O_2$ consumption at several submaximal exercise intensities, with the subsequent calculation of a regression equation relating these two variables. However, this direct determination of the HR/$O_2$ consumption relationship for each individual requires elaborate equipment and extensive testing. Thus, it is more feasible for the practitioner to use universal or even population-specific prediction equations for prescribing aerobic exercise intensity for individuals.

The two most common methods used to compute THR without direct determination of the HR/$O_2$ consumption relationship are the straight percentage technique and the Karvonen formula. With the straight percentage technique, THR is computed simply as a chosen percentage of the maximal HR (i.e., 220 − Age × %). In comparison, the Karvonen formula computes THR in the following manner:

$$\text{THR} = [(\text{Maximal HR} - \text{Resting HR}) \times \%] + \text{Resting HR}$$

It is obvious that for either of these two methods to be effective in computing the proper THR required to elicit the desired aerobic exercise intensity, you must have an accurate measurement or prediction of maximal HR and substantiation of the submaximal HR/$O_2$ consumption relationship.

Early work from Robinson suggested that maximal HR in adults peaked at about 200 bpm and declined approximately one bpm with each progressing year. Subsequent research studies produced results that seemed to match the results Robinson produced. These data have probably led to the *a priori* use of the equation, 220 − Age, for predicting maximal HR in adults. In addition, a separate and distinct maximal HR prediction equation (Maximal HR = 200 − 50% Age) for obese individuals (body fat >30% or BMI >30) is suggested. Once maximal HR has been determined, either the straight percentage technique or Karvonen's formula may be used to calculate the THR, which is subsequently used for monitoring aerobic exercise intensity.

## DETERMINING EXERCISE INTENSITY

Validity in monitoring HR during exercise as an indicator of aerobic intensity depends upon the relationship between HR and $O_2$ consumption. Research reports over the last three decades have examined this relationship for different segments of the adult population and found that the relationship between relative submaximal $O_2$ consumption level and relative submaximal HR was somewhat different for men and women, exercise mode, and various patient groups. Table 14.8 is a comprehensive look at the relationship between %$\dot{V}O_{2max}$ and %$HR_{max}$ based on approximately 20 research studies.

The recommended intensity level of 60% $\dot{V}O_{2max}$ corresponds to about 70% $HR_{max}$. Using the relationship between $O_2$ consumption and HR, you can calculate THR for any individual if the $HR_{max}$ is known. For example, the THR for a normal weight 40-year-old woman to train at 60%$\dot{V}O_{2max}$ is calculated as follows.

$$HR_{max} = 220 − 40 = 180 \text{ bpm}$$

$$60\% \, \dot{V}O_{2max} \text{ corresponds to } 70\% \, HR_{max}$$

$$70\% \, HR_{max} = 0.70 \times 180 = 126 \text{ bpm}$$

Similar calculations can be made for any combination of age and relative $O_2$ consumption level.

The straight percentage technique for calculating THR is easy to use, but it does not take into account variance in fitness levels among individuals. Nor does the straight percentage technique provide much leeway for THR in the elderly. For example, if an 80-year-old woman was to exercise at 50% of $\dot{V}O_{2max}$ (corresponding to 60% $HR_{max}$), her THR would be 84 bpm according to the straight percentage technique. However, Karvonen's technique for calculating THR would yield far different results. If her resting HR was 85 bpm, using the Karvonen equation presented above would yield a THR of 118 bpm [THR = (140 − 85)0.60 + 85]. In this example, the straight percentage method underestimates the Karvonen method for calculating THR. The biggest advantage of the straight percentage technique is its simplicity, i.e., the only information needed for calculating THR is the subject's age.

To alleviate the perceived weakness of the straight percentage technique, Karvonen and associates arbitrarily set resting HR at zero, arguing that one's HR will never go below its resting level. They then calculated THR relative to the HR reserve (HRR; maximal HR minus resting HR). In doing this, the theoretical assumption was that a one-to-one correspondence between relative $O_2$ consumption level and relative HR would be achieved. In other words, 60% $\dot{V}O_{2max}$ would correspond to 60% of HRR, 70% $\dot{V}O_{2max}$ would correspond to 70% HRR, and so forth.

Because one of the benefits of cardiovascular fitness is a decrease in resting HR, you can see how THR is adjusted in Karvonen's formula according to variances in resting HR for different fitness levels. Another example of how you would calculate THR using Karvonen's equation is given below for a 20-year-old obese man with a resting HR of 80 bpm who is to exercise at 50% of $\dot{V}O_{2max}$:

$$HR_{max} = 200 − (0.50 \times 20) = 190 \text{ bpm}$$

$$HRR = 190 − 80 = 110 \text{ bpm}$$

$$THR = (0.50 \times 110) + 80 = 135 \text{ bpm}$$

### Relationship Between %HRmax and %$\dot{V}O_2$max

Knowledge of the rectilinear relationship between %$HR_{max}$ and %$\dot{V}O_{2max}$ is essential to formulate an aerobic training routine. The relationship between %$HR_{max}$ and %$\dot{V}O_{2max}$ allows the use of HR (a variable easy to measure) rather that $\dot{V}O_2$ (a complicated and impractical variable to measure) to set exercise intensity along prescribed metabolic ($\dot{V}O_2$) limits. Since one goal of aerobic training to achieve effective equivalent metabolic loads (intensity) for training, HR serves as a useful index of $\dot{V}O_2$ with the HR measured during exercise indirectly indicating an exercise $\dot{V}O_2$ response along a continuum of low to moderate to heavy exercise.

Using the coefficients provided in Table 14.8, the relationship between $\dot{V}O_{2max}$ and $HR_{max}$ can also be used to calculate either of these variables when only one is known. The usual method in using these equations involves prescribing a metabolic load for a specific exercise mode (i.e., 75%$\dot{V}O_{2max}$ for treadmill exercise), entering this value into an appropriate equation, and then calculating the X variable (%$HR_{max}$, i.e., 85%) from the known Y variable (%$\dot{V}O_{2max}$). For example, if a 30-year-old individual's $HR_{max}$ is approximately 190 bpm, a training HR of approximately 162 bpm (85% of 190) is needed to reach the desired metabolic load of 75% $\dot{V}O_{2max}$. However, as you will see next, this technique is not quite appropriate.

The chief variable of interest in prescribing cardiovascular exercise is the metabolic stimulus, $\dot{V}O_2$. Therefore, the main goal in prescribing aerobic exercise intensity is to select the metabolic load in terms of relative oxygen cost (as %$\dot{V}O_{2max}$) and to accurately match this with a target HR (as %$HR_{max}$). To do this, a proper exercise training stimulus (%$\dot{V}O_{2max}$) is first determined (how this is determined is presented in the clinical section of the book). This value is then used to ascertain, via regression, the %$HR_{max}$, which serves as an index of the targeted metabolic stimulus and is used to approximate the metabolic response during exercise.

Since HR serves as an indicator of metabolic load, and not vice versa, regression equations should be constructed in a

| Table 14.8 | PUBLISHED REGRESSION EQUATIONS FOR THE RELATIONSHIP BETWEEN HEART RATE AND OXYGEN CONSUMPTION |
|---|---|

| Study | Slope | Intercept | Mode | Male | Female | AHY | HRCI |
|---|---|---|---|---|---|---|---|
| **Method 1: Using $\dot{V}O_{2max}$ as the Y variable and $\%HR_{max}$ as the X variable** | | | | | | | |
| 1 | 1.41 | −42.0 | LCE | ✓ | | ✓ | |
| 1 | 1.32 | −35.2 | LCE | ✓ | | | CD |
| 2 | 1.30 | −36.3 | LCE | ✓ | | ✓ | |
| 3 | 1.39 | −44.8 | LCE | ✓ | | ✓ | |
| 4 | 1.31 | −43.5 | LCE | ✓ | | ✓ | |
| 5 | 1.41 | −45.1 | LCE | ✓ | | ✓ | |
| 4 | 1.32 | −37.8 | ACE | ✓ | | ✓ | |
| 2 | 1.20 | −29.3 | ACE | ✓ | | ✓ | |
| 6 | 1.41 | −46.2 | ACE | ✓ | | ✓ | |
| 6 | 1.31 | −37.0 | ACE | ✓ | | | HLPSCI |
| 6 | 1.23 | −30.9 | ACE | ✓ | | | LLPSCI |
| 7 | 0.95 | +0.49 | ACE | ✓ | ✓ | | HLQSCI |
| 7 | 1.04 | −5.96 | ACE | ✓ | ✓ | | LLQSCI |
| 7 | 1.37 | −38.2 | ACE[a] | ✓ | ✓ | | HLQSCI |
| 7 | 1.05 | −6.8 | ACE[a] | ✓ | ✓ | | LLQSCI |
| 8 | 1.37 | −41.0 | TM | ✓ | | ✓ | |
| 9 | 1.20 | −34.0 | TM | ✓ | | | |
| 10 | 1.50 | −52.0 | TM | ✓ | | | |
| 11 | 1.25 | −24.0 | TM | ✓ | | | |
| 12 | 1.20 | −24.5 | TM | | ✓ | | |
| 13 | 1.11 | −19.0 | TM | ✓ | ✓ | ✓ | |
| 13 | 1.15 | −23.0 | TM | ✓ | ✓ | | OB |
| 14 | 1.30 | −34.5 | TM | ✓ | | ✓ | |
| 5 | 1.27 | −34.4 | Skier | ✓ | | ✓ | |
| 5 | 1.20 | −26.9 | Shuffle | ✓ | | ✓ | |
| 5 | 1.22 | −28.4 | Stepper | ✓ | | ✓ | |
| 5 | 1.18 | −21.0 | Rower | ✓ | | ✓ | |
| 15 | 1.46 | −49.6 | DWR | ✓ | | | |
| 15 | 1.66 | −67.9 | DWR | | ✓ | | |
| 16 | 1.53 | −54.5 | DWR | ✓ | | | AG |
| 16 | 1.59 | −62.4 | DWR | | ✓ | | AG |
| **Method 2: Using $\%HR_{max}$ as the Y variable and $\%\dot{V}O_{2max}$ as the X variable** | | | | | | | |
| 17 | 0.55 | +43.2 | TM | ✓ | ✓ | | PU |
| 18 | 0.64 | +36.8 | TM | ✓ | | ✓ | |
| 18 | 0.63 | +39.0 | TM | | ✓ | ✓ | |
| **Method 3: Using $\%HRR$ as the Y variable and $\%\dot{V}O_2 R$ as the X variable** | | | | | | | |
| 19 | 1.00 | −0.1 | LCE | ✓ | ✓ | ✓ | |
| 20 | 1.03 | +1.5 | TM | ✓ | ✓ | ✓ | |
| **Method 4: Using $\%HRR$ as the Y variable and $\%\dot{V}O_{2max}$ as the X variable** | | | | | | | |
| 19 | 1.12 | −11.6 | LCE | ✓ | ✓ | ✓ | |
| 20 | 1.10 | −6.1 | TM | ✓ | ✓ | ✓ | |

[a]Represents ACE in the supine position. LCE, leg cycle ergometer; ACE, arm cycle ergometer; TM, treadmill; DWR, deep water running (wet-vest supported); CD, cardiac patients; HLPSCI, high lesion paraplegia spinal cord injury; LLPSCI, low lesion paraplegia spinal cord injury; HLQSCI, high lesion quadriplegia spinal cord injury; LLQSCI, low lesion quadriplegia spinal cord injury; OB, obese subjects; AG, aged subjects; PU, pulmonary patients; AHY, apparently healthy, younger; HRCI, high risk or chronically ill.

way that places $\%HR_{max}$ in the Y variable position in the equation. This arrangement recognizes that a given level of whole-body $O_2$ consumption requires (i.e., predicts, in the language of regression analysis) a certain HR response (refer back to the Fick equation presented in Chapter 7 to see how HR and $\dot{V}O_2$ are related). The regression equations shown in Table 14.8 (method 1 equations), while describing the relationship between metabolism and HR adequately, trans-pose the equation, in effect making $\dot{V}O_2$ dependent on HR when physiologically the opposite is true. *HR is dependent on the metabolic rate ($\dot{V}O_2$) during exercise.* Because of this and because HR is the variable most likely to be monitored during training sessions, the prediction of $\%HR_{max}$ by a regression equation that uses $\%\dot{V}O_{2max}$ data as the independent variable in the regression analysis is a better way to design these regression equations.

A common mistake in the use of these regression equations occurs when the independent variable (X or $\%HR_{max}$) is predicted instead of the dependent variable (Y or $\%\dot{V}O_{2max}$) by first starting with a desired value for the dependent variable ($\%\dot{V}O_{2max}$). Most of the original equations (Table 14.8, method 1 equations) use $\%HR_{max}$ in the independent variable (X variable) position and then proceed to calculate $\%HR_{max}$ during exercise prescription from a Y variable ($\%\dot{V}O_{2max}$) that was decided *a priori*. In the procedure typically used, the equation is transposed, i.e., the actual predictor variable (X or $\%HR_{max}$) is itself being predicted (calculated). This is a faulty use of regression theory and has been cited as a problem; it was subsequently corrected (Table 14.8, method 2 equations) by using $\%HR_{max}$ as the dependent variable (3). A better practice is one in which the metabolic load is prescribed (chosen) and an equation which uses $\%\dot{V}O_{2max}$ as the predictor (X variable) is selected to calculate the criterion or dependent variable ($\%HR_{max}$). Using these equations, it is the criterion variable (Y variable) that should always be predicted from a value of the independent variable (i.e., X variable), which is chosen based on a predetermined prescribed training intensity (i.e., $\%\dot{V}O_{2max}$).

## Relationship Between %HRR and %V̇O₂R

Another key relationship with implications for the way exercise intensity is formulated is the association between HRR and $\dot{V}O_2$ reserve ($\dot{V}O_2R$; the difference between maximal and resting $\dot{V}O_2$). The longstanding theoretical assumption has been that %HRR is equivalent to $\%\dot{V}O_{2max}$. This assumption was tested and found to be true in a study of 122 obese females (baseline body mass prior to training, averaged 103 kg), in which the relationship between %HRR and $\%\dot{V}O_{2max}$ followed the line of identity (i.e., a slope of 1.0 and an intercept of 0) (4). However, following training and calorie-restricted diet with an average body mass loss of 20 kg, the relationship between %HRR and $\%\dot{V}O_{2max}$ no longer was one to one but had shifted upward and produced a discrepancy of 10 percentage points between the variables.

More recent research contradicts the equivalency assumption, showing that these variables, although highly correlated for both cycle and treadmill exercise (r = 0.99), are not absolutely equivalent (i.e., the regression line differs significantly from the line of identity) for younger and elderly subjects (5,6). The discrepancy between the corresponding percentages of HRR and $\dot{V}O_{2max}$ is especially large for light to moderate exercise intensity and in older, less fit subjects compared with the discrepancy produced in younger, fit individuals (5). Thus, the discrepancy between these variables is inversely proportional to exercise intensity (as the intensity increases, the discrepancy decreases) and fitness level (less fit individuals produce greater discrepancies). *Figure 14.9* presents the regression lines of the relationship between %HRR and $\%\dot{V}O_2R$ or $\%\dot{V}O_{2max}$ from Swain, clearly showing that the regression lines for %HRR and $\%\dot{V}O_2R$ are more closely associated with the line of identity. While in the case of cycling, the regression of %HRR on

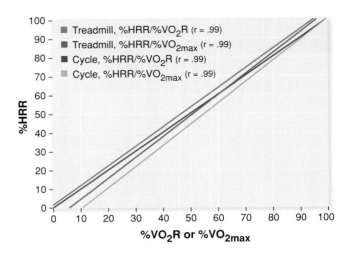

**FIGURE 14.9.** Regression lines depicting the relationship between % heart rate reserve (%HRR) and $\%\dot{V}O_2R$ or $\dot{V}O_{2max}$ during treadmill and cycle ergometer exercise: treadmill, $\%HRR/\%\dot{V}O_2R$ (r = 0.99); treadmill, $\%HRR/\%\dot{V}O_{2max}R$ (r = 0.99); cycle $\%HRR/\%\dot{V}O_2R$ (r = 0.99); and cycle, $\%HRR/\%\dot{V}O_{2max}$ (r = 0.99). Data from Swain et al (5,6).

$\%\dot{V}O_2R$ was not significantly different from the line of identity, treadmill exercise produced a %HRR on $\%\dot{V}O_2R$ regression that was significantly different (the slope and intercept are different from 1 and 0, respectively) from the identity line. This difference was not likely based on exercise mode but was probably due to the higher ambient laboratory temperatures the subjects experienced in the treadmill study.

Selecting exercise intensity in terms of $\%\dot{V}O_2R$ instead of $\%\dot{V}O_{2max}$ reduces the errors associated with the discrepancies between $\%\dot{V}O_{2max}$ and %HRR that occur at low to moderate intensities and in very deconditioned subjects, such as the frail elderly, cardiac patients, renal failure patients, pulmonary patients, and obese individuals. In consideration of this, Swain suggests at least three advantages to prescribing exercise based on $\%\dot{V}O_2 R$, rather than $\%\dot{V}O_{2max}$.

- The close association between %HRR and $\%\dot{V}O_2 R$ provides a more accurate intensity than does the relationship between %HRR and $\%\dot{V}O_{2max}$ when exercise intensity is based on HR value.
- For individuals of different fitness levels, $\dot{V}O_2 R$ provides an equivalent relative intensity allowing any given patient/client to make a similar adjustment in relative effort (i.e., when selecting exercise intensity at $40\%\dot{V}O_2 R$, both high fit and low fit individuals have to adjust their relative efforts above rest to the same degree).
- Selecting exercise intensity based on $\%\dot{V}O_2 R$ utilizes net (or reserve) values while $\dot{V}O_{2max}$ is a gross term. However, it is the net calorific expenditure that should be considered for weight-loss purposes, rather than gross expenditure (rest + exercise). Refer back to Chapter 5 for a discussion of these concepts.

Table 14.9 illustrates the advantages listed above. Refer to Case Study 14.2 for another illustration of the use of $\%\dot{V}O_2R$ in aerobic exercise prescription.

| Table 14.9 | EQUIVALENT AEROBIC EXERCISE INTENSITIES USING %HRR, % $\dot{V}O_2$ R, AND % $\dot{V}O_2$ DIFFERENTIATED BY FITNESS LEVEL | | | |
|---|---|---|---|---|

| | | | %$\dot{V}O_{2max}$ | |
| %HRR | %$\dot{V}O_2$ R | 5 MET capacity | 10 MET capacity | 20 MET capacity |
|---|---|---|---|---|
| 0% (rest) | 0% | 20% | 10% | 5% |
| 40% | 40% | 52% | 46% | 43% |
| 50% | 50% | 60% | 55% | 53% |
| 85% | 85% | 88% | 87% | 86% |
| 100% | 100% | 100% | 100% | 100% |

From rest to maximal exercise, %HRR and %$\dot{V}O_2$ R units provide equivalent intensities. For the same intensity to be achieved during submaximal exercise, units of %$\dot{V}O_{2max}$ must be adjusted upward. The greater the fitness level of the individual, the less adjustment there is needed in %$\dot{V}O_{2max}$ units, especially at light exercise levels. HRR, heart rate reserve; MET, metabolic equivalents.

## CASE STUDY 14.2: *USE OF %$\dot{V}O_2R$ IN AEROBIC EXERCISE PRESCRIPTION*

### CASE

George is a 50-year-old former high school football player who has been sedentary for the last 25 years. He is 178 cm tall and weighs 118 kg with 26% body fat. He has a family history of heart disease, and his resting blood pressure is currently 155/95. Due to a complaint of shortness of breath, he was given a stress test. On the test, he achieved a maximal heart rate of 160 beats per minute and an estimated aerobic capacity from the treadmill test of 6 metabolic equivalents (21 mL·kg$^{-1}$·min$^{-1}$). During the test, George experienced shortness of breath, but otherwise the test was normal except for indicating that the subject was deconditioned.

### DESCRIPTION

In *ACSM's Guidelines for Exercise Testing and Prescription*, the concept of the $\dot{V}O_2$ R was introduced as a replacement for the $\dot{V}O_{2max}$ as a way to establish exercise intensity for aerobic exercise prescription. Basing exercise prescriptions on the reserve value rather than the maximal value reduces the error inherent in the % heart rate reserve (%HRR)/$\dot{V}O_{2max}$ relationship, as this case study illustrates.

### INTERVENTION

In the clinical foundation section of the text, a detailed examination of exercise prescriptions is provided for a number of patient groups. The following serves to illustrate the difference in prescribing aerobic exercise based on older criteria, i.e., $\dot{V}O_{2max}$ versus current criteria, i.e., $\dot{V}O_2$ R. The recommended threshold intensity for low fitness level adults is 40% $\dot{V}O_2$ R. Using this value, a target metabolic load ($\dot{V}O_2$) can be calculated as follows:

$$\text{Target } \dot{V}O_2 = (\text{Intensity fraction})(\dot{V}O_{2max} - 3.5) + 3.5$$

$$= 0.40(21 - 3.5) + 3.5$$

$$= 10.5 \text{ mL·kg}^{-1}\text{·min}^{-1}$$

The target metabolic load is 10.5 mL·kg$^{-1}$·min$^{-1}$. Using the appropriate metabolic equation from Table 5.5 in Chapter 5 of the text, we can estimate what his equivalent exercise workload would be on the Monark cycle ergometer using the following equation:

$$\dot{V}O_2 = 0 + (10.8 \cdot W \cdot M^{-1}) + 7.0$$

$$10.5 = (10.8W \div 118) + 7.0$$

$$1.5 = 10.8W \div 118$$

$$413 = 10.8W$$

$$38.24 = W$$

We convert the power output unit to kgm·min$^{-1}$ by multiplying by 6.12; hence, 38.24W × 6.12 = 234 kgm·min$^{-1}$. This power output on the cycle ergometer would give George the exercise intensity needed to begin his aerobic conditioning program. *But what if 40% $\dot{V}O_{2max}$ had been chosen instead of 40% $\dot{V}O_2$ R? In this case, the target $\dot{V}O_2$ would have been 0.40 × 21.0 = 8.4 mL·kg$^{-1}$·min$^{-1}$. What would be the difference in the power output on the cycle ergometer?*

$$\dot{V}O_{2max} = 0 + (10.8 \cdot W \cdot M^{-1}) + 7.0$$

$$8.4 = (10.8W \div 118) + 7.0$$

$$1.4 = 10.8W \div 118$$

$$165.2 = 10.8W$$

$$15.3 = W \text{ or } 93.6 \text{ kgm·min}^{-1}$$

This exercise load on the cycle ergometer is about 40% of the initial stimulus he needs in his exercise prescription.

## Rating of Perceived Exertion and Exercise Intensity

Sometimes a person's rating of perceived exertion (RPE) may be more indicative of true exercise intensity than actual HR, especially in situations in which medication or disease state may alter the normal HR response to exercise. RPE scales designed for this purpose have been shown to be valuable tools in monitoring training programs. Support for the use of RPE scales for monitoring exercise intensity centers around the idea that the RPE integrates information coming from the peripheral working muscles and joints, central cardiovascular and respiratory functions, and central nervous system.

The two most commonly used RPE scales are shown in *Figure 14.10*. One is a 15-point scale ranging from 6 to 20 with a verbal description provided at every odd number. The other is similar but uses a scale rating from 0 to 10. The proposed advantage of the 10-point scale (category-ratio) is that it allows for more finely tuned subjective evaluation of exercise stress because there are no absolute limits. When using this scale, people are permitted to use decimals and also go beyond 10 or below 0.5 on either end of the scale. For example, if an increase in exercise intensity feels 20% harder than it did at 10, the RPE would be 12. The 15-point scale is probably best for most applications, whereas the 10-point scale may be especially sensitive for determining subjective symptoms, such as breathing difficulties, aches, and pain.

The RPE can also be used in conjunction with HR prescription methods for monitoring exercise intensity. At the beginning of a training program, the participant can be instructed to exercise at the prescribed HR and to monitor RPE and HR simultaneously. When the participant can identify the relationship between HR and RPE, HR can be monitored less frequently while the RPE is used for self-monitoring during exercise. The RPE can be similarly used as a built-in safety point during the exercise session. A value on the RPE scale can be set as a stop point for exercise or as a signal to reduce exercise intensity. Use of the RPE in this manner may reduce the risk of a participant exerting too much effort in an attempt to reach a predetermined THR.

## ENDURANCE TRAINING TECHNIQUES

Every exercise session should be divided into three phases: warmup, conditioning, and cooldown. The focus thus far in this chapter has been the conditioning phase of the exercise session. This is the phase of the exercise session that is governed by the guidelines established for mode, frequency, duration, and intensity. During conditioning, blood pressure increases, HR is elevated, and metabolic rate rises to meet the demand for energy. These physiologic responses to exercise are a form of stress response. Generally this exercise stress is good for the body. The adaptation or adjustment to exercise stress or overload is what increases fitness

| RPE Scale | %VO$_{2max}$ | Category-ratio RPE Scale |
|---|---|---|
| 6 | 0% (rest) | 0 Nothing at all |
| 7 Very, Very Light | | 0.5 Very, Very Weak |
| 8 | < 30% | |
| 9 Very Light | | 1 Very Weak |
| 10 | | |
| 11 Fairly Light | 30-49% | 2 Weak |
| 12 | | 3 Moderate |
| 13 Somewhat Hard | 50-74% | 4 Somewhat Strong |
| 14 | | |
| 15 Hard | 75-84% | 5 Strong |
| 16 | ≥ 85% | 6 |
| 17 Very Hard | | 7 Very Strong |
| | | 8 |
| 18 | | 9 |
| 19 Very, Very Hard | | 10 Very, Very Strong |
| 20 | 100% | Maximal |

**FIGURE 14.10.** Exercise intensity relative to ratings of perceived exertion.

level and exercise capacity. However, abrupt changes in the physiologic parameters controlling muscular activity may result in injury or provoke a disease response.

## Warm up and Cool down

Warm up before the conditioning phase of exercise helps the body adjust gradually to the overload and reduces any possible risks from exercise. The purpose of the warm up period before aerobic exercise is to slowly increase the aerobic energy production so it approaches the level prescribed for intensity under the exercise prescription. The best way to increase aerobic energy production during the warm up is to do an aerobic type of exercise at low intensity. Individuals should start out slowly and gradually work up to a level close to the prescribed THR or RPE over a period of 5 to 10 minutes. It is acceptable to incorporate stretching exercises into the warm up period, but stretching should not constitute the whole warm up.

A good indicator of whether warm up has been effective is the onset of perspiration. This means that body temperature has risen slightly, the muscles are warm, and metabolism has increased closer to the level prescribed in the training regimen. At this point, the individual can now progress directly into the conditioning phase of the workout.

When the conditioning phase has been completed, the subject should gradually cool down by either reducing greatly the intensity of exercise that was used for conditioning or by continuing with some other low-intensity aerobic exercise. The principle objective of the cool down is to return pooled blood from the exercised muscles back to the central circulation. The length of the cool down should be determined by the environment, fitness level, and speed of recovery for the individual participant. The best reference to determine when the cool down is complete is HR. A good rule of thumb is to monitor HR during the cool down period; when the HR reaches 100 bpm or within 20 beats of the resting HR, the cool down is complete. Stretching exercises can also be incorporated into the cool down period, but they should be done near the end of the cool down when the system has recovered somewhat from the higher intensity work of the conditioning phase. *How do you know when you are cooled down?* A good guide is when HR is below 100 bpm or within 20 beats of the resting HR.

## Performance Training

Interval training for aerobic endurance involves the performance of repeated exercise bouts at a high intensity interspersed with active rest intervals of low-intensity exercise. Interval training designed to improve $\dot{V}O_{2max}$ should use intervals longer than 60 seconds so that the aerobic energy pathways are stressed. Interval training is generally not recommended for the general population nor is interval training necessary to meet the training objectives of health and fitness. Usually interval training is most beneficial for competitive athletes who are concerned with maximal performance and training for competition near

maximal aerobic capacity. There is conflicting evidence as to whether continuous or interval training regimens are more effective in improving biochemical, physiologic, and performance measures related to endurance exercise. Research shows that interval training produces greater increases in $\dot{V}O_{2max}$ and in maximal exercise capacity, whereas continuous training is more effective at increasing muscle oxidative capacity and delaying the accumulation of blood lactate during endurance exercise (7). The following example illustrates the type of weekly training in which a competitive marathon runner may engage.

- Day 1: 4- to 5-mile easy run (morning) and lower body light resistance training (afternoon)
- Day 2: 8- to 10-mile easy run
- Day 3: 12- to 15-mile road run (moderate)
- Day 4: 5 mile-morning easy run and vigorous track interval work (afternoon); intervals may be 3 × 1000 m, 1 × 5000 m, 2 × 1000 m all at 110% race pace with a 5-minute rest period between each work interval
- Day 5: 1-hour run at desired pace
- Day 6: Rest
- Day 7: 4- to 5-mile run (morning) and upper body light resistance training (afternoon)

▶ *INQUIRY SUMMARY.* The proper stimulus during endurance training is based on frequency, duration, and intensity. Of these three, intensity is the most important and can be precisely controlled by a target HR that takes into account age and resting HR. Since HR and metabolic rate are linearly related, a prescribed metabolic training stimulus (%$\dot{V}O_{2max}$ or %$\dot{V}O_2$ R) can be achieved by considering %HRmax or %HRR. Current research has shown that %$\dot{V}O_2$ R and %HRR vary in a one-to-one relationship and that prescribing aerobic exercise according to this relationship has several advantages. Do you think the one-to-one relationship between %$\dot{V}O_2$ R and %HRR is constant across all populations?

## *Summary*

The principle of specificity relates to the type of activity while the overload principle dictates that when dosage parameters are adjusted regularly, continual gains in performance can be realized. General physical fitness can be achieved when attention is given to the musculoskeletal and cardiorespiratory systems in training. For enhanced musculoskeletal function, training programs first focus on strength gains and, depending on the sport-specific goals, power and speed may then be specifically addressed with appropriate programs. Progressive overload for gains in these areas requires that strict attention be given to mode, duration, frequency, and intensity of training. These same dosage parameters are necessary to follow when improvements in cardiorespiratory fitness are sought. Particularly important is the intensity variable. For cardiorespiratory fitness, heart rate and metabolic load ($\%\dot{V}O_2R$ or $\%\dot{V}O_{2max}$) are the two main variables of interest. Regression equations have shown that heart rate (as a percentage of the heart rate reserve) is most closely associated with metabolic load when $\dot{V}O_2$ is expressed as a percentage of its reserve capacity (i.e., $\%\dot{V}O_2R$). The rating of perceived exertion may also be used to gauge intensity of aerobic activity.

## SUMMARY KNOWLEDGE

1. Why is knowledge of the bioenergetic system used in an exercise or sport task important regarding the principle of specificity?
2. Why is the activity continuum important in exercise training?
3. Why is it important to know the difference between dynamic and static exercises?
4. Why is the concept of cross-training important to consider in exercise training for athletic performance?
5. How does dynamic resistance exercise training affect sports performance?
6. Why may free-weight resistance training be better than machine resistance training as an adjunct to sport-specific training routines?
7. Why is overload an important principle of training?
8. Why is the $\%\dot{V}O_2R$ method for determining endurance exercise intensity superior to the $\%\dot{V}O_{2max}$ method?

### References

1. Tesch PA, Colliander EB, Kaiser P. Muscle metabolism during intense, heavy-resistance exercise. *Eur J Appl Physiol Occup Physiol* 1986;55:362–366.
2. Keul J, Haralambie G, Bruder M, et al. The effect of weight lifting exercise on heart rate and metabolism in experienced weight lifters. *Med Sci Sports* 1978;10:13–15.
3. Swain DP, Abernathy KS, Smith CS, et al. Target heart rates for the development of cardiorespiratory fitness. *Med Sci Sports Exerc* 1994;26:112–116.
4. Jakicic JM, Donnelly JE, Pronk NP, et al. Prescription of exercise intensity for the obese patient: the relationship between heart rate, $\dot{V}O_2$ and perceived exertion. *Int J Obes Relat Metab Disord* 1995;19:382–387.
5. Swain DP, Leutholtz BC. Heart rate reserve is equivalent to $\%\dot{V}O_2$ reserve, not $\%\dot{V}O_{2max}$. *Med Sci Sports Exerc* 1997;29:410–414.
6. Swain DP, Leutholtz BC, King ME, et al. Relationship between %heart rate reserve and $\%\dot{V}O_2$ reserve in treadmill exercise. *Med Sci Sports Exerc* 1998;30:318–321.
7. Gorostiaga EM, Walter WB, Foster C, Hickson RC. Uniqueness of interval and continuous training at the same maintained exercise intensity. *Eur J Appl Physiol Occup Physiol* 1991;63:101–107.

### Suggested Readings

Masterson GL, Brown SP. The effects of weighted rope jump training on power performance in collegians. *J Strength Cond Res* 1993;7:108–114.
Swain DP, Leutholtz BC. Heart rate reserve is equivalent to $\%\dot{V}O_2$ reserve, not $\%\dot{V}O_{2max}$. *Med Sci Sports Exerc* 1997;29:410–414.
Swain DP, Leutholtz BC, King ME, et al. Relationship between %heart rate reserve and $\%\dot{V}O_2$ reserve in treadmill exercise. *Med Sci Sports Exerc* 1998;30:318–321.

### On the Internet

Visit the textbook's accompanying website at **http://connection.lww.com/go/brownexphys** to find live Internet links for excellent content on aspects of physical training:

Sports Performance Journal. Available at: **http://www.athletesperformance.com/spj/**. Accessed June 02, 2005.
Plyometrics. Available at: **http://www.brianmac.demon.co.uk/plymo.htm**. Accessed June 02, 2005.
Sports Fitness Advisor: Sports training tips and programs to build peak sports fitness. Available at: **http://www.sport-fitness-advisor.com/index.html**. Accessed June 02, 2005.
Georgia State University Department of Kinesiology and Health: Strength training main page. Available at: **http://www2.gsu.edu/**~wwwfit/strength.html. Accessed June 02, 2005.
Sports Coach. Available at: **http://www.brianmac.demon.co.uk/siteindx.htm**. Accessed June 02, 2005.
Do It Sports: Virtual training. Available at: **http://www.doitsports.com/virtualtraining/virtualtraining.tcl**. Accessed June 02, 2005.
Personal Training on the Net. Available at: **http://www.ptonthenet.com/**. Accessed June 02, 2005.
Exercise Prescription on the Net. Available at: **http://www.exrx.net/**. Accessed June 02, 2005.
Sportscience. Available at: **http://www.sportsci.org/index.html?jour/03/03.htm**. Accessed June 02, 2005.
Shape Up America! Available at: **http://shapeup.org/**. Accessed June 02, 2005.

## Writing to Learn

The concept of the $\dot{V}O_2R$ is changing the way exercise intensity is being viewed and prescribed for aerobic fitness. Research and write a paper on how this concept may alter the exercise prescription process for the following clinical populations: cardiac patients, pulmonary patients, and patients with a neuromuscular disorder.

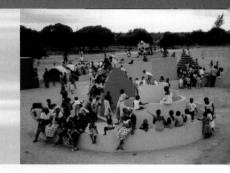

# 15 Pediatric Exercise Physiology

*Although most degenerative diseases, like cardiovascular disease, manifest themselves in adulthood, their genesis may be traced to unhealthy behaviors in earlier years. The dismal health statistics for adults are just a reflection of those seen for children. For example, today's children show an increase of more than 100% in the prevalence of obesity compared to their counterparts of only a few decades ago. The National Children and Youth Fitness Studies have revealed that a large percentage of today's youth do not participate in physical activity appropriate for long-term health promotion. Consequently conservative estimates indicate that eight to nine million school-aged children may be at increased risk for degenerative diseases because of insufficient physical fitness.* How can health professionals promote physical activity in a society that encourages a sedentary lifestyle?

## CHAPTER OUTLINE

GROWTH, DEVELOPMENT, AND MATURATION
- Anthropometric Growth and Development
- Physiologic Development

EVALUATING FITNESS AND PHYSICAL ACTIVITY IN CHILDREN
- Fitness Testing of Children
- Clinical Exercise Testing of Children
- Assessing Physical Activity in Children

Activity Questionnaires
Pedometers
Accelerometers
Heart-Rate Monitoring
Activity Diaries

CHILDHOOD RESPONSES TO PHYSICAL ACTIVITY AND EXERCISE TRAINING
- Exercise Capacities of Children Versus Adults
- Exercise Injuries in Children
- Emotional Distress in Young Athletes
- Behavior Carryover

EXERCISE PRESCRIPTION, GUIDELINES, AND RECOMMENDATIONS FOR CHILDREN

---

The importance of a physically active lifestyle in reducing the risk of premature morbidity and mortality is well established. Conventional wisdom suggests that developing an active lifestyle during childhood can help a child achieve or maintain a healthy body weight, healthy blood lipid profile, insulin sensitivity, and active lifestyle into adulthood. However, controversies remain about how much exercise or activity is necessary to achieve and maintain health in children and adolescents, even though guidelines on the amount of physical activity required to produce health benefits in youth and adults have been published and subsequently revised. Also undetermined is if the benefits of an active childhood carry over into adulthood. Some of these controversies are based in the understanding of the physiologic differences between children and adults, the difficulties in evaluating fitness in children, the difficulties in monitoring activity in children, and the risks associated with exercise training in children. This chapter addresses these and other issues relevant to pediatric exercise physiology.

## Growth, Development, and Maturation

**Growth**, **development**, and **maturation** are terms that describe the changes that occur in the body throughout life. Although these terms are related, they are not synonymous. Growth refers to an increase in size, development refers to specialization, and maturation refers to functional adulthood. As the healthy child matures physically, growth and development of the tissues brings about physiologic changes that allow the child to sustain the demands of exercise seen in the capable adult. When studying pediatric exercise physiology, one must consider how all three of these parameters affect the systems that are called upon during acute and chronic exercise.

Growth, development, and maturation can be defined by the system or function being measured. For example, growth of the male genitals during puberty is associated with development of the reproductive system and maturation of the boy into manhood. Each of these processes (growth, development, and maturation) has landmark indicators that can be used to determine the state of progress. However, the rate of change in each of these parameters is different among children and within a child. Thus, it becomes difficult to pick a time point when comparisons among children or comparisons between children and adults can be made.

The period of life from birth to adulthood is divided into phases. Each phase is defined by chronologic age or by a band of time. Since it is difficult to measure physiologic parameters for exercise in children under the age of 6, we have defined the chronologic phases of growth, development, and maturation into three distinct time periods for the purpose of this chapter. Children are in the age range of 6 to 12 years, adolescents 13 to 18 years, and adults more than 18 years of age.

## ANTHROPOMETRIC GROWTH AND DEVELOPMENT

**Anthropometry** is the science of measuring the human body and its parts. Professionals in the field of anthropometry have studied extensively how changes in height and weight are related to development and maturation. Scientists have also studied, with keen interest, anthropometric changes in childhood populations throughout the world to learn more about the rise in childhood obesity that has occurred during the past two decades.

The National Center for Health Statistics, in collaboration with the National Center for Chronic Disease Prevention and Health Promotion, has compiled data from a large number of children to produce growth charts that represent the normal growth patterns of children (*Figs. 15.1 and 15.2*). Health care professionals reference these charts to identify the percentage of the population norm in which a particular child lies. Monitoring the growth of a child over time, in reference to the population norm, may allow the identification of abnormalities in growth and development that may be corrected if detected early.

Height increases most rapidly during the first 2 years of life. A child will reach approximately 50% of his/her height by age 2. Thereafter, growth curves for both boys and girls are fairly linear until they flatten out at the time of sexual maturation. Full height is reached at about 16.5 years of age for girls and about 18.0 years for boys. The plot of weight change over time generally parallels changes in height. Referring back to Figures 13.18 and 13.19, the plot of body mass index (BMI) change over time shows a slightly different curve than those of height and weight. BMI declines after infancy and continues to decline until the child reaches 4 to 6 years of age. Thereafter, BMI begins a gradual rise and continues to rise throughout most of adulthood.

BMI is less accurate in predicting childhood overweight than in adults. BMI for children is gender specific and changes throughout growth and development, whereas BMI for adults is neither gender nor age specific. A child's BMI-for-age at or above the 95th percentile is considered overweight, and between the 85th and 95th percentiles is considered at risk for overweight. The term overweight rather than obesity is the preferred designation for describing large children and adolescents because the comorbidities associated with obesity in adults have not yet manifested themselves in overweight children. Therefore, health professionals are being cautious not to prematurely label a large child as being diseased. A childhood BMI below the 5th percentile is considered underweight.

Standards for the assessment of body fat content in children have been developed because of the concern about the relationship between childhood body fatness and adult obesity (refer to Table 13.8). These standards are only guidelines to be used by health professionals since the health risks associated with different levels of fatness in children have not been established clearly (1). Girls of all ages carry more body fat content than boys, but the difference is small before the onset of puberty. Six- to 8-year-old boys average 13% to 15% body fat, while girls of the same age average 16% to 18%. Postpubescent boys, ages 14 to 16 years, average 10% to 12% fat, compared with girls that age averaging 21% to 23%. By late adolescence, males average 13% fat and females 24% (2). The optimal percent body fat for boys of all ages is 10% to 20% and for girls is 15% to 25%. Since the relationship between skinfold thickness and percent fat changes only slightly with age and hydrostatic weighting tends to overestimate body fat content in children, the standards associated with skinfold measures can be used for children between 6 and 18 years of age (2).

## PHYSIOLOGIC DEVELOPMENT

Parallel to the growth of the body and its parts is the physiologic development of tissues, organs, and systems. The physiologic development of tissues, organs, and systems brings them into maturity and increases their functional capacities. The systems that are most integrated into our ability to perform exercise are the pulmonary, cardiovascular, and musculoskeletal systems. The physiologic development of these systems allows for a greater capacity to perform both anaerobic and aerobic exercise. In other words, as physiologic development occurs, our capacity to withstand the metabolic demands of exercise increases.

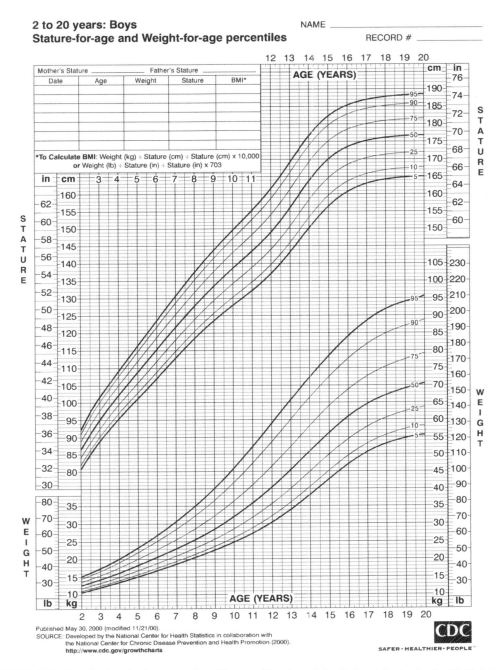

**2 to 20 years: Boys**
**Stature-for-age and Weight-for-age percentiles**

NAME _____

RECORD # _____

**FIGURE 15.1.** Growth chart for boys ages 2 to 20 years. (Courtesy of the National Center for Health Statistics.)

The development of the pulmonary system parallels overall body growth. All lung volumes increase until growth is complete. However, the development of the alveoli is complete by 6 years of age. Throughout childhood and adolescence, growth in lung size increases the available surface area for gas exchange such that arterial blood gas values in children are similar to those for adults. Changes in lung volumes, airway resistance, and compliance of the respiratory system allow for increased maximal minute ventilation. The maximal minute ventilation of a child increases from 30 to 40 L·min$^{-1}$ at age 6 to 100 to 140 L·min$^{-1}$ by maturity.

Parallel to changes in the pulmonary system are those that occur in the cardiovascular system. Heart volume, relative to body size, is larger in children than in adults, meaning that body growth is proportionately greater than cardiac growth. Cardiac contractility does not change during growth and development. Resting heart rate is higher in children than adults because the resting heart rate is generally negatively related to body size. Blood pressure at rest and during exercise is lower in children than adults because children have a lower peripheral resistance than adults. Stroke volume, at any given workload, is lower in

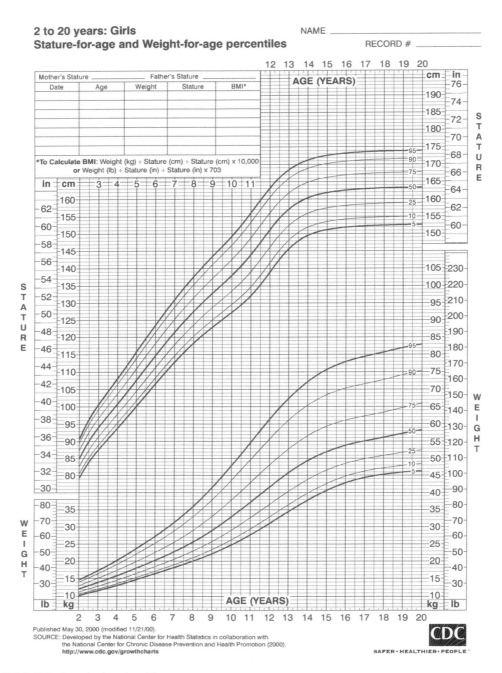

**2 to 20 years: Girls**
**Stature-for-age and Weight-for-age percentiles**

NAME _____

RECORD # _____

AGE (YEARS)

*To Calculate BMI: Weight (kg) ÷ Stature (cm) ÷ Stature (cm) x 10,000
or Weight (lb) ÷ Stature (in) ÷ Stature (in) x 703

Published May 30, 2000 (modified 11/21/00).
SOURCE: Developed by the National Center for Health Statistics in collaboration with
the National Center for Chronic Disease Prevention and Health Promotion (2000).
http://www.cdc.gov/growthcharts

CDC
SAFER • HEALTHIER • PEOPLE™

**FIGURE 15.2.** Growth chart for girls ages 2 to 20 years. (Courtesy of the National Center for Health Statistics.)

children than adults. However, the higher heart rate, for a given workload, does not completely compensate for the smaller stroke volume. Therefore, cardiac output, at any given exercise intensity, is lower in children than adults. To maintain the same $\dot{V}O_2$ with the lower $O_2$ delivery due to the lower cardiac output, the arterial-to-venous difference is greater in the child.

The development of the pulmonary and cardiovascular systems allows for greater $O_2$ delivery to the exercising muscles. This means that the capacity for aerobic exercise increases as the child grows and develops. Maximal $O_2$

consumption ($\dot{V}O_{2max}$) increases throughout childhood and adolescence for both boys and girls. Most of the increase in $\dot{V}O_{2max}$ is due to increased muscle mass, particularly in the lower body. Boys generally have a higher $\dot{V}O_{2max}$ than girls because they are generally larger than girls. When children reach puberty, the aerobic capacity for boys continues to rise, but the rate of increase is diminished for girls. Much of the gender difference in $\dot{V}O_{2max}$ is due to increased muscularity in boys and increased adiposity in girls after puberty. Another factor that contributes to the sex difference in $\dot{V}O_{2max}$ of adolescents is the decreased hemoglobin concentration following the onset of menses in girls. Lower hemoglobin levels diminish the $O_2$-carrying capacity of the blood, which decreases $\dot{V}O_{2max}$.

Much, but not all, of the increase in anaerobic work capacity seen during adolescence is due to increased muscle mass. Both strength and power output increase from age 6 to 18 for both genders. Boys demonstrate greater anaerobic capacities than girls due to the increase in male hormone production with the onset of puberty. Other factors that contribute to higher anaerobic capacities for both sexes are related to rapid glycolysis. Glycolytic enzyme capacity is lower in children than adults. Lactate production, the lactate threshold, and the ability to buffer lactic acid are all lower in children compared with adults. Muscle glycogen stores are lower and the glycogenolytic rate is also lower in children. Muscle ATP concentration is the same in children and adults, but the smaller muscle mass in children greatly reduces the power output of children.

▶ **INQUIRY SUMMARY.** Growth, development, and maturation are terms that describe the changes occurring in the body throughout life. The science of studying growth of the body and its parts is called anthropometry. As scientists and health professionals examine the growth of a child over time, in reference to the population norm, they can identify abnormalities in growth and development that may be corrected if detected early. As the child grows and develops, physiologic changes occur in the tissues, organs, and systems. Changes in the pulmonary, cardiovascular, and musculoskeletal systems allow for greater exercise capacities as the child develops. Changes in these systems allow for a greater aerobic capacity because of increased $O_2$ delivery and utilization in the tissues. Greater muscle mass and improved glycolytic capacity allow for increased strength and power output in adults compared with children. *Identify clinical tests or evaluations that could be administered to a child to see if he/she was growing and developing his or her capacity for exercise in a normal way.*

## Evaluating Fitness and Physical Activity in Children

Understanding the relationships among childhood physical activity, physical fitness, and health has been hampered by the lack of satisfactory instruments for measuring these variables in children. Traditionally physical fitness tests have been used to monitor the health and physical well-being of the nation's children. However, fitness tests often focus on evaluating speed, muscular power, and agility. Whereas these traits are important for athletic success and are primarily determined by genetics, aerobic power, body composition, joint flexibility, and muscular strength and endurance are health-related traits that are only partially influenced by heredity and can be changed significantly by appropriate exercise and activity patterns. Nonetheless, criterion-referenced health standards for these traits have not been adequate for the task (3). Therefore, it is difficult to determine if today's children are more or less fit than those of previous decades because our evaluation tools may be invalid (3).

Most definitions of fitness, old or new, are framed in terms of what fitness enables one to do (e.g., run long distances rapidly) or in terms of what capacities one should possess (e.g., specific relative $\dot{V}O_{2max}$). Although the physiologic states required for the desired capabilities are often assumed to have some relationship to one's level of physical activity, under these definitions certain children may be categorized as "fit" even though they may have never undergone a real "training effect" (3). In other words, a child may have inherent athletic ability that was never trained or developed which allows the child to perform well in fitness tests based on muscular power or agility. This problem is not as prevalent in adult fitness testing because most adult assessment tests are not rooted in fundamentals of sport performance such as agility. If the level of physical activity in which a child engages has nothing to do with whether he/she can meet the physical fitness test standards, then there is a problem with either the standards or our concept of fitness. Regardless of whether the evaluation tools are revisions of traditional fitness tests, criterion-referenced health standards, or newly designed evaluators, the tools must be able to distinguish between active and inactive populations of children. The evaluation tools must also demonstrate an effectual relationship between test achievement scores and optimal functional capacity and health.

Another point to consider when evaluating fitness and health is the concept or assumption that physical fitness is a product of physical activity. If this was true, then the critical variable to be considered would be the amount of physical activity necessary to produce the physiologic responses associated with optimal health. Once again, our methods of evaluation may be inadequate. First of all, an accurate method for measuring physical activity in children has not been developed. Secondly, questions related to the physiologic responses of children to various types of exercise remain unanswered because fewer scientists are studying children and exercise than are studying adults and exercise. One reason that data are lacking may be that few scientists would puncture a child's artery, take a muscle biopsy from a child, or expose a child to harsh environments just to satisfy scientific curiosity. Another reason for insufficient data is that most **hypokinetic diseases** are clinically manifest among adults, not children. Therefore, many of the conclusions about physical activity, physiologic adaptation, and health in children are extrapolated from data derived from adults. Box 15.1 introduces James Sallis, who has studied extensively how environmental factors affect physical activity.

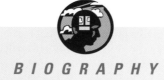

BIOGRAPHY

## James F. Sallis, PhD

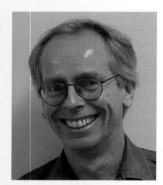

James F. Sallis, PhD, received his doctorate in clinical psychology in 1981 from Memphis State University, with an internship at Brown University. He was a post-doctoral fellow in cardiovascular disease prevention and epidemiology at the Stanford Center for Research in Disease Prevention. He is currently a professor of psychology at San Diego State University. Dr. Sallis has spent much of his career studying how the environment (school, social, community, geography) affects physical activity levels in children and adolescents. Most of his research is concerned with applying behavioral science to physical activity, although he also studies nutrition and behavior. His current primary interest is to improve the understanding of how environments and policies contribute to the epidemic of physical inactivity.

Dr. Sallis has received awards from the Division of Health Psychology of the American Psychological Association, as well as from the American Alliance of Health, Physical Education, Recreation, and Dance. He was elected to the Board of Trustees of the American College of Sports Medicine and International Council for Physical Activity and Fitness Research. Dr. Sallis is the author of more than 300 scientific publications and is on the editorial boards of several journals. He served on the editorial committee for the 1996 United States Surgeon General's Report, *Physical Activity and Health*. Dr. Sallis is coauthor of *Physical Activity and Behavioral Medicine* (Sage, 1999).

Dr. Sallis has directed or codirected numerous grants from the National Institutes of Health, Centers for Disease Control and Prevention, California Department of Health Services, and International Life Sciences Institute to study the effects of physical activity interventions and other health promotion programs. He directs the "Active Living Policy and Environmental Studies" program for the Robert Wood Johnson Foundation.

James F. Sallis, PhD

Dr. Sallis and colleagues are working to use research-based programs to improve physical activity throughout the nation and internationally. He is a frequent consultant to government agencies, research programs, health organizations, and corporations throughout the world.

## FITNESS TESTING OF CHILDREN

Assessing the functional capacity of children generally involves fitness testing rather than clinical exercise testing (*Fig. 15.3*). Clinical exercise testing is usually reserved for children with symptoms of disease, established disease, or suspected medical abnormalities (4). In spite of the previously mentioned weaknesses of some fitness test batteries, data from fitness tests can be used to describe the health and fitness status of children. Assessment of physical fitness in children is most often performed in school-based physical education programs. The two most common physical fitness test batteries come from the President's Council on Physical Fitness and Sport (President's Challenge) and the Cooper Institute in Dallas, Texas (FITNESSGRAM). These test batteries are similar in nature, but the scores from the President's Challenge are compared with national norms, whereas the scores from the FITNESSGRAM are compared to researched and developed health standards.

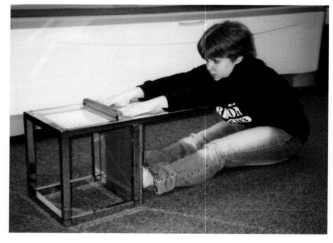

FIGURE 15.3. An adolescent performing the sit-and-reach fitness test for flexibility.

The difference between national normative data and health standards is that national norms are simply a collection of descriptive data that portray the child and adolescent populations. Normative data do not tell us anything about the health status of a child or adolescent. Placement of a child or adolescent within the norms just tells where the child stands in relation to his/her peers. This may lead some children who are actually healthy to perceive themselves as unfit, while others who are unhealthy but physically skilled perceive themselves as healthy and fit.

Health standards, on the other hand, are carefully researched criteria. By using these criterion-referenced standards, a professional knows if a child meets the minimum recommendation for being fit on each test item. Furthermore, the criteria for each test item are based on health-related physical fitness and not skill performance. Thus, the scores are not skewed by individual differences in athletic prowess.

The President's Challenge, a physical fitness awards program that recognizes children for their levels of physical fitness, consists of five fitness tests: 1) curlups or partial curlups, 2) shuttle run, 3) endurance run/walk, 4) pullups, right angle pushups, or flex-arm hang, and 5) V-sit reach or sit and reach (*Fig. 15.4*).

The program offers three levels of awards for children, depending on their level of fitness. The Presidential Physical Fitness Award is given to boys and girls who score above the 85th percentile on all five tests (Table 15.1). The National Physical Fitness Award is given to boys and girls who score above the 50th percentile in all five tests (Table 15.2), while a Participant Physical Fitness Award is given to participants who fall below the 50th percentile. A description of each of the five tests in the President's Challenge can be found in Table 15.3.

Recently the President's Council on Physical Fitness and Sport added a new award to the President's Challenge. The Presidential Health Fitness Award focuses on helping children develop health-related fitness rather than athletic

PHYSICAL FITNESS

THE PRESIDENT'S CHALLENGE PHYSICAL FITNESS SCORECARD **FOR THE ADMINISTRATOR**

Name__________ School/Organization __________ Gender _____

Instructions: The Scorecard has been designed so that it may be copied onto heavy stock paper. If copied on both sides, this card will keep testing information for a student from age 6 through 17.

| | | TEST ___ | TEST ___ | TEST ___ | TEST ___ | TEST ___ | TEST ___ |
|---|---|---|---|---|---|---|---|
| The President's Challenge<br>Physical Fitness Events | | Date___<br>Age___<br>Grade___<br>Ht.___<br>Wt.___ | Date___<br>Age___<br>Grade___<br>Ht.___<br>Wt.___ | Date___<br>Age___<br>Grade___<br>Ht.___<br>Wt.___ | Date___<br>Age___<br>Grade___<br>Ht.___<br>Wt.___ | Date___<br>Age___<br>Grade___<br>Ht.___<br>Wt.___ | Date___<br>Age___<br>Grade___<br>Ht.___<br>Wt.___ |
| **1. Curl-ups** (# of reps. within 1 min.) **or Partial Curl-ups** (#) | Raw score | | | | | | |
| | Level | Pr N Pa | Pr N Pa | Pr N Pa | Pr N Pa | Pr N Pa | Pr N Pa |
| **2. Shuttle Run** (seconds xx.x) | Raw score | | | | | | |
| | Level | Pr N Pa | Pr N Pa | Pr N Pa | Pr N Pa | Pr N Pa | Pr N Pa |
| **3. V-sit** (inches) **or Sit & Reach** (centimeters) | Raw score | | | | | | |
| | Level | Pr N Pa | Pr N Pa | Pr N Pa | Pr N Pa | Pr N Pa | Pr N Pa |
| **4. Endurance run/walk** 1/4 mile 6-7 yr. old; 1/2 mile 8-9 yr. old; 1 mile 10-17 yr. old (min:sec) | Raw score | | | | | | |
| | Level | Pr N Pa | Pr N Pa | Pr N Pa | Pr N Pa | Pr N Pa | Pr N Pa |
| **5. Pull-ups or Rt. Angle Push-ups** (#) **or Flexed-Arm Hang** (sec) | Raw score | | | | | | |
| | Level | Pr N Pa | Pr N Pa | Pr N Pa | Pr N Pa | Pr N Pa | Pr N Pa |
| AWARD EARNED (Check one & instructor sign) | **PRES** | | | | | | |
| | **NAT'L** | | | | | | |
| | **PART** | | | | | | |
| **COMMENTS** | | | | | | | |

*Pr = Presidential N = National Pa = Participant*

This form may be photocopied.

FIGURE 15.4. The President's Challenge Physical Fitness scorecard. (Courtesy of the President's Challenge, a program of The President's Council on Physical Fitness and Sport, 2004.)

**Table 15.1    PRESIDENTIAL PHYSICAL FITNESS AWARD STANDARDS (85TH PERCENTILE)**

**Boys**

| Age | Muscular endurance | | Agility | Flexibility | | Cardiorespiratory endurance | | Muscular strength | |
|---|---|---|---|---|---|---|---|---|---|
| | Curlups (# in 1 min) | Partial Curlups | Shuttle run (sec) | V-sit reach (in) | Sit & reach (cm) | 1-mile run* | (min:sec) | Pullups (#) | Pushups (#) |
| 6 | 33 | 22 | 12.1 | 3.5 | 31 | 10:15 | *1:55 | 2 | 9 |
| 7 | 36 | 24 | 11.5 | 3.5 | 30 | 9:22 | *1:48 | 4 | 14 |
| 8 | 40 | 30 | 11.1 | 3.0 | 31 | 8:48 | *3:30 | 5 | 17 |
| 9 | 41 | 37 | 10.9 | 3.0 | 31 | 8:31 | *3:30 | 5 | 18 |
| 10 | 45 | 35 | 10.3 | 4.0 | 30 | 7:57 | | 6 | 22 |
| 11 | 47 | 43 | 10.0 | 4.0 | 31 | 7:32 | | 6 | 27 |
| 12 | 50 | 64 | 9.8 | 4.0 | 31 | 7:11 | | 7 | 31 |
| 13 | 53 | 59 | 9.5 | 3.5 | 33 | 6:50 | | 7 | 39 |
| 14 | 56 | 62 | 9.1 | 4.5 | 36 | 6:26 | | 10 | 40 |
| 15 | 57 | 75 | 9.0 | 5.0 | 37 | 6:20 | | 11 | 42 |
| 16 | 56 | 73 | 8.7 | 6.0 | 38 | 6:08 | | 11 | 44 |
| 17 | 55 | 66 | 8.7 | 7.0 | 41 | 6:06 | | 13 | 53 |

**Girls**

| Age | Muscular endurance | | Agility | Flexibility | | Cardiorespiratory endurance | | Muscular strength | |
|---|---|---|---|---|---|---|---|---|---|
| 6 | 32 | 22 | 12.4 | 5.5 | 32 | 11:20 | *2:00 | 2 | 9 |
| 7 | 34 | 24 | 12.1 | 5.0 | 32 | 10:36 | *1:55 | 2 | 14 |
| 8 | 38 | 30 | 11.8 | 4.5 | 33 | 10:02 | *3:58 | 2 | 17 |
| 9 | 39 | 37 | 11.1 | 5.5 | 33 | 9:30 | *3:53 | 2 | 18 |
| 10 | 40 | 33 | 10.8 | 6.0 | 33 | 9:19 | | 3 | 20 |
| 11 | 42 | 43 | 10.5 | 6.5 | 34 | 9:02 | | 3 | 19 |
| 12 | 45 | 50 | 10.4 | 7.0 | 36 | 8:23 | | 2 | 20 |
| 13 | 46 | 59 | 10.2 | 7.0 | 38 | 8:13 | | 2 | 21 |
| 14 | 47 | 48 | 10.1 | 8.0 | 40 | 7:59 | | 2 | 20 |
| 15 | 48 | 38 | 10.0 | 8.0 | 43 | 8:08 | | 2 | 21 |
| 16 | 45 | 49 | 10.1 | 9.0 | 42 | 8:23 | | 1 | 24 |
| 17 | 44 | 58 | 10.0 | 8.0 | 42 | 8:15 | | 1 | 25 |

Only one test score is necessary for the categories of muscular endurance, flexibility, cardiorespiratory endurance, and muscular strength. *Scores for the distance option for 6- to 7-year-olds are for the quarter mile and 8- to 9-year-olds for the half-mile. Data taken from the President's Challenge, a program of The President's Council on Physical Fitness and Sports (Available at: http://www.fitness.gov/. Accessed November 01, 2004).

| Table 15.2 | NATIONAL PHYSICAL FITNESS AWARD STANDARDS (50TH PERCENTILE) |
|---|---|

**Boys**

| Age | Muscular endurance | | Agility | Flexibility | | Cardiorespiratory endurance | | Muscular strength | | |
|---|---|---|---|---|---|---|---|---|---|---|
| | Curlups (# in 1 min) | Partial Curlups (#) | Shuttle run (sec) | V-sit reach (in) | Sit & reach (cm) | 1-mile run* | (min:sec) | Pullups (#) | Pushups (#) | Flexed arm hang (sec) |
| 6 | 22 | 10 | 13.3 | 1.0 | 26 | 12:36 | *2:21 | 1 | 7 | 6 |
| 7 | 28 | 13 | 12.8 | 1.0 | 25 | 11:40 | *2:10 | 1 | 8 | 8 |
| 8 | 31 | 17 | 12.2 | 0.5 | 25 | 11:05 | *4:22 | 1 | 9 | 10 |
| 9 | 32 | 17 | 11.9 | 1.0 | 25 | 10:30 | *4:14 | 2 | 12 | 10 |
| 10 | 35 | 24 | 11.5 | 1.0 | 25 | 9:48 | | 2 | 14 | 12 |
| 11 | 37 | 26 | 11.1 | 1.0 | 25 | 9:20 | | 2 | 15 | 11 |
| 12 | 40 | 32 | 10.6 | 1.0 | 26 | 8:40 | | 2 | 18 | 12 |
| 13 | 42 | 39 | 10.2 | 0.5 | 26 | 8:06 | | 3 | 24 | 14 |
| 14 | 45 | 40 | 9.9 | 1.0 | 28 | 7:44 | | 5 | 24 | 20 |
| 15 | 45 | 40 | 9.7 | 2.0 | 30 | 7:30 | | 6 | 30 | 28 |
| 16 | 45 | 37 | 9.4 | 3.0 | 30 | 7:10 | | 7 | 30 | 28 |
| 17 | 44 | 42 | 9.4 | 3.0 | 34 | 7:04 | | 8 | 37 | 30 |
| **Girls** | | | | | | | | | | |
| 6 | 23 | 10 | 13.8 | 2.5 | 27 | 13:12 | *2:26 | 1 | 6 | 5 |
| 7 | 25 | 13 | 13.2 | 2.0 | 27 | 12:56 | *2:21 | 1 | 8 | 6 |
| 8 | 29 | 17 | 12.9 | 2.0 | 28 | 12:30 | *4:56 | 1 | 9 | 8 |
| 9 | 30 | 20 | 12.5 | 2.0 | 28 | 11:52 | *4:50 | 1 | 12 | 8 |
| 10 | 30 | 24 | 12.1 | 3.0 | 28 | 11:22 | | 1 | 13 | 8 |
| 11 | 32 | 27 | 11.5 | 3.0 | 29 | 11:17 | | 1 | 11 | 7 |
| 12 | 35 | 30 | 11.3 | 3.5 | 30 | 11:05 | | 1 | 10 | 7 |
| 13 | 37 | 40 | 11.1 | 3.5 | 31 | 10:23 | | 1 | 11 | 8 |
| 14 | 37 | 30 | 11.2 | 4.5 | 33 | 10:06 | | 1 | 10 | 9 |
| 15 | 36 | 26 | 11.0 | 5.0 | 36 | 9:58 | | 1 | 15 | 7 |
| 16 | 35 | 26 | 10.9 | 5.5 | 34 | 10:31 | | 1 | 12 | 7 |
| 17 | 34 | 40 | 11.0 | 4.5 | 35 | 10:22 | | 1 | 16 | 7 |

Only one test score is necessary for the categories of muscular endurance, flexibility, cardiorespiratory endurance, and muscular strength. *Scores for the distance option for 6- to 7-year-olds are for the quarter mile and 8- to 9-year-olds for the half-mile. Data taken from the President's Challenge, a program of The President's Council on Physical Fitness and Sports (Available at: http://www.fitness.gov/. Accessed November 01, 2004).

| **Table 15.3** | **TESTING INSTRUCTIONS FOR THE PRESIDENT'S PHYSICAL ACTIVITY AND FITNESS AWARDS PROGRAM** |
|---|---|
| **Test** | **Instructions** |
| Curlups | Child lies on back with knees flexed about 12 inches from buttocks. Partner holds feet. Arms are crossed over chest with hands on opposite shoulders. Child curls up and touches thighs with elbows and then returns until the shoulder blades touch the floor. Score is the number performed in 1 minute. |
| Partial Curlups | Child lies on back with knees flexed about 12 inches from buttocks. Feet are not held. Partner places his/her hands under the child's head. Child curls up slowly, sliding fingers up the legs until fingertips touch the knees and returns until his/her head touches the partner's hands. One curl is performed every 3 seconds until the child cannot keep the rhythm or reaches the target for the award. Record the number done with proper rhythm. |
| Shuttle run | Two lines are marked 30 feet apart and two blocks of wood are placed behind one of the lines. The child starts from behind the opposite line and runs to the blocks, picks up the first block, returns it to the starting line, runs to the second block, and returns it to the starting line. Blocks are placed, not thrown across the line. Score is the time to the nearest tenth of a second. |
| V-sit reach | A straight line is marked as a baseline. A perpendicular line crosses the baseline and is marked in half-inches for two feet on either side of the baseline. The child sits with no shoes while legs straddle the measuring line and heels are at the baseline about 12 inches apart. Legs are held flat by a partner and the child holds hands together with palms down. Child reaches forward as far as possible, keeping fingers on the measuring line. Three practice attempts are made, and the fourth attempt is held for 3 seconds. Score is recorded to the nearest half-inch. Positive scores are measured beyond the baseline, while negative scores are measured behind the baseline. |
| Sit & reach | A sit & reach box is constructed so that a platform with a measuring scale reaches over the child's feet and lower legs. Shoes are removed and the feet are placed against the base of the box, which is measured at 23 cm. Three practice attempts are allowed, after which the fourth trial is held for measurement. Score is measured in cm. |
| 1-mile run | Child is encouraged to run/walk 1 mile as quickly as possible. Score is time in minutes and seconds. Alternatively, 6- to 7-year-olds can cover a one-fourth–mile course and 8- to 9-year-olds can cover a one-half–mile course. |
| Pullups | Child hangs from a horizontal bar with arms extended and feet not touching the floor. An overhand or underhand grip can be used. Child raises himself/herself until chin clears the bar and then lowers the body to the starting position. Score is the number performed correctly. |
| Pushups | Child lies face down on a mat with hands under shoulders, fingers and legs straight, and toes supporting feet. Child pushes up to where arms are straight, keeping back and knees straight. Child then lowers himself/herself to the point that was predetermined at which the elbow joint is at 90 degrees. Pushups are done to a rhythm of one per 3 seconds. One pushup is performed every 3 seconds until the child cannot keep the rhythm or reaches the target for the award. Record the number done with proper rhythm. |
| Flexed arm hang | Using either the overhand or underhand grip, the child hangs on a horizontal bar with the arms flexed and chin above the bar. The child holds this position as long as possible. The test ends when the child's chin touches or falls below the bar. Score is time in seconds. |

Taken from the President's Challenge, a program of The President's Council on Physical Fitness and Sports (Available at: http://www.fitness.gov/. Accessed November 01, 2004).

skills (Table 15.4). The tests for cardiorespiratory endurance, muscular strength and endurance, and flexibility are identical to those in the Presidential Physical Fitness Award and National Physical Fitness Award. However, the scoring standards for the Health Fitness Award are lower than those for the other two awards. In addition, the Health Fitness Award has standards for body fatness as evaluated by BMI.

 *Experiences in Work Physiology Lab Exercise 13: Fitness Testing and Activity Monitoring provides experience in fitness testing and activity monitoring in children.*

The FITNESSGRAM is a health-related battery of test items selected to assess important aspects of a child's health rather than athletic skill or agility. Children's scores

| Table 15.4 | PRESIDENTIAL HEALTH FITNESS AWARD STANDARDS |
|---|---|

**Boys**

| Age | Muscular endurance Partial curlups (#) | Body composition BMI range | Flexibility V-sit reach (in) | Flexibility Sit & reach (cm) | Cardiorespiratory endurance 1-mile run* (min:sec) | | Muscular strength Pullups (#) | Muscular strength Pushups (#) |
|---|---|---|---|---|---|---|---|---|
| 6 | 12 | 13.3–19.5 | 1 | 21 | 13:00 | *2:30 | 1 | 3 |
| 7 | 12 | 13.3–19.5 | 1 | 21 | 12:00 | *2:20 | 1 | 4 |
| 8 | 15 | 13.4–20.5 | 1 | 21 | 11:00 | *4:45 | 1 | 5 |
| 9 | 15 | 13.7–21.4 | 1 | 21 | 10:00 | *4:35 | 1 | 6 |
| 10 | 20 | 14.0–22.5 | 1 | 21 | 9:30 | | 1 | 7 |
| 11 | 20 | 14.0–23.7 | 1 | 21 | 9:00 | | 2 | 8 |
| 12 | 20 | 14.8–24.1 | 1 | 21 | 9:00 | | 2 | 9 |
| 13 | 25 | 15.4–24.7 | 1 | 21 | 8:00 | | 2 | 10 |
| 14 | 25 | 16.1–25.4 | 1 | 21 | 8:00 | | 3 | 12 |
| 15 | 30 | 16.6–26.4 | 1 | 21 | 7:30 | | 4 | 14 |
| 16 | 30 | 17.2–26.8 | 1 | 21 | 7:30 | | 5 | 16 |
| 17 | 30 | 17.7–27.5 | 1 | 21 | 7:30 | | 6 | 18 |

**Girls**

| Age | Muscular endurance Partial curlups (#) | Body composition BMI range | Flexibility V-sit reach (in) | Flexibility Sit & reach (cm) | Cardiorespiratory endurance 1-mile run* (min:sec) | | Muscular strength Pullups (#) | Muscular strength Pushups (#) |
|---|---|---|---|---|---|---|---|---|
| 6 | 12 | 13.1–19.6 | 2 | 23 | 13:00 | *2:50 | 1 | 3 |
| 7 | 12 | 13.1–19.6 | 2 | 23 | 12:00 | *1:40 | 1 | 4 |
| 8 | 15 | 13.2–20.7 | 2 | 23 | 11:00 | *5:35 | 1 | 5 |
| 9 | 15 | 13.5–21.4 | 2 | 23 | 10:00 | *5:25 | 1 | 6 |
| 10 | 20 | 13.8–22.5 | 2 | 23 | 10:00 | | 1 | 7 |
| 11 | 20 | 14.1–23.2 | 2 | 23 | 10:00 | | 1 | 7 |
| 12 | 20 | 14.7–24.2 | 2 | 23 | 10:30 | | 1 | 7 |
| 13 | 25 | 15.5–25.3 | 3 | 25 | 10:30 | | 1 | 7 |
| 14 | 25 | 16.2–25.3 | 3 | 25 | 10:30 | | 1 | 7 |
| 15 | 30 | 16.6–26.5 | 3 | 25 | 10:00 | | 1 | 7 |
| 16 | 30 | 16.8–26.5 | 3 | 25 | 10:00 | | 1 | 7 |
| 17 | 30 | 17.1–26.9 | 3 | 25 | 10:00 | | 1 | 7 |

Only one test score is necessary for the categories of flexibility, cardiorespiratory endurance, and muscular strength. *Scores for the distance option for 6- to 7-year-olds are for the quarter mile and 8- to 9-year-olds for the half-mile. Data taken from the President's Challenge, a program of The President's Council on Physical Fitness and Sports (Available at: http://www.fitness.gov/. Accessed November 01, 2004). BMI, body mass index.

are compared to health fitness standards, not to national norms. Although the FITNESSGRAM claims to be a better health-related evaluation for the child than the President's Challenge, the items in the FITNESSGRAM are almost identical to those found in the President's Challenge. FIT-NESSGRAM test items are as follows:

- Aerobic capacity (select one)
  - The pacer, a 20-m progressive, multistage shuttle run set to music
  - One-mile run/walk
  - Walking test (secondary students only)
- Body Composition (select one)
  - Percent body fat calculated from triceps and calf skinfold measures
  - BMI
- Upper body strength (select one)
  - 90-degree pushups
  - Pullups
  - Flexed arm hang
  - Modified pullups

- Flexibility (select one)
  - Sit and reach
  - Shoulder stretch
- Abdominal Strength
  - Curlups
- Trunk extensor strength and flexibility
  - Trunk lift

The FITNESSGRAM was developed commercially, and as such, it must be purchased from the Cooper Institute. Information about the FITNESSGRAM can be found at the Cooper Institute website (5). An example of how physical fitness tests can be used to help monitor a child's health during a developmental stage can be seen in Case 15.1.

## CLINICAL EXERCISE TESTING OF CHILDREN

Clinical laboratory exercise testing of children can be useful for those with medical symptoms, established disease, or suspected medical abnormalities. The tests can reveal information relevant to physical therapy, prevention, and medical intervention. Clinical exercise testing of children

---

## CASE STUDY 15.1: *FITNESS AND STRENGTH DURING PUBERTY*

### CASE

You are a health educator working for a public school district in your state. A mother of one of the students in your school district comes to you for help and advice. Amanda is an 11-year-old girl in middle school who loves to play soccer and basketball. Amanda's mother is confused about how to guide Amanda through her pubertal development while she is competing in middle-school athletics. The mother asks if there are any measures you can monitor during Amanda's 3 years in middle school to ensure that Amanda is maintaining health but also not losing any athletic potential.

### DESCRIPTION

There is a tremendous amount of cultural pressure for girls to be slim. Female athletes in particular receive daily messages that they need to have a low body fat percentage to be competitive. Young girls are often confused about how body composition changes during normal growth and development relate to athletic success. Parents are oftentimes caught in a quandary about how to best monitor their child's eating and exercise habits.

### EVALUATION/INTERVENTION

Discussions with Amanda and her mother lead you to several conclusions: (a) Amanda and her mother want Amanda to

be a successful athlete, (b) mother and daughter recognize the pressure from society for girls to restrict their food consumption, (c) Amanda and her mother want Amanda to remain lean so she does not lose any competitive edge, and (d) they both realize that changes in Amanda's body will occur as she passes through puberty. You tell Amanda and her mother that there are several physical tests that can be performed periodically to evaluate both Amanda's nutritional status as well as her physical fitness or athletic potential.

You all decide that measurements every 6 months will be adequate to determine if Amanda is maintaining her ability to perform physically without jeopardizing her health. Since the school system regularly performs the fitness tests in the President's Challenge, you decide that some of those tests can be used to monitor Amanda's status.

The specific tests of interest are: (a) shuttle run to evaluate agility, which is a good indicator of athletic potential, (b) 1-mile run to evaluate cardiorespiratory capacity, which is important for both soccer and basketball, (c) pullups to evaluate upper body muscular strength, which would tend to decrease if Amanda gained too much body fat during development, and (d) body mass index (BMI) to evaluate body fatness.

Over the next 3 years you record the following for the parameters being measured.

***Case Study 15.1, continued***

| Test | Score 1 | Score 2 | Score 3 | Score 4 | Score 5 | Score 6 |
|------|---------|---------|---------|---------|---------|---------|
| Shuttle run (sec) | 10.6 | 10.5 | 10.4 | 10.2 | 10.2 | 10.2 |
| 1-mile run (min:sec) | 8:08 | 8:14 | 8:00 | 7:58 | 7:55 | 7:50 |
| Pullups (#) | 2 | 2 | 3 | 3 | 3 | 4 |
| BMI | 16.0 | 16.3 | 16.5 | 16.5 | 16.8 | 17.0 |

BMI = body mass index.

Your assessment during the 3 years is that Amanda is in excellent physical condition and that her health was not jeopardized. Amanda scored better than the 85th percentile for almost all of her fitness tests. Her shuttle run scores decreased with age, which is normal for maturing girls. Her 1-mile times were exceptional at all ages and continued to decline throughout her development. Her pullup scores increased, whereas pullups decrease through puberty for most girls. Thus, Amanda was able to increase her strength during puberty. However, Amanda's health did not appear to be jeopardized because as she increased her physical fitness levels, her BMI also increased. This increase in BMI through puberty followed the normal curve for girls her age. Amanda's BMI hovered just below the 50th percentile. This means that Amanda's fantastic 1-mile scores were truly due to a high level of cardiovascular fitness and not due to her carrying an emaciated body weight. Furthermore, Amanda's increasing strength scores also suggest that Amanda was maintaining a strong, lean body. Otherwise, lean body tissue loss would have been reflected in lower strength scores.

primarily deals with the cardiorespiratory capacity, but sometimes evaluations of anaerobic capacity are performed. The aerobic exercise test can be performed on either a treadmill or cycle ergometer. Younger children do not perform as well on a cycle ergometer because the test may be limited by peripheral muscular discomfort due to their underdeveloped knee extensors. Young children are also more easily distracted during cycle ergometry tests than during treadmill testing. Testing protocols for children are similar to or modified from adult protocols (see Chapter 19). Children generally handle changes in treadmill grade easier than changes in treadmill speed. The Bruce protocol has been used successfully for children, but the American College of Sports Medicine (ACSM) recommends a modified Balke protocol in which speed is held constant and grade is increased at 2-minute intervals (4). The McMaster cycle protocol, in which the initial workload is set according to the child's height, is the preferred test for children.

A recent research study produced a prediction equation for estimating the metabolic cost of walking in children (6). Metabolic information obtained from the use of this equation can be used to prescribe exercise interventions for children or to assist in a nutritional program for a child. In this study, girls and boys underwent yearly treadmill testing at ages 6, 7, 8, 9, and 10 years. Each year the child completed six 5-minute treadmill-walking bouts at 40.2, 53.6, 67, 80.4, 93.8, and 107.2 $m \cdot min^{-1}$. Walking speeds were presented in ascending order with a 5-minute rest period in between bouts. During the last 2 minutes of each exercise bout, expired air was collected and indirect calorimetry was used to determine energy expenditure ($\dot{V}O_2$). The following prediction equation was produced:

$$\dot{V}O_2 = 24.852 + 0.003214(\text{walking speed})^2 - 0.995(\text{age}) - 0.263(\text{walking speed})$$

($\dot{V}O_2$ is expressed in $mL \cdot kg^{-1} \cdot min^{-1}$, walking speed in $m \cdot min^{-1}$, and age in years.) The error in predicting energy expenditure using this equation is $\pm 1.0$ metabolic equivalents (MET). At the range of speeds used during testing, this represents an error of $\pm 35\%$ at low speeds and $\pm 10\%$ at fast speeds.

Energy expenditure in caloric equivalents ($kcal \cdot min^{-1}$) can be estimated by multiplying the $\dot{V}O_2$ derived from the equation by the child's weight (kg) and then multiplying this number by 0.005. The information obtained from this equation can be used clinically to manipulate the energy balance of the child to achieve a desired objective. An example of how this equation can be used for an 8-year-old child weighing 30 kg and walking at a speed of 70 $m \cdot min^{-1}$ is shown below.

Example:

$$\dot{V}O_2 = 24.852 + 0.003214(70 \ m \cdot min^{-1})^2 - 0.995(8 \ yr) - 0.263(70 \ m \cdot min^{-1})$$

$$\dot{V}O_2 = 14.23 \ mL \cdot kg^{-1} \cdot min^{-1}$$

$$kcal \cdot min^{-1} = 14.23 \ mL \cdot kg^{-1} \cdot min^{-1}(30 \ kg)(0.005 \ kcal \cdot L^{-1} \ O_2)$$

$$kcal \cdot min^{-1} = 2.13$$

Thus, if this child was to participate in a walking program in which the speed of walking was 70 m·min$^{-1}$ for 30 minutes per day, the energy cost of the exercise period would be 64 kcal.

## ASSESSING PHYSICAL ACTIVITY IN CHILDREN

It is difficult to determine exactly how much physical activity to recommend for children so they can receive the associated health benefits. The ACSM, Centers for Disease Control, and United States Surgeon General have all made recommendations. The original recommendation was for youth and adults to participate in 20 to 60 minutes of continuous exercise at a moderate to high intensity 3 or more days per week. That recommendation was changed in 1996 to suggest that persons over 2 years of age accumulate at least 30 minutes of moderate-intensity physical activity on most but preferentially all days of the week. The 1996 recommendation was again revised by the Institute of Medicine in 2002 to what is now suggested: children and adults should accumulate 60 minutes of activity on most but preferably all days of the week. Note that this newest recommendation calls for twice the volume of activity as the previous recommendation.

Some professionals are calling this new recommendation unfounded (7). They state that there is no research to support the notion that increasing daily activity from 30 to 60 minutes will substantially increase fitness or health in children. They also feel that this recommendation was made simply in the hope of attenuating the childhood obesity epidemic. In other words, since the previous recommendation of 30 minutes of moderate activity per day did not slow the rise in the prevalence of childhood obesity, 60 minutes may have an effect. Wishful thinking, but how this recommendation will affect children's behavior, the family environment, physical education, and health policy remains to be seen.

Physical activity recommendations are generally derived from information in adults, based on the amount of activity thought to provide health benefits (7). Guidelines for children and adolescents are based either on adult recommendations or arbitrary activity recommendations (7). The recent recommended increases in volume of activity are based on the observation that youth may already meet the adult guidelines and that activity levels of youth decrease over time; therefore, to achieve the recommended amount of physical activity as an adult, children should start at a greater amount of physical activity (7). The recommended increases may also be a frenzied effort to curb the increasing prevalence of obesity throughout the world.

Furthermore, the National Association for Sport and Physical Education (NASPE) released the first physical activity guidelines for infants, toddlers, and preschoolers in 2002 (8). NASPE attests that confining babies and young children to strollers, play pens, and car and infant seats for hours at a time delays physical and cognitive development. NASPE also contends that such restrictions can begin the path to sedentary preferences and childhood obesity. To the contrary, adopting a physically active lifestyle early in life increases the likelihood that infants and young children will learn to move more skillfully and ensures healthy development and later participation in physical activity. NASPE gives five guidelines for physical activity that parents and caregivers should implement (Table 15.5).

---

### Table 15.5   PHYSICAL ACTIVITY GUIDELINES FOR INFANTS, TODDLERS, AND PRESCHOOLERS

**Guidelines for infants**

- Infants should interact with parents and/or caregivers in daily physical activities that are dedicated to promoting the exploration of their environments.
- Infants should be placed in safe settings that facilitate physical activity and do not restrict movement for prolonged periods of time.
- Infants' physical activity should promote the development of movement skills.
- Infants should have an environment that meets or exceeds recommended safety standards for performing large-muscle activities.
- Individuals responsible for the well-being of infants should be aware of the importance of physical activity and facilitate the child's movement skills.

**Guidelines for toddlers and preschoolers**

- Toddlers should accumulate at least 30 minutes daily of structured physical activity; preschoolers at least 60 minutes.
- Toddlers and preschoolers should engage in at least 60 minutes and up to several hours per day of unstructured physical activity and should not be sedentary for more than 60 minutes at a time except when sleeping.
- Toddlers should develop movement skills that are building blocks for more complex movement tasks; preschoolers should develop competence in movement skills that are building blocks for more complex movement tasks.
- Toddlers and preschoolers should have indoor and outdoor areas that meet or exceed recommended safety standards for performing large-muscle activities.
- Individuals responsible for the well-being of toddlers and preschoolers should be aware of the importance of physical activity and facilitate the child's movement skills.

Courtesy of the National Association for Sport and Physical Education, Washington DC, 2002.

Regardless of one's personal philosophy on the exact volume of exercise or physical activity that is needed for children, most professionals agree that children have become less active over the past few decades. NASPE has developed the Physical Best program to educate, challenge, and encourage all children to develop the knowledge, skills, and attitudes for a healthy and fit life. The goal of the program is to move students from dependence to independence for their own fitness and health by promoting regular, enjoyable lifelong physical activity. The focus of Physical Best is to educate all children regardless of athletic talent or physical and mental abilities or disabilities (9).

Physical Best is a comprehensive, health-related physical education program for use in K–12 physical education curricula. When combined with the FITNESSGRAM/ACTIVITYGRAM, it provides a complete physical education/assessment program with teacher training and resources. The emphasis is on students working and maintaining a healthful level of aerobic fitness, muscular fitness, flexibility, and body composition. It is noncompetitive and inclusive, positive and individualized, with ready-to-use practical information and activities. It is research based (incorporates the latest youth fitness research and practices) and standards based (incorporates health and fitness standards). Physical Best workshops are available where professionals can certify as Physical Best Health-Fitness Specialists (9).

The ability to measure and monitor physical activity in children seems imperative so that appropriate preventive and therapeutic exercise interventions can be created for both individuals and the population. Children's patterns of physical activity have been assessed by a number of methods, including direct observation, activity questionnaires, heart-rate monitoring, pedometers, accelerometers, and metabolic measures. Each method has its own advantages and disadvantages. Direct observation provides an objective assessment of activity by a trained professional, but it can be intrusive to the child. Activity questionnaires are nonintrusive but somewhat unreliable. Heart-rate monitoring is objective and reliable but complex. Pedometers and activity monitors are objective, but they are also complex and have not been well validated in children. Metabolic measures are valid but expensive and often intrusive. Therefore, the best assessment tool for physical activity in children depends upon the characteristics of the child, the environment in which activity is to be measured, and the resources available.

Professionals need to understand that they may not obtain totally accurate results when using these physical activity monitoring tools. One way to overcome some of the possibility of getting an inaccurate physical activity measure is to use two or more tools simultaneously to measure physical activity. This way, if the results from the tools correspond, more confidence can be placed in the results. If the results don't correspond, the professional can look for possible sources of error in measurement. Another way to avoid potential inaccuracies is to become familiar with the normal values for the population being studied. If the professional is familiar with what values to expect from a particular tool in the population he/she is measuring and he/she obtains a value that is outside the ranges of expectation, then he/she will recognize this as a faulty value and can make a reassessment.

## Activity Questionnaires

The most plausible field tests for measuring physical activity in children are activity questionnaires, heart-rate monitoring, pedometers, and activity monitors. Activity questionnaires generally require a recall or observational report of the child's activity. Some questionnaires include reports from the child as well as parents and teachers. Some of the most common questionnaires are the Seven-Day Physical Activity Recall, Modifiable Activity Questionnaire for Adolescents, Previous Day Physical Activity Recall (PDPAR), and National Children and Youth Fitness Study Questionnaire (10,11). Correlations between questionnaire scores and other activity measures range from approximately 0.20 to 0.90. This is quite variable, from being a rather poor indicator of actual physical activity to being a relatively good measure of physical activity. Nonetheless, these are the best tools we currently have available.

## Pedometers

Pedometers have been around for several decades (*Fig. 15.5*). The pedometer itself is designed to measure steps taken by the child during the day. The accumulation of these steps is converted to a distance, and energy expenditure is estimated. Pedometer measures correlate moderately well with metabolic measures, but only the total amount of activity is recorded without any reference to exercise intensity or activity patterns.

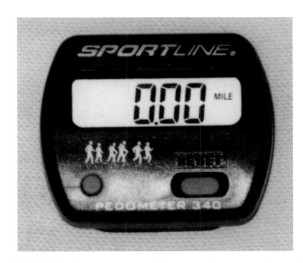

**FIGURE 15.5.** A pedometer used for measuring distance traveled.

## Accelerometers

Activity monitors are fairly new to the field and work on a principle different than pedometers. Activity monitors are really accelerometers that continuously measure the intensity, frequency, and duration of movement for extended periods *(Fig. 15.6)*. Activity counts from the accelerometer can be downloaded to a computer, which provides estimates for exercise intensity and energy expenditures. Activity monitors have been validated against indirect calorimetry for adults and children. However, activity monitor thresholds for exercise intensity in children have not yet been derived. Correlations between accelerometer measures and calorimetry measures range from about 0.60 to 0.85, which are fairly high correlations. Accelerometers are therefore probably one of the best tools for measuring childhood activity.

Some accelerometers only provide a value for activity counts, which is a unit of measure specific to that particular accelerometer. In this case, comparisons can be made only within-accelerometer, and no reference to metabolism can be inferred. Other accelerometers have employed regression equations, which are accelerometer specific and can be used to predict metabolic variables. In this case, estimates of metabolic rates can be made and utilized for exercise or nutritional interventions. Cross comparisons among accelerometers and across populations can also be made with the metabolic data.

Figure 15.7 shows the data from a 24-hour recording of a 14-year old girl. In this illustration, the recording day was a Saturday. This girl awoke at 7:00 AM, played in a soccer game between 11:00 AM and 1:00 PM, remained active during the afternoon, but felt sick and slept from 6:00 until 11:00 PM. When she awoke at 11:00 PM, she ate and took some medicine. Values from the recording reveal that this girl spent 1007 kcal in sedentary activity and 431 kcal in physical activity throughout the 24-hour period. Her estimated energy expenditure for the day was 1428 kcal.

### Heart-Rate Monitoring

Heart rate is strongly related to $O_2$ consumption and energy expenditure across a wide range of values. Heart-rate monitors can accumulate data from short or long bouts of activity throughout the day *(Fig. 15.8)*. An extensive review of heart-rate data on children has revealed that adolescents ages 13 to 18 attain more than 60 minutes per day of low-intensity physical activity; children 12 years of age and younger attain 2 hours or more of activity at low intensity; while children of all ages attain 30 minutes per day of activity at or above 50% of **heart-rate range** (7). The continuous assessment of usual activity patterns in children has provided the observation that children attain maximal voluntary physical activity in very brief periods, rather than in one or two prolonged periods (7). If the goal is to match intensity of youth recommendations to those for adults and the intensity criteria is for moderate-intensity exercise, then most children attain 1 to 2 hours per day of activity at that level now.

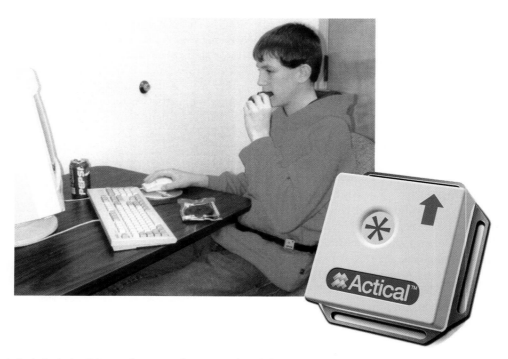

**FIGURE 15.6.** The Actical physical activity monitor or accelerometer. This adolescent boy is downloading and reading the data from the accelerometer. The accelerometer can be worn on the hip, waist, or wrist, and is the size of a wristwatch.

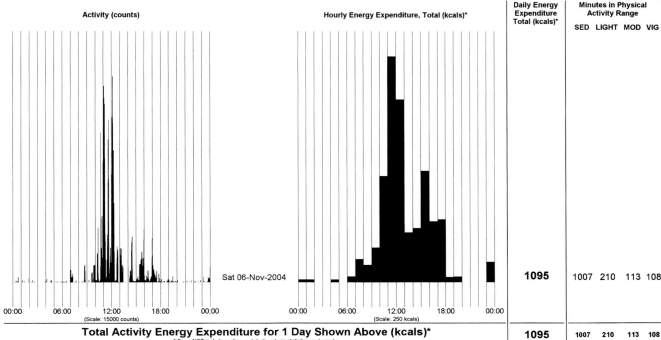

**ActiCal Activity and Energy Expenditure Report (AEE)**

| **Subject Identity** | Jackie | | | | |
|---|---|---|---|---|---|
| **Subject Height** | 137.2 cm (54.0 in) | **Weight** | 61.2 kg (134.9 lbs) | **Gender** | Female |
| | | | | **Age** | 14 years |

| **Data Collection Start Time** | Sat, 06-Nov-2004, 00:00 | **Data Collection End Time** | Mon, 08-Nov-2004, 12:00 | **Device Serial Number** | C841371 |
|---|---|---|---|---|---|
| **Energy Expenditure Output Type** | Activity Energy Expenditure (AEE) | **Regression Model** | Single (1R) | **Age Level** | Adolescent |
| **Light/Moderate Cut-point** | 0.010 kcals/min/kg | **Moderate/Vigorous Cut-point** | 0.050 kcals/min/kg | **Device Location** | Hip |

Activity (counts) — Hourly Energy Expenditure, Total (kcals)*

| | Daily Energy Expenditure Total (kcals)* | Minutes in Physical Activity Range SED LIGHT MOD VIG |
|---|---|---|
| Sat 06-Nov-2004 | **1095** | 1007  210  113  108 |

00:00   06:00   12:00   18:00   00:00
(Scale: 15000 counts)

00:00   06:00   12:00   18:00   00:00
(Scale: 250 kcals)

| **Total Activity Energy Expenditure for 1 Day Shown Above (kcals)*** | **1095** | 1007  210  113  108 |
|---|---|---|

\* Does NOT include resting metabolic rate in statistics and graphs

**A person of this age, gender, weight, and height needs <u>1428</u> calories to maintain their normal bodily functions.**

(Based on Harris J, Benedict F. A biometric study of basal metabolism in man. Washington D.C. Carnegie Institute of Washington. 1919)

Printed: Mon, 08-Nov-2004  12:45          Mini Mitter Company, Inc.          Page 1 of 1

**FIGURE 15.7.** Data output from an accelerometer. The panel on the left gives the number of activity counts registered by the accelerometer, and the panel on the right gives the estimated energy expenditure in kcal for each hour during the 24-hour recording.

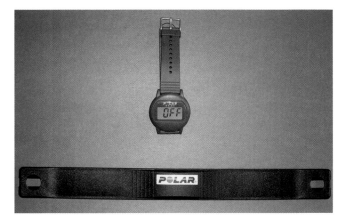

**FIGURE 15.8.** A heart-rate monitor used for estimating energy expenditure associated with physical activity.

## Activity Diaries

Physical activity diaries are commonly used to assess physical activity in children and adolescents because these diaries are inexpensive, unobtrusive, and easily administered. One such instrument, which has become very popular for assessing physical activity in adolescents, is the PDPAR (11). The PDPAR was designed to provide accurate data on mode, frequency, intensity, and duration of physical activities; which is then used to estimate physical activity energy expenditure.

The PDPAR is an activity diary that is segmented into seventeen 30-minute intervals. The youth completing the questionnaire is provided with a list of 35 different activities in which youth normally engage. The youth then records the number of the activity in which he/she participated for any given 30-minute interval of the previous day.

For the selected activity, he/she also records the appropriate intensity using the following descriptors: very light (slow breathing and little or no movement), light (normal breathing and movement), medium (increased breathing and moderate movement), and hard (hard breathing and quick movement). From the recorded data, an estimated MET value is derived for each activity within the given time frame (e.g., 3:00 PM to 11:30 PM).

Test-retest reliability for the PDPAR is 0.98. The correlation between energy expenditure (kcal·kg$^{-1}$·min$^{-1}$) and pedometer counts was 0.88, while the correlation between the PDPAR and accelerometer counts was 0.77. The correlation between percentage heart-rate range and mean energy expenditure from the PDPAR was 0.53 (11). Thus, the PDPAR is one of the most valid and reliable physical activity questionnaires for adolescents available. Box 15.2 discusses the differences between structured childhood physical activities and unstructured physical activities.

▶ *INQUIRY SUMMARY.* The science underlying fitness assessment and activity monitoring in children is not as advanced as with adults. Traditional fitness tests have been criticized as being evaluations of athletic ability rather than health-related fitness. Measuring health-related fitness in children, on the other hand, is difficult because most hypokinetic diseases are not manifest until adulthood. The President's Challenge and FITNESSGRAM are the most common tools used for childhood fitness assessment. Activity monitoring in children is also difficult, and the activity threshold-health relationship has not been well established. *What method of fitness assessment and activity monitoring would you want for your child?*

## Childhood Responses to Physical Activity and Exercise Training

Childhood obesity is rising dramatically in the United States, as well as in many other countries. This is of particular concern because childhood obesity is associated with high blood pressure and elevated cholesterol levels, both of which are manifest in many children even at the ages of 5 or 6 years. Since regular physical activity can play a major role in preventing coronary heart disease, hypertension, and glucose insensitivity, it becomes imperative to know how children respond to exercise interventions aimed at reducing the risk of these degenerative diseases. Interpretation of the available data is difficult, however, because the growth process itself may interact with the effects of regular exercise.

A perusal of the literature on the effects of fitness and activity on childhood cardiovascular disease risk reveals a consensus that fit and active children tend to have lower blood triglyceride and higher high-density lipoprotein cholesterol levels than unfit, inactive children. Exercise studies on children generally show little change in blood pressure, glucose tolerance, body fatness, and metabolic profile for children whose profiles fall within the normal range, while the profile for these variables improves following exercise training in obese or hypertensive children. The most logical conclusion that can be made at this time is that regular physical activity in children can reduce the incidence of cardiovascular disease risk factors and attenuate the symptoms of degenerative diseases only if these conditions are already manifest. Furthermore, increasing

**Box 15.2**

*PERSPECTIVE*

# The Physical Activity Paradox

The perception of most professionals is that our children are not as physically active as they were in decades past. It is often stated that children spend too much time watching television and playing computer games when they could be outside playing games and sports. However, participation in youth sports programs has skyrocketed over the past two decades, and heart-rate monitoring research has shown that the levels of physical activity in our children are above that which is suggested for the attainment and maintenance of health. *How can you explain this apparent paradox?* One possible explanation is unstructured activity. Our society and communities may be programming inactivity into our lives. For example, in a straight-line distance, it may be only one-

half mile from a child's home to the shopping mall. However, because of the way the community is structured, there are no bike path, sidewalk, or straight-line street accesses to the mall. The distance to the mall via the only possible route is one and a half miles through winding neighborhood roads. This may necessitate the child being driven to the mall rather than walking or biking. Another example is structured sports. Let's take two children, one from two decades past and one from today. The child from two decades past would ride his/her bike or walk to the neighborhood schoolyard or park to participate in soccer practice. The child of today has his parent bring him/her in the car to the soccer practice. *How much inactivity is programmed into your life?*

evidence that disease risk factors have a fair persistency over years warrants the promotion of physical activity in children.

## EXERCISE CAPACITIES OF CHILDREN VERSUS ADULTS

Adolescence is marked by stages of unprecedented physiologic changes in the musculoskeletal, cardiorespiratory, and reproductive systems. In both sexes, but particularly in boys, there is a substantial gain in lean body mass during puberty. Muscle mass accounts for approximately 40% of body composition in boys at age 5 and increases to approximately 55% by age 17. With girls, the change is less dramatic, from 40% at age 5 to 45% at age 17. In contrast, the body consists of about 15% body fat in girls at age 6 and increases to about 25% by age 17. Boys have about 10% body fat at age 6 and around 15% at age 17. The changes in body size and composition are preceded by or accompanied by dramatic changes in the hormonal milieu of the body. All of these changes during growth and development can have a dramatic effect on how the individual responds to the metabolic demand of physical activity.

Physiologic markers that are used to define metabolic fitness are different for children and adults and change as children develop physically. While values for $\dot{V}O_{2max}$ increase at the same rate in both boys and girls, values for girls tend to be lower. The $\dot{V}O_{2max}$ values for girls plateau at about age 14, whereas the plateau does not occur for boys until age 18. The power output during high-intensity anaerobic exercise is lower in adolescents than in adults. This could be due to underdeveloped metabolic pathways, differences in hormonal influences, differences in muscle fiber distribution, and lower glycogen stores. The result is lower maximal blood lactate levels and a lower ratio of inorganic phosphate to phosphocreatine in exercised youth compared with adults.

Maximal heart rate is stable through childhood and adolescence at about 200 beats per minute. Children have a markedly lower stroke volume during all levels of exercise than adults. The lower exercise stroke volume is compensated in part by a higher heart rate, but the end result is still a lower cardiac output at any metabolic workload. The lower cardiac output in children correlates with their lower exercise blood pressure compared with adults since blood pressure = $\dot{Q} \times R$ (refer back to Chapter 6). Oxygen consumption is maintained in working muscles of children by a higher **arterio-mixed venous $O_2$ difference** at submaximal workloads. Although absolute levels of maximal pulmonary ventilation are lower in children than adults, ventilatory volumes are the same in children, adolescents, and adults when expressed relative to body size. The ventilatory volume needed to supply a given amount of $O_2$ to the tissues is high in young children, but it decreases with age. This means that as the child ages, the efficiency of ventilation improves.

## EXERCISE INJURIES IN CHILDREN

Many children and adolescents participate in organized sports and personal fitness programs designed to develop athletic skills and increase fitness. However, new injury patterns are developing as the focus of these programs shifts from free play to regimented competition. An estimated 50% of all injuries that are sustained by children and adolescents while playing organized sports are likely preventable (12). The major portion of responsibility for injury prevention in youth lies not with the youth, but with the adults (i.e., parents, coaches, athletic trainers, sports officials). Hence, adults must take responsibility to assure that everything feasible is done to prevent the occurrence of exercise-induced injuries in children.

To provide the safest environment for children participating in exercise and sport, adults need to understand how and when children are most susceptible to injury and whether intense training during childhood and adolescence leads to inordinate physical stresses on the cardiorespiratory and/or musculoskeletal systems of young athletes. First, children and adults involved in endurance sports such as running and swimming respond similarly to training. If the training regimen is employed properly and the training volume increased gradually, the risk of injury to the cardiorespiratory system is minimal in adults and even lower in children. In fact, moderate amounts of physical activity have been associated with optimal growth patterns in children. On the other hand, children are at higher risk than adults for overuse injury to the musculoskeletal system.

The growing bones of a child are more susceptible to certain types of mechanical injury than mature bones because of the presence of **growth cartilage**. Growth cartilage is present at the **growth plate** (epiphyseal plate), joints, and sites of major tendon insertions (Fig. 15.9). The growth plate, or epiphysis, is at risk of disruption from the shearing forces produced during some types of intense exercises. Disruption of the epiphysis is of particular concern because this can interrupt the bone growth process. It is known that the cartilage of the growth plate is at its weakest point during the most intensive phases of growth. Growth plates ossify or harden with calcium when the child matures, and the growth cartilage is replaced with mature cartilage, which is less susceptible to injury. Therefore, children are at greatest risk for musculoskeletal injury when they are participating in very intense exercise during a growth phase. The concern then for children doing heavy aerobic training (e.g., running) and/or heavy resistance training (e.g., weightlifting) is that the constant repetitive forces applied to the bone during training create microtrauma to the growth plate, causing the growth plate to ossify prematurely. Although preliminary evidence suggests heavy exercise training can cause premature closure of the growth plate in young animals, there are no data to indicate that intense training will cause this to happen in children. Nonetheless, until data become available, it would be wise to practice caution.

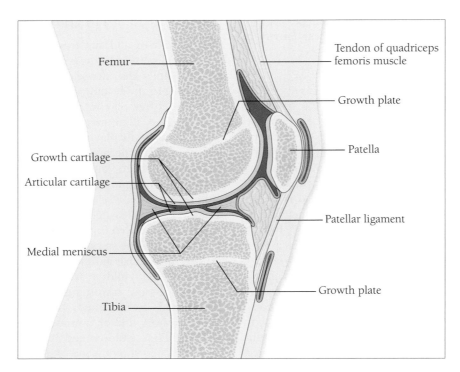

**FIGURE 15.9.** The growth plates associated with the bones of the knee joint.

Disruption of bone growth in children can also be caused by certain behaviors that are associated with, but not directly related to, physical activity. Most young athletes feel the pressure to compete and win. This drive to win is often accompanied by participation in unhealthy behaviors, such as extreme dieting and substance abuse. Although the detrimental effects of extreme dieting have been discussed in other chapters of this book, we will reiterate here that extreme dieting can cause retardation in the growth process and significantly affect bone health.

Substance abuse can be separated into two categories: 1) substance abuse to enhance exercise performance and 2) substance abuse to escape psychologic distress. Many young athletes who are competing at high levels or who feel extreme pressure to win at any level are turning to drugs and alcohol for reprieve. The demands of physical training, coupled with the psychologic pressure to perform well, is the driving force behind the use of drugs and alcohol as an escape mechanism. Competitive athletes, who are mature in years, often get themselves trapped into using drugs and alcohol to escape the pressures of competition they face every day. Young athletes, who have developing and fragile psyches are even more vulnerable to the stressors of athletic competition.

Substance abuse to enhance exercise performance is becoming more common among young athletes. The most common substance abused is anabolic steroids. Children as young as 10 years old have reported using anabolic steroids to enhance athletic performance (13). Varied sources report that 2% to 5% of middle school and high school children have used anabolic steroids. Along with a long list of other side effects of steroid use, anabolic steroids cause early growth plate closure in the bones of otherwise growing children.

Another location in the skeletal system where children are particularly susceptible to injury is at the **articular cartilage**. Articular cartilage of growing bone is of greater depth than that of adult bone, and the impact of repetitive microtrauma to this area can cause degenerative changes in the ossification centers of the growing bone of the ankle, knee, or elbow of some children. The microtrauma of overuse can also result in an inflammation of the **cartilaginous apophysis** (projection point of the bone such as a tuberosity or tubercle that is still not completely ossified in children). Untreated inflammation of these areas can cause a tearing away of the tendon from the bone that can only be repaired through surgery. Common areas for this type of inflammation in adolescents are at the tibial tubercle, as with Osgood-Schlatter disease *(Fig. 15.10)*, and at the calcaneus (Sever disease). Risks of these types of injury diminish as the child matures and the bone becomes ossified.

*Is there an optimal level of training for children above which injuries occur?* The apparent answer to this question is yes, but the volume of training at which injury risk increases is not well defined. Clinical evidence indicates that rapid loading of the muscles, tendons, and bone associated with explosive and intensive movements in exercise can lead to injury of the growing bone and connective tissue. These overuse injuries can be prevented by following some prudent guidelines set forth by the ACSM (Table 15.6) (14).

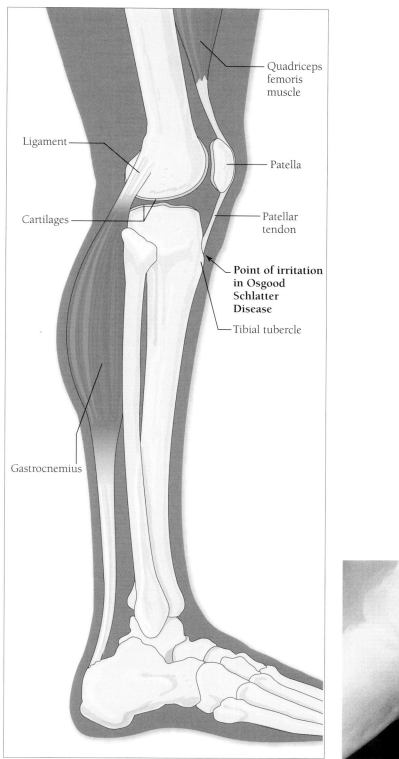

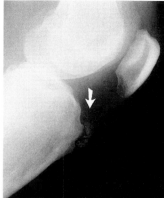

**FIGURE 15.10.** The site of tibial tubercle apophysitis or Osgood-Schlatter disease.

Prepubescent children can generally regulate body temperature in thermoneutral or warm environments, but exercise in hot environments presents a higher risk for heat injuries in children than adults. Contributing to this increased risk is the tendency for children to exhibit a greater O₂ cost and heat production for a standard submaximal exercise workload. Compared to adults, children also have lower sweating rates, lower rates of sweat production per eccrine gland, and lower sensitivities of eccrine glands to changes in core temperature. Accordingly, children

| Table 15.6 | GUIDELINES FOR PREVENTING OVERUSE INJURIES IN ADOLESCENTS AND CHILDREN |
|---|---|

- Emphasize to young participants that general fitness is the basis for all sports participation.

- Encourage children to participate in several different sports, rather than specializing in a single sport at an early age.

- Allow children to play and have fun. When children control the intensity of the activity themselves, they seem likely to stay within the safe ranges for intensity and volume of exercise.

- Counsel children to participate in sports that are realistic to the individual's body type and match competitors for age, height, weight, maturity, and skill.

- Design and enforce game rules that encourage safe play.

- Increase training volume gradually. Each week there should be no more than a 10% increase in the amount of training time, distance, or repetitions performed in the activity.

Adapted from American College of Sports Medicine. Physical fitness in children and youth. *Med Sci Sports Exerc* 1988;20:422–423.

exercising in warm to hot weather should be monitored closely, and fluid replacement should be encouraged, if not coerced. More information on fluid balance and heat tolerance in children can be found in Chapter 8.

Weight training is gaining popularity in all segments of society. Increasing numbers of children and adolescents are using weight training to improve their appearance, strength, and sports skills. There is substantial evidence to show that improper weight training can cause musculoskeletal injuries in children, such as ruptured intervertebral discs and damage to epiphyseal growth plates. However, few injuries occur in programs that are carefully supervised and involve proper instruction on technique. Table 15.7 contains some prudent guidelines for weight training in children and adolescents.

## EMOTIONAL DISTRESS IN YOUNG ATHLETES

There appear to be increasing numbers of children who specialize in sports at an early age and train year-round for their sport to compete on a higher level. Competition at high levels requires training regimens for children that could be considered extreme even for adults. The ever-increasing requirements for success create a constant pressure for athletes to train longer, harder, more intelligently, and often at an earlier age (15). Athletes of all ages and competition levels are vulnerable to psychologic stress and psychiatric disorders. Psychiatric illness in child athletes may arise from (a) coincidence (meaning the child would have developed the illness regardless of participating in a sport), (b) a predisposing pathology that first attracted the athlete to the sport (e.g., a sport like gymnastics may foster an obsessive-compulsive disorder because of the need to repeat a move over and over), or (c) a psychopathology caused by the sport itself (meaning the child would not have developed the disorder if he/she had not participated in the sport). Regardless of the cause, there are stressors that are particular to competitive athletes which put the child athlete at high risk for psychiatric illness.

| Table 15.7 | GUIDELINES FOR PREVENTING WEIGHT-TRAINING–RELATED INJURIES IN CHILDREN AND ADOLESCENTS |
|---|---|

- Be sure the child can understand and follow directions.

- Weight training should not be started without instruction on proper technique and safety. Proper techniques should be demonstrated first, followed by the gradual addition of resistance. Proper breathing techniques (no breath holding) should be taught.

- All exercise sessions should be supervised by trained personnel (including the use of spotters).

- Exclude lifting of maximal weight and weightlifting competitions.

- Children and prepubescents should not lift more weight or resistance than the amount with which they can complete at least eight repetitions in good form.

- Progressive resistance should be achieved by increasing repetitions first and then increasing weight.

- No matter how big or strong the youth appears, remember that he/she is physiologically immature.

- Perform full-range, multi-joint exercises as opposed to single-joint isolated exercises.

- Balance the exercise bout by performing exercises that work both the agonist and antagonist muscles.

- Limit strength training sessions to twice per week and allow for at least one rest day between exercise days.

Pressure to win or perform at a high standard is probably the greatest stressor inducing psychiatric illness in young athletes. The consequence of this pressure to excel is most often manifest in excessive stress. Children who are more susceptible to excessive stress are those who:

- Have low self-esteem
- Have low internal performance expectations in an environment of high external expectations
- Worry frequently about failure
- Are perfectionists
- Are depressed
- Fear competition
- Worry about adult expectations
- Are overtraining

Parents, coaches, and other adults working with child athletes need to know their athletes so they can recognize the signs and symptoms of stress. Each child will experience different signs of stress, but some of the most frequent manifestations of excessive stress are:

- Moodiness
- Worry
- Emotional outbursts
- Nervousness
- Headaches
- Limited attention span

The American Academy of Pediatrics suggests that children do not train intensively and that children do not specialize in sports until after adolescence (15). The academy encourages children to participate in a variety of different activities and develop a wide range of skills. Children are encouraged to participate in sports at a level consistent with their abilities and interests. Pushing children beyond these limits is discouraged. Coaches of child athletes should be knowledgeable about proper training techniques, equipment, and unique physiologic and emotional characteristics of young competitors. Parents and coaches should be aware of the symptoms of excessive stress and should be monitoring the child for such symptoms. Parents, coaches, and a pediatrician should also monitor the child's physical and emotional growth. The nutritional needs of the child should be adequately met, and signs and symptoms of heat disorders and dehydration should be monitored during training.

## BEHAVIOR CARRYOVER

Participation in organized sports and physical education during childhood and adolescence is often publicized as likely to promote more active lifestyles in adulthood (*Fig. 15.11*). The assumption is that **behavior carryover** will occur, meaning an active lifestyle during youth will persist into adulthood. However, public policy has not vigorously supported participation in school sports and physical education. The National Children and Youth Fitness Study indicated that only about one-third of ele-

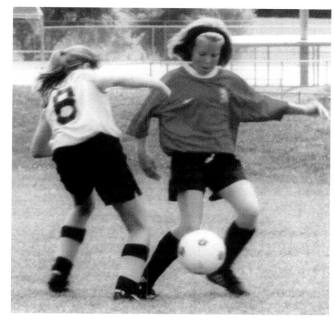

**FIGURE 15.11.** Some children in the United States are getting more than the suggested amount of activity to attain optimal health.

mentary and secondary schools offer daily physical education classes (1), while the Youth Risk Behavior Survey indicated only 32% of high school students participated in daily physical education classes (16). Furthermore, only a handful of studies have addressed the association between childhood and adult physical activity patterns (17).

One possible reason an association between participation in school physical education and adult activity patterns has not been established is that the physical education curricula has been off the mark. Baseline data from one study revealed that students in physical education did not move for half the time available for activity and that continuous movement averaged only 2.2 minutes per class period (18). These statistics become even more embarrassing for the physical education program in that the same study showed identical students spending more than 70% of their recess time moving (18).

A possible explanation for this paradox found by the researchers was that teachers were certified by the state to teach physical education, but none had received training in fitness-oriented physical education. This explanation was supported when researchers also observed that many of the classes were organized for only one or a few children to participate at once, while other students were watching or not staying on task. Another explanation was that although the facilities seemed to be adequate for aerobic activity, teachers lacked sufficient equipment.

Another factor that is often put forth as a promoter of activity in children is parental modeling. The theory behind this is that children's behavior is a reflection of parental behavior. This does not seem to be the case, however, in that patterns of exercise in middle school students were found to be very weakly correlated with exercise patterns of their fathers (r = 0.13) and mothers (r = 0.07) (19). In addition, no association was observed between children's perception of parental exercise patterns and the children's own exercise habits.

Although the research has shown that traditional physical education classes and parental role models have not automatically nurtured our children into more physically active lifestyles, the home and school are still important avenues in which healthy lifestyle development of children can occur. In the area of childhood obesity, for example, research has shown that lifestyle exercise, programmed aerobic exercise, and calisthenics will each reduce body weight to the same degree in overweight children during an intensive weight-loss phase (20–22). During follow-up, however, the children doing lifestyle exercise lost additional weight or maintained weight loss better than the children doing programmed aerobic exercise or calisthenics. Fitness changes, as measured by heart rate during submaximal exercise and recovery, were also maintained better in the children doing lifestyle exercises. These data suggest that if children are taught lifestyle exercise and rewarded appropriately for healthy behaviors, behavioral as well as physiologic goals can be reached (20–22). Traditional examples of lifestyle activities are swimming, walking, bicycling, and hiking. On the other hand, recreational activities such as tennis, badminton, and golf are also considered lifestyle activities.

Short-term studies indicate that physical activity tracks at low to moderate levels in the transition from early to middle childhood (17). Correlations between activity patterns in adolescence and young adulthood are fairly low (r = ~0.05 to 0.20). On the other hand, being forced or strongly encouraged to participate in physical activity during preteen and teen years is negatively related to adult exercise habits (r = −0.05 to −0.20).

Tracking physical fitness from childhood into adulthood is somewhat better (17). The correlation for tracking strength fitness from young teens to young adults is about 0.33, but greater from late teens into young adults (0.66). Correlations for tracking of flexibility fitness from early and late teens into young adulthood is much better than that for strength, 0.68 and 0.82, respectively. Cardiorespiratory fitness tracking does not seem to correlate as well. The correlation from childhood to early adolescence is about 0.50, but drops to about 0.30 when tracking from early to late adolescence. The associations remain at this level as one tracks cardiorespiratory fitness from adolescence into young adulthood (r = 0.30 to 0.50). The presently available data indicate low to moderate relationships among childhood, adolescent, and adulthood physical activity as well as health-related physical fitness (17). Nonetheless, the data suggest the importance of a childhood lifestyle that tracks into adulthood.

 *LINKUP:* **Research Highlight: Physical Fitness and Physical Activity During Adolescence,** *found at http://connection.lww.com/go/brownexphys and on the Student Resource CD-ROM, summarizes a study into the relationship between physical fitness and physical activity during adolescence and cardiovascular disease risk factors in adulthood.*

With this in mind, the President's Council on Fitness and Sport has issued the President's Challenge for both adults and children to maintain an active lifestyle. The President's Active Lifestyle Award is given to anyone who can demonstrate that they are maintaining an active lifestyle. An active lifestyle is defined as participating in any activity that causes all or most of the body parts to move, resulting in an increased heart rate and breathing. Activities can be done alone, in school, in organized sports, or with family and friends. To receive the award, a person needs to accumulate 60 minutes of activity 5 days per week for 6 continuous weeks. The award can also be achieved when girls accumulate 11,000 pedometer steps and boys accumulate 13,000 steps on each of the 5 days per week for 6 continuous weeks. Participants are encouraged to continue earning awards by repeating the program over and over.

▶ *INQUIRY SUMMARY.* Childhood responses to physical activity and exercise training are different from adults because children's cardiorespiratory, musculoskeletal, hormonal, and metabolic systems are underdeveloped. Nonetheless, the child's physiologic systems respond to exercise training similarly to the way adults respond. Special safety precautions should be considered when encouraging physical activity and exercise training for children and adolescents because the underdevelopment of some of their physiologic systems puts them at higher risk for injury. If children develop an active lifestyle and high level of physical fitness, there is only a fair chance that these behaviors will carry into adulthood. Think back to the activity patterns and fitness level you had as a child and adolescent. *Have they tracked into your adulthood?*

## Exercise Prescription, Guidelines, and Recommendations for Children

As seen throughout this chapter, there are very little scientific data on children and exercise from which we can make definitive recommendations as to type, frequency, duration, and intensity of exercise. Most of the available literature is descriptive in nature and deals with either fitness testing and evaluation or sports participation; even in these reports, much of the text is devoted to either what is lacking in the literature or what should be done in the future. Specific physiologic recommendations regarding exercise prescription and participation for children in relation to health parameters are sparse. The ACSM itself devotes only a few pages in its Guidelines for Exercise Testing and Prescription manual to children, and most of this deals with the benefits of exercise and safety, not with prescription (4). ACSM's Resource Manual for Guidelines for Exercise Testing and Prescription only devotes one page to children, and this section only deals with safety for resistance training. The lack of definitive physiologic, medical, or health-related data leaves the exercise professional almost empty handed when trying to prescribe exercise for children using the familiar parameters of type, frequency, duration, and intensity. However, it might be more appropriate to follow general guidelines that encourage lifestyle activity and just let children have fun rather than prescribe regimented fitness programs (18–20).

The optimal amount and type of exercise to recommend for children should be based on individual maturity, health status, skill level, and prior exercise experience (4). The emphasis should be placed on active play that is enjoyable for the child. Creative activities that keep the child engaged for prolonged periods of time are also suggested. Exercise intensity should not be prescribed because children are at low cardiac risk and they have a good ability to adjust intensity by their own perceived exertion (4). Children should be encouraged to participate in a wide variety of activities that are both aerobic and anaerobic in nature, as well as activities that are weight bearing (4). Young children should try to accumulate 1 to 2 hours of physical activity a day at low to moderate levels of intensity (4). Adolescents

can be encouraged to participate in more vigorous activities for 30 minutes per day, three times per week for greater health and fitness benefits (4). Safety should always be prominent. The guidelines provided in Table 15.8 represent a conglomeration of scientific guidelines, prudent principles for practice, and projective reasoning that can help provide the best exercise experience for the child.

▶ **INQUIRY SUMMARY.** Specific guidelines regarding type, frequency, duration, and intensity of exercise in children have not been clearly delineated. However, the most important guideline for children is that they participate in physical activity on a daily basis and that they do so in an enjoyable and safe environment. *What things could you do to encourage a 10-year-old child who loves TV and video games to be more active?*

## Summary

The science underlying fitness assessment and activity monitoring in children is not as advanced as in adults. Traditional fitness tests have been criticized as being evaluations of athletic ability rather than health-related fitness. On the other hand, tests like the President's Challenge and FITNESSGRAM have been reconstructed or designed so that health-related fitness is the primary concern. Several methods for monitoring physical activity in children are utilized. Each method carries its own strengths and weaknesses, and each method has been shown to be reliable and valid to one degree or another.

Childhood responses to physical activity and exercise training are different from adults because children's cardiorespiratory, musculoskeletal, hormonal, and metabolic systems are underdeveloped. Nonetheless, the child's physiologic systems respond to exercise training similarly to those of adults. Special safety precautions should be considered when encouraging physical activity and exercise training for children. The two biggest safety issues for exercising children deal with the physical environment and resistance training. Specific guidelines regarding type, frequency, duration, and intensity of exercise in children are not prerequisites to the development of health-related fitness. The most important guideline for children is that they participate in physical activity on a daily basis and that they do so in an enjoyable and safe environment. If children are taught proper training techniques and are monitored safely, they can enjoy an active lifestyle that has a good chance of carrying over into adulthood.

| Table 15.8 | **EXERCISE PRESCRIPTION FOR ADOLESCENTS AND CHILDREN: PRINCIPLES FOR PRACTICE** |
|---|---|

- Encourage daily activity at a moderate level for at least 60 minutes per day, with the intensity and duration set by the child himself/herself.

- Increase the quantity of exercise gradually.

- Focus on overall health and fitness to ensure adequate strength, flexibility, and endurance.

- Assure proper body mechanics during exercise and activity.

- Assure proper footwear, appropriate running surfaces, and safe equipment.

- Take appropriate safety precautions, especially in hot environments.

- Offer praise, show interest, and give encouragement.

- Set a good example, as adults, by being physically active.

- Encourage informal activity as well as exercise activity.

- Reward exercise behaviors rather than fitness achievement or athletic accomplishments.

### SUMMARY KNOWLEDGE

1. What are some things to consider when evaluating the appropriateness of a fitness test for children?
2. Under which conditions would you perform a clinical exercise test for a child?

3. What are some of the strengths and weaknesses of different methods for assessing physical activity in children?

4. How do the physiologic differences between children and adults affect how a child might respond to exercise training or a fitness test?

5. What precautions should be taken in providing an exercise or activity program for children?

6. What things can be done to maximize the potential for an active lifestyle to carry over from childhood into adulthood?

7. What would be some key components in an exercise program or activity plan for a 6- to 8-year-old, 12-year-old, and 16-year-old? How do these differ with age?

## References

1. Ross JG, Pate RR. The national children and youth fitness study II: summary and findings. *JOPERD* 1987;58:51–56.

2. Lohman TG. The use of skinfold to estimate body fatness on children and youth. *JOPERD* 1987;58:99–102.

3. Updyke WF. In search of relevant and credible physical fitness standards for children. *Res Q Exerc Sport* 1992;63:112–119.

4. American College of Sports Medicine. *ACSM's guidelines for exercise testing and prescription.* 6th ed. Baltimore: Lippincott Williams & Wilkins, 2000:217–223.

5. The Cooper Institute: FITNESSGRAM/ACTIVITYGRAM. Available at: http://www.cooperinst.org/ftgmain.asp. Accessed September 10, 2004.

6. Morgan DW, Tseh W, Caputo JL, et al. Prediction of the aerobic demand of walking in children. *Med Sci Sports Exerc* 2002;34:2097–2102.

7. Epstein LH, Paluch RA, Kalakanis LE, et al. How much activity do youth get? A quantitative review of heart-rate measured activity. *Pediatrics* 2001;108:E44.

8. National Association of Sports and Physical Education: NASPE releases first ever physical activity guidelines for infants & toddlers. Available at: http://www.aahperd.org/NASPE/template.cfm?template=toddlers.html. Accessed October 22, 2004.

9. Physical Best: Discover how you can implement health-related physical education effectively. Available at: http://www.american-fitness.net/Physical%5FBest/. Accessed November 01, 2004.

10. Pereira MA, Fitzgerald SJ, Gregg EW, et al. A collection of physical activity questionnaires for health related research. *Med Sci Sports Exerc* 1997;29:S5–S205.

11. Weston AT, Petosa R, Pate RR. Validation of an instrument for measurement of physical activity in youth. *Med Sci Sports Exerc* 1997;29:138–143.

12. American College of Sports Medicine. Physical fitness in children and youth. *Med Sci Sports Exerc* 1988;20:422–423.

13. Faigenbaum AD, Zaichkowsky LD, Gardner DE, et al. Anabolic steroid use by male and female middle school students. *Pediatrics* 1998;101:e6.

14. Current comment from the American College of Sports Medicine. August 1993. The prevention of sport injuries of children and adolescents. *Med Sci Sports Exerc* 1993;25(Suppl):1–7.

15. American Academy of Pediatrics Committee on Sports Medicine and Fitness. Intensive training and sports specialization in young athletes. *Pediatrics* 2000;106:154–157.

16. Grunbaum JA, Kann L, Kinchen SA, et al. Youth risk behavior surveillance—United States, 2001. *MMWR Surveill Summ* 2002; 51:(SS04) 1–62.

17. Malina RM. Physical activity and fitness: pathways from childhood to adulthood. *Am J Hum Biol* 2001;13:162–172.

18. Parcel GS, Simons-Morton BG, O'Hara NM, et al. School promotion of healthful diet and exercise behavior: an integration of organizational change and social learning theory interventions. *J Sch Health* 1987;57:150–156.

19. Godin G, Shephard RJ, Colantonio A. Children's perception of parental exercise: influence of sex and age. *Percept Mot Skills* 1986;62:511–516.

20. Epstein LH, McCurley J, Wing RR, et al. Five-year follow-up of family-based behavioral treatments for childhood obesity. *J Consult Clin Psychol* 1990;58:661–664.

21. Epstein LH, Wing RR, Koeske R, et al. A comparison of lifestyle change and programmed aerobic exercise on weight and fitness changes in obese children. *Behav Ther* 1982;13:651–665.

22. Epstein LH, Wing RR, Koeske R, et al. A comparison of lifestyle exercise, aerobic exercise, and calisthenics on weight loss in obese children. *Behav Ther* 1985;16:345–356.

## Suggested Readings

Bar-Or O. New and old in pediatric exercise physiology. *Int J Sports Med* 2000;21:S113–S117.

Naughton G, Farpour-Lambert NJ, Carlson J, et al. Physiological issues surrounding the performance of adolescent athletes. *Sports Med* 2000;30:309–325.

Sirard JR, Pate RR. Physical activity assessment in children and adolescents. *Sports Med* 2001;31:439–454.

Sothern MS, Loftin M, Suskind RM, et al. The health benefits of physical activity in children and adolescents: implications for chronic disease prevention. *Eur J Pediatr* 1999;158:271–274.

## On the Internet

The President's Council on Physical Fitness and Sports. Available at: **http://www.fitness.gov/.** Accessed May 16, 2005.

KidSource Online: Promoting physical activity and exercise among children. Available at: **http://www.kidsource.com/kidsource/content4/promote.phyed.html.** Accessed May 16, 2005.

Consumer Product Safety Commission: Prevent injuries to children from exercise equipment. Available at: **http://www.cpsc.gov/cpscpub/pubs/5028.html.** Accessed May 16, 2005.

The President's Challenge. Available at: **http://www.presidentschallenge.org/.** Accessed May 16, 2005.

Centers for Disease Control: National Center for Chronic Disease Prevention and Health Promotion: Nutrition & physical activity. Available at: **http://www.cdc.gov/nccdphp/dnpa/.** Accessed May 16, 2005.

Kidnetic.com. Available at: **http://www.kidnetic.com.** Accessed May 16, 2005.

## Writing to Learn

*The State Health Department has come to you as a health professional for assistance in progressing toward the health goals set forth in Healthy People 2010. Specifically they want you to become part of a team to evaluate how much physical activity children in your state are receiving each day. After the initial assessment, you are to help them design a plan they can implement to help children become more active. Your first planning meeting with the team is within the next 2 weeks. Make an outline of things you think they need to consider in assessing physical activity in children and in designing a plan to encourage more physical activity for children.*

# CHAPTER

# 16   Geriatric Exercise Physiology

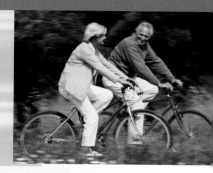

*The Swiss gerontologist Frederick Verzar wrote, "Old age is not an illness. It is a continuation of life with decreasing capacities for adaptation." The study of exercise physiology is largely about how the body adapts to the stress of acute and chronic exercise.* How do you think the "decreasing capacities for adaptation" of the older individual affect their capacity for exercise?

The question posed in the chapter opening has important and far-reaching societal consequences. *Aging is a normal biologic process, but are we all automatically consigned to a final few years of progressive loss of functional capacity that ultimately leads to disability? Or is there a more optimal level of function that we can achieve, even in the eighth or ninth decade of life, that allows us to be relatively free of serious disability?* Since this text is concerned with the physiology of exercise, we will answer the last question by focusing on the physiologic responses and adaptations to exercise under the condition of normal aging. These questions are of particular concern to exercise physiology students because aging demographics dictate that therapists and other health care personnel who provide exercise and related services will likely intersect with an elderly population that is becoming more numerous.

## Aging

Statistics on aging are startling. In the year 1900, 4% of the population (3 million people) was aged older than 65 years; today approximately 13% (38 million people) are older than 65. This represents more than a 12-fold increase in the number of people in this age category since the end of the 19th century. This increase is much greater than the rate of increase for the total United States population (from 75 million to 290 million, almost a four-fold increase) during the same time period.

Table 16.1 shows that the absolute and proportional increases in the aged population are expected to continue well into the 21st century. For example, by the year 2050 the number of individuals over age 65 is expected to be almost 87 million people, which is more than double what it was in the year 2000. Due to the demographics of birthrates from the 1960s through the first decade of the 21st century, most of the growth in individuals over age 65 will likely occur between the years 2010 and 2030. Notice also that the median age of the older population increased during the last two decades of the 20th century and will continue to do so. The median age of the 65-and-over population in the United States was 73.3 years in 1990, up from 71.9 years in 1960. Table 16.1 also shows that since 1980 the proportion of the aged who are 65 to 74 years old has been getting smaller. This trend will continue until the year 2010. The proportion of people aged 75 to 84 years is getting larger, with this trend

| Table 16.1 | THE NUMBER AND PROPORTION OF THE ELDERLY | | | | | |
|---|---|---|---|---|---|---|
| | | | **Projections** | | | |
| | **1980** | **1990** | **2000** | **2010** | **2020** | **2050** |
| ≥65 years (millions) | 25.6 | 31.1 | 34.7 | 40.2 | 54.6 | 86.7 |
| % total population | 11.3 | 12.5 | 12.6 | 13.2 | 16.3 | 20.6 |
| Increase in preceding decade (%) | — | 21.6 | 11.7 | 15.9 | 35.8 | 8.3 |
| **% Distribution of the Population Age ≥65** | | | | | | |
| 65–74 years (%) | 61.0 | 58.1 | 52.3 | 52.9 | 58.2 | 43.8 |
| 75–84 years (%) | 30.3 | 32.2 | 35.4 | 31.9 | 28.5 | 32.2 |
| ≥85 years (%) | 8.7 | 9.7 | 12.3 | 15.2 | 13.3 | 24.1 |

Note: These middle-series Census Bureau projections are based on the following assumptions: total fertility rate equals 2.25; life expectancy in 2050 is 82.0 years; and annual net immigration is 820,000. Source: United States Bureau of the Census, Statistical Abstract of the United States: 2003 (Washington, DC: U.S. Government Printing Office, 2003), Tables 3 and 12.

also continuing until year 2010. The oldest-old (≥85 years) is the most rapidly growing elderly age group. This group will number about 21 million in the year 2050, or 24.1% of elderly Americans and about 5% of all Americans.

These statistics indicate what we have heard most of our lives—that the population is getting older. By the end of the current decade, the old people living among us will likely be the oldest they have ever been as a group. Besides living longer, these individuals are also healthier than at any previous time in history, yet many of these individuals have patterns of activity that are not conducive to optimal health.

There has been great progress in the reduction of mortality as reflected by an increase in the average **life expectancy**, which measures changes in survivorship. Life expectancy is the average length of life of a person. However, **gerontologists** are especially interested in assessing progress in survivorship for those aged 65 and older. A statistic for doing this is termed the **age-specific life expectancy**, which is the average duration of life for an individual of a given age. Table 16.2 presents age-specific life expectancy data by sex and race at various elderly ages in the United States. As you can

see, gains in life expectancy for aged males have not kept pace with those of aged females.

## DEFINITION OF AGING

An important place to begin the study of geriatric exercise physiology is to define aging. Verzar's remark concerning old age provides us with a good starting point for this definition. However, even with this start, aging is not easily defined since it is genetically determined and environmentally modulated. Of necessity, our definition should distinguish between three important aspects of aging: **chronologic aging**, **biologic aging**, and **pathologic aging**.

### Chronologic Aging

An intuitive definition is that aging is simply the process of *becoming older*. Viewed this way, aging is the passage of time, or what is referred to as chronologic aging. A useful way of designating age by time is to divide people into broad age categories such as young, middle, and old age. However, when dealing with people over the age of 55 years,

| Table 16.2 | YEARS OF LIFE EXPECTANCY AT AGES 65 AND 75 | | | |
|---|---|---|---|---|
| | **White** | | **African American** | |
| **Year and age** | **Male** | **Female** | **Male** | **Female** |
| ***1900–1902**** | | | | |
| 65 years | 11.5 | 11.2 | 10.4 | 11.4 |
| 75 years | 6.8 | 7.3 | 6.6 | 7.9 |
| ***1995*** | | | | |
| 65 years | 15.7 | 19.1 | 13.6 | 17.1 |
| 75 years | 9.7 | 12.0 | 8.8 | 11.1 |
| ***2000*** | | | | |
| 65 years | 16.3 | 19.4 | 14.2 | 17.7 |
| 75 years | 10.1 | 12.3 | 9.2 | 11.6 |

*Death registration states only. Data from the National Center for Health Statistics.

gerontologists like to assign less broad category designations. One useful way of viewing age categories among older individuals is to make a distinction between the young-old (55 to 74 years), the old-old (75 to 84 years), and the oldest-old (85 years and older). Although our definition carries Verzar's idea of "continuation of life," astute readers will catch the circularity. The phrase "becoming older" that formed the basis of our definition of chronologic aging is itself synonymous with the term "aging." This is akin to saying that aging is aging. Also, two individuals may be the same age yet be so remarkably different as to make age by chronology almost meaningless. This necessitates that we focus our definition on the innate physiologic makeup of individuals and consider the biology of aging.

## Biologic Aging

An individual who is 75 years old chronologically may have the biologic age of a 55-year-old and vice versa. While this example may seem extreme, it points to the fact that aging, as a biologic phenomenon, is not simply the passage of time but is the accumulation of biologic events that occur over a span of time. The concepts of chronologic and biologic aging are related but not necessarily highly related for a given individual, as shown in the example above of the disparity between biologic and chronologic age. Because of this, it is hard to say at what point in life a person is considered biologically old, since genetic and prenatal influences coupled with the postnatal environment (demographic, economic, psychologic, and social) act to modify the aging sequence differently in all individuals. Biologic aging is a developmental process that has more to do with physiology than with chronology. Biologic age is also closely associated with functional abilities and capacities, which helps explain why some individuals feel younger than their chronologic age, while others feel older than their chronologic age. The connection between biologic age and function is in concert with Verzar's definitional emphasis on "capacities for adaptation." Therefore, it can be said that biologic aging is a measure of one's success for adaptation. Individual variation in the ability to adapt with age helps explain the differing rates of biologic aging for different individuals. The mechanisms to explain this are varied and complex; however, one thing is becoming clear: increasing physical activity is a powerful factor that many believe attenuates the process of biologic aging.

## Pathologic Aging

Like Verzar, we are loath to consider aging pathologic, yet aging may be entirely due to the effects of disease processes in the body. There is a strong association between biologic aging and pathology. That is, biologic deterioration with aging may create susceptibility to disease. The opposite may also be true; disease processes may lead to biologic deterioration (aging). Therefore, changes that occur as a result of disease processes define pathologic aging. However, most scientists try to separate the aging process from disease, since people age even when no disease is afflicting the body. Diseases can be classified in three ways related to their connection to aging (1).

1. Some diseases are practically universal and inevitable with age and are indistinguishable from normal aging in many respects. Atherosclerosis, a chronic disease of the blood vessels, is an example.
2. Some diseases are age related but are neither universal nor inevitable. Cancer risk increases with age, but not all elderly people contract cancer.
3. Some diseases are not age related, but their impact is greater as individuals age. Death rates from respiratory diseases are higher in older age groups than in younger or middle-aged groups.

Diseases represent the chief barriers to extended health and longevity. *Why do people become old? Is there any way to stop the aging process?* These two questions are almost as old as mankind. The upper age limit for survival seems to be approximately 120 to 125 years, if we arrive at this figure based on experience alone. The longest-lived persons validated by science are Shirechiyo Izumi of Japan and Jeanne Calmet of France, both of whom reached 122 years before dying. This figure effectively represents the maximum **lifespan**, perhaps until someone extends it further. Human longevity refers to the age beyond which no one can expect to live.

*Is the human lifespan an absolute standard, or can we expect a significant extension of the length of life?* People who think the human lifespan can be extended are proponents of **prolongevity**, the significant extension of the length of life by human action. Others insist that new medical treatments, improved technology, and better health habits may continue to increase life expectancy but that the human lifespan is unlikely to increase. A key factor for substantially increasing life expectancy at birth and at specific ages (i.e., 65 and 75) appears to be eliminating deaths from cardiovascular disease. Table 16.3 shows that ending major cardiovascular-renal disease would provide far greater gains in life expectancy than eliminating deaths from infective and parasitic diseases, diabetes mellitus, influenza and pneumonia, accidents, and even cancer.

## THEORIES OF AGING

Regardless of whether lifespan can be increased, we are still left with our original question—*how is aging explained?* Most biologic theories of aging to date are not mutually exclusive but can be grouped within two general, yet overlapping, perspectives used to explain the mechanism of aging: aging as random events and aging as programmed (genetic) events.

Aging as random events asserts that biologic changes result from the accumulation of randomly occurring insults from the environment. Over time, the accumulation of these "injuries" is incompatible with life. This perspective postulates the older "wear and tear" theory of aging that says we are progressively worn down by environmental factors that affect us at the organ and cellular levels. Our

| Table 16.3 | GAIN IN LIFE EXPECTANCY IF VARIOUS CAUSES OF DEATH WERE ELIMINATED | |
|---|---|---|
| | **Gain in years** | |
| **Various causes of death** | *At birth* | *At age 65* |
| Major cardiovascular-renal disease | 11.8 | 11.4 |
| Malignant neoplasms | 2.5 | 1.4 |
| Accidents | 0.7 | 0.1 |
| Influenza and pneumonia | 0.5 | 0.2 |
| Diabetes mellitus | 0.2 | 0.2 |
| Infective and parasitic diseases | 0.2 | 0.1 |

Data from the United States Public Health Service.

body's maintenance and repair systems do not compensate for the effects of normal wear and tear, and the excess brought on by an unhealthy (or overly active) lifestyle. Compensation is effective when we are young, but the ability to repair damage is lost the older we become. This theory also posits an inverse relationship between rate of living and length of life—those who live hard and fast cannot expect to live very long. The body simply wears out with use over time. Examples of insults that produce "wear and tear" include sun exposure, smoking, accidents, and radiation. These factors may cause damage to human organs over time through a variety of mechanisms. Other theories in the random-event perspective include free radicals, somatic mutation and DNA repair, error theory, protein modification, and waste product accumulation.

Aging as programmed events states that there is a sequence of events written into our genetic material that determines our maximal lifespan. For example, in the late 1950s Leonard Hayflick discovered that the doubling capacity of cells is limited and different for each species—the "Hayflick limit." It is now being postulated that the Hayflick limit may be based on telomere shortening. Telomeres, found at the end of chromosomes, shorten with each cell division and when they become too short, the cell can no longer divide.

Telomeres may represent the "aging program." The telomere theory is of interest to cancer research. Found at the tip of each chromosome, telomeres are nothing more than long chains of repeated DNA sequences and are the genetic elements essential for proper chromosome structure and function. Telomeres shorten with each cell division unless the cell also contains telomerase, an enzyme that prevents or reverses this shortening process. The length of the telomere may determine longevity. This can be seen in children who are born with progerias, a group of genetic disorders that appear to cause premature aging. These children have abnormally short telomeres. The relative "immortality" of many cancer cells may be related to their ability to produce telomerase, which would allow them to keep their telomeres from shortening. Researchers have focused on how to arrest telomerase in cancer cells and how to prevent the telomere shortening in normal cells to lengthen life.

- *Is it possible to extend telomere length without causing cancer?*
- *Will telomere extension increase lifespan?*
- *Will cancer one day be treated by arresting telomerase production?*

Other theories in the programmed-event perspective include those involving the neuroendocrine and immunologic systems and longevity genes. Researchers in aging are also focusing on aging in an evolutionary framework, but this is outside the scope of this chapter to explore. For a review of specific aging theories not covered in this chapter, consult the feature *On the Internet* at the end of the chapter.

▶ *INQUIRY SUMMARY.* Statistics on aging attest to the phenomenon referred to as the "graying of America." While this phenomenon has been viewed in purely chronologic terms, aging itself is more complex. In this regard, our definition of aging should also focus on the biology and pathology of aging. When viewed in this way, two 75-year-old individuals may not really be the same "age." *What are the implications of this definitional emphasis for our nation's policies on the "elderly?"*

## Aging, Physical Inactivity, and Disability

As we have seen, any chronologic criterion for determining old age is too narrow and rigid and assumes that everyone ages in the same way and at the same time. However, we know that one person may be biologically old at 45 and another biologically young at 60. For individuals who are biologically younger than their chronologic age, consistent and appropriate physical activity throughout life is thought to be a key factor. Much of the health problems and physical deterioration experienced in old age results from disuse of body systems. Employing simple exercises throughout life and even starting an exercise program at a later point in one's life produces positive physical and mental outcomes. Some exercise is better than none. For example, older people, including the frail and ill, will gain mobility, improve the quality of life, and prolong independence when performing regular strength and flexibility exercises. Loss of mobility is a significant cause of loss of independence among elderly men and women. This problem is especially acute among elderly females. As a group, elderly females have a longer life expectancy but also a longer period of dependent living (*Fig. 16.1*).

The relationship between lifetime physical activity and longevity was shown in the classic study of Harvard alumni

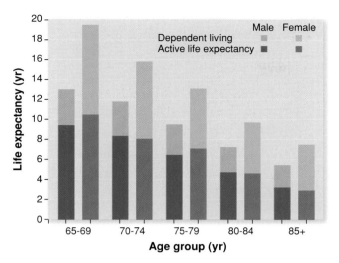

FIGURE 16.1. Life expectancy and active life expectancy for males and females. Total life expectancy is shown by each bar, which is then divided into active life expectancy and dependent living. Data from Katz S, Branch LG, Branson MH, et al. Active life expectancy. *N Engl J Med* 1983;309:1218–1224.

(2). The Harvard study tracked the health and lifestyles of 16,936 men who entered Harvard from 1916 to 1950. The subjects were followed until 1978 at which time 1413 had died. The results showed that men who walked more than 9 miles a week ($\geq$900 kcal·wk$^{-1}$ expended) had a 21% lower risk of death than those who walked less than 3 miles a week. The optimum energy expenditure was about 3500 kcal·wk$^{-1}$, which produced half the risk of death of those who did little or no exercise. Also shown in the study was that a lifetime of physical activity reduced the negative health effects of cigarette smoking or high blood pressure and was even effective in offsetting an inherited tendency toward early death.

## AGING, HEALTH STATUS, AND FUNCTIONAL CAPACITY

Rather than rely on strict medical criteria to determine health, one's **functional ability** to perform normal life roles or activities more effectively defines health status during the aging process (3). As will be shown in Chapter 19, there is a clear association between a loss of functional ability/capacity and the onset of disability. Limitation in the ability to perform various **activities of daily living** (ADL) and/or various **instrumental activities of daily living** is prevalent in the elderly population. Since aging and declining health often go hand-in-hand, the maintenance of physiologic functional capacity through regular physical activity is an important concept in any discussion of geriatric exercise physiology. Therefore, the underlying premise in this chapter is that physical activity (or exercise) is necessary for the maintenance of functional capacity (health) and reduces the prevalence of disability with aging.

 **LINKUP:** *We owe a good deal of our present knowledge in such fields as the physiology of aging and exercise prescription to the work of Dr. Michael L. Pollock. See his biography at http://connection.lww.com/go/brown-exphys and on the Student Resource CD-ROM.*

The aging process causes deterioration in functional capacity. More than 80% of individuals older than 75 years have functionally limited mobility or agility. An important question is can regular exercise training throughout life reduce the age-related decline toward disability. *Do you think disability with old age is inevitable?*

One of the main effects of aging is a loss of functional capacity, but the extent and rate of this loss is different for different individuals. The loss of functional capacity with age is itself caused by three main factors: increased age, reduced physical activity, and disease (*Fig. 16.2*). The relationship between disease and functional limitations/disability during aging defines the concept of **secondary aging**. However, **primary aging** is the deterioration of physiologic processes in the absence of factors that cause secondary aging (i.e., diseases).

Although disease modification associated with the adoption of physical activity can retard premature death by 1 to 2 years, a long-term physically active lifestyle will not alter primary aging or the lifespan. As we will see, physiologic

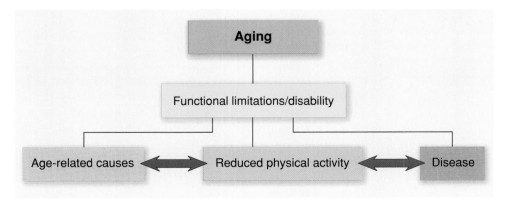

FIGURE 16.2. The interaction among aging, disease, and physical inactivity with the loss of functional capacity.

decline leading to functional decline is inevitable, but the decline may be accentuated by pathologic processes and reduced physical activity. Theoretically, in the absence of these latter two factors, biologic aging may be attenuated.

Therefore, in describing these relationships, physical activity is seen as modifying the rate of onset of functional limitations and disability by reducing the occurrence of disease and attenuating loss of function purely due to aging. This has been eloquently demonstrated in a longitudinal study of 11 men who exercised regularly over a 33-year time period. In this study, the age-associated decline in maximal aerobic capacity ($O_2$ consumption, $\dot{V}O_2max = 0.27$ mL·min$^{-1}$·kg$^{-1}$·yr$^{-1}$) was less than one-half of that experienced by aging sedentary men (4). While the decline in aerobic power with age is inevitable, it appears that the rate of the decline can be attenuated with vigorous exercise training throughout life. *Can you name some of the more obvious functional benefits that would result from regular exercise?*

Age is significantly related to becoming dependent. For many older individuals, the principle cause of dependency is a loss of functional capacity that progresses with age and that precludes participation in ADL. In terms of $\dot{V}O_2max$, the threshold for independency appears to be around 18 mL·kg$^{-1}$·min$^{-1}$ in men and about 15 mL·kg$^{-1}$·min$^{-1}$ in women (5). Since physical activity, especially vigorous exercise, increases $\dot{V}O_2max$, we have a clear picture of the efficacy of exercise training to reduce the slide to dependency in old age. It has been suggested that the 20% increase in $\dot{V}O_2max$ and strength produced by regular exercise training is the equivalent of a 20-year reversal in these aspects of functional aging (6).

Physical inactivity is a behavioral risk factor influencing the development of disability. The reason for this is that inactivity leads to decreases in physiologic capacity and function, such as losses in cardiorespiratory fitness (i.e., reducing self-selected walking speed), muscle mass (i.e., reducing strength), and joint flexibility (i.e., limiting mobility). Physical inactivity inevitably leads to loss of function and a downward spiral towards disability as aging occurs. As individuals become disabled with age, dependency ensues. A *Lancet* editorial expresses this thought well:

> "A large and rapidly increasing number of people live perilously close to functional thresholds of physical ability, needing only a minor illness to render them dependent. If crossing of thresholds for independence could be prevented or postponed, the quality of many lives would be improved and the social and economic costs of supporting an infirm aged population would be reduced" (7).

The major conditions causing activity limitations include heart disease, spine and back disorders, arthritis, lower-extremity disorders, asthma, diabetes, and mental illness. Approximately 40 million noninstitutionalized adults in the United States report having, on average, almost two disabilities per person. These conditions are responsible for most disabilities and institutionalizations. The main causes of the loss of disability-free life expectancy are specific medical conditions, such as circulatory, locomotor, and respiratory disorders.

Regular exercise training can impact most of the conditions shown, and even small increases in aerobic power, strength, and flexibility can lead to large improvements in quality of life for persons who already have one or more disabilities. Since the population is getting older, reducing the slide to dependency has the obvious potential of reducing the burden of aging on a society in which health care costs are astronomic. For example, 13% of the United States population is ≥65 years, yet this group represents an inordinate proportion of total hospital stays (37%) and days of care in hospitals (50%). Silverstone (8) has documented that increased health care dollars are expended in persons older than 75 years old.

The overall impact of lifestyle on the decline to dependency is astonishing. Health care professionals who prescribe exercise and other lifestyle interventions are well positioned to reduce the burden on society that dependency produces. A final quote illustrates how regular physical activity and other lifestyle factors are powerful tools to maintain independent living:

> "The cumulative influence of regular physical activity, control of body mass, and cessation of smoking can bring about a 40% increase in aerobic power, the equivalent of approximately 40 years of aging, sufficient to correct the functional problems encountered in most frail elderly men and women" (7).

Independence is a quality that can be measured using instruments specifically designed for this task. See Box 16.1 for information on how to measure independent living in elderly individuals.

The decline in physical function with age is a multifactorial problem, becoming more insidious with advanced age. The extent to which physical function can be preserved with regular exercise is complex and poorly elucidated in older adults. However, biologic aging can be attenuated by maintaining a regular exercise program. The rest of this chapter describes how normal aging affects the acute and chronic responses to exercise in various physiologic systems. Before reading these sections, review Table 16.4, which briefly outlines the physiologic effects of aging on various body systems.

 **LINKUP:** *Peripheral skeletal muscle abnormalities figure prominently in exercise tolerance associated with congestive heart failure.* **Access** *Research Highlight: Randomized Trial of Progressive Resistance Training to Counteract the Myopathy of Chronic Heart Failure, found at http://connection.lww.com/go/brownexphys and on the Student Resource CD-ROM, for a summary of recent research in this area.*

▶ *INQUIRY SUMMARY.* Independent living in old age requires that functional reserves be great enough to cope with sudden illness or injury. While exercise training does

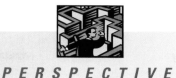

*P E R S P E C T I V E*

## *Measuring Independence*

Since health status may be defined in terms of functional capacity, it is important to have measurement tools that assist in quantifying tasks and activities related to daily living to assess the functional health (i.e., independence) of individuals. In this regard, independence is defined in relation to the ability to perform functional tasks. These tasks of daily living are divided into two categories: activities of daily living (ADL) and instrumental activities of daily living (IADL). ADL refers to activities that are related strongly to self-care: eating, dressing, grooming, toileting, and transfers, while IADL refers to more complex activities: cooking, cleaning, using the telephone, and financial management. In all of these tasks, and many others of like nature, the level of independence is an important measurement to make in assessing health status. Three methods have traditionally been used for assessing independence via the performance of ADL or IADL tasks:

- Self-reports by the patient
- Ratings based on observations of the patient's behavior by a rater or an attendant
- Direct examination of the individual's performance by a trained professional, such as an occupational therapist or physical therapist

Whereas the first two methods provide the total level of independence of the individual, they fail to provide the detailed objective profile that is often necessary to plan a specific treatment program. To correct this problem, the Maquire Trilevel ADL Assessment (MTAA) instrument was developed. This tool divides ADL tasks into six categories: communication, eating, mobility, hygiene, dressing, and organization, with each category further divided into three environmental levels: personal, home or sheltered environment, and the community.

**LINKUP: See Perspective: Example of Use of MTAA Instrument for Individual with Rheumatoid Arthritis,** found at *http://connection.lww.com/go/brownexphys* and on the Student Resource CD-ROM.

The instrument is scored according to the following guidelines:

1. Rate each task in each of the six categories (communication, eating, mobility, hygiene, dressing, and organization) by answering two questions: 1) is the patient totally independent or does the patient require some assistance or supervision and 2) does the patient require equipment for functioning or safety? Use I, S, A, D, or NA ratings as shown on the form and check whether any equipment is needed (list the equipment).
2. A quantitative score is provided for each environmental level (personal, home, community) of the six categories. Score each environmental level with the appropriate score shown on the form (4, 3, 2, 1, 0).
3. Transfer the score of each level to the MTAA score sheet (end of form). An average score for each category is calculated.

A problem with the MTAA instrument is that no validity or reliability studies have ever been conducted on it. Therefore, whether you are measuring the patient's actual ability or some other trait needs to be answered before completely accepting the results of this instrument.

### *REFERENCE*

Maquire GH. Activities of daily living. In: Lewis CB, ed. *Aging: the health care challenge*. Philadelphia: FA Davis Co, 1996:47–78.

---

not guarantee that individuals will always be able to live independent lives, the preponderance of evidence suggests that disability is far more common in older people who do not lead lifestyles that include some exercise or other forms of vigorous physical activity. *What are some hindrances to being physically active that older people face?*

## Exercise Physiologic Changes with Aging

When you are considering aging and the exercise response, it is important to differentiate the physiologic responses to exercise in normal aging from those responses that are the consequences of a disease state. As shown in Table 16.4, several key physiologic changes occur with aging that result in a loss of function. These key losses ultimately result in reduced functional ability, but many of the age-related changes may be reversed or slowed with exercise training. In this section we start with the cardiopulmonary system and look in detail at the physiologic principles related to aging and exercise. However, because muscle strength and power are also important to maintain as we age, we turn our attention in the last part of this section to aspects of the neuromuscular system in aging and exercise.

| Table 16.4 | PHYSIOLOGIC EFFECTS OF AGING |
|---|---|
| **Category and change produced** | **Functional significance** |
| **Cardiovascular system** | |
| ↓ capillary/fiber ratio | ↓ muscle blood flow |
| ↓ cardiac muscle and heart volume | ↓ maximal SV and $\dot{Q}$ |
| ↓ elasticity of blood vessels | ↑ TPR, MAP, and cardiac afterload |
| ↓ myocardial myosin-ATPase | ↓ myocardial contractility |
| ↓ sympathetic stimulation of SA node | ↓ maximal HR |
| **Pulmonary system** | |
| ↓ elasticity | ↑ work of breathing and ↓ lung elastic recoil |
| ↑ size of alveoli | ↓ diffusion capacity and ↑ dead space |
| ↓ number of pulmonary capillaries | ↓ ventilation / perfusion |
| **Musculoskeletal system** | |
| ↓ muscle mass (↓ number or type IIa & IIb fibers); | |
| ↓ size of motor units; ↓ total | ↓ strength and power |
| **Protein and [$N_2$]** | |
| ↓ size and number of mitochondria & ↓ oxidative enzymes | ↓ oxidative capacity |
| ↑ muscle and joint stiffness | ↓ flexibility, mobility, and stability |
| ↓ lactate dehydrogenase | ↓ glycolysis |
| ↓ water content in intervertebral cartilage | ↑ chance of fractures of the spine |
| ↓ bone minerals | ↑ risk of fracture due to osteoporosis and ↓ bone mass |
| ↑ kyphosis | ↓ height |
| **Metabolic system** | |
| ↑ percent body fat | ↓ mobility and ↑ disease risk |
| ↓ glucose tolerance | ↑ risk of diabetes and heart disease |

SV, stroke volume; $\dot{Q}$, cardiac output; TPR, total peripheral resistance; MAP, mean arterial blood pressure; HE, heart rate; ↓, decrease; ↑, increase.

## THE CARDIOVASCULAR SYSTEM

The cardiovascular system is perhaps the most important bodily system to consider in our discussion of geriatric exercise physiology. Heart disease remains the principal cause of death among the elderly and also accounts for a great deal of morbidity, disablement, and inactivity in older people. Therefore, to understand geriatric exercise physiology, you must have a sound grasp of how the cardiopulmonary system adapts to the combined effects of aging and exercise.

### Cardiac Reserve

Aging generally brings about a reduction in the cardiac reserve capacity, which is the amount of cardiac output ($\dot{Q}$) remaining above that required for ADL. Cardiac reserve is the heart's ability to adjust to the immediate demands placed on it. For example, running to catch a bus would cause an increase in $O_2$ demand, which must be balanced by increased blood circulation. This is achieved by an increase in either stroke volume (SV) or heart rate (HR) or both. Approached another way, cardiac reserve is the maximum percentage that $\dot{Q}$ can increase above normal. In the normal young adult, the cardiac reserve is 300% to 400%, or about four times the normal $\dot{Q}$. In the athletically trained person, cardiac reserve is occasionally as high as 500% to

600%. In the elderly person, cardiac reserve may be as low as 200%, or just two times the normal $\dot{Q}$.

The concept of differences in cardiac reserve among different individuals is depicted in *Figure 16.3* as a reduction in $\dot{Q}_{max}$ due to normal aging, deconditioning, and/or disease processes. Cardiac reserve is reduced with aging as a function, primarily, of the decline in maximal HR. The decline in maximal HR affects both maximal cardiac output ($\dot{Q}max$) and $\dot{V}O_2max$, as can be demonstrated using the Fick equation (discussed below).

HR reserve (maximum HR − resting HR) is also affected by the decrease in maximal HR with age, although resting HR is not changed with aging. Maximal HR is controlled by input from the sympathetic nervous system. This input declines by about 5% per decade as we age. As in younger individuals, exercise training reduces resting HRs of older individuals, but maximal HR is not affected. Thus, there is a biologic determinism at work in aging that leads to an automatic reduction in work capacity as a direct result of physiologic decline. *Can you explain this reduction in work capacity in terms of $\dot{V}O_2max$?*

A loss in cardiac reserve impinges on the functional ability of individuals by reducing, for instance, ambulation speed at a given relative $O_2$ cost (i.e., % $\dot{V}O_2max$). If the $\dot{V}O_2max$ is reduced enough (through normal aging or

**Normal Athlete 18-20 years old**                       $\dot{Q}$ = 24 L · min$^{-1}$ maximum

| Rest 4-6 L · min$^{-1}$ | Required for ADL | Reserve Capacity |
|---|---|---|

**Effects of Normal Aging > 60 years old**              $\dot{Q}$ = 18-20 L · min$^{-1}$ maximum

| Rest 4-6 L · min$^{-1}$ | Required for ADL | Reserve Capacity | Aging loss |
|---|---|---|---|

**Effects of Normal Aging and Deconditioning > 60 years old**    $\dot{Q}$ = 14 L · min$^{-1}$ maximum

| Rest 4-6 L · min$^{-1}$ | Required for ADL | Reserve Capacity | Deconditioning loss | Aging loss |
|---|---|---|---|---|

**Effects of Age, Deconditioning, and Disease**          $\dot{Q}$ = 10 L · min$^{-1}$ maximum

| Rest 4-6 L · min$^{-1}$ | Required for ADL | Reserve Capacity | Ischemia/infarction loss | Deconditioning loss | Aging loss |
|---|---|---|---|---|---|

**FIGURE 16.3.** Effects of aging, deconditioning, and disease on cardiac output ($\dot{Q}$) reserve. The four bar graphs show the $\dot{Q}$ of different hypothetical individuals. Maximal values are systematically reduced by normal aging, deconditioning, and the effects of disease. ADL, activities of daily living.

disease processes), a given ambulation pace may require the individual to access anaerobic as well as aerobic energy sources. For example, someone with a 4 metabolic equivalents (MET) functional capacity is already at 25% (1 MET ÷ 4 MET) of this functional limit at rest, and even a 2 mi·hr$^{-1}$ walking pace would place this individual at approximately 65% (2.5 MET) of $\dot{V}O_2$max. Individuals with impairments leading to diminished mechanical efficiency will experience a higher energy cost at a given ambulation speed. With aging, deconditioning, and/or disease, the normal walking pace may then approximate the maximal aerobic capacity. An understanding of this scenario is vital when prescribing exercise to older individuals. For example, differentiating **dyspnea** produced normally by exercise from that produced by a lowered functional capacity from aging and/or pathology is critical to understanding the exercise response in elderly individuals.

## Fick Equation

Maximal HR, SV, and $\dot{Q}$ decrease progressively with age regardless of gender or training status, resulting in a decline in $\dot{V}O_2$max of 6% to 10% per decade after the age of 25 years (9). The decline accelerates to approximately 15% per decade after age 60 due to diminishing central cardiac function in addition to the decline in maximal HR (10). The decline in $\dot{V}O_2$max with aging is attenuated in older subjects who continue a vigorous exercise program throughout life, but the reason for this attenuated decline is still the subject of ongoing research. The Fick equation can be used to isolate the factors responsible for the decline in $\dot{V}O_2$max with aging. *If the decline in maximal HR is biologically determined and not reversed by exercise training, what other factors may explain the attenuated decline in $\dot{V}O_2$max with aging for the individual who continues to exercise throughout life?*

The Fick equation is presented below and may be expressed in either resting, submaximal, or maximal exercise values.

$$\dot{V}O_2 = (SV \times HR)(a - \bar{v}O_2 \Delta)$$

In the equation $(a - \bar{v} O_2 \Delta)$ is the arterial (a) and mixed venous ($\bar{v}$) blood $O_2$ difference and represents peripheral $O_2$ extraction by the tissues. The term $(SV \times HR)$ represents central delivery of $O_2$. The product of HR and SV in the equation is $\dot{Q}$. To allow for factors pertaining to hemodynamic properties to be used in the equation, $\dot{Q}$ can be alternately solved as (mean arterial pressure [MAP] ÷ total peripheral resistance [TPR]), producing the following version of the Fick equation.

$$\dot{V}O_2 = (MAP \div TPR)(a - \bar{v}O_2 \Delta)$$

These two equations can then be combined.

$$(SV \times HR)(a - \bar{v}O_2 \Delta) = \dot{V}O_2$$
$$= (MAP \div TPR)(a - \bar{v}O_2 \Delta)$$

Finally $(a - \bar{v}O_2 \Delta)$ can be expressed in terms of $O_2$ content: $(CaO_2 - C\bar{v}O_2 \Delta)$. This is read as the difference in $O_2$ content between arterial and mixed venous blood, producing the final equation.

$$(SV \times HR)(CaO_2 - C\bar{v}O_2 \Delta) = \dot{V}O_2$$
$$= (MAP \div TPR)(CaO_2 - C\bar{v}O_2 \Delta)$$

*Figure 16.4* uses this equation to show the effects of age on the cardiorespiratory limitations to exercise. The Fick equation, first presented in Chapter 7, shows that whole-body metabolism ($\dot{V}O_2$) is a function of central cardiac dynamics (SV × HR) and peripheral extraction of $O_2$ ($CaO_2 - C\bar{v}O_2\Delta$). The right side of the equation shows that cardiac function can also be represented as MAP and TPR. The rest of this section presents some key research

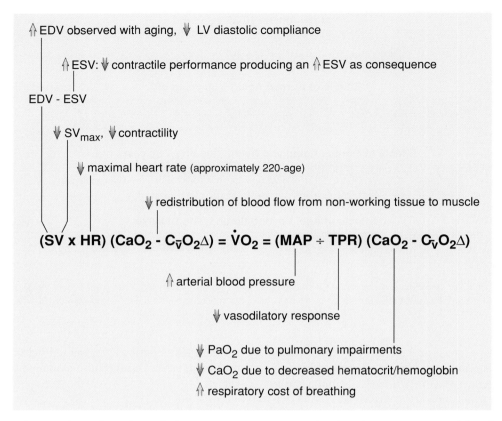

$\Uparrow$ EDV observed with aging, $\Downarrow$ LV diastolic compliance

$\Uparrow$ ESV: $\Downarrow$ contractile performance producing an $\Uparrow$ ESV as consequence

EDV - ESV

$\Downarrow$ SV$_{max}$, $\Downarrow$ contractility

$\Downarrow$ maximal heart rate (approximately 220-age)

$\Downarrow$ redistribution of blood flow from non-working tissue to muscle

$$(SV \times HR)\,(CaO_2 - C_{\bar{v}}O_2\Delta) = \dot{V}O_2 = (MAP \div TPR)\,(CaO_2 - C_{\bar{v}}O_2\Delta)$$

$\Uparrow$ arterial blood pressure

$\Downarrow$ vasodilatory response

$\Downarrow$ PaO$_2$ due to pulmonary impairments
$\Downarrow$ CaO$_2$ due to decreased hematocrit/hemoglobin
$\Uparrow$ respiratory cost of breathing

**FIGURE 16.4.** Effects of age on the cardiorespiratory limitations to exercise as expressed in the Fick equation. EDV, end-diastolic volume; ESV, end-systolic volume; LV, left ventricular; PaO$_2$, partial pressure of arterial oxygen.

studies related to the variables of the Fick equation that help explain how the decline in $\dot{V}O_2$ can be attenuated with age.

### Effects of Exercise Training

A chronic increase in blood volume leading to enhanced diastolic filling rates has been the primary adaptive response for increasing SV$_{max}$, $\dot{Q}_{max}$, and thus $\dot{V}O_2$max in trained younger men. However, it is not clear if improvements in central cardiac factors alone is the mechanism chiefly responsible for attenuating the decline in $\dot{V}O_2$max in trained older people. Other possible causes for the attenuated decline in cardiovascular functional capacity in older people who train include a maintenance of maximal peripheral extraction of O$_2$ (CaO$_2$ − C$\bar{v}$O$_2\Delta$) with aging, secondary to maintenance of muscle oxidative capacity and capillary density and/or maintenance of lean body mass and relative percent fat. The reason the decline in $\dot{V}O_2$max is slowed in older individuals who exercise throughout life is a complex issue. This question is beginning to be answered in the research arena. One thing we know is that the reduced rate of decline does not have anything to do with HR since the maximal HR of endurance-trained older men and women is the same as their sedentary counterparts.

*LINKUP: Refer to* **Research Highlight: Cardiovascular Performance of Endurance-Trained Older Men,** *found at http://connection.lww.com/go/brownexphys and on the Student Resource CD-ROM, for one possible answer to this complicated research question.*

Because HR$_{max}$ does not differ between older endurance-trained athletes and their sedentary peers, the ability to resist the decline in $\dot{V}O_2$max with aging may, to a large degree, rely on a higher SV$_{max}$ and $\dot{Q}_{max}$. Blood volume expansion has been shown to be the key factor in increasing cardiac performance in younger men after training. Since older trained men, like younger men, have larger maximal SV and $\dot{Q}$ values than their sedentary counterparts, it would seem likely that this same mechanism would be important in increasing **diastolic function**, and thus SV$_{max}$ and $\dot{V}O_2$max, in older individuals as well. However, plasma, red cell, and total blood volumes tend to be lower in older individuals matched for body composition and physical activity habits with their younger counterparts. Although exercise-induced hypervolemia has been demonstrated in trained older individuals, it was only very recently that training-induced blood volume-mediated improvements in cardiac function were shown to be operative in older trained men (11).

Hagberg and colleagues (11) demonstrated that plasma and total blood volume were independent predictors of $\dot{V}O_2$max, $SV_{max}$, and end-diastolic volume (EDV) in older men (11). These older male master athletes had peak exercise $\dot{Q}$ and SV indexes that were 25% and 31% higher, respectively, than their sedentary counterparts. *Was this a result of improved diastolic function or systolic function?* Although the importance of diastolic function was stressed in a study of older men, a review of Hagberg's results indicates that **systolic function** may play a significant role as well (11). For example, when measuring the change from rest to peak exercise, end-systolic volume (ESV) was reduced to a greater degree in master athletes ($-25.4$ mL) versus lean sedentary men ($-13.2$ mL), a 92% difference between groups. However, the difference between groups was 66% for EDV. Therefore, the training response in diastolic and systolic functions in this sample of older men tended to be equally distributed, but an argument could be made for the primacy of improved systolic versus diastolic function in this study. Although the authors downplayed the importance of systolic functional improvements in the study, they did stress that improvements in contractility, as evidenced by reductions in ESV, have been shown elsewhere.

An age-related decrease in contractile reserve due to a decrease in beta-adrenergic receptor responsiveness of cardiac tissue may contribute to the age-related change in the ability of the ventricle to reduce its ESV, thus improving SV. However, the results of studies by Hagberg and colleagues (11) and Schulman and colleagues (12) indicate that a training adaptation may also attenuate the reduction in contractile reserve. Myocardial contractility has been shown to be higher in older endurance-trained men compared with a younger group. Also, in a study investigating the cardiovascular adaptations with aging in endurance-trained women, systolic function was maintained across age (9). It is apparent that improved systolic function is an important adaptive response to endurance training, but the preponderance of evidence still points to diastolic functional improvements as being chiefly responsible for attenuating the decline in $\dot{V}O_2$max seen in aging. Additional evidence for this is that in endurance-trained women across four age groups (age ranges for the groups = 20 to 29, 40 to 45, 49 to 54, 58 to 63 years), left ventricular diastolic filling rate (an index of improved diastolic function) averaged approximately 37% faster than left ventricular emptying rate (an index of improved systolic function) (9). Like in younger and older men, blood volume was maintained with age in endurance-trained women, a primary adaptation necessary for improvements in diastolic function. In addition, due to declining maximal HR with age, there is a likely shift away from a dependence on catecholamine-mediated increases in HR and **inotropy** (because of the decreased beta-adrenergic responsiveness in aging) to the use of the Frank-Starling mechanism.

Weibe and coauthors (9) investigated an alternative hypothesis by looking at the peripheral extraction portion of the Fick equation, $CaO_2 - C\bar{v}O_2\Delta$, to explain the age-related reduced decline in $\dot{V}O_2$max. Since there were no differences across the four groups, the maintenance of $CaO_2 - C\bar{v}O_2\Delta$ in endurance-trained women is another mechanism that slows the decline in $\dot{V}O_2$max with age. Weibe and colleagues also stressed that improved diastolic function through blood volume maintenance with age was the key adaptive response. The younger and older women in this study also demonstrated the ability to continue increasing SV to maximal exercise levels. However, there are equivocal results on this ability in other older subjects (13). Finally, there also appears to be some evidence that older men and women adapt differently to chronic endurance training. Spina (14) concluded that two-thirds of the training-induced increase in $\dot{V}O_2$max in older men is due to augmented $\dot{Q}$ and one-third is due to a wider $\Delta CaO_2 - C\bar{v}O_2$, while older women rely more on an increase in $\Delta CaO_2 - C\bar{v}O_2$ to improve $\dot{V}O_2$max.

## THE PULMONARY SYSTEM

The pulmonary system also changes with age, as depicted in Table 16.4. The three important changes of an aged pulmonary system are an increase in alveolar size, less elastic support structure, and respiratory muscle weakening. Like cardiac reserve, pulmonary reserve capacity decreases with age so moderate to strenuous physical activities can be demanding due to pulmonary changes alone. This is especially true if individuals smoke or are chronically exposed to airborne contaminants. The changes that occur in the pulmonary system with age ultimately lead to a greater difficulty in ventilating the alveoli so that during exercise, ventilation differs between young and older individuals. In older individuals, for example, there is an increased dependence on breathing frequency versus tidal volume as exercise intensity increases. The loss of tidal volume reserve, therefore, serves as the primary mechanism for the overall loss of pulmonary reserve with aging. The primary factor for the decreased dependence on tidal volume during exercise of increasing intensity is the structural disintegration that comes from a gradual loss of lung support structure elasticity.

Along with these pulmonary structural and functional changes, there is also a decline in the strength of the respiratory muscles and a reduced ventilatory efficiency with age. Ventilatory efficiency is the ratio of the change in ventilation to the change in $\dot{V}CO_2$ at low to moderate exercise intensities. The end result is a potential impairment in the $O_2$ transport capacity. However, because of the large reserve capacity of the lungs, there does not appear to be a compromise in the ability of the elderly to ventilate the lungs in normal aging. Therefore, ventilation, for young or old subjects, does not limit endurance performance.

## THE NEUROMUSCULAR SYSTEM

Maintaining adequate functional capacity of the neuromuscular system is important to remaining independent with advancing age. The neuromuscular benefits of

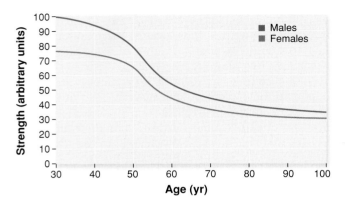

**FIGURE 16.5.** Proposed strength curves from a compilation of findings on the changes in voluntary strength (isometric and dynamic contractions from several limb muscles) with increasing age. As shown, males are stronger than females throughout life, but the difference in strength becomes less with advanced age. Data from Rice CL, Cunningham DA. Aging of the neuromuscular system: influences of gender and physical activity. In: Shephard RJ. *Gender, physical activity, and aging*. London: CRC Press, 2002:121–150.

exercise in elderly people are perhaps the most substantial because they can reduce the number of falls that occur, which can significantly affect the rest of individuals' lives. The ability of older persons to perform ADL is largely dependent on the maintenance of muscle mass, strength, and power, factors that are essential if elderly individuals are to maintain functional abilities and quality of life.

Starting about age 30 muscle strength declines at a rate of 10% to 15% per decade (15). At about the seventh or eighth decade of life the decline in strength has reached its lowest point (50% of the strength level of young adults). Further loss with aging beyond the eighth decade is usually less drastic. As shown in *Figure 16.5*, strength levels may be maintained fairly well to about age 50, with an accelerated decline over the next 25 years. With the decline in strength, there is also a loss of speed of movement, which affects the ability of older individuals to generate power. The rate of loss in power-generating capacity may be twice as great as the decline in strength after age 65, resulting in more serious difficulties with daily activities than is accounted for by strength loss alone. Elderly people show large and functionally important gains in isometric and dynamic strength, power, and force control following strength training. Although elderly people rely more on neural changes to improve strength than do younger subjects, muscle hypertrophy and muscle protein turnover does occur.

## Sarcopenia

Sarcopenia is the loss of muscle mass with aging. This section provides a discussion on the effect exercise training may have in attenuating muscle loss in the elderly. Since strength is related to muscle cross-sectional area, the occurrence of sarcopenia with aging is also associated with

strength deficits. Two major factors account for loss of muscle mass with aging:

- Decrease in individual fiber size (atrophy)
- Reduction in muscle fiber number

The loss of fiber size comes about primarily through reductions in type II fiber cross-sectional area. This, in turn, is accounted for by **motor unit remodeling** with age. Motor unit remodeling in older individuals occurs as a result of alterations in the normal turnover of synaptic connections at neuromuscular junctions. In elderly (as in younger) individuals, the turnover of synaptic junctions occurs as a consequence of a cyclic denervation, axonal sprouting, and reinnervation of the muscle. In aging, a large amount of reinnervation of muscle fibers occurs by collateral axonal sprouting from adjacent type I fibers. In this situation, some denervated type II fibers become reinnervated by axonal sprouting from adjacent innervated type I fibers. Thus, with aging there is a decrease in type II fiber number and a concomitant increase in type I fibers. The loss in type II fiber number is a direct consequence of some of these fibers remaining denervated with atrophy occurring and some type II fibers being reinnervated by type I α-motor neurons. Some type II fibers, therefore, become (or approximate) type I fibers with respect to their physiologic and biochemical properties. When this occurs, whole-muscle performance is altered as resistance to fatigue is increased due to the proliferation of type I fibers, while peak torque is reduced due to the reduction in type II fibers. Remodeling ultimately leads to a reduction in the number of motor units with age. The number of motor units decreases by about 1% per year beginning in the third decade and accelerates beyond age 60. It is presently not known if remodeling can be altered with exercise training.

The functional decline with age is a common consequence of sarcopenia, but loss of muscle mass and gross structural adaptations do not fully explain the fact that age-related weakness ensues. For example, there are other changes in the neuromuscular system occurring with age. Central drive, the ability to activate muscle voluntarily, decreases with age due to the progressive increase of the corticospinal tract's threshold of excitability. There is also a decrease in motoneuron conduction velocity and an increase in electrical resistance of the sarcolemma. Sarcopenia and neural changes that accompany aging ultimately lead to strength and power deficits. Falls, a consequence of these functional deficits, are the primary cause of injury, morbidity, and mortality in elderly individuals. However, there is increased evidence that progressive resistance exercise can improve the functional status of elderly individuals apart from changes in central cardiac function. Case study 16.1 shows how resistance-exercise training improves the functional abilities of individuals with congestive heart failure. If resistance training is performed throughout life, older men are generally similar to their younger sedentary counterparts in dynamic strength, maximum voluntary isometric strength, muscle cross-sectional

## CASE STUDY 16.1: *CLINICAL BENEFITS OF RESISTANCE EXERCISE*

### CASE

Frank is a 73-year-old male with a history of ischemic and nonischemic congestive heart failure (CHF). Frank presented with a significant history of chronic obstructive pulmonary disease, permanent pacemaker (1992), implanted cardiac defibrillator, chronic atrial fibrillation, post-myocardial infarction, coronary artery bypass graft surgery (five grafts in 1990), and noninsulin-dependent diabetes mellitus. Frank also has an extensive social history for smoking (30 pack years). Frank has been weight stable at 220 lb (100 kg) for the past 3 months and is currently taking the following medications: isosorbide mononitrate, albuterol, metformin, albuterol/ipratropium, temazepam, fosinopril, warfarin, digoxin, and furosemide daily.

Frank was referred by a local cardiologist to be a participant in an exercise-training research study. Resting ejection fraction was 10%, resting heart rate was 78 beats per minute (bpm) (paced), and resting blood pressure was 102/58. The entry exercise test consisted of a modified Naughton protocol on which Frank exercised for 4.5 minutes and stopped due to fatigue and shortness of breath. $\dot{V}O_2$peak was 14.0 mL·kg$^{-1}$·min$^{-1}$, peak respiratory exchange ratio was 1.06, and peak rating of perceived exertion (RPE) was 17. Peak heart rate was 116 bpm with a peak blood pressure of 126/58. Frank experienced chest pain and dyspnea upon cessation of the exercise test and requested to assume a supine position during recovery. Water was given ad labitum. Sublingual nitroglycerin was administered, and symptoms resolved within 2 minutes of supine recovery. Frank was sent back to the cardiologist because of the chest pain.

### EVALUATION/INTERVENTION

As part of a research study examining if resistance exercise can increase the functional ability of CHF patients, Frank was randomized into the project's experimental group. Frank was studied at baseline for mixed-muscle, whole-body, and plasma protein synthesis rates. Stable isotopes were used during a 10-hour study at baseline and post-exercise. Frank performed exercise for 12 weeks at 80% of one repetition maximum (1 RM). He was carefully monitored for the first six sessions for changes in heart rate and rate-pressure product. Frank was familiarized for the first six sessions at 50% of 1 RM. As a result of the experimental study, Frank's strength increased 90% over 12 weeks. Total work expressed in joules increased by 125%. Functional measures for timed walking speed and stair ascent increased 45% from baseline to post-exercise. Percent body fat decreased by 17% after 12 weeks and Frank lost 4.5 kg body weight. Mixed-muscle protein synthesis increased 90% during training. Frank self-reported that he felt better, was less fatigued, and was sleeping better. Frank also reported that he and his wife went on a walking tour of northern Italy. Frank's metformin dosage was cut in half midway through the exercise study.

A post-exercise exit treadmill test revealed a significant improvement in exercise tolerance from 8.0 minutes to 17.0 minutes on the modified Naughton protocol. $\dot{V}O_2$peak increased from 10.5 to 16.5 mL·kg$^{-1}$·min$^{-1}$, RPE was 13 to 14, and Frank had no symptoms of chest pain following the test.

Used with permission from Charles Cortes, PhD, Department of Surgery, Metabolism Unit, The University of Texas Medical Branch at Galveston.

---

area, and power. It is possible, therefore, to preserve muscle function similar to that of younger sedentary adults if an active lifestyle is maintained during aging.

Several studies demonstrate that elderly people can increase muscle protein synthesis following resistance training, thus attenuating sarcopenia and increasing functional abilities In one study, a group of elderly male and female subjects ($\geq$76 years old) resistance trained 3 days per week for 3 months at 65% to 100% of one repetition maximum (1 RM) (16). Following training, subjects had a significantly greater mixed muscle protein synthesis rate, increased muscle mass, and greater isokinetic strength at an angular velocity of 60 degrees·sec$^{-1}$. This study and others refute the idea held previously that elderly subjects gain strength only through neural adaptations, i.e., improvements in motor unit recruitment and activation patterns. It is probably the case, however, that longer periods of training are needed to demonstrate hypertrophy in elderly subjects. In a 2-year trial of resistance-exercise training 2 days

per week at 80% of 1 RM, elderly subjects increased their muscle cross-sectional area by 8.7% with no change observed in the control group (17). The following list shows the types of functional improvements demonstrated in frail elderly subjects participating in resistance training.

- Increased dynamic and static strength
- Increased gait velocity
- Improved stair-climbing power
- Increase in the level of spontaneous physical activity
- Improved power at several joints, i.e., knee, elbow, shoulder, and ankle

▶ *INQUIRY SUMMARY.* The reduction in $\dot{V}O_2$ with age is a normal consequence of a reduced maximal HR and $\dot{Q}$. Even though the pulmonary system does demonstrate structural and functional changes, pulmonary reserve with normal aging is great enough to rule out the pulmonary system limiting maximal aerobic power. The loss of aerobic power that does occur can be attenuated with age as a

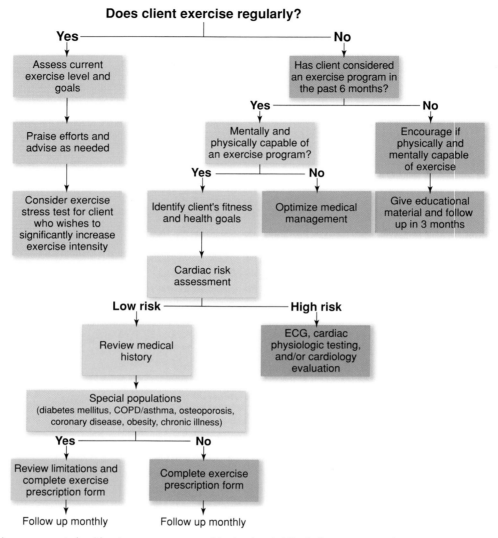

**FIGURE 16.6.** Exercise assessment algorithm to gauge current activity level and ability before recommending an exercise program to older clients. Reprinted with permission from Brennan FH Jr. Exercise prescriptions for active seniors. A team approach for maximizing adherence. *Phys Sportsmed* 2002;30:19–29, copyright 2005. The McGraw-Hill Companies. All rights reserved.

consequence of primary physiologic adaptations in central cardiac function that arise as a result of the expanded blood volume and improved diastolic and systolic function following endurance training. Sarcopenia and neural changes are an inevitable result of aging. With sarcopenia, there is a progressive loss of functional capacity that ultimately leads to dependency. An effective countermeasure to sarcopenia is regular resistance training, which leads to increased muscle protein synthesis, improved motor unit activation, and increases in functional abilities. *In what way might the physiologic changes brought on by exercise reduce the incidence of disability in older individuals? How do you think the attenuation of sarcopenia and the increase in aerobic power with exercise training complement one another to improve the functional abilities of elderly individuals?*

## *Exercise Training for the Elderly*

Elderly individuals of all ages can adapt and respond to endurance and strength training. Besides the benefits for the cardiovascular, pulmonary, and neuromuscular systems just reviewed, additional benefits from regular exercise include improved bone health, reduction in risk for osteoporosis, improved postural stability, more optimal body composition, and increased flexibility and range of motion.

### EXERCISE GUIDELINES FOR OLDER ADULTS

The American College of Sports Medicine lists the following goals for older adults engaging in an exercise program:

1. Maintenance of functional capacity for independent living

2. Reduction in the risk of cardiovascular disease
3. Retardation of the progression of chronic disease
4. Promotion of psychologic well-being
5. Provision of opportunities for social interaction

These goals can best be met when programs are tailored to the individual. Three considerations are especially important to follow for the elderly client: exercise assessment, risk assessment, and exercise prescription. When you are considering exercise assessment, an algorithm is helpful in determining an individual's ability to start an exercise program (*Fig. 16.6*). At the same time the exercise assessment algorithm is being used, a cardiovascular risk assessment algorithm should also be followed (*Fig. 16.7*). These algorithms can be used with the Physical Activity Readiness Questionnaire presented in Chapter 20. Taken together, these devices give both client and exercise personnel confidence that the individual is ready to participate.

When you are beginning an exercise program, guidelines to formulate the exercise prescription, such as the one presented in *Figure 16.8*, can be used. When the individual has known cardiac or moderate to severe valvular disease, symptoms suggestive of disease, or two or more cardiac risk factors (advanced age is one), cardiac physiologic testing, electrocardiogram, echocardiogram, and/or cardiology consultation before starting a vigorous exercise prescription should be sought. Pulmonary function testing and medical consultation should be sought for individuals with a history of pulmonary disease. When elderly individuals have low to moderate risk, there is generally no need for medical examination or a stress test before beginning a low- to moderate-intensity exercise program.

For the elderly individual, the following guidelines are recommended:

- Mode of activity: the program should be comprehensive and should incorporate cardiovascular, strength, and flexibility training. The individual should enjoy the activities, and the activities should be safe within the physical limitations of the individual. Aquatic exercise and other exercises during which weight is supported may be especially suited to elderly individuals with reduced ability to tolerate weight-bearing activity. Elderly individuals should be willing to comply with the program.
- Duration of activity: continuous or performed in short bouts throughout the day, gradually increasing session time by as little as 5 minutes per week to reach a final goal of 30 to 40 minutes of total exercise for that day.

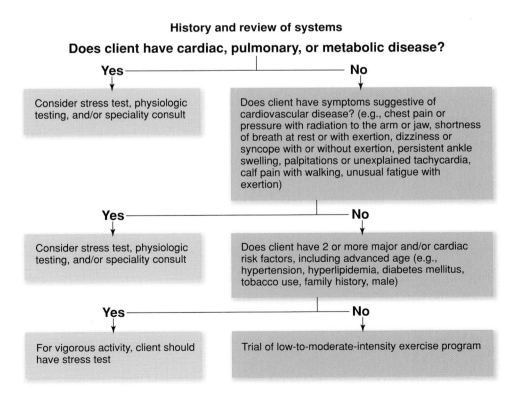

**History and review of systems**

**Does client have cardiac, pulmonary, or metabolic disease?**

Yes ——————————— No

Consider stress test, physiologic testing, and/or speciality consult

Does client have symptoms suggestive of cardiovascular disease? (e.g., chest pain or pressure with radiation to the arm or jaw, shortness of breath at rest or with exertion, dizziness or syncope with or without exertion, persistent ankle swelling, palpitations or unexplained tachycardia, calf pain with walking, unusual fatigue with exertion)

Yes ——————————— No

Consider stress test, physiologic testing, and/or speciality consult

Does client have 2 or more major and/or cardiac risk factors, including advanced age (e.g., hypertension, hyperlipidemia, diabetes mellitus, tobacco use, family history, male)

Yes ——————————— No

For vigorous activity, client should have stress test

Trial of low-to-moderate-intensity exercise program

**FIGURE 16.7.** Cardiovascular risk assessment algorithm for older adults to evaluate and assess potential cardiovascular risks for those about to begin an exercise program. *The choice of a particular test depends on the patient's baseline electrocardiogram and physical ability. Reprinted with permission from Brennan FH Jr. Exercise prescriptions for active seniors. A team approach for maximizing adherence. *Phys Sportsmed* 2002;30:19–29,

Name: _____    Age: _____    Date: ___ / ___ / ___

**I. Mode of Activity:**    ☐ Jogging    ☐ Water aerobics    ☐ Rowing    ☐ Walking
                           ☐ Cycling    ☐ Swimming    ☐ Racket sports    ☐ _____

**II. Duration**    ☐ 20 minutes    ☐ 40 minutes    ☐ _____ minutes

**III. Frequency:**    _____ times per week

**IV. Intensity**    ☐ low    ☐ moderate    ☐ vigorous

Low-intensity exercise: < 40% $\dot{V}O_2$reserve (Borg 10 = < 40% HRR)
Moderate-intensity exercise: 40% to 60% $\dot{V}O_2$reserve (Borg 13 = 60% HRR)
Vigorous-intensity exercise: > 60% $\dot{V}O_2$reserve (Borg 16 = 80% HRR)

Calculating Cardiovascular Training Zone:
    A. Calculate client's maximal heart rate (Max HR).* 220-age in years = Max HR =_____ beats per minute (bpm)
    B. Take clients's resting heart rate (RHR) and record = _____ bpm
    C. Heart Rate Reserve (HRR) = maximum heart rate-resting heart rate = _____ bpm
    D. Estimate cardiovascular training zone = HRR x % intensity (e.g., 40%) + RHR = Target Heart Rate in bpm
    E. Cardiovascular training zone: **Try to keep the heart rate within 10 bpm of the calculated number**

* Consider buying a heart rate monitor as a guide

**V. Progression of Conditioning**
    ☐ Initial Phase
    ☐ Duration: 4 to 6 weeks
    ☐ Goal is to increase frequency, proper form, and form "good habits"

    ☐ Improvement Phase
    ☐ Duration: 4 to 6 months
    ☐ Goal is to gradually increase duration and intensity of exercise

    ☐ Maintenance Phase
    ☐ Occurs after 6 months
    ☐ Goal is to maintain cardiovascular fitness while avoiding overuse injuries

**Borg Relative Perceived Exertion Scale**

| 6 | | |
|---|---|---|
| 7 | Very, very light | |
| 8 | | Low intensity |
| 9 | Very light | |
| 10 | | |
| 11 | Fairly light | |
| 12 | | |
| 13 | Somewhat hard | Moderate intensity |
| 14 | | |
| 15 | Hard | |
| 16 | | |
| 17 | Very hard | Vigorous intensity |
| 19 | | |
| 20 | Very, very hard | |

**VI. Special Precautions**
    Coronary heart disease _____
    Diabetes mellitus _____
    Osteoarthritis _____
    Asthma _____
    Pulmonary disease _____
    Obesity _____
    Chronic illness _____
    Other _____

**VII. Follow-up Appointment**
    Primary Care Provider: _____
    Office Phone Number: _____

**FIGURE 16.8.** Worksheet of exercise prescription for active seniors. Reprinted with permission from Brennan FH Jr. Exercise prescriptions for active seniors. A team approach for maximizing adherence. *Phys Sportsmed* 2002;30:19–29, copyright 2005. The McGraw-Hill Companies. All rights reserved.

- Frequency: the current recommendation is to exercise most days of the week; however, in some instances when clients have very poor functional capacities, frequency should be increased while training duration and intensity are decreased.
- Intensity: the difficulty level can be low, moderate, or high, depending on the individual's fitness level and ultimate goals. In general, a low- to moderate-intensity program is best for elderly individuals. The level of intensity depends to a large extent on the individual. For some sedentary clients, aerobic exercise as low as 20% to 30% $\dot{V}O_{2max}$ is a sufficient intensity stimulus. The goal is to maintain their interest, avoid overuse injuries, and avoid triggering a cardiovascular event.
- Progression: slow progression is key for the elderly exerciser due to a slower physiologic rate of adaptation.
- Timely follow up: since elderly clients need to be encouraged, regular monitoring of progress is necessary. Encouragement should come in the form of how to advance their training, what to expect as they exercise, and who to contact if any questions or concerns arise.

The algorithms and exercise prescription forms increase client safety when carefully followed. More will be said about exercise prescription for elderly people in Chapter 19. Also, the last section of the book details specific exercise recommendations for clinical populations.

Because mode of activity for elderly individuals should be comprehensive, a resistance-training program is recommended in addition to the aerobic exercise prescription. This type of program need not be elaborate and may consist of about eight to ten basic resistance exercises working major muscle groups. Flexibility exercises should also be incorporated into each exercise session, primarily as warmup and cooldown activities, with special attention to stretching the hamstrings and muscles in the low back. Strength and flexibility training guidelines for older individuals are as follows.

1. Light warmup and cooldown of 5 to 10 minutes involving active range of motion activities that stretch the major joints. It is recommended that activity to increase circulation precede stretching warmups. Ballistic movements should be avoided.
2. Work large muscle groups (quadriceps, gluteals, hamstrings, deltoids, biceps, triceps, latissimus dorsi, and abdominal muscles). The best exercises to perform are multijoint movements.
3. Use weights that can be lifted 10 to 15 times with "fairly light" to "somewhat hard" exertion. Avoid excessive straining during lifting and breathe freely during the lift (normal breathing pattern). When that weight becomes too easy, increase the weight slightly, but keep the number of repetitions the same.
4. Lift the weight in a fairly slow, deliberate manner working the muscles through their normal range of motion (do not do partial lifts or movements). Ballistic movements should be avoided.
5. Perform one to two sets, 2 to 3 days per week. Rest for 1 to 2 seconds between repetitions and 1 to 2 minutes between sets of exercises.
6. Rest 48 hours between sessions for recovery.
7. Stop immediately and sit or lie down if chest pain or pressure, dizziness, abnormal heartbeats, or unusual shortness of breath are experienced. If symptoms are not relieved after 1 or 2 minutes of rest, get assistance. Report any symptoms to a physician before resuming exercise.
8. Exercise with training partner(s).
9. Drink plenty of fluids before, during, and after resistance training.
10. Avoid fast transitions from one type of movement to another to avoid postural hypotension, which may produce dizziness, fainting, or falling.

▶ *INQUIRY SUMMARY.* The general recommendations for beginning an exercise program for senior clients apply to adults of all ages. Key to these recommendations is the necessity of a comprehensive program of endurance, resistance, and flexibility exercises. *Why is a comprehensive program recommended?*

## Summary

Physical inactivity leads to an increased rate of physiologic aging and ultimately to a greater prevalence of disability across the population. This in turn broadens the socioeconomic impact of aging. This impact can be lessened and the quality of life can be improved in individuals who engage in chronic exercise training. Exercise training produces significant physiologic adaptations in the cardiopulmonary and neuromuscular systems that lead to functional improvements and increase the functional abilities of people as they age. Trained elderly individuals are often similar to their younger untrained counterparts in terms of the functional capacities of the muscular and cardiopulmonary systems. The rate of decline in aerobic power and muscular strength and power is attenuated when people engage in exercise training throughout life.

### SUMMARY KNOWLEDGE

1. Define primary and secondary aging and discuss the interrelationship between these two terms.
2. Define aging and distinguish between the chronologic, biologic, and pathologic components.
3. Explain how exercise helps maintain independent living.
4. Why does maximal heart rate decline with age and what effect does this have on aerobic power?
5. Why is maintenance of strength necessary in old age?
6. Why is the process of sarcopenia an important concept in the study of the physiology of aging?

7. Why is blood volume expansion with aerobic training important in attenuating the decline in aerobic power with aging?

8. What is the relationship between disability and independence?

9. Discuss the neuromuscular consequences of aging and the impact this has on the functional capacity of the muscular system.

10. How is it possible to improve the functional capacity of individuals without improving central cardiac function?

### References

1. Kohn RR. Aging and age-related diseases: normal processes. In: Johnson HA, ed. *Relations between normal aging and disease*. New York: Raven Press, 1985:1–43.

2. Lee IM, Hsieh CC, Paffenbarger RS Jr. Exercise intensity and longevity in men. The Harvard alumni health study. *JAMA* 1995;273:1179–1184.

3. Maquire GH. Activities of daily living. In: Lewis CB, ed. *Aging: the health care challenge*. Philadelphia: FA Davis Co, 1996:47–78.

4. Kasch FW. Thirty-three years of aerobic exercise adherence. *Quest* 2001;53:362–365.

5. Paterson DH, Cunningham DA, Koval JJ, et al. Aerobic fitness in a population of independently living men and women aged 55–86 years. *Med Sci Sports Exerc* 1999;31:1813–1820.

6. Shephard RJ. Conclusions: implications for health and society. In: Shephard RJ, ed. *Gender, physical activity, and aging*. London: CRC Press, 2002:265–281.

7. Physical activity in old age. *Lancet* 1986;2:1431.

8. Silverstone B. Public policies on aging: reconsidering old-age eligibility. *Gerontologist* 1994;34:724–725.

9. Wiebe CG, Gledhill N, Jamnik VK, et al. Exercise cardiac function in young through elderly endurance trained women. *Med Sci Sports Exerc* 1999;31:684–691.

10. Fleg JL, Bos AG, Brant LH, et al. Longitudinal decline of aerobic capacity accelerates with age. *Circulation* 2000;102 (suppl II):602. Abstract 108262.

11. Hagberg JM, Goldberg AP, Lakatta L, et al. Expanded blood volumes contribute to the increased cardiovascular performance of endurance-trained older men. *J Appl Physiol* 1998;85:484–489.

12. Schulman SP, Fleg JL, Goldberg AP. Continuum of cardiovascular performance across a broad range of fitness levels in healthy older men. *Circulation* 1996;94:359–367.

13. Proctor DN, Beck KC, Shen PH, et al. Influence of age and gender on cardiac output-$VO_2$ relationships during submaximal cycle ergometry. *J Appl Physiol* 1998;84:599–605.

14. Spina RJ. Cardiovascular adaptations to endurance exercise training in older men and women. *Exerc Sport Sci Rev* 1999; 27:317–332.

15. Lindle RS, Metter EJ, Lynch NA, et al. Age and gender comparisons of muscle strength in 654 women and men aged 20–93 years. *J Appl Physiol* 1997;83:1581–1587.

16. Yarasheski KE, Pak-Loduca J, Hasten DL, et al. Resistance exercise training increases mixed muscle protein synthesis rate in frail women and men ≥76 years old. *Am J Physiol* 1999;277:E118–E125.

17. McCartney N, Hicks AL, Martin J, et al. A longitudinal trial of weight training in the elderly: continued improvements in year 2. *J Gerontol A Biol Sci Med Sci* 1996;51:B425–B433.

### Suggested Readings

Beissner KL, Collins JE, Holmes H. Muscle force and range of motion as predictors of function in older adults. *Phys Ther* 2000;80:556–563.

Lewis CB, ed. *Aging: the health care challenge*. Philadelphia: FA Davis Co, 1996.

Shephard RJ, ed. *Gender, physical activity, and aging*. London: CRC Press, 2002.

Evans WJ. Exercise training guidelines for the elderly. *Med Sci Sports Exerc* 1999;31:12–17.

### On The Internet

University of Texas Southwestern Medical Center: Shay/Wright Laboratory: Facts about telomeres and telomerase. Available at: **http://www.swmed.edu/home_pages/cellbio/shay-wright/intro/facts/sw_facts.html**. Accessed June 14, 2005.

University of Texas Southwestern Medical Center: Shay/Wright Laboratory. Available at: **http://www.swmed.edu/home_pages/cellbio/shay-wright/index.html**. Accessed June 14, 2005.

United States Administration on Aging. Available at: **http://www.aoa.dhhs.gov/**. Accessed June 14, 2005.

Institute of Gerontology at Wayne State University. Available at: **http://www.iog.wayne.edu/**. Accessed June 14, 2005.

United States Census Bureau. Available at: **http://www.census.gov/**. Accessed June 14, 2005.

## Writing to Learn

1. There is a gradual change in body composition with age as muscle mass progressively declines and fat mass increases. At the same time there is a progressive reduction in $\dot{V}O_2$ with age. Write a paper describing how the change in body composition affects the $\dot{V}O_2$ as a person ages.

2. Design a study to determine the validity and reliability of the Maguire Trilevel ADL Assessment instrument.

# CHAPTER

# 17 Female-Specific Issues

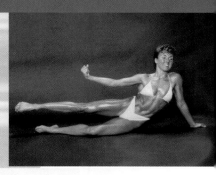

*Although it is now well accepted that exercise is beneficial for women as well as men, this was not the case just a generation or two ago. Until the last one-third of the 20th century, women were considered too weak or fragile to participate in vigorous exercise, and society thought it was doing women a favor by protecting them against the stresses and physiologic risks associated with exercise and athletics. Young girls who enjoyed sports a generation ago were sometimes called "Tomboys" rather than female athletes. Young boys who had not yet developed the motor skills or athletic abilities of their peers might have heard things like "you throw like a girl." As more teenage and older women began participating in athletics, scientists began studying the physiology of exercise in girls and women.* Are there any special considerations for girls or women who want to exercise train and participate in athletic competition?

## CHAPTER OUTLINE

COMPARISONS BETWEEN THE SEXES
- Morphologic Differences
- Physiologic Differences
- Trainability
GYNECOLOGIC CONSIDERATIONS
- Menstruation
- Pregnancy
  - Exercise and Fetal Well-Being
  - Exercise and Obstetric Outcome
  - Exercise and Maternal Well-Being
  - Exercise and Post-Partum Athletic Performance

- Lactation
- Menopause
NUTRITIONAL ISSUES
- Osteoporosis
- Iron Deficiency
- Eating Disorders
- Female Athlete Triad
- Excessive Exercise Disorder
- Special Nutritional Needs for Women
  - Nutritional Concerns During Pregnancy
  - Nutritional Concerns for Lactation
  - Nutritional Needs Post-Menopause

Because most of the epidemiologic research on exercise and health has been performed on men rather than women, many of the conclusions about exercise and health for women may be intrinsically biased. Only in the past 30 years or so have exercise scientists been studying female-specific issues related to exercise training. Although still in its infancy, the science of exercise physiology for women has given us insights into the inherent physiologic differences between males and females, how females respond to exercise training, the risks of exercise training for females, exercise and the female reproductive system, and nutritional factors that are specific to the female athlete. These and other issues relevant to the exercising female are discussed in this chapter.

## Comparisons Between the Sexes

*Are women different from men, and are boys different from girls?* The overall answer to this question may seem obvious, but the answer could be either yes or no in the realm of exercise physiology. Anatomically, it is quite apparent that females are different from males. These anatomic differences are generally a reflection of hormonal differences between the sexes, which in turn are really due to the sex-specific **genotype** expression for each sex. *The questions for exercise scientists then are: What are the inherent differences between the sexes, and how do these differences affect the exercise response?* Box 17.1 profiles a prominent researcher in this area.

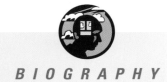

### BIOGRAPHY

# Barbara L. Drinkwater

Barbara L. Drinkwater received her BS degree from Douglass College, her master's degree from the University of North Carolina at Greensboro, and her PhD from Purdue University. Both Douglass College and the University of North Carolina have awarded her their Distinguished Alumni Awards. DeMontfort University in the United Kingdom and the University of Toronto in Canada have awarded Drinkwater honorary doctorates.

Drinkwater's research has revolved around the response of women to exercise as mediated by environmental factors and aging. Special areas of interest have been the female athlete, the female athlete's performance under environmental stressors such as heat and altitude, the effect of athletic amenorrhea on bone health, and the role of calcium and exercise in preventing osteoporosis. Drinkwater currently serves as a member of the Scientific Advisory Board of the National Osteoporosis Foundation.

Although Drinkwater has served in many professional organizations, she has been particularly active in the American College of Sports Medicine (ACSM). She has served on the

Board of Trustees, as Vice-President for Education, and as President. In 1984 she received the ACSM Citation Award and in 1996, the prestigious ACSM Honor Award.

The early years in Drinkwater's career were spent at the Institute of Environmental Stress at the University of California at Santa Barbara (1969–1982). She then had a brief stint at the

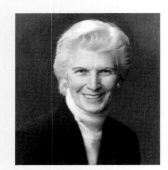

Barbara L. Drinkwater, Ph.D.

Department of Kinesiology at the University of Washington (1982–1984). She finished her career as a research physiologist in the Department of Medicine at the Pacific Medical Center in Seattle, Washington. Drinkwater has not only made a significant contribution to our understanding of female-specific issues in exercise physiology but has distinguished herself as one of the premier exercise physiologists of our time.

## MORPHOLOGIC DIFFERENCES

Probably the most obvious differences between the sexes in regard to athletic performance or exercise training are those of inherent size and body composition. These differences between the sexes are quite small and of minimal consequence during exercise or athletic performance throughout childhood. However, from adolescence forward, girls cannot compete with boys because they do not have the muscle mass and strength of boys. After puberty, girls have broader hips than boys, whereas boys have broader shoulders with longer arms and legs than girls (*Fig. 17.1*). Compared with the average adult male, the average female is about 8 to 10 cm shorter, is 11 to 14 kg lighter in total body mass, has 5 to 7 kg more adipose tissue, and has 18 to 20 kg less lean body mass (1). Furthermore, men have greater muscle mass and heart volumes than women, while women have smaller blood and lung volumes than men (Table 17.1) (2–4).

These structural differences impose significant limitations for women competing in athletic events in which per-

formance is based primarily on strength, power, leverage, and/or aerobic capacity. This fact is illustrated in *Figure 17.2* where it is shown that the woman-to-man fitness score ratios for cardiorespiratory capacity ($\dot{V}O_{2max}$), muscular strength, and muscular endurance are far below the line of equality. On the other hand, the woman-to-man comparative ratio for flexibility and body fat is much greater than the line of equality.

The point can be further illustrated in competitive athletics. The world records for sports such as track and field or speed skating are better for men than for women. The inherent morphologic differences between men and women are also considered when they participate in sports. For example, the net height for men's volleyball is 8 ft (2.438 m), whereas the net height for women's volleyball is 7.3 ft (2.235 m). The difference in net height takes into consideration the fact that women are shorter than men and have a lower capacity for developing power. The circumference for a man's basketball is 29.5 in (74.9 cm) versus 28.5 in (72.4 cm) for a women's basketball. The size difference takes into account the smaller hand size of

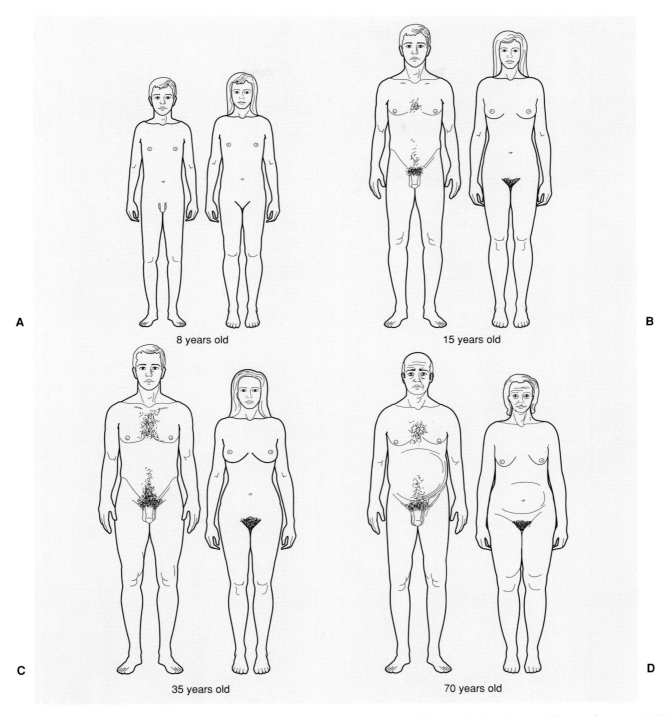

**A** 8 years old

**B** 15 years old

**C** 35 years old

**D** 70 years old

**FIGURE 17.1.** Male/female morphologic differences. **A.** 8-year-old boy and girl. **B.** 15-year-old boy and girl. **C.** 35-year-old man and woman. **D.** 70-year-old man and woman.

women. The tee-off location for women on a golf course is several meters closer to the hole than it is for men, again taking into consideration the woman's lesser ability to generate power. These adjustments are made because the morphologic differences between men and women affect their physical capacities and abilities to perform.

## PHYSIOLOGIC DIFFERENCES

Overall, women are about two-thirds as strong as men, but this ratio varies depending upon the muscle groups tested and how strength is expressed (*Fig. 17.3*). Disparity between the genders in absolute muscle strength (total force

| *Table 17.1* | INHERENT MORPHOLOGIC AND PHYSIOLOGIC DIFFERENCES BETWEEN GENDERS* | |
| --- | --- | --- |
| **Variable** | **Male** | **Female** |
| Slow-twitch fiber size ($\mu$m$^2$) | 5699 | 3875 |
| Fast-twitch fiber size ($\mu$m$^2$) | 4965 | 4193 |
| Vital capacity (mL) | 4800 | 3200 |
| Residual volume (mL) | 1200 | 1000 |
| Total lung capacity (mL) | 6000 | 4200 |
| Heart volume (mL) | 785 | 560 |
| Left ventricular mass (g) | 189 | 115 |
| Resting stroke volume (mL) | 118 | 92 |
| Maximal stroke volume (mL) | 134 | 100 |
| Maximal cardiac output (L·min$^{-1}$) | 24.1 | 18.5 |
| $\dot{V}O_{2max}$ (L·min$^{-1}$) | 3.79 | 2.41 |
| $\dot{V}O_{2max}$ (mL·kg$^{-1}$·min$^{-1}$) | 55.4 | 42.4 |
| $\dot{V}O_{2max}$ (mL·kg$^{-1}$LBM·min$^{-1}$) | 63.1 | 55.1 |
| Hemoglobin (g·dL$^{-1}$) | 15.3 | 13.6 |
| Blood volume (L) | 5.25 | 4.07 |
| Resting $\Delta a - \overline{v}O_2$ (mL·dL$^{-1}$) | 6.9 | 5.0 |
| Maximal $\Delta a - \overline{v}O_2$ (mL·dL$^{-1}$) | 17.0 | 14.3 |

*Values do not reflect extremes seen with adaptations to athletic training. $\Delta a$-$\overline{v}O_2$, arterial $-$ mixed venous $O_2$ difference.

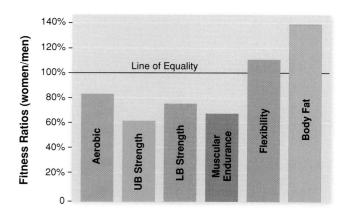

FIGURE 17.2. Comparisons of fitness ratios at the 50th percentile for males and females aged 20 to 29 years. Aerobic, cardiorespiratory fitness ($\dot{V}O_{2max}$ as mL·kg$^{-1}$·min$^{-1}$); UB strength, bench press·body weight$^{-1}$; LB strength, leg press·body weight$^{-1}$; muscular endurance, pushups; flexibility, sit & reach; body fat, % body fat. Line of equality is where scores between the genders are equal. Data from American College of Sports Medicine. *ACSM's guidelines for exercise testing and prescription.* 6th ed. Baltimore: Lippincott Williams & Wilkins, 2000:57–90.

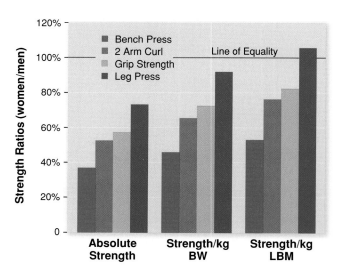

FIGURE 17.3. Comparison of strength ratios between untrained females and males. BW, body weight; LBM, lean body mass. Line of equality is where scores between the genders are equal. Data from Wilmore JH. Alterations in strength, body composition and anthropometric measurements consequent to a 10-week weight training program. *Med Sci Sports* 1974;6:133–138.

generated) diverges when muscle groups in the upper body are compared. On the other hand, the disparity between genders in absolute strength converges when muscle groups in the lower body are compared (5). Since it is generally accepted that muscle strength is directly related to muscle size, the differences in strength between men and women continue to converge as strength is expressed relative to body weight and lean body mass (Fig. 17.3). This convergence is depicted in the figure as the bars get progressively closer to 100% (i.e., when viewing strength as absolute versus relative to body mass or lean body mass), the point at which there is no strength difference. For example, bench-press strength depicted as absolute strength has a ratio of 0.35, that is, women's strength is only 35% of men's strength in the bench-press exercise. However, the ratio becomes 45% when strength is viewed relative to body mass and slightly more than 50% when viewed relative to lean body mass.

With this in mind, the relative strength differences between men and women are simply a reflection of muscular hypertrophy. This hypertrophy is due to the larger size (15% to 30%) of the individual muscle fibers in men since the number of muscle fibers within a specific muscle is the same between men and women (6) and there is no definitive evidence to support hypertrophy resulting from fiber type splitting in humans. The mechanism underlying greater skeletal muscle hypertrophy in men compared with women may be due to the effect of **androgens** stimulating protein synthesis in men, albeit no gender differences in smooth muscle structure and function have been demonstrated. Although the inherent muscle size of men is greater than women, this does not necessarily mean that both genders do not respond to strength training similarly (see Trainability below).

Flexibility is one area of fitness in which women consistently score higher than men. The data consistently show that women are more flexible than men across all age groups (*Fig. 17.4*) (7). However, it has not yet been determined whether or not women are more trainable in flexibility than men.

The heart volume of women, whether expressed in absolute terms or relative to body mass, is only 70% to 75% of men (Table 17.1) (1). Correspondingly, women have an absolute left ventricular mass that is only 60% of men and a ventricular mass to lean body mass ratio which is 93% of men (*Fig. 17.5*). The smaller ventricular volume for women results in lower maximal cardiac output. Moreover, women have a lower arterial $O_2$ content at rest and during maximal exercise, a lower hemoglobin concentration, and a lower arterial venous $O_2$ difference than men. All of these factors may contribute to the lower **$O_2$ pulse** in women.

The $O_2$ pulse is a measure of the respiratory efficiency of the heart. It is calculated by dividing $O_2$ consumption (mL·min$^{-1}$) by heart rate. At similar workloads, the $O_2$ pulse of boys and girls is equal up until about 15 years. At

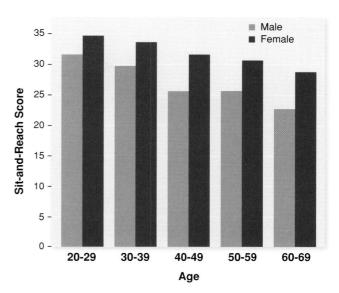

**FIGURE 17.4.** Sit & reach scores for males and females by age groups and gender. Scores are based on a sit & reach box in which the "zero" point is set at 26 cm. Data from American College of Sports Medicine. *ACSM's guidelines for exercise testing and prescription.* 6th ed. Baltimore: Lippincott Williams & Wilkins, 2000:88.

this age, the $O_2$ consumption plateaus in females while it improves rapidly in males until the early 20s (Table 17.2).

As mentioned in earlier chapters, the physiologic measurement most closely related to endurance exercise performance is maximal $O_2$ consumption ($\dot{V}O_{2max}$). When $\dot{V}O_{2max}$ is expressed as L·min$^{-1}$, values for women are about 40% less than those for men (*Fig. 17.6*). If the measurement is normalized by body mass (mL·kg$^{-1}$·min$^{-1}$), the gender difference is reduced to about 20%. Even when $\dot{V}O_{2max}$ is expressed relative to lean body mass and normalized for training status, there remains a 15% difference between the sexes (8). This remaining difference is thought to be the consummation of the inherent biologic differences heretofore mentioned.

Lower $\dot{V}O_{2max}$ values for women are probably inconsequential when exercise training for health or fitness is being undertaken because the qualitative response to dynamic exercise training is the same for both sexes. On the other hand, in the world of athletic performance, the relationship between $\dot{V}O_{2max}$ and body mass is critical because movement of the total body mass of the athlete constitutes most of the energy load during most competitive activities. Hence, the woman remains at a competitive disadvantage aerobically.

Women are also at a disadvantage in competition that relies primarily upon the lactic acid energy system (rapid glycolysis). Females tend to have lower lactic acid levels in their blood following maximal exercise than do males. This lower lactic acid level following maximal exercise in women suggests that they have a lower capacity for glycolytic production of ATP. However, blood lactic acid content is an absolute measurement, and if lactic acid were

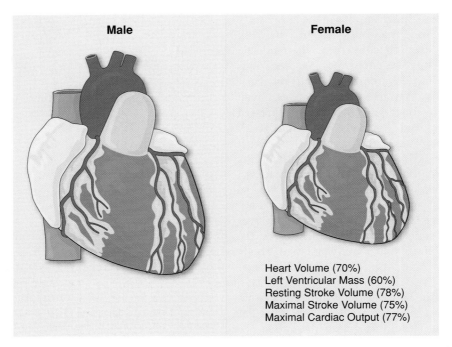

**FIGURE 17.5.** Physiologic differences in cardiac structure and function between males and females. Heart volume, 70%; left ventricular mass, 60%; resting stroke volume, 78%; maximal stroke volume, 75%; maximal cardiac output, 77%. Percentages represent the woman-to-man ratio.

| Table 17.2 | AGE-RELATED IMPROVEMENTS IN AEROBIC PARAMETERS FOR WOMEN | |
|---|---|---|
| | $\dot{V}O_{2max}$ | Maximal cardiac output |
| Young (19–31 years) | 12% | 11% |
| Middle aged (34–48 years) | 11% | 10% |
| Older (51–54 years) | 8% | 10% |

Data from Kilbom A. Physical training in women. *Scand J Clin Lab Invest Suppl* 1971;119:1–34.

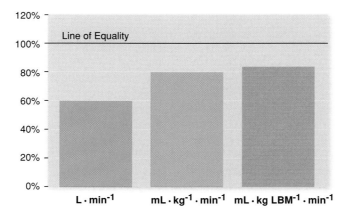

**FIGURE 17.6.** A comparison of $\dot{V}O_{2max}$ values for males and females. L/min, $\dot{V}O_{2max}$ expressed in L of $O_2$ per minute; $mL \cdot kg^{-1} \cdot min^{-1}$, $\dot{V}O_{2max}$ expressed as mL of $O_2$ per kg of body weight per minute; $mL \cdot kg$ $LBM^{-1} \cdot min^{-1}$, $\dot{V}O_{2max}$ expressed as mL of $O_2$ per kg of lean body mass per minute. Line of equality is where scores between the genders are equal.

expressed per kg of muscle mass, the gender difference would be minimized.

Athletic performance ratios (women's record divided by men's record) are closest to unity (a value of 1.0) in 100-meter (1.064) and 200-meter (1.082) sprints, which rely primarily on the ATP-PC energy system (Table 17.3) (1). Although the concentration of ATP and PC are similar between men and women, total phosphagen available for use during exercise is less for women because of their smaller muscle mass. When maximal power output is expressed relative to body mass, men and women are similar.

The role of **estrogen** and **progesterone** in the hormonal and metabolic responses to exercise in women is unclear despite several years of research (3). Although some animal and human studies have shown that women may utilize more fatty acids as energy sources during submaximal exercise than men, the data are not conclusive because these studies have not been able to control confounding variables such as menstrual status, training status, diet, and body composition. Another hormonal factor that has not been considered is the metabolic consequences of chronic exercise in highly trained women whose hormonal milieu may be altered because of menstrual irregularities.

## TRAINABILITY

Regardless of the inherent morphologic or physiologic differences between men and women, the question not yet addressed is if women respond to chronic exercise training in the same manner as men. The biologic gender differences portrayed in the previous discussion denote two areas in which training response may be gender specific; these are muscular strength and aerobic capacity.

Muscular strength in both men and women increases with heavy resistance training. The relative increase (% change) in strength of college-aged men and women following a 10-week progressive resistance program performed 2 days per week was greater for women in all muscle groups trained, except the biceps (*Fig. 17.7*) (5). Body composition analysis revealed, however, that lean body mass increased to a greater extent in men, whereas body fat loss was greater for women. These differences in training response may be explained in part by the lower initial strength of women. In other words, the greater improvements in strength for women could be due to the fact that they were less experienced with strength training or athletics than men and therefore had a greater margin for improvement than men. Strength gains for leg extension in older men and women, who were both untrained and inactive, were similar in magnitude following a strength-training program (*Fig. 17.7*) (9).

Coincidentally, when nationally prominent track-and-field athletes between the ages of 16 and 23 years were strength trained, they showed a 30% to 40% improvement in both upper- and lower-body strength after 6 months (10). The data from these two studies suggest that the trainability of the female for strength is equivalent to that of the male.

Results from early studies implied that the hypertrophic response to heavy resistance training is practically

| **Table 17.3** | **SELECTED MEN'S AND WOMEN'S WORLD RECORDS THROUGH 2004** | | |
|---|---|---|---|
| Event | Women | Men | Difference* |
| **Weightlifting (63-kg woman vs. 62-kg man)** | | | |
| Snatch (kg) | 115.0 | 152.5 | 75% |
| Clean and jerk (kg) | 135.0 | 177.5 | 76% |
| **Track and field** | | | |
| High jump (m) | 2.09 | 2.45 | 15% |
| Long jump (m) | 7.52 | 8.95 | 16% |
| Pole vault (m) | 4.92 | 6.14 | 20% |
| 100 m | 10.49 | 9.78 | 7% |
| 200 m | 21.34 | 19.32 | 10% |
| 400 m | 47.60 | 43.18 | 10% |
| 1500 m (min:sec) | 3:50.46 | 3:26.00 | 13% |
| 10,000 m (min:sec) | 29:31.78 | 26:20.31 | 12% |
| Marathon (hr:min:sec) | 2:15:25 | 2:04:55 | 8% |
| **Swimming** | | | |
| 50 m free (sec) | 23.59 | 21.10 | 12% |
| 200 m free (min:sec) | 1:54.04 | 1:41.10 | 13% |
| 50 m breast (sec) | 29.96 | 26.20 | 14% |
| 200 m breast (min:sec) | 2:17.75 | 2.02.92 | 12% |
| 50 m fly (sec) | 25.36 | 22.71 | 12% |
| 200 m fly (min:sec) | 2:04.04 | 1:50.73 | 12% |

*Percentage difference computed as women's divided by men's.

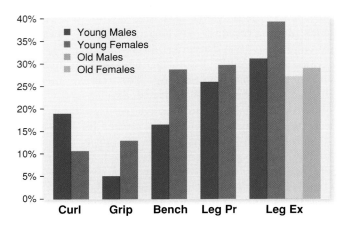

**FIGURE 17.7.** Relative increases in strength of men and women following progressive resistance-exercise training. Data from Wilmore JH. Alterations in strength, body composition and anthropometric measurements consequent to a 10-week weight training program. *Med Sci Sports* 1974;6:133–138 and from Lemmer JT, Hurlbut DE, Martel GF, et al. Age and gender responses to strength training and detraining. *Med Sci Sports Exerc* 2000;32:1505–1512.

insignificant for women when compared with men. Upper-body girth improvements, following 10 weeks of strength training in untrained men and women, were only 0.1 to 0.6 cm for women compared with 0.5 to 1.2 cm for men (5). Moreover, there was a strong correlation between strength and muscle girth for men (r = 0.63 to 0.77) but not for women (r = 0.09 to 0.42). Similarly, athletic women showed analogous hypertrophic responses (0.2 to 0.5 cm) following a 6-month strength-training program (10). However, more recent studies have confirmed that women who weight train receive similar strength gains (percentage increase from pretraining values) as men. Research has also revealed that women undergo a similar degree of myofiber and whole-muscle hypertrophy as that observed in men (11). The discrepancy in hypertrophic response between the early research and more recent research findings is because in the later studies skinfold thickness had been reduced, which nullified any increase in circumference area. It now seems that although women have less initial strength and smaller myofibers than men, relative increments in strength and fiber size induced by strength training are similar between genders if the same exercise stimulus is presented to both (11). Thus, in absolute terms (i.e., girth or cross-sectional area), men show greater hypertrophy than women; however, in relative terms (percentage increase in myofiber size), both sexes respond the same.

Kilbom (12) studied the adaptations to aerobic exercise training in several groups of women aged 19 to 64 years. The training protocol was bicycle exercise 2 to 3 days per week for 7 weeks at 73% to 77% of $\dot{V}O_{2max}$. Maximal cardiac output and $\dot{V}O_{2max}$ improved to the same extent in all age groups, suggesting that girls and women of all ages respond similarly to aerobic exercise training. This magnitude of adaptation in $\dot{V}O_{2max}$ for females is comparable to

that seen for males. Other studies in which men and women trained identically for 7 weeks on an interval-training program produced a magnitude of increase in $\dot{V}O_{2max}$ that was the same for both sexes (1). It must be remembered, though, that if the initial $\dot{V}O_{2max}$ for a woman in these studies was lower than that of a man, her relative improvement due to training would be comparatively greater.

Thus far in this chapter, we have seen that there are certain innate structural and physiologic differences between males and females that affect their respective maximal exercise capacities, and that in relative terms, the magnitude of adaptation to exercise training is similar between the sexes. A question that has not been answered is if the physiologic response to acute submaximal exercise is the same in performance-matched or physiologically matched males and females.

Costill and coworkers (13) initially addressed this question when they studied male and female runners who were matched for $\dot{V}O_{2max}$, training mileage, and muscle fiber type distribution. Biopsies from the gastrocnemius muscle revealed that succinate dehydrogenase and carnitine palmitoyl transferase (two mitochondrial enzymes) activities were 50% and 30% higher, respectively, in the men than the women. The capacity for palmitoyl coenzyme A oxidation was also about 33% higher in the men. During 60 minutes of exercise at 70% of $\dot{V}O_{2max}$, however, the respiratory exchange ratio for the two groups was identical, suggesting that the fat-derived energy production for the two groups was similar.

Further insight into this question has been provided by Pate and associates (14). Subjects in their study were male and female runners who were originally matched for training history and performance on a 15-mile road race. Laboratory testing also revealed that they were matched for $\dot{V}O_{2max}$, cardiorespiratory response to submaximal exercise, submaximal respiratory exchange ratio, and percent body fat. The only difference found between the groups was that the men had higher hematocrit and hemoglobin levels. Except for a few anomalies, the data from these two studies suggest that when men and women have similar training patterns and performance capacities, their physiologic profiles are equivalent.

Although research concerning women and exercise is still in its infancy and there are many questions to be answered, the current knowledge indicates that there is little reason to limit the healthy female from active participation in endurance or power sports. Notwithstanding, there are several specific concerns related to female participation in vigorous exercise training.

*Experiences in Work Physiology Lab Exercise 14: Comparison of Fitness Evaluations Between Genders provides experience in fitness testing for women, while allowing you to make some firsthand comparisons between men and women.*

▶ *INQUIRY SUMMARY.* The anatomic differences between the sexes are generally a reflection of the expression of hormonal differences that arise during the maturation process. The result is that females have a smaller body frame, lower muscle mass, lower lean body mass to fat mass ratio, less absolute strength, lower cardiorespiratory capacity, and less muscle hypertrophy than males. Nonetheless, the trainability of females is similar to that of males. This is not surprising in that the metabolic processes of both genders are controlled in the same manner. *Accordingly, in which activities would you suspect that females could perform at the same level as males?*

## Gynecologic Considerations

There are three developmental phases in a female's life when significant hormonal changes affect her metabolically: the onset of menarche, pregnancy, and menopause. All three of these phases are directly related to the woman's reproductive cycle and present special considerations for exercise. As a girl passes through puberty, growth and development of the reproductive organs is accompanied by great changes in the musculoskeletal system. Body fat is redistributed, the pattern of bone mineralization and maturation is established, and the metabolic response to exercise is affected by a new hormonal milieu. The major concern during this phase is that exercise training not compromise the development of the reproductive system or the integrity of the menstrual cycle.

During pregnancy, the hormonal milieu changes again, and the woman has special metabolic demands to meet the developing fetus' need for energy and nutrients. The concern during this phase is that the increased metabolic demand of exercise not compromise either the woman's or the child's health. As a woman passes through menopause, the hormonal milieu changes one more time, and the primary concern becomes maintaining the integrity of the musculoskeletal system so she can preserve her functional capacity. Thus, the effect of exercise training on menstruation, pregnancy, and menopause should be of prominent interest to any female who intends to be physically active throughout her life.

### MENSTRUATION

Research into the effects of exercise training on the menstrual cycle has focused on two areas, delayed menarche and cessation of menses. **Primary amenorrhea** is defined as the delay of menarche beyond 16 years of age, whereas **secondary amenorrhea** is when the menses ceases in women who have previously been menstrual.

Early observations of 729 Hungarian female athletes showed that there was no disturbance of the onset of menarche; the age of menarche was even slightly early for Swedish swimmers when compared to nonathletes. In con-

trast, numerous studies in the United States have shown that menarche occurs later in athletes than nonathletes. There could be several factors contributing to the discrepancies in the literature.

1. The early studies were performed more than 40 years ago, and training programs are much different now in scope and intensity than they were then.
2. Retrospective sampling procedures utilized in many studies to compare the age of menarche in groups that began training before and after menarche have been shown to be inherently biased.
3. Although some research has shown that age of menarche has been delayed by several months in athletic girls, the mean age of menarche of all these athletic populations is still younger than 16 (not considered primary amenorrhea) and within the normal distribution.
4. Although menarche may occur later in athletes than nonathletes, this may be due to social rather than physiologic influences.
5. None of the data are conclusive enough to show that exercise delays menarche in anyone.

The mean age of menarche in the United States is about 13 years with a standard deviation of 1.2 years. This means that 99% of all girls in the United States reach menarche before 16 years.

Over the past several years, there have been numerous reports of female athletes experiencing a cessation of menses, commonly called **athletic amenorrhea**. This type of secondary amenorrhea, often seen in athletes, is generally defined as less than four menses per year or the cessation of menses beyond 90 days. Although the exact cause of athletic amenorrhea is not known, it may be related to intensity of training and/or nutritional deficiencies in susceptible individuals. For example, it has been reported that the incidence of amenorrhea was 34% in a group of runners, 23% in a group of joggers, while being only 4% in a nonrunning control group (15). On the other hand, a cross-sectional study of endurance runners, who were well matched for age, body fat, weight, and training volume, showed that the amenorrheic runners had significantly higher scores on scales of restrictive eating disorders (16). This presents the possibility that it may have been the restrictive eating (poor nutrition) that caused the higher prevalence of amenorrhea in these athletes, or a combination of restrictive eating with intense exercise training.

Psychologic causes of athletic amenorrhea may be related to the stress of competition, the stress of being a student athlete, or other more serious psychologic disorders. It is also likely that the cause(s) of amenorrhea is different for each female and that the threshold for inducement of amenorrhea is variable among females (Fig. 17.8).

Although no causal relationship between exercise itself and amenorrhea has been established, some of the earlier hypotheses have been discounted. Cross-sectional studies have established that athletic amenorrhea is not caused

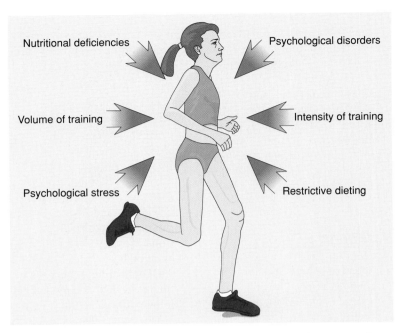

**FIGURE 17.8.** Factors that contribute to the development of athletic amenorrhea.

by **hyperandrogenism**, **hyperprolactinemia**, premature menopause, or inadequate body fatness, even though the last hypothesis continues to receive widespread publicity in the popular press.

Only one study has shown that athletic amenorrhea may be related to exercise itself (17). In this study, a strenuous training program was imposed upon a group of regularly menstruating women. Within the first month of training, the luteinizing hormone surge, follicular and luteal development, and ovulation were suppressed in a large portion of the subjects. As training continued, these irregularities were manifested in a greater number of women. It could not be determined whether the actual cause of these irregularities could be attributed to the type of exercise, the energy cost of the exercise, or an energy imbalance.

It is not known for sure if menstrual disorders perceptible in exercising women subside when exercise training is reduced or discontinued. Based on limited evidence, it is presumed that once training stops, the menstrual cycle resumes to a normal pattern and the reproductive functions of the woman are not prejudiced in any way. In any event, it would be wise for physicians, physical therapists, athletic trainers, coaches, and others involved with female athletic health care and counseling to maintain a conservative approach. A girl or woman should not be led to believe that menstrual irregularities are normal responses to training. Accurate records of menstrual cycles should be kept; if athletic amenorrhea occurs, the athlete should see a gynecologist to determine if exercise itself or some aspect associated with training is responsible for the hormonal changes associated with the menstrual disorder.

The early position of some in the medical community was that participation in sports, particularly swimming, while menstruating was unhealthy. The reality is that there is no bacterial contamination of pool water or increased risk of bacterial infection of the reproductive organs when participating in swimming or any other sport during menses. The consensus of medical experts is that there is little reason to discourage a healthy female athlete from training or competing during menses, provided her own experience demonstrates that there are no abnormal symptoms while doing so.

## PREGNANCY

Available evidence supports the existence of both risks and benefits of exercise conditioning during human pregnancy. The ability to preserve maternal-fetal well-being in the face of the metabolic and environmental stresses encountered during exercise depends on an adequate level of maternal-fetal physiologic reserve. Therefore, from a theoretical viewpoint, acute bouts of exercise may represent a significant challenge to maternal-fetal well-being. Conversely, chronic exercise, if properly prescribed, has the potential of enhancing physiologic reserve and can be fetoprotective.

### Exercise and Fetal Well-Being

Three different mechanisms have been proposed to explain how fetal growth and development may be altered by exposure to maternal exercise, **acute fetal hypoxia**, **fetal hypoglycemia,** and elevated fetal temperature (*Fig. 17.9*). Acute fetal hypoxia results from a redistribution of blood flow from the viscera to the working muscles. Several lines of evidence indicate that the fetus may indeed experience transient hypoxia during maternal exercise. These include a reduction in uterine blood flow during maternal exercise;

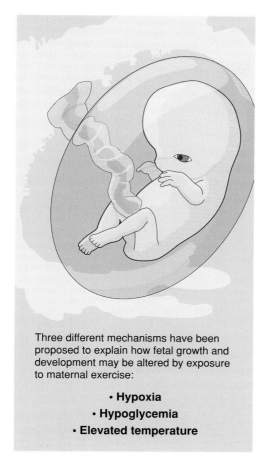

Three different mechanisms have been proposed to explain how fetal growth and development may be altered by exposure to maternal exercise:

- **Hypoxia**
- **Hypoglycemia**
- **Elevated temperature**

**FIGURE 17.9.** Possible fetal risks during maternal exercise.

a moderate increase in fetal heart rate (5 to 25 beats per minute) during exercise, followed by a return to baseline post-exercise; and an exercise-induced fetal bradycardia, which is an initial protective cardiovascular reflex to acute hypoxia. Although there has been conflicting results in the literature surrounding fetal hypoxia during maternal exercise, the studies reporting reduced uterine blood flow during exercise may be inherently biased because these studies used subjects with complicated pregnancies and also supine exercise. Supination itself occludes venous return because the weight of the fetus is resting on the inferior vena cava.

The second proposed mechanism for altered fetal growth and development resultant from maternal exercise is fetal hypoglycemia. During exercise, maternal blood glucose concentration may be reduced because of increased carbohydrate use by the working muscles and reduced glycogenolysis in the liver. Since the fetus relies primarily on glucose for metabolic fuel, maternal hypoglycemia could lead to fetal undernutrition. The exact cause of maternal hypoglycemia is not yet known, and more research needs to be done in this area.

The third mechanism postulated for fetal risk in exercising mothers is an increase in maternal body temperature which is transferred to the fetus, resulting in pathologic changes in fetal development, especially during the first trimester. Research investigating thermoregulatory function during aerobic exercise through 32 weeks of gestation reveals that exercising women were able to regulate core temperature effectively in temperate environments into the third trimester. This suggests that temperature regulation is not impaired in the pregnant woman, but prudence discourages prolonged high-intensity, long-duration exercise or exercise in hot environments because of innate risks of hyperthermia and dehydration.

## Exercise and Obstetric Outcome

It is difficult to determine from the literature if exercise training during pregnancy affects obstetric outcome because virtually all of the existing studies on human subjects have either used retrospective questionnaires for data collection, employed only a limited subject sample, involved possible group selection biases, or failed to control potential confounding variables such as age, nutritional status, smoking, and alcohol consumption. Some of the early studies on obstetric outcome deduced that physically active mothers gained less body mass (2 to 5 kg), delivered significantly earlier (5 to 8 days), had fewer spontaneous abortions, had fewer surgical deliveries, had shorter labors, had reduced indicators of fetal distress (17% versus 50%), delivered lighter infants (300 to 500 g) with about 220 g less fat mass, and had shorter hospital stays than nonexercising mothers or mothers who stopped exercise training during the early stages of gestation.

However, a meta-analysis performed several years ago, which included all prospective research studies reported to that time, found no significant differences between exercising and nonexercising groups for maternal weight gain, gestational age at birth, length of labor, or infant birth weight (18). More recent studies support the meta-analytical results and also show no difference in the incidence of spontaneous versus induced labor, mode of delivery, or frequency of labor complications between exercising and nonexercising mothers. It may be that the benefits of exercise for the pregnant women have to do with her personal health and not obstetric outcome.

Only one study has examined the effects of strength training itself on pregnancy outcomes (19). In this study, 50 **primiparous** women participated in a strength-training program for at least 12 weeks into gestation. Exercise sessions were held twice a week for 60 minutes and included exercises to strengthen the arms, legs, abdomen, and perineal muscles. Mean values for infant birth weight and gestational age at delivery were similar between the strength-training mothers and 50 nonexercising controls. Maternal weight gain was 1.5 kg less in the exercising mothers.

Although the research does not always concur that exercising during pregnancy yields an advantageous obstetric outcome, the research does indicate that moderate aerobic and/or strength training conditioning does not jeopardize fetal development or complicate labor.

## Exercise and Maternal Well-Being

Most of the postulated benefits of exercise during pregnancy seem to be associated with maternal well-being. Of particular concern is whether or not exercise conditioning increases maternal fitness, decreases the stress and discomforts of pregnancy, or prevents gestational complications. With respect to maternal fitness, one complicating factor for researchers is that direct measurement of $\dot{V}O_{2max}$ has been avoided in most studies because of concerns for maternal and fetal safety. Another factor to consider is that aerobic conditioning effects may be masked in late gestation by other hemodynamic effects of pregnancy itself, particularly those affecting venous return. Ignoring these methodologic limitations, the research suggests that maternal $\dot{V}O_{2max}$ as expressed in absolute terms ($L \cdot min^{-1}$) can be increased substantially with conditioning during pregnancy and that $\dot{V}O_{2max}$ relative to body mass ($mL \cdot kg^{-1} \cdot min^{-1}$) can be maintained or augmented slightly. It also appears that the aerobic conditioning effects during pregnancy become more apparent with increasing intensity of exertion. Research into the stress and discomforts of pregnancy and gestational complications suggest that these are reduced with exercise conditioning. Table 17.4 depicts the common maternal benefits associated with exercise training during pregnancy.

*LINKUP:* **Research Highlight: Effect of Pregnancy on Heart Rate/Oxygen Consumption Calibration Curves,** *found at http://connection.lww.com/go/brownexphys and on the Student Resource CD-ROM, presents some interesting data on how the heart rate/ $\dot{V}O_2$ relationship during exercise changes for women who are pregnant.*

| Table 17.4 | MATERNAL BENEFITS FROM EXERCISE DURING PREGNANCY |
|---|---|

Increased $\dot{V}O_{2max}$

Decreased submaximal exercise heart rate

Decreased submaximal exercise perceived exertion

Increased fat metabolism

Decreased submaximal ventilatory demand

Increased self-esteem

Decreased incidence of backache

Decreased physical discomforts

Decreased post-partum resting heart rate

Increased postpartum stroke volume

More rapid post-partum recovery

## Exercise and Post-Partum Athletic Performance

In contrast to determining the effects that exercise training has on pregnancy and obstetric outcome, it seems important to consider what effects pregnancy and childbirth have upon exercise performance. Champion athletes have competed successfully during their first 3 or 4 months of pregnancy. Furthermore, 46% of the female athletes who competed in the Olympics before pregnancy and then continued competition after becoming mothers improved their performance within the first year after childbirth. An additional 31% of these athletes improved their performances between the first and second year after childbirth (20). It must be remembered, nonetheless, that this research was performed 40 years ago and that intensity of training for elite athletic competition has changed since then. The physiologic profiles of today's female athlete have changed as well.

Pregnancy often becomes a strong motivator for a woman to change some of her unhealthy lifestyle habits. Notwithstanding, the historical position of the American College of Obstetricians and Gynecologists was for a woman not to initiate a new aerobic sport during pregnancy and not to intensify any training effort. They further counseled that previously sedentary women should probably not engage in any aerobic activity more strenuous than walking. It is not surprising that such recommendations tended to be conservative in light of the bewildering scientific data. On the other hand, more recent scientific data do tend to indicate that healthy previously inactive women can participate in progressive, individually prescribed aerobic exercise regimens without increased risk to themselves or their developing fetuses. The position of the American College of Obstetricians and Gynecologists has progressed over the years from permitting limited amounts of exercise during pregnancy to encouraging women to engage in 30 minutes or more of moderate-intensity exercise on most, if not all, days of the week. The only exercise exceptions for the pregnant woman are to not engage in scuba diving because the fetus is at risk for decompression sickness, and not to engage in activities that present an increased risk for abdominal trauma, such as lacrosse, soccer, and kickboxing.

The decision for any woman to either initiate an exercise program or to continue with a previous training regimen should be based upon the woman's history, the surrounding circumstances, and in accordance with prudent medical advice. It should be remembered though, that the greatest risks for exercise during pregnancy lie within the first and third trimesters. During the first trimester, exercise-induced hyperthermia may affect the closure of the neural tube, causing serious defects in the central nervous system of the fetus. During the third trimester, competition between maternal and fetal physiologic needs becomes the greatest. Hence, if the choice were to initiate or expand an exercise program during pregnancy, it should be done during the second trimester.

If a pregnant woman is initiating an exercise program, altering an existing program, or continuing with her current regimen, she should follow the process outlined below for exercising during pregnancy:

1. Medical screening: Medical screening should be done by or in conjunction with a physician or obstetrician. The primary purpose of medical screening is to determine if there are any contraindications for exercise during pregnancy (Table 17.5). Absolute contraindications prohibit any exercise participation. Relative contraindications are when the risks may exceed the benefits of exercise, and the decision whether or not to exercise during pregnancy should be made in accordance with a physician or obstetrician.

2. Exercise prescription: The exercise prescription should consist of specific individual guidelines for warmup, conditioning, and cooldown. Unfortunately, widespread disagreement exists with regard to the optimal target range for exercise intensity, duration, and frequency. The American College of Sports Medicine recommends an appropriate frequency of 3 to 5 days per week, with a duration of 15 to 30 minutes. Monitoring exercise intensity during pregnancy becomes difficult in that resting heart rate decreases during the third trimester. Therefore, the use of conventional heart rates for target zones to prescribe exercise intensity is less reliable than for nonpregnant women. Available data suggest that perception to exertion remains stable re-

| Table 17.5 | CONTRAINDICATIONS FOR EXERCISE DURING PREGNANCY |
|---|---|

**Absolute contraindications**

Heart disease
Peripheral vascular disease
Ruptured membranes
Incompetent cervix
Premature labor
Multiple pregnancy
Bleeding or placenta previa
History of three or more spontaneous abortions or miscarriages
Toxemia or pre-eclampsia in current pregnancy

**Relative contraindications**
Hypertension
Anemia (Hb <10 g·dL$^{-1}$) or other blood disorders
Thyroid disease
Diabetes
Palpitations or irregular heart rhythms
Breech presentation in third trimester
Excessive obesity
Extreme underweight or history of anorexic behaviors
Significant pulmonary disease
Extremely sedentary lifestyle
History of bleeding during pregnancy
History of precipitous labor
History of intrauterine growth retardation
Presence of twins (after 24 weeks of gestation)

| Table 17.6 | SAFETY PRECAUTIONS FOR EXERCISE DURING PREGNANCY |
|---|---|

Avoid high ambient temperatures and humidities

Avoid supine exercise after the fourth month

Avoid sports or activities with a high risk of injury

Avoid bouncing or ballistic movements

Avoid deep flexion or extension of joints because of connective tissue laxity

Precede each exercise session with an adequate warmup

Conclude each exercise session with an adequate cooldown

Consume liquids liberally before and after exercise

Avoid Valsalva maneuver

Avoid exercising to exhaustion

Prefer nonweight-bearing activities

Increase exercise quantity and quality gradually

gardless of pregnancy status and therefore use of rating of perceived exertion (RPE) scales is highly recommended. A target intensity of approximately 12 to 14 on the 6 to 20 point Borg RPE scale is appropriate for most pregnant women. The revised Borg RPE scale runs from 1 (exertion while standing) to 10 (exertion at maximal capacity). A pregnant woman should attempt to maintain a work level between 3 and 5. The intensity maintained on either scale is described as bring moderate to somewhat hard.

3. Safety precautions: After passing the medical screening and receiving the exercise prescription, the pregnant woman should be advised of certain safety precautions specific to exercising during pregnancy (Table 17.6).

4. Reasons to discontinue exercise: Each exercising mother should be advised to discontinue exercise if certain signs or symptoms are manifest such as those listed in Table 17.7.

The key for a woman who exercises during her pregnancy is to work at her own level of comfort. All conditioning programs should include exercises for strength, flexibility, and aerobic fitness, with an adequate warm up and cool down. With regard to flexibility, pregnant women should be cautious as the hormones that facilitate delivery can also allow for overstretching. Pregnant women should not stretch beyond the point that they could reach before conception.

## LACTATION

Mothers who nurse their children have a physiologic demand placed upon their body that mothers who bottle-feed do not incur. Nursing mothers are providing their infants

| Table 17.7 | *REASONS TO DISCONTINUE EXERCISE DURING PREGNANCY* |
|---|---|
| Pain or bleeding | |
| Dizziness or faintness | |
| Pubic pain | |
| Palpitations | |
| Back pain | |
| Rapid heart rate | |
| Shortness of breath | |
| Difficulty walking | |
| Persistent contractions (>6 per hour) | |
| Absence of fetal movement | |
| Insufficient weight gain (<1.0 kg·month$^{-1}$ during last 6 months) | |
| Persistent, severe headaches and/or visual disturbances | |

with all of the essential nutrients for growth and development. This not only includes adequate vitamins and minerals but also includes an adequate supply from the energy-yielding nutrients. Breastfeeding adds approximately 500 kcal to the mother's daily energy intake needs. Since exercise also places an excess energy demand upon the mother, the question arises as to whether the excess energy demand of breastfeeding and exercise can jeopardize the health of either the mother or infant. The health concerns surrounding the compatibility of exercise and lactation center on three issues: (a) the influence of exercise on the lactating mother's health, (b) the influence of exercise on the mother's milk, and (c) the influence of exercise on the infant's feeding and growth.

Only a handful of studies have examined the effects of exercise on maternal health during lactation. With regard to fitness level, women who exercised regularly during pregnancy and lactation had a 53% greater $\dot{V}O_{2max}$ than women who were sedentary. Women who were sedentary during pregnancy and then began an exercise-training program while breastfeeding increased their $\dot{V}O_{2max}$ by 13% to 25%. Lactating women who exercise report expending from 400 to 800 kcal·d$^{-1}$ more than sedentary mothers, but their higher energy expenditure is compensated for by an increase in energy intake by 300 to 700 kcal·d$^{-1}$. These and other data suggest that a return to prepregnancy body weight is most likely to occur in lactating women who exercise.

Maternal estrogen levels are maintained at a low level during lactation, while maternal calcium demand is elevated. These two factors generally decrease bone mineral density of the lactating mother. Only two studies have examined bone density of lactating mothers who exercise.

Neither of these studies provides sufficient evidence as to whether exercise is beneficial or detrimental to the bone health of the lactating mother.

Although there are no prospective studies investigating the psychologic health of lactating mothers who exercise versus lactating mothers who are sedentary, results from more general research on the effects of exercise on maternal psychologic health can probably be applied to lactating mothers. Mothers who exercise score better on measures of post-partum adaptation such as satisfaction with life circumstances, confidence in mothering tasks, and quality of relationship with partner compared to sedentary women. Exercising mothers are more likely to participate in activities of personal fulfillment such as entertainment, hobbies, and socializing than sedentary mothers.

A series of studies have been performed to determine how acute exercise and exercise training during lactation affect milk composition and volume. Findings on the effects of exercise training on milk composition are consistent across studies. No differences have been found in protein, lactose, lipid, or energy content of milk from exercising mothers versus sedentary controls. Moreover, an acute bout of submaximal exercise does not alter the calcium, phosphorus, magnesium, sodium, potassium, ammonium, urea, or lipid content of mother's milk. Lactic acid, in contrast, may be elevated in mother's milk following an acute bout of exercise. The majority of studies that investigated lactic acid content of milk following a single bout of exercise report that maximal exercise increases milk lactic acid levels, possibly to the point of affecting the taste of the milk. However, lactating mothers do not routinely perform maximal graded exercise tests. Submaximal exercise, at intensities routinely prescribed for lactating mothers (50% to 75% $\dot{V}O_{2max}$), does not elevate lactic acid concentration. Therefore, a lactating mother should be able to participate in an exercise-training program without worry as to lactic acid accumulation in her milk.

In addition, there is no evidence to suggest that exercise training or an acute exercise bout compromises the volume of milk production. Studies on lactating women who exercise regularly show that their milk production is the same compared with nonexercising controls. Women who performed a single exercise bout also produced milk in the same amount following exercise as they did under the nonexercising condition.

Cross-sectional studies reported that growth of infants consuming breast milk of exercising mothers was not different from that of infants consuming milk from sedentary mothers. Even when lactating mothers who were exercising reduced their energy intake post-partum in an effort to lose weight, their infants' growth was not compromised. Furthermore, the evidence shows that infant acceptance of post-exercise milk is unchanged even following maximal exercise in which lactic acid content may be elevated. It can only be concluded from the limited data available that maternal cardiovascular and psychologic health are improved with exercise, and that when maternal exercise is coupled with an adequate diet, there is no impairment in infant growth, mammary gland development, milk production, milk composition, or milk acceptance by the infant.

## MENOPAUSE

**Menopause** is the period of development in a woman's life when the concentrations of circulating reproductive hormones decrease to the point at which she no longer menstruates. The menopausal years are preceded by **perimenopause**, a period of a few years before the permanent cessation of menses. It is during this perimenopausal era when the patterns of self-care can have a significant impact on post-menopausal health. Many women begin to experience the symptoms of menopause during perimenopause, such as hot flashes, fatigue, irritability, headaches, and forgetfulness. Women's percent body fat increases after menopause, due to a decline in lean body mass and an increase in body fat (*Fig. 17.10*). The fat distribution also changes, with more fat becoming centrally located. This redistribution of body fat is important because it may put the woman at higher risk for chronic diseases such as cardiovascular disease, diabetes, and some types of cancer. Therefore, maintaining a regular exercise program is of great importance to the menopausal woman.

About 75% of all perimenopausal women experience physical symptoms such as hot flashes. However, regular exercise has the tendency to decrease the incidence and severity of hot flashes. Weight-bearing exercises can decrease the risk of **osteoporosis** and bone fractures and help maintain lean body mass. Physical activity can have psychologic benefits also. Women who exercise regularly report improved mood states, decreased depression, better self-perceived health, and decreased stress. On the other hand, increased levels of stress due to menopausal symptoms during the transition can reduce a woman's motiva-

tion to exercise. Thus, the paradox is that exercise can improve a menopausal woman's health, but the symptoms of menopause reduce her motivation to exercise. An example of how one woman struggled to initiate an exercise program after menopause is given in Case Study 17.1.

▶ *INQUIRY SUMMARY.* The onset of menarche, pregnancy, and menopause are three developmental phases in a female's life when significant hormonal changes affect her metabolically. Exercise throughout a woman's life, particularly during these developmental stages, is healthful and desirable. Although some of the literature shows that the onset of menarche may be delayed by a few months in female athletes, the delay is not beyond what would be considered normal. Some girls and women experience athletic amenorrhea, and the exact cause is not well understood. However, it seems that there are no long-lasting negative side effects to a woman's reproductive system due to extensive exercise training. Exercise through perimenopause and menopause can help a woman maintain her functional capacity and decrease risk of chronic disease. *Can you think of any personal concerns a woman may have about exercise during any one of these developmental phases? How might her concerns be rectified?*

## *Nutritional Issues*

Exercise and nutritional issues are inseparably connected. As you have learned previously in this book, nutrients provide the means by which the metabolic requirements of exercise are met. If the nutritional needs of the body are not met, exercise can drain the body of vital nutrients, and this can lead to serious health problems.

Women are at higher risk than men for developing osteoporosis and **iron-deficiency anemia** because of their different hormonal profile and reduced hemoglobin concentration. Thus, any effect, positive or negative, that exercise or nutrition has on bone mineral content or hemoglobin concentration should be of particular interest to women.

There are certain psychologic factors that place girls and women at higher risk for developing exercise- and nutrition-related disorders. It is well known that the prevalence of eating disorders is much higher in females than males; female athletes are at particularly high risk for developing eating disorders. Exercise conditioning, whether for athletic competition or fitness, is generally seen as a positive behavior. Nevertheless, some girls and women go beyond what is necessary for fitness or athletic competition and compulsively exercise for several hours a day. This type of **excessive exercise disorder** can induce serious health consequences. If a female develops an eating disorder, such as **anorexia nervosa**, along with the symptoms of amenorrhea and osteoporosis, she has entered the **female athlete triad**. Recovering from the female athlete triad is very difficult because the behaviors that lead to the disease (exercise and weight control) are

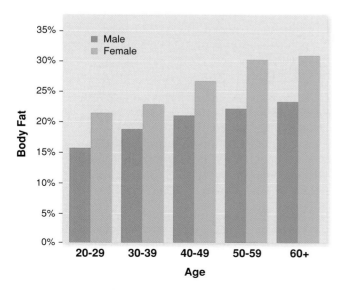

**FIGURE 17.10.** Body fat percentages for males and females by age.

## CASE STUDY 17.1: *POST-MENOPAUSAL EXERCISE TRAINING*

### CASE

You are a physical therapist with a master's degree in exercise physiology who assists with an outpatient community exercise rehabilitation program. A post-menopausal woman named Trudy has entered your program. Trudy had a myocardial infarction (MI) 2 years ago but never followed up with rehabilitative exercise. She recently fractured her hip and has recovered from surgery. Trudy's bone scan (dual-energy x-ray absorptiometry [DXA]) shows that she has osteoporosis. These two conditions have motivated her enough to enroll in your rehabilitation program.

### DESCRIPTION

Some women are sedentary throughout their lives until they reach menopause. Then after menopause, they develop a serious health problem that can be improved or eliminated with regular exercise training. These women, who have not exercised in their younger years, are often intimidated by the whole idea of exercise training. Working with these women is difficult because you have to help them overcome the tangible barriers to exercise (e.g., time, place, knowledge) and the intangible barriers to exercise (e.g., preconceived notions, emotional ties to noncompliant behaviors).

### EVALUATION/INTERVENTION

Your review of Trudy's medical chart reveals that her MI was a minor event and that she has not presented any symptoms since the original occurrence. Trudy is totally compliant in taking her heart medication. Her DXA scan does show that her bone mineral density is more than two standard devia-

tions below the average for a 68-year-old woman (osteoporosis). You administer a graded exercise test to maximal capacity on a treadmill, with gas analysis. Her vital signs show that Trudy responds normally to increased exercise intensity. Trudy's maximal oxygen uptake on the treadmill was 23.0 mL·kg$^{-1}$·min$^{-1}$, which places her between the 20th and 30th percentiles for her age. Trudy's sit & reach score is 17 cm, below the 10th percentile. Her upper-body strength is above the 50th percentile, but various lower-body strength assessments show her to be very weak.

The exercise program you design for Trudy consists of cardiorespiratory exercise, strength-training exercises, and flexibility development. The cardiorespiratory exercise program consists of water aerobics prescribed at an initial intensity at which her heart rate corresponds to 50% of her treadmill $\dot{V}O_{2max}$. The buoyancy of the water will reduce the stress on the hip as she develops strength in the pelvic area. Intensity will be increased as she responds to conditioning. The strength and flexibility training are targeted specifically at the lower body to help with her recovery from surgery and to maintain or gain bone mineral density.

As Trudy progresses in her conditioning program, you should also explore any tangible and intangible barriers to exercise. Possible areas for exploration are (a) conflicts: potential conflicts in priorities, conflicts with lifestyle, perceptual conflicts, conflicts with competing behaviors; (b) personal experience: past negative as well as positive experiences with exercise; and (c) emotional barriers: distorted thinking patterns, emotional links to sedentary behaviors, such as depression. As you explore and uncover barriers to exercise compliance, you can then decide how to overcome those barriers *Do you need help from other members of the health care team?*.

---

seen as positive behaviors when not taken to the extreme. In this last section of the chapter, we will discuss how exercise and nutrition for the female can relate to physiologic and psychologic disorders.

## OSTEOPOROSIS

Osteoporosis is a condition in which the bones become thin and brittle due to loss of mineral content and are more susceptible to fractures. This condition has recently become a concern for exercising women who develop amenorrhea because estrogen levels are reduced during amenorrhea and osteoporosis is related to estrogen deficiency. More importantly, osteoporosis is especially common in post-menopausal women because of the reduced levels of estrogen during menopause. **Type I osteoporosis** is eight times more common in women than men and is related to vertebral and distal radius fractures in women 50

to 65 years old. Type I osteoporosis is the cause of hip, pelvic, and distal humerus fractures in women over age 70.

The National Osteoporosis Foundation has outlined five steps to promote bone health and prevent osteoporosis:

1. Get the daily recommended amounts of calcium and vitamin D (calcium: 1000 to 13000 mg·d$^{-1}$; vitamin D: 400 to 800 IU·d$^{-1}$).
2. Engage in regular weight-bearing exercise.
3. Avoid smoking and excessive alcohol consumption.
4. Talk to your physician about bone health.
5. Have a bone density test and take medication when appropriate.

It has become evident that exercise promotes an increase in bone mass. Examination of active and sedentary populations at single points in time generally supports a positive correlation between activity level and bone mineral content. Moreover, increased activity may be associated with a slower rate of age-related bone loss. However, the changes in bone density are less impressive in **prospective studies** than are reported in **cross-sectional studies**. This may be due to the fact that the optimal mode of exercise, along with the optimal threshold for duration and frequency of exercise for bone health, has not been elucidated. It also remains to be determined whether or not the skeletal response to exercise is site specific. In any case, it seems that the skeletal system is dynamic in nature and responds to both weight-bearing and nonweight-bearing exercise training and to inactivity.

The American College of Sports Medicine has concluded that weight-bearing physical activity has beneficial effects on bone health across the age spectrum. Physical activities that generate relatively high-intensity loading forces, such as plyometrics, gymnastics, and high-intensity resistance training, augment bone mineral accrual in children and adolescents. Gains in bone mass that are induced through exercise in childhood are maintained into adulthood. Although quantitative dose-response studies are lacking, the following are guidelines for exercise prescription to augment bone mineral content in children and adolescents:

- Mode of exercise: impact activities such as gymnastics, plyometrics, jumping, moderate-intensity resistance training, sports that involve running and jumping
- Intensity of exercise: high in terms of bone-loading forces—resistance training should be <60% one repetition maximum (1 RM)
- Frequency of exercise: at least 3 days per week
- Duration of exercise: 10 to 20 minutes, two times per day

The primary goal for adults is to maintain bone mass. However, it is still unclear if adults can increase bone density through exercise. Observational studies suggest that the age-related decline in bone mineral density is attenuated and the relative risk for fracture is reduced in people who are physically active, even when the activity is not particularly vigorous. However, as with children and adolescents, there have been no large randomized, controlled trials to confirm these observations. Moreover, although physical activity may counteract the age-related decline in bone mass, there is no strong evidence to suggest that even vigorous physical activity will reduce the menopause-related loss of bone mass in women. The following exercise prescription is recommended to help preserve bone health during adulthood:

- Mode of exercise: weight-bearing endurance activities such as stair climbing, tennis, jogging, and hiking; activities that involve jumping such as volleyball and basketball; resistance exercises such as weightlifting
- Intensity of exercise: moderately high in terms of bone-loading forces
- Frequency of exercise: weight-bearing endurance activities three to five times per week; resistance exercises two to three times per week
- Duration of exercise: 30 to 60 minutes per day of a combination of activities

## IRON DEFICIENCY

The capacity for $O_2$ transport in the blood is directly related to blood **hemoglobin** content or to the capacity of the heme (iron) entity on the hemoglobin to bind $O_2$. Iron-deficiency anemia refers to a low red blood cell count resultant from inadequate iron intake and/or absorption. It has already been mentioned that women inherently have a lower hemoglobin content than men. Women are also more susceptible to iron-deficiency anemia than men because of iron loss during menstruation. Female athletes may be even more susceptible because of the possibility of a greater iron need during exercise training. Thus, it becomes important for the exercise physiologist, physical therapist, or clinician to recognize that a significant number of exercising women are iron deficient and consequently are at risk for developing anemia. Evaluations of dietary intake, blood hemoglobin, and iron should be used routinely to assist the exercising woman to avoid iron-deficiency anemia. A dietary recall or diet history can reveal whether or not a woman is receiving adequate iron. Blood tests that reveal hemoglobin counts below 11 to 12 $g \cdot dL^{-1}$ are considered to be indicative of anemia.

## EATING DISORDERS

Eating disorders affect more than 8 million people in the United States, of whom 97% are females. The causes of eating disorders vary and are too complex to detail in this chapter, but the overall cause is psychologic. The underlying psychologic disturbance causing eating disorders manifests itself in a distorted perception of body weight or body image. The disease is manifest when the patient obsesses over "fixing" what he/she perceives as a physical ailment by participating in unhealthy eating and exercise behaviors. The patient's attempt to heal the perceived physical problem is, in reality, a misguided attempt to heal the emotional being.

It seems that individuals with eating disorders have unconsciously, over time, turned to food or eating rituals, rather than people, for meeting certain emotional needs. The problem is that neither food nor food rituals work, since these behaviors do not provide the necessary responsiveness or self-growth. The result is that the person repeatedly turns to food ritual behaviors in an attempt to fulfill a need, whether it is a sense of calm, control, accomplishment, or love. An example can be seen with anorexia nervosa. Dieting to lose weight may not seem harmful initially, but in the individual with anorexia, dieting becomes the purpose of life and a secure and safe place to go. Dieting turns into an artificial world where the anorexic individual can go to cope with feelings of meaninglessness, low self-esteem, failure, dissatisfaction, the need to be unique, or the desire to be special, to be a success or to be in control.

The three types of eating disorders that are most common in female athletes are anorexia nervosa, **bulimia**, and **binge-eating disorder**. The American Psychiatric Association has defined certain diagnostic criteria for each of these eating disorders. Those criteria for anorexia are displayed

| Table 17.8 | DIAGNOSTIC CRITERIA FOR ANOREXIA NERVOSA |
|---|---|

Body weight remains below 85% of that expected for age and height
Intense fear of gaining weight or becoming fat
Distorted body image
Amenorrhea in post-pubescent females (i.e., the absence of at least three consecutive menstrual cycles)

**Subtypes**
Restricting: does not engage in binge eating or purging behavior
Binge eating/purging: engages in binge eating and/or purging behavior

Source: American Psychiatric Association. *Diagnostic and statistical manual of mental disorders*. 4th ed. Washington, DC: American Psychiatric Association, 1994.

in Table 17.8. To be diagnosed with anorexia, a person has to meet all of the diagnostic criteria. For example, just being skinny and lightweight does not make a woman anorexic. She would also have to be afraid to become fat, have a distorted body image, and be amenorrheic.

Many anorexic girls and women cannot maintain their restrictive dieting behaviors and turn to bulimia as a coping mechanism. It is estimated that about 50% of bulimic individuals were previously anorexic. Similar to anorexia, bulimia is characterized by an intense fear of gaining weight and becoming fat (Table 17.9). However, the true root to either of these eating disorders is psychologic and not physiologic. Girls and women who have periods of uncontrollable eating that are not associated with anorexic or bulimic behaviors can be classified as binge eaters (Table 17.10). Diagnosis of binge-eating disorder does not require that the person be fearful of gaining weight or becoming fat.

*What predisposes a person to developing an eating disorder?* The answer to that question is not known. Profession-

| Table 17.9 | DIAGNOSTIC CRITERIA FOR BULIMIA NERVOSA |
|---|---|

Episodes of binge eating (eating an extremely large amount of food in a discrete period of time, while feeling out of control)

Use of compensatory behaviors to prevent weight gain
The binge/compensatory behaviors occur at least twice a week for 3 months

Self-esteem is based on a distorted body image
The disorder is not always associated with anorexia

**Subtypes**
Purging: compensates by self-induced vomiting or the misuse of laxatives or diuretics
Nonpurging: compensates without purging, such as fasting or exercising excessively

Source: American Psychiatric Association. *Diagnostic and statistical manual of mental disorders*. 4th ed. Washington, DC: American Psychiatric Association, 1994.

| Table 17.10 | DIAGNOSTIC CRITERIA FOR BINGE-EATING DISORDER |
|---|---|

Episodes of binge eating (eating an extremely large amount of food in a discrete period of time, while feeling out of control)

The binge-eating episodes are associated with at least three of the following: eating very rapidly, eating until feeling stuffed, overeating when not hungry, eating in secret, feeling bad about oneself after overeating, feeling distressed over binge-eating behaviors, binging 2 days a week for at least 6 months, binging is unaccompanied by anorexia, bulimia, or compensatory behaviors

Source: American Psychiatric Association. *Diagnostic and statistical manual of mental disorders*. 4th ed. Washington, DC: American Psychiatric Association, 1994.

als have inferred that there are some general predisposing factors common to these eating disorders. The most commonly referenced are: (a) adolescent turmoil in which the development of an individual identity has not been achieved, (b) controlling parents who are denying, emotionally unhealthy, and frustrated in their own aspirations, (c) alienation towards one's body caused by a society in which the female body is a sex symbol and commodity, (d) a competitive environment in which slimness is emphasized, and (e) pressure to be perfect.

Of the three eating disorders, binge-eating disorder carries with it the least severe physiologic consequence, being overweight. Anorexia and bulimia, in contrast, are characterized by some serious clinical symptoms, even death (Table 17.11). It is estimated that 5% to 10% of anorexic

| Table 17.11 | CLINICAL SIGNS OF ANOREXIA AND BULIMIA |
|---|---|

Emaciation

Dry, yellow skin

**Lanugo**

Cold peripheries

Hormonal disturbances

Electrocardiogram changes

Hypotension

Dental erosion

Anemia

Bone loss

Bradycardia

Amenorrhea

Edema

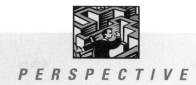

**Box 17.2**

## *P E R S P E C T I V E*

# *Helping a Friend with an Eating Disorder*

Many of us know of a friend, relative, or coworker who is struggling with an eating disorder. Our concern for this individual strongly motivates us to want to help this person. You may think: *Maybe it's my imagination—she really doesn't have an eating disorder. How do I approach her? What do I say? What if I say the wrong thing? Where can I get help for her?*

These are valid questions that need to be answered before you make any attempt to help an eating-disorder victim. First of all, eating disorders are different from physiologic disorders, and the thought process of the eating disorder patient is distorted. Nonetheless, you can help an eating-disorder victim. However, your goal as a friend, loved one, or colleague is not to challenge them, scare them, or to force them into treatment. Your goal is to love them into treatment.

The eating-disorder patient is almost always in denial about the problem. Eating disorders are secretive diseases in which the victim hides her behaviors. Challenging this person by pointing out that she has a problem only pushes her deeper into the disease and into denial. Persons with eating disorders generally do not trust anyone—not themselves or other people. You cannot help them until you gain their trust. Not until you gain the person's trust will she be ready to come out of denial and seek help.

*How do you gain trust?* Show love and concern. However, the manner in which you show love and concern is crit-

ical. Statements like, *You look like you have lost a lot of weight, are you sure you are eating enough?* only push the person away from you and deeper into the disease because that type of question challenges her disorder. Better statements would be ones like, *You look like you are not feeling well—are you OK? Lately I have noticed that you don't have the same zip you used to—is everything OK? It seems like we haven't spent as much time together lately as we have in the past. I miss hanging with you.* These types of statements are not challenging to the eating-disorder victim because they don't challenge the disorder—they show concern for the individual. By constantly showing genuine concern for the individual, you develop trust. Then when she is ready, the eating-disorder victim will open up a little to see if it is safe to let you see inside.

At the point the person with an eating disorder begins to open up, you need to nurture that trust. Do not expect to get her to accept help the first time she lets you into her emotional self. It may take you weeks or months until she trusts you enough to come out of denial about her eating disorder. In the meantime, you can be checking the resources in your community for professional services relevant to eating disorders. Most university student health services provide help. Many agencies can provide help. Check around. Be patient with your friend and let her guide herself into accepting treatment.

individuals die within 10 years of contracting the disease, while 20% die within 20 years. Only about 50% recover fully, while the remainder struggle in and out of treatment for the rest of their lives. Box 17.2 shows you some things you can do to try and help a friend or relative with an eating disorder.

## FEMALE ATHLETE TRIAD

Possibly even more devastating than developing an eating disorder is when an eating disorder is coupled with amenorrhea and bone mineral loss. This condition is almost exclusively found in female athletes and has therefore been termed the female athlete triad (*Fig. 17.11*). Girls and women who train intensely and try to lose weight often develop disordered eating behaviors. The poor nutritional

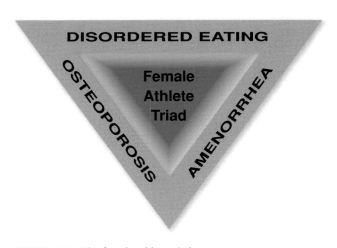

**FIGURE 17.11.** The female athlete triad.

state caused by the eating disorder and intense exercise training lead to amenorrhea. The occurrence of amenorrhea removes the protective effect of estrogen on bone mineral health, and osteoporosis develops. As the restrictive dieting and intense exercise training continue, the problem is magnified. The beneficial effects of exercise on bone density are offset by the persistent amenorrhea, and bone health is further jeopardized. The risk of musculoskeletal injuries is increased, and the athlete may train harder and restrict food intake even more in an attempt to gain back athletic prowess. One can see that each one of the triad's prongs feeds back maliciously upon the other until the individual is trapped into a downward spiral of deteriorating health (Fig. 17.11).

**LINKUP: Perspective: Eating Disorders,** *found at* **http://connection.lww.com/go/brownexphys** *and on the Student Resource CD-ROM, shows an evaluation of a woman who was anorexic for more than 25 years.*

Treatment for a woman caught in the female athlete triad should include psychologic counseling to deal with the issues relevant to the eating disorder, a reduction in training volume by 10 to 20%, an increase in food consumption that will restore body weight or maintain body weight at a normal level, and a daily intake of calcium that exceeds 1500 mg. Even after successful therapy, bone mass may remain reduced and the woman could be at increased risk for osteoporosis and bone fractures the rest of her life. A reduction in bone mineral content of only 5% increases the risk of bone fracture by 40%.

## EXCESSIVE EXERCISE DISORDER

Along with the increase in the number of people with eating disorders, there has been a rise in the number of people with excessive exercise disorder. Some girls and women have become addicted to exercise, while others have replaced or accompanied their ritualistic disordered eating with compulsive exercise. Some bulimic and binge-eating individuals use exercise as their purging or compensatory behavior for binge eating. Regardless, these individuals perform hours of daily exercise and refuse to stop exercising when injured, exhausted, counseled, or threatened. Case Study 17.2 provides some insights into some of the difficulties professionals face when treating an eating-disorder patient who insists upon exercising.

Psychiatrists have not yet officially accepted excessive exercise disorder as a psychologic disease, so there is not yet consensus about the signs, symptoms, and risks associated with the disorder. People who develop this disorder are generally hard-working, task-oriented, high-achieving individuals with a tendency to be dissatisfied with themselves. Certain factors may predispose an individual to excessive exercise disorder, such as: (a) a society that places a high value on achievement, being fit, and being thin; (b)

family role models who present athletic success as the ultimate achievement; and (c) individuals who are unstable in their own self-worth and/or relationships with others. The key in determining if a person has an excessive exercise disorder is to determine if they insist on exercising while presenting the symptoms of overtraining (Table 17.12).

## SPECIAL NUTRITIONAL NEEDS FOR WOMEN

The nutritional needs of girls and women are generally the same as those of boys and men. When nutrient needs differ between the genders, it is usually due to the average larger body size of males compared to females. Nonetheless, there are certain periods of a woman's life when special attention should be given to nutrition. These periods of the life cycle for the woman include pregnancy, lactation, and post-menopause. Exercise in and of itself does not jeopardize the nutritional health of the woman. However, if a woman's nutritional status is questionable to begin with, she may be jeopardizing her health or her baby's health if she continues to exercise under conditions of poor nutritional care.

### Nutritional Concerns During Pregnancy

A pregnant woman requires additional energy to grow and maintain the developing fetus as well as to support the increasing growth of the placenta, breast tissue, and fat stores of her own. In addition to the increased energy to support growth of the tissues, vitamins and minerals are needed to support differentiation and regulatory processes within the fetus. It has been estimated that the pregnant woman needs to consume an additional 300 kcal of energy each day to support a healthy pregnancy during the second and third trimesters. However, this estimate is just an approximation that may not be accurate for all women because there is a wide variation in energy expended by pregnant women. Some women expend less energy during pregnancy than prior to conception, while other women expend over 25% more energy during pregnancy than prior to conception.

The amount of energy expended during pregnancy depends on factors other than those associated with growth and development. Changing behaviors is one factor that can affect energy expenditure during pregnancy. A woman who is conservative in her approach to pregnancy may change her accustomed lifestyle behaviors to actually getting more sleep, resting more during the day, and doing fewer activities of daily living than before pregnancy, in spite of maintaining an exercise program. Other women may become more health conscious during pregnancy and therefore adopt a more active lifestyle. Adjustments in a woman's metabolism may also compensate for the increased energy demand of a growing child. Such adjustments may include minimizing fat deposition, minimizing the thermic effect of food, and reducing the cost of physical activity. Since all of the factors associated with energy expenditure of the pregnant woman are not easily measured, and some of them are

## CASE STUDY 17.2:  *EXERCISE TRAINING FOR AN EATING-DISORDER PATIENT*

### CASE

You are an exercise physiologist working in a university health and wellness program. The Student Counseling Center has referred to you Jen, a student who is anorexic. Jen is receiving counseling at the center. Although Jen is in treatment for anorexia, she insists that she maintain an exercise program to stay in shape. The referring psychologist and Jen have made a contract in which Jen agrees to only exercise at your facility and follow your recommendations. (This may seem strange, but the counselor feels that if Jen insists upon exercising anyway, it would be in her best interest if she exercised in a facility where she would be monitored by a clinical exercise physiologist who understands women's issues.) Jen is a 21-year-old junior who has been anorexic for 4 years.

### DESCRIPTION

The tremendous amount of environmental pressure to be thin causes many girls and women to succumb to anorexia. A large proportion of these anorexics couple their restrictive dieting behaviors with exercise in an effort to enhance or maintain weight loss. Since exercise is seen as a positive health behavior, anorexics who are compulsive exercisers can often go unnoticed in fitness facilities. Furthermore, some anorexics in treatment conceal their compulsive exercise routines from their therapist.

### EVALUATION/INTERVENTION

Your initial meeting with Jen is scheduled for an intake interview. During that first interview, Jen fills out the routine paperwork, including a medical history and consent forms for fitness testing. You and Jen discuss the rules for her participating in an exercise program under your supervision. Listed below is a summary of the rules specific to Jen's condition.

1. Jen will only exercise in your facility and will not exercise at home, on campus, or anywhere else without your approval.
2. Jen will only be allowed to perform the exercise program prescribed by you. She is not allowed to add anything to her exercise program without your approval. This includes increasing exercise time, exercise volume, sets, repetitions, number, or type of exercises performed, etc.
3. Jen will check in with you and/or one of your staff members each time she comes to the facility and will not begin her exercise for that day until she has checked in.
4. Jen agrees that she will submit to regularly scheduled testing and evaluations at your facility.
5. Jen agrees that she will allow you (or staff member) to monitor her vitals during exercise.
6. Jen agrees that she will stop exercising at any time you or your staff member thinks it is in her best interest.

7. Jen is to bring a sports drink to every one of her workouts. The sports drink cannot be a diet drink, meaning it must contain calories. The sports drink will be consumed while Jen is at your facility, and it will be consumed in the presence of you or your staff member.
8. Jen is not allowed to weigh herself at any time while in your facility.
9. If Jen does not abide by all of these rules, she will be dismissed immediately from the program.

Your next meeting with Jen is to perform her fitness assessment and design her program. Jen's cardiorespiratory capacity and flexibility are all within the normal range for her age and gender. Her muscular strength and endurance values are in the 10th percentile for her age. Jen has an extremely low body weight (90 lb, 41 kg). Her percent body fat is 8.9%. All other health indicators indicate that Jen is cleared to participate in an exercise program.

The program you design for her is one for flexibility and strength training. You do not allow Jen to participate in an aerobic exercise program because aerobic conditioning will likely cause additional weight loss. Strength training and flexibility exercises do not have as strong a tendency to promote weight loss as aerobic training. Plus you want to increase Jen's lean tissue mass since she is emaciated.

Prohibiting aerobic exercise does not seem reasonable to Jen at first, but you agree to reconsider in 1 month, based on her progress in treatment. Jen becomes angry at the rule to drink a calorie-containing sports drink at her workouts, but you reassure her that her body needs the sugar to maintain the exercise bout and that further weight loss will not be tolerated. She concedes. If Jen refuses to abide by the rules, you must release her from the program because your job is to monitor and protect Jen's health the best you can.

The types of rules you have set down for Jen may seem harsh and extremely rigid, but individuals with anorexia are in emotional turmoil, and they become obsessive about maintaining their compulsive anorexic behaviors. They will do almost anything to maintain certain routine behaviors they think will help them lose weight. Consequently, their obsession about the need to lose weight causes them to act in ways that are manipulative, compulsive, and deceitful. These negative behavioral characteristics are not an inherent part of the anorexic's personality. It is the eating disorder that causes them to behave this way, in spite of their own moral code of ethics. Eating-disorder therapy will help Jen change her distorted thinking patterns, her distorted body image, and her obsessive/compulsive behaviors; but in the mean time, you need to ensure that Jen's exercise program does not support these distortions and does not jeopardize her health.

| Table 17.12 | SYMPTOMS OF OVERTRAINING |
|---|---|
| Overall fatigue |
| Reduction in performance |
| Decreased ability to concentrate |
| Loss of emotional vigor |
| Increased compulsiveness |
| Soreness, stiffness |
| Decreased $\dot{V}O_{2max}$ |
| Decreased heart rate response to exercise |
| Hormonal imbalance |
| Muscle wasting |
| Weight loss |

only hypothesized factors, the best indicator of adequate energy intake for the pregnant woman is weight gain.

Most women who eat a balanced diet can meet their nutrient needs for pregnancy without supplementation. The recommended increase in nutrient needs for pregnancy range from 0 to 10% for most vitamins and minerals, and from 10 to 30% for most other nutrients. The vitamin $B_6$ need is 46% over baseline, folate 50% above baseline, and iron 100% above baseline. Even so, the Institute of Medicine Nutrient Supplement Subcommittee suggests that the pregnant woman only supplements her diet with iron and folate. Other than that, the recommended diet for a pregnant woman is similar to what is recommended for the general population. The only added advice is for the woman to consume at least three servings of dairy products each day and to avoid alcohol consumption.

## Nutritional Concerns for Lactation

The energy needs of the lactating mother are also elevated in comparison with the nonpregnant, nonlactating woman. The recommended dietary allowance for lactating woman is 500 extra kcal per day. However, just as with pregnancy, this estimate is not accurate for all women. Also, as with pregnancy, the best indicator of adequate energy intake is the woman's body weight. Although many women are anxious to lose the extra body weight gained during pregnancy, weight loss of more than 0.5 kg per week can reduce milk production. Furthermore, an energy intake of less than 1500 kcal per day can reduce milk production to a level below what can support infant growth and development.

Breast milk contains a substantial amount of protein, especially the premature milk the baby receives during the first few weeks of nursing. The amount of milk given to the baby through the first 6 to 12 months of nursing ranges from 12 to 15 g a day. This means that the nursing mother

needs to increase her pre-pregnancy intake of protein by 15 g per day. Supplementation of protein is not suggested because most American women consume an abundance of dietary protein.

The need for some vitamins and minerals is greater during lactation than pregnancy, while the need for others is lower than during pregnancy. Iron and folate needs, for which the woman may have been supplementing during pregnancy, are reduced during breastfeeding. Therefore, breastfeeding women do not generally need vitamin and/or mineral supplementation. However, there is one nutrient that needs to be consumed in abundance and that often is neglected—water. A nursing mother should drink at least 2 L of water each day, and drink a cup of water every time she breastfeeds her baby. Caffeinated beverages should be limited to 2 cups a day because caffeine passes into the breast milk and can affect the baby. Caffeinated beverages should not replace other fluids consumed by the mother. If the mother is exercising, she needs to increase her fluid consumption beyond 2 L a day to replace fluid loss during perspiration. Other than these simple recommendations, a diet abundant in vegetables will supply all the micronutrient requirements for the nursing mother.

## Nutritional Needs Post-Menopause

The most recent dietary reference intake charts for adults have expanded categories to include women ages 51 to 70 and older than 70. This is a needed expansion since life expectancy for women has increased to the late seventies and the nutrient needs of older women are different from young women. The energy expenditure of older women is reduced by about 13% when compared to young women. This means that for the older woman to receive adequate nutrition and maintain a healthy weight, her diet needs to be more nutrient dense. The problem is further complicated, because as we age, our ability to absorb and utilize certain micronutrients is reduced.

Protein is the only energy-yielding nutrient that is of concern for the older woman. The protein need for women does not change with age. This means that if a woman reduces her energy intake to maintain a healthy weight as she ages, she will have to eat more protein or eat foods with a higher protein content than she had earlier in life. The micronutrients that are of concern for older women are vitamin D, vitamin $B_{12}$, vitamin $B_6$, and folate. Key minerals for the older women are calcium, zinc, magnesium, and iron.

The recommended intake of vitamin D for postmenopausal women is two to three times that recommended for younger women. This is because older women have reduced synthesis rates of vitamin D and generally receive less sunlight exposure. The ability to absorb protein-bound vitamin $B_{12}$ is often reduced in older women. Since the absorption of vitamin $B_{12}$ is easiest in fortified foods and supplements, these are recommended for older women. The recommendation for vitamin $B_6$ is only slightly higher for older women than younger women.

Therefore, supplementation of this vitamin may not be necessary. Adequate folate, as well as adequate vitamins $B_{12}$ and $B_6$, can help prevent risk of cardiovascular disease in older women. The folate requirement for older women is twice that of younger women. However, adequate folate intake can be obtained rather easily because enriched cereal grains are now fortified with folate.

Maintaining adequate calcium intake will help reduce the age-related rate of bone loss in older women. Older women lose some capacity to absorb calcium because of a loss in vitamin D receptors in the gut. Therefore, the recommendation for calcium intake in older women is 200 mg more than that for younger women. Zinc deficiencies in older women are not common, but many older women have borderline intake of zinc. Similarly, magnesium deficiencies are uncommon but have occurred in older women. The recommended dietary allowance for iron in women post-menopause drops to that of men. Therefore, an adequate diet can provide the amount of iron needed for older women. The biography for this chapter presents information on Barbara Drinkwater, who has studied many aspects of women and exercise, including training response, athletics, and the female athlete triad.

▶ *INQUIRY SUMMARY.* Nutrition and exercise are inseparably connected. Girls and women who exercise need to be aware of some nutritional issues to which they are more susceptible than boys and men. Females are at higher risk for developing osteoporosis and iron-deficiency anemia than males because of the different hormonal changes that females pass through during development as compared with males. Females are also more susceptible than males to psychologic problems of eating disorders, excessive exercise disorder, and the female athlete triad because the cultural expectations for females are different than that of males. Regardless of the physiologic and psychologic problems that can arise in exercising females, exercise training and athletic competition provide many benefits. *Who do you think is responsible for educating girls and women about their nutritional needs while exercising?*

## Summary

Girls are different from boys and women are different from men when comparisons are made in exercise physiology. On average, females are not as strong as males because of their smaller body size and proportionately higher fat-to-lean tissue ratio. However, the strength differences between the sexes are reduced when strength is expressed in relative terms. The metabolic capacity of females may be less than males, but this is probably due to the smaller organ sizes of the female (e.g., heart volume).

Regardless of the inherent morphologic or physiologic differences between genders, females respond to exercise training in the same manner as males. Exercise training

during pregnancy, however, presents special needs. The pregnant woman should monitor her exercise volume, exercise intensity, hydration status, and perceived exertion more closely than the nonpregnant woman. Exercise post-menopause presents very little risk compared with its health benefits. An emotionally healthy female, who is cognizant of her nutritional needs while exercise training, should be encouraged to exercise throughout her life unless certain contraindications arise.

### SUMMARY KNOWLEDGE

1. What morphologic or structural differences should be considered when comparing exercise performance in males and females?
2. What are some contraindications for exercising during pregnancy?
3. What health outcomes might a woman expect who exercises during perimenopause and menopause?
4. What is osteoporosis and how does it develop?
5. As an exercise professional, how would you deal with a female athlete who presents with amenorrhea?
6. What are some signs and symptoms of an eating disorder?
7. What are the symptoms of iron-deficiency anemia?
8. Why is the female athlete triad such a destructive disorder?
9. What are some signs and symptoms of excessive exercise disorder?

### References

1. Fox EL, Bowers RW, Foss ML. *The physiological basis for exercise and sport.* 5th ed. Dubuque, Ia: Brown & Benchmark, 1993:368–408.
2. Åstrand PO, Cuddy TE, Saltin B, et al. Cardiac output during submaximal and maximal work. *J Appl Physiol* 1964;19:268–274.
3. Mitchell JH, Tate C, Raven P, et al. Acute response and chronic adaptation to exercise in women. *Med Sci Sports Exerc* 1992;24 (6 Suppl):S258–S265.
4. George JD, Fisher AG, Wehrs PR. *Laboratory experiences in exercise science.* Boston: Jones & Bartlett Publishers, 1994:224.
5. Wilmore JH. Alterations in strength, body composition and anthropometric measurements consequent to a 10-week weight training program. *Med Sci Sports* 1974;6:133–138.
6. Costill DL, Daniels D, Evans W, et al. Skeletal muscle enzymes and fiber composition in male and female track athletes. *J Appl Physiol* 1976;40:149–154.
7. American College of Sports Medicine. *ACSM's guidelines for exercise testing and prescription.* 6th ed. Baltimore: Lippincott Williams & Wilkins, 2000:85–88.
8. Sparling PB. A meta-analysis of studies comparing maximal oxygen uptake in men and women. *Res Q Exerc Sport* 1980;51:542–552.
9. Lemmer JT, Hurlbut DE, Martel GF, et al. Age and gender responses to strength training and detraining. *Med Sci Sports Exerc* 2000;32:1505–1512.
10. Brown CH, Wilmore JH. The effects of maximal resistance training on the strength and body composition of women athletes. *Med Sci Sports* 1974;6:174–177.
11. Deschenes MR, Kraemer WJ. Performance and physiologic adaptations to resistance training. *Am J Phys Med Rehabil* 2002;81(11 Suppl):S3–S16.

12. Kilbom A. Physical training in women. *Scand J Clin Lab Invest Suppl* 1971;119:1–34.

13. Costill DL, Fink WJ, Getchell LH, et al. Lipid metabolism in skeletal muscle of endurance-trained males and females. *J Appl Physiol* 1979;47:787–791.

14. Pate RR, Barnes C, Miller W. A physiological comparison of performance-matched female and male distance runners. *Res Q Exerc Sport* 1985;56:245–250.

15. Dale E, Gerlach DH, Wilhite AL. Menstrual dysfunction in distance runners. *Obstet Gynecol* 1979;54:47–53.

16. Myerson M, Gutin B, Warren MP, et al. Resting metabolic rate and energy balance in amenorrheic and eumenorrheic runners. *Med Sci Sports Exerc* 1991;23:15–22.

17. Bullen BA, Skrinar GS, Beitins IZ, et al. Induction of menstrual disorders by strenuous exercise in untrained women. *New Engl J Med* 1985;312:1349–1353.

18. Lokey EA, Tran ZV, Wells CL, et al. Effects of physical exercise on pregnancy outcomes: a meta-analytic review. *Med Sci Sports Exerc* 1991;23:1234–1239.

19. Beckmann CRB, Beckmann CA. Effect of a structured antepartum exercise program on pregnancy and labor outcome in primiparas. *J Reprod Med* 1990;35:704–709.

20. Zaharieva E. Survey of sportwomen at the Tokyo Olympics. *J Sports Med Phys Fitness* 1965;2:215–219.

### Suggested Readings

Brown W. The benefits of physical activity during pregnancy. *J Sci Med Sport* 2002;5:37–45.

Clapp JF 3rd, Kim H, Burciu B, et al. Beginning regular exercise in early pregnancy: effect on fetoplacental growth. *Am J Obstet Gynecol* 2000;183:1484–1488.

Cussler EC, Lohman TG, Going SB, et al. Weight lifted in strength training predicts bone change in postmenopausal women. *Med Sci Sports Exerc* 2003;35:10–17.

Dook JE, James C, Henderson NK, et al. Exercise and bone mineral density in mature female athletes. *Med Sci Sports Exerc* 1997;29: 291–296.

Greydanus DE, Patel DR. The female athlete: before and beyond puberty. *Pediatr Clin North Am* 2002;49:553–580.

Hawkins SA, Schroeder ET, Dreyer HC, et al. Five-year maintenance of bone mineral density in women master runners. *Med Sci Sports Exerc* 2003;35:137–144.

Kohrt WM, Bloomfield SA, Little KD, et al, for the American College of Sports Medicine. American College of Sports Medicine position stand: physical activity and bone health. *Med Sci Sports Exerc* 2004;36:1985–1996.

Loucks AB. Physical health of the female athlete: observations, effects, and causes of reproductive disorders. *Can J Appl Physiol* 2001;26 Suppl:S176–S185.

Lumbers ER. Exercise in pregnancy: physiological basis of exercise prescription for the pregnant woman. *J Sci Med Sport* 2002;5:20–31.

Otis CL, Drinkwater B, Johnson M, et al. American College of Sports Medicine position stand: the female athlete triad. *Med Sci Sports Exerc* 1997;29:i–ix.

Vincent KR, Braith RW. Resistance exercise and bone turnover in elderly men and women. *Med Sci Sports Exerc* 2002;34:17–23.

Warren MP, Stiehl AL. Exercise and female adolescents: effects on the reproductive and skeletal systems. *J Am Med Womens Assoc* 1999;54:115–120.

West RV. The female athlete. The triad of disordered eating, amenorrhea and osteoporosis. *Sports Med* 1998;26:63–71.

### On the Internet

TeensHealth Answers & Advice: Female athlete triad. Available at: **http://www.kidshealth.org/teen/food_fitness/sports/triad.html**. Accessed June 16, 2005.

Family Practice Notebook.com: Female athlete triad. Available at: **http://www.fpnotebook.com/SPO36.htm**. Accessed June 16, 2005.

Women's Exercise Network. Available at: **http://www.womensexercisenetwork.com/**. Accessed June 16, 2005.

Association of Women for the Advancement of Research and Education: Project AWARE: Managing menopause: exercise. Available at: **http://www.project-aware.org/Managing/exercise.shtml**. Accessed June 16, 2005.

Fit to Deliver Prenatal Fitness Program. Available at: **http://www.fit-todeliver.com**. Accessed June 16, 2005.

4 Girls Health. Available at: **http://www.4girls.gov**. Accessed June 16, 2005.

## Writing to Learn

*Females respond to exercise training the same as males. However, special attention should be given to the changing needs of the exercising female. The stages of childhood, adolescence, pregnancy, and post menopause bring with them particular concerns relevant to exercise and nutrition. Design a table that lists the stages of childhood, adolescence, pregnancy, and post menopause in rows and then make a column for exercise and nutritional concerns and another column for exercise and nutritional remedies. Fill in the cells for the table.*

# Exercise Physiology for Clinical Populations

*Part 3 of the text continues the applied approach, but now centers on clinical issues related to exercise testing and training. This part of the book is especially important for physical and occupational therapy students, and for those students pursuing other health professions. This part of the book is also critical for exercise physiologists who will be working with special populations.*

*Section 1 begins with two chapters presenting content usually not covered in depth in other exercise physiology texts. Our treatment of pharmacology and pathophysiology in Chapter 18 is a foundation for the remaining chapters of Part 3. Additionally, Chapter 19 presents the disablement process, essential material for the health professions student studying therapeutic exercise. Chapter 20 contains a detailed presentation of exercise testing.*

*The text ends with Section 2, which covers clinical exercise for several chronic disorders that the exercise professional encounters frequently: cardiopulmonary disorders (Chapter 21), obesity (Chapter 22), and oncological and neuromusculoskeletal disorders (Chapter 23).*

# CHAPTER

# 18 Introduction to Pharmacology and Pathophysiology

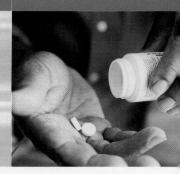

*Individuals with active pathology are often on a course of both medication and exercise prescription. Patients must adhere appropriately to both for therapy to be effective.* What are common difficulties faced by patients trying to adhere to either of these regimens?

## CHAPTER OUTLINE

This chapter, which combines concepts of pharmacology and pathophysiology, provides the necessary information to relate to the remaining chapters focusing on clinical foundations in exercise physiology. Most individuals in clinical exercise programs will be on a course of prescriptive drug therapy and will have some sort of pathophysiologic involvement. Understanding these concepts is vital for therapists who use prescriptive exercise training to enhance individuals' physical abilities within their pathophysiologic limitations.

## Basic Pharmacology

As a health care professional, the individuals you will most often encounter in clinical exercise programs are usually older adults, and quite often they are on a course of multiple medications. Older individuals ($\geq$65 years) consume 30% of the prescribed and from 40% to 50% of the over-the-counter medications taken in this country, yet they make up only 13% of the United States population. This **polypharmacy** has several features:

- Medications are given that are not always necessary
- Duplicate medications are often given
- Persons are often on a course of concurrently interacting medications
- Individuals are taking inappropriate dosages
- When adverse **drug** reactions occur, drug treatment often follows
- Once the course of polypharmacy is discontinued, improvement follows

The combination of physiologic changes accompanying aging, the negative effects of polypharmacy, and the physiologic responses to acute exercise place older patients at risk for adverse effects during therapeutic exercise training. Because exercise and medications, often working in opposition, alter the magnitude and direction of physiologic variables, **pharmacology** is an important topic for a clinical exercise physiology text. Your responsibility as a health care professional is to understand the effects and potential side effects of the drug regimen of your patients and how exercise training interacts with medication regimens. In this section, an introduction to basic pharmacology is provided before we move to specific classes of drugs.

 *LINKUP: Elderly individuals often experience adverse effects of both exercise and drugs and are at an increased risk for both individually and in combination. Perspective: Adverse Effects of Drugs and Exercise in Elderly Patients, found at http://connection.lww.com/ go/brownexphys and on the Student Resource CD-ROM, discusses this dual problem.*

## DEFINITION OF PHARMACOLOGY

Pharmacology is defined as the study of the interactions between physiologic processes and drugs. Drugs, by definition, alter function by interactions, starting at the molecular and cellular level, and then progressing to the organ and finally the systemic level. A complicating factor in the prescription of medication is that of interindividual variability. Not all individuals react the same way to a given drug dosage because drug metabolism is variable among individuals. The goal of the physician is to prescribe appropriate therapeutic dosages to improve the medical status of their patients. Therefore, the goal of drug therapy is to fit the right kind of medication and an appropriate dose to the individual needs of the patient at a given moment in time (see Case Study 18.1).

## PHARMACOKINETICS AND PHARMACODYNAMICS

The foundation of medical prescription rests on two important concepts within pharmacology: **pharmacokinetics**

## CASE STUDY 18.1: *ANTIARRHYTHMIA PRESCRIPTION*

### CASE

Bill is a 65-year-old manager who complained to his physician about what felt like flutters accompanied by lightheadedness. Three years earlier he suffered a lateral wall myocardial infarction and has since been on a course of isosorbide dinitrate, atenolol, and diltiazem. He experienced these symptoms while in the doctor's office; the attending nurse, while palpating his pulse, could not feel a pulse after every other beat. The physician promptly ordered Bill to be placed on a 24-hour Holter monitor to "capture" such episodes on tape. Subsequent analysis showed that Bill experienced an irregular heart rhythm known as ventricular bigeminy (premature ventricular contractions [PVCs] every other beat), with occasional couplets of PVCs. Chapter 20 explains arrhythmias in detail.

### DESCRIPTION

Cardiac arrhythmia is an alteration in rhythm or rate of the heart beat and may be serious enough to warrant medical intervention. An arrhythmia is a change from the normal rate or control of the heart's contractions. Where the changes are under the influence of the sinoatrial (SA) node, the term sinus arrhythmia is used. Sometimes rhythms are generated outside of the SA node. These are separated into supraventricular and ventricular, depending on their origin. In Bill's case, the locus was in the ventricle. In ventricular rhythms, the depolarization wave spreads through the ventricles by an irregular and therefore slower pathway. The QRS complex is thus wide and abnormal. Repolarization pathways are also different, causing the T wave to have an unusual morphology. Above 120 beats per minutes, this rhythm is termed ventricular tachycardia and may pose a serious threat.

### INTERVENTION

Bill's physician prescribed quinidine to control the ventricular ectopy. However, Bill could not tolerate the quinidine well and experienced gastrointestinal symptoms. He was taken off the quinidine and placed on procainamide, which alleviated the gastrointestinal problems. After months on this regimen, Bill again began to have symptoms of flutter and dizziness. His physician again ordered Holter monitoring, which showed that his original ventricular ectopy had returned. Bill also began to notice joint pain, which caused him to cease the exercise prescription on which he had been placed. The physician stopped the procainamide treatment and Bill was admitted to the hospital, where he underwent exercise thallium testing to determine the extent of myocardial perfusion during exercise and to determine if the ectopy was ischemia induced. The test was negative for ischemia but positive for anterior wall **dyskinesis**, consistent with a ventricular aneurysm. Bill also underwent electrophysiologic testing to induce ventricular tachycardia. Bill subsequently began a course of mexiletine. Bill was retested in an attempt to reinduce the ventricular tachycardia, which was unsuccessful. Bill was discharged on mexiletine and was to resume his monitored cardiac rehabilitation program.

and **pharmacodynamics**. Pharmacokinetics, how the body handles drugs, has five aspects:

1. Absorption: how and where the drug is introduced to the body
2. **Bioavailability**: the availability of a particular amount of a drug at the site of drug action
3. Distribution: how the drug moves to different locations in the body
4. Metabolism: how the drug is transformed from its active to its inactive state
5. Excretion: how the drug passes out of the body

Pharmacodynamics is concerned with processes involved in the interaction between a drug and an effector organ that results in a clinical response, either a therapeutic (efficacious) or adverse (toxic) effect. Pharmacodynamics measures the intensity, peak, and duration of action of a medication. *Figure 18.1* shows the interaction of these two concepts in the patient. Note that the pharmacokinetic effect precedes, and largely causes, the pharmacodynamic effect.

Absorption and bioavailability are affected by dosage and route of administration of a drug. Typically three variables are taken into account for dosage:

1. Amount of the drug given at one time
2. Method and route of administration
3. Duration of drug prescription (1)

Methods of drug administration includes *continuous* (e.g., wearing a transcutaneous nitroglycerin patch) or *intermit-*tent (the time interval between doses taken by any route) input. Likewise, there are two basic access routes of administration: **enteral** or **parenteral**. Enteral means that the drug enters the gastrointestinal (GI) system before it enters the circulation. It can enter the GI system by mouth or through the rectum. Parenteral means that the drug enters via a route other than the intestinal route. In this access route, the drug can enter through any of the following means:

- Intravenous
- Subcutaneous injection
- Intramuscular injection
- Intrathecal injection (spinal)
- Intraperitoneal injection
- Sublingual
- Inhalational

## Pharmacokinetics and Age-Related Physiologic Changes

Because clinical exercise programs are most often populated with older individuals, it is necessary to review the interactions between age-related physiologic changes and the concept of pharmacokinetics (2). A brief review of pharmacokinetics altered by age-related physiologic changes is presented in *Table 18.1*.

In older adults, GI motility is decreased, which may prolong the absorption phase of the drug as it stays in one locale within the intestinal tract for a longer time period. The likelihood of a decreased mucosal cell count in elderly in-

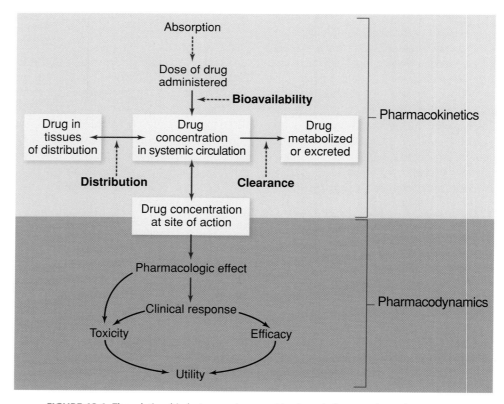

**FIGURE 18.1.** The relationship between pharmacokinetic and pharmacodynamic processes.

| **Table 18.1** | **PHARMACOKINETICS ALTERED BY AGE-RELATED PHYSIOLOGIC CHANGES** |
| --- | --- |

**System Change**

**Gastrointestinal**
Acid production unchanged
Drug-drug interaction alters absorption
Splanchnic blood flow decreases with no effect on drug absorption

**Liver**
Decrease in hepatic blood flow often associated with decreased first-pass metabolism
Phase I drug metabolism decreased
Phase II drug metabolism unaffected

**Fluid and tissue compartments**
Decrease in total body water
Decrease in plasma volume
Decrease in extracellular fluid
Increase in fat compartment
Decrease in muscle mass

**Plasma drug-binding proteins**
Decrease in serum albumin
No change in $\alpha$-acid glycoprotein
Decrease in plasma globulin

**Kidneys**
Decrease in renal blood flow
Decline in creatine clearance
Decline in tubular secretion
Decrease in glomerular filtration rate

**Cardiorespiratory**
Decrease in cardiac index
Decrease in vital capacity
Decrease in cardiac output
Decrease in splanchnic and renal blood flow

dividuals coupled with reduced intestinal blood flow may also affect absorption in elderly individuals. This increases the bioavailability of the drug by reducing its availability to the hepatic portal circulation where it first passes before entering the systemic circulation. Box 18.1 provides additional information about hepatic portal circulation.

Bioavailability refers to the proportion of a drug that reaches the systemic circulation unchanged after a particular route of administration. When drugs are taken by mouth, their bioavailability is determined by factors in the drug, including the nature of the molecule, its stability, and the formulation administered. Bioavailability is also determined by factors in the patient such as a reduced intestinal surface area as a result of celiac disease or intestinal resection. Whether or not the drug is taken with a meal also affects bioavailability. If less of the drug is sent to the liver because of poor portal circulatory uptake, there is the potential for reduced inactivation of the drug by the liver and for greater bioavailability due to a reduced **first-pass effect** of the drug. The liver primarily dictates the magni-

tude of the first-pass effect. In addition, this effect may also be enhanced by the reduced renal function seen with aging. As kidney competency declines with age due to reduced renal blood flow, drug accumulation and the potential for **toxicity** ensues. Bioavailability is also increased by the parenteral routes of administration. Typical among these are intravenous, injection, and sublingual administration, which are particularly fast acting.

After absorption, drugs enter the general circulation and are distributed. Solubility in lipid and the extent of protein binding dictate distribution. Distribution refers to the amount of drug that is free to bind to its specific receptor site at the plasma membrane of the target tissue. Thus, if too much protein binding occurs, less of the drug is available for action at target tissues. To be pharmacologically active, higher free drug levels must exist. Given these facts, many elderly people are susceptible to increased pharmacologic activity. For example, the dietary protein intake of many elderly individuals is often less than adequate. In this situation, these people may become **hypoproteinemic** and have lower levels of albumin (plasma protein), resulting in higher plasma free drug concentration and an increased pharmacologic effect. This effect, however, may be countered by the reduced cardiac output seen in elderly individuals. Lower cardiac output leads to a decreased peripheral blood flow, less distribution of the drug, and lower pharmacologic effect.

Drug metabolism takes place in the liver. In older individuals, drug metabolism is slow due to a smaller liver mass and less hepatic blood flow. This increases drug bioavailability. Drug metabolism by the liver is classified into phase I and phase II metabolism during which the drug is first converted to a more easily excreted metabolite (phase I), and then the drug or its metabolite is coupled with an endogenous substrate (phase II). As shown in Table 18.1, phase I metabolism is decreased with age, which allows more of the biologically active drug to remain to have a pharmacologic effect. Phase II metabolism is unaltered by age. The changes in phase I metabolism with age allow drug **half-life** to increase in older individuals. Half-life is the time it takes for a drug to be reduced to 50% of its initial plasma concentration. If half-life increases, the effects of the drug will be longer lasting, increasing bioavailability. Drug half-life dictates the frequency of its administration. Typically the following frequencies are commonly prescribed:

- qid: four times per day
- tid: three times per day
- bid: twice per day
- qd: once daily

Because these frequencies are linked to the half-life of the drug, medications should always be taken at consistently regular intervals. If these intervals are adhered to inconsistently, drug plasma concentrations will be altered and the proper therapeutic dose will be lost.

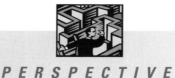

**Box 18.1**

## PERSPECTIVE

# Hepatic Portal Circulation

There are three types of blood circulatory systems, two of which (systemic circulation and pulmonary circulation) depend on the heart to pump blood. The third type of circulation is known as a portal system, which consists of specialized channels connecting one capillary bed site to another but not depending directly on a central pump. The largest of these in the human is the hepatic portal system connecting the intestines to the liver. Normally there is only one capillary bed for each branch of a circuit; however, there are a few instances where there are two capillary beds, one after each other, in series. These are known as portal systems or portal circulations. Part of the blood supply to the liver is venous blood coming directly from the gastrointestinal tract and spleen via the hepatic portal vein. This arrangement enables the digested and absorbed substances from the gut to be transported directly to the liver, where many of the body's metabolic requirements are synthesized. Thus, there are two micro-circulations in series, one in the gut and the other in the liver. The hepatic portal circulation serves the intestines,

spleen, pancreas, and gall bladder. The liver receives its blood from two main sources: the hepatic artery, which as a branch of the aorta, supplies oxygenated blood to the liver; and the hepatic portal vein, which is formed by the union of veins from the spleen, stomach, pancreas, duodenum, and colon. The hepatic portal vein transports the following to the liver:

- Absorbed nutrients from the duodenum
- White blood cells (added to the circulation) from the spleen
- Poisonous substances, such as alcohol, which are absorbed in the intestines
- Waste products, such as carbon dioxide, from the spleen, pancreas, stomach, and duodenum

The hepatic artery and hepatic portal vein open into the liver sinuses where the blood is in direct contact with the liver cells. The deoxygenated blood, which still retains some dissolved nutrients, eventually flows into the inferior vena cava via the hepatic veins.

---

The renal system is chiefly responsible for clearing or eliminating a drug from the body. Unfortunately, this system is affected by age because of decreases in kidney mass by about 20% by the eighth decade of life and the 10-$mL \cdot min^{-1}$ per decade reduction in renal blood flow after age 30. Reduced elimination because of decreased kidney function means that bioavailability is increased in elderly individuals.

### Pharmacodynamic Processes

Pharmacodynamics is concerned with the intensity, peak, and duration of action of a drug. At the effector organ, a drug's effect is dictated by receptors, which are membrane-bound macromolecules. Receptors are of four general types: regulatory proteins, enzymes, transport proteins, or structural proteins. Receptors function in a nonspecific manner common to many cells; therefore, drugs produce multiple effects at many sites of action. These effects are classified as primary, secondary, and side effects. An individual's tolerance for the drug is determined by considering all possible effects so that toxicity is avoided.

While a drug's activity is nonspecific, a particular drug does prefer one group or subgroup of receptors if the con-

centration is great enough. This selectivity is based on the traditional "lock and key" complementary relationship formed between the drug and receptor, much like the enzyme-receptor complementary relationship. Receptor sites are found all over the body. For example, common receptor sites for cardiac medications are found in the autonomic nervous system, kidneys, and vascular smooth muscle. Receptors of the autonomic nervous system are specific to one of its two branches: sympathetic and parasympathetic. Recall that sympathetic branch activity secretes norepinephrine (adrenaline) and parasympathetic branch activity secretes acetylcholine from their respective post-ganglionic fibers. Therefore, the receptors for each of these branches are referred to as adrenergic and cholinergic, respectively. Subdivisions of these receptor types are classified as follows:

- Adrenergic receptors: alpha ($\alpha_1$ and $\alpha_2$), beta ($\beta_1$ and $\beta_2$), and dopamine
- Cholinergic receptors: muscarinic ($M_1$ and $M_2$) and nicotinic

There is less distinct division of the alpha adrenergic receptors than there is of the beta adrenergic receptors.

Alpha receptors are activated more strongly by norepinephrine than by **isoproterenol**, and the opposite of this is true of beta receptors. **Phenoxybenzamine** can be used to block alpha adrenergic receptors and **propranolol** can be used to block beta adrenergic receptors. Other selective antagonists are also available for the adrenergic receptors.

The assignment of muscarinic receptors into subtypes is still tentative. The cholinergic receptors are so-named because of the chemicals that can activate them to the exclusion of the other. Muscarine is a poison from toadstools that activates only muscarinic cholinergic receptors (these receptors are blocked by **atropine**), while nicotine activates only nicotinic cholinergic receptors (these receptors are blocked by **curare**). Obviously, acetylcholine activates both types of cholinergic receptors. Nicotine receptors are found in the ganglia (sympathetic and parasympathetic connections that arise from nerves coming out of the spinal cord and connecting to peripheral nerves going to effector organs) and at the neuromuscular junction. The muscarinic receptors are found everywhere that parasympathetic nerve terminals synapse at a tissue.

These major receptors are classified by their sensitivity to **agonist** and **antagonist** drugs. An agonist drug is one that produces biochemical and physiologic changes within the cell, and antagonist drugs interact with receptors to block a response. Drugs that mimic the activity of sympathetic neurotransmitters (i.e., epinephrine, norepinephrine, and dopamine) are called **sympathomimetics** (adrenergic agonists). Drugs that block sympathetic nervous system action are called **sympatholytics** (adrenergic antagonists). Likewise, drugs that simulate parasympathetic activity are known as **parasympathomimetics** (cholinergic agonists), and drugs that block cholinergic activity are called **parasympatholytics** (cholinergic antagonists). *Table 18.2* summarizes the autonomic receptor types, locations, and functions.

The following sections highlight several major classes of drugs encountered most often in therapeutic exercise programs. Pulmonary and cardiovascular physiology are altered by disease in such a way as to disrupt the attempt of normal homeostatic mechanisms to return function to normal. Because of this, drugs are used to help restore normal function. The available pharmaceuticals used in the treatment of the conditions presented in this section are extensive; therefore, only a basic overview will be given of a few of the most important classes of drugs. You are advised to consult other texts that present more comprehensive information for a more complete understanding of the use of a given medication in clinical practice.

▶ *INQUIRY SUMMARY.* Pharmacology, the study of the interactions between living systems and molecules, has two basic components: (a) pharmacokinetics, how the drug moves within the body (as dictated by drug absorption, bioavailability, distribution, metabolism, and excretion) and (b) pharmacodynamics, how the drug produces effects within the body. Since the aging process produces physiologic changes that impact both of these components and since most clinical exercise programs are populated by older individuals, clinical exercise personnel must be aware of the interactions between drugs and exercise in older people. *A problem encountered in the aged population is polypharmacy; how might regular exercise training help older individuals overcome the problems inherent in chronic polypharmacy?*

## Table 18.2 AUTONOMIC RECEPTOR TYPES AND FUNCTIONS

| Receptor Type | Location | Function |
|---|---|---|
| Cholinergic muscarinic | CNS neurons, atrial myocardium, SA and AV node smooth muscle, smooth muscle of secretory glands, bronchi | Decrease contractility, decrease heart rate, decrease peripheral vascular resistance, bronchoconstriction |
| Cholinergic nicotinic | Skeletal muscle endplates, autonomic ganglion cells | Stimulation of neuromuscular junction |
| Adrenergic alpha | Vascular smooth muscle, papillary dilator muscle, pilomotor smooth muscle; smooth muscle of bronchi, GI tract, uterus, and bladder | Vasoconstriction, iris dilatation, intestinal relaxation, intestinal sphincter contraction, pilomotor contraction, bladder sphincter contraction |
| Adrenergic beta | Heart; fat cells; respiratory, uterine, and vascular smooth muscle; skeletal muscle; liver | Vasodilation ($\beta_2$), cardioacceleration ($\beta_1$), increased myocardial strength ($\beta_1$), intestinal relaxation ($\beta_2$), uterus relaxation ($\beta_2$), calorigenesis ($\beta_2$), glycogenolysis ($\beta_2$), lipolysis ($\beta_1$), bladder wall relaxation ($\beta_2$) |

AV, atrioventricular; CNS, central nervous system; GI, gastrointestinal; SA, sinoatrial.

# Commonly Encountered Medications in Clinical Exercise Programs

Modern pharmacotherapy for patients with chronic illnesses has been very successful and has contributed to longevity of elderly persons. For example, the management of cardiac and pulmonary dysfunction involves the prescription of a multifaceted drug regimen in an attempt to produce an efficacious clinical response in patients with disease and disability. Clearly the use of prescriptive medications has allowed many people to live much longer with chronic diseases. The next two sections are provided to familiarize you with medications likely to be encountered in clinical exercise programs.

## CARDIOVASCULAR MEDICATIONS

Physiologic side effects may occur in patients as exercise responses and drugs interact in a synergistic fashion. For example, patients may develop symptoms when medications that cause peripheral vasodilation are taken with aerobic exercise interventions that also produce peripheral vasodilation. The symptoms, e.g., hypotension, dizziness, and **syncope**, may be present only when both exercise and drug intervention occur simultaneously. In a similar manner, drugs may blunt the physiologic effects of exercise, as is the case when taking beta-blocking medications. Beta blockers limit the normal increase in heart rate that occurs with an imposed exercise load. In addition, health care professionals who provide exercise therapy need to be alert to the potential side effects of cardiovascular medications, some of which can be exacerbated by exercise (3). *Table 18.3* lists common side effects of cardiopulmonary drugs and the proper patient response.

The goal of pharmacologic treatment of coronary artery disease (CAD) is to prevent myocardial ischemia and infarction and to maximize and improve cardiovascular function. *Table 18.4* presents the major medical conditions with the commonly prescribed cardiovascular medications used in treatment. The following brief descriptions highlight many of these drugs.

**LINKUP:** *Beta-blocker medications blunt the heart rate response to endurance exercise, yet not all cardiovascular responses are blunted by beta-adrenergic blockade. Men and women may also respond differently. Research Highlight: Changes in Stroke Volume with Beta Blockade, found at http://connection.lww.com/go/ brownexphys and on the Student Resource CD-ROM, presents one study that demonstrates this phenomenon.*

## Organic Nitrates

Common nitrates are those that are longer acting, such as isosorbide mononitrate (e.g., Imdur) and isosorbide dinitrate (e.g., Isordil), and those that are rapidly acting, such

| Table 18.3 | COMMON SIDE EFFECTS OF CARDIOPULMONARY DRUGS AND THE PROPER PATIENT RESPONSES |
| --- | --- |

| Side Effect | Action |
| --- | --- |
| Abdominal pain | Visit physician |
| Asthmatic attack | Visit physician |
| Bradycardia | Visit physician |
| Cough | None |
| Dehydration | None |
| Difficulty breathing or swallowing | Visit physician |
| Dizziness or fainting | Visit physician |
| Drowsiness | None |
| Easy bruising | None |
| Fatigue | None |
| Headache | None |
| Insomnia | Call physician |
| Joint pain | Visit physician |
| Loss of taste | None |
| Muscle cramps | Call physician |
| Nausea | None |
| Nightmares | Call physician |
| Orthostatic hypotension | Call physician |
| Palpitations | Call physician |
| Paralysis | Visit physician |
| Sexual dysfunction | Call physician |
| Skin rash | Call physician |
| Stomach irritation | Call physician |
| Swelling of feet or abdomen | Call physician |
| Symptoms of congestive heart failure (shortness of breath, swollen ankles, coughing up blood) | Visit physician |
| Tachycardia | Call physician |
| Unexplained swelling, unusual or uncontrolled bleeding | Call physician |
| Vomiting | Call physician |
| Weakness | None |

| *Table 18.4* | *COMMONLY PRESCRIBED CARDIOVASCULAR MEDICATIONS* |
|---|---|
| **Condition** | **Drug Class** |
| Angina pectoris | Organic nitrates<br>Beta blockers<br>Calcium channel blockers |
| Arrhythmia | Beta blockers<br>Calcium channel blockers<br>Agents prolonging depolarization |
| Congestive heart failure | Positive inotropes (digitalis)<br>Diuretics<br>ACE inhibitors<br>Vasodilators |
| Hypertension | Diuretics<br>Beta blockers<br>ACE inhibitors<br>Vasodilators<br>Calcium channel blockers |

ACE, angiotensin-converting enzyme.

as nitroglycerin (e.g., Nitro-Time). The purpose of nitrate administration, as shown in *Figure 18.2*, is to: (a) redistribute blood flow along collateral channels and from epicardial to endocardial regions, (b) relieve coronary artery spasm, and (c) induce peripheral vasodilation to unload the heart by reducing afterload (reduced blood pressure) and preload (d). The vasodilatory effect of nitrates on the peripheral vasculature causes pooling of blood. This lowers the venous return and ventricular volume, which reduces preload. Because the ventricle is now on a reduced stretch, mechanical stress on the myocardial walls is also lower, thereby reducing myocardial $O_2$ demand.

Organic nitrates act directly on arterial and vascular smooth muscle to produce arterial and venous vasodilation. By reducing preload and afterload, nitrates reduce myocardial $O_2$ consumption and restore the balance between $O_2$ supply and demand. However, coronary blood flow is unaltered. Concomitant with a decrease in mean blood pressure is the activation of the sympathetic nervous system. Increases in heart rate and **contractility** partially reverse the decrease in myocardial $O_2$ consumption produced by arterial and venous vasodilation. In patients with variant angina, organic nitrates can prevent or reverse

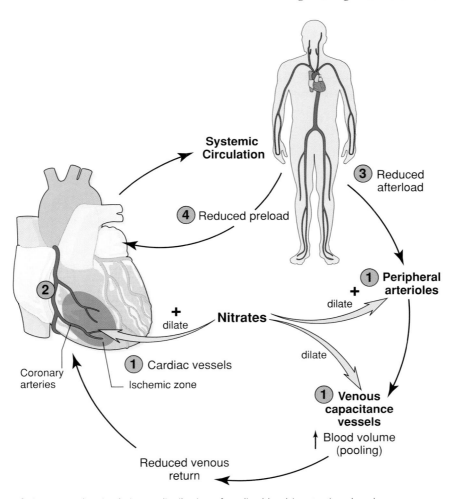

**FIGURE 18.2.** The effects of nitrates on the circulation: redistribution of cardiac blood (see text), reduced coronary spasm, reduced afterload, and reduced preload. The major effect of nitrates is on venous capacitance vessels, but there are also coronary and peripheral arteriolar dilation effects.

coronary artery spasm. Generally side effects of nitrates are direct extensions of their therapeutic effect. They include severe headache, syncope, flushing, hypotension, and reflex tachycardia. Nitrates increase the exercise capacity of patients with angina because they reduce cardiac workload during exercise.

Individuals with CAD should be administered sublingual nitrate at the onset of chest pain. Blood pressure should be monitored, and the patient should be recumbent to prevent hypotension. The patient should return to the upright position slowly after administration. If pain is not relieved, emergency medical care should be implemented immediately.

## Beta Blockers

Beta-blockade therapy attempts to strike a balance between $O_2$ supply and demand in the ischemic heart. To do this, beta blockade produces negative **chronotropic**, **dromotropic**, and **inotropic** effects on the sinus node, on the atrioventricular (AV) node, and on myocardial contraction, respectively (*Fig. 18.3*) (5). The consequent reduction in myocardial $O_2$ demand is subsequently therapeutic for angina pectoris. As shown in *Figure 18.4*, beta blockade decreases the heart's demand for $O_2$ by reducing wall stress. There is a large reduction in $O_2$ demand and a negligible increase in $O_2$ supply. Wall stress is reduced through qualitative changes in the factors shown in Figure 18.4. As a result, there is less $O_2$ deficit and decreased reliance on anaerobic metabolism. Beta-blockade therapy to control atrial and ventricular **tachyarrhythmias** is also ef-

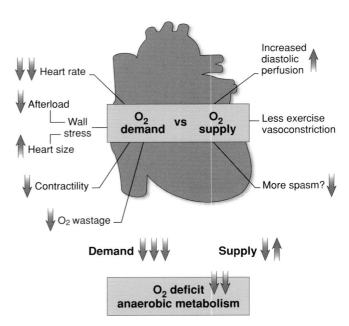

**FIGURE 18.4.** Effects of beta blockade on the ischemic heart. Beta blockers reduce angina by deceasing demand for $O_2$ not supply of $O_2$.

fective, with three proposed mechanisms: inhibiting phase 0 depolarization (class I), inhibiting spontaneous depolarizations (class II), and increasing the duration of the cardiac action potential (class III) (*Fig. 18.5*).

Beta blockers are not prescribed for patients with hypotension, congestive heart failure (CHF), bradycardia, AV blocks, and chronic obstructive pulmonary disease (COPD). The common side effects of beta blockers are

- Dizziness or lightheadedness due to hypotension— change body position more slowly
- Bronchospasm
- Tiredness, cold hands and feet, headache, nightmares, difficulty sleeping, heartburn, constipation, and gas
- Sudden weight gain
- Increased shortness of breath; wheezing; difficulty breathing; skin rash; slow, fast, or irregular heartbeat; swelling of feet and lower legs
- Chest (heart) pain or even heart attack with abrupt cessation
- Severe vomiting or diarrhea
- Depression

Beta blockers increase the exercise capacity of patients with angina. Higher levels of activity can be attained before the ischemic threshold is reached. Patients on beta-blocker drugs will have a lower heart rate than usual at the same level of exercise. If exercise testing and prescription are given, any change in the drug dosage may necessitate a repeat test and prescription.

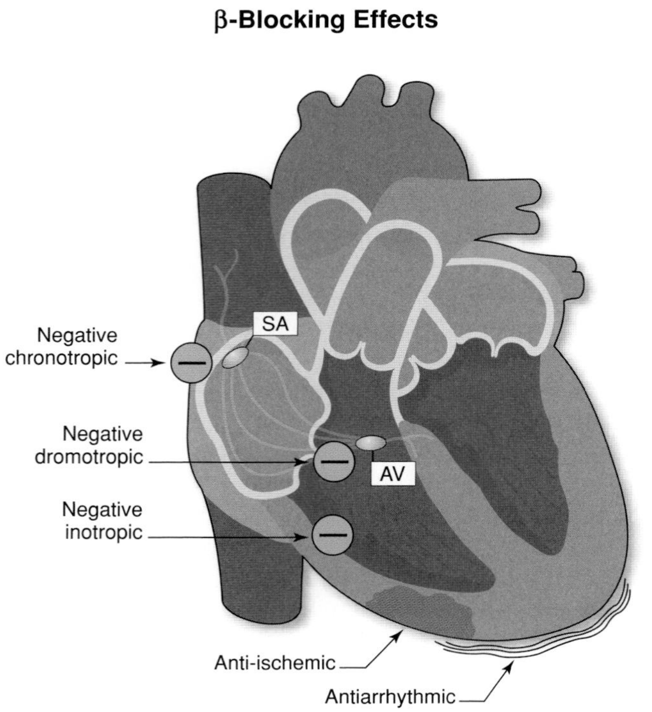

## Calcium Channel Blockers

Calcium channel blockers work by blocking the entry of $Ca^{2+}$ through the $Ca^{2+}$ channels in smooth muscle and

### β-Blocking Effects

![heart diagram] Negative chronotropic — SA, Negative dromotropic — AV, Negative inotropic, Anti-ischemic, Antiarrhythmic

**FIGURE 18.3.** Cardiac effects of beta-adrenergic blocking drugs at the levels of the sinoatrial (SA) node, atrioventricular (AV) node, conduction system, and myocardium.

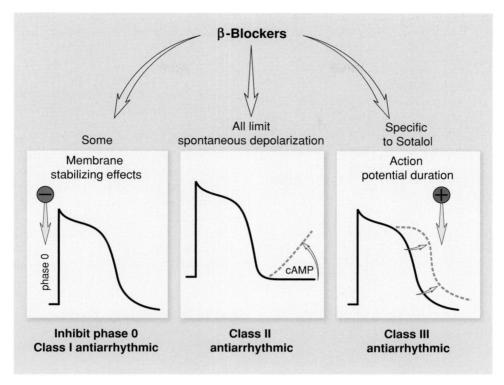

FIGURE 18.5. Antiarrhythmia properties of class I, II, and III beta blockers.

myocardium (6). Muscle contraction is thus attenuated, which produces vasodilation in smooth muscle and a negative inotropic effect (reduced myocardial strength of contraction) in cardiac muscle. The vasodilatory effect reduces peripheral vascular resistance (decreased afterload), which helps in the medical management of angina pectoris, hypertension, and coronary spasm. These effects increase $O_2$ supply more than they decrease $O_2$ demand, and like the action produced by beta blockers, the heart relies less on anaerobic metabolism (decreased $O_2$ deficit). Mechanisms of the anti-ischemic effect of $Ca^{2+}$ channel blockade are shown in *Figure 18.6*.

Calcium channel blockers are of two general classifications: those that dilate peripheral arterioles end with "pine" (amlodipine [Norvasc], felodipine [Plendil], nisoldipine [Sular], and nifedipine [e.g., Procardia]). Those that

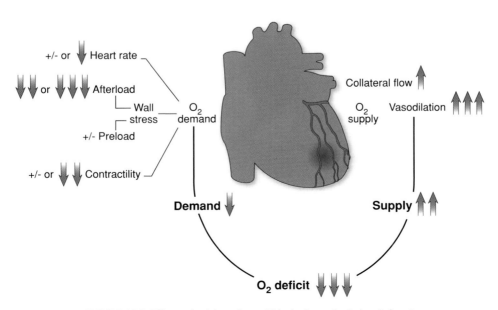

FIGURE 18.6. Effects of calcium channel blockade on the ischemic heart.

dilate coronary arteries are verapamil [e.g., Isoptin] and diltiazem [e.g., Cardizem]. Side effects are divided into common, less common, and rare:

- Common side effects: feeling tired; flushing; swelling of the abdomen, ankles, or feet; heartburn
- Less common side effects: very fast or very slow heartbeat; wheezing, coughing, or shortness of breath; trouble swallowing; dizziness, numbness or tingling in the hands or feet; upset stomach; constipation (especially when taking verapamil)
- Rare side effects: headache, fainting, chest pain, yellowing of the skin or eyes (jaundice), fever, rash, bleeding, swollen or tender gums, vivid dreams

Calcium channel blockers increase the exercise capacity of patients with angina because the drug decreases myocardial $O_2$ demand and increases myocardial blood supply. As with other medications that lower blood pressure, patients should be observed for postural hypotension.

## Positive Inotropes

Positive inotropes improve the pumping capacity of the heart in chronic or **acute heart failure** (7). In **chronic heart failure**, positive inotropes are not used until pump failure is severe. However, positive inotropic therapy is commenced immediately in acute heart failure. Digitalis (e.g., Digoxin) is an important drug to improve pump function during CHF. It has both neural and myocardial cellular effects (*Fig. 18.7*). Digitalis activates the parasympathetic nervous system and inhibits the sympathetic nervous system. This results in a slower heart rate and conduction through the AV node. The positive inotropic effect of digitalis comes about through sodium-calcium exchange (Fig. 18.7 insert), whereby cy-

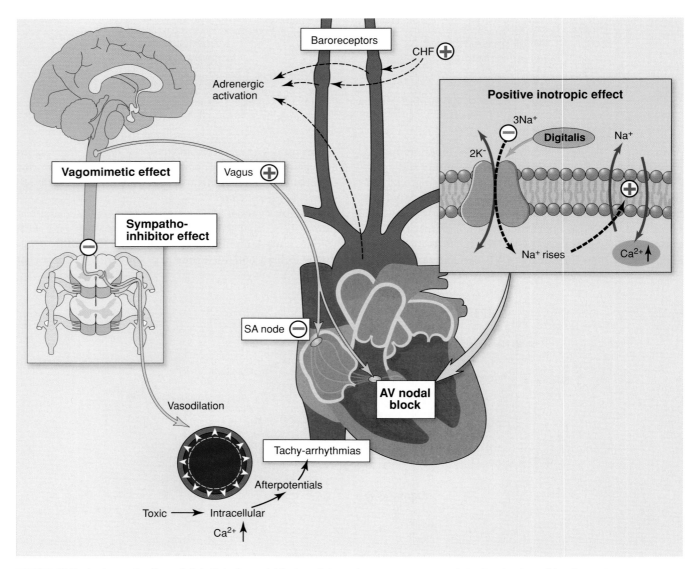

**FIGURE 18.7.** The inotropic effect of digitalis is due to inhibition of the sodium pump in myocardial cells whereby $Ca^{2+}$ influx to the cytosol via exchange with sodium is promoted. Digitalis also slows the heart rate, inhibits the atrioventricular node, and decreases sympathetic drive.

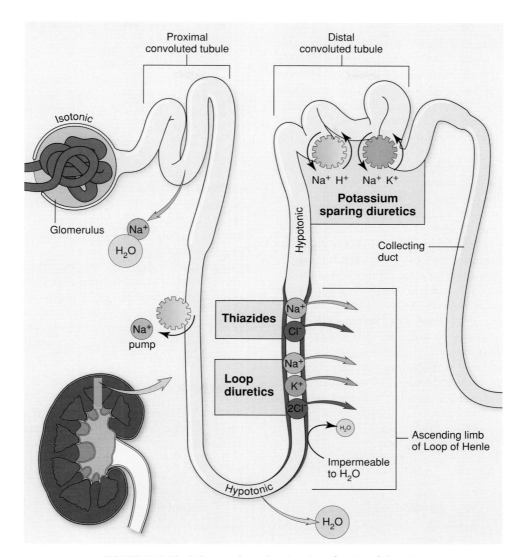

**FIGURE 18.8.** The kidney nephron showing sites of action of diuretics.

tosolic $Ca^{2+}$ concentration is increased, which enhances myocardial contractility and pump performance.

Digitalis increases the exercise capacity of patients with CAD because of improved ventricular performance. Exercise personnel should be aware of the effects of digitalis on the electrocardiogram, such as sagging ST segment, which mimics the ST depression seen in ischemia. Side effects of digitalis include toxicity leading to ST depression and **arrhythmias**. Other side effects include nausea, vomiting, drowsiness, fatigue, and confusion. Patients on digitalis should check their pulse daily and report significant bradycardia or sustained tachycardia.

## Diuretics

Diuretics are used to treat symptomatic heart failure, primarily to control pulmonary and peripheral symptoms of congestion, and they are also important in the treatment of hypertension (8). The three major groups of diuretics are the loop diuretics, thiazides, and potassium-sparing diuretics, each acting at different sites of the nephrons in the kidneys (*Fig. 18.8*).

Loop diuretics constitute a family of drugs that remove water from the body. They are used to lower blood pressure in people with hypertension and to reduce the amount of work the heart has to do, allowing it to pump more efficiently in people with CHF. The most widely used loop diuretic is furosemide (e.g., Lasix). The "loop" refers to the drug's action on the loop of Henle, a structure of the kidney involved in reabsorbing water. Kidneys control the extracellular fluid (ECF) volume by adjusting sodium chloride (NaCl) and water excretion. Each day the kidney filters more than 22 mol of $Na^+$. To maintain NaCl balance, approximately 1.4 kg of NaCl must be reabsorbed by the renal tubules on a daily basis. Thus, the body maintains blood pressure at the expense of ECF volume. When NaCl intake is greater than output (as in CHF or renal failure), edema develops. Loop diuretics act primarily by blocking the $Na^+/K^+/Cl^-$ cotransporter in the membrane of the thick ascending limb of the Henle loop. Because this is the same site responsible for concentrating and diluting urine, loop diuretics decrease maximal urinary concentrating and diluting. The thick ascending limb is a major site of $Ca^{2+}$ and $Mg^{2+}$ reabsorption, processes that are dependent on normal $Na^+$ and $Cl^-$ reabsorption. Therefore, loop diuretics increase urinary water, $Na^+$, $K^+$, $Ca^{2+}$, and $Mg^{2+}$ excretion.

Loop diuretics are more potent than thiazide diuretics, but thiazides are the most commonly prescribed class of diuretics. They inhibit $Na^+$ and $Cl^-$ transport in the cortical thick ascending limb and early distal tubule. They have a milder diuretic action than do the loop diuretics because this nephron site reabsorbs less $Na^+$ than the thick ascending limb. Potassium-sparing diuretics act in the distal tubules of the nephron and are often given to avoid the hypokalemia (decreased $K^+$ concentration) that accompanies the agents previously described. They should never be given in the setting of hyperkalemia (increased $K^+$ concentration) or in patients on drugs or with disease states likely to cause hyperkalemia.

Side effects associated with diuretics include fluid and electrolyte imbalances, which may lead to muscle weakness and spasms, dizziness, headache, incoordination, and nausea. Diuretics increase the exercise capacity of patients with CHF.

## Angiotensin-Converting Enzyme Inhibitors

Angiotensin-converting enzyme (ACE) inhibitors interrupt the molecular messengers that constrict blood vessels (9). These drugs have dual vasodilatory actions, working principally through the renin-angiotensin-aldosterone system but also having an effect on the bradykinin system (*Fig. 18.9*). Working through the renin-angiotensin-aldosterone system, ACE inhibitors inhibit the normal vasoconstriction that follows angiotensin II release. Working through bradykinin, ACE inhibitors lead to the formation of vasodilatory nitric oxide and prostaglandins. ACE inhibitors improve heart function in individuals with heart failure and are also used to treat hypertension. The most common ACE inhibitors are captopril (Capoten), enalapril (Vasotec), lisinopril (Zestril, Prinivil), ramipril (Altace), and moexipril (Univasc). Common side effects are cough; hypotension; rash; swelling of face, lips, and tongue; GI disturbances; headache; dizziness; lightheadedness; and fatigue. Patients on diuretic therapy may be more prone to hypotension with ACE inhibitor therapy so those patients need to be cautioned to change body position slowly. ACE inhibitors increase the exercise capacity of patients with CHF.

## PULMONARY MEDICATIONS

Three major categories of drugs are used in chronic pulmonary disease: anti-inflammatory agents, bronchodila-

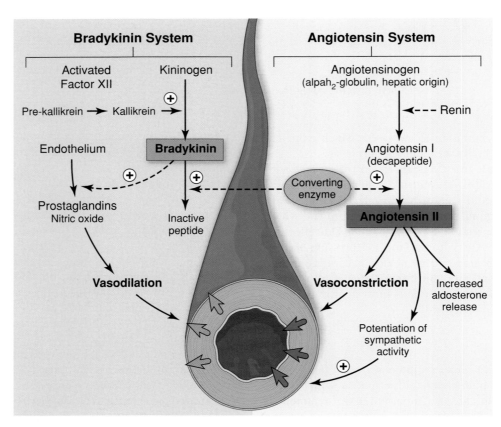

**FIGURE 18.9.** The dual vasodilatory actions of angiotensin-converting enzyme (ACE) inhibitors.

tors, and cromolyn sodium. The goal of therapy with these drugs is to dilate air passages, which promotes improved alveolar ventilation, a more optimal breathing pattern, and the removal of secretions. This results in improved functional abilities for patients limited by pulmonary disease.

## Anti-Inflammatory Agents

A major problem in obstructive pulmonary disease is the inflammatory response within airways. Inflammation results in swelling and increased secretion by the mucous glands. As a result, the airway is decreased in size and ventilation is reduced. One goal of therapy, therefore, is to arrest the inflammation process. Corticosteroids are the most potent anti-inflammatory drugs available and are used to treat many health conditions. This drug class is mainly used for treating **asthma**, but it has also been used for treating COPD. Oral corticosteroids decrease the inflammation in the lungs that is associated with asthma and COPD. They may take longer to work than inhaled corticosteroids because they have to travel through the circulation before they get to the lungs. Corticosteroids are only used in COPD patients who do not respond well to other standard therapies. Types of corticosteroids include oral dexamethasone (e.g., Decadron), fludrocortisone acetate (Florinef Acetate), oral hydrocortisone (Cortef, Hydrocortone), methylprednisolone (e.g., Medrol), oral prednisolone (e.g., Orapred), oral prednisone (e.g., Deltasone), and oral triamcinolone (e.g., Atolone).

Some people with COPD who respond well to oral corticosteroids can be maintained on long-term inhaled steroids. The use of these drugs is widespread, despite little evidence of efficacy in the treatment of COPD. Inhaled corticosteroids do not slow the decline in lung function. They do, however, decrease the frequency of exacerbations and improve disease-specific and health-related quality of life issues for some people with COPD. Inhaled corticosteroids have fewer side effects than oral steroids, but they are less effective than oral steroids, even at high doses.

The side effects of corticosteroids are dependent on dosage, duration of therapy, and route of administration. Side effects are not likely to manifest with short-term usage, but long-term usage may result in bruising, delayed wound healing, elevated cholesterol, GI irritation, headache, hypertension, increased susceptibility to infection, muscle atrophy, and osteoporosis. Exercise activities that produce muscle hypertrophy and enhance bone strength are desirable, but excessive stress to skeletal structures is not desirable.

## Bronchodilators

Bronchoconstriction is the major functional problem in most obstructive pulmonary diseases. Drugs that dilate the bronchi, therefore, are often the first line of defense to correct breathing difficulties in these patients. Bronchodilators act by several means:

- Increasing the concentration (or blocking the decrease) of cyclic adenosine monophosphate (cAMP), which de-

creases intracellular $Ca^{2+}$ concentration and results in smooth muscle relaxation and bronchodilation
- Blocking cyclic guanosine monophosphate (cGMP), a vasoconstrictor agent
- Decreasing inflammatory response, a cause of bronchi narrowing
- Blocking mast cell release

The following classes of vasodilator drugs are especially important:

- Sympathomimetics (epinephrine, ephedrine, isoproterenol, albuterol [e.g., Proventil]) dilate the bronchi by stimulating beta adrenergic receptors in the bronchial smooth muscle cell. The side effects are tachycardia, **palpitations**, angina, GI distress, nervousness, muscle tremor, headache, dizziness, anxiety, sweating, and insomnia. There is an elevated resting heart rate while taking systemic sympathomimetics so exercise personnel should take this into consideration when monitoring and prescribing exercise.
- Sympatholytics (phentolamine) reduce alpha stimulation and thus promote bronchodilation.
- Parasympatholytics (atropine) block parasympathetic stimulation, preventing an increase in cGMP and producing an increase in cAMP, which promotes bronchodilation.
- Methylxanthines (theophylline) inhibit the action of phosphodiesterase, the enzyme that degrades cAMP. Side effects, which may appear at very low serum concentration levels, include headache, restlessness, anxiety, insomnia, and hyperactivity. As in the use of sympathomimetics, there is often an elevated resting heart rate; therefore, caution should be used when formulating an exercise prescription.
- Glucocorticoids (oral use [prednisone] or inhalational route [dexamethasone sodium phosphate]) block or inhibit substances that cause vasoconstriction. Very common side effects are weight gain and mood swings. Common side effects are mild weakness in limbs, easy bruising of skin, impaired wound healing, acne, osteoporosis (glucocorticoids double the risk of developing osteoporosis of the hip and quadruple the risk of developing vertebral fractures), cataracts (30% of patients on glucocorticoids develop posterior subcapsular cataracts), immunosuppression, and hypothalamic-pituitary-adrenal axis suppression. Occasional side effects are high blood pressure, elevated blood sugar (worsening of diabetes mellitus), red/purple stretch marks, and stomach irritation (ulcers).

## Cromolyn Sodium

Cromolyn sodium (Intal) is indicated as a component of therapy in the treatment of mild persistent and moderate persistent asthma. Cromolyn is of little benefit during an acute exacerbation of asthma. The mechanism of action of cromolyn consists of inhibition of the degranulation of sensitized and nonsensitized mast cells, which occurs after exposure to specific antigens. The drug also inhibits the release of histamine from the mast cell. These actions serve to inhibit the early asthmatic response through stabilization of the mast cell membrane. Cromolyn also inhibits the late asthmatic response. Long-term prophylaxis of 6 to 12 weeks is necessary to prevent the increased airway hyperactivity associated with specific allergen exposure. Cromolyn has no intrinsic bronchodilator, antihistaminic, anticholinergic, vasoconstrictor, or anti-inflammatory activity. Cromolyn is extremely safe and is one of the least toxic drugs used in the management of asthma. More common side effects may include cough, nasal congestion or irritation, nausea, sneezing, throat irritation, and wheezing.

### Other Common Agents

Expectorants are drugs that loosen and clear mucus and **phlegm** from the respiratory tract. They act by liquefying mucus, that is, they are decongestants. Expectorants may keep mucus from sticking to the airways, making the mucus easier to cough up. Therefore, they are used in the treatment of coughs to help expel secretions. Antitussives are agents that specifically inhibit or suppress the act of coughing. However, they should not be used to suppress productive coughing. Expectorants and antitussives are most commonly used in the symptomatic treatment of the common cold or **bronchitis**. An example of an expectorant is guaifenesin (e.g., Fenesin). The side effects of guaifenesin in some individuals are nausea, vomiting, dizziness, rash, and itching. Side effects of antitussives are slowed or difficulty breathing, severe drowsiness, and rash or itching. The following are less serious side effects of antitussives: drowsiness, dizziness, constipation, upset stomach, nervousness, or restlessness.

Decongestants are drugs that dry up nasal, sinus, and bronchial secretions. They open sinus drains and help evacuate mucus from the sinus cavities. Common side effects of decongestants include dry mouth or throat, tachycardia, insomnia, anxiety, and difficulty in urinating (especially in men >50 years old). In asthma, decongestants can make secretions in the lungs harder to clear. Decongestants can be safely used by individuals with asthma who have post-nasal drip, colds, and sinus infections. If asthma becomes more active than usual, decongestants should be stopped until the asthma is better controlled. An example of a decongestant is pseudoephedrine (e.g., Sudafed).

Mucolytics thin mucus to make it less sticky and easier to cough up from the lungs and bronchial tubes. Mucolytics are used in the reduction of sputum viscosity and thus are given to help expectoration in chronic asthma and bronchitis. An example of a mucolytic is acetylcysteine (e.g., Mucomyst). Acetylcysteine can produce these side effects: sudden tightness of the airways (bronchospasm), nausea, fever, and drowsiness.

▶ *INQUIRY SUMMARY.* Cardiovascular and pulmonary medications are commonly encountered in clinical exercise programs due to the pervasiveness of cardiovascular and pulmonary disease in the population. The goal in the medical management of cardiovascular disease is to prevent myocardial ischemia and infarction and to maximize and improve cardiovascular function. The goal in the medical management of pulmonary disease is to create a more optimal breathing pattern by dilating air passages and removing secretions. *A great array of cardiovascular and pulmonary medications is available today to help these patients—how might other therapeutic regimens complement these two goals?*

## Overview of Cardiovascular Pathophysiology

Cardiovascular disease is the leading cause of death in industrialized nations, with an estimated prevalence rate of one of every 4.7 deaths. About 13.5 million people currently have a history of cardiovascular disease. Each year approximately 1.25 million Americans have heart attacks, with about one-third of these fatal. About half of the deaths are sudden and unexpected. Approximately 2 million Americans suffer from CHF at any given time, with 400,000 new cases annually, requiring 900,000 hospitalizations per year. Despite these grim statistics, over the last few decades there has been a steady decline in mortality from cardiovascular disease. During the last 50 years, it is estimated that the 73% decline in total death rate was mostly due to the 56% decrease in heart disease death rate and the 70% decrease in stroke death rate.

### SIGNS AND SYMPTOMS OF CARDIOVASCULAR DISEASE

The signs and symptoms associated with cardiovascular disease may be grouped by the organ system affected. *Table 18.5* shows the systems affected and the symptoms produced. The following symptoms are usually considered common.

- Chest pain: pain radiating to the neck, jaw, upper trapezius muscle, upper back, shoulder, or arms. Chest pain of cardiac origin may be secondary to angina, myocardial infarction, pericarditis, mitral valve prolapse, or dissecting aortic **aneurysm**. Case study 18.2 differentiates noncardiac from cardiac chest pain. The pattern of chest pain is usually specific to the condition (*Figs. 18.10, 18.11,* and *18.12*).

*Experiences in Work Physiology Lab Exercise 15: Discussing Differential Diagnosis of Chest Pain presents a laboratory exercise in which students learn to distinguish chest pain patterns.*

- Palpitation: an irregular (arrhythmic) heart beat can have several origins ranging from benign (mitral valve prolapse, anxiety) to severe (CAD, cardiomyopathy, AV valve disease) conditions. The physical sensation is often referred to as a pounding in the chest and may produce

**Table 18.5**   **CARDIOVASCULAR SIGNS AND SYMPTOMS BY ORGAN SYSTEM**

| System | Symptoms | System | Symptoms |
|---|---|---|---|
| General | Weakness<br>Fatigue<br>Weight change<br>Poor exercise tolerance | Genitourinary | Urinary frequency<br>Nocturia<br>Concentrated urine<br>Decreased urinary output |
| Integumentary | Pressure ulcers<br>Loss of body hair<br>Cyanosis (lips and nail beds) | Musculoskeletal | Chest, shoulder, neck,<br>jaw, or arm pain<br>Myalgias<br>Muscular fatigue |
| Central nervous | Headaches<br>Impaired vision<br>Dizziness or syncope | | Muscle atrophy<br>Edema<br>Claudication |
| Respiratory | Labored breathing<br>Productive cough | Gastrointestinal | Nausea and vomiting<br>Ascites (abdominal distension) |

## CASE STUDY 18.2: DIFFERENTIATING CHEST PAIN

### CASE

Sally is a 60-year-old woman employed at a sawmill (repetitive shoulder flexion and extension and lifting tasks). She is also undergoing a divorce and child custody hearing. She was diagnosed with left anterior chest pain after a history of hysterectomy and was found to be a four pack per day smoker for 30 years. She describes her chest pain as sudden, crushing, and radiating down the left arm. Tests after treatment in the emergency room were negative for cardiac involvement. Blood pressure was 195/115 mm Hg upon admittance. The diagnosis at this time was stress-induced chest pain. In an earlier pain episode, she described radiating pain around the chest, under the armpit, and in the upper back. No numbness or tingling was noticed, and the pain did not radiate down the arm.

### DESCRIPTION

There are many different causes of chest pain, most of which are not related to cardiac problems. In clinical practice, clues must be gathered to help differentiate one origin of chest pain from another. For example, the following are broad categories under which chest pain may be caused, followed by an example in each category and specific clues that may distinguish each (the clues are not comprehensive):

- Cancer: mediastinal tumors
  - Weight loss though chronically inactive
  - Pain that does not respond to treatment
  - Nocturnal pain
- Pleuropulmonary: pulmonary hypertension
  - Pain not palpable
  - Pain worsens in the lying position
  - Presence of associated signs and symptoms, such as persistent cough or dyspnea
- Epigastric: esophageal spasm
  - Symptoms relieved by antacids
  - Symptoms are not reproduced or aggravated by effort or exertion

- Presence of associated signs and symptoms of nausea, vomiting, dark urine, jaundice, indigestion, abdominal fullness or bloating
- Breast: mastitis
  - Report of lump, nodule, skin puckering
  - Recent childbirth and/or breastfeeding
  - Association between painful symptoms and menstrual cycle
- Neuromusculoskeletal: Tietze syndrome
  - Symptoms associated with words like aching, burning, hot
  - Pain is unrelated to effort and lasts for hours or weeks to months
  - Symptoms are relieved by heat and stretching
- Cardiac: myocardial infarction
  - Pain associated with physical activity
  - Pain related to temperature changes, emotional reactions, or large meal
  - Associated symptoms such as dyspnea, arrhythmias, syncope

### INTERVENTION

Sally underwent a neurologic screen, which was negative. Other tests included deep tendon reflexes (within normal limits) and strength testing (limited by pain); no changes in sensation, two-point discrimination, or proprioception were observed. Left pectoral palpation revealed pain with tenderness and swelling at the second, third, and fourth costochondral joints. Resisted shoulder horizontal adduction produced pain and radiating symptoms. Active shoulder range of motion was normal but painful on the left. Pain in the chest, arm, and upper back region was not altered by respiratory movements (deep breathing or coughing). The supine position did not produce pain. The diagnosis was Tietze syndrome secondary to repetitive motion and exacerbated by emotional stress. The patient also had shoulder impingement syndrome. The pain and movement dysfunction were relieved after 6 weeks of physical therapy.

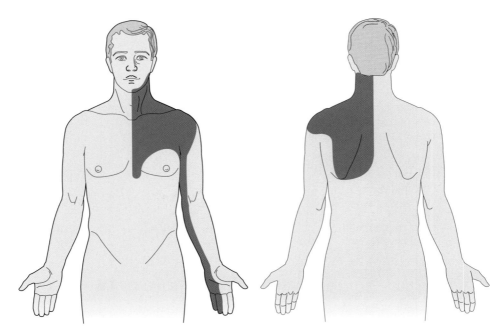

**FIGURE 18.10.** Angina chest pain pattern. Left: The area of substernal discomfort projected to the left shoulder and arm over the distribution of the ulnar nerve. Right: Anginal pain may radiate to the back (left scapula).

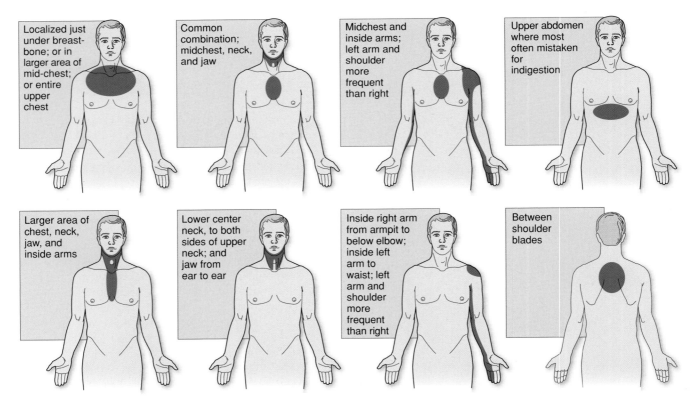

Localized just under breast-bone; or in larger area of mid-chest; or entire upper chest

Common combination; midchest, neck, and jaw

Midchest and inside arms; left arm and shoulder more frequent than right

Upper abdomen where most often mistaken for indigestion

Larger area of chest, neck, jaw, and inside arms

Lower center neck, to both sides of upper neck; and jaw from ear to ear

Inside right arm from armpit to below elbow; inside left arm to waist; left arm and shoulder more frequent than right

Between shoulder blades

**FIGURE 18.11.** Myocardial infarction chest pain pattern.

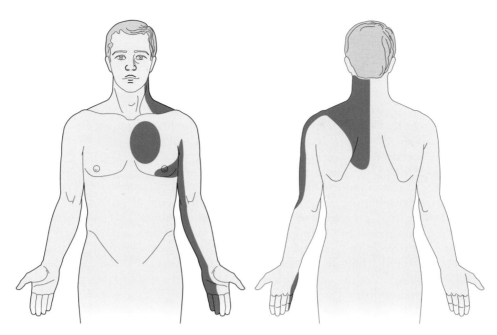

**FIGURE 18.12.** Pericarditis chest pain pattern. Left side: Substernal pain (dark oval) associated with pericarditis may radiate anteriorly to the costal margins, neck, upper back, upper trapezius muscle, and left supraclavicular area or down the left arm. The lighter area shows the referral pattern anteriorly and posteriorly (right side).

lightheadedness. The duration and frequency of occurrence are significant to observe, i.e., from less than six per minute (benign) to lasting several hours (pathologic when occurring with pain, shortness of breath, fainting, or severe lightheadedness).

- **Dyspnea**: shortness of breath; can be of cardiovascular or pulmonary pathologic origin, or it may occur in relatively benign conditions, such as with fever, medications, allergies, poor physical conditioning, or obesity. When of cardiovascular origin, dyspnea is related to poor left ventricular pumping capability, resulting in fluid backup to the lungs and shortness of breath.
- Syncope: fainting, caused by reduced $O_2$ delivery to the brain; can be caused by various cardiovascular conditions, such as arrhythmias, **orthostatic hypotension** (sudden drop in blood pressure), poor ventricular function, CAD, and vertebral artery insufficiency. Noncardiac conditions may also cause syncope via a vasovagal maneuver from hyperventilatory responses initiated by anxiety or emotional stress.
- Fatigue: may be cardiac in origin when accompanied by symptoms such as dyspnea, chest pain, palpitations, or headache. Fatigue may also be secondary to neurologic, muscular, metabolic, or pulmonary conditions. Fatigue may also be due to deconditioning.
- Cough: associated with pulmonary or cardiac conditions with associated pulmonary complications. In CHF, a cough is the result of fluid backup to the lungs.
- **Cyanosis**: discoloration of the lips and nail beds due to a lack of $O_2$, usually of pulmonary or cardiac origin.
- **Edema**: may be of cardiac origin when symptoms of right-sided CHF include swelling of the ankles, ab-

domen, and hands; dyspnea; fatigue; and dizziness. Most often the cause of right heart failure is left heart failure.
- **Claudication**: leg pain occurs in peripheral vascular disease as arteries or veins become narrowed due to the process of atherosclerosis. Skin discoloration occurs also.

*LINKUP:* **Resistance exercise involves an increase in both systolic and diastolic blood pressure. Sometimes these increases are quite large; therefore, individuals with cardiovascular problems must take precautions when performing such exercise. Case Study: Resistance Exercise and Aneurysm,** *found at http://* **connection.lww.com/go/brownexphys and on the Student Resource CD-ROM, presents an individual with a history of abdominal aneurysm who wants to engage in resistance training.**

## CARDIOVASCULAR DISORDERS

The following three tables present three categories of cardiac disease: diseases affecting heart muscle, diseases affecting heart valves, and defects of the cardiac nervous system. Following these presentations, occlusive heart disease and CHF are discussed in more detail.

### Disorders Affecting the Heart Muscle

In most cases, a cardiac pathologic condition can be traced to one of three processes: (a) obstruction or restriction, (b) inflammation, or (c) dilation or distension.

Combinations of these problems can cause pain in the chest, neck, back, and/or shoulder. *Table 18.6* presents six specific pathologic processes with associated signs and symptoms.

### Disorders Affecting Heart Valves

*Table 18.7* presents conditions that occur secondary to impairment of the valves caused by disease (e.g., rheumatic fever), infection (e.g., endocarditis), or congenital deformity (e.g., mitral valve prolapse). Three types of valvular deformity affect the aortic, mitral, tricuspid, or pulmonic valves: stenosis, regurgitation, or prolapse. Stenosis refers to a narrowing that prevents the valve from opening fully. Regurgitation refers to the improper closure of the valve that allows blood to flow back into the heart chamber. Prolapse, specific only to the mitral valve, refers to the bulging backward of the valve leaflets into the left atrium. These conditions increase the work of the heart by requiring the heart to pump harder to force blood through a stenosed valve or to maintain adequate flow if blood is reentering an atrium.

### Disorders Affecting the Cardiac Nervous System

The heart's nervous system can fail to conduct normal electrical impulses, leading to a cardiac arrhythmia. Arrhythmias can induce fast rates (tachycardia) or slow rates (bradycardia) and may cause extra beats and fibrillations. All these problems may cause circulatory dynamics to change, leading to mild or severe symptoms (*Table 18.8*).

### Occlusive Heart Disease

Atherosclerotic occlusive disease refers to processes that result in arterial obstruction by the formation of lesions, leading to reduced perfusion of arteries that supply blood to the myocardium (CAD) or to the extremities (peripheral vascular disease). The result is tissue ischemia, which can affect the heart and skeletal muscle. Myocardial ischemia is one of the 10 most common primary pathologies leading to cardiac muscle dysfunction and ultimately heart failure. The major disorders caused by insufficient blood supply to the myocardium are angina pectoris, CHF, and myocardial infarction. Occlusive heart disease (also known as CAD)

| **Table 18.6** | **DISEASES/DISORDERS AFFECTING THE HEART MUSCLE** | |
|---|---|---|
| **Disease/Disorder** | **Underlying Pathologic Process** | **Clinical Signs and Symptoms** |
| Coronary artery disease | Atherosclerotic process leading to narrowing of coronary artery lumen, which restricts blood flow to the muscle | Asymptomatic until a critical deficit of blood supply is reached; symptoms usually appear when the artery narrows by 75% |
| Angina pectoris | Imbalance between myocardial $O_2$ demand and supply caused by advanced atherosclerosis and leading to myocardial ischemia | Chest pain radiating to the left shoulder and arm, and less commonly to the neck, jaw, teeth, upper back, and abdomen. Burning indigestion may be present as well as nausea, dyspnea, and exercise intolerance. May be relieved by rest and nitrates. See Figure 18.10. |
| Myocardial infarction (MI) | Sudden decrease in coronary perfusion leading to myocardial tissue death | Same as angina except that pain is not relieved by rest or nitrates. Syncope is common. See Figure 18.11. |
| Pericarditis | Inflammation of the pericardium as caused by a number of different diseases (secondary pericarditis); also may be primary pericarditis | Chest pain (patterned after MI but aggravated by deep breathing and trunk movements), dyspnea, increased pulse rate, and increased core temperature. See Figure 18.12. |
| Congestive heart failure | Decreased pump function secondary to intrinsic myocardial disease or structural defects; left-sided heart failure is the principle cause of right-sided heart failure | Left-sided heart failure causes fatigue and dyspnea upon exercise and is associated with persistent cough, orthopnea, tachycardia, edema, and decreased renal function. Right-sided heart failure causes fatigue and is associated with dependent edema (i.e., feet and ankles), cyanosis of the nail beds, and distended neck veins. |
| Aneurysm | Weakened vessel wall created from a trauma, congenital vascular disease, infection, or atherosclerosis; can occur in thoracic, abdominal, and peripheral arteries | Chest pain, awareness of pulsating mass in abdomen (with abdominal and back pain), extreme pain along the base of the neck, along the back between the scapular blades, groin and leg pain (with leg weakness), tachycardic rate, and systolic hypotension (<100 mm Hg). Refer to Case Study: Resistance Exercise and Aneurysm, found at http://connection.lww.com/go/brownexphys and on the Student Resource CD-ROM. |

## Table 18.7 — DISEASES/DISORDERS AFFECTING THE HEART VALVES

| Disease/Disorder | Underlying Pathologic Process | Clinical Signs and Symptoms |
|---|---|---|
| Rheumatic fever | Streptococcal bacteria infection resulting in scarring and deformity of the heart valves | Fever and sore throat followed by migratory joint symptoms in the knees, shoulders, feet, ankles, elbows, fingers, or neck; weakness, malaise, weight loss, and anorexia may accompany the fever |
| Endocarditis | Bacterial infection inflaming the cardiac endothelium, damaging the tricuspid, aortic, or mitral valve | Musculoskeletal symptoms, including arthralgia, arthritis, low back pain, and myalgias; dyspnea; chest pain; and cold and painful extremities |
| Mitral valve prolapse | Slight variation in the shape of the mitral valve causing prolapse upon closing | Common "triad" of symptoms include palpitations, fatigue, and dyspnea; other symptoms include tachycardia, anxiety, depression, panic attacks, migraine headaches, and chest pain |

results from a complex genetic makeup and interactions with the environment. Environmental interactions include nutrition, activity levels, and history of smoking. The underlying disease process is atherosclerosis, a progressive disease that begins in childhood and occurs in any artery in the body but most commonly in medium-sized arteries of the heart, brain, kidneys, and legs.

*LINKUP: **Atherosclerosis (from atherosis [lipid deposit in the intima of arteries, producing fatty streaking] and sclerosis [hardening process that reduces vessel compliance]), a form of arteriosclerosis (vascular damage leading to progressive thickening and loss of resiliency of the artery wall), is a vascular disorder that plays a major role in CAD (due to atherosclerosis of the coronary arteries) and stroke (due to atherosclerosis of the cerebral arteries). See Perspective: Etiology of Atherosclerosis, found at http://connection.lww.com/go/brownexphys and on the Student Resource CD-ROM, for additional information about this disorder.***

## Congestive Heart Failure

CHF is a major health care problem today. CHF leads to the inability of the heart to maintain normal blood pressure and tissue perfusion via a reduced cardiac output. *Figure 18.13* shows the process of neurohumoral adaptation in CHF. The reduced organ perfusion is especially important for kidney function as renal ischemia sets in, which results in enhanced renin release. Enhanced renin release is also potentiated from the increase in sympathetic discharge that comes about because of the baroreceptor reflex activated by hypotension. Sympathetic discharge stimulates $\beta_1$ renal receptors involved in renin release. This reflexive neurohumoral activation leads to peripheral vasoconstriction via the increased formation of angiotensin II (see Fig. 18.9), which increases peripheral vascular resistance and cardiac afterload. This scenario causes left ventricular function to fall further. With the increased afterload, the ventricle is not able to empty properly which leads to an increased preload (ventricular dilation). In the face of the high preloads and afterloads,

## Table 18.8 — DISEASES/DISORDERS AFFECTING THE CARDIAC NERVOUS SYSTEM

| Disease/Disorder | Underlying Pathologic Process | Clinical Signs and Symptoms |
|---|---|---|
| Arrhythmia | Disorders of the heart rate and rhythm caused by disturbances in the conduction system; may be due to underlying coronary artery disease | Fibrillation may be felt as palpitations, sensations of fluttering, skipping, or pounding; dyspnea, chest pain, anxiety, pallor, nervousness, and cyanosis are often the outcome |
| Sinus tachycardia | Normal physiologic response to conditions such as fever, exertion, hypotension, hypovolemia, congestive heart failure, shock, anemia, anxiety, and thyrotoxicosis; especially problematic in patients with organic myocardial disease | Rapid rate (>100 bpm) may produce palpitations, restlessness, chest pain or discomfort, agitation, anxiety |
| Sinus bradycardia | Normal in fit individuals, but could be a result of sinus node pathology | Reduced rate (<60 bpm) may produce syncope |

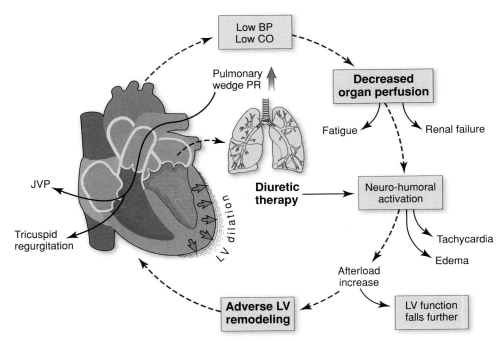

**FIGURE 18.13.** Neurohumoral adaptation in congestive heart failure. When the left ventricle (LV) fails, there is inability to maintain normal blood pressure and normal organ perfusion. The failed LV leads to an increase in the pulmonary wedge pressure with consequences through the right heart. LV failure also eventually leads to neurohumoral activation in an effort to compensate. However, this scenario inevitably leads to abnormal left ventricular hypertrophy.

ventricular wall stress is increased according to the law of LaPlace:

$$\text{Wall stress} = (\text{Pressure} \times \text{Radius}) \div (2 \times \text{Wall thickness})$$

CHF leads to a progressive ventricular dilation, the ventricle undergoing wall remodeling, leading to further loss of function. Wall stress is one of the major determinants of myocardial $\dot{V}O_2$, and a key point of medical therapy for CHF is to improve myocardial $O_2$ balance by reducing the radius of the left ventricle, which decreases wall stress and $O_2$ demand. As pulmonary edema increases, pulmonary capillary wedge pressure increases, leading to backflow into the right heart and eventually right heart failure.

### Peripheral Vascular Disorders

Peripheral vascular disease (PVD) can affect the arterial, venous, or lymphatic circulatory system. The underlying process is usually atherosclerosis causing disturbances of circulation to the extremities, resulting in significant loss of function in either the upper or lower extremities. Other causes of PVD are embolism, thrombosis, trauma, vasospasm, inflammation, or autoimmunity. *Table 18.9* summarizes seven peripheral vascular disorders, along with their associated underlying pathologic processes and clinical signs and symptoms.

▶ *INQUIRY SUMMARY.* Cardiovascular diseases are the leading cause of death and illness in the United States, yet the incidence rate of these diseases has decreased over the last three decades. Health care professionals who use exercise therapy should be familiar with the basic pathophysiology of heart and vascular diseases as well as the clinical signs and symptoms of the many disorders comprising this disease category. *Why is knowledge of the signs and symptoms of cardiovascular disorders important information for the therapist?*

## Overview of Pulmonary Pathophysiology

Obstructive lung disease is defined as a decrease in exhaled airflow caused by a narrowing or obstruction of the airways, such as with asthma, **emphysema**, and chronic bronchitis. Restrictive lung disease is defined as a decrease in the total volume of air that the lungs are able to hold. Often this is due to a decrease in the elasticity or **compliance** of the lungs themselves or a problem in the expansion of the chest wall during inhalation. Pulmonary disease is ranked among the leading causes of death in the United States, with cigarette smoking and air pollution among major preventable factors associated with it. However, like heart disease in the last 20 years, the death rate from respiratory diseases has fallen. The following sections cover both obstructive and restrictive pulmonary conditions.

| **Table 18.9 PERIPHERAL VASCULAR DISORDERS** | | |
|---|---|---|
| **Disease/Disorder** | **Underlying Pathologic Process** | **Clinical Signs and Symptoms** |
| Occlusive arterial disease | Atherosclerotic process leading to disturbances in circulation to the extremities and peripheral ischemia | Loss of hair on the toes, intermittent claudication producing deep muscle pain or cramping due to ischemia, which increases during exercise and is relieved by rest. Pain location is determined by site of major arterial occlusion. Other symptoms include decreased skin temperature; dry, scaly, or shiny skin; poor nail and hair growth; ulcerations and possible gangrene on weight-bearing surfaces. |
| Raynaud disease | Vasomotor disorder associated with hypersensitivity of the digital arteries to cold, release of serotonin, disposition to vasospasm | Digital pallor increasing to cyanosis with cold, numb, red, and painful digits |
| Thrombophlebitis | May be superficial (often iatrogenic, associated with insertion of intravenous catheters) or deep (one-third of individuals older than 40 who have had major surgery or MI). Associated with venous stasis, hypercoagulability, or injury to the venous wall. | Venous distension with a palpable, hard cord running with the vein. Other signs include redness, warmth, and swelling. |
| Lymphedema | Excessive accumulation of fluid in tissue spaces secondary to an obstruction of the lymphatic system from trauma, infection, radiation, or surgery | Symptoms include edema of the dorsum of the foot or hand and decreased range of motion. Usually worsens after prolonged dependency. |
| Hypertension | Essential hypertension is of unknown origin or no identifiable cause. Secondary hypertension may have a number of underlying causes, such as renal artery stenosis, oral contraceptive use, hyperthyroidism, adrenal tumors, and medication use. | May be entirely asymptomatic in early stages, but may include the following symptoms: occipital headache, dizziness, flushed face, vision changes, spontaneous nosebleeds, and increased nocturnal urinary frequency |
| Transient ischemic attack | Hypertension | Sudden difficulty with speech, temporary blindness, paralysis or extreme weakness affecting one side of the body |
| Orthostatic hypotension | May occur as a normal consequence of aging or secondary to the effects of drugs such as antihypertensives, diuretics, and antidepressants | Lightheadedness, syncope, visual blurring, sense of weakness |

MI, myocardial infarction.

## CHRONIC OBSTRUCTIVE PULMONARY DISEASES

COPD is a spectrum of chronic respiratory disorders characterized by airflow limitation and persistently impaired gas exchange. COPD is really three basic pathologies:

- Asthma: the bronchioles are obstructed by muscle spasm, swelling of mucosa, and thick secretions
- Bronchitis: the membranes lining the bronchial tubes are affected, resulting in inflammation of the lining
- Emphysema: the air spaces beyond the terminal bronchioles are affected, resulting in breakdown of the alveolar walls and enlargement of the air spaces

Clinical signs and symptoms of each of these disorders are listed below.

- Asthma: dyspnea, wheezing, cough, pursed-lip breathing, flared nostrils, unusual pallor, hunched-over body posture, cough occurring 5 to 10 minutes after exercise
- Bronchitis: acute form involves mild fever, malaise, back and muscle pain, sore throat, cough with sputum production; chronic form involves persistent cough with sputum production, reduced chest expansion, wheezing, fever, dyspnea, cyanosis, decreased exercise tolerance

- Emphysema: shortness of breath, dyspnea on exertion, orthopnea immediately after assumption of the supine position, chronic cough, barrel chest, weight loss, malaise, use of accessory respiratory muscles, prolonged expiratory period, wheezing, pursed-lip breathing, increased expiratory rate, peripheral cyanosis

These conditions are also associated with a decrease in expiratory flow rates and an increase in residual volume, the major pulmonary tests providing physicians with a definitive diagnosis (*Fig. 18.14*). Over time the lungs become hyperinflated and the individual has trouble exhaling air due to airway obstruction. The major risk factors for COPD are listed in *Table 18.10*, along with the major structural and pathophysiologic signs. Whether the lung disorder is obstructive or restrictive dictates if the resultant spirometric volume measurement is normal, increased, or decreased.

## RESTRICTIVE LUNG DISEASE

In obstructive disease, the lungs become hyperinflated. The opposite is true of restrictive disease in which lung expansion is diminished. As in obstructive disease, pulmonary ventilatory measures and functional variables can be used to understand the pathophysiology of restrictive lung disease. Three important variables assisting our understanding of the pathophysiology of restrictive disease are compliance, lung volume, and work of breathing.

Compliance refers to the capacity of the lung and chest wall to expand, allowing airflow to the respiratory exchange surfaces. Compliance is the measurement of how much pressure is needed to overcome the elastic forces of a structure. With reduced compliance (either in the lung, chest wall, or both), the normal pressure flow relationship is altered and gas exchange is reduced. Lung compliance is the change in lung volume divided by the change in lung pressure ($\Delta VL/\Delta PL$). Chest wall compliance is the change in lung volume divided by the change in trans-chest wall pressure ($\Delta VL/\Delta PCW$). Respiratory system compliance is the change in lung volume divided by the change in trans-respiratory system pressure ($\Delta VL/\Delta PRS$) (10). As compliance decreases, there must be a greater trans-pulmonary pressure to expand a lung that has become stiffer due to pathologic changes. For both lungs, compliance is about 200 mL of air per cm water trans-pulmonary pressure. This

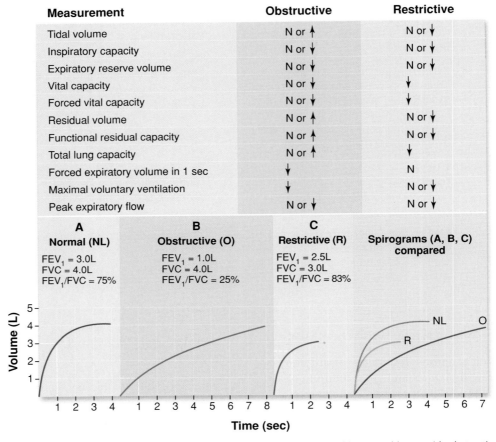

| Measurement | Obstructive | Restrictive |
|---|---|---|
| Tidal volume | N or ↑ | N or ↓ |
| Inspiratory capacity | N or ↓ | N or ↓ |
| Expiratory reserve volume | N or ↓ | N or ↓ |
| Vital capacity | N or ↓ | ↓ |
| Forced vital capacity | N or ↓ | ↓ |
| Residual volume | N or ↑ | N or ↓ |
| Functional residual capacity | N or ↑ | N or ↓ |
| Total lung capacity | N or ↑ | ↓ |
| Forced expiratory volume in 1 sec | ↓ | N |
| Maximal voluntary ventilation | ↓ | N or ↓ |
| Peak expiratory flow | N or ↓ | N or ↓ |

| A | B | C | |
|---|---|---|---|
| **Normal (NL)** | **Obstructive (O)** | **Restrictive (R)** | **Spirograms (A, B, C) compared** |
| $FEV_1 = 3.0L$ | $FEV_1 = 1.0L$ | $FEV_1 = 2.5L$ | |
| $FVC = 4.0L$ | $FVC = 4.0L$ | $FVC = 3.0L$ | |
| $FEV_1/FVC = 75\%$ | $FEV_1/FVC = 25\%$ | $FEV_1/FVC = 83\%$ | |

**FIGURE 18.14.** Spirometric comparisons of forced expiratory breathing maneuvers in normal lungs and lungs with obstructive and restrictive diseases. Patients with obstructive disease have trouble exhaling; the maximal amount of air exhaled is roughly equal to normal, but patients take much longer to exhale the air. Patients with restrictive disease can perform the maneuver in about the same time frame as individuals without disease; however, since their restriction is in the amount of air that the lung can hold in inhalation, their maximal exhalation is reduced. $FEV_1$, forced expiratory volume over the first second; FVC, forced vital capacity; $FEV_1/FVC$, ratio of forced expiratory volume over the first second to forced vital capacity (expressed as a percentage by multiplying by 100).

| **Table 18.10** | **MAJOR RISK FACTORS AND SIGNS OF CHRONIC OBSTRUCTIVE PULMONARY DISORDER** | |
| --- | --- | --- |
| **Risk Factor** | **Structural Signs** | **Pathophysiological Signs** |
| Cigarette smoking | Diffuse distention and over-aeration of alveoli | Disturbed ventilation |
| Air pollution | Disruption of interalveolar septa | Altered airflow and blood flow |
| Genetic factors | Loss of pulmonary elasticity | Frequently partial obstruction of bronchi |
| Bronchial inflammation | Restructuring of alveoli into large air sacs resulting in poor, uneven alveolar ventilation and inadequate perfusion of underventilated alveoli | Inspiration and expiration are labored (wheezing) and more work is required of breathing |
| Chronic respiratory tract infections | Increased lung volumes | Resulting hypoxia and hypercapnia |
| Old age | Barrel-shaped chest as the chest wall expands (increased lung volume and increased use of accessory shoulder and abdominal muscles) | Chronic productive cough with mucus Minor respiratory infections of no consequence to young individuals with normal lungs are fatal or near fatal for the elderly |

means that for every 1 cm water increase in trans-pulmonary pressure, the lungs expand 200 mL. *Figure 18.15* demonstrates this concept by showing that a greater trans-pulmonary pressure is needed to inflate the diseased lung to total lung capacity than is true of the normal lung. These graphs are referred to as compliance curves, and as you can see, the curve is shifted to the right and downward in restrictive lung disease.

Because of reduced compliance, patients with restrictive lung disease have to work harder to ventilate the lungs. This is referred to as increased work of breathing. Work of breathing refers to the mechanical processes of pulmonary ventilation. In restrictive disease, pulmonary ventilation is achieved at a reduced tidal volume (VT) and a higher breathing frequency. All lung volumes and capacities even-

tually become lower as the disease progresses (*Fig. 18.16*). The lower VT results from lower pulmonary compliance. To maintain pulmonary ventilation at adequate levels, breathing frequency increases to compensate for the lower VT. However, when frequency increases too much, energy is wasted in breathing as all of the respiratory muscles must work harder to overcome reduced lung compliance. The $O_2$ cost of breathing by this extra muscular work is increased from a normal level of 5% of whole-body $\dot{V}O_2$ to more than 25%. This increase reduces the available $\dot{V}O_2$ needed to perform normal activities of daily living. Because of this, these patients are forced to limit their activity. In severe cases, patients can experience respiratory muscle fatigue and even failure.

Some of the signs and symptoms of restrictive lung disease are as follows:

- Increased breathing frequency
- Dyspnea
- Hypoxemia
- Cough
- **Muscle wasting**
- Weight loss
- Decreased diffusing capacity

### RESPIRATORY ACIDOSIS AND ALKALOSIS

The purpose of breathing is to provide $O_2$ to the cells and remove $CO_2$ from the cells. If ventilation is altered by some pathologic state, such as COPD, acid–base balance in the body is thrown off and disorders arise. **Respiratory acidosis** is a clinical disturbance that is due to alveolar hypoventilation. Production of $CO_2$ occurs rapidly, and failure of ventilation promptly increases the $PaCO_2$. Alveolar hypoventilation leads to an increased $PaCO_2$ (i.e., hypercapnia). The increase in $PaCO_2$ in turn decreases the

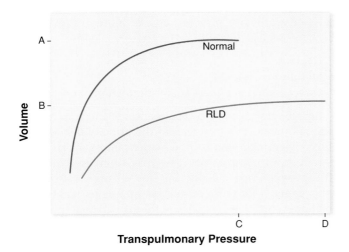

**FIGURE 18.15.** Compliance curves in normal lungs and lungs with restrictive disease. A and B, point of maximal lung volume; C and D, point of maximal trans-pulmonary pressure. RLD, restrictive lung disease.

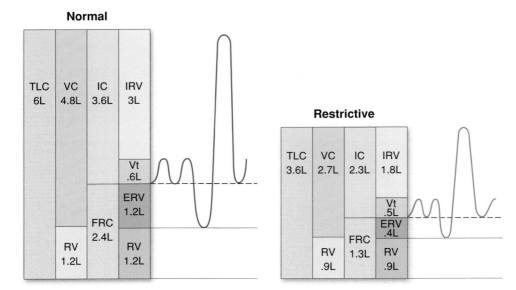

**FIGURE 18.16.** Comparison of lung volumes and capacities in normal lungs and those with restrictive disease. TLC, total lung capacity; VC, vital capacity; IC, inspiratory capacity; IRV, inspiratory reserve volume; VT, tidal volume; RV, residual volume; FRC, functional residual capacity; ERV, expiratory reserve volume.

$HCO_3^-/PaCO_2$ ratio and decreases pH. Hypercapnia and respiratory acidosis occur when impairment in ventilation occurs and the removal of $CO_2$ by the lungs is less than the production of $CO_2$ in the tissues.

Respiratory acidosis can be acute or chronic. In acute respiratory acidosis, the $PaCO_2$ is elevated above the upper limit of the reference range (i.e., >47 mm Hg) with an accompanying acidemia (pH <7.35). In chronic respiratory acidosis, the $PaCO_2$ is elevated above the upper limit of the reference range, with a normal or near-normal pH secondary to renal compensation and an elevated serum bicarbonate ($HCO_3^-$ >30 mm Hg). Acute respiratory acidosis occurs when an abrupt failure of ventilation occurs. This failure in ventilation may be caused by depression of the central respiratory center by cerebral disease or drugs, inability to ventilate adequately due to neuromuscular disease (e.g., myasthenia gravis, amyotrophic lateral sclerosis, Guillain-Barre syndrome, muscular dystrophy), or airway obstruction related to asthma or COPD. Chronic respiratory acidosis may be secondary to many disorders, including COPD. Hypoventilation in COPD involves multiple mechanisms, including decreased responsiveness to hypoxia and hypercapnia, increased ventilation-perfusion mismatch leading to increased dead space ventilation, and decreased diaphragm function secondary to fatigue and hyperinflation.

Chronic respiratory acidosis may be secondary to obesity hypoventilation syndrome (i.e., Pickwickian syndrome), neuromuscular disorders such as amyotrophic lateral sclerosis, and severe restrictive ventilatory defects as observed in interstitial fibrosis and thoracic deformities.

Lung diseases that primarily cause abnormality in alveolar gas exchange usually do not cause hypoventilation but tend to cause stimulation of ventilation and hypocapnia

secondary to hypoxia. Hypercapnia only occurs if severe disease or respiratory muscle fatigue occurs.

**Respiratory alkalosis** is one of many acid–base disorders found among critically ill patients. It is detected by arterial blood gas and electrolyte levels, which are monitored frequently. To diagnose respiratory alkalosis or assess the severity of the condition, the acid–base balance must be understood. Alkalosis, by definition, is a pathologic state that causes or tends to cause an increase in blood pH. One can have an alkalosis with normal pH if compensation has occurred. Alkalemia is defined as a blood pH above 7.44. The term respiratory in respiratory alkalosis refers to the primary respiratory mechanism responsible for the change.

Hypocapnia (low $PCO_2$) develops whenever $CO_2$ output from the lungs exceeds its production by tissues because of ventilatory stimulus. One or more of three basic mechanisms usually underlie respiratory alkalosis.

- Hypoxia
- **Metabolic acidosis**
- Direct central nervous system stimulation of respiration

In respiratory acid–base disturbances, changes in ventilation, and hence $PCO_2$, represent the primary disturbance, and compensation occurs by alterations in plasma $HCO_3^-$.

In chronic respiratory alkalosis, increased urinary $HCO_3^-$ excretion resists the pH change caused by hypocapnia. This renal compensation begins within several hours and takes several days for the maximal response. In acute respiratory alkalosis, an initial small decrease may occur in plasma $HCO_3^-$ concentration because of chemical mass action. Hypocapnia leads to increased formation of carbonic acid, lowered plasma hydrogen ion concentration (alkalemia), and concomitant reduced plasma $HCO_3^-$ con-

| Table 18.11 | CHARACTERISTICS OF PRIMARY ACID–BASE DISTURBANCES | | | |
|---|---|---|---|---|
| | pH | H⁺ | PaCO₂ | HCO₃⁻ |
| Normal | 7.4 | 40 nEq/L | 40 mm Hg | 24 mEq/L |
| Respiratory acidosis | ↓ | ↑ | ⇑ | ↑ |
| Respiratory alkalosis | ↑ | ↓ | ⇓ | ↓ |
| Metabolic acidosis | ↓ | ↑ | ↓ | ⇓ |
| Metabolic alkalosis | ↑ | ↓ | ↑ | ⇑ |

The double arrows indicate the primary event causing the acidosis or alkalosis. $PaCO_2$ is the compensation variable when the condition is of metabolic origin, and $HCO_3^-$ is the compensation variable when the condition is of respiratory origin.

centration. This is quantitatively less profound than renal compensation and is not related to change in $HCO_3^-$ excretion. Formulas for estimating appropriate compensation in simple respiratory alkalosis (limit of compensation is $[HCO_3^-]$ of approximately 15) include the following:

Acute alkalosis:
$$\text{Change in pH} = (\text{Change in } PCO_2) \times 0.08$$

Chronic alkalosis:
$$\text{Change in pH} = (\text{Change in } PCO_2) \times 0.003$$

*Table 18.11* shows the characteristics of primary acid–base disorders. Signs and symptoms of respiratory acidosis include decreased ventilation, confusion, sleepiness, **diaphoresis**, shallow and rapid breathing, restlessness, and cyanosis. Blood $K^+$ concentration increases (hyperkalemia) as the body exchanges the circulating $H^+$, with possible cardiac electrical abnormalities ensuing. Signs and symptoms for respiratory alkalosis include hyperventilation; lightheadedness; dizziness; numbness and tingling of the face, fingers, and toes; and syncope.

▶ *INQUIRY SUMMARY.* Pulmonary diseases can be broadly placed into two general categories: those that obstruct air from leaving the lungs and those that restrict air from entering the lungs. *The symptoms of each are similar, but how might exercise tolerance be different between these two pathologies?*

## Overview of Metabolic Pathophysiology

Metabolic activity in the body functions largely through the regulatory role of the neuroendocrine system. The combined neuroendocrine system functions through fast-acting (nervous system) and slow-acting (endocrine system) responses. Working together, both systems process biochemical information to regulate metabolism, fluid bal-

ance, blood pressure, and responses to stressors. This section concentrates on several major disorders related to metabolic dysfunction (*Table 18.12*).

### DIABETES MELLITUS

Diabetes mellitus is a chronic condition characterized by deficient insulin or defective mechanisms to utilize insulin in the body. This metabolic disease leads to **hyperglycemia** as a result of the ineffective use of insulin (or lack of insulin), resulting in altered energy metabolism. Diabetes is classified as type 1 when it is contracted early in life and there is little or no insulin produced. The much more common type 2 is usually contracted later in life (>age 35). *Table 18.13* presents the differences between these two disorders. Individuals can also be susceptible to developing diabetes due to years of altered glucose tolerance characterized by transiently abnormal elevations in serum glucose.

Individuals with diabetes often develop physical complications such as **diabetic neuropathy**, **periarthritis**, hand stiffness, **microvascular disease**, **macrovascular disease**, and infections. Individuals with diabetes in poor control also have to deal on a daily basis with the effects of hyperglycemia, consistent levels of which may lead to **ketoacidosis**. The hyperglycemic state is characterized by blood glucose levels >300 mg·dL⁻¹ and associated signs and symptoms. The **hypoglycemic** state is defined by blood glucose levels <70 mg·dL⁻¹.

### METABOLIC ACIDOSIS AND ALKALOSIS

The primary difference between metabolic and respiratory acidosis is the origin of the acidosis. In respiratory acidosis, hypoventilation leads to an increase in $PaCO_2$ with renal compensation (↑ $HCO_3^-$), but in metabolic acidosis there is a decrease in $HCO_3^-$ with respiratory compensation in the form of an increase in ventilation (↓ $PaCO_2$). Metabolic acidosis is caused by diarrhea, diabetes mellitus, and chronic renal failure. In the case of alkalosis, the compensatory responses are opposite to those of acidosis. In respiratory alkalosis, there is an increased pH (↓ $H^+$) caused by a decrease in plasma $PaCO_2$ due to hyperventilation. Reduction in $PaCO_2$ leads to a reduced rate of $H^+$ secretion by the renal tubules, which leads to a greater excretion of $HCO_3^-$ in the urine, reducing plasma concentration of $HCO_3^-$ as well. This last effect is the compensatory response. In **metabolic alkalosis**, the increase in pH and decrease in $H^+$ are caused by a rise in extracellular $HCO_3^-$. Compensation is in the form of hypoventilation, which increases $PaCO_2$. A simple stepwise progression can be used to determine acid–base disorders.

1. Determine pH value for acidosis or alkalosis.
2. Determine $PaCO_2$ and $HCO_3^-$ values to determine whether there is a respiratory or metabolic component to the acidosis or alkalosis.
3. Determine if compensation is present.

## Table 18.12 CLINICAL SIGNS AND SYMPTOMS OF METABOLIC DISEASES/DISORDERS

| Disease/Disorder/Condition | Clinical Signs and Symptoms |
|---|---|
| Diabetes mellitus | **Polyuria**, **polydipsia**, **polyphagia**, weight loss, hyperglycemia, **glycosuria**, **ketonuria**, fatigue, blurred vision, irritability, recurring infections, numbness in the hands and feet, cuts and bruises that are difficult to heal |
| Diabetic ketoacidosis | Thirst, hyperventilation, fruity odor to breath, lethargy/confusion, coma, muscle and abdominal cramps, dehydration, flushed face/hot dry skin, elevated temperature, blood pH <7.3 |
| Hyperglycemia | Thirst, severe dehydration, lethargy/confusion, coma, seizures, abdominal pain and distension |
| Hypoglycemia (insulin shock) | Sympathetic symptoms: pallor, perspiration, increased heart rate, palpitation, irritability/nervousness, weakness, hunger, shakiness; CNS symptoms: headache, double/blurred vision, slurred speech, fatigue, numbness of lips/tongue, confusion, convulsion/coma |
| Dehydration | Thirst and weight loss early progressing to poor skin turgor; dryness of the mouth, throat, and face; absence of sweat; increased body temperature; low urine output; postural hypotension; dizziness when standing; confusion; and increased **hematocrit** |
| Edema | Weight gain, excess fluid, dependent fluid collection, pitting edema |
| Potassium depletion | Muscle weakness, fatigue, cardiac arrhythmias, abdominal distension, nausea and vomiting |
| Metabolic acidosis | Headache, fatigue, drowsiness, nausea, diarrhea, muscular twitching, convulsions, coma, rapid and deep breathing |
| Metabolic alkalosis | Nausea, prolonged vomiting, diarrhea, confusion, irritability, agitation, muscle weakness, convulsions, slow and shallow breathing |

## Table 18.13 DIFFERENCES BETWEEN TYPE 1 AND TYPE 2 DIABETES MELLITUS

| Factor | Type 1 | Type 2 |
|---|---|---|
| Age of onset | Usually <20 years | Usually >35 years |
| Type of onset | Abrupt | Gradual |
| Insulin production | Little or none | Below normal or above normal |
| Incidence | 10% | 90% |
| Ketoacidosis | May occur | Unlikely |
| Insulin injections | Required | Needed in 20% to 30% of patients |
| Body weight at onset | Normal or thin | 80% are obese |
| Management | Diet, exercise, insulin | Diet, exercise, oral hypoglycemic agents or insulin |
| Etiology | Viral/autoimmune | Obesity-associated insulin receptor resistance |
| Hereditary | Yes | Yes |

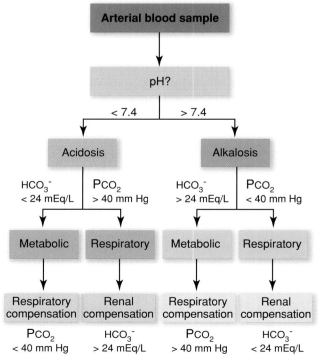

FIGURE 18.17. Algorithm for determining acid–base disorders.

*Figure 18.17* shows these steps as a simple flowchart. Full ventilatory compensation of primary metabolic disorders usually takes from 6 to 12 hours, and metabolic compensation of primary respiratory disorders usually take from 3 to 5 days. When compensation is not present, there are two or more underlying causes for the acid–base disorder, which is then classified as a mixed acid–base disorder. In these instances, there is usually both metabolic and respiration causes of the acid–base disorder.

▶ *INQUIRY SUMMARY.* This section has been limited to a discussion of diabetes mellitus and acid–base disorders. Diabetes prevents the normal use of glucose for metabolism; when the disease is uncontrolled, ketoacidosis can result. There are several causes of respiratory and metabolic acidosis and alkalosis. These conditions are often present in clinical populations in which exercise therapy is recommended. *How may exercise recommendations change in the presence of some of the physiologic perturbations caused by these conditions?*

## Summary

Pharmacology is the science that deals with the chemistry, effects, and uses of drugs. It includes pharmacokinetics, the activity and fate of drugs in the body over a period of time, and pharmacodynamics, the study of the physiologic effects of drugs. Use of drugs in clinical practice is important from the standpoint of patient care because medications help normalize physiologic function in individuals with chronic disorders. Cardiovascular and pulmonary pathophysiology, including the signs and symptoms of many different manifestations of these diseases, are a major cause of hospitalizations. Health care professionals who use exercise training should have a clear understanding of the effects of cardiovascular and pulmonary drugs and have a sound grasp of the pathology underlying major clinical conditions.

### SUMMARY KNOWLEDGE

1. Compare and contrast pharmacodynamics with pharmacokinetics.
2. Describe how polypharmacy is potentially disruptive to the use of therapeutic exercise training.
3. Why are elderly individuals at risk for adverse effects of drugs and exercise training?
4. Why is knowledge of membrane receptors important to understand pharmacologic effects?
5. Describe the pathophysiology of cardiovascular disease and list typical signs and symptoms.
6. Describe the pathophysiology of pulmonary disease and list typical signs and symptoms.
7. Compare and contrast metabolic and respiratory acidosis and alkalosis.
8. List typical signs and symptoms of diabetes mellitus.

### References

1. Grimes K, Cohen M. Cardiac medications. In Hillegass EA, Sadowsky HS, eds. *Essentials of cardiopulmonary physical therapy*. Philadelphia: WB Saunders Co., 1994:481–529.
2. Timiras ML, Luxenberg J. Pharmacology and drug management in the elderly. In Timiras PS, ed. *Physiological basis of aging and geriatrics*. 3rd ed. New York: CRC Press, 2003:407–414.
3. Goodman CC, Snyder TEK. *Differential diagnosis in physical therapy*. Philadelphia: WB Saunders Co., 2000.
4. Thadani U, Opie LH. Nitrates. In Opie LH, ed. *Drugs for the heart*. 4th ed. Philadelphia: WB Saunders Co., 1995:31–49.
5. Opie LH, Sonnenblick EH, Frishman W, et al. Beta-blocking agents. In Opie LH, ed. *Drugs for the heart*. 4th ed. Philadelphia: WB Saunders Co., 1995:1–30.
6. Opie LH, Frishman W, Thadani U. Calcium channel antagonists (calcium entry blockers). In Opie LH, ed. *Drugs for the heart*. 4th ed. Philadelphia: WB Saunders Co., 1995:50–82.
7. Marcus FI, Opie LH, Sonnenblick EH, et al. Digitalis and acute inotropes. In Opie LH, ed.. *Drugs for the heart*. 4th ed. Philadelphia: WB Saunders Co., 1995:145–172.
8. Opie LH, Kaplan NM, Poole-Wilson PA. Diuretics. In Opie LH, ed. *Drugs for the heart*. 4th ed. Philadelphia: WB Saunders Co., 1995:83–103.
9. Opie LH, Poole-Wilson PA, Sonnenblick E, et al. Angiotensin-converting enzyme inhibitors. Contrasts with conventional vasodilators. In Opie LH, ed. *Drugs for the heart*. 4th ed. Philadelphia: WB Saunders Co., 1995:105–142.
10. Castro M. Mechanical aspects of breathing. In Berne RM, Levy MN, eds. *Principles of physiology*. 3rd ed. Philadelphia: Mosby, 2000:311–322.

### Suggested Readings

Goodman CC, Snyder TEK. *Differential diagnosis in physical therapy*. Philadelphia: WB Saunders Co., 2000.

Grimes K, Cohen M. Cardiac medications. In Hillegass EA, Sadowsky HS, eds. *Essentials of cardiopulmonary physical therapy*. Philadelphia: WB Saunders Co., 1994.

### On the Internet

Cardiovascular Physiology Concepts: Pathophysiology of heart failure. Available at: **http://www.cvphysiology.com/Heart%20Failure/HF003.htm**. Accessed June 20, 2005.

Heart Spring: Heart attack symptoms. Available at: **http://heartspring.net/heart_attack_symptoms.html**. Accessed June 20, 2005.

Become an Expert in Spirometry. Available at: **http://www.spirxpert.com/test5.htm**. Accessed June 20, 2005.

The National Emphysema Foundation. Available at: **http://nef-usa.org/**. Accessed June 20, 2005.

Queen's University at Kingston Department of Pathology: The pathology of restrictive interstitial lung disease. Available at: **http://www.path.queensu.ca/present/boag/resp/PH2ILD.htm**. Accessed June 20, 2005.

The National Women's Health Information Center: Lung disease overview. Available at: **http://www.4woman.gov/faq/lung_disease.htm**. Accessed June 20, 2005.

## Writing to Learn

*The typical patient in cardiopulmonary rehabilitation programs is usually on a number of medications for their condition(s). Very common among these drugs is a class of medications called beta blockers. Research and write a paper that addresses the effects of these medications on performing a graded exercise test that elicits $\dot{V}O_{2max}$.*

# CHAPTER

# 19 Disablement and Exercise Prescription

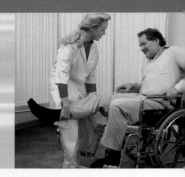

*Disability, the result of physical or mental impairment, prevents individuals from performing their socially defined roles. The role of therapeutic exercise is to prevent the decline to disability and also to rehabilitate patients from disability. What types of physical adaptations have to occur for individuals with disabilities to move from the ranks of the disabled?*

## CHAPTER OUTLINE

CONCEPTUALIZATION OF DISABILITY
- A Public Health Initiative
- Pathway to Disablement

DISABLEMENT MODELS
- The Nagi Model of Disablement
- A New Perspective on the Disablement Process Model

DISABILITY AND THE EXERCISE PRESCRIPTION
- Passive Stimulus-Response Paradigm
  - Group-Mediated Cognitive-Behavioral Intervention

EXERCISE PRESCRIPTION INTERVENTION TRIAD
- Functional Status
- Activity and Dosage

You have probably come in contact with someone with a physical disability. Perhaps a parent or grandparent, aunt or uncle, brother or sister, or maybe an acquaintance has an ailment that limits his or her involvement in social activities. Disability does not respect age, striking the young and old alike. Disability is sometimes the result of sudden accidental trauma; however, for many of those with physical disability, it is the result of chronic disease processes. Regardless of the origin and circumstances of the people that disability strikes, there is growing awareness that physical activity is an important health behavior leading to a reduction in physical disability, a concept that is essential for the practice of preventive and rehabilitative exercise.

## Conceptualization of Disability

**Disability** is defined as the inability to engage in age- and gender-specific roles in a particular social context and physical environment. There are three general categories of disability: **developmental**, **injury related**, and **chronic disease/aging related**. Cerebral palsy is an example of a disorder of movement and posture that leads to developmental disability, paralysis from traumatic spinal cord injury is an example of an injury-related disability, and arthritis is an example of a disease process leading to

chronic disease/aging disability. Developmental disabilities account for only about 1% of all disabilities in the United States regardless of age, while chronic conditions cause almost half of all disabilities among older adults.

There is a higher prevalence of disabling conditions in older individuals, primarily in the category of chronic disease (*Fig. 19.1*). Between 1984 and 1995 the prevalence of all major chronic diseases increased among persons older than age 70. Yet, in spite of the increased prevalence of chronic disease in the older population, disability rates for older Americans have been declining. In 1982 there were 6.4 million older Americans with disabilities. In 1999 this total numbered 7 million, which is less than a quarter of the increase that might have been expected (*Fig. 19.2*).

Reasons for the lower than expected number of chronically disabled individuals include the following:

- Improved management and treatment of chronic diseases
- Increased use of devices: canes, walkers, walk-in showers, support rails, and accessible facilities
- Changes in health behavior

### A PUBLIC HEALTH INITIATIVE

Many individuals remain healthy and functionally independent well into their ninth decade. The three factors

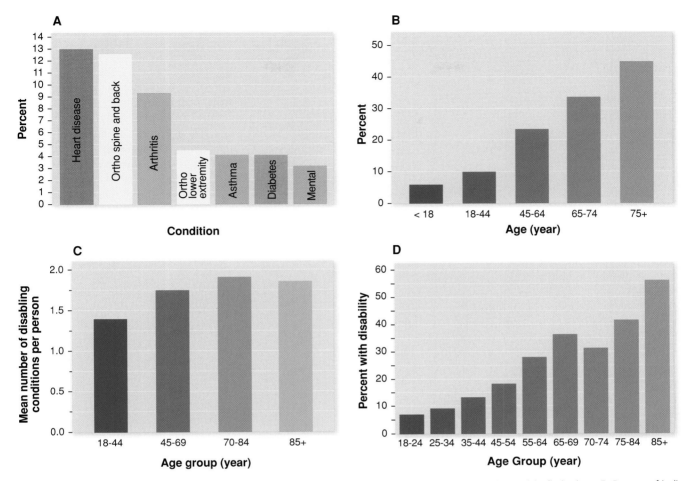

**FIGURE 19.1.** Disabling chronic conditions in older individuals. **A.** Prevalence of the major conditions causing activity limitations. **B.** Percent of individuals in each age group limited in activities because of chronic conditions. **C.** The mean number of conditions per person causing an activity limitation. **D.** Percentage of persons with activity limitations by age group.

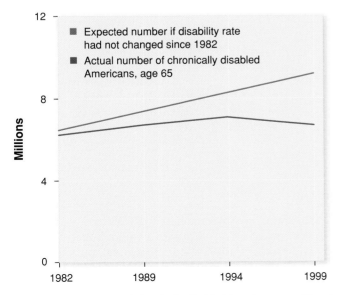

**FIGURE 19.2.** Number of chronically disabled Americans age 65 and older is less than projected.

mentioned above enable older individuals to stay independently active despite physical limitations. Habitual physical activity is a particularly important reason for the delay in general debility in some elderly individuals. Being physically active can postpone disability by as much as 20 years by reducing the impact of circulatory, locomotor, and respiratory disorders. These disorders represent the main causes of the observed loss of disability-free life expectancy (1). The connection is easy to grasp. Physical inactivity is a powerful causative factor for disability because it increases the risk of **active pathology**, **impairment**, and **functional limitation**, the precursors to disability (discussed below). Although the prevalence of disability is not as high as expected, disability remains a major problem for senior citizens with chronic diseases. An important goal, therefore, is to reduce the degree of disability experienced by older individuals. This can best be accomplished through prevention, and when necessary, rehabilitation programs.

The extent of disability in America can be seen in the following statistics:

- The average American elderly man is affected by some form of disability for 11 years (14 years for elderly women)
- About one in seven Americans have one or more disabling conditions that interfere with their daily activities
- Nine million Americans cannot work, attend school, or maintain a household
- Annual disability-related costs to the nation total more than $180 billion

Modern medical care has greatly increased the survival rate of catastrophic medical conditions and injuries. However, this victory has not come without costs. Individuals are often left with disabling conditions that result in a diminished quality of life and the need for continuing support services.

By the year 2020 about 55 million people will be over age 65. Projections indicate that by the year 2040 the number of people in the United States with chronic conditions will increase by 50% from what it was during the past decade (*Fig. 19.3*). With increased age, there is an increased risk of cardiovascular disease, arthritis, other chronic disorders, and the likelihood of disability. A key public health goal then is to increase the number of disability-free years in the lengthened lifespan. This can best be attained with effective primary, secondary, and tertiary prevention programs targeted to an aging population.

- Primary prevention (avoiding disease before it starts) may include a senior exercise program on a college campus or a hospital-based risk factor reduction program
- Secondary prevention involves using screening tests or examinations to detect early disease before it is clinically evident (i.e., giving a stress test to diagnose heart disease in people with a certain risk profile); screening tests are considered "secondary" because they are aimed at keeping the pathologic process from continuing to an adverse outcome (i.e., catching the disease at a treatable stage)

- Tertiary prevention focuses on reducing further disability in already established (symptomatic) disease through the rehabilitative process

The 1979 United States Surgeon General's *Report on Health Promotion and Disease Prevention, Healthy People* established the healthy people initiative. Under this initiative, the United States health plan is updated every 10 years. The Office of Disease Prevention and Health Promotion of the United States Department of Health and Human Services furthered this initiative by creating health behavior targets for the year 2000 (*Healthy People 2000*). *Table 19.1* shows how well these year 2000 targets were achieved for the older population. As indicated in Table 19.1, the nation met only four of the ten *Healthy People 2000* targets. This national effort continues in the form of *Healthy People 2010*, which has the following overarching goals:

- Help individuals of all ages increase life expectancy and improve their quality of life
- Eliminate health disparities among different segments of the population

Examining the health status of people with disabilities is an emerging public health activity. Within the *Healthy People* initiative, there are ten leading health indicators that represent the top health issues in America. These top ten issues include health care access, immunization, overweight and obesity, physical activity, tobacco use, mental health, substance use, sexual behavior, injury, and environmental quality. People with disabilities are represented in 12 of the 22 objectives used to track progress for these ten indicators. Currently, compared to people without disabilities, people with disabilities are less likely to have health insurance and engage in physical activity 3 or more days a week, and are more likely to be obese and smoke cigarettes. Clearly, as the population ages, these preventive health initiatives will become more important.

 **LINKUP:** *Prolonged physical inactivity is associated with long-term risks of disease in persons with or without disability.* **Perspective: Disabling Consequences of Inactivity,** *found at http://connection.lww.com/go/ brownexphys and on the Student Resource CD-ROM, describes these risks and how physical activity can help individuals with specific disabling conditions.*

## PATHWAY TO DISABLEMENT

Disablement has been conceptualized as a sequential, stepwise process that starts with a pathophysiologic disorder and proceeds through a unidirectional, causal progression to disability. This sequential disablement model, best viewed as a main pathway to disability, was discussed briefly in Chapter 1 (see Fig. 1.8). The conceptual scheme shown in Figure 1.8 demonstrates that various factors

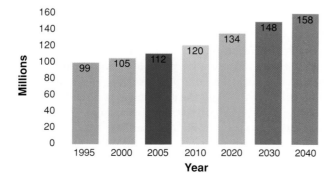

**FIGURE 19.3.** The number of people with chronic conditions.

| Table 19.1 | THE NATIONAL REPORT CARD ON HEALTHY AGING |

| Indicator | Current Data for Persons ≥65 Years | *Healthy People 2000* Target | Grade |
|---|---|---|---|
| **Health behaviors** | | | |
| No physical activity during leisure time in past month (%) | 34.6 (2000) | No more than 22% people age ≥65 with no leisure-time physical activity | Fail |
| Overweight (%) | 37.1 (1999) | No more than 20% people age ≥20 who are overweight (BMI ≥27.3)* | Fail |
| Eating 5+ fruits/vegetables daily (%) | 31.8 (2000) | At least 50% people age ≥2 who eat 5+ servings of fruit/vegetables a day* | Fail |
| Current smoker (%) | 11.1 (1997/1998) | No more than 15% people age ≥18 who smoke* | Pass |
| **Preventive care and cancer screening** | | | |
| Flu vaccine in past year | 64 (2000) | At least 60% of people ≥65 who had a flu shot within the past year | Pass |
| Ever had pneumonia vaccine | 53 (2000) | At least 60% of people ≥65 who had received a pneumonia vaccination | Fail |
| Mammogram within past 2 years | 68 (2000) | At least 60% of women ≥70 who had a mammogram within the past 2 years* | Pass |
| Ever had colorectal screening | 48.5 (1999) | At least 40% people age ≥50 who have ever received a sigmoidoscopy* | Pass |
| **Fall-related deaths and injuries** | | | |
| Hip fractures | 863 (1998) | No more than 607 per 100,000 hospitalizations for hip fractures, adults ≥65 | Fail |
| Fall-related deaths | 162.7 (1998) | No more than 105 per 100,000 deaths from falls and fall-related injuries, adults ≥85 | Fail |

*No specific target for people age ≥65 identified. From the Gerontological Society of America report entitled "The State of Aging and Health in America," 2003.

impact the pathway to disability. These factors comprise the totality of an individual's life experiences:

1. Biologic factors (congenital conditions, genetic predispositions)
2. Demographic factors (age, sex, education, income)
3. Psychologic factors (coping mechanism, social support)
4. Individual factors (comorbidities, lifestyle habits)
5. Environmental factors (medical and rehabilitative care, medications, physical and social environment)

As shown, these five factors may be positively influenced by prevention and the promotion of health, wellness, and fitness.

The main pathway to disablement progresses through the following stages:

1. Active pathology: Interruption or interference with normal processes and efforts of the organism to regain normal state
2. Impairment: Anatomic, physiologic, mental, or emotional abnormalities or loss
3. Functional limitation: Limitation in performance at the level of the whole person
4. Disability: Limitation in performance of socially defined roles and tasks within a sociocultural and physical environment

Figure 1.8 shows arrows pointing in both directions along the main pathway. The focus of this bidirectionality assumes that there are the potential positive effects of prevention and rehabilitation programs at any stage in the main pathway. Improvement in one component has an effect on the development or progression of a preceding component in the pathway to disability. Even in cases of a diagnosed pathology and impairment, disability does not have to be inevitable if the disablement process can be limited by timely therapy, rehabilitation, or lifestyle adjustments (2). For example, low physical work capacity, an impairment in the disablement model, is reversible with regular **exercise training**. Although regular exercise may not completely restore the functional capacity lost through damage or disease, improvement is possible for many individuals with disability and for older adults who have functional loss through years of sedentariness.

A major premise of the disability model is that active pathology is the necessary starting point to the entire disablement process. The thought is that a disability cannot occur without a pathologic process. However, recent evidence has shown that low physical fitness leads to functional limitations *independent* of disease processes (3). Morey and coworkers (3) demonstrated that within the pathway to disablement, lack of physical fitness is considered an impairment even when pathology does not exist.

This is clinically relevant because exercise is a key factor in preventing functional limitations and disabilities, whether they are caused by chronic disease or not. Therefore, the emphasis of any prevention program should be on developing interventions that can prevent pathology from becoming impairment, impairment from becoming functional limitation, functional limitation from becoming disability, and any of these conditions from causing **secondary conditions**. In the next sections of this chapter, we discuss in more detail the classical (shown earlier) and current viewpoints of the disablement process model. Concepts of how the **exercise prescription** for older individuals is affected when incorporated within the context of a disablement model are also presented.

▶ *INQUIRY SUMMARY.* Disability affects the abilities of individuals to function within their social and physical environments. Disability affects a large percentage of the population and becomes particularly prevalent with advancing age. Disability usually begins with active pathology that progresses to impairment and functional limitation. However, the disablement process should not be viewed as a rigid, causal relationship. Instead, the pathway may be reversed, and disability need not be inevitable. In this regard, physical activity allows individuals to remain functionally independent to old age and may help in the disablement process at any step. *List some chronic conditions likely to be positively affected by physical activity.*

## Disablement Models

Disablement is a global term that refers to the various impacts of chronic and acute conditions on the functioning of specific body systems, on basic human performance and activities, and on how well people function within their spheres of influence within society (4). Disability models are tools with which health care professionals devise strategies for meeting the needs of disabled individuals. Two basic models of disability are prevalent: the medical and social models of disablement.

For the majority of the 20th century disability was defined within the context of a medical model. This model describes disability as a direct result of pathology and impairment, and not the result of features of our society and environment, even though such features may often be changed, thus lessening disability. Thus, the medical model defines disabling conditions as principally the products of physical and/or mental impairments that constrain performance. The medical model influenced the development of most of the nation's disability-related policies and programs. However, the medical model of disability has been criticized for leading individuals with disabilities to internalize the negative message inherent in the medical model, i.e., that all the problems of individuals with disabilities stem from not having "normal" bodies. These individuals often believe that their impairments automati-

cally prevent them from participating in social events, making them less likely to challenge their exclusion from mainstream society. The consequences of the heavy emphasis placed by the medical model on the individual's impairment are, therefore, thought to be mostly negative.

In contrast to the medical model, the social model views disability as the result of a dynamic process involving complex interactions among biologic, behavioral, psychologic, social, and environmental factors. Both views of disability affect the way people with disabilities think about themselves. The social model enables people with disabilities to look at themselves in a more positive way, which increases their self-esteem and independence. The social model advocates looking beyond a person's impairment and functional limitation to all the relevant factors that affect his or her ability to be a full and equal participant in society. This encouragement to independence is an important concept within the social model of disablement because incapacity and dependence lead to social and economic isolation (5). In contrast, it has been argued that the medical model encourages the marginalization of individuals with disabilities within the constraints of the social environment. Within this context, these individuals simply assume an inability to engage in various activities, thereby engaging in a self-fulfilling prophecy, saying to themselves: *I am disabled; therefore, I am unable to participate.* The social model, rather than denying the existence of impairments and physiologic differences between those individuals who are disabled and those who are not, addresses impairments and physiologic differences without attaching value judgments to them. For example, the medical model would say that the inability to carry out activities is the natural product of an impairment (i.e., you are not mobile because you have a spinal injury). In contrast, the social model places physical or mental impairments in social and environmental contexts that contribute to the inability of individuals with impairments to carry out activities. Thus, the social model views disability not in purely medical/clinical terms but partly as a social construction shaped by environmental factors, including physical characteristics built into the environment, cultural attitudes and social behaviors, and the institutionalized rules, procedures, and practices of private entities and public organizations.

### THE NAGI MODEL OF DISABLEMENT

In the early 1960s Saad Nagi, a sociologist, developed a model of disablement (main pathway shown earlier) which incorporated the prevailing medical model of disability (pathology and impairment) but also added a social construct. This model, which has since become one of the most influential in **gerontology** and **geriatric medicine**, greatly influenced the social model by developing the idea that disability is the expression of a physical or mental limitation in a *social context*. To Nagi, disability is the gap between a person's capabilities and the demands created by social and physical environments. Nagi's model, which forms the main pathway to disability, challenged the traditional medical model for our understanding of the genesis of disability by recognizing distinctions between impairments, functional limitations, and disabilities (2). Because of these distinctions, aspects of the environment are incorporated into the concept of disability by the Nagi model. Nagi focused on how expectations for the individual were affected by the impairment *and* by characteristics of the environment, including physical and sociocultural barriers. In Nagi's view, disability is not inherent in the individual but is a product of the interaction of the individual with the environment.

As shown earlier, Nagi's disablement model includes four distinct but interrelated concepts. These are shown again below with an example for each:

1. *Active pathology* may result from infection, metabolic imbalance, degenerative disease processes, trauma, or other factors. An example is coronary artery disease manifesting itself as stable angina pectoris (as a rule, not all active pathologies are associated with impairments).
2. *Impairment* is tissue-level loss of function. An example of an impairment associated with coronary artery disease is cardiopulmonary deconditioning, i.e., low aerobic power, secondary to inactivity (as a rule, impairments do not necessarily lead to functional limitations).
3. *Functional limitation* is loss of function at the level of the whole person. An example of a functional limitation associated with coronary artery disease and stable angina pectoris is the inability to perform basic functional tasks such as ascending a flight of stairs (as a rule, if a functional limitation is present, an impairment, i.e., tissue-level dysfunction, is always present).
4. *Disability* refers to social rather than organismic functioning. An example of a disability that may be associated with coronary artery disease is the inability to socialize with friends and relatives in certain social contexts, i.e., attending a party (as a rule, not all impairments and functional limitations precipitate disability).

Within this model, **therapeutic exercise** interventions work at the level of impairment, functional limitation, and disability, with a view to improving functional capacity. In contrast, the traditional medical diagnosis begins with pathology in the treatment of disease processes. Using the example of coronary artery disease mentioned above, when stable angina is manifested, the impairment associated with this pathology is with the onset of severe myocardial ischemia at a workload-dependent anginal threshold. Aerobic exercise conditioning for this individual is an intervention at the impairment level in an attempt to increase the amount of work that can be accomplished at the anginal threshold point (i.e., a greater rate pressure product is achieved, effectively increasing the anginal threshold). Treating this impairment directly influences function by increasing the pain threshold and reducing pain during an activity of daily living (i.e., climbing stairs). As functional limitations decrease, so does the amount of disability.

An important aspect of Nagi's model is that it distinguishes between functional limitations (how disease and impairment work to produce movement dysfunction) and disabilities (how individuals' basic human performances and roles in society are altered by acute and chronic conditions). Functional limitations are the most basic manifestations of disease as they indicate difficulty performing basic physical activities. Functional limitations, therefore, are primarily reflective of reduced physical performance caused by impairments, while disabilities are primarily reflective of how the individuals' social responsibilities and relationships suffer because of functional limitations. For example, functional limitation in ascending and descending stairs may produce disability in the following manner:

- Social interaction is lost when the person is restricted to the home
- Social activity is limited when the person cannot climb stairs leading to the front door of a church or other social outlet
- Social role suffers when the person cannot fulfill his/her economic obligations (i.e., cannot work when climbing stairs is a necessary part of the job)

To reiterate, in Nagi's model, disability is the inability of individuals to perform socially defined roles and tasks expected of them within a sociocultural and physical environment. These roles and tasks are organized in spheres of life activities such as those of the family or other interpersonal relations; work, employment, and other economic pursuits; and education, recreation, and self-care. The Nagi model is important because it extends the scope of practice of therapists along a continuum of health care services—from the medical aspects of practice to the social aspects of practice, thereby encompassing all of the stages of the disablement process (i.e., from disease to disability). The Nagi model places a broad perspective onto professional practice. That is, understanding the functional limitations and disabilities of individuals is as critical to medical care as is identifying and treating the underlying pathologies. By understanding the functional capacities of patients, caregivers are better able to judge disease severity, the impact of multiple morbidities, and the need for rehabilitation and support services. Therefore, understanding the genesis of disability is the key to effective therapeutic or rehabilitation programs, including therapeutic exercise intervention.

The following illustration should help your understanding of disability and the terms of the disablement model. Paraplegia is an example of a disabling condition that can result from the accidental fracture of the lumbar vertebra and crush-injury of the spinal cord (the *pathology*). This injury results in the flaccid paralysis of the muscles of the lower limbs (paraplegia, an *impairment*). This leaves the individual unable to walk or drive a car (*functional limitations*). Public transportation, sidewalks, washrooms, and work environments often do not accommodate wheelchairs, which may result in unemployment and being deprived of social and cultural activities (*disability*).

*Do functional limitations inexorably lead to disability?* As we have seen, the answer to that question is no. For example, two patients may have Parkinson disease with almost identical clinical profiles showing moderate impairments (rigidity) and similar functional limitations (slow, shuffling gait, deliberate movement patterns). However, their disability profiles may be drastically different with one person needing help dressing and restricting all outside activities and social contact, and the other person fully engaged in a social life, such as attending church, maintaining telephone contact, and showing independence in daily activities.

As we have seen, Saad Nagi introduced the disablement model as a theoretic framework to describe clinical practice. His model has since undergone repeated modifications, but the basic framework remains. Box 19.1 presents Nagi's reflections on the development of his model.

## A NEW PERSPECTIVE ON THE DISABLEMENT PROCESS MODEL

The Nagi model of disability advances two key concepts: disease is the underlying cause of disability (medical model) and disability is also the result of interactions between people and their social/physical environments (social model). Therefore, Nagi's conceptualization reinforced the prevailing medical model of disability but also laid the groundwork for the social model of disability.

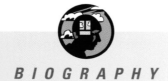

**Box 19.1**

## BIOGRAPHY

# Saad Z. Nagi

Saad Z. Nagi was born in Samalig, Menufia, Egypt and came to the United States in 1953 to pursue graduate studies in sociology. Nagi received his doctorate from Ohio State University in 1958 and immediately received a faculty appointment at this institution, which he held until his retirement in 1990. During this time period Nagi became one of America's top researchers in medical sociology and a key policy analyst in the field of disability.

In the early 1960s Nagi was working on plans for a large-scale study entitled "Decision-Making on Disability Benefits and Rehabilitation Potential." At the time, the Social Security Administration made decisions about benefits, while the state-federal programs of vocational rehabilitation made decisions concerning potential (i.e., who could get benefits). Central to such a study was the meaning of disability and how this concept was applied in related programs. While the main focus was on the two agencies of concern in the study, Nagi tried to learn as much as possible about other federal agencies and clinical settings that dealt with disability including workers' compensation, veterans' programs, rehabilitation facilities, and others. This search revealed that the concept of disability was used either without attempts to define it, or used definitions that were confusing the meaning of disability with related but independent concepts. It was also revealed that such confusion constituted an impediment to advancing systematic knowledge about disability. Significant questions were raised about the criteria used in decisions on benefits and services.

A turning point in this road to discovery occurred in 1963 when Nagi was invited to a conference on "Sociological Theory and Rehabilitation," held in Carmel, California. Nagi comments:

"My assignment was to comment on a paper to be given the second day of the meetings. Listening to the first day's proceedings—papers, comments, and questions—I noticed problems in communication stemming from the lack of clarity in concepts. That night I stayed in my hotel room and drafted the basic elements of a conceptual framework and attempted to specify the meaning of the component concepts: pathology, impairment, functional limitations, and disability. This was presented on the second day of meetings. The organizers of the conference asked for an article, which appeared in the book of proceedings published in 1964."

The conceptual framework that Nagi developed at this conference was used in plans, data collection, and analysis for the study of decision making mentioned above. It was also used in plans for the national disability surveys conducted by the Social Security Administration, National Center for Health Statistics, and United States Census Bureau, and for other surveys in the United States and other countries. It has been utilized in a number of monographs dealing with disability, including one on disability prevention recently published by the National Academy of Sciences. Nagi's model of the process of disablement has had a profound impact on physical therapists and has provided the theoretic underpinnings for the description of physical therapy practice.

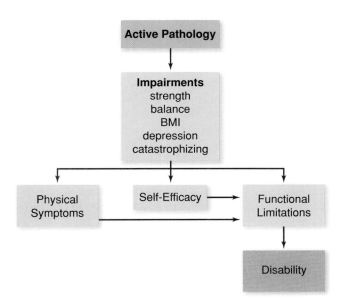

**FIGURE 19.4.** Revised model of the main pathway to disability. (Redrawn with permission from Rejeski WJ, Focht BC. Aging and physical disability: on integrating group and individual counseling with the promotion of physical activity. *Exerc Sport Sci Rev* 2002;30:166–170.)

Current thinking on disablement process models places added emphasis on psychologic processes and incorporates physical symptoms of impairment into the main pathway. Both psychologic factors and physical symptoms can impact the rate at which disability progresses over time. As we saw in the disablement model depicted in Figure 1.8, psychologic factors are placed externally to the main disablement pathway. This notion is currently being challenged and a revised disablement model is being advocated. The revised model is presented in *Figure 19.4* (6).

The revised disablement model incorporates into the main pathway physical symptoms (e.g., knee pain in individuals with arthritis) and **self-efficacy** beliefs, which were shown to be independent predictors of performance (7). The revised model views functional limitations as being moderated by symptoms and self-efficacy *within* the disablement model, not external to it. In the revised model, physical symptoms are shown as having a direct effect on functional limitations or an indirect effect via self-efficacy.

Self-efficacy is related to health behaviors. Individuals with high pre-existing self-efficacy have lower perceived effort during exercise tasks and feel better during exercise than individuals with lower self-efficacy. This has important clinical consequences. For example, it has been demonstrated that high self-efficacy beliefs of heart attack victims and their spouses (i.e., positive beliefs towards patients' cardiac capacities) result in greater improvement in cardiac function 6 months into recovery. Self-efficacy plays a powerful role in determining the choices people make, the effort they will expend, how long they will persevere

in the face of challenge, and the degree of anxiety or confidence they will bring to a functional task. Often what we do and how we behave are better predicted by our beliefs about our capabilities than by what we are actually capable of accomplishing. Efficacious beliefs evolve from the individual's perception of competence in performing a behavior, while inefficacious beliefs result from failing to meet personal performance expectations.

The disablement model serves as an important starting point when therapeutic exercise intervention is planned in the context of **patient/client** management. Using the disablement model as a guide, health professionals may prescribe therapeutic exercise to improve the physical function and health status of patients with documented impairments and functional limitations or of individuals who just want to feel better performing their daily routines (*Fig. 19.5*). The goal of therapeutic exercise intervention is to reduce the severity of the disablement process at any point along the main pathway and to prevent secondary conditions from occurring.

▶ *INQUIRY SUMMARY.* Two models of disability have been prevalent: the medical and social models. Nagi's approach effectively combined these, stressing both pathology and impairment and the social and environmental consequences that lead from functional limitations to disability. The main pathway to disability should not assume a unidirectional, causal progression without the possibility of reversal. At any point in the main pathway, the effects of exercise intervention may produce positive functional outcomes. A new perspective incorporates other precursors to functional limitations (i.e., physical symptoms and self-efficacy beliefs) into the main pathway. These further explain how impairment affects functional ability. *Why are physical symptoms a precursor to functional limitations in the new perspective model of disablement?*

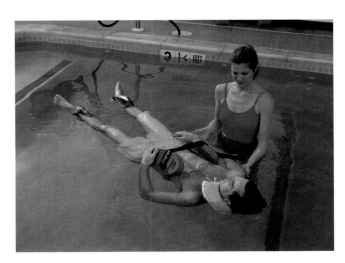

**FIGURE 19.5.** Aquatic therapy.

# *Disability and the Exercise Prescription*

Exercise prescription provides the parameters by which therapeutic exercise can be systematized into a training routine. These parameters are provided below in the section introducing the exercise prescription intervention triad. Exercise training is the repeated use of the exercise prescription to improve the general physical fitness and athletic performance of well clients and to reduce functional limitations and/or disabilities of patients. Exercise training is systematic in nature and involves an organized sequence of exercises, physical activities, or movement patterns that result in positive outcomes for the individual. Over time, exercise training produces physiologic **adaptations**, which result when training is performed above an accustomed level and enough recovery time is allowed to avoid **overtraining**.

The objectives of exercise prescription and training are often the same whether you are working with a patient seeking therapeutic intervention or a client seeking to enhance his/her sport, recreational activity, or job performance. Regardless of the status of the individual, therapeutic exercise can be used to better functional status and physical performance, and it is based on the personal goals of individuals developed in consultation with a health care professional. The desired outcome is always optimal functioning in the home, workplace, school, or recreational/sport setting. Accordingly, the goals of therapeutic exercise training are to:

1. Improve physical function, health status, and the sense of well-being in patients diagnosed with impairments, functional limitations, or disabilities
2. Prevent complications and decrease the use of health care resources
3. Improve or maintain physical function or health status of well individuals
4. Prevent or minimize future impairments, functional limitations, or disabilities for any individual (8)

These goals are best achieved when the disablement model is used to guide practitioners.

In 1997 the Institute of Medicine referred to disablement as the "enabling-disabling" process to acknowledge that disabling conditions develop and progress but also may be reversed through the application of rehabilitation and other forms of therapeutic intervention (*Fig. 19.6*). Since disability is the result of both impairment and environment, reducing disability requires attention to physical, behavioral, and sociocultural needs.

In Figure 19.6, the environment is depicted as a circle and represents both physical space and social structures, such as family, community, and society. If the symbolic person shown in the figure fits into circle (A), disability is not manifested and the person is fully integrated into society through social opportunities (employment, education, parenthood, leadership roles, etc.) and physical space (housing, workplaces, transportation, etc.). However, if

the symbolic person does not fit into circle (B), disability is manifested and the individual has increased needs (the person's size symbolically increases) which cannot be met by the environment. In this case, the individual eclipses the environment (i.e., his/her needs are too great to be adequately accommodated).

When disability occurs, two alternative routes may be taken. First, functional restoration may be accomplished through rehabilitation and/or other interventions. This places the rehabilitated individual back into their previous environmental circumstances (C). Second, there may be expanded access to the environment through appropriate environmental modifications (D). As shown in the figure, when this happens, the person is still enlarged, but now their environment is also expanded to accommodate their functional limitation(s). It is important to note that both approaches to disability may be taken singly or in combination. However, this text stresses restoration through physical rehabilitation using exercise intervention.

## PASSIVE STIMULUS-RESPONSE PARADIGM

Exercise prescription has been traditionally conceptualized under the rubric of a passive stimulus-response paradigm. This paradigm suggests that the best way to prescribe exercise that individuals are willing to initiate and maintain is through the traditional dose-response model delivered at exercise centers (clinical or recreational) and/or via home-based activities. This model has the following characteristics:

- Physical activity dosage (stimulus) is prescribed with intensity, frequency, and duration being key parameters
- Patient consistently adheres to the parameters of the exercise (dosage) prescription
- Patient's tolerance (physiologic responses or clinical signs and symptoms associated with dosage) to the exercise prescription is noted and recorded
- Exercise prescription is progressed or regressed as dictated by patient tolerance and functional improvement or decline, respectively

This paradigm is described as passive in that the individual participant usually has little initial input into the process. Adherence and compliance with the recommendation are assumed. Since the exercise prescriptive process is designed to reduce the decline to functional limitation and disability, it is important that the activity prescription be implemented in a manner appropriate for the intended target population. Adherence to the dose-response model is necessary for positive clinical outcomes to be realized. Therefore, any approach that improves adherence may be considered clinically superior.

### Group-Mediated Cognitive-Behavioral Intervention

The prevalence of many disabilities can be reduced using intervention strategies involving exercise. For exercise training to be effective, however, participants must adhere

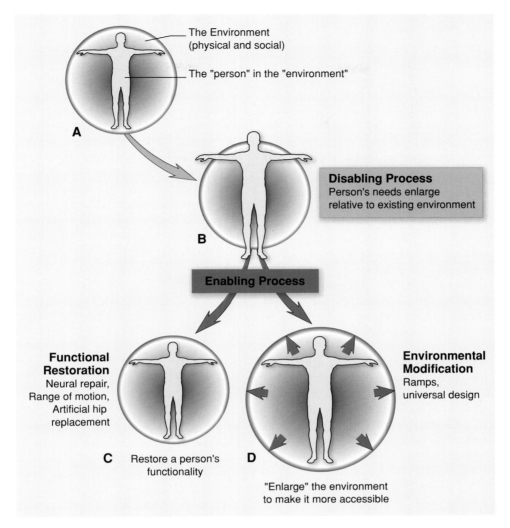

**FIGURE 19.6.** Conceptual overview of the enabling-disabling process. **A.** Person without disability. **B.** Person with disability. **C.** Disabled person has function restored through the rehabilitative (enabling) process. **D.** Disabled person has access to environment expanded through environmental manipulation. (Redrawn with permission from Mathiowetz N, Wunderlich GS, eds. Survey measurement of work disability: summary of a workshop. Washington, DC: National Academy of Sciences, National Academy Press, 2000.)

to the general guidelines of the exercise prescription based on the traditional dose-response model. The problem is that about 50% of all individuals discontinue exercise within 6 months of starting. The high **recidivism** inherent in exercise programs is a major roadblock to primary and tertiary prevention efforts. In addition, there is evidence that traditional approaches to increase adherence do not work well in the elderly population, a group of particular interest because of the high prevalence of disability. Delivering an exercise prescription to people most in need of exercise intervention requires a concerted effort to adopt strategies that enhance the likelihood of success. Success in this context usually means that the individual continues with his/her exercise prescription (sustained frequency and duration of exercise) after concluding a formal intervention program. Because of high recidivism, deviation

from the traditional dose-response model may be necessary for some groups.

Different strategies to increase adherence have been tried, with varying degrees of success. One such strategy used to encourage adherence to physical activity among older individuals is a group-mediated cognitive-behavioral (GMCB) intervention (9). This intervention involves the use of a group setting to teach participants how to identify, monitor, and achieve valued outcomes associated with physically active lifestyles. The goal of this intervention is to produce individuals who maintain lifestyles of physical activity. The group setting involves a certain amount of social pressure and employs motivation and support tactics to encourage participants toward cognitive and behavioral changes. The cognitive and behavioral changes produced by GMCB are thought to enhance adherence to physically active lifestyles once participation in a formal exercise program is over.

GMCB intervention uses instructional techniques to teach cognitive-behavioral skills and group interaction/participation skills. In a recent research study using formal exercise combined with GMCB, participants were more able to adhere to a home-based exercise regimen following the conclusion of the formal program than the group that did not receive the cognitive-behavioral intervention. The following strategies are typical of those used in GMCB.

- Promote and develop group identity; tactics may include naming the group, creating a group logo, designing t-shirts
- Promote positive talk; for example, the group agrees that it will have an "above average" success rate in changing individual members' behaviors
- Teach self-regulatory skills (self-monitoring of effort, symptoms and behavior, and goal setting); the tactic is to use a group discussion format to create a motive within the group to be successful at self-monitoring and goal setting
- Fostering social support (emotional and esteem support); using group discussions on dealing with failure to attain goals and develop tactics relevant to individual participants to deal with these failures; use of pairing (buddy system) to practice, motivate, and check on each other's efforts at self-monitoring
- Goal setting: develop specific goals for increasing active time and decreasing sedentary time at home (i.e., reduce time spent watching television); the goals must be personally achievable yet contribute to group success for increasing activity and breaking up sedentary time; for goals to be realized, accurate self-monitoring of decreases in sedentary activities and increases in active living is important
- Discuss relevant topics; these may include (a) activity logs for recording physical activity, (b) age-appropriate norms for activity and sedentary time, (c) use of self-regulatory instruments (i.e., activity counters) to track the amount of activity performed each day, (d) failure support, (e) how to become an independent exerciser, (f) designing and planning safe and effective home-based physical activity, (g) use of self-reinforcement when goals are achieved, (h) relapse prevention
- Group participation: members share their experiences and develop solutions to the problems faced by the members

The goal of these group sessions is to develop a plan for eventually becoming independent of the group exercise program. The intervention presented by Brawley and coworkers (9) is a 3-month program in which participants wean themselves from the structured program. The group setting can be a particularly effective model to promote an independent lifestyle of physical activity in elderly individuals.

For adults with or without chronic disease, there should be flexibility in physical activity programming rather than strict adherence to the passive stimulus-response paradigm. For example, individuals should be active participants rather than passive adherents to exercise prescriptions. Accordingly, Rejeski and Focht (6) recommend *negotiating* the physical activity prescription, whereby the participant willingly "contracts" the prescriptive guidelines based on his/her self-efficacy beliefs, affective responses, and physical symptoms. As part of the activity prescription, participants should be taught to integrate physical activity into their daily lives. Using the cognitive-behavioral intervention strategy to enhance adherence to exercise, exercise prescription personnel are less tightly bound to a passive stimulus-response paradigm that may be less effective for some individuals (6).

 **LINKUP:** *Cognitive-behavioral intervention appears to be effective in enhancing adherence to physical activity once the exercise intervention program concludes. The synopsis of a research study demonstrating this can be found in* **Research Highlight: Increasing Adherence to Physical Activity in Older Adults,** *found at http://connection.lww.com/go/brownexphys and on the Student Resource CD-ROM.*

▶ *INQUIRY SUMMARY.* Functional limitations and disabilities may be rehabilitated by exercise interventions using appropriately applied exercise prescriptions, which are only effective when individuals adhere to prescribed parameters. However, the prevailing passive stimulus-response paradigm may not be appropriate for all populations. Therefore, exercise personnel should be skilled enough to alter the dose-response model for a given population. In this way, the desired functional outcomes may be achieved. *Why should special attention be given to the elderly population to increase exercise intervention adherence?*

## Exercise Prescription Intervention Triad

To prescribe therapeutic exercise, the following components must be considered:

- Functional and health status of the individual
- Dosage or amount of therapeutic exercise given
- Activity or type of therapeutic exercise given (10)

This triad of factors is shown in *Figure 19.7*. The exercise prescription is a plan for physical activity formulated to achieve specific beneficial outcomes while minimizing the accompanying risks associated with exercise (see Case Study 19.1). The exercise prescription is an essential tool in the management of patients with impairments or functional limitations and is also important in primary prevention efforts for apparently healthy clientele. Regardless of the ultimate goal, a properly written and conducted

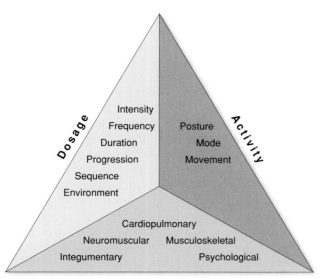

**Functional Status of Psycho-Physiological Systems**

FIGURE 19.7. The exercise prescription intervention triad.

exercise prescription ensures a safe level of exercise. With the safety issue in mind, exercise prescription and training must be done properly to avoid situations in which the health of the individual is compromised. Exercise prescriptions may involve too much or too little exercise, resulting in overtraining or undertraining (no therapeutic benefit produced), respectively. These are important considerations in rehabilitating patients toward functional improvements, in training athletes for competition, or in conducting general health-promotion efforts for a defined group of individuals. To minimize risks and maximize rehabilitation or training benefit, therapeutic exercise prescriptions should be individualized to the particular needs of the individual.

The idea of individualization is paramount in prescribing therapeutic exercise. The personal behaviors of individuals often dictate the success of the rehabilitative effort. Therefore, an awareness of the psychosocial aspects of behavioral change is a necessary part of the successful exercise prescription (see Case Study 19.2). Whether you are working

## CASE STUDY 19.1: *THE RISKS OF EXERCISE*

### CASE

Hank, a 54-year-old post-myocardial infarction patient, was referred to the local cardiac rehabilitation program. His family history revealed that his father and two brothers died of heart attacks in their 40s. Hank progressed through the 12-week phase III program and was in his last week without incident, but he was a fragile patient throughout his time in the program. Hank was exercising on the cycle ergometer at his usual heart rate prescription without apparent difficulty and was being continuously monitored with electrocardiogram telemetry. With no warning, he went into ventricular tachycardia. The nurse and exercise physiologist on duty quickly responded to the patient but arrived to late to stop his fall from the ergometer. Cardiopulmonary resuscitation, nasal cannula oxygen, and transport to the emergency room were initiated immediately. The physician on duty administered drugs, and advanced cardiac life support was started. The patient did not recover, as an agonal rhythm persisted until asystole.

### DESCRIPTION

Vigorous exercise is associated with a seven-fold increase in the risk of cardiovascular complications resulting in death compared with the death rate from heart disease while engaging in sedentary activities (1). This mortality rate is far

greater in individuals with coronary artery disease. The relative risk of myocardial infarction not resulting in death is somewhat less, about two to six times greater during vigorous exercise than during other activities. Habitual exercise has been shown to reduce risk. Sedentary men are 56 times as likely to have cardiac arrest during exercise compared to other times, but physically active men have only five times the risk of cardiac arrest during exercise compared with other times. In addition, there is an inverse relationship between the number of exercise sessions engaged in per week and the relative risk of a cardiovascular event. Finally, recent studies have shown that regular exercise training protects against cardiac events while exercising. Health professionals who conduct therapeutic exercise sessions should be aware of these risks. However, the data show that even in the best clinical exercise programs, risks will not be totally ameliorated.

### INTERVENTION

Immediate steps were taken to review the basic emergency procedures of the cardiopulmonary rehabilitation program. This case is included in this text to illustrate that exercise, while important for overall health, does not come without risks—sometimes serious risks for certain individuals. Health professionals are aware of these risks, and clinical exercise programs are designed to reduce risks as much as possible.

## CASE STUDY 19.2: *COMPLIANCE AND SAFETY**

### CASE

Steve is a middle-aged former athlete who underwent meniscal trimming under arthroscopic procedures. While recovering, Steve made the claim to his family and therapist/trainer that he would be able to run and jump on the healing knee cartilage within a few weeks. The therapist/trainer had difficulty gearing down the program for him. Each time Steve was given exercise instructions to perform at home, he increased the repetitions of each set of exercises. The extra work caused significant stresses to the knee joint area, with more swelling, stiffness, and pain. Steve is now limping on the limb with walking and refuses to go back to the crutches for weight-bearing relief.

### DESCRIPTION

Patient compliance is a major factor in any rehabilitation, wellness, and exercise programs, because it deals directly with the underlying motivations of why and how one should or should not participate in wellness activities. Historically, only approximately 22% to 28% of the adult population are engaged in regular exercise programs. Researchers in the area of change management have found that certain key steps usually precede a change in one's thinking, later reflected in his or her behavior. Usually an awareness of the problem surfaces first, then a precontemplation stage occurs as one ponders how to approach the issue, then fuller contemplation and planning occurs, then action or change is set in motion, and finally a re-evaluation of the effects of changed thinking or behavior. The risks of on-again, off-again exercise are not fully documented, yet we do know that benefits of habitual long-term exercise are manifold. We also know that the effects of exercise training are not "storable" for more than 7 to 14 days. One model suggests that the exerciser is placing him or herself at more risk for orthopedic injuries by doing infrequent and intense exercise or when being overly zealous in his/her approach to exercise or rehabilitation. Additionally, more researchers are finding that the social aspects of exercise help with compliance.

Surgical procedures, rehabilitation, and exercise training regimens have changed over time. These have all combined to speed rehabilitation and recovery from injuries or surgeries. Combining the above with pride in one's past athletic abilities may lead to an overzealous approach to recovery, which is further complicated by the old adage: "no pain, no gain." People may be especially at risk if they do not follow the medical or training team's recovery timelines and advice. The rate and total time required for various tissues to heal remain roughly unchanged if some significant surgical trauma has occurred. Some patients, in an effort to regain their function as quickly as possible, have been observed in clinic to overuse the area that is undergoing healing. The effect of weight bearing or exercising too much at certain early stages of healing can have deleterious results since the body is using its resources to heal and to adapt to a rehabilitation regimen. Also, aging effects can dampen or slow the person's ability to heal from tissue damage.

### INTERVENTION

Steve needs careful and empathetic confrontation regarding the overuse of his joint. His self-worth should be preserved to maintain the relationship and yet temper his prideful expectations. Explaining the new context of circumstances that he is now under may help him see that his body is now aged and his knee tissue after surgery will not heal as quickly as a muscle pull or skin laceration. Pointing out the cause and effect of the tissue overuse and current symptoms should be done. A possible approach may be to find a testimonial person of like age and surgical history to add credibility to the therapist/trainer's case. If the patient does not heed further advice, the physician may need to be brought in as a "coach" image to try to transmit the idea and use the inherent authority of the relationship to urge the patient to stop overdoing his therapeutic exercise program. Redefining what success and winning is to him may go a long way to eventual long-term recovery.

*Used with permission of Sam Coppoletti, Program Director, Physical Therapy Assistant Program, Shawnee State University, Portsmouth, OH.

with a patient or a well client, individualizing the exercise prescription is necessary for at least three reasons. First, physiologic and perceptual responses to acute exercise therapy vary among and within individuals across the lifespan or in individuals performing different types of exercises. Second, the magnitude and rate of development of chronic adaptations to exercise training vary among individuals. Third, therapeutic exercise programs considerably different in structure and makeup may still achieve desired outcomes

in individual clients. These factors necessitate the need to consider individual interests, abilities, and limitations when writing the exercise prescription (11).

Because of these factors, the dose-response relationship during the **titration** of the exercise prescription must be monitored closely. Titrating the exercise prescription is accomplished by carefully monitoring acute physiologic responses, signs and symptoms, and the overall progress being made as the dosage and activity components of the exercise prescription intervention triad are manipulated during the course of therapy or training. The three components (limbs) of the triad are the parameters around which the exercise prescription is built and individualized for different individuals. For all individuals, the exercise prescription is influenced by a variety of factors, including needs, goals, physical and health status, available time to exercise, personal preferences, and practical considerations, such as cost, equipment, and the availability of adequate training or clinical facilities. The same parameters are used regardless of whether the client is a young athlete, older athlete, or patient.

The way in which the exercise prescription is applied to different patients or clients and the rate of physiologic adaptation they attain must be followed closely and, as much as possible, be based on objective test data. The overriding concern is for patient/client safety; however, as previously stated, the well-formulated exercise prescription must also provide a therapeutic or training benefit while minimizing risks. Specific goals and interventions to reduce impairments and functional limitations or to improve the fitness levels of well clients are typical parts of the exercise prescription intervention plan. The plan is followed closely as individuals progress (or sometimes regress) through the course of their treatment or training program. Monitoring must be constant and involves the evaluation of changes in the status of the individual to assess functional improvements and to achieve effective and efficient results.

## FUNCTIONAL STATUS

The exercise prescription intervention triad is used to assist the development of a therapeutic exercise program. The first stage of the decision-making process regarding patient/client management involves three important factors:

1. Identify the impairments or functional limitations to be treated
2. Relate the impairments and functional limitations to the appropriate physiologic system(s) (or to the individual's psychologic profile)
3. Prioritize the physiologic (or psychologic) systems involved (10)

Impairment in any of the systems shown at the base of the exercise prescription intervention triad may produce movement dysfunctions. For example:

- Cardiopulmonary impairments can result in irregular breathing patterns (i.e., excessive use of accessory breathing muscles) and produce movement dysfunction due to decreased aerobic endurance and altered bioenergetics
- Neuromuscular impairments can alter motor control patterns and result in movement dysfunction due to altered gait

- Musculoskeletal impairments can alter static and dynamic kinetics and kinematics and result in movement dysfunction due to altered muscle length-tension properties, force capability, or arthrokinematics
- Integumentary impairments can alter skin, muscle, and fascia properties and result in movement dysfunction due to altered limb mobility
- Psychologic impairments can alter the emotional state and result in movement dysfunction due to depression and a loss of motivation to be physically active.

Conceptually therapeutic exercise prescriptions are based on dose and activity, which are prescribed after careful consideration of the disability profile (functional status) of the individual. This profile is developed via the diagnostic process in which impairments and related functional limitations and disabilities are discovered and documented. Assessing the functional status of the systems shown on the horizontal limb (base) of the triad defines the medical and functional conditions of the patient. Impairments related to the systems shown at the base of the triad help guide the clinician in designing the dosage and activity parameters of the exercise prescription. For example, dosage and activity prescription may be substantially different if the impairment is in the musculoskeletal versus cardiopulmonary system. Determining the functional status of the individual is the foundation of a properly written exercise prescription and a well-designed therapeutic exercise program. For this reason, the base of the triad is the most important consideration in developing a therapeutic exercise program for an individual. Once the functional status of the affected psychophysiologic systems has been identified, the next stage is to develop the activity and dosage parameters of the exercise prescription.

## ACTIVITY AND DOSAGE

The activity component of the exercise prescription intervention triad involves selecting appropriate movements, postures, exercises, or physical activities for the type of impairment identified and the functional goal desired. A list of appropriate activities for impairments and functional limitations or for improving general physical fitness includes many of the following:

- Aerobic activities, such as weight-supported (arm ergometry, leg ergometry, rowing, chair exercise, and/or aquatic exercise) or weight-bearing (walking, jogging, running, and/or stepping) activities
- Muscular strength and endurance activities, such as static or dynamic resistance exercise, manual resistance, elastic bands or tubing and/or pulleys (the type of muscle contraction intended, i.e., eccentric, concentric, static, dynamic, and isokinetic, is often an important consideration for muscular strength and endurance activities)
- Passive or active **joint flexibility** exercises, such as stretching and range of motion activities

■ Specialized activities, such as ergonomics, posture awareness, movement and balance activities, breathing exercises, and gait training

Once chosen, the activity must be given defining parameters according to the activity limb of the triad. For example, in choosing aerobic exercise to rehabilitate a cardiac patient, the mode may be leg ergometer exercise, the posture is the seated position upon a friction-braked ergometer while maintaining a properly erect upper body, and the movement may involve a pedal frequency of 50 revolutions per minute.

The dosage component of the exercise prescription intervention triad involves factors that amplify the physiologic responses to the exercise prescription. Dosage components include:

1. Intensity (amount of difficulty needed)
2. Frequency (number of exercise therapeutic sessions in a given time period, e.g., 4 days per week, two times per day, etc.)
3. Duration of the activity or technique (number of sets and repetitions, time involvement, or length of the training session)
4. Training progression (progressively overloading the patient so that further adaptations are realized)
5. Sequencing of the exercise session (warmup, stimulus activity, cooldown)
6. Environmental considerations (humidity, temperature, and air quality if exercising outdoors)

Physical activity causes an increase in energy release from the working muscles and results in a disruption in homeostasis, which manifests as acute changes in resting physiologic variables. Individuals' acute psychophysiologic responses (both magnitude and direction) to exercise depend on how the variables presented in the list above are prescribed and the type of activity chosen. For example, dosage manipulation involving a bout of endurance exercise causes acute cardiorespiratory and metabolic responses that are quantitatively and qualitatively different than those caused by resistance exercise. Clinicians should be aware of these differences when prescribing exercise. In the last section of the text, specific examples of exercise prescription are covered using the general scheme outlined above. Many individuals who have functional limitations and disabilities are confined to a wheelchair. Some of these chairs are motorized, therefore allowing no exercise benefit while using the wheelchair. However, many of these individuals use manual wheelchairs, allowing a degree of arm activity throughout the day.

*Experiences in Work Physiology Lab Exercise 16: The Relationship Between V̇O₂ and Heart Rate During Wheelchair Exercise establishes the relationship between heart rate and V̇O₂ for wheelchair ambulation in a group of healthy college-aged students. This exercise also provides practical experience formulating regression equations.*

▶ *INQUIRY SUMMARY.* Exercise is systematically prescribed for all individuals (patients or well clients) following a model that includes an intervention triad. The intervention triad involves first assessing the functional status of five psychophysiologic systems. Based on this assessment, activities are selected and a therapeutic dosage is identified. This model of exercise prescription works best in clinical programs when practitioners are guided by a disablement model that allows therapists to intervene at the level of impairment, functional limitation, and disability. The goals and objectives for therapeutic exercise training may be different depending on the client. *Considering therapeutic exercise training, how might goals in terms of functional outcomes be different for a 60-year-old cardiac patient compared to a 17-year-old track athlete?*

## Summary

Disability has been conceived as a causal pathway that starts with pathology and progresses to impairments and functional limitations. Disability results when individuals are unable to meet social obligations. Disability occurs in many individuals, but the prevalence of chronic disease and the aging population make elderly people especially susceptible to functional limitations and disabilities. The disablement model is an important clinical concept because it guides practitioners' use of exercise intervention. It is also important to realize that disablement is the result of physical impairment and socio-environmental influences. Many individuals with functional limitations and disabilities may respond to appropriate exercise prescription. When planned and systematized, exercise training may be transformed from a hit-or-miss proposition to one that provides individuals with a degree of certainty regarding their therapeutic goals. The goals of therapeutic exercise change depending on individual needs. A therapist can guide individuals to their desired outcomes using the exercise prescription intervention triad. The triad dictates that activity and dosage prescriptions are based on the functional capacities of the various psychophysiologic systems of the body. Impairments and functional limitations found in any system dictate the nature of the subsequent therapeutic exercise program.

### SUMMARY KNOWLEDGE

1. Why is the prevalence of disability not as high today as it could be?
2. What is the main pathway to disability?
3. What is the essential difference between the medical and social models of disability?
4. Why have physical symptoms and self-efficacy beliefs been added as precursors to functional limitations in the disablement model?

5. Describe the passive stimulus-response paradigm of exercise prescription.
6. How might adherence to an active lifestyle be promoted after a formal intervention program concludes?
7. Why is the exercise prescription intervention triad important in therapeutic exercise programs?

### References

1. Robine JM, Ritchie K. Healthy life expectancy: evaluation of global indicator of change in population health. *Br Med J* 1991;302: 457–460.
2. *Guide to physical therapist practice.* 2nd ed. Alexandria, Va: American Physical Therapy Association, 2001.
3. Morey MC, Pieper CF, Cornoni-Huntley J. Physical fitness and functional limitations in community-dwelling older adults. *Med Sci Sports Exerc* 1998;30:715–723.
4. Verbrugge L, Jette AM. The disablement process. *Soc Sci Med* 1994;38:1–14.
5. Scotch RK. Models of disability and the Americans with Disabilities Act. *Berkeley J Employ Labor Law* 2000;21:213–222.
6. Rejeski WJ, Focht BC. Aging and physical disability: on integrating group and individual counseling with the promotion of physical activity. *Exerc Sport Sci Rev* 2002;30:166–170.
7. Rejeski WJ, Craven T, Ettinger WH Jr, et al. Self-efficacy and pain in disability with osteoarthritis of the knee. *J Geron B Psychol Sci Soc Sci* 1996;51:P24–P29.
8. Hall C. Introduction to therapeutic exercise and the modified disablement model. In: Hall CM, Brody LT, eds. *Therapeutic exercise: moving towards function.* Baltimore: Lippincott Williams & Wilkins, 1999.
9. Brawley LR, Rejeski WJ, Lutes L. A group-mediated cognitive-behavioral intervention for increasing adherence to physical activity in older adults. *J Appl Biobeh Res* 2000;5:47–65.
10. Hall C. Patient management. In: Hall CM, Brody LT, eds. *Therapeutic exercise: moving towards function.* Baltimore: Lippincott Williams & Wilkins, 1999.
11. Franklin BA, ed. *ACSM's guidelines for exercise testing and prescription.* 6th ed. Baltimore: Lippincott Williams & Wilkins, 2000.

### Suggested Readings

Hall C, Brody LT, eds. *Therapeutic exercise: moving towards function.* Baltimore: Lippincott Williams & Wilkins, 1999.
Nagi S. Disability concepts revisited: implications for prevention. In: Pope A, Tarlov A, eds. *Disability in America: toward a national agenda for prevention.* Washington, DC: Institute of Medicine, National Academy Press, 1991.

### On the Internet

Disability Resources on the Internet. Available at: **http://www. disabilityresources.org/**. Accessed June 24, 2005.
National Center for the Dissemination of Disability Research. Available at: **http://www.ncddr.org/**. Accessed June 24, 2005.
National Rehabilitation Information Center. Available at: **http://www. naric.com/**. Accessed June 24, 2005.

## Writing to Learn

*The disablement process is an important concept to grasp if your goal is to work with individuals with chronic disease. Consider, for example, the pathology of congestive heart failure (CHF). The abnormal heart rate response to increased $O_2$ demand is an associated impairment, the inability to perform activities of daily living because of the abnormal heart rate response (along with other impairments) is the functional limitation, and the disability is the inability to work. Someone with CHF could simultaneously be in all of these stages at one time. The exercise prescription and some of the treatment goals would be targeted toward correcting the impairment and ultimately minimizing or alleviating the disability. These categories are not discrete and exclusive. Research and write a paper on the potential impairments, functional limitations, and disabilities in these patients, and then describe how the exercise prescription could minimize the impairments, functional limitations, and disabilities.*

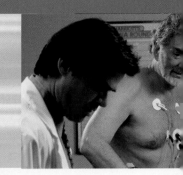

## CHAPTER

# 20 Clinical Exercise Testing

*The proper starting point for designing exercise prescriptions is to determine functional capacity by means of clinical exercise testing. Once functional capacity is known, exercise prescriptions can be written that will result in an increase in cardiovascular endurance, ultimately reducing functional limitations and disabilities.* Is objective test data always needed for writing exercise prescriptions?

## CHAPTER OUTLINE

MEASURING CARDIOVASCULAR ENDURANCE
- Ventilatory and Lactate Threshold
- Determining $\dot{V}O_{2max}$

PRINCIPLES OF EXERCISE TESTING
- Sensitivity, Specificity, and Predictive Accuracy of Exercise Testing
- Health Screening and Risk Stratification Prior to Exercise Testing

SELECTING THE GRADED EXERCISE PROTOCOL
- Treadmill Protocols
- Leg and Arm Ergometer Protocols
- Field and Submaximal Exercise Testing

EXERCISE ELECTROCARDIOGRAPHY
- The 12-Lead Electrocardiogram
  - The Limb Leads
  - The Chest Leads
  - Three Laws of Electrocardiography

- Recognizing Ischemic Responses
  - Subendocardial Ischemia
  - Transmural Ischemia
- Recognizing Arrhythmias
  - Normal Sinus Rhythm
  - Sinus Bradycardia
  - Sinus Tachycardia
  - Sinus Arrhythmia
  - Atrial Premature Beats and Junctional Premature Beats
  - Paroxysmal Supraventricular Tachycardia
  - Atrial Flutter and Atrial Fibrillation
  - Ventricular Arrhythmias

THE GRADED EXERCISE TEST
- Preparation for Testing
- Components of the Graded Exercise Test
- Relative Indications
- Interpreting Results

Many patients requiring therapeutic exercise intervention have functional deficits in three fundamental areas of physical fitness: muscular strength, muscular endurance, and cardiovascular endurance. Physiologic decline that produces these functional deficits is usually the result of the combined effects of inactivity, aging, and/or chronic disease. Regardless of the causative factor, reduced physical fitness hampers patients' abilities to adequately perform activities of daily living. The progressive functional decline in the muscular and cardiorespiratory systems that occurs as a person ages, and that which is exacerbated by chronic illness, can be attenuated by exercise training. Exercise training ultimately allows individuals to maintain functional abilities and more productive lives. However, to provide individualized exercise training programs for individuals with chronic conditions, assessment procedures on which to base exercise prescriptions are necessary. This chapter provides these assessment procedures as the necessary foundation for further therapeutic intervention.

## Measuring Cardiovascular Endurance

Chapter 1 defined physical activity as bodily movements that substantially increase energy expenditure, while exercise, a subclass of physical activity, was defined as planned, structured, and repetitive bodily movements to improve or maintain one or more of the components of physical fitness. The concepts of physical activity and physical fitness are interrelated in that physical fitness is the organic capacity for performing physical activity. As a component of physical fitness, endurance is generally defined as the physical quality that allows an individual to exercise for long periods of time with a minimal amount of fatigue. For example, muscular endurance is a subclass of endurance that involves the muscles' ability to contract repeatedly and exert force against a resistance (e.g., weighted objects). However, when exercise is performed in a continuous and rhythmic manner for a prolonged time, endurance involves the capacity of the cardiopulmonary system to sustain elevated levels of $O_2$ metabolism. Therefore, cardiovascular endurance, another subclass of endurance, is the degree to which an individual is able to marshal cardiovascular, pulmonary, and muscular (metabolic) reserves to deliver and utilize $O_2$ during exercise.

Cardiovascular endurance is usually quantified as the maximal volume of $O_2$ consumed in mitochondrial respiration during prolonged maximal effort exercise ($\dot{V}O_{2max}$, also referred to as aerobic power or aerobic capacity). The level of fitness (i.e., the amount of endurance) of the three key physiologic systems mentioned above largely determines such things as biologic age, disease risk, general health, and the ability to perform daily physical tasks, such as climbing stairs. The ability to walk vigorously, perform household or employment tasks, or simply to recreate without becoming fatigued requires an adequate level of cardiovascular endurance.

Being able to accurately determine cardiovascular endurance is extremely important in populations as diverse as patients with pulmonary disease and heart disease and marathon runners. For these and other population groups, knowledge of maximal **functional capacity** helps to determine clinical or sport-specific training parameters. $\dot{V}O_{2max}$ is the variable that most directly defines the concept of cardiovascular endurance, one of the five components of health-related physical fitness (refer back to Case Study 1.1). $\dot{V}O_{2max}$ is accepted as the criterion measure of cardiovascular endurance and provides the clinician with knowledge of the individual's functional ability, which is necessary for devising exercise prescriptions for the patient or the trained athlete.

## VENTILATORY AND LACTATE THRESHOLD

While $\dot{V}O_{2max}$ has been the gold standard for determining cardiovascular endurance, it is not the only standard, and it may not be the best indicator in all instances when the functional ability of individuals is important to assess. For example, although $\dot{V}O_{2max}$ represents the available $O_2$ consumption possible during maximal exercise, it is not possible to exercise at maximal exercise intensities for much more than 1 minute due to rapidly developing acidosis and muscle fatigue. A better measure of cardiovascular endurance may be the ability to sustain submaximal exercise for prolonged periods of time while remaining under the threshold of acidosis.

**Ventilatory threshold** or **lactate threshold** is thought to be a better indicator of functional cardiorespiratory capacity because it is associated with an increase in blood lactate accumulation and the attendant onset of muscle fatigue. For example, low ventilatory threshold scores reflect early acidosis onset at lower workloads with an attendant reduction in prolonged work ability. For the endurance-trained athlete, the training intensity at the ventilatory threshold reflects an individual's maximally sustained steady-state intensity or race pace. This makes the ventilatory threshold (i.e., the pace at which acidosis sets in) highly correlated with race performance (1). This concept holds true for many clinical populations as well. For example, the ventilatory threshold, not the $\dot{V}O_{2max}$, is a better indicator of functional performance in daily tasks for individuals with congestive heart failure who also have a left ventricular assist device (2). Refer to Case Study 20.1 for insights into this clinical population.

The clinical value of the ventilatory threshold as an indicator of functional performance can be equal to that of the $\dot{V}O_{2max}$. Ventilatory threshold is a phenomenon whereby minute ventilation deviates from a strictly linear response to a curvilinear response with increasing workloads. At the point of the ventilatory threshold, a hyperventilatory drive increases the **ventilatory equivalent for $O_2$** ($\dot{V}E/\dot{V}O_2$). This is followed shortly thereafter by an increase in the **ventilatory equivalent for $CO_2$** ($\dot{V}E/\dot{V}CO_2$). Ventilatory response after the ventilatory threshold represents an appropriate increase in breathing that is due to an increase in blood acidosis and $PaCO_2$. The ventilatory threshold is detected by plotting $\dot{V}E$, $\dot{V}E/\dot{V}O_2$, and/or $\dot{V}E/\dot{V}CO_2$ against a measure of exercise intensity (e.g., $\dot{V}O_2$, running velocity, watts) and pinpointing the break from linearity in the developed curve, that is, the point at which the rate of increase in $\dot{V}E$ exceeds the rate of increase in $\dot{V}O_2$ (*Fig. 20.1*). This breakpoint represents the point at which exercise intensity (expressed as %$\dot{V}O_{2max}$) can be sustained without developing lactate acidosis. This assumes that the ventilatory threshold is identical to the lactate threshold, an assumption that cannot be made under certain conditions, i.e., altered carbohydrate nutrition, enzyme deficiency diseases, exercise training, or altered states of sympathetic stimulation. For individuals with cardiopulmonary disease, the two thresholds are similar.

## DETERMINING $\dot{V}O_{2max}$

Regardless of the objectives of the therapeutic exercise program, $\dot{V}O_{2max}$ is still accepted as the single most important measure of cardiovascular endurance impairment. For this reason, direct measurement or at least valid estimation of $\dot{V}O_{2max}$ is essential to the successful administration of preventive and rehabilitative exercise programs. The purposes for determining $\dot{V}O_{2max}$ (or $\dot{V}O_{2peak}$) include:

- Providing data that are helpful in the development of exercise prescriptions and training regimens
- Collecting baseline and follow-up data that allow for evaluation of progress in program participants

## CASE STUDY 20.1: *LEFT VENTRICULAR ASSIST DEVICE*

### CASE

Bob, a 64-year-old male with ischemic cardiomyopathy, had a New York Heart Association (NYHA) functional class of III, which made him eligible for heart transplantation. While Bob was hospitalized and awaiting transplantation, inotropic therapy failed to maintain ventricular function; therefore, he was maintained with the aid of a left ventricular assist device (LVAD), which was implanted 1 month after hospitalization. Eight weeks before and 5 weeks after LVAD implantation, exercise tests were performed. $\dot{V}O_{2peak}$ was 13.5 mL·kg$^{-1}$·min$^{-1}$ preimplantation and 13.9 mL·kg$^{-1}$·min$^{-1}$ post-implantation (both measured directly by expired gas analysis). After the first exercise test, the patient was engaged in 13 weeks (only 3 to 4 weeks of exercise training was done while the LVAD was implanted) of progressive exercise training (treadmill exercise [intensity range of 11 to 13 on the 20-point Borg scale], resistance exercise using elastic bands, and light hand weights). By the second test, the patient was exercising on the treadmill at 5.5 metabolic equivalents (MET) (2.5 mi·hr$^{-1}$ at 7.5% grade) for 20 minutes with no handrail support. This intensity was well tolerated. Based on these data, the post-implantation $\dot{V}O_{2peak}$ of 4.0 MET was lower than anticipated. Gas analysis of the patient's steady-state exercise training session was conducted to verify the treadmill workload used during training. This was also duplicated in an age-matched healthy control subject. The following table shows the results from these studies. The MET response is to a workload of 2.5 mi·hr$^{-1}$ at 7.5% grade.

| Subject | Estimated MET | Actual MET | Deficit [1 − (Actual ÷ Estimated) × 100 |
|---|---|---|---|
| LVAD aided | 5.4 | 3.5 | 35% |
| Healthy | 5.4 | 5.3 | 2% |

### DESCRIPTION

Patients with congestive heart failure (CHF) have at least two traditional routes of health care: to be treated medically with drugs to improve ventricular function and, if warranted, to undergo heart transplantation. A third alternative exists today for individuals who may not qualify for transplantation. LVADs assist the left ventricle in providing an adequate cardiac output by diverting blood flow from the left ventricle through a pump attached to the apex of the ventricle. Cardiac output can be increased to 10 L·min$^{-1}$ during exercise with these devices, enough outflow for moderate exercise. Among the criteria used to assess whether transplantation is needed is a severely impaired $\dot{V}O_{2peak}$. A $\dot{V}O_{2peak}$ of 14 mL·kg$^{-1}$·min$^{-1}$ is the minimum threshold for transplantation. *How does the patient aided with an LVAD perform*

*during exercise testing?* Evidence suggests that conventional exercise testing does not accurately reflect the functional capabilities of patients with an LVAD undergoing exercise training (see the citation below). This fact causes doubt in the utility of the $\dot{V}O_{2peak}$ to classify the status of these patients in functional terms. For example, these patients can often exercise train at higher workloads (expressed as MET) than they achieved during exercise testing. Thus, it seems that either the training MET is overestimated or the exercise testing peak MET is underestimated in these patients. Recently, a case report was published (see reference below) that compared the steady-state $\dot{V}O_2$ response during exercise training in a patient with an LVAD with the $\dot{V}O_2$ response in an age-matched individual with normal left ventricular function.

### INTERPRETATION

The patient with the LVAD implanted maintained a steady-state response $\dot{V}O_2$ that was 35% lower than the expected (estimated) value, while the healthy person's estimated and actual values were very similar. The difference between the $O_2$ requirements apparently needed for steady-state exercise and the actual $O_2$ used is referred to as the $O_2$ deficit. While CHF patients do perform steady-state exercise with $O_2$ deficits, the deficits normally disappear as CHF patients take longer to reach steady state at a given workload. Apparently CHF patients implanted with LVADs persist in these deficiencies, yet they are also able to tolerate this disparity at reasonable perceived exertion levels.

Neither the use of handrail support (subjects were instructed against overly relying on the handrail) nor the instrumentation (age-matched control subjects under identical conditions were used) could explain the observed results. Therefore, we must look to a physiologic explanation for these results. One possibility is that physiologic adaptations to chronic CHF results in impaired aerobic metabolism and improved anaerobic mechanisms in a compensatory attempt to normalize functional capability as much as possible. How much the LVAD contributed to these results is speculative since the patient trained only 3 to 4 weeks with the device.

A key point in this case is the fact that there was a fundamental difference between estimated values and the patient's actual functional ability. Though the patient was classified as NYHA functional class III and Weber class C (moderately to severely limited), the patient demonstrated considerably more functionality in the therapeutic exercise program. The paradigm that gas exchange data is closely associated with cardiopulmonary dysfunction is built on the assumption that there is little reserve beyond the aerobic pathways for patients to draw upon. However, in patients with chronic central limitations, compensatory adaptation of anaerobic mechanisms in chronically $O_2$-deprived peripheral

**Case Study 3.1, continued**

musculature allows these individuals to meet the demands of daily physical tasks. This compensatory adaptation may well also include a greater ventilatory threshold, which was documented at 95% in this patient, well above that seen in healthy, untrained individuals.

One of the most important lessons learned from this case is that while exercise testing gives valuable data about the exercise capacity in these patients, it may not reflect the patient's true functional capabilities. Therefore, therapists should evaluate cardiopulmonary test data in balance with clinical assessment of the patient's self-reported ability and replication of functional tasks.

Humphrey R. Cardiopulmonary exercise response in a patient with a left ventricular assist device: inability of conventional cardiopulmonary exercise testing to identify capabilities. *Phys Ther Case Rep* 1998;1:172–177.

- Increasing motivation for entering and adhering to exercise programs
- Assisting in diagnosis and treatment of hypokinetic diseases
- Educating participants about the benefits of cardiovascular fitness and endurance exercise

Knowing a given patient's $\dot{V}O_{2max}$ allows the clinician to identify vocational and leisure activities that may be included or excluded based on the individual's functional capacity. Decisions to allow return to work or to classify as disabled may also be justified using the $\dot{V}O_{2max}$ score. For example, a $\dot{V}O_{2max}$ below 15 mL·kg$^{-1}$·min$^{-1}$ defines a moderately impaired respiratory system in pulmonary patients (3). For purposes of employment, a score <15 mL·kg$^{-1}$·min$^{-1}$ is considered to be indicative of physical impairment (4). The $\dot{V}O_{2max}$ test can also predict with accuracy the endurance performance in a large group of individuals with a wide range of $\dot{V}O_{2max}$ scores.

Measuring $\dot{V}O_{2max}$ is usually performed by open-circuit spirometry (Chapter 5) and relies on several closely monitored physiologic variables to ascertain whether the individual actually achieves the maximal exercise state. These variables are heart rate (HR), $\dot{V}O_2$, and the respiratory exchange ratio (RER). The test should ideally last between 8 to 12 minutes. Shorter test durations can produce premature fatigue due to excessively large incremental increases in intensity.

Excessively long or short test durations can lower the $\dot{V}O_{2max}$ score attained. An attendant problem in testing for $\dot{V}O_{2max}$ is knowing when the person has actually achieved his/her maximal exercise capacity. Accordingly, the criterion of a plateau in $\dot{V}O_2$ response as work intensity increases is usually the gold standard for knowing when $\dot{V}O_{2max}$ has been achieved (*Fig. 20.2*). In addition, HR and RER provide valuable information during the test. An RER of about 1.15 and a HR that approximates the age-predicted maximal level (220 − Age) are additional indirect evidence that a valid measure of $\dot{V}O_{2max}$ has been achieved. Attaining two of these three criteria is usually considered necessary for achieving $\dot{V}O_{2max}$. However, not all healthy individuals, and even fewer chronically ill individuals, can meet these three criteria. In such cases, other terminology is used, such as $\dot{V}O_{2peak}$ or symptom-limited $\dot{V}O_{2max}$. The most direct evidence that confirms achievement of $\dot{V}O_{2max}$ is an actual plateau in $\dot{V}O_2$. If this one criterion is missing, the others are probably not very meaningful.

 **LINKUP:** *Clinicians are usually more concerned with measuring $\dot{V}O_{2peak}$ than $\dot{V}O_{2max}$. The reasons for this are many and are addressed in Perspective: $\dot{V}O_{2peak}$ or $\dot{V}O_{2max}$?, found at http://connection.lww.com/go/brownexphys and on the Student Resource CD-ROM. In this chapter, the two terms are used interchangeably, but technically they are not synonymous. When either $\dot{V}O_{2peak}$ or $\dot{V}O_{2max}$ is meant, the correct symbol is used.*

$\dot{V}O_{2max}$ can also be accurately estimated without relying on direct measurement, which requires expensive laboratory equipment. When $\dot{V}O_{2max}$ is estimated based on valid and reliable methods, there is a close statistical relationship between the estimated and actual $\dot{V}O_{2max}$ values obtained. Estimating $\dot{V}O_{2max}$ saves the time and expense of performing direct measurements of $\dot{V}O_{2max}$. The absence or presence of the following factors affects the association between estimated and actual $\dot{V}O_{2max}$:

- Habituation: Familiarization with the testing ergometer improves the association between predicted and actual values, and the variability between these scores decreases
- Fitness: Increased fitness level decreases the variability between actual and predicted scores, although $\dot{V}O_{2max}$ still tends to be overpredicted for well-trained individuals and $\dot{V}O_{2max}$ tends to be underpredicted in untrained individuals
- Heart disease: Predicted values are higher than actual values in these patients
- Handrail holding (treadmill protocols): $\dot{V}O_{2max}$ is overpredicted as predicted values are greater than actual values
- Exercise protocol: As the exercise testing protocol becomes more demanding (i.e., the incremental stages of the test progress more vigorously in intensity from stage to stage), $\dot{V}O_{2max}$ is overpredicted and variability increases (5)

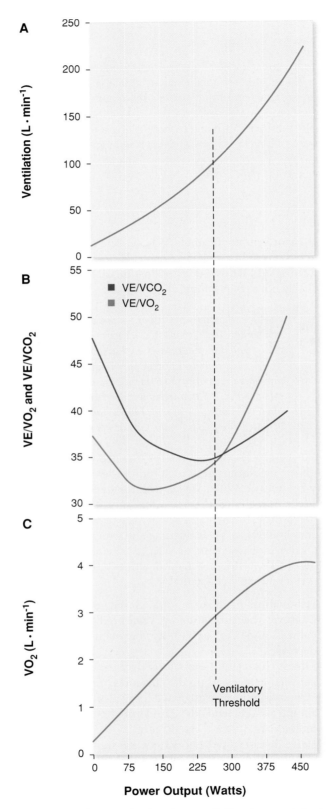

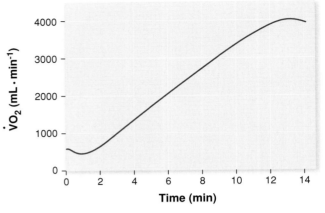

FIGURE 20.2. During an incremental exercise test, $\dot{V}O_2$ increases in a linear fashion with workload until high workloads at which time the rate of increase in $\dot{V}O_2$ slows, eventually plateauing at a level that defines the maximal aerobic power of the individual in terms of $\dot{V}O_{2max}$ and workload.

Choosing when to measure $\dot{V}O_{2max}$ versus when to estimate it can be difficult. $\dot{V}O_{2max}$ can be predicted using submaximal or maximal laboratory or field exercise tests and associated prediction equations; a sample is listed in *Table 20.1*. For research purposes, the measurement of $\dot{V}O_{2max}$ is required. However, measurement of $\dot{V}O_{2max}$ for clinical purposes is not as vital when there are valid and reliable ways to estimate its value. Clearly, if prediction techniques significantly over- or underestimate the actual value of a patient's functional aerobic capacity, subsequent exercise prescriptions will not be as precise as they could be.

 **LINKUP:** *The popular American College of Sports Medicine (ACSM) equations used to estimate steady-state $\dot{V}O_2$ response to exercise have sometimes been used to estimate $\dot{V}O_{2max}$ by using the final grade and speed (treadmill), power output (leg or arm ergometer), or step rate and height (stepping) achieved in a conventional graded exercise test. Since steady state is not achieved in the final stage of a maximal graded exercise test, using these equations in this manner results in an overestimation of the actual $\dot{V}O_2$ response.* **Research Highlight: Accuracy of $\dot{V}O_{2max}$ Prediction Equations in Older Adults,** *found at http://connection.lww.com/go/brownexphys and on the Student Resource CD-ROM, presents a study that investigated this problem in older men and women.*

▶ *INQUIRY SUMMARY.* Ventilatory threshold is a commonly used marker for monitoring respiratory function during exercise. However, $\dot{V}O_{2max}$ (functional aerobic power) is the single best indicator of cardiovascular endurance. Measuring $\dot{V}O_{2max}$ and/or ventilatory threshold gives important clinical information that can be subsequently used for devising the exercise prescription. *What are other reasons for knowing the individual's actual $\dot{V}O_{2max}$ and ventilatory threshold?*

FIGURE 20.1. Three graphs show how ventilation changes during incremental exercise performed to volitional fatigue. **A.** Pulmonary ventilation increases in a linear fashion until the break point identified as the ventilatory threshold. **B.** Ventilatory equivalent for $O_2$ and $CO_2$ (ventilatory equivalent for $CO_2$ also experiences a breaking point). **C.** Linear increase in $\dot{V}O_2$ as work rate increases.

| Table 20.1 | EQUATIONS PREDICTING $\dot{V}O_{2max}$ |
|---|---|

| Exercise Mode | Equation |
|---|---|
| **Using maximal tests** | |
| Treadmill ergometry ($mL \cdot kg^{-1} \cdot min^{-1}$) | |
| Bruce Protocol | $14.8 - 1.379$(Time in minutes) $+ 0.451$(Time$^2$) $- 0.012$(Time$^3$)<br>Generalized equation<br>$2.282$(Time in minutes) $+ 8.545$<br>Handrail support<br>$3.9$(Time in minutes) $- 7.0$<br>Standardized Bruce ramp |
| Individualized ramp<br>Protocol (Myers) | $0.72x + 3.67$ |
| x is the predicted based on peak speed/grade using the ACSM walking equation (refer to Chapter 5 for this equation) | |
| Individualized ramp<br>Protocol (Foster) | $0.694x + 3.33$ |
| x is the predicted based on peak speed/grade using the ACSM walking equation (refer to Chapter 5 for this equation) | |
| Balke protocol | $1.51$(Time in minutes) $+ 11.12$<br>Healthy males |
| Cycle ergometry ($mL \cdot min^{-1}$) | |
| Storer | $10.51$(watts) $+ 6.35$(kg mass) $- 10.49$(Age) $+ 519.3$<br>Healthy males<br>$9.39$(watts) $+ 7.7$(kg mass) $- 5.88$(Age) $+ 136.7$<br>Healthy females |
| **Using submaximal tests** | |
| Treadmill ergometry ($mL \cdot kg^{-1} \cdot min^{-1}$) | |
| Ebbeling | $15.1 + 21.8$(Walk speed [$mi \cdot hr^{-1}$]) $- 0.327$(HR) $- 0.263$(Speed)(Age) $+$<br>$0.00504$(HR)(Age) $+ 5.989$(Sex [F $= 0$, M $= 1$])<br>Male/female |
| Cycle ergometry ($L \cdot min^{-1}$) | |
| Siconolfi | $0.348$ (O$_2$ [Åstrand]) $- 0.035$(Age) $+ 3.011$<br>Healthy males<br>$0.302$ (O$_2$ [Åstrand]) $- 0.019$(Age) $+ 1.593$<br>Healthy females |
| Step ergometry ($mL \cdot kg^{-1} \cdot min^{-1}$) | |
| McArdle | $0.42$(Recovery HR) $+ 111.33$<br>Healthy males<br>$0.1847$(Recovery HR) $+ 65.81$<br>Healthy females |
| Field tests ($mL \cdot kg^{-1} \cdot min^{-1}$) | |
| Rockport walking test (1 mile walk) | $132.853 - 0.1692$(kg mass) $- 0.3877$(Age) $+ 6.315$(Sex [F $= 0$, M $= 1$]) $-$<br>$3.2649$(Time in minutes) $- 0.1565$(HR at end of walk) |
| 1.5-Mile run test | $3.5 + (483 \div$ Time in minutes) |

ACSM, American College of Sports Medicine; HR, heart rate.

## *Principles of Exercise Testing*

There are three major purposes for clinical exercise testing:

1. Therapeutic application: Exercise prescription is based on a determination of functional aerobic capacity (i.e., cardiovascular endurance or $\dot{V}O_{2max(peak)}$)
2. Diagnostic application: Determines the presence of disease
3. Prognostic application: Determines the probable outcome of the disease

These general purposes, while distinct, are not mutually exclusive. For example, knowledge of an individual's functional capacity is useful information for both diagnostic and prognostic purposes. The first application, functional testing, is valuable for activity counseling, exercise prescription, and/or disability assessment. The second application, diagnostic testing, is the initial test of choice to evaluate individuals with at least an intermediate probability of significant coronary artery disease. And in the third application, exercise testing may be employed as a tool for prognostic assessment using several indices and the Duke

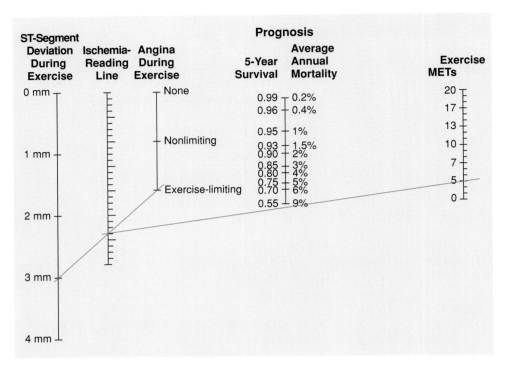

**FIGURE 20.3.** The Duke nomogram. Patient prognosis can be determined in a process that uses data from an exercise test. ST-segment depression, angina, and functional aerobic capacity in MET are determined during exercise testing. ST-segment depression and the presence or absence of angina are documented on their respective lines on the nomogram, and a straight line connecting these points is drawn. The intersecting point on the ischemia reading line is then connected to the point signifying exercise tolerance (MET) with a straight line. This line intersects the prognosis line, which signifies the 5-year survival and average annual mortality rate. (From Mark DB, Shaw L, Harrell FE Jr, et al. Prognostic value of a treadmill exercise score in outpatients with suspected coronary artery disease. *N Engl J Med* 1991;325:849–853.)

nomogram (*Fig. 20.3*). Prognosis is related to functional capacity as either measured by $\dot{V}O_{2max}$ or estimated by metabolic equivalents (MET) for the work rate performed. In this regard, clinically significant MET for maximal exercise capacity are related to prognosis in the following fashion:

- <5 MET: Poor prognosis; functional capacity is usually limited immediately after myocardial infarction (MI); peak cost of basic activities of daily living
- 10 MET: Good prognosis with medical therapy; as good as coronary bypass surgery
- 13 MET: Excellent prognosis regardless of other exercise responses
- 18 MET: Indicative of elite endurance athletes
- 20 MET: Indicative of world-class endurance athletes

In general, exercise testing is very effective in the following ways:

- Evaluation of coronary artery disease and pulmonary symptoms
- Evaluation of the effects of cardiopulmonary procedures and the effects of therapy
- Evaluation of whether further, more definitive testing is required
- Basis on which to prescribe a safe level of exercise and physical activity for the apparently healthy, asympto-

matic population and for individuals with chronic disease

## SENSITIVITY, SPECIFICITY, AND PREDICTIVE ACCURACY OF EXERCISE TESTING

The chief diagnostic tool used in exercise testing is the electrocardiogram (ECG). The ECG indicates if the myocardium is receiving enough $O_2$ during exercise. Therefore, in exercise testing, the ECG is used to define test outcome as either positive (abnormal) or negative (normal) for ischemia. As is demonstrated below, the criterion for a positive exercise ECG test is usually an ST segment that is depressed ≥1 mm below the isoelectric line and stays depressed for at least 0.08 seconds beyond the J point. However, for the ECG to be effective as a diagnostic tool during exercise testing, an effective exercise protocol must be selected. As we will see in the section on selecting the exercise protocol, matching the exercise protocol to a patient is an important preliminary function.

Both the ECG and the testing protocol impact test **specificity** and **sensitivity**. That is to say, exercise testing may be useful in *confirming* (specificity) and *ruling out* (sensitivity) disease. The key to successful exercise testing is to stress the cardiopulmonary system sufficiently with an exercise mode that is correctly selected and applied to the patient. When this is done, potential underlying disease may be revealed as indicated by ECG ischemic responses. In this way, the exercise protocol and ECG work in concert to maximize test specificity and sensitivity.

While one of the goals of exercise testing is to help diagnose disease, it is not designed to provide a definitive diagnosis but only to provide an estimate of the probability of the presence of disease. In addition, exercise testing *alone* cannot establish the estimated probability of disease. There must also be an understanding of the prevalence of cardiovascular disease (CVD) in the population being tested before the test is given. This is postulated in Bayes' theorem, which states that the post-test probability that a person has disease is the product of the pretest probability of disease presence and the probability that the test result is a true result. There are four possible outcomes to diagnostic exercise testing:

1. True positive: A positive test result in an individual with CVD
2. False positive: A positive test result in an individual without CVD
3. True negative: A negative test result in an individual without CVD
4. False negative: A negative test result in an individual with CVD

Theoretically, sensitivity and specificity percentages are best applied to population characteristics and not individuals. The ability of a test to detect disease and help the clinician make a correct diagnosis is determined by test sensitivity, specificity, and predictive accuracy. As sensitivity and specificity approach 100%, the ability of the test to discriminate, i.e., differentiate diseased from nondiseased populations, improves.

Sensitivity refers to the percent of patients tested who have CVD and who also test positive. *Does the test have the ability to detect disease when it is present?* This is the basic question related to sensitivity. Sensitivity, the percentage of CVD patients who produce an abnormal ECG test result, is quantified as follows:

$$Sensitivity = TP \div (TP + FN)$$

TP is the true positive (abnormal ECG exercise test in the presence of CVD) and FN is the false negative (normal ECG exercise test in the presence of CVD). Therefore, sensitivity is equal to all those with truly positive tests divided by all those with disease. As you can see, some individuals with disease will test negative. Sensitivity of exercise testing averages about 68% in controlled studies. This means that 68% of those individuals with disease will have a TP exercise ECG and 32% will have an FN exercise ECG. Exercise test sensitivity increases in patients with multivessel disease.

Specificity is the exact opposite of sensitivity since it focuses on healthy subjects who test negative for CVD. Specificity is the ability of the exercise ECG test to correctly exclude disease when it is absent. Another way of saying this is that specificity is equal to all those with truly negative tests divided by all those without disease. Specificity is quantified as follows:

$$Specificity = TN \div (TN + FP)$$

TN is the true negative (normal ECG exercise test and no CVD) and FP is the false positive (abnormal ECG exercise test and no CVD). Specificity of exercise testing averages about 77% in controlled studies. This means that 77% of those individuals without disease will have a TN exercise ECG and 23% will have an FP exercise ECG.

To understand the likelihood that any single individual patient has coronary heart disease requires the use of another statistic—predictive accuracy. Predictive accuracy is a measure of how accurately exercise testing identifies the presence or absence of coronary artery disease in patients. Therefore, predictive accuracy applies to both positive and negative tests in the following manner:

Positive tests: Predictive accuracy = $TP \div (TP + FP)$

Negative tests: Predictive accuracy = $TN \div (TN + FN)$

The strength of exercise testing to predict disease depends on the population being tested. If the likelihood of disease in patients is high based on the presence of CVD symptoms (i.e., typical angina), most of the positive tests will be true positives and not many will be false positives. The converse is also true. When CVD is not likely present, more of the positive tests will be false positives than true positives. Predictive accuracy falls in this case. Also of predictive value is the level of cardiovascular stress attained by the patient during testing. Unless the patient has attained 85% or more of predicted maximal HR during the test, a test should not be classified as negative. The reason for this is that ischemic responses do not appear unless the individual is stressed sufficiently. The 85% predicted maximal HR appears to be a reliable threshold to produce negative results if disease is present.

## HEALTH SCREENING AND RISK STRATIFICATION PRIOR TO EXERCISE TESTING

Prior to clinical exercise testing and prescription, an appraisal of the individual's health status should be conducted via a well-planned, comprehensive health risk appraisal. Health risk appraisal is an analysis of all that is known about a person's entire life situation, including personal and family medical history, occupation, and social environment, so that an estimate, compared with national averages, can be made of his or her risk of disability or death. Health status is usually assumed to be good in situations when exercise programming is designed for strength, power, and speed development for apparently healthy, younger individuals. Competitive and recreational athletes training for strength, power, and/or speed are not considered part of the "high risk" population. However, this assumption may change as weight training is gaining popularity among middle-aged to older individuals who may be part of the Senior Olympics movement.

Health risk appraisal is necessary when working with the general population, and it becomes critical when working with certain subsets of that population, such as obese individuals, the elderly, or chronically ill patients. At least three purposes of health screening for exercise testing and prescription have been identified:

1. To avoid exercising individuals with medical contraindications
2. To identify individuals who should be medically evaluated and undergo exercise testing prior to starting an exercise program
3. To identify individuals who should participate only in a medically supervised exercise program

Health care professionals should have established appraisal procedures for the population(s) with which they are working. A first step is to use a validated, self-administered questionnaire as a preparticipation screening tool to identify those adults who should not participate in physical activity programs or those who should seek medical advice prior to participation. For example, the Physical Activity Readiness Questionnaire (PAR-Q) was constructed for this purpose (*Fig 20.4*) (9). The PAR-Q has been found to have a sensitivity of 100% (it is able to detect all individuals with disease) and a specificity of 80% (only 20% of individuals without disease are excluded from exercise) for detecting medical conditions that would preclude participation in exercise. After the PAR-Q has been given, it is important to screen for CVD risk factors and signs and symptoms of chronic disease (see Chapter 18). Once these are determined, individuals can be stratified based on the likelihood of untoward events occurring during exercise. Stratification should be completed prior to participation in exercise testing and training.

Decisions regarding whether particular individuals need to have a current medical examination and be exercise tested prior to entering an exercise program are important. In addition, it is important for health care professionals to know the likelihood that an individual may experience an untoward event during exercise. For these reasons, individuals may be stratified for such a likelihood into one of three risk classifications advocated by the ACSM:

1. Low risk: Men <45 years old and women <55 years old who are asymptomatic and have a maximum of one risk factor for coronary artery disease
2. Moderate risk: Men ≥45 years old and women ≥55 years old or individuals who have two or more risk factors for coronary artery disease
3. High-risk individuals with signs and symptoms of cardiovascular and pulmonary disease or those who have been diagnosed with cardiovascular, pulmonary, or metabolic disease

The ACSM risk strata can be used to provide general guidelines on the need for a medical examination and exercise testing prior to participation in a moderate or vigorous exercise program and the need to have a physician supervise the exercise test (9). *Table 20.2* presents these guidelines from the ACSM.

Further classification consisting of four levels stratified by risk of complications during exercise is recommended by the American Heart Association for use with the cardiac population:

1. Class A: Apparently healthy; defined as individuals <age 40 with no CVD symptoms, major risk factors, or known disease, or individuals of any age with no known CVD disease or major risk factors and who have a normal exercise test; *no activity restrictions*
2. Class B: Documented stable CVD; not at increased risk during moderate physical activity; *risk during vigorous physical activity is low but present*
3. Class C: Documented stable CVD; *risk is present during exercise*
4. Class D: Documented unstable CVD; *physical activity is contraindicated, and ADL must be individually prescribed based on an assessment of each person*

Apparently healthy men (<45 years) and women (<55 years) do not necessarily need a diagnostic exercise test prior to participation in a moderate (40% to 60% $\dot{V}O_{2max}$) or even a vigorous (>60% $\dot{V}O_{2max}$) exercise program. Moreover, if these individuals are given an exercise test (maximal or submaximal), physician supervision is generally not necessary. Apparently healthy older men and women can also participate in moderate exercise programs without an exercise test, but vigorous exercise programs should not be attempted without an exercise test evaluation. If the exercise test requires maximal effort, a physician needs to supervise the test. Under these guidelines, exercise testing and prescription are safe for most of the apparently healthy population.

Clinicians weigh the risks of exercise testing versus the benefit to the patient before deciding to conduct a test. A general rule is that exercise tests should not be done on an emergent basis, that is, when the individual's condition is in flux. Before testing can be done, unstable conditions must be treated and corrected first. There are two ways to classify conditions that may preclude exercise testing: absolute contraindications and relative contraindications.

Absolute contraindications are unstable medical conditions needing stabilization before testing is performed. Thus, exercise testing is *absolutely contraindicated* until the conditions are stabilized. These conditions include the following:

- A recent significant change in the resting ECG suggesting significant ischemia, recent (within 2 days) MI, or other acute cardiac event
- Unstable angina

Physical Activity Readiness
Questionnaire - PAR-Q
(revised 2002)

# PAR-Q & YOU

**(A Questionnaire for People Aged 15 to 69)**

Regular physical activity is fun and healthy, and increasingly more people are starting to become more active every day. Being more active is very safe for most people. However, some people should check with their doctor before they start becoming much more physically active.

If you are planning to become much more physically active than you are now, start by answering the seven questions in the box below. If you are between the ages of 15 and 69, the PAR-Q will tell you if you should check with your doctor before you start. If you are over 69 years of age, and you are not used to being very active, check with your doctor.

Common sense is your best guide when you answer these questions. Please read the questions carefully and answer each one honestly: check YES or NO.

| YES | NO | |
|---|---|---|
| ☐ | ☐ | **1. Has your doctor ever said that you have a heart condition and that you should only do physical activity recommended by a doctor?** |
| ☐ | ☐ | **2. Do you feel pain in your chest when you do physical activity?** |
| ☐ | ☐ | **3. In the past month, have you had chest pain when you were not doing physical activity?** |
| ☐ | ☐ | **4. Do you lose your balance because of dizziness or do you ever lose consciousness?** |
| ☐ | ☐ | **5. Do you have a bone or joint problem (for example, back, knee or hip) that could be made worse by a change in your physical activity?** |
| ☐ | ☐ | **6. Is your doctor currently prescribing drugs (for example, water pills) for your blood pressure or heart condition?** |
| ☐ | ☐ | **7. Do you know of any other reason why you should not do physical activity?** |

**If you answered**

## YES to one or more questions

Talk with your doctor by phone or in person BEFORE you start becoming much more physically active or BEFORE you have a fitness appraisal. Tell your doctor about the PAR-Q and which questions you answered YES.

- You may be able to do any activity you want — as long as you start slowly and build up gradually. Or, you may need to restrict your activities to those which are safe for you. Talk with your doctor about the kinds of activities you wish to participate in and follow his/her advice.
- Find out which community programs are safe and helpful for you.

## NO to all questions

If you answered NO honestly to all PAR-Q questions, you can be reasonably sure that you can:

- start becoming much more physically active – begin slowly and build up gradually. This is the safest and easiest way to go.
- take part in a fitness appraisal – this is an excellent way to determine your basic fitness so that you can plan the best way for you to live actively. It is also highly recommended that you have your blood pressure evaluated. If your reading is over 144/94, talk with your doctor before you start becoming much more physically active.

**DELAY BECOMING MUCH MORE ACTIVE:**

- if you are not feeling well because of a temporary illness such as a cold or a fever – wait until you feel better; or
- if you are or may be pregnant – talk to your doctor before you start becoming more active.

**PLEASE NOTE:** If your health changes so that you then answer YES to any of the above questions, tell your fitness or health professional. Ask whether you should change your physical activity plan.

Informed Use of the PAR-Q: The Canadian Society for Exercise Physiology, Health Canada, and their agents assume no liability for persons who undertake physical activity, and if in doubt after completing this questionnaire, consult your doctor prior to physical activity.

**No changes permitted. You are encouraged to photocopy the PAR-Q but only if you use the entire form.**

NOTE: If the PAR-Q is being given to a person before he or she participates in a physical activity program or a fitness appraisal, this section may be used for legal or administrative purposes.

"I have read, understood and completed this questionnaire. Any questions I had were answered to my full satisfaction."

NAME ____________________

SIGNATURE ____________________ DATE ____________________

SIGNATURE OF PARENT
or GUARDIAN (for participants under the age of majority) ____________________ WITNESS ____________________

**Note: This physical activity clearance is valid for a maximum of 12 months from the date it is completed and becomes invalid if your condition changes so that you would answer YES to any of the seven questions.**

 Supported by: Health Canada Santé Canada

continued on other side...

...continued from other side

# PAR-Q & YOU

Physical Activity Readiness
Questionnaire - PAR-Q
(revised 2002)

Canada's Physical Activity Guide to Healthy Active Living

**Physical activity improves health.**

Every little bit counts, but more is even better – everyone can do it!

Get active your way – build physical activity into your daily life...

- at home
- at school
- at work
- at play
- on the way

...that's active living!

**Choose a variety of activities from these three groups:**

**Endurance**
4-7 days a week
Continuous activities for your heart, lungs and circulatory system.

**Flexibility**
4-7 days a week
Gentle reaching, bending and stretching activities to keep your muscles relaxed and joints mobile.

**Strength**
2-4 days a week
Activities against resistance to strengthen muscles and bones and improve posture.

Starting slowly is very safe for most people. Not sure? Consult your health professional.

For a copy of the *Guide Handbook* and more information: **1-888-334-9769**, or **www.paguide.com**

Eating well is also important. Follow *Canada's Food Guide to Healthy Eating* to make wise food choices.

## Get Active Your Way, Every Day–For Life!

Scientists say accumulate 60 minutes of physical activity every day to stay healthy or improve your health. As you progress to moderate activities you can cut down to 30 minutes, 4 days a week. Add-up your activities in periods of at least 10 minutes each. Start slowly... and build up.

**Time needed depends on effort**

| Very Light Effort | Light Effort *60 minutes* | Moderate Effort *30-60 minutes* | Vigorous Effort *20-30 minutes* | Maximum Effort |
|---|---|---|---|---|
| • Strolling<br>• Dusting | • Light walking<br>• Volleyball<br>• Easy gardening<br>• Stretching | • Brisk walking<br>• Biking<br>• Raking leaves<br>• Swimming<br>• Dancing<br>• Water aerobics | • Aerobics<br>• Jogging<br>• Hockey<br>• Basketball<br>• Fast swimming<br>• Fast dancing | • Sprinting<br>• Racing |

**Range needed to stay healthy**

**You Can Do It – Getting started is easier than you think**

Physical activity doesn t have to be very hard. Build physical activities into your daily routine.

- Walk whenever you can – get off the bus early, use the stairs instead of the elevator.
- Reduce inactivity for long periods, like watching TV.
- Get up from the couch and stretch and bend for a few minutes every hour.
- Play actively with your kids.
- Choose to walk, wheel or cycle for short trips.
- Start with a 10 minute walk – gradually increase the time.
- Find out about walking and cycling paths nearby and use them.
- Observe a physical activity class to see if you want to try it.
- Try one class to start – you don t have to make a long-term commitment.
- Do the activities you are doing now, more often.

| Benefits of regular activity: | Health risks of inactivity: |
|---|---|
| better health<br>improved fitness<br>better posture and balance<br>better self-esteem<br>weight control<br>stronger muscles and bones<br>feeling more energetic<br>relaxation and reduced stress<br>continued independent living in later life | premature death<br>heart disease<br>obesity<br>high blood pressure<br>adult-onset diabetes<br>osteoporosis<br>stroke<br>depression<br>colon cancer |

Health Canada Santé Canada — Canadian Society for Exercise Physiology

Source: Canada's Physical Activity Guide to Healthy Active Living, Health Canada, 1998 http://www.hc-sc.gc.ca/hppb/paguide/pdf/guideEng.pdf



**FITNESS AND HEALTH PROFESSIONALS MAY BE INTERESTED IN THE INFORMATION BELOW:**

The following companion forms are available for doctors' use by contacting the Canadian Society for Exercise Physiology (address below):

The **Physical Activity Readiness Medical Examination (PARmed-X)** – to be used by doctors with people who answer YES to one or more questions on the PAR-Q.

The **Physical Activity Readiness Medical Examination for Pregnancy (PARmed-X for Pregnancy)** – to be used by doctors with pregnant patients who wish to become more active.

References:
Arraix, G.A., Wigle, D.T., Mao, Y. (1992). Risk Assessment of Physical Activity and Physical Fitness in the Canada Health Survey Follow-Up Study. **J. Clin. Epidemiol.** 45:4 419-428.
Mottola, M., Wolfe, L.A. (1994). Active Living and Pregnancy, In: A. Quinney, L. Gauvin, T. Wall (eds.), **Toward Active Living: Proceedings of the International Conference on Physical Activity, Fitness and Health.** Champaign, IL: Human Kinetics.
PAR-Q Validation Report, British Columbia Ministry of Health, 1978.
Thomas, S., Reading, J., Shephard, R.J. (1992). Revision of the Physical Activity Readiness Questionnaire (PAR-Q). **Can. J. Spt. Sci.** 17:4 338-345.

For more information, please contact the:

Canadian Society for Exercise Physiology
202-185 Somerset Street West
Ottawa, ON K2P 0J2
Tel. 1-877-651-3755 • FAX (613) 234-3565
Online: www.csep.ca

The original PAR-Q was developed by the British Columbia Ministry of Health. It has been revised by an Expert Advisory Committee of the Canadian Society for Exercise Physiology chaired by Dr. N. Gledhill (2002).

Disponible en français sous le titre «Questionnaire sur l'aptitude à l'activité physique - Q-AAP (revisé 2002)».

 Supported by: Health Canada Santé Canada

FIGURE 20.4. The revised Physical Activity Readiness Questionnaire form. (Reprinted with permission from the Canadian Society for Exercise Physiology, Inc., 2002.)

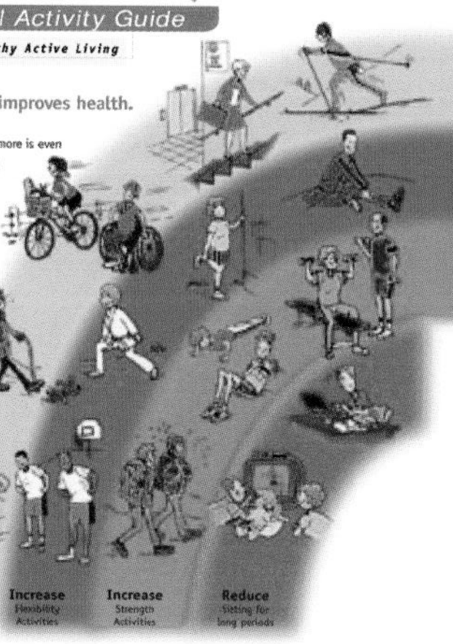

| Table 20.2 | *GENERAL GUIDELINES ACCORDING TO RISK STRATIFICATION, LEVEL OF EXERCISE INTENSITY, AND TYPE OF EXERCISE TEST FOR RECOMMENDING (A) CURRENT (WITHIN 1 YEAR) MEDICAL EXAMINATION AND EXERCISE TESTING AND (B) PHYSICIAN SUPERVISION OF EXERCISE TESTS* | | |
|---|---|---|---|
| | **Low Risk** | **Moderate Risk** | **High Risk** |
| **A** | | | |
| Moderate exercise | Not necessary | Not necessary | Recommended |
| Vigorous exercise | Not necessary | Recommended | Recommended |
| **B** | | | |
| Submaximal test | Not necessary | Not necessary | Recommended |
| Maximal test | Not necessary | Recommended | Recommended |

Moderate exercise for the purposes of these guidelines may be defined quantitatively as a relative exercise intensity of about 40% to 60% $\dot{V}O_{2max}$. Moderate exercise may also be defined qualitatively as an intensity well within the individual's capacity, noncompetitive, gradually initiated and progressed, and one which can be comfortably sustained for a prolonged period of time (~45 minutes). Vigorous exercise is defined as activities requiring >6 metabolic equivalents or >60% $\dot{V}O_{2max}$. (Adapted from Franklin BA, ed. *ACSM's guidelines for exercise testing and prescription*. 6th ed. Baltimore: Lippincott Williams & Wilkins, 2000.)

- Uncontrolled cardiac arrhythmias causing symptoms or hemodynamic compromise
- Severe symptomatic aortic stenosis
- Uncontrolled symptomatic heart failure
- Acute pulmonary embolus or pulmonary infarction
- Acute myocarditis or pericarditis
- Suspected or known dissecting aneurysm
- Acute infections

When benefits of exercise testing outweigh the risks of testing, relative contraindications can be superceded. This means that exercise testing is *contraindicated* unless the *relative* risk of testing is less than the benefit to be achieved from testing. These relative contraindications include the following conditions:

- Left main coronary stenosis
- Moderate stenotic valvular heart disease
- Electrolyte abnormalities (e.g., hypokalemia, hypomagnesemia)
- Severe arterial hypertension (i.e., systolic blood pressure >200 mm Hg and/or diastolic blood pressure >110 mm Hg) at rest
- Tachyarrhythmias or bradyarrhythmias
- Hypertrophic cardiomyopathy and other forms of outflow tract obstruction
- Neuromuscular, musculoskeletal, or rheumatoid disorders that are exacerbated by exercise
- High degree atrioventricular block
- Ventricular aneurysm
- Uncontrolled metabolic disease (e.g., diabetes, thyrotoxicosis, or myxedema)
- Chronic infectious disease (e.g., mononucleosis, hepatitis, AIDS)

▶ *INQUIRY SUMMARY.* Exercise testing may be used for diagnostic, prognostic, and functional assessments. Of particular interest for the therapist is the use of these tests to assess functional capacity. For proper diagnostic and prognostic values, test sensitivity and specificity must be as high as possible. Health screening and risk stratification are two pivotal activities in medical practice. *How do health screening and risk stratification relate to patient safety during testing?*

## Selecting the Graded Exercise Protocol

Choosing an appropriate exercise test involves matching the proper exercise mode and **exercise protocol** to the patient. Proper attention must be paid to the physical limitations of the patient and the reason for testing. Individuals must be able to perform the exercise mode chosen so that the cardiopulmonary system can be adequately stressed. In some instances, it may be appropriate to match exercise mode to the job task of the individual, which is especially important when testing for job-related fitness. Treadmill tests, versus other kinds of testing scenarios, are extremely popular because most individuals are more accustomed to walking than other exercise modes. However, patients may have orthopedic limitations that preclude one test versus another.

Mode selection is easy when obvious physical limitations are present. For example, when a patient has severe arthritis in both knees, leg exercise modes such as treadmill walking or cycle ergometer exercise are not warranted. Treadmill walking may also be precluded because of postural instability, neuromuscular disease, paraplegia, or stroke. In these cases, leg or arm ergometry may be a viable alternative. However, most individuals (especially chronic disease patients) are relatively unfamiliar with cycling exercise; therefore, cycling may be a second choice to be used only when absolutely necessary. The reason for this is that most individuals do not participate in cycling, and thus they may experience local muscular fatigue and have to end the test prior to a work rate being achieved that can adequately stress the cardiopulmonary system. The diagnostic value of the test in such instances is reduced. Similar problems are present when arm ergometry is selected as the test mode.

In some circumstances, it may also be necessary to select nontraditional exercise modes to evaluate the patient, as when assessing task-specific function and symptomatology (*Box 20.1*). In these instances, patients can carry heavy objects, climb stairs, or wear weighted belts. It is often within the therapist's professional discretion to devise such tests to properly assess patients' physiologic and symptomatic responses. *How would you devise a test if a patient informs you that he/she only gets chest pain when shoveling snow?* Movement tasks may be so unique and symptoms so task specific that therapists must use creativity in devising test procedures and conditions to adequately evaluate patients.

Various graded exercise protocols have been designed and successfully used during the past half century. These tests are either continuous or discontinuous, with the majority of tests using walking, running, or cycling as the mode of exercise. Generally there is a strong correlation between $\dot{V}O_{2max}$ values obtained from continuous and discontinuous tests when performed with the same mode of exercise, but the values obtained for cycling are approximately 10% lower than those for treadmill protocols.

Discontinuous loading (rest periods interspersed with exercise periods) is used when patients cannot tolerate continued exercise with increasing work intensities. A common example of this is arm ergometer testing. However, when patients can tolerate uninterrupted exercise, continuous loading is preferred. In continuous loading, stages last approximately 2 to 3 minutes each, which is usually enough time for the cardiovascular system to adjust to steady state with each exercise load (stage). Both types of protocols are graded in that each stage has a MET value (1 MET = 3.5 mL·kg$^{-1}$·min$^{-1}$ O$_2$ consumed) assigned to it based on the workload of the stage. That is, these tests begin at one level of exertion or metabolic intensity (i.e., MET level) and advance in different degrees of exertion over time from stage to stage. If the protocol has large increases in intensity between stages, each stage should be longer to allow the cardiovascular system time to adjust to the new workload. This allows a more precise determination of the cardiovascular responses to a given stage, and the exercise dose is more precisely matched to a physiologic response. This is very important to achieve in clinical testing when functional capacity needs to be determined and exercise prescriptions are written.

Another type of continuous protocol is ramp loading. Here the protocol progresses more rapidly because each stage is shorter in duration (typically 1 minute). Work intensity on the treadmill or cycle ergometer is changed every minute. For instance, treadmill speed may be held constant with gradual changes in grade (1% to 3%) every minute, whereas on the cycle ergometer, power output may change by 5 to 25 watts every minute. The jumps in workload are small which is tolerated well by patients, but there is no allowance for the attainment of physiologic steady state with each stage because stage duration is too short. However, since physiologic steady state is not achieved, it is harder to define the individual's functional aerobic capacity in terms of workload achieved. Continu-

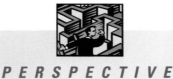

*PERSPECTIVE*

**Box 20.1**

# *Nontraditional Exercise Tests*

Exercise testing using modes of activity designed to recreate patterns of activity occurring in patients' daily lives is often useful and necessary. These kinds of exercise tests are referred to as task-specific tests, and they are useful to verify work capacity for job-related functions and to evaluate symptoms that occur only with specific types of exercise. Jobs that require individuals to carry heavy tools and boxes, get in and out of different body positions repeatedly, climb stairs, or walk through viscous material such as water or mud can be simulated in the lab or the test can be field based. Carrying objects while walking on a treadmill has been an alternative and useful mode of testing for years.

Such testing is useful for evaluating reproducible exertional symptoms, which are specific to one type of exercise.

For example, individuals often complain of exertional symptoms when lifting objects (i.e., performing pressure-loaded exercise such as weightlifting). In addition, the activity pattern may not be reproducible in the laboratory and trying to reproduce the symptoms in field testing may be impractical. In such situations, monitoring of the actual activity performed in the daily life of the patient is preferable. This can be accomplished by means of devices such as a Holter monitor that is capable of capturing electrocardiographic evidence as symptoms are documented by the individual. Health care personnel should be cognizant of these alternative methods of testing to best understand patients' symptomology in relation to their specific exertional pattern.

ous ramp protocols are best used when $\dot{V}O_{2max}$ is being determined by direct measurement. Various graded exercise protocols are now briefly described below. All of these protocols may be used to directly (actual measurement) or indirectly (estimated measurement) determine $\dot{V}O_{2max}$.

## TREADMILL PROTOCOLS

The Bruce protocol is one of the most widely used of all the treadmill protocols (*Table 20.3*). With this protocol, treadmill speed and grade are changed every 3 minutes. The advantage of this protocol is that the test is relatively short. However, since the incremental increases in intensity are large (approximately 3 MET per stage), this protocol is not recommended for subjects with very low functional capacities. The beginning stage of the Bruce protocol is usually inappropriately difficult for most individuals with chronic disease; therefore, a modified version has been adopted. The modified Bruce protocol allows these individuals to "warm up" for stage 1 with two less intense workloads (stages). Even with this change in the protocol, the rapid advance in intensity may be too rigorous for most patients who may then fatigue early in the protocol, prior to the development of significant electrocardiographic changes or symptoms that may help in the diagnosis of heart disease. Other protocols have been developed to help overcome these problems.

The Balke protocol uses a constant walking speed with increasing intensity as the grade is elevated by 2.5% every 2 minutes. This format results in a constant increase in $\dot{V}O_2$ of about 1 MET per increment (*Table 20.4*). The modified Balke protocol is very popular in clinical settings, where

| Table 20.4 | BALKE PROTOCOL FOR TREADMILL GRADED EXERCISE TESTING | | | |
|---|---|---|---|---|
| Stage | Speed (mi·hr$^{-1}$) | Grade (%) | Duration (minutes) | MET |
| 1 | 3.0 | 2.5 | 2 | 4.3 |
| 2 | 3.0 | 5.0 | 2 | 5.4 |
| 3 | 3.0 | 7.5 | 2 | 6.4 |
| 4 | 3.0 | 10.0 | 2 | 7.4 |
| 5 | 3.0 | 12.5 | 2 | 8.5 |
| 6 | 3.0 | 15.0 | 2 | 9.5 |
| 7 | 3.0 | 17.5 | 2 | 10.5 |
| 8 | 3.0 | 20.0 | 2 | 11.6 |
| 9 | 3.0 | 22.5 | 2 | 12.6 |

MET, metabolic equivalents.

patients with low functional capacities are tested, because MET values in the initial stages of the test are very low (*Table 20.5*). For example, a 12-minute maximal test on the modified Balke protocol requires a functional capacity of 6 MET. Contrast this with the Bruce protocol, which requires 7 MET by stage 2. Clearly the Balke protocol is a superior testing tool for individuals with very low functional capacities. During the Balke protocol, treadmill speed is initially set at 2.0 mi·hr$^{-1}$ while grade increases by 3.5% at each stage for the first five stages. At this point, treadmill

| Table 20.3 | BRUCE PROTOCOL FOR TREADMILL GRADED EXERCISE TESTING* | | | |
|---|---|---|---|---|
| Stage | Speed (mi·hr$^{-1}$) | Grade (%) | Duration (minutes) | MET |
| 0 | 1.7 | 0 | 3 | 1.7 |
| 0.5 | 1.7 | 5 | 3 | 2.9 |
| 1 | 1.7 | 10 | 3 | 4.7 |
| 2 | 2.5 | 12 | 3 | 7.1 |
| 3 | 3.4 | 14 | 3 | 10.2 |
| 4 | 4.2 | 16 | 3 | 13.5 |
| 5 | 5.0 | 18 | 3 | 17.3 |
| 6 | 5.5 | 20 | 3 | 20.4 |
| 7 | 6.0 | 22 | 3 | 23.8 |

*Stages 0 and 0.5 represent additions (called the modified version) to the Bruce protocol, which actually begins at stage 1. MET, metabolic equivalents.

| Table 20.5 | MODIFIED BALKE PROTOCOL FOR TREADMILL GRADED EXERCISE TESTING | | | |
|---|---|---|---|---|
| Stage | Speed (mi·hr$^{-1}$) | Grade (%) | Duration (minutes) | MET |
| 1 | 2.0 | 0 | 3 | 2.5 |
| 2 | 2.0 | 3.5 | 3 | 3.5 |
| 3 | 2.0 | 7.0 | 3 | 4.5 |
| 4 | 2.0 | 10.5 | 3 | 5.4 |
| 5 | 2.0 | 14.0 | 3 | 6.4 |
| 6 | 2.0 | 17.5 | 3 | 7.4 |
| 7 | 3.0 | 12.5 | 3 | 8.5 |
| 8 | 3.0 | 15.0 | 3 | 9.5 |
| 9 | 3.0 | 17.5 | 3 | 10.5 |
| 10 | 3.0 | 20.0 | 3 | 11.6 |
| 11 | 3.0 | 22.5 | 3 | 12.6 |

MET, metabolic equivalents.

speed increases to 3.0 mi·hr$^{-1}$ and treadmill grade is reset to 12.5% and subsequently incremented by 3.5% at each stage. This protocol may be a bit cumbersome for the subject who is approaching $\dot{V}O_{2max}$, as both the speed and grade are being readjusted simultaneously.

A standardized treadmill ramp protocol, the Pepper protocol, was developed recently for older adults at the Duke University Claude D. Pepper Older Americans Independence Center/Center of Aging and Human Development. As shown in *Table 20.6*, this protocol uses small incremental increases in metabolic requirements that range from 0.2 to 0.9 (at later stages) MET as the test progresses. The test was designed so that maximal effort is reached in about 8 to 12 minutes. The assigned MET values derived from the ACSM treadmill walking equation are approximate values as the Pepper protocol does not allow the attainment of steady state with each stage.

| Table 20.7 | TREADMILL PROTOCOL FOR MAXIMAL GRADED EXERCISE TESTING OF HIGHLY FIT INDIVIDUALS | | |
|---|---|---|---|

| Stage | Grade (%) | MET | | |
| | | 6.0 mi·hr$^{-1}$ | 8.0 mi·hr$^{-1}$ | 10.0 mi·hr$^{-1}$ |
|---|---|---|---|---|
| 1 | 0 | 10.2 | 12.3 | 16.3 |
| 2 | 2.5 | 11.2 | 13.6 | 18.0 |
| 3 | 5.0 | 12.3 | 15.0 | 19.8 |
| 4 | 7.5 | 13.3 | 16.4 | 21.5 |
| 5 | 10.0 | 14.3 | 17.8 | 23.2 |
| 6 | 12.5 | 15.4 | 19.1 | 24.9 |
| 7 | 15.0 | 16.4 | 20.5 | 26.7 |

Each stage is 2 minutes in duration. MET, metabolic equivalents.

| Table 20.6 | PEPPER PROTOCOL FOR TREADMILL GRADED EXERCISE TESTING | | |
|---|---|---|---|

| Stage | Duration (minutes) | Speed (mi·hr$^{-1}$) | Grade (%) | MET |
|---|---|---|---|---|
| 1 | 0–1 | 1.5 | 0 | 2.1 |
| 2 | 1–2 | 1.5 | 2 | 2.6 |
| 3 | 2–3 | 1.5 | 4 | 3.0 |
| 4 | 3–4 | 2.0 | 3 | 3.4 |
| 5 | 4–5 | 2.0 | 5 | 3.9 |
| 6 | 5–6 | 2.0 | 6 | 4.2 |
| 7 | 6–7 | 2.0 | 7 | 4.5 |
| 8 | 7–8 | 2.0 | 8 | 4.7 |
| 9 | 8–9 | 2.0 | 9 | 5.0 |
| 10 | 9–10 | 2.5 | 8 | 5.7 |
| 11 | 10–11 | 2.5 | 10 | 6.4 |
| 12 | 11–12 | 2.5 | 12 | 7.0 |
| 13 | 12–13 | 2.5 | 14 | 7.7 |
| 14 | 13–14 | 3.0 | 12 | 8.3 |
| 15 | 14–15 | 3.0 | 13 | 8.7 |
| 16 | 15–16 | 3.0 | 14 | 9.1 |
| 17 | 16–17 | 3.3 | 14 | 9.9 |
| 18 | 17–18 | 3.3 | 16 | 10.8 |
| 19 | 18–19 | 3.3 | 18 | 11.7 |
| 20 | 19–20 | 3.3 | 20 | 12.6 |

MET, metabolic equivalents.

None of the protocols thus far described is suited for testing fit individuals or highly trained athletes. If these persons were to be tested with the previously mentioned protocols, test length would become unreasonable and treadmill grade unmanageable. A better approach is a continuous running test, such as the following, for highly trained individuals:

After a 10-minute warmup at 3.5 mi·hr$^{-1}$ and 0% grade, the subject begins running at 6.0, 8.0, or 10.0 mi·hr$^{-1}$ at 0% grade. Grade is then incremented by 2.5% every 2 minutes until the subject terminates the test due to exhaustion.

$\dot{V}O_{2max}$ values from this test protocol correlate well with those obtained with a multisession discontinuous grade protocol. *Table 20.7* shows the treadmill protocol used for highly trained individuals.

## LEG AND ARM ERGOMETER PROTOCOLS

Leg ergometer testing is a valuable alternative to treadmill testing, especially for patients who may have difficulty ambulating on a treadmill. The same general guidelines used for treadmill testing apply to leg ergometer testing. Power output for leg ergometers is expressed as kg·m·min$^{-1}$ or watts (1 watt = 6.12 kg·m·min$^{-1}$). Pedal rate is held constant at 50 to 60 rev·min$^{-1}$ for the low to average fit individual and 70 to 100 rev·min$^{-1}$ for the highly fit person. Leg ergometer protocols usually begin with a warmup phase, with little or no resistance, followed by work stages lasting 2 to 3 minutes that are incremented by 25 (individuals weighing <70 kg) to 50 (individuals weighing >70 kg) watts per stage (150 to 300 kg·m·min$^{-1}$). Since work output on a leg ergometer is not dependent on body mass, the relative $\dot{V}O_2$ for an individual can be calculated by dividing the $\dot{V}O_2$ by body mass (kg). This results in changing the $\dot{V}O_{2max}$ value to mL·kg$^{-1}$·min, which can be converted into MET by dividing by 3.5. The protocol should be adjusted so that the test will be over in approximately 8 to 10 minutes after a suitable warmup period of about 5 minutes.

Patients with disorders that will not allow treadmill or leg ergometer exercise may be evaluated with arm ergometer testing. Arm exercise results in $\dot{V}O_{2max}$ that is 30% to 40% lower than that determined by leg exercise. Arm exercise protocols may be continuous or discontinuous, but discontinuous formats seem to be tolerated the best. Work stages last 2 to 3 minutes and are incremented by 12.5 watts.

## FIELD AND SUBMAXIMAL EXERCISE TESTING

The actual measurement of $\dot{V}O_{2max}$ is time consuming and requires complicated laboratory procedures. The physical therapist, exercise physiologist, athletic trainer, or coach is often faced with the need to assess a person's aerobic fitness without sophisticated laboratory equipment. In some cases, the clinician may not want to expose older individuals and those at high risk to exhausting maximal workloads. In other cases, however, a field test may actually require that the individual give a maximal exertion (i.e., during a 12-minute run/walk, the subject will give a maximal effort for 12 minutes). Field tests are also useful for testing large numbers of people and when extreme accuracy is not required. For these reasons, simple submaximal exercise tests have been designed for estimating $\dot{V}O_{2max}$. The basis of these submaximal tests is an established relationship between HR and $\dot{V}O_2$ at similar rates of power output. Field tests are usually based on time or distance.

One of the most popular field tests for estimating $\dot{V}O_{2max}$ is Kenneth Cooper's 12-minute run test (Cooper Protocol). During this test, the subject is instructed to run/walk over as much distance as possible in 12 minutes. Fitness category and $\dot{V}O_{2max}$ are assigned according to distance traveled. The original 12-minute time used in this test can be altered based on the individual or group being tested. For example, a 6-minute test has been developed for patients or elderly adults with low aerobic capacities, with the hospital hall serving as the track during the test. These tests are often used to assess functional exercise capacity (6).

 **LINKUP: The 6-minute walk test has been used for many years to test the functional exercise capacity of individuals, such as those with chronic heart failure and chronic obstructive pulmonary disease.** Research Highlight: Reliability and Intensity of the 6-Minute Walk Test in Healthy Elderly Subjects, *found at http://connection.lww.com/go/brownexphys and on the Student Resource CD-ROM, discusses an investigation performed to test the reliability of this test in healthy elderly subjects.*

Other tests are also designed to score the time it takes to cover a specific distance. During the 1-mile walk test, sub-

jects are instructed to walk as fast as possible around a quarter-mile track for a total distance of 1 mile. HR is determined immediately upon termination of exercise. A regression equation for predicting $\dot{V}O_{2max}$ has been derived:

$$\dot{V}O_{2max}\ (L \cdot min^{-1}) = 6.9652 + (0.0091 \times Weight)$$
$$- (0.0257 \times Age) + (0.5955 \times Sex)$$
$$- (0.224 \times Time) - (0.0115 \times HR)$$

Weight = body weight in lb, age = years, sex = 0 for female and 1 for male, time = walking time expressed as minutes:hundredths, and HR = HR immediately post-exercise (7).

More recently a submaximal treadmill jogging test has been designed for estimating $\dot{V}O_{2max}$ in relatively fit individuals (8). The treadmill test requires subjects to sustain a comfortable submaximal jogging pace (4.3 to 6.5 $mi \cdot hr^{-1}$ for women and 7.5 $mi \cdot hr^{-1}$ for men; 0% grade) for at least 3 minutes until steady-state HR is achieved ($\leq 180$ beats per minute [bpm]). $\dot{V}O_{2max}$ is subsequently calculated from a prediction equation:

$$\dot{V}O_{2max}\ (mL \cdot kg^{-1} \cdot min^{-1}) = 54.07$$
$$+ (7.062 \times Sex) - (0.1938 \times Weight)$$
$$+ (4.47 \times Speed) - (0.1453 \times HR)$$

Sex = 0 for female and 1 for male, weight = body mass in kg, speed = treadmill speed in $mi \cdot hr^{-1}$, and HR = steady-state HR.

The 3-minute step test is one of the easiest field tests to administer for estimating $\dot{V}O_{2max}$. The premise behind this test is that submaximal steady state will be reached within 3 minutes and that fit individuals will have a lower exercise and recovery HR than unfit individuals. The test is performed on a 12-inch high bench with a stepping rate of 24 $st \cdot min^{-1}$. Immediately following 3 minutes of exercise, a pulse count is taken for 1 minute. The pulse count is subsequently used to determine a qualitative rating of fitness (*Table 20.8*), with lower scores being better. Data in this table are 1-minute pulse counts. For example, a count of 117 for a 37-year-old woman gives a fitness rating of average.

The most popular submaximal cycle ergometer test for estimating $\dot{V}O_{2max}$ is probably the Åstrand-Ryhming test. This test is different from other submaximal tests in that $\dot{V}O_{2max}$ is estimated from the HR response to a single submaximal workload lasting approximately 6 minutes. The subject begins by cycling with a pedal rate kept constant at 50 $rev \cdot min^{-1}$ at a workload selected according to gender and level of fitness (*Table 20.9*). HR is monitored during the last portion of the fifth and sixth minute. If the HR is between 125 and 170 bpm, with the fifth and sixth minute counts within 5 bpm of each other, the test is terminated and the average HR for the fifth and sixth minute is used to predict $\dot{V}O_{2max}$. If the difference between the two rates exceeds 5 bpm, the duration of the test is continued until a constant HR is attained for 2 consecutive minutes.

This HR and work rate are then used to obtain a $\dot{V}O_{2max}$ value with the Åstrand-Ryhming nomogram (*Fig. 20.5*).

| Table 20.8 | RATINGS FOR SCORES FROM THE 3-MINUTE STEP TEST | | | | | |
|---|---|---|---|---|---|---|
| | Age | | | | | |
| Rating | 18–25 | 26–35 | 36–45 | 46–55 | 56–65 | >65 |
| **Excellent** | | | | | | |
| Men | ≤80 | ≤81 | ≤84 | ≤86 | ≤85 | ≤87 |
| Women | ≤85 | ≤88 | ≤90 | ≤94 | ≤94 | ≤89 |
| **Good** | | | | | | |
| Men | 81–89 | 82–89 | 85–96 | 87–97 | 86–97 | 88–96 |
| Women | 86–98 | 89–100 | 91–102 | 95–103 | 95–104 | 90–101 |
| **Above average** | | | | | | |
| Men | 90–99 | 90–99 | 97–103 | 98–106 | 98–103 | 97–102 |
| Women | 99–108 | 101–110 | 103–109 | 104–114 | 105–111 | 102–115 |
| **Average** | | | | | | |
| Men | 100–105 | 100–107 | 104–111 | 107–116 | 104–112 | 103–113 |
| Women | 109–117 | 111–119 | 110–118 | 115–120 | 112–118 | 116–122 |
| **Below average** | | | | | | |
| Men | 106–116 | 108–117 | 112–119 | 117–122 | 113–120 | 114–120 |
| Women | 118–126 | 120–128 | 119–128 | 121–126 | 119–128 | 123–128 |
| **Poor** | | | | | | |
| Men | 117–128 | 118–128 | 120–130 | 123–132 | 121–129 | 121–130 |
| Women | 127–139 | 129–138 | 129–140 | 127–135 | 129–138 | 129–134 |
| **Very poor** | | | | | | |
| Men | ≥129 | ≥129 | ≥131 | ≥133 | ≥130 | ≥131 |
| Women | ≥140 | ≥139 | ≥141 | ≥136 | ≥139 | ≥135 |

For example, an unconditioned 40-year-old male starts cycling at 600 kg·m·min$^{-1}$ (100 watts). HR during the fifth minute is 135 bpm and the sixth minute is 144. The test is extended another minute and the HR recorded is 146 bpm. Average HR for the test then becomes 145, which is the average of the last 2 minutes of the test when steady state was attained. $\dot{V}O_{2max}$ is estimated with the nomogram at about 2.45 L·min$^{-1}$. Using *Table 20.10*, the correction factor for a 40-year-old male is 0.83. The corrected $\dot{V}O_{2max}$ value becomes 2.034 L·min$^{-1}$ (0.83 × 2.450). *Why do you think these correction factors decrease with increasing age?*

▶ *INQUIRY SUMMARY.* Selecting the appropriate exercise protocol for a particular individual is an important early task

| Table 20.9 | GUIDELINES FOR THE ÅSTRAND-RYHMING CYCLE ERGOMETER TEST |
|---|---|
| **Suggested power output: kg·m·min$^{-1}$ (watts)** | |
| Unconditioned males | 300 (50) or 600 (100) |
| Conditioned males | 600 (100) or 900 (150) |
| Unconditioned females | 300 (50) or 450 (75) |
| Conditioned females | 450 (75) or 600 (100) |

in clinical exercise testing. There are many different types of exercise protocols; however, when any of these do not meet the needs for testing, therapists may devise their own exercise protocol. *What do you think are the necessary conditions that would cause a therapist to devise a new exercise testing protocol for a patient rather than use an existing one?*

## Exercise Electrocardiography

Information collected from the ECG is arguably the most fundamental of all response variables measured during exercise testing. Whether the exercise test is ultimately judged positive or negative is determined largely by analysis of ECG waveforms (*Fig. 20.6*). With the ECG, the clinician is able to determine if the myocardium is becoming ischemic during and after exercise. The exercise ECG is also used to analyze rhythm disturbances elicited during testing and other problems such as conduction disturbances. Given this importance, allied health personnel involved in exercise testing and training must be competent interpreters of the resting and exercise ECG.

### THE 12-LEAD ELECTROCARDIOGRAM

The ECG is a graphical representation of cardiac electrical signals gathered at the chest surface by **electrodes** attached

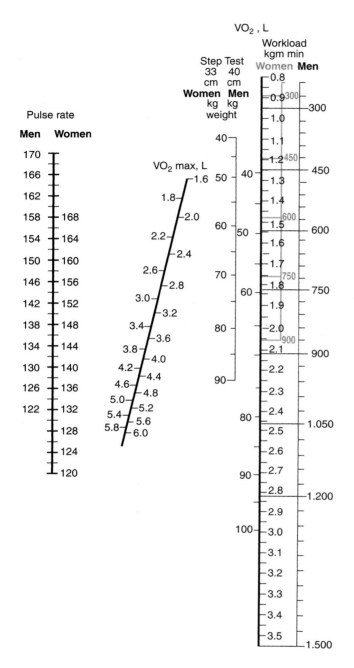

Males: $\dot{V}O_2$max (mL/kg/min) =
111.33 − [0.42 × recovery HR (beats/min)]

**FIGURE 20.5.** Åstrand-Ryhming nomogram showing two examples of how to extrapolate $\dot{V}O_{2max}$ from steady-state pulse rate and work rate. (From Åstrand P-O, Ryhming I. A nomogram for calculation of aerobic capacity (physical fitness) from pulse rate during submaximal work. *J Appl Physiol* 1954;7:218–221.)

| Table 20.10 | AGE CORRECTION FACTOR FOR PREDICTED $\dot{V}O_{2max}$ VALUES FROM THE ÅSTRAND-RYHMING CYCLE ERGOMETER TEST | | |
|---|---|---|---|
| **Age** | **Factor** | **Age** | **Factor** |
| 15 | 1.10 | 45 | 0.78 |
| 20 | 1.05 | 50 | 0.75 |
| 25 | 1.00 | 55 | 0.71 |
| 30 | 0.92 | 60 | 0.68 |
| 35 | 0.87 | 65 | 0.65 |
| 40 | 0.83 | 70 | 0.62 |

ercise or during pathologic disturbances). The ECG is an electrical snapshot or picture of the heart. However, as any single photographic representation of an individual's features can give us a distorted picture of the person's overall appearance, a full representation of the electrical "photograph" of the heart can only be obtained by taking multiple ECGs from many different perspectives. One view is not enough. By convention, current standard practice is to record a 12-lead ECG. This is equivalent to 12 electrical "photos" of the heart, which let us "see" the heart from an electrical standpoint more clearly.

The ability to detect coronary artery disease increases with the number of ECG leads used. As originally developed, ECG electrodes were placed on the extremities at the wrists and ankles. However, this scheme of electrode placement for exercise studies has given way to the Mason-Likar placement configuration, in which the electrodes are moved up to the torso (*Fig. 20.7*). *What do you think was the reason for moving the electrodes to the torso?* The 10 electrodes are configured by the electrocardiograph into the 12-lead system. In this system, several of the electrodes are used more than once to produce the 12 leads. For example, as shown below, leads I and II both use the right arm (RA) electrode.

### The Limb Leads

The recorded leads represent the differences in voltage (i.e., potential) between two electrodes placed on the surface of the body or between a single electrode and a zero potential inside the electrocardiograph. *Figure 20.8* shows an example of the 12 leads recorded as a complete ECG. These leads are divided into two groups: six extremity (limb) leads shown in the two columns to the left (leads I, II, III and leads $aV_R$, $aV_L$, $aV_F$) and six precordial (chest) leads shown in the two columns to the right ($V_{1-6}$). The limb leads can be further divided into two groups, bipolar leads (I, II, III) and unipolar leads ($aV_R$, $aV_L$, $aV_F$). These 12 leads view the same cardiac event (the P-QRS-T cycle) from different angles or perspectives, thus giving the clinician a more complete picture of how the heart is working electrically.

to **ECG leads** and inscribed on recording paper by the **electrocardiograph**. These electrical signals are the depolarization and repolarization events produced by the heart and occurring in cyclic fashion approximately 60 to 100 times per minute at rest (or whatever the HR is during ex-

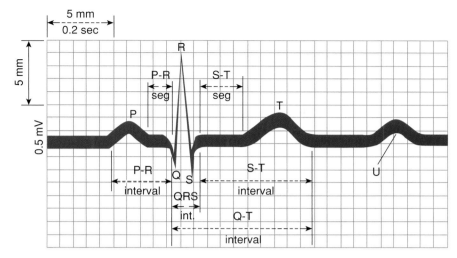

**FIGURE 20.6.** A typical electrocardiogram (ECG) tracing on standard graph paper showing all the waves, complexes, and intervals. The graph paper is divided into 1-mm squares and the speed of the paper output from the machine is such that 5 mm advance each 0.2 seconds. The basic ECG is in three phases: atrial depolarization (P wave), ventricular depolarization (QRS complex), and ventricular repolarization (T wave). Segment refers to a length on the isoelectric line and interval refers to and includes major events (P, QRS, or T) of the cardiac electrical cycle on the ECG. (Reprinted with permission from Pillitteri A. *Maternal and child health nursing: care of the childbearing and childrearing family.* 4th ed. Philadelphia: Lippincott Williams & Wilkins, 2002.)

The electrocardiograph always records the six limb leads first. The voltages produced by the heart travel through the torso where they are detected by the various electrodes. *How does the electrocardiograph turn these voltages into the common ECG configurations recorded on paper?* Remember that the leads basically show the difference in voltage between electrodes placed on the body or between

a single electrode and a zero potential in the electrocardiograph. These voltage differences change with each lead being viewed. Therefore, each ECG from the different leads will appear in a slightly different shape (morphology) while keeping the same basic appearance. Let's look more closely at how this works.

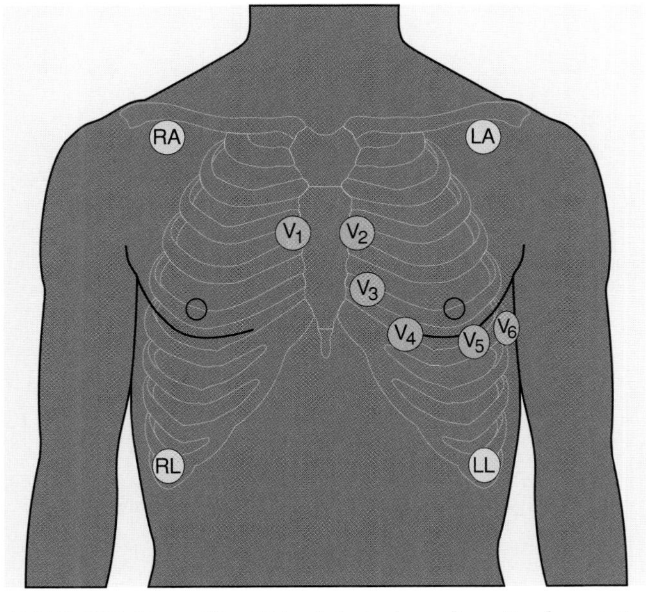

The bipolar leads are so named because they record electrical voltage differences between two extremities (electrodes) in the following manner. Refer to Figure 20.7 for acronym labels:

$$\text{Lead I} = \text{LA} - \text{RA}$$

$$\text{Lead II} = \text{LL} - \text{RA}$$

$$\text{Lead III} = \text{LL} - \text{LA}$$

These voltage subtractions are performed by the electrocardiograph to produce the ECGs from the three bipolar leads shown in Figure 20.8. The three bipolar leads are related according to the Einthoven equation:

$$\text{Lead I} + \text{Lead III} = \text{Lead II}$$

The Einthoven equation shows that the voltage of the R wave in lead II is equal to the voltages of the R waves in leads I and III combined. These three leads and their representative electrodes are presented schematically in *Figure 20.9*, which shows the spatial arrangement of the three bipolar leads, known as the Einthoven triangle. This arrangement is named after Willem Einthoven, the Dutch physician who invented the electrocardiograph about 100 years ago. Modern electrocardiographic practice has kept Einthoven's convention. Notice in the Einthoven triangle that the positive and negative signs relate to the electrodes

**FIGURE 20.7.** Mason-Likar 12-lead electrode configuration for exercise testing showing the proper electrode placements on the chest and abdomen. These are then connected to the subject (patient) with electrocardiogram leads. RA, right arm; LA, left arm; RL, right leg; LL, left leg; V, voltage.

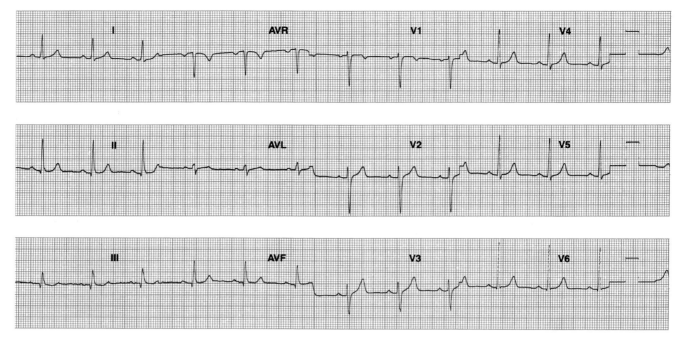

**FIGURE 20.8.** Sample electrocardiogram showing the 12 standard leads. (Reprinted with permission from Davis D. *Quick and accurate 12-lead ECG interpretation*. 4th ed. Philadelphia: Lippincott Williams & Wilkins, 2004.)

placed at the RA, LA, and LL positions. In electrocardiography, the electrocardiograph alternately makes the different electrodes either positive or negative depending on which lead is being recorded. In the bipolar system invented by Einthoven, the RA electrode is always negative and the LL electrode is always positive, while the LA elec-

trode is positive when recording lead I and negative when recording lead III. Notice that the RL electrode serves as an electrical ground only and is not designated either positive or negative. Figure 20.9B shows how the Einthoven triangle can be redrawn so that the leads intersect, resulting in a triaxial array.

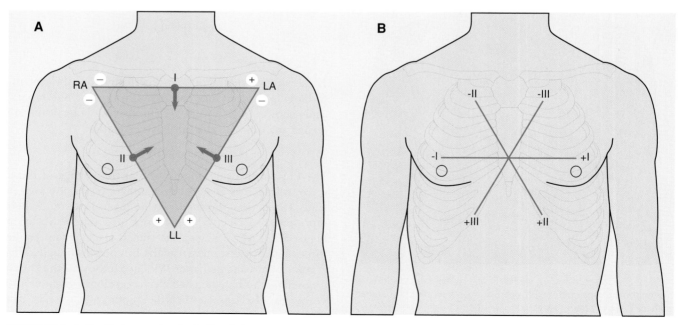

**FIGURE 20.9. A.** The Einthoven triangle. **B.** The Einthoven triangle converted to a triaxial array.

*LINKUP:* **A brief biography of Willem Einthoven can be accessed at http://connection.lww.com/go/brownex phys and on the Student Resource CD-ROM.**

In the 1930s and 1940s nine more ECG leads were added to complete the current complement of 12 leads. These unipolar leads include three unipolar extremity leads and six unipolar chest leads. The unipolar nature of these leads refers to the recording of electrical voltages at one location (the electrodes on the body are all assigned a positive charge) relative to a zero potential found inside the electrocardiograph. This configuration differs from the bipolar leads, which are reflective of a voltage difference between two surface electrodes. The lower case "a" in the three unipolar extremity leads stands for augmented because the voltages detected at each extremity have been increased 50% over their actual value to make the leads more readable

(the size of the waveform is increased) when they are recorded on paper. The augmented voltage leads also have a spatial orientation similar to that of the bipolar leads. These spatial relationships are drawn in *Figure 20.10*, which shows the triaxial diagrams of the bipolar leads (A), the unipolar extremity leads (B), and how these converge to form the hexaxial diagram (C). The three augmented voltage leads are related according to the following equation:

$$aV_R \ aV_L + aV_F = 0$$

That is, the sum of the QRS wave voltages (positive and negative deflections) of these leads equals zero.

The hexaxial diagram in Figure 20.10 shows that the six extremity leads have a specific *orientation* and *polarity*. Orientation refers to the direction in which the leads point—always toward their positive poles, demonstrating directionality. For example, leads II, III, and $aV_F$ point downward or

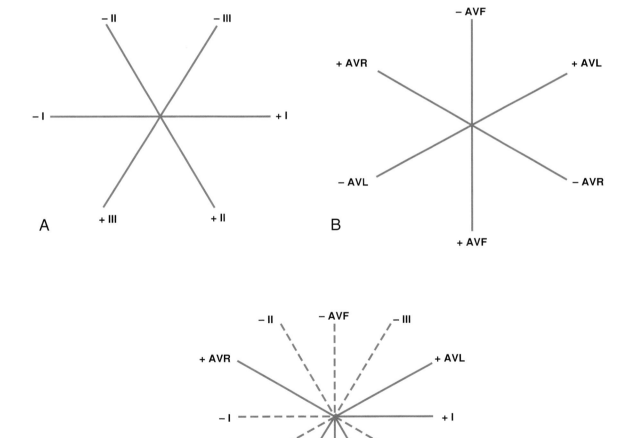

**FIGURE 20.10. A.** Triaxial array of the bipolar leads. **B.** Triaxial array of the unipolar leads. **C.** The two diagrams are combined into a hexaxial array showing the relationship of all six extremity leads. The negative pole of each lead is indicated by a dashed line. (Reprinted with permission from Davis D. *Quick and accurate 12-lead ECG interpretation*. 4th ed. Philadelphia: Lippincott Williams & Wilkins, 2004.)

inferiorly (notice that II and III have a diagonal orientation as well), Leads I and $aV_L$ point laterally to the left (notice that $aV_L$ also has a diagonal orientation), and lead $aV_R$ points laterally to the right with a diagonal orientation. Polarity refers to the placement position of the positive electrode on the body in the lead configuration. Orientation and polarity determine lead **vector**. A vector has both direction and magnitude, which gives the six extremity leads an angular designation (*Fig. 20.11*). Using the hexaxial lead array, it becomes possible to determine the average direction (*mean QRS axis*) that the ventricles are pointing electrically in the frontal plane of the body. Knowing the mean electrical axis of the ventricles helps in the diagnosis of a number of disorders (Case Study 20.2). Vector analysis of the QRS determines the average direction of the QRS complex or mean QRS electrical axis. This important information helps electrocardiographic diagnosticians determine the presence or absence of cardiac or pulmonary disease.

 *See Experiences in Work Physiology Lab Exercise 17: Vector Analysis of the Mean QRS Axis. This exercise explains a simple, three-step method for determining the mean of several vectors to establish the general direction in which the frontal plane the QRS complex is predominantly pointed.*

### The Chest Leads

The conventional placement of the six ECG chest electrodes is shown below (refer again to Fig. 20.7 for an illustration of the placement of these electrodes):

- V1: Fourth intercostal space just to the right of the sternum

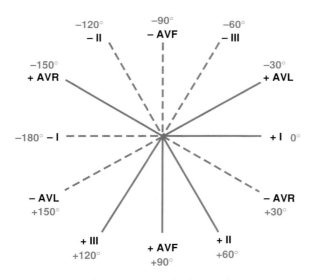

**FIGURE 20.11.** The hexaxial array with the angular designations. All leads above lead I have negative angular values, and the leads below it have positive values. (Reprinted with permission from Davis D. *Quick and accurate 12-lead ECG interpretation*. 4th ed. Philadelphia: Lippincott Williams & Wilkins, 2004.)

- V2: Fourth intercostal space just to the left of the sternum
- V3: On a line midway between leads V2 and V4
- V4: On the midclavicular line in the fifth interspace
- V5: On the anterior axillary line at the same level as V4
- V6: On the midaxillary line at the same level as lead V4

With the chest leads, it is possible to discern the ventricular depolarization process that occurs sequentially over two phases (*Fig. 20.12*). After a slight pause, the atrioventricular (AV) node releases the electrical signal down the bundle branches through the interventricular septum to the ventricles. The first phase of ventricular activation begins in the left to right depolarization of the interventricular septum. The vector of septal depolarization is depicted by the rightward pointing arrow in the figure. Using the three basic laws of electrocardiography, we can interpret the deflections produced following septal depolarization as a septal R wave in V1 and a septal Q wave in V6. The same electrical event has produced a different response in these two leads.

The second step in ventricular activation is shown in Figure 20.12 as a vector (arrow 2) for the left ventricular myocardial mass. Notice that this line is a heavier arrow. Remember that vectors represent both direction and magnitude. Since the left ventricle is a much larger muscle mass than the septal or right ventricular mass, the resulting voltages produced are larger deflections. Therefore, when the left ventricle is activated last in the ventricular activation sequence, there is a large S wave produced in V1 and a large R wave produced in V6. This pattern of activation is recorded across the precardium by the chest leads to produce progressively larger R waves and progressively smaller S waves. Normal R wave progression results in an R wave in V3 or V4 that is equal in amplitude to the S wave. The point at which the R:S ratio is 1 (equal R and S amplitudes) is called the normal transition zone (*Fig. 20.13*). Early transition (electrical counterclockwise rotation) occurs in lead V2 and late transition (electrical clockwise rotation) occurs in V5. Analysis of R wave progression across the precardium aids the diagnosis of medical abnormalities. For example, abnormal R wave progression helps physicians diagnose anterior wall MI, a condition that results in a loss of normal R wave progression. Diagnosis of left or right ventricular hypertrophy is also aided by interpreting R wave progression across the precardium.

### Three Laws of Electrocardiography

There are three basic laws of electrocardiography that determine why the various ECGs produced by the 12 leads are shaped differently. The three laws are depicted graphically in *Figure 20.14*.

1. A downward or negative deflection appears in any lead when the wave of depolarization spreads toward the negative pole of that lead (i.e., away from the positive pole; Fig. 20.14A)
2. A biphasic deflection appears in any lead when the wave of depolarization spreads at right angles (perpendicular) to that lead (Fig. 20.14B)

## CASE STUDY 20.2: *MITRAL VALVE STENOSIS*

### CASE

Mary, age 55, has been complaining of fatigue during the infrequent times she engages in physical activity and was subsequently given a maximal exercise test and resting echocardiogram (ECG). The exercise test revealed an extremely low functional aerobic capacity ($\dot{V}O_{2max}$ = 19 mL·kg$^{-1}$·min$^{-1}$) but was negative for ischemic heart disease (no ST segment depression). Her ECG revealed mitral valve stenosis.

### DESCRIPTION

The ECG below also reveals right ventricular hypertrophy (i.e., relatively tall R waves in lead $V_1$ with right axis deviation). *How might mitral valve stenosis be related to right axis deviation?* The answer lies in the central hemodynamic effect of the stenotic mitral valve. When the left atrium cannot fully empty its contents into the left ventricle with each beat, a back pressure builds into the left atrium and eventually into the pulmonary circuit. The higher pulmonary circuit pressure causes the right ventricle to pump against a chronically elevated pressure, and right ventricular compensatory hypertrophy ensues. The mean electrical axis then gradually shifts to the right, accounting for the greater right ventricular muscle mass.

After studying Experiences in Work Physiology Lab Exercise 20, determine the mean electrical axis of the ECG below.

### INTERVENTION

A stenotic mitral valve impedes left ventricular outflow, thus reducing cardiac output and exercise performance. It was decided in this case not to correct the condition surgically and to manage the patient medically. Mary was placed on antibiotic prophylaxis and anticoagulation medication and was told to engage in no severe exercise or competitive sports. Mary was also given an exercise prescription of mild to moderate exercise to improve her functional aerobic capacity.

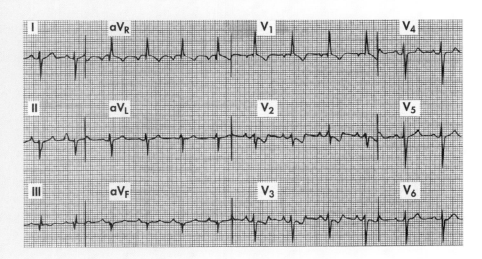

3. An upward or positive deflection by the recording pen of the electrocardiograph is produced in any lead when a wave of depolarization spreads toward the positive pole of that lead (Fig. 20.14C).

Because of these principles, a single cardiac electrical cycle will look different when viewed from the perspective of different leads. Notice in *Figure 20.14* the average current flow depicted by the vector (large arrow). ECGs A, B, and C, represented by their respective leads, are shaped the way they appear because of the three laws just mentioned. To check your understanding at this point, match each of the three laws with a specific ECG in Figure 20.14.

The six extremity (limb) leads record electrical voltages transmitted onto the frontal plane of the body. Figure 20.15 shows this by superimposing the hexaxial diagram onto the body of an individual. As we have seen, these frontal plane leads record heart voltages directed upward and downward and to the right and left. However, since the heart is a three-dimensional structure sending out its electrical currents in all directions and across many different planes, there is a need to have recording leads that capture voltages directed in other planes as well. This has been accomplished with the six chest or precordial leads which record voltages transmitted onto the horizontal plane (*Fig. 20.16*). These leads record heart voltages directed anteriorly (front) and posteriorly (back) and to the right and left in the horizontal plane. More leads could be used, and sometimes physicians alter the placement of one or two of the chest leads to examine the ECG from a slightly different horizontal perspective. However, these 12 leads are usually enough to

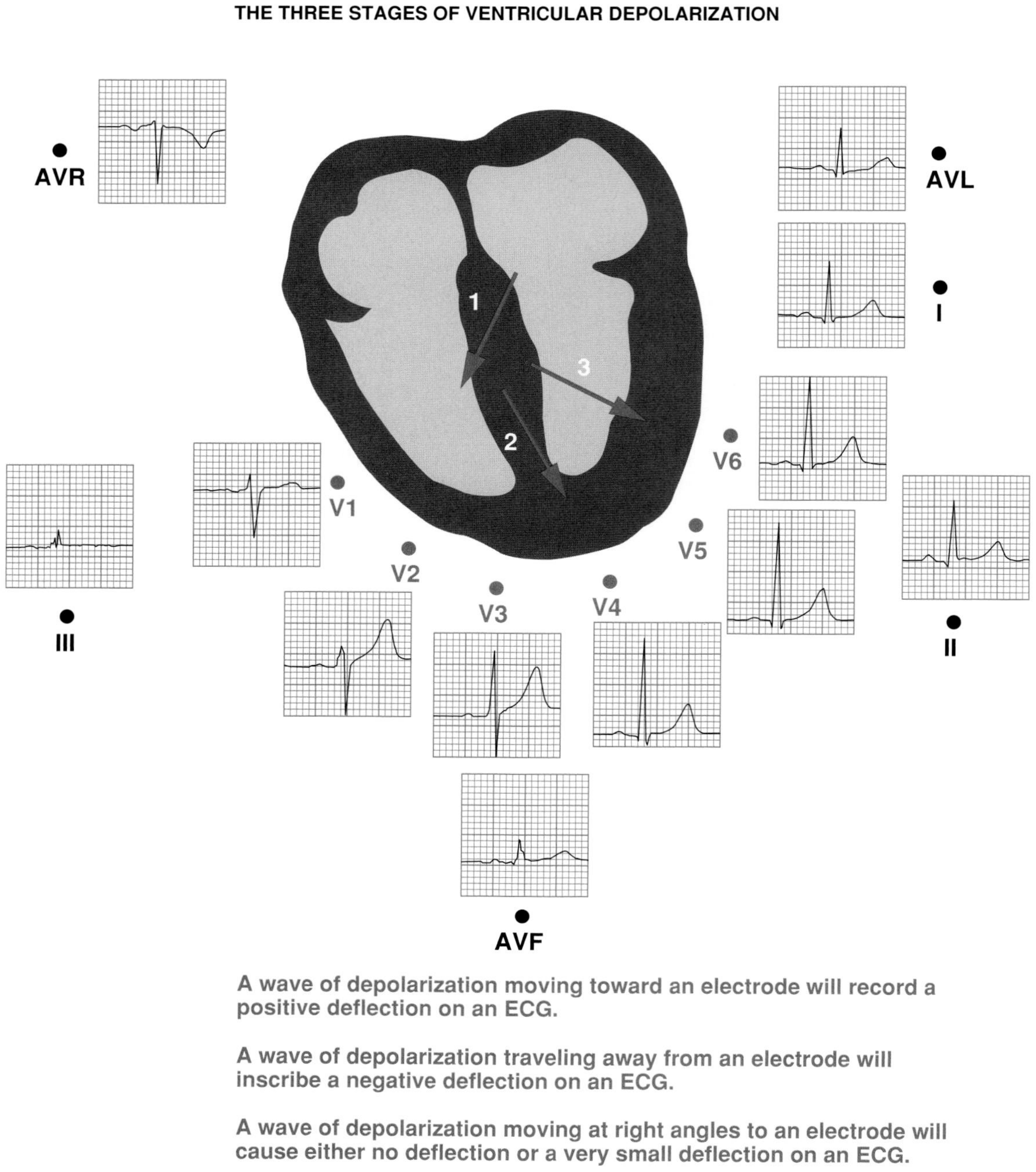

**THE THREE STAGES OF VENTRICULAR DEPOLARIZATION**

**A wave of depolarization moving toward an electrode will record a positive deflection on an ECG.**

**A wave of depolarization traveling away from an electrode will inscribe a negative deflection on an ECG.**

**A wave of depolarization moving at right angles to an electrode will cause either no deflection or a very small deflection on an ECG.**

**FIGURE 20.12.** The first phase of ventricular activation depolarizes the septum from left to right (*arrow 1*). The second phase depolarizes the main bulk of the ventricles. The arrow points to the left ventricle because it is electrically predominant. (Reprinted with permission from Davis D. *Quick and accurate 12-lead ECG interpretation*. 4th ed. Philadelphia: Lippincott Williams & Wilkins, 2004.)

provide a clear three-dimensional picture of atrial and ventricular depolarizations and repolarizations.

## RECOGNIZING ISCHEMIC RESPONSES

The main purpose of exercise electrocardiography is to detect the presence of ischemic heart disease. Exercise produces normal changes to the ECG, such as a minor shortening of the P-R and QRS durations and progressive shortening of the Q-T interval. Minor J point depression

may also occur. However, these changes do not occur because of myocardial ischemia. The main ischemic responses depicted on the ECG are ST-T changes, including ST depression, ST elevation, and T waves that are hyperacute, flattened, or inverted.

### Subendocardial Ischemia

ST segment changes are widely accepted criteria for myocardial ischemia and injury. Normally, the ST segment is

## PRECORDIAL LEAD CONFIGURATIONS

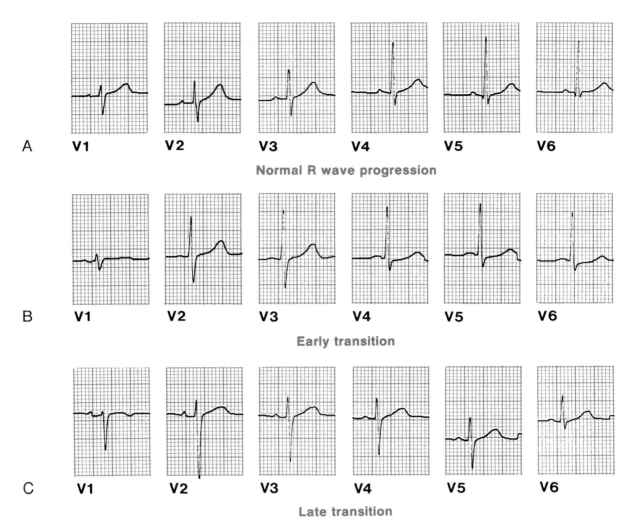

**FIGURE 20.13.** Three sets of chest lead electrocardiograms showing different patterns of R wave progression. **A.** Normal. **B.** Early transition. **C.** Late transition. (Reprinted with permission from Davis D. *Quick and accurate 12-lead ECG interpretation*. 4th ed. Philadelphia: Lippincott Williams & Wilkins, 2004.)

**isoelectric.** However, if the myocardium becomes ischemic, the ST segment may become significantly depressed, i.e., drop below the isoelectric line. The following criteria have been established for significant ST depression: J point 1 mm below isoelectric and the ST segment remaining depressed 80 ms after the J point. There are three types of ST depression: upsloping, horizontal, or downsloping; the clinical condition worsens with each respective type. Judging ST-T changes during exercise may be difficult due to movement artifact and the fact that some J point depression occurs normally. It is usually necessary to have a reasonably stable isoelectric line and observe the changes in three consecutive ECG complexes for sound clinical judgment. Also, in the discussion to follow, it will be important to clearly distinguish between myocardial ischemia and MI. Ischemia literally means to hold back blood, and this condition may be transient as in the case of patients who experience angina pectoris with exercise. Ischemia of this nature produces significant J point and ST segment depression. However, when ischemia becomes too severe, necrosis (death) of a portion of the heart muscle may occur. This, by definition, is MI, which produces ST elevation.

Of the three types of ST segment depression, an upsloping morphology is the least threatening. However, upsloping depression is of two types, rapid and slow. Of the two, a rapidly upsloping depression (>1 mV/s with <1.5-mm ST depression) is normal during exercise. However, a slowly upsloping depression (>1.5-mm ST depression maintained for 80 ms) of the ST segment beyond the J point is at least borderline and probably abnormal in individuals with a pretest likelihood of coronary artery disease. Horizontal depression with the criteria of at least 1-mm depression maintained for 80 ms beyond the J point is next in line of severity, followed by downsloping ST depression.

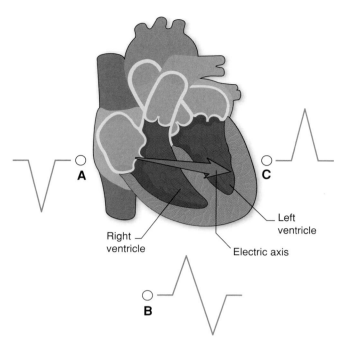

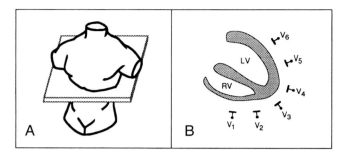

**FIGURE 20.16.** The horizontal plane of the body and the spatial relationships of the six chest leads. (Reprinted with permission from Lilly L. *Pathophysiology of heart disease: a collaborative project of medical students and faculty.* 3rd ed. Philadelphia: Lippincott Williams & Wilkins, 2002.)

**FIGURE 20.14.** The three basic laws of electrocardiography are demonstrated by the positioning of electrodes A, B, and C. The average ventricular vector of the typical heart is shown by the arrow. The direction is due to the larger mass of the left ventricle. The negative deflection in A is because the current flow is away from the electrode. The current flow is perpendicular to electrode B. The positive deflection in C is because the current flow is toward the electrode.

ST segment depression produces a different current of injury vector from that of ST segment elevation (*Fig. 20.17*). This factor relates to the area of the myocardium becoming ischemic. Notice in this figure that, when ischemia is isolated to the subendocardial area of the myocardium, the vector is away from the recording electrode (i.e., $V_5$) and ST depression occurs. However, when acute transmural ischemia occurs, the current of injury is towards $V_5$, resulting in ST elevation. Transmural ischemia is much worse clinically than is subendocardial ischemia. Transmural ischemia involving ST elevation is indicative of acute transmural MI (Q-wave infarct patterns), while subendocardial ischemia is indicative of acute subendocardial infarction (non-Q-wave infarct patterns) or angina pectoris.

### Transmural Ischemia

Transmural ischemia producing ST elevation can be localized via the various ECG lead orientations while subendocardial ischemia generally cannot be localized. For example, *Figure 20.18* shows an acute inferior wall transmural MI. The infarction can be localized to the inferior wall because the leads showing ST elevations (II, III, and $aV_F$) point inferiorly. Notice also that there is ST segment depression in several of the leads. For an acute transmural MI, this is referred to as *reciprocity*. When the transmural MI is located anteriorly and laterally, reciprocity occurs in the inferior leads, and when the MI is located inferiorly, reciprocity occurs anteriorly and laterally. Reciprocal changes do not have to be extensive, i.e., reciprocity need only involve one or two of the leads just mentioned.

One characteristic of transmural MIs is their evolving nature. Within minutes of the onset of infarction, the classic current of injury appears on the ECG manifesting as ST elevations and reciprocal depressions. Tall peaked T waves may also be present. After hours to days the ST elevations start to return to normal (isoelectric line), T waves become inverted in the leads showing ST elevations, and finally new Q waves appear after 1 or more days following the infarction. The Q waves are in the leads that showed ST elevations and are a result of the necrotic myocardium's

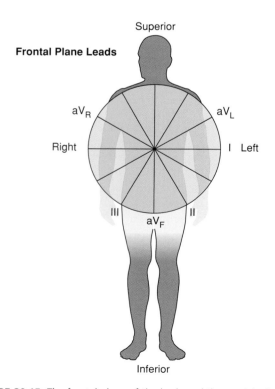

**FIGURE 20.15.** The frontal plane of the body and the spatial relationships of the six extremity leads in the hexaxial array.

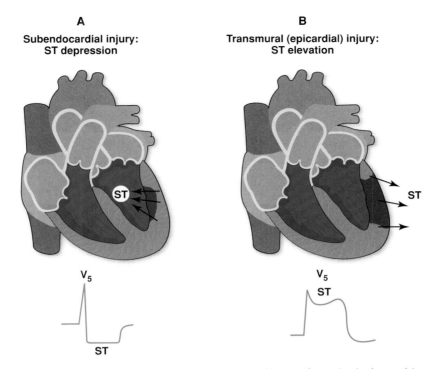

**A**
**Subendocardial injury:**
**ST depression**

**B**
**Transmural (epicardial) injury:**
**ST elevation**

FIGURE 20.17. **A.** Acute subendocardial ischemia produces ST depression in the overlying lead. **B.** Acute transmural ischemia produces ST elevation in the overlying lead.

**INFERIOR INFARCTION**

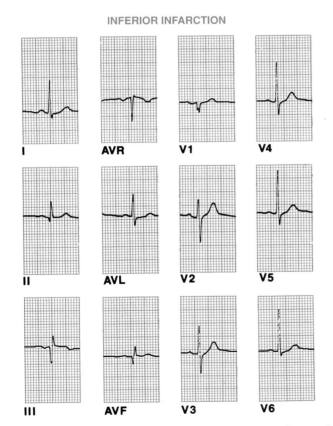

FIGURE 20.18. Extremity leads showing acute transmural inferior wall myocardial infarction. Notice the ST elevation. (Reprinted with permission from Davis D. *Quick and accurate 12-lead ECG interpretation.* 4th ed. Philadelphia: Lippincott Williams & Wilkins, 2004.)

inability to conduct electricity. The new Q wave becomes a permanent marker of an old transmural MI in a localized area of the heart. These local areas may be narrowly defined as follows:

- Anteroseptal: QS complex in $V_1$ and $V_2$; left anterior descending coronary artery or one of its branches is implicated
- Strictly anterior: QS or QR complex in $V_3$ and $V_4$; left anterior descending coronary artery is implicated
- Anterolateral or anteroapical: QS or QR complex in $V_5$ and $V_6$; left circumflex coronary artery is implicated
- Extensive anterior: QS or QR complex in leads $V_1$ to $V_5$ or $V_6$; multiple coronary arteries are implicated
- Inferior wall: QR complex in leads II, III, and $aV_F$; right coronary artery is implicated
- Posterior wall: Tall R waves and ST depressions in leads $V_1$ and $V_2$

Given the preceding discussion, the diverse ECG changes produced by ischemic heart disease can be depicted in the scheme presented in *Figure 20.19.* As can be seen, there are noninfarctional and infarctional ischemic patterns each characterized by particular ST-T morphology.

## RECOGNIZING ARRHYTHMIAS

Cardiac arrhythmias are of two general types. Supraventricular arrhythmias originate above the ventricles, and ventricular arrhythmias originate in the ventricles. For each of the following cardiac rhythms, an ECG recording is

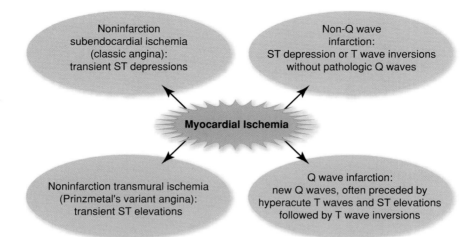

**FIGURE 20.19.** Summary of the diverse electrocardiogram changes seen with ischemic heart disease.

provided with a description of the features of each rhythm. Rhythms arising above the ventricles and from the sinus node are included first.

## Normal Sinus Rhythm

The normal cardiac rhythm is called normal sinus rhythm because it begins with an impulse from the sinoatrial (SA) node and conducts through normal pathways to the AV node. Normal sinus rhythm has the following characteristics (*Fig. 20.20*):

- P waves are negative in lead aVR and positive in lead II
- Rate is between 60 and 100 bpm

## Sinus Bradycardia

Sinus bradycardia is a sinus rhythm with an HR of less than 60 bpm (*Fig. 20.21*). If sinus bradycardia is moderate, no symptoms are apparent, but very slow rates may produce symptoms such as lightheadedness and syncope. Sinus bradycardia may occur with the following conditions:

- Normal variant such as in individuals who exercise train

- Drugs that increase vagal tone (digitalis) or decrease sympathetic tone (beta blockers)
- Hypothyroidism
- Hyperkalemia
- Sick sinus syndrome
- Sleep apnea syndrome

## Sinus Tachycardia

Sinus tachycardia is a sinus rhythm with an HR of more than 100 bpm, usually between 100 and 180 bpm (*Fig. 20.22*). The following conditions are commonly associated with sinus tachycardia:

- Fever
- Congestive heart failure
- Anxiety, excitement, pain
- Physical exertion
- Drugs that increase sympathetic tone or block vagal tone
- Acute MI
- Hyperthyroidism
- Bleeding, vomiting, diarrhea, or dehydration resulting in intravascular volume loss

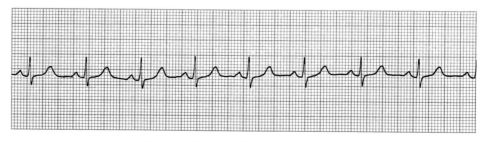

**Sinus rhythm at 82 beats per minute**

**FIGURE 20.20.** Normal sinus rhythm is best understood by looking at leads II and aV_R. (Reprinted with permission from Davis D. *Quick and accurate 12-lead ECG interpretation.* 4th ed. Philadelphia: Lippincott Williams & Wilkins, 2004.)

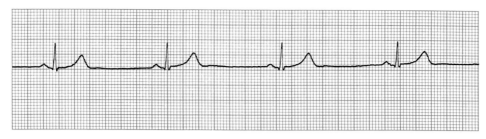

Sinus bradycardia at 43 beats per minute

**FIGURE 20.21.** Sinus bradycardia. (Reprinted with permission from Davis D. *Quick and accurate 12-lead ECG interpretation.* 4th ed. Philadelphia: Lippincott Williams & Wilkins, 2004.)

## Sinus Arrhythmia

Sinus arrhythmia is an irregularity in rhythm in which the impulse is initiated by the SA node, but the rate is not perfectly maintained. Instead, there is an accentuated beat-to-beat variation in rate that is caused most commonly by the respiratory cycle (*Fig. 20.23*). Sinus pause occurs when the SA node fails to initiate an impulse for one cycle. This figure shows that sinus pause can be associated with escape beats arising out of the atria, AV node, or ventricles (*Fig. 20.24*).

## Atrial Premature Beats and Junctional Premature Beats

Atrial premature beats (APB) and junctional premature beats (JPB) are very common and result from ectopic stimuli in the atria or AV junction (node) (*Fig. 20.25*). The majority of APB and JPB are benign; therefore, their presence does not infer cardiac disease. The following characteristics are common to these supraventricular arrhythmias:

- Premature, occurring before the next normal P wave
- QRS complex preceded by a visible P wave that has a different shape and/or different PR interval (either longer or shorter) than the P wave seen with normal sinus beats
- Compensatory pause before the normal sinus beat resumes

- QRS complex is identical to previous normal sinus beats
- Some APB may be blocked due to an AV junction that is refractory

## Paroxysmal Supraventricular Tachycardia

Paroxysmal supraventricular tachycardia is a sudden run (increased rate) of three or more beats. These may be nonsustained (up to 30 seconds) or sustained for minutes, hours, or longer. There are three types of sudden supraventricular tachycardias: atrial tachycardia (AT), atrioventricular nodal re-entrant tachycardia (AVNRT), and atrioventricular re-entrant tachycardia (AVRT). These may cause symptoms of palpitation, lightheadedness, or syncope if sustained at a fast rate. These tachycardias are depicted in *Figure 20.26.*

AT is defined as three or more consecutive APB. AVNRT is caused by a rapidly circulating impulse in the AV node area, as shown in Figure 20.26. Re-entry is a term that describes situations in which a cardiac impulse literally spins around and around a given set of cells. These arrhythmias are also called circus movement tachycardias and can appear in any part of the heart. APB can sometimes cause AVNRTs. These arrhythmias can cease spontaneously, but sometimes they require treatment. An increase in vagal tone, slowing impulses to the vagus nerve and thus halting the re-entrant circuit, can be accomplished in one of several ways: a Val-

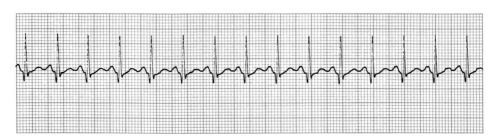

Sinus tachycardia at 149 beats per minute

**FIGURE 20.22.** Sinus tachycardia. (Reprinted with permission from Davis D. *Quick and accurate 12-lead ECG interpretation.* 4th ed. Philadelphia: Lippincott Williams & Wilkins, 2004.)

## RESPIRATORY SINUS ARRHYTHMIA

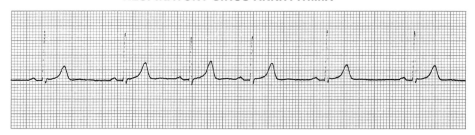

**Heart rate increases with inspiration and decreases with expiration.**

**FIGURE 20.23.** Sinus arrhythmia caused by the respiratory cycle. (Reprinted with permission from Davis D. *Quick and accurate 12-lead ECG interpretation.* 4th ed. Philadelphia: Lippincott Williams & Wilkins, 2004.)

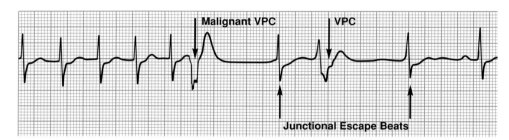

**Supraventricular tachycardia followed by a malignant VPC, followed by a junctional escape beat, a VPC, and another junctional escape beat and reverting to sinus rhythm**

**FIGURE 20.24.** A junctional escape beat is shown after a period of sinus pause. (Reprinted with permission from Davis D. *Quick and accurate 12-lead ECG interpretation.* 4th ed. Philadelphia: Lippincott Williams & Wilkins, 2004.)

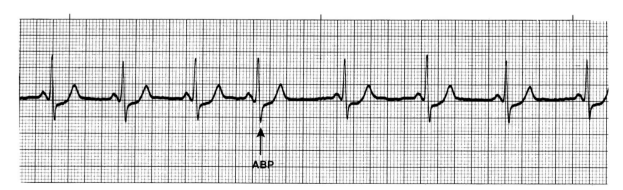

**FIGURE 20.25.** The atrial premature beat is shown after the fourth sinus beat. (Reprinted with permission from Huff J. *ECG workout: exercises in arrhythmia interpretation.* 4th ed. Philadelphia: Lippincott Williams & Wilkins, 2001.)

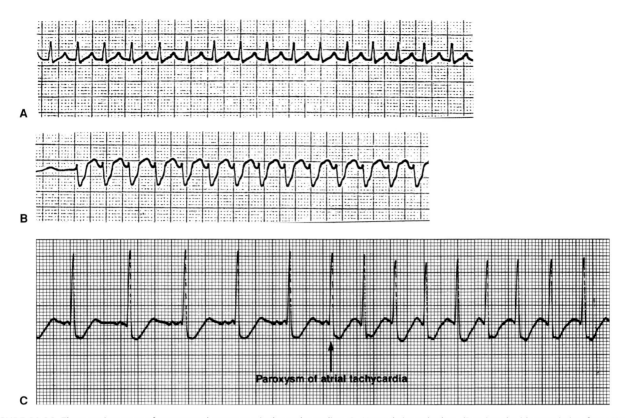

**FIGURE 20.26.** Three major types of paroxysmal supraventricular tachycardias. **A.** Normal sinus rhythm. (Reprinted with permission from Harwood-Nuss A, Wolfson AB, Linden CH, et al. *The clinical practice of emergency medicine*. 3rd ed. Philadelphia: Lippincott Williams & Wilkins, 2001.) **B.** Atrial tachycardia showing a focus outside the sinoatrial node fires automatically at a rapid rate. (Reprinted with permission from Harwood-Nuss A, Wolfson AB, Linden CH, et al. *The clinical practice of emergency medicine*. 3rd ed. Philadelphia: Lippincott Williams & Wilkins, 2001.) **C.** Atrioventricular nodal re-entrant tachycardia showing the wave of excitation originating and spinning around the atrioventricular nodal area. (Reprinted with permission from Nettina S. *The Lippincott manual of nursing practice*. 7th ed. Philadelphia: Lippincott Williams & Wilkins, 2001.)

salva maneuver or carotid sinus massage. Other treatments may involve drugs to interrupt the re-entrant mechanism or electric cardioversion to depolarize the heart, interrupt abnormal rhythms, and allow the sinus node to regain control of the cardiac electrical cycle. Another similar rhythm, AVRT, uses a bypass tract that connects the atria and ventricles. These last two arrhythmias are very similar.

A group of arrhythmias that arise out of the AV node, but which are not re-entrant, are the AV junctional rhythms. These occur when the AV junction becomes the heart's pacer and the atria are stimulated in a retrograde (backward) fashion. This retrograde activity produces ECG morphologies that are abnormal.

## Atrial Flutter and Atrial Fibrillation

Two other forms of supraventricular arrhythmias are atrial flutter and atrial fibrillation (Fig. 20.27). Atrial flutter stimulates the atria to contract at a rate of about 300 bpm. The ventricles respond to the rapid rate of AV electrical bombardment by conducting less of the stimulation than it receives. This means that the ventricular rate with atrial flutter is slower, usually either 150, 100, or 75 bpm. The ventricular rate in atrial flutter is usually stable but does sometimes

change in a stepwise fashion. There is a regular irregularity to atrial flutter that is not present with atrial fibrillation.

With atrial fibrillation, the baseline is undulating due to the fibrillation waves compared with the flutter waves produced in atrial flutter. Because the atrial rate is much faster in atrial fibrillation, the AV node is only able to conduct a small fraction of the stimulation it receives and it conducts this in an irregular fashion. Therefore, atrial fibrillation is an irregularly irregular rhythm. Atrial fibrillation is more dangerous clinically than is atrial flutter. This is due to altered hemodynamics as a result of ineffective atrial pumping. This results in a decreased cardiac output because the atria are not effectively delivering blood to the ventricles. Also there is an inverse relationship between the ventricular rate found with atrial fibrillation and the level of cardiac output. That is, the higher the ventricular rate, the lower will be the cardiac output. With high ventricular rates and low cardiac output, patients may become hypotensive or experience congestive heart failure.

## Ventricular Arrhythmias

Ventricular arrhythmias are ectopic (nonsinus) beats that arise in the ventricles themselves. Examples of ventricular

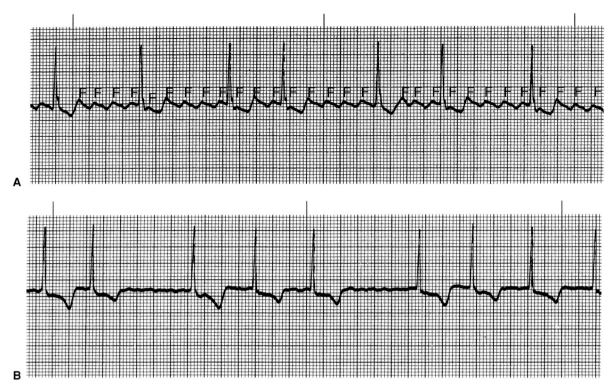

**FIGURE 20.27.** Atrial flutter **(A)** and atrial fibrillation **(B)**. The "sawtooth" waves of flutter are regular and the fibrillatory waves of fibrillation are irregular. (Reprinted with permission from Huff J. *ECG workout: exercises in arrhythmia interpretation*. 4th ed. Philadelphia: Lippincott Williams & Wilkins, 2001.)

arrhythmias are premature ventricular contraction (PVC), ventricular tachycardia (VT), and ventricular fibrillation (VF). There are several features of PVCs that are important to mention. These are frequency, compensatory pause, uniform and multiform PVCs, and the R on T phenomenon.

Frequency refers to the number of PVCs arising per minute. PVCs may occur in various combinations. For example, two consecutive PVCs are referred to as a couplet (*Fig. 20.28*). When one PVC follows each normal beat, ventricular bigeminy is present; when one PVC follows two normal beats, ventricular trigeminy is present (*Fig. 20.29*). Compensatory pause refers to the pause before the next normal beat following a PVC (*Fig. 20.30*). When the

PVC falls almost exactly between two normal beats, the PVC is said to be interpolated (*Fig. 20.31*).

PVCs may be uniform (same) or multiform (different) in appearance in any particular lead (*Fig. 20.32*). PVCs of the same appearance in a particular lead originate from the same ectopic site and are therefore unifocal in origin. However, PVCs of different appearance in a particular lead may originate from different ectopic sites, but not always. Therefore, multiform PVCs are not necessarily multifocal in origin.

The R on T phenomenon refers to PVCs that are timed in their appearance that they fall near the peak of the T wave of the preceding normal beat (*Fig. 20.33*). This is a dangerous electrical occurrence because VT or VF could

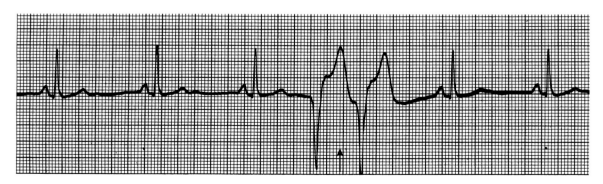

**FIGURE 20.28.** Two premature ventricular contractions (V) together are referred to as a pair or couplet. (Reprinted with permission from Huff J. *ECG workout: exercises in arrhythmia interpretation*. 4th ed. Philadelphia: Lippincott Williams & Wilkins, 2001.)

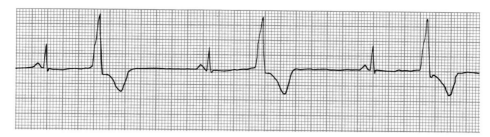

VPCs in bigeminy

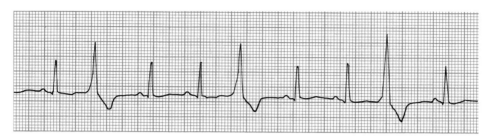

VPCs in trigeminy

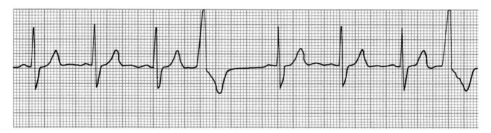

VPCs in quadrigeminy

**FIGURE 20.29.** Ventricular bigeminy, trigeminy, and quadrigeminy. (Reprinted with permission from Davis D. *Quick and accurate 12-lead ECG interpretation*. 4th ed. Philadelphia: Lippincott Williams & Wilkins, 2004.)

easily be precipitated. In all, PVCs are very common arrhythmias, occurring in normal and diseased hearts. General principles that govern when PVCs are of concern help guide clinicians. First, frequent PVCs often accompany underlying cardiac disease and/or valvular problems. For example, PVCs are common with mitral valve prolapse and are the most common arrhythmia seen with acute MI. PVCs are also caused by numerous cardiac stimulants and are also seen in patients with electrolyte disturbances.

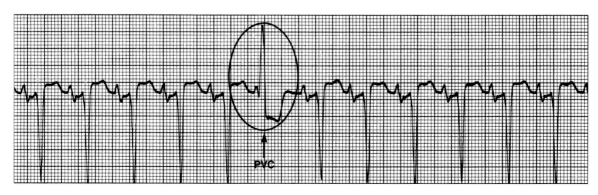

**FIGURE 20.30.** A premature ventricular contraction is characterized as occurring early, has a wide aberrant shape, and usually occurs with a compensatory pause prior to the next normal beat. (Reprinted with permission from Nettina S. *The Lippincott manual of nursing practice*. 7th ed. Philadelphia: Lippincott Williams & Wilkins, 2001.)

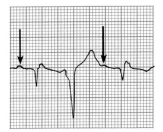

Interpolated VPC

**FIGURE 20.31.** Some premature ventricular contractions are interpolated and thus do not have a compensatory pause prior to the next beat. (Reprinted with permission from Davis D. *Quick and accurate 12-lead ECG interpretation*. 4th ed. Philadelphia: Lippincott Williams & Wilkins, 2004.)

VT is a run of three or more consecutive PVCs that may be nonsustained or sustained (>30 seconds in duration). Examples of two incidences of nonsustained VT are found in *Figure 20.34*. VT that is sustained and very rapid may lead to syncope or sudden death. Dangerous VT of this nature is usually associated with structural cardiac abnormalities such as prior MI, cardiomyopathy, and/or ventricular enlargement. A common cause of VT is coronary artery disease with prior MI. VT can digress to VF. VF is a condition in which the ventricles do not beat but rather experience an asynchronous quivering when no cardiac output and blood pressure are possible. VF requires immediate defibrillation with an unsynchronized direct current shock. VF is the most common cause of sudden cardiac death.

▶ *INQUIRY SUMMARY.* Therapists who prescribe exercise for clinical populations should have a basic understanding of exercise electrocardiography. This includes a solid understanding of the 12-lead system, ischemia patterns, and recognizing arrhythmias. *How can an understanding of electrocardiography help the physical therapist or exercise physiologist be a better clinician?*

*LINKUP: ECG interpretation is fundamental knowledge for health care professionals who assist in clinical exercise testing. Perspective: ECG Interpretation, found at http://connection.lww.com/go/brownexphys and on the Student Resource CD-ROM, presents basic information on how to interpret an ECG.*

## The Graded Exercise Test

Besides the more obvious medical purposes for performing a stress test, i.e., determining a diagnosis and prognosis, the graded exercise (or stress) test is also a useful tool for evaluating the functional capacity of patients for performing endurance exercise. Testing of this nature is important for patients/clients before they enter medically supervised exercise programs because it provides a noninvasive means to measure cardiovascular and pulmonary responses to increased activity. Exercise testing involves systematically and progressively increasing $O_2$ demand and evaluating patients' physiologic responses to the increased demand. In this regard, clinical exercise testing is usually ordered by a physician who may want to further evaluate the patient prior to starting an exercise program.

Further evaluation prior to exercise training is a prudent decision because people who enter exercise programs are often sedentary, overweight, hypercholesterolemic, and middle-aged; they also frequently smoke and suffer from chest pain during exertion. All of these conditions, and others, place individuals at higher than normal risk for coronary artery disease and sudden death due to an untoward cardiac event when exercising. Testing prior to exercise participation helps the physician and exercise specialist assess the risks involved and provide a basis for sound exercise prescriptions.

### PREPARATION FOR TESTING

The client preparing for clinical exercise testing must follow some explicit instructions regarding their legal rights, test preparation, and personal safety. First, before the individual is allowed to undergo testing, he/she must provide informed consent for the procedure. Informed consent is an ethical and legal requirement of all medical testing. The word *informed* implies that the person has been told and understands all pertinent facts, knowledge of material risks, and benefits associated with the test. Proper communication implies that the person is of a lawful age, is not mentally incapacitated, knows and fully comprehends the importance and relevance of the material risks, and gives his/her consent voluntarily and not under any mistake of

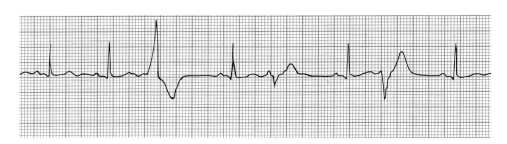

Sinus rhythm with three isolated multifocal VPCs

**FIGURE 20.32.** Multiform premature ventricular contractions have different shapes in the same lead. (Reprinted with permission from Davis D. *Quick and accurate 12-lead ECG interpretation*. 4th ed. Philadelphia: Lippincott Williams & Wilkins, 2004.)

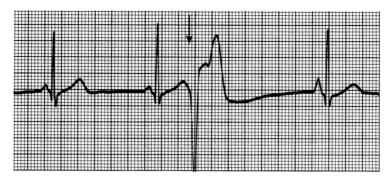

**FIGURE 20.33.** The R on T phenomenon (premature ventricular contraction [PVC] labeled is falling near the peak of the T wave of the preceding beat) predisposes to ventricular tachycardia or ventricular fibrillation. (Reprinted with permission from Huff J. *ECG workout: exercises in arrhythmia interpretation*. 4th ed. Philadelphia: Lippincott Williams & Wilkins, 2001.)

fact or duress (9). A sample informed consent form is provided in *Figure 20.35*.

Patient preparation also involves the collection of preliminary medical data. This may include the following information from recent and past medical history:

- Disclosure of all medical diagnoses
- Findings of previous medical examinations
- History of symptoms
- Recent illnesses or hospitalizations, new medical diagnoses or surgical procedures
- Any orthopedic problems that may hamper test performance
- Medication use, drug allergies
- Indications of habitual use of caffeine, alcohol, tobacco, or illicit drugs
- Exercise history
- Work history with emphasis on physical demands
- Family history of chronic disease

Sometimes it may be necessary to perform a physical examination of the patient prior to the clinical exercise test. In this case, the following information should be obtained by a physician or other trained health care professional:

- Body weight and body composition (if warranted)

- Apical pulse rate and rhythm
- Resting blood pressure
- Lung auscultation
- Palpation of the cardiac apical impulse
- Auscultation of the heart
- Palpation and auscultation of the carotid, abdominal, and femoral arteries
- Evaluation of the abdomen for bowel sounds, masses, and tenderness
- Palpation and inspection of the lower extremities for edema and presence of arterial pulses
- Inspection of the skin
- Tests of neurologic function
- Follow-up examination of any orthopedic or other medical condition that would limit exercise testing

Prior to arriving to the clinic to undergo testing, the patient must be instructed to adhere to the following:

- Abstain from food, tobacco, alcohol, and caffeine for at least 3 hours before testing
- Wear comfortable clothing, including proper footwear, for exercise
- Female clients should wear a sports bra
- Continue to take prescribed medications, unless otherwise instructed by a physician

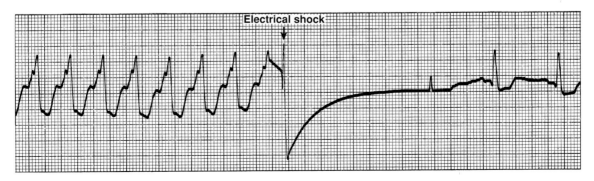

**FIGURE 20.34.** Sustained ventricular tachycardia converted to normal sinus rhythm by direct current cardioversion. (Reprinted with permission from Huff J. *ECG workout: exercises in arrhythmia interpretation*. 4th ed. Philadelphia: Lippincott Williams & Wilkins, 2001.)

# Informed Consent for an Exercise Test

### 1. Purpose and Explanation of the Test

You will perform an exercise test on a cycle ergometer or a motor-driven treadmill. The exercise intensity will begin at a low level and will be advanced in stages depending on your fitness level. We may stop the test at any time because of signs of fatigue or changes in your heart rate, ECG, or blood pressure, or symptoms you may experience. It is important for you to realize that you may stop when you wish because of feelings of fatigue or any other discomfort.

### 2. Attendant Risks and Discomforts

There exists the possibility of certain changes occurring during the test. These include abnormal blood pressure, fainting, irregular, fast or slow heart rhythm, and in rare instances, heart attack, stroke, or death. Every effort will be made to minimize these risks by evaluation of preliminary information relating to your health and fitness and by careful observations during testing. Emergency equipment and trained personnel are available to deal with unusual situations that may arise.

### 3. Responsibilities of the Participant

Information you possess about your health status or previous experiences of heart-related symptoms (e.g., shortness of breath with low-level activity, pain, pressure, tightness, heaviness in the chest, neck, jaw, back, and/or arms) with physical effort may affect the safety of your exercise test. Your prompt reporting of these and any other unusual feelings with effort during the exercise test itself is very important. You are responsible for fully disclosing your medical history, as well as symptoms that may occur during the test. You are also expected to report all medications (including nonprescription) taken recently and, in particular, those taken today, to the testing staff.

### 4. Benefits to Be Expected

The results obtained from the exercise test may assist in the diagnosis of your illness, in evaluating the effect of your medications or in evaluating what type of physical activities you might do with low risk.

### 5. Inquiries

Any questions about the procedures used in the exercise test or the results of your test are encouraged. If you have any concerns or questions, please ask us for further explanations.

### 6. Use of Medical Records

The information that is obtained during exercise testing will be treated as privileged and confidential as described in the Health Insurance Portability and Accountability Act of 1996. It is not to be released or revealed to any person except your referring physician without your written consent. However, the information obtained may be used for statistical analysis or scientific purposes with your right to privacy retained.

### 7. Freedom of Consent

I hereby consent to voluntarily engage in an exercise test to determine my exercise capacity and state of cardiovascular health. My permission to perform this exercise test is given voluntarily. I understand that I am free to stop the test at any point if I so desire.

I have read this form, and I understand the test procedures that I will perform and the attendant risks and discomforts. Knowing these risks and discomforts, and having had an opportunity to ask questions that have been answered to my satisfaction, I consent to participate in this test.

_____          _____
Date                                                 Signature of Patient

_____          _____
Date                                                 Signature of Witness

_____          _____
Date                                                 Signature of Physician or Authorized Delegate

**FIGURE 20.35.** Sample informed consent. (Used with permission from Whaley MH, ed. *ACSM's guidelines for exercise testing and prescription.* 7th ed. Baltimore: Lippincott Williams & Wilkins, 2006.)

Once the patient has arrived for testing and all questions have been answered, the patient is ready for the test. Test sequence occurs in three parts: pretest, test, and post-test. During these three distinct time sequences, the main variables that will be assessed are: 12-lead ECGs (resting during the pretest and post-test periods and exercise ECG during the testing period), HR and blood pressure in the pretest and post-test periods and during exercise, and rating of perceived exertion (RPE) during exercise. The testing area should be 22°C or less and humidity 60% or less, if possible. Oral temperature should be taken to avoid testing during periods of acute systemic infection.

## COMPONENTS OF THE GRADED EXERCISE TEST

The testing sequence mentioned above is standard for all formal clinical exercise tests. Conducting the actual test is the same for all protocols and modes, with only minor differences that are mostly related to working the specific ergometer and protocol during the test. If there is any doubt as to the benefit of testing or the safety of testing for a given patient/client and on a given day, the test should not be performed at that time. The pretest sequence requires that a 12-lead ECG be recorded in the supine and exercise postures. The clinician should note any ECG changes between the supine and exercise positions. Resting blood pressure should also be documented in these positions (supine first). Once resting data are collected, the patient can be moved to the testing ergometer and the test may commence immediately. The 12-lead ECG should be recorded during the last 15 seconds of each stage of the test and at the peak exercise moment. If any arrhythmia is observed, a 3-lead recoding of it should be made of each occurrence. The 3-lead ECG should be continually observed on the monitor during the test. Blood pressure should be measured during the last minute of each stage and verified, if necessary. The RPE rating should also be taken from the patient. Other rating scales such as the ones for dyspnea and angina can also be employed for those patients likely to be limited by these symptoms (*Fig. 20.36*). The recovery or post-test protocol is followed in a sequential fashion:

- Record a 12-lead ECG immediately after exercise (to capture the peak exercise stress point) and then record a 12-lead ECG every 2 minutes until exercise-induced ECG and hemodynamic changes return to baseline
- Blood pressure measures should be made in a like manner to what was previously outlined for the ECG
- As long as symptoms persist after exercise, symptomatic ratings should be obtained using appropriate scales (Fig. 20.36)

*When should the exercise test be terminated?* This key question is decided by either the patient, who has the right to terminate the test at any time, or the clinician, who uses clinical judgment to terminate the test when an abnormal finding is presented or when a predetermined end point has been reached. Several medical/physiologic indications, grouped according to clinical, hemodynamic, and ECG responses, may arise that will help indicate to the test supervisor that the test should be halted. These include absolute and relative indications for terminating the test:

### ABSOLUTE INDICATIONS

- Drop in systolic blood pressure of ≥10 mm Hg from baseline blood pressure despite an increase in workload, when accompanied by other evidence of ischemia
- Moderate to severe angina
- Increasing nervous system symptoms (e.g., ataxia, dizziness, or near syncope)
- Signs of poor perfusion (cyanosis or pallor)
- Technical difficulties monitoring the ECG or systolic blood pressure
- Subject's desire to stop

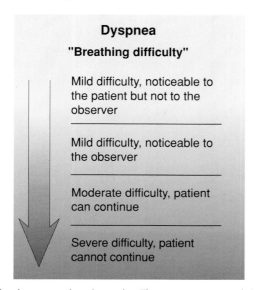

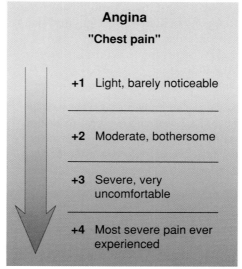

**FIGURE 20.36.** The dyspnea and angina scales. The two are presented side-by-side to save space. One symptom should not be construed as being tied to or caused by the other.

- Sustained VT
- ST elevation (≥1.0 mm) in leads without diagnostic Q waves (other than $V_1$ or $aV_R$)

### RELATIVE INDICATIONS

- Drop in systolic blood pressure of ≥10 mm Hg from baseline blood pressure despite an increase in workload in the absence of other evidence of ischemia
- ST or QRS changes such as excessive ST depression (>2-mm horizontal or downsloping ST segment depression) or marked axis shift
- Arrhythmias other than sustained VT, including multifocal PVCs, triplets of PVCs, supraventricular tachycardia, heart block, or bradyarrhythmias
- Fatigue, shortness of breath, wheezing, leg cramps, or claudication
- Development of bundle branch block or intraventricular conduction delay that cannot be distinguished from VT
- Increasing chest pain
- Hypertensive response, i.e., systolic blood pressure of more than 250 mm Hg and/or a diastolic blood pressure of more than 115 mm Hg

### INTERPRETING RESULTS

Usually in the clinical arena the test of cardiopulmonary functional capacity is symptom limited in that the end point of the test is dictated by the medical/physiologic condition of the patient and not the achievement of $\dot{V}O_{2max}$. Clinical exercise tests should not be halted for an arbitrary criterion, such as predicted maximal HR or when 85% of age-adjusted maximal HR has been reached. Rather, what is important is that a true functional capacity within the patient's symptomatic limitations has been achieved. When viewed this way, functional capacity can be defined as the peak metabolic/physiologic responses and ergometric workload achieved on the test. The clinician should always interpret functional capacity in light of the signs and symptoms occurring at the termination point. Case Study 20.3 presents results of exercise testing to determine the functional capacity of the individual.

 *LINKUP:* **Case Study: Chronic Obstructive Pulmonary Disease,** *found at http://connection.lww.com/go/brownex phys and on the Student Resource CD-ROM, presents another case study showing exercise testing to determine functional capacity of individuals. These case studies can be used as guides to interpret future patient tests.*

▶ *INQUIRY SUMMARY.* The graded exercise test is an important tool in clinical exercise programs because it provides vital information regarding patient metabolic and physiologic responses to exercise in a controlled environment. In this setting, the main purpose of the test is to determine functional capacity. In so doing, the clinician determines peak metabolic and physiologic variables, the ergometric workload at which these peak variables are achieved, and the associated signs and symptoms at this point. This is very useful, clinically relevant information that will be vital to the treatment plan of the patient. *Why is knowledge of functional capacity important?*

## Summary

This chapter introduces concepts and principles of clinical exercise testing. Patients with comorbidities more than likely have functional deficits in the cardiopulmonary system requiring the therapist to test the functional capacity of this system to develop an appropriate treatment plan. This is best accomplished via a formal graded exercise test. This test yields values (predicted or measured) of $\dot{V}O_{2max}$, the single best indicator of cardiovascular endurance or fitness. There are several types of clinical exercise tests, some more suited for particular patients than others. Care must be taken to match a test protocol and mode with the medical needs of the patient being tested. Prior to testing, health screening and risk stratification helps determine if an exercise test is needed prior to enrolling a patient in a fitness program and if a physician is needed to conduct the test. For clinical populations, exercise testing has proven to be sensitive and specific enough to be of predictive value, i.e., its accuracy in correctly identifying the presence or absence of coronary artery disease is significant. Clinical exercise testing, therefore, has both diagnostic and prognostic purposes alongside its use in functional assessment. Therapists who use clinical exercise testing as a tool in assessing cardiopulmonary deficits need to have a sound understanding of electrocardiography and should have basic skills of ECG interpretation. These skills involve a basic understanding of 12-lead ECGs, ischemic responses, and arrhythmia recognition. The ECG is one of the main output variables collected during the graded exercise test sequence, i.e., the pretest, exercise, and post-test phases. The other variables include blood pressure, RPE, dyspnea, and angina pain ratings (if necessary), and related signs and symptoms.

### SUMMARY KNOWLEDGE

1. Why are $\dot{V}O_{2max}$ and $\dot{V}O_{2peak}$ not synonymous terms?
2. What are some differences and similarities between ST depression and ST elevation?
3. Describe the difference between test sensitivity and specificity.
4. Why are there 12 leads in electrocardiography, and what do they depict?
5. What is the purpose of exercise electrocardiography?
6. Why is the mean QRS electrical axis important?
7. What is the difference between a contraindication and an indication?

## CASE STUDY 20.3: *CARDIAC BYPASS GRAFT SURGERY*

### CASE

Stuart (57-year-old male, weight 81.8 kg, height 172 cm) has a history of coronary artery disease and coronary artery bypass grafts (CABG). He had a history of experiencing angina upon exertion prior to the CABG surgery. He is on dipyridamole, has a body fat of 30 percent, and an age-adjusted maximum heart rate (HR) of 163 beats per minute (bpm).

### DESCRIPTION

Coronary artery disease produces a narrowing of the coronary arteries and restricts the flow of blood to the heart. The purpose of CABG surgery is to correct this situation by improving the flow of blood and $O_2$ to the heart. Following surgery, Stuart was given a stress test prior to entering a fitness program as recommended by his physician. The results of his stress test are shown below.

Resting electrocardiogram (ECG): slight ST-T flattening; no arrhythmias present

Resting blood pressure (BP): 123/84

Resting HR: 75 bpm; protocol: Bruce

Terminal HR: 135 bpm; terminal BP: 170/88; terminal MET: 10.2; terminal RPP: 230; terminal RPE: 8; test terminated due to significant ischemic response, +3 dyspnea, and fatigue.

### INTERVENTION

This test is positive for ischemia as ST/T changed from a flattening at rest to 2.5 mm of horizontal depression in the inferior leads at maximal exercise. Angina was not experienced. The return to baseline took 8 minutes. No arrhythmias were present at rest, exercise, or recovery. The physiologic responses to exercise were equivocal. HR and systolic BP both increased and diastolic BP was stable; however, systolic BP failed to increase in a linear fashion from stage 2 to stage 3. Total exercise duration was 8 minutes on the Bruce protocol. The ending stage of Bruce produces a MET response of 10.2 if at steady state. However, Stuart was not at physiologic steady state; therefore, his functional aerobic capacity based on the generalized Bruce equation (see Table 20.1) was 8.9 MET. Stuart's functional aerobic capacity is formally documented as:

8.9 MET at an HR of 135, BP of 170/88, RPE of 8, and with significant ECG evidence of inferior wall ischemia (without angina) and symptoms of dyspnea and fatigue. Peak workload was 3.4 mi·hr$^{-1}$ at 14% grade.

Stuart will likely not be cleared to enter the fitness program until the ischemic response to exercise is rectified. He clearly is more suited for a clinical exercise program such as phase III cardiopulmonary rehabilitation.

| Stage | HR | BP | MET | RPE | Comments and reason for termination |
|---|---|---|---|---|---|
| 1 | 96 | 3/10 | | | |
| | 94 | | | 3 | |
| | 96 | 158/86 | 4.7 | 4 | +2 dyspnea |
| 2 | 110 | | | 4 | |
| | 118 | | | 5 | |
| | 118 | 168/86 | 7.1 | 6 | +2 dyspnea, fatigue, ECG showed 1-mm ST/T horizontal depression |
| 3 | 125 | | | 8 | |
| | 135 | 170/88 | 10.2 | 8 | +3 dyspnea, fatigue, ECG showed 2.5-mm ST/T horizontal depression |

**References**

1. Joyner MJ. Modeling optimal marathon performance on the basis of physiological factors. *J Appl Physiol* 1991;70:683–687.
2. Jaski BE, Kim J, Maly RS, et al. Effects of exercise during long-term support with a left ventricular device. *Circulation* 1997;95:2401–2406.
3. Brannon FJ, Foley MW, Starr JA, et al. *Cardiopulmonary rehabilitation: basic theory and application.* 3rd ed. Philadelphia: FA Davis Co, 1998.
4. American Thoracic Society. Evaluation of impairment secondary to respiratory disease. *Am Review Resp Dis* 1982;126:945–951.
5. Froelicher VF, Follansbee WP, Labovitz AJ. *Exercise and the heart.* 3rd ed. St. Louis: Mosby, 1993.
6. Kervio G, Carre F, Ville NS. Reliability and intensity of the six-minute walk test in healthy elderly subjects. *Med Sci Sports Exerc* 2003;35:169–174.
7. Kline GM, Porcari JP, Hingemeister R, et al. Estimation of V̇O$_{2max}$ from a one-mile track walk, gender, age, and body weight. *Med Sci Sports Exerc* 1987;19:253–259.
8. George JD, Vehrs PR, Allsen PE, et al. Development of a submaximal treadmill jogging test for fit college-aged individuals. *Med Sci Sports Exerc* 1993;25:643–647.
9. Franklin BA, ed. *ACSM's guidelines for exercise testing and prescription.* 6th ed. Baltimore: Lippincott Williams & Wilkins, 2000.

### Suggested Readings

Robergs RA. An exercise physiologist's "contemporary" interpretations of the "ugly and creaking edifices" of the $O_{2max}$ concept. *J Exerc Physiol online* 2001;4:1–44.

Schairer JR, Brawner CA, Levine SD. Peripheral arterial disease: case report from the Henry Ford Hospital. *Clin Exerc Physiol* 2001;3:194–198.

Schairer JR, Levine SD, Brawner CA. Emphysema: case report from the Henry Ford Hospital. *Clin Exerc Physiol* 2001;3:133–136.

Seelig CB. *Simplified EKG analysis: a sequential guide to interpretation and diagnosis.* Philadelphia: Hanley & Belfus, Inc, 1992.

### On the Internet

Centenary Cardiology Associates. Available at: **http://www.centenarycardiology.com/index2.html**. Accessed July 28, 2005.

Michigan Heart & Vascular Institute: Cardiovascular Diagnostic Tests. Available at: **http://www.mhvi.org/owners_manual/diag_stress.asp**. Accessed July 28, 2005.

Cincinnati Children's Hospital Medical Center: The Heart Center Encyclopedia. Available at: **http://www.cincinnatichildrens.org/health/heart-encyclopedia/**. Accessed July 28, 2005.

Heart1.com: Diagnostics. Available at: **http://www.heart1.com/care/diag10.cfm**. Accessed July 28, 2005.

12-Lead ECG: The Art of Interpretation. Available at: **http://www.12leadecg.com/full/**. Accessed July 28, 2005.

## Writing to Learn

*Do a literature search of case study preparations (minimum of three cases) involving clinical exercise testing of either cardiac or pulmonary patients (one or the other, not both). Write a paper detailing the findings of these three cases and critically evaluate the reported case regarding these findings.*

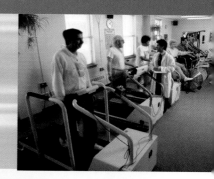

# 21 Exercise for Cardiopulmonary Disorders

*Movement, whether viewed as therapeutic mobilization for the acutely ill patient or therapeutic exercise training for the chronically ill patient, is essential for the maintenance of proper function of individuals with cardiopulmonary and cardiovascular dysfunctions. The individuals pictured are exercising as part of a regular program of cardiopulmonary rehabilitation following myocardial infarction or some other cardiac problem.* What do you think are the advantages of an exercise program for these individuals?

## CHAPTER OUTLINE

CARDIOVASCULAR ENDURANCE, PHYSICAL ACTIVITY, AND HEALTH

THE EXERCISE PRESCRIPTION
* The Exercise Prescription Intervention Triad
* Exercise Prescription for Cardiovascular Endurance Impairment

CARDIOPULMONARY REHABILITATION

THE EXERCISE SESSION
* Sequencing
* Environment and Feedback

Exercise and health go hand-in-hand. For the general population, regular exercise will prevent or delay the onset of chronic disease, and exercise is a key ingredient in physiologic rehabilitation for those individuals with chronic disease. This chapter focuses on exercise prescription, emphasizing the process of cardiopulmonary rehabilitation. In this chapter, we show how data generated from exercise testing are used to develop individualized exercise and physical activity prescriptions for various patient groups, and how exercise training leads to higher functional levels for these individuals.

## Cardiovascular Endurance, Physical Activity, and Health

Physical inactivity is epidemic in Western society and is arguably the largest public health crisis being faced today, given the association between physical inactivity and a plethora of chronic, degenerative diseases. Most notable of the chronic health problems are the cardiovascular diseases (CVD) that remain the leading cause of death despite a decline in their incidence rate over the last 35 years. The benefits of regular physical activity and exercise are evident in preventing chronic diseases, yet only about 25% of adults engage in physical activity of a type, frequency, and intensity likely to convey health benefits (*Fig. 21.1*).

Cardiovascular diseases are of multifactorial **etiology** and are related to the **risk factors** shown in *Table 21.1*. Of the risk factors shown in Table 21.1, physical inactivity is a particularly powerful causative factor. Consider the following statistics. Individuals who adopt a lifestyle of physical activity reduce their risk of heart attacks by 50%. This is compared with a 40% reduced risk when individuals quit smoking and a 35% reduced risk when high blood pressure is medically controlled. Adding a combination of any of these risk factors in your lifestyle involves greater risk of disease than if any single factor was present. Likewise, when you remove a combination of any of these factors from your life, there is a larger reduction of risk than when only a single factor is removed. In particular, the message concerning exercise and physical activity is clear: *regular participation protects against disease. But what is the relationship among physical activity, cardiovascular endurance, and health?* We now turn to a discussion of this question.

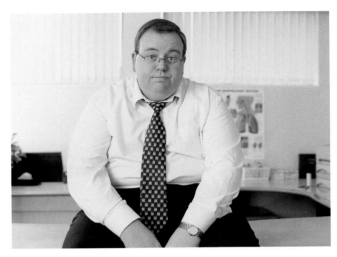

**FIGURE 21.1.** Physical inactivity is the most direct cause of obesity in America and is also linked to many other lifestyle diseases.

Physical inactivity is related to a wide variety of health problems, including:

- CVD: According to year 2000 estimates, CVD is the leading cause of death in the United States (claimed 945,836 lives in the year 2000; 39.4% of all deaths or one of every 2.5 deaths) with nearly 60 million Americans having one or more forms of CVD, such as
  - Ischemic heart disease—7.6 million people with myocardial infarction (MI) and 6.6 million people with angina pectoris

| *Table 21.1* | **RISK FACTORS FOR CARDIOVASCULAR DISEASES** |
|---|---|
| **Factor** | **Defined as** |
| Family history | Coronary disease in male first-degree relative <55 years old or in female first-degree relative <65 years old |
| Smoking | <6 months since quitting |
| Increased cholesterol | Total cholesterol >200 mg·dL$^{-1}$ or HDL <35 mg·dL$^{-1}$ |
| Hypertension | Systolic blood pressure ≥140 mm Hg or diastolic blood pressure ≥90 mm Hg |
| Physical inactivity | No regular participation in physical activity as recommended by the United States Surgeon General's report |
| Obesity | BMI ≥30 kg·m$^{-2}$ or waist girth >100 cm |
| Impaired fasting glucose | Fasting blood glucose ≥110 mg·dL$^{-1}$ |

BMI, body mass index; HDL, high-density lipoprotein.

- Hypertension—one in five Americans has high blood pressure
- Stroke—nearly 5 million people have been diagnosed
- Peripheral vascular disease—affects 10 million people in the United States, including 5% of the over-50 population
- Congestive heart disease—5 million Americans are now living with heart failure, and 550,000 new cases are diagnosed each year
- Cancer: Second leading cause of mortality in the United States
- Diabetes mellitus: Sixth leading cause of mortality in the United States
- Obesity: One of every three adults over age 20 is affected
- Osteoporosis: 15 to 20 million Americans affected

The following statistics help put the burden of these diseases in perspective. National health expenditures are projected to total $2.2 trillion and reach 16.2% of the gross domestic product (GDP) by the year 2008. This growth in health spending is projected to average 1.8% above the GDP growth rate for the decade from 1998 to 2008. In the year 2000 medical costs for people with chronic conditions totaled $774 billion, a figure projected to rise to $1.7 trillion by the year 2020. For a person with a chronic condition, total annual medical expenditures are $6032, which increases to $16,245 if that individual also has functional limitations. However, a healthy person's annual medical expenditures average only $1105. A Medicare beneficiary with a chronic condition visits, on average, eight different physicians. Furthermore, 80% of Medicare beneficiaries have one or more chronic conditions accounting for 99% of total spending for the Medicare program.

Besides those mentioned above, the following statistics give us a better perspective on CVD:

- One in three males can expect to develop some major CVD before age 60, and the odds for women are one in 10
- More than 2600 Americans die each day of CVD—an average of one death every 33 seconds
- If all forms of CVD were eliminated, life expectancy would rise by almost 7 years, compared with 3 years if all forms of cancer were eliminated (as of year 2001, male life expectancy at birth was 74.4 years compared with 79.8 years for females)
- The probability at birth of eventually dying from major CVD is 47% but only 22% from cancer and 0.7% from the human immunodeficiency virus/acquired immunodeficiency syndrome

Even with these grim statistics, death rates from CVD declined 17% from 1990 to 2000.

Sedentary living is a major factor in the etiology of the above disorders. Furthermore, our understanding of the fundamental relationship among these (and other) health problems, physical activity, and health-related physical fitness has shifted the key question from *"should a person exercise,"* to *"what type and how much exercise should we do to reap maximal health benefits?"* This shift now places the emphasis on the dose-response relationship and the best recommendations for health promotion, disease prevention, and rehabilitation. *Is there a threshold dose of exercise below which no health benefits will be achieved? A related question is: do health benefits still accrue if the exercise dose does not convey physical fitness?*

The preceding questions can be rephrased. *Is an exercise dose sufficient enough to increase aerobic capacity (i.e., cardiovascular endurance) the minimum requirement needed to receive the health benefits of exercise, or may there be gains in health apart from gains in cardiovascular endurance?* This key question has large implications for the average person who may find it difficult to exercise with the intensity necessary to achieve an increase in cardiovascular endurance, defined as an increase in $\dot{V}O_{2max}$. Fortunately health benefits are achieved even if aerobic power is not improved, or even when performing other types of exercise besides endurance activities. The key is to engage in some form of physical activity over most days of the week. The reason is intuitive. Physical activity involves bodily movement, and movement, especially physical activity intense enough to produce a significant increase in energy expenditure, is inherently healthful for your limbs and the organ systems of your body.

This is true even when considering the rehabilitative process. For example, when providing movement stress through early mobilization intervention after an acute episode of cardiopulmonary dysfunction and through chronic exercise training once the acute period is resolved, the body adapts to higher levels of function in several key organ systems. Although functional decline is inevitable with a combination of aging and progressively developing disease pathology, the adaptations achieved through exercise training reduce the *rate* of physical decline through the decades of life, effectively maintaining individuals' functional status for longer periods of time.

There are four possible relationships among physical activity, health-related fitness, and health (1).

1. Physical activity may improve fitness, thereby improving health
2. Physical activity may improve health and fitness through separate mechanisms
3. Physical activity may improve some aspect of health but not necessarily fitness
4. Physical activity may improve fitness but not certain aspects of health

These complex relationships are shown interactively in *Figure 21.2.* Physical activity leads to health through the development of physical/physiologic fitness. However, health and fitness also may impact physical activity. Providing more complexity to the model is the fact that many other factors (shown in the lower box) can impact physical activity, fitness, and health. Since the question is now "how much should we exercise" not "should we exer-

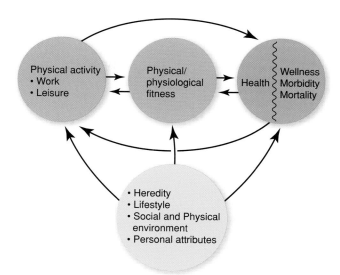

**FIGURE 21.2.** Model depicting the interactions among physical activity, fitness, and health. (Modified with permission from Bouchard C, Shephard RJ. Physical activity, fitness, and health: the model and key concepts. In Bouchard C, Shephard RJ, Stephens T, eds. *Physical activity, fitness, and health: international proceedings and consensus statement.* Champaign, Ill: Human Kinetics Publishers, 1994.)

cise," research has focused on the dose of physical activity needed.

The dose of activity received and the response (health benefit) generated is a concept that has important public health consequences. Benefits accrue at a rapid rate with increasing exercise dose (*Fig. 21.3*). As you move from sedentary living to higher and higher levels of physical activity, health benefits become greater but level off at very high activity levels at which the health return for time invested is not as great. Dose (X-axis of Fig. 21.3) is the prescribed amount of activity given, i.e., *type, frequency, duration,* and *intensity,* while response or benefit (Y-axis of Fig. 21.3) is the effect of the activity. These effects may be changes in $\dot{V}O_{2max}$, resting blood pressure, insulin sensitivity, blood lipid levels, body composition, mood states, exercise economy, or any other physiologic or psychologic change brought about by mobilization and exercise training.

Regular physical activity and cardiovascular endurance (fitness) are closely associated with health outcomes and a reduction in functional limitations. The innate physical fitness of individuals and the volume of chronic physical activity they routinely perform have been studied extensively with regard to health outcomes. Higher levels of all forms of physical activity and physical fitness are associated with better health, physical function, and longevity across a wide age range. For example, the Harvard alumni study demonstrated in 17,000 males aged 35 to 74 that those individuals expending greater than 8.4 mJ of energy per week in exercise (walking, stair climbing, sports play) had a 25% to 30% lower mortality rate than those with lower weekly

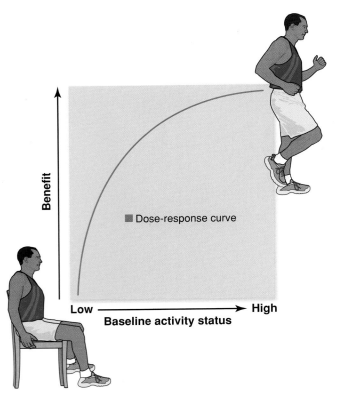

FIGURE 21.3. Estimated dose-response curve for exercise prescription. The amount of activity (dose) is related to the benefit (response) achieved in a curvilinear fashion.

cular endurance is arguably the most important component of physical fitness. This is true because risk of chronic disease and physical disability is strongly tied to the diminution, over time, in $\dot{V}O_{2max}$.

Although the concept of improving cardiovascular endurance through an increase in $\dot{V}O_{2max}$ is important, exercise intensities sufficient to increase $\dot{V}O_{2max}$ (usually defined as vigorous) are not necessary for reaping health benefits. It is now known, for example, that moderately intense physical activity also leads to health benefits. The recommendations of the publication *Healthy People 2000* center on this thought as stated in objective A, "by 2000, the proportion of Americans who regularly participate in moderately intense physical activities, such as walking for three or more times per week, 30 or more minutes per occasion, should be increased from 50% to 60%." *Healthy People 2000*

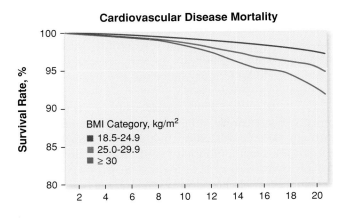

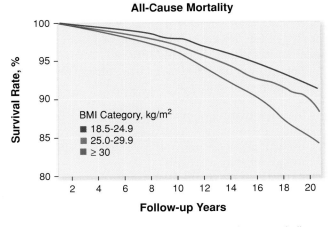

FIGURE 21.4. Survival curves for cardiovascular disease and all-cause mortality by body mass index (BMI) categories. Data are from 25,714 men with 1025 all-cause deaths and 439 cardiovascular disease deaths during 258,781 man-years of observation. Obese men had a 2.6 times higher risk for cardiovascular disease and a 1.9 times higher risk for all-cause mortality compared with normal-weight men. In this study, exercise tolerance (maximal metabolic equivalents) was inversely related to BMI category. (Modified with permission from Wei M, Kampert JB, Barlow CE, et al. Relationship between low cardiorespiratory fitness and mortality in normal-weight, overweight, and obese men. *JAMA* 1999;282:1547–1553.)

energy expenditures (2). A 23% lower mortality rate was also associated with moderately vigorous sports play initiated in middle age (3).

Similarly, studies investigating the effect of physical fitness on all-cause mortality have been performed, leading to the conclusion that the least fit male versus the most fit male has a 3.5 times greater risk of mortality. The same comparison in women showed that least fit women had 4.5 times greater risk (4). In addition, other risk factors added to low habitual physical activity and physical fitness exacerbate the problem. For example, *Figure 21.4* shows how being overweight or obese potentiates mortality rates in men with low cardiovascular fitness. However, just because a person is lean does not provide immunity. Lean people who are unfit have death rates two to three times higher than obese people who are moderately fit.

These studies demonstrate that physical activity and physical fitness are independently related to reduced mortality. The reduction in mortality rate is related to a myriad of physiologic adaptations that occur with regular exercise training. However, benefits also accrue when extra physical activity apart from formal exercise is performed. Although it is independently related to disease risk, note that the key physiologic marker linking physical activity and cardiovascular fitness is $\dot{V}O_{2max}$, which is increased by engaging in endurance activities. Cardiovas-

is a document managed by the Office of Disease Prevention and Health Promotion, United States Department of Health and Human Services. This document lists goals and objectives that originally were to be met in the year 2000 and have been updated for the year 2010.

Although vigorous activity of the kind and intensity that promote an increase in cardiovascular fitness (i.e., $\dot{V}O_{2max}$) is still advocated in *Healthy People 2000* (objective B), it is noteworthy that vigorous is defined in the 2000 objectives as an intensity equal to 50% or greater of maximal cardiorespiratory capacity. This is a level that is 10% lower than the intensity specified as vigorous in the 1990 objectives. This clear trend toward a recommendation of moderate as opposed to vigorous exercise recognizes the importance of getting a large percentage of the population to be physically active. Most people are more likely to adhere to moderate but not vigorous exercise. Even though the likelihood of realizing gains in $\dot{V}O_{2max}$ (i.e., cardiovascular endurance) is less for moderately intense exercise, this is rightly seen as inconsequential because health benefits are still achievable when exercising at a moderate intensity level.

Although cardiovascular endurance has a genetic component that explains 25% to 40% of the variation in fitness among individuals, habitual physical activity is the major determinant of this component of physical fitness. Therefore, for all practical purposes, cardiovascular endurance can only be attained through a program of prescribed physical activity that applies the training principles of specificity and overload to activities that stress the physiologic systems involved in $O_2$ transport and metabolism. When these principles are applied to endurance training programs, the body adapts by increasing its ability to deliver and utilize $O_2$. As we saw in Chapter 14, specificity refers to the type of activity chosen to reach a defined goal, and overload refers to the manipulation of exercise training activity over a period of time (e.g., months) to systematically increase physiologic stress so that physiologic systems undergo a gradual adaptation. Both of these concepts are revisited in this chapter, which covers cardiopulmonary exercise prescription.

▶ *INQUIRY SUMMARY.* Physical fitness and regular physical activity confer tangible health benefits to individuals. If enough people were more active, the overall increase in the health of the population would be of great benefit to society. However, even with this knowledge the large majority of individuals still do not exercise regularly. *What are some ways in which a health care professional can advocate for increased exercise awareness?*

## The Exercise Prescription

Exercise is a key ingredient in cardiopulmonary rehabilitation. However, the status of the patient with regard to the course of the disease, i.e., the **acute**, **subacute**, or **chronic** state, dictates how exercise is used. In the acute phase, early mobilization is a key aspect of the rehabilitative process. However, in the management of subacute and chronic cardiopulmonary and cardiovascular dysfunctions, therapeutic exercise training becomes a vital aspect of rehabilitation. Mobilization is the therapeutic and prescriptive application of low-intensity exercise or other movements designed to produce gravitational and mild exercise stimuli. The goal of early mobilization is to exploit the acute effects of exercise and gravitational stress to optimize $O_2$ transport. However, exercise training focuses on chronic physiologic adaptations in the long-term management of cardiopulmonary disorders. The goal of exercise training is to exploit the cumulative effects of and adaptation to long-term exercise to optimize the function of all steps in the $O_2$ transport system. For both mobilization and exercise training, a properly developed prescription is an essential therapeutic intervention.

Mobilization prescription in a patient with acute cardiopulmonary dysfunction is a key component of cardiopulmonary physical therapy when managing the acutely ill patient. Mobilization prescription per se is different than exercise prescription in that the acutely ill patient cannot be exercise tested in the conventional manner and therefore a typical exercise prescription based on a graded exercise test cannot be written.

 **LINKUP:** *See* **Perspective: Mobilization Prescription for Acute Cardiopulmonary Dysfunction,** *found at http:// connection.lww.com/go/brownexphys and on the Student Resource CD-ROM, describes the unique needs of these acutely ill patients.*

As we saw in Chapter 19, an exercise prescription is a plan for physical activity formulated to achieve specific beneficial outcomes while minimizing accompanying risks. Exercise prescriptions have at least three primary functions.

1. Increase functional capacity
2. Improve health by reducing risk factors for chronic disease
3. Ensure safety during exercise

A properly conceived exercise prescription is an important tool in the management of the acute and chronic disease patient, and the apparently healthy adult or child. Inappropriate exercise for a given individual and a lack of sound counseling about exercise can lead to dangerous situations in which the health and sometimes the life of the person can be compromised. While these three common functions of the exercise prescription should be considered in every activity plan, each should be weighted differently with regards to the particular needs of the individual client. "The art of exercise prescription is the successful integration of exercise science with behavioral techniques that result in long-term program adherence and attainment of the individual's goals." (5)

## THE EXERCISE PRESCRIPTION INTERVENTION TRIAD

The exercise prescription intervention triad (refer to Fig. 19.7), introduced in Chapter 19, serves as the conceptual framework in this chapter for developing exercise prescription interventions. The triad is a comprehensive conceptual framework that applies to any of the systems shown on its base. As a comprehensive model, not all of its many components may be easily fitted to the rehabilitation of a given psycho-physiologic system. The focus of Chapters 20 and 21 is on exercise testing and training to rehabilitate patients with specific cardiopulmonary dysfunctions. However, as you can see from the base of the triad, testing for cardiopulmonary impairment gives us only one aspect of the total functional status of a given patient or client. A given individual may have functional limitations in a number of the different systems shown on the base of the triad. Therapeutic intervention following assessment of the functional status of these systems is directed toward specific problems identified, and a total rehabilitation approach is possible when multiple limitations are found. Oftentimes for the chronic patient, the cardiopulmonary system represents the *limiting* system for performing activities of daily living; therefore, prime attention is usually given to improving the functional capacity of the $O_2$ transport system. Toward that end, assessing the functional status of the cardiopulmonary system was addressed in Chapter 20. To effect physiologic rehabilitation of the cardiopulmonary system, we now address the two ascending limbs of the triad, *dosage* and *activity*.

## EXERCISE PRESCRIPTION FOR CARDIOVASCULAR ENDURANCE IMPAIRMENT

The activity limb of the triad relates to the type of activity chosen to rehabilitate a particular impairment associated with a system shown on the base of the triad. Since this chapter is concerned only with the rehabilitation of subacute and chronic cardiopulmonary disorders, the activity chosen will necessarily pertain to that goal. For example, if aerobic activity is chosen, the mode can be cycling, swimming, walking, or any similar mode of rhythmic movement that stresses the $O_2$ transport system. However, if the focus of rehabilitation is on an impairment of the neuromuscular system, balance and coordination training may be chosen, with the mode being a balance board, balance beam, or computerized balance device. The mode chosen will determine posture (e.g., standing, sitting, supine, prone, etc.). Further, the movement needs to be specifically defined. Posture and movement are two aspects of activity prescription that may be concerned more specifically with rehabilitating systems other than the cardiopulmonary system shown on the base of the triad. In this chapter, we concentrate on the use of aerobic exercise training to rehabilitate the cardiopulmonary system.

The dosage limb of the triad has eight components. Of these, feedback, environment, and sequence are covered in the section of the chapter entitled the Exercise Session. Speed and contraction are more properly related to rehabilitation of neuromuscular and musculoskeletal impairments and are not covered in this chapter. The other three components of dosage, **intensity**, **duration**, and **frequency**, relate specifically to intervention for decreased cardiovascular endurance and are the items inherent to the traditional exercise prescription.

**LINKUP:** *Physical therapists must take into account individual impairments and abilities in establishing exercise prescriptions.* **Perspective: Exercise Prescription for Various Clinical Populations Typically Seen by Physical Therapists,** *found at http://connection.lww.com/go/brownexphys and on the Student Resource CD-ROM, presents several impairments that a physical therapist may encounter.*

The dose of exercise can be characterized, as in prescription of medicine, in terms of potency, slope, maximal effect, variability, and side effects. Potency relates to the power of a dose of exercise to cause a given physiologic response. As dose increases, potency increases and produces a corresponding physiologic effect. Slope relates to the change in response (effect) of the health-related outcome for a given change in dose. Over a wide range of effective dosages (i.e., frequency, duration, and intensity of activity), the response will be a linear increase; however, with increasing dosage, slope occurs as the response tapers off and plateaus. Diminishing return is a characteristic of the prescription of exercise *and* medicine. At some point more dosage is not better. Slope is also related to the particular response variable being studied, as some health-related benefits may take months to realize while others occur more quickly.

Maximal effect relates to the effect dose has on outcomes. For example, strenuous exercise (high dosage) increases $\dot{V}O_{2max}$ and modifies risk factors, while light exercise (low dosage) usually does not increase $\dot{V}O_{2max}$ but does change risk factors. Variability refers to the variable responses among individuals to exercise training. Not everyone will respond alike or to the same degree to exercise training. Side effects refer to the fact that exercise can produce both positive and negative (side) effects. A side effect of exercise may be sudden death or something less severe like sore muscles.

The American College of Sports Medicine generally recommends three to five exercise sessions per week of 20 to 60 minutes per session and an intensity of about 55%/65% to 90% of maximal heart rate, which relates to about 40%/50% to 85% of heart rate (HR) reserve or $\dot{V}O_2R$. The achievement of an energy expenditure of approximately 200 to 300 kcal should be the minimum goal for any client. Individuals with very low functional capacities, such as debilitated cardiopulmonary patients, will not be able to achieve this exercise dosage from the outset of their reha-

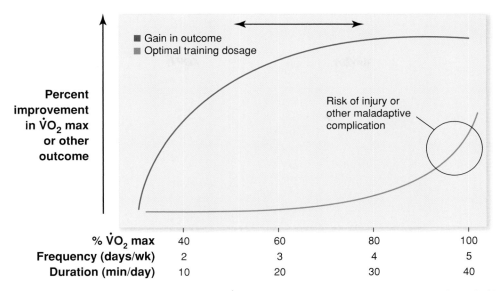

FIGURE 21.5. As exercise dosage increases, both functional status ($\dot{V}O_{2max}$) and health outcomes increase in a curvilinear fashion. As the top curve shows, the patient and therapist can expect diminishing returns, and the curve can be moved to the left (for the patient) or to the right (for the trained athlete).

bilitative effort, but this energy expenditure can serve as an attainable goal. Over time, dosage variables can be manipulated and exercise increased to allow patients who are adapting well to the exercise prescription to achieve this level of energy expenditure. Patients will realize gains in cardiovascular fitness and achieve positive health outcomes when the cardiopulmonary system is overloaded in an effective and safe manner.

As shown in *Figure 21.5*, intensity, frequency, and duration (X-axis) are related to functional improvement or health outcomes (Y-axis). The therapist can manipulate these dosage variables for any given individual to achieve his/her functional and health-related goals. The optimal training dosage shown in the figure applies to most individuals. However, care should be taken when applying this optimal dosage to patients with cardiopulmonary and/or cardiovascular dysfunctions. The top curve may be moved to the left for cardiopulmonary patients, indicating that the plateau in functional or health gains may occur earlier on the X-axis. Health outcomes and $\dot{V}O_{2max}$ can even be improved with lighter exercise dosages for individuals starting with low fitness levels. Also shown in Figure 21.5, risks associated with increasing exercise dosage may include orthopedic, or worse, cardiac complications.

While frequency and duration can be effectively manipulated to progressively overload the cardiopulmonary system, intensity more precisely defines the overload imposed on the cardiopulmonary system to bring about a positive adaptive response. Therefore, intensity is the most important dosage component in the rehabilitation of cardiopulmonary and cardiovascular dysfunctions. Because of its relative importance in the dosage limb of the triad, intensity should be prescribed very carefully.

There have been recent advances in our understanding of exercise intensity prescription. Case Study 21.1 presents an example of using % $\dot{V}O_2R$ in prescribing exercise intensity, and Case Study 21.2 follows up on a case presented in Chapter 20 by providing an exercise prescription for the patient. As you review these cases, keep the exercise prescription intervention triad in mind. The triad is an important model that should help you visualize the relationships among the components of the exercise prescription.

 *LINKUP:* **Case Study: Exercise Prescription for a Patient with Chronic Obstructive Pulmonary Disease,** *found at http://connection.lww.com/go/brownexphys and on the Student Resource CD-ROM, provides an exercise prescription for the patient with chronic obstructive pulmonary disease introduced in Chapter 19.*

▶ *INQUIRY SUMMARY.* The exercise prescription is an important aspect of the rehabilitation of cardiopulmonary patients. Key components of the exercise prescription are activity and dosage. Through exercise prescription, the therapist progressively manipulates dosage variables to effect gradual physiologic improvement. Of all the variables in the dosage component, exercise intensity must be precisely prescribed. *Why is exercise intensity the most important component of dosage in prescribing exercise?*

## Cardiopulmonary Rehabilitation

The term cardiopulmonary rehabilitation is used here to refer to programs that enhance the quality of life for cardiac

## CASE STUDY 21.1: *MYOCARDIAL INFARCTION PATIENT*

### CASE

Frank, a 46-year-old, 180-pound sales-man, was admitted to the hospital complaining of chest pain, which was late diagnosed as acute inferior wall myocardial infarction (MI). After catheterization, it was determined that Frank's left anterior descending coronary artery was 95% blocked. Frank immediately underwent a percutaneous transluminal coronary angioplasty procedure to dilate the artery. This procedure was successful with only mild damage to the left ventricle. Echocardiography showed a short time later that Frank's left ventricular performance was normal (ejection fraction +53%). Frank was allowed to convalesce for 2 weeks following which he was given a symptom-limited graded exercise test. The following were the outcomes:

- Normal sinus rhythm and no ischemic responses
- Resting heart rate (HR) of 64 beats per minute (bpm)
- Maximal HR of 158 bpm
- Resting blood pressure of 130/78 mm Hg
- Maximal blood pressure of 165/85 mm Hg
- $\dot{V}O_{2max}$ of 6.5 metabolic equivalents (MET) after finishing 7 minutes of the Bruce protocol

### INTERPRETATION AND EXERCISE PRESCRIPTION

A peak MET level of 6.5 represents Frank's functional aerobic capacity, a low level for his age. The American College of Sports Medicine recommends that the intensity prescription can begin as low as 40% of $\dot{V}O_2R$. Given Frank's relatively young age and successful medical treatment, you decide to provide a target HR based on 50% to 70% $\dot{V}O_2R$, equivalent to 50% to 70% HR reserve (HRR). The following calculation gives Frank's target MET:

$$
\begin{aligned}
\text{Target } \dot{V}O_2 &= (\% \text{ intensity})(\dot{V}O_{2max} - \dot{V}O_{rest}) + 1 \\
&= 0.50(6.5 - 1) + 1 \\
&= 0.50(5.5) + 1 \\
&= 2.8 + 1 \\
&= 3.8 \text{ MET or } 13.3 \text{ mL·kg}^{-1}\text{·min}^{-1} \text{ at 50\%} \\
&\quad \dot{V}O_2R
\end{aligned}
$$

and

$$
= 4.9 \text{ MET or } 17.2 \text{ mL·kg}^{-1}\text{·min}^{-1} \text{ at 70\%}\ \dot{V}O_2R
$$

The corresponding target HR at this metabolic load would be:

$$
\begin{aligned}
\text{Target HR} &= (\% \text{ intensity})(HR_{max} - HR_{rest}) + HR_{rest} \\
&= 0.50(158 - 64) + 64 \\
&= 0.50(94) + 64 \\
&= 47 + 64 \\
&= 111 \text{ bpm at 50\% HRR}
\end{aligned}
$$

and

$$
= 130 \text{ bpm at 70\% HRR}
$$

Based on this metabolic training load, calculate appropriate treadmill and cycle ergometer workloads that would represent this $\dot{V}O_2$ and HR prescription. *How would you prescribe exercise duration for this patient at the beginning of phase II, and how would you progress the patient through the course of phase II?* The answers to these questions relate to the inverse relationship between exercise intensity and duration. Early in the course of phase II, Frank needs to stay on the low end of the intensity prescription so that his physiologic responses can be monitored to make sure he is tolerating this load well. His exercise duration therefore can be lengthened to a time that he can conformably endure without becoming exhausted. Duration will be derived by trial and error with prudent attention paid to the patient's signs and symptoms during exertion. As he becomes fit, he may be progressed initially in such a way that increases the duration of activity at the same exercise intensity (i.e., 50% $\dot{V}O_2R$). An interesting caveat to this is that as Frank's functional capacity increases, he will have to perform greater ergometric workloads to maintain the same relative intensity of work (i.e., %HRR and % $\dot{V}O_2R$). In this regard, his exercise intensity prescription will naturally increase, allowing him to do a higher ergometric workload at the same relative exercise intensity. Indeed, there may never be a real need to increase Frank's exercise intensity prescription given this naturally occurring increase in ergometric workload. After the phase II period, Frank should progress into phases III and IV. If weight loss is a goal, he should concentrate on activities that maximally optimize caloric expenditure and work up to expending at least 1000 kcal per week.

and/or pulmonary patients. The same general model used for the rehabilitation of the cardiac patient is applicable to the pulmonary patient. However, many of these programs are dichotomized, that is, the program may see only cardiac patients or pulmonary patients but not both. In this chapter, we treat them together while recognizing their vital differences. One obvious difference is that the course of the disease for the cardiac and pulmonary patient may be quite different. For example, the cardiac patient usually experiences a sudden event (e.g., MI) around which medical

management and the rehabilitative effort are focused. Pulmonary disease, however, is much more subtle, taking longer to emerge as a hindrance in the life of the person. The rehabilitation effort in such a case may start well after the disease course has caused considerable damage, thereby ultimately assuring that rehabilitation will be less effective.

Cardiopulmonary rehabilitation is a multidisciplinary program of education, risk factor modification, and exercise intervention to assist individuals with cardiopulmonary and

## CASE STUDY 21.2: *EXERCISE PRESCRIPTION FOR A PATIENT WITH CARDIAC BYPASS GRAFT SURGERY*

 This patient was introduced in Chapter 20. The following is a sample exercise prescription for this individual based on his functional capacity of 8.9 metabolic equivalents (MET) at a heart rate (HR) of 135 beats per minute (bpm) and a peak workload of 3.4 mi·hr$^{-1}$ at 14% grade on the treadmill (not steady rate). Stuart has a good exercise capacity for his age and medical status; therefore, he qualifies for a phase III program. He should begin with an exercise intensity range of approximately 50% to 70% $\dot{V}O_2R$ (50% to 70% HR reserve [HRR]). If his resting $\dot{V}O_2$ is 3.5 mL·kg$^{-1}$·min$^{-1}$, the target metabolic intensity is calculated to be:

Target $\dot{V}O_2$ = (% intensity)($\dot{V}O_{2max}$ − $\dot{V}O_{2rest}$) + 1
$$= 0.50(98.9 - 1) + 1$$
$$= 0.50(7.9) + 1$$
$$= 4.0 + 1$$
$$= 5.0 \text{ MET (17.5 mL·kg}^{-1}\text{·min}^{-1}) \text{ at 50\% } \dot{V}O_2R$$

and

$$= 6.5 \text{ MET (22.8 mL·kg}^{-1}\text{·min}^{-1}) \text{ at 70\% } \dot{V}O_2R$$

The corresponding target heart rate at this metabolic load would be:

Target HR = (% intensity)(HR$_{max}$ − HR$_{rest}$) + HR$_{rest}$
$$= 0.50(135 - 75) + 75$$
$$= 0.50(60) + 75$$
$$= 30 + 75$$
$$= 105 \text{ bpm at 50\% HRR}$$
or
$$= 117 \text{ bpm at 70\% HRR}$$

Comparing this exercise intensity prescription with the results of his stress test shows that Stuart would be exercising at a likely dyspnea rating of +2 and will likely experience a 1-mm ST horizontal depression. These are acceptable responses given his overall exercise tolerance and the fact that he did not experience angina during the test. The key for Stuart is to increase his exercise tolerance gradually and work up to an acceptable caloric expenditure for weight reduction. He should begin on a 3 d·wk$^{-1}$ routine at 20 to 30 min·d$^{-1}$ (this may be continuous or discontinuous as tolerated). As he progresses, the therapist should increase exercise duration as tolerated until Stuart is able to exercise continuously for 45 to 60 minutes. Over time this will positively impact his body composition and weight. Stuart should also be referred to a clinical dietitian for nutrition education and weight reduction. Stuart's systolic blood pressure should be monitored, and he should have electrocardiograms to check for ischemic responses during each visit.

cardiovascular dysfunctions to achieve optimal physical, psychologic, and functional status within the limitations of their disease. Positive functional outcomes are realized because improvements in central and peripheral circulation, pulmonary ventilation, and the autonomic nervous system increase patients' tolerance for work. Psychologic benefits also arise from the improved emotional stability and self-esteem that stem from the rehabilitative effort.

Cardiopulmonary rehabilitation programs encompass a four-phase approach tied to patient status. The process of recovery starts from the time of the acute event and extends through the subacute and chronic phases of recovery. For the purpose of classifying patient status, cardiopulmonary rehabilitation is divided into inpatient (acute status, phase I) and outpatient (subacute status, phase II; chronic status, phases III and IV) rehabilitation. Acute patients are hospitalized and are initially placed in the intensive or coronary care unit. When the medical condition of the patient becomes stable, the patient is placed in the stepdown unit and phase I cardiopulmonary rehabilitation usually begins at this point. A team of professionals such as physicians, nurses, physical therapists, dietitians, and respiratory therapists is usually involved in all phases of cardiopulmonary

rehabilitation. Phase I may last as long as the patient is in the hospital, which may be several days to as long as 2 weeks. Longer hospital courses are generally associated with patients that have more complications, which in turn result in higher morbidity and mortality rates. The activity plan in phase I stresses early mobilization and light exercise and/or movement activity. The general goal of phase I is to prepare the patient for living at home with little assistance after discharge and to effect early physiologic adaptation for a smooth entrance into phase II, early outpatient rehabilitation. The following are more immediate goals of phase I cardiopulmonary rehabilitation:

- Evaluate physiologic responses to self-care and ambulation activities
- Provide feedback to physicians and nurses regarding physiologic responses
- Prevent further deconditioning
- Prepare and identify safe guidelines for progression of activity through convalescence
- Provide patient and family education regarding disease progression, risk factor modification, self-monitoring techniques, and general home activity guidelines

*Table 21.2* presents a typical activity plan for progressing a stable patient through phase I, which ends when the patient is discharged from the hospital.

*LINKUP: When considering exercise intensity, the relationship between %HR_{max} and %\dot{V}O_{2max} is an important consideration. Knowledge of the rectilinear relationship between HR and \dot{V}O_2 is essential to formulate the exercise intensity prescription. This linear relationship allows the clinician to use HR (a variable easy to measure) rather that \dot{V}O_2 (a variable complicated and impractical to measure) to set exercise intensity along prescribed metabolic (\dot{V}O_2) limits. Consult* **Perspective: Principles of Regression and Exercise Prescription,** *found at http://connection.lww.com/go/brownexphys and on the Student Resource CD-ROM, for a better understanding of current issues regarding the relationship between %HR_{max} and % \dot{V}O_{2max}.*

The subacute phase of rehabilitation, phase II, begins as early as 24 hours after hospital discharge and lasts up to 6 weeks. Specific goals of all outpatient phases of cardiopulmonary rehabilitation include the following:

- Improve functional capacity through an individualized exercise prescription
- Provide education so that the patient can understand the disease for better lifestyle management of risk factors
- Improve confidence and self-reliance to become independent in all areas of care
- Teach behaviors that are consistent with attaining and maintaining good health

Additional goals for pulmonary patients and strategies to meet these goals include the following:

- Improve respiratory symptoms by mobilizing respiratory secretions (to enhance airway clearance) and em-

ploying strategies to relieve shortness of breath and strengthen respiratory muscles
- Improve nutritional status by maintaining optimal body weight and composition
- Improve psychologic status by treating stress and depression that accompany severe pulmonary disease

Outpatients in phase II are closely supervised and monitored during the exercise program. They may report to the outpatient clinic (hospital or other formal clinical setting) as many as 3 days per week. Trained health care personnel provide supervision, and monitoring is provided in the form of electrocardiogram (ECG), blood pressure, HR, arterial $O_2$ saturation, signs and symptoms of exercise intolerance, and other variables as needed.

The subacute status progresses to the chronic status (phases III and IV) with continued healing and improved exercise tolerance. To achieve this status, patients are independent in performing self-monitoring techniques, medically stable, and no longer require frequent ECG monitoring. In phases III and IV, the chronic patient undergoes continual exercise training to further physiologic adaptation. Phase III lasts for about 6 weeks, and the goal is to improve on the physiologic gains made during phase II. Monitoring and supervision are less intrusive. For example, ECG monitoring in phase II is continual but is only intermittent as needed in phase III. Patients in phase III are gradually weaned from intense monitoring with a goal being to become a more independent exerciser in a phase IV program. The supervision and monitoring involved in phase III is therefore purposefully reduced to achieve this goal. Phase III exercise sessions are usually conducted 3 to 5 days per week.

Heart disease requires active intervention for life; therefore, the successful phase IV program should be considered a "maintenance" phase. However, this term can be misleading because the phase IV patient can and does continue to improve physiologically and does not just maintain the

| Table 21.2 | ACTIVITY GUIDE AND FUNCTIONAL CLASSIFICATION FOR INPATIENT CARDIOPULMONARY REHABILITATION | |
|---|---|---|
| **Functional Class** | **Inpatient Activities** | |
| I | Sits up in bed with assistance; does own self-care activities (seated or may need assistance); stands at bedside with assistance; sits up in chair for 15–30 minutes 2–3 times per day | |
| II | Sits up in bed independently; stands independently; does own self-care activities in bathroom, seated; walks in room and to bathroom | |
| III | Sits and stands independently; does own self-care activities in bathroom, seated or standing; walks in halls with assistance for short distances (50–100 feet) as tolerated up to 3 times per day | |
| IV | Does own self-care and bathes; walks in halls for short distances (150–200 feet) with minimal assistance 3–4 times per day. | |
| V | Walk in halls independently for moderate distances (250–500 feet) 3–4 times per day | |
| VI | Independent ambulation on unit 3–6 times per day or as desired | |

| Table 21.3 | NEW YORK HEART ASSOCIATION CLASSIFICATIONS WITH GUIDELINES FOR EXPECTED EXERCISE CAPACITIES AND PERMISSIBLE WORKLOADS | | | |
|---|---|---|---|---|
| **Status** | **Characteristics** | **Maximal Capacity (MET)** | **Maximal Permissible Workload (kcal/min and MET\*)** | |
| | | | Continuous | Intermittent |
| I | Can walk without symptoms or limitation; can do most light effort activities; 0–15% impairment | 6.5 | 4.0/3.2 | 6.0/4.9 |
| II | Has symptoms with light work; slight limitation of physical activity; comfortable at rest; ordinary physical activity results in fatigue, palpitations, dyspnea, or angina; 15–30% impairment | > 4.5 < 6.5 | 3.0/2.5 | 4.0/3.2 |
| III | Has symptoms with minimal effort; marked limitation of physical activity; comfortable at rest; less than ordinary physical activity results in fatigue, palpitations, dyspnea, or angina; 30–70% impairment | 3.0 | 2.0/1.6 | 3.0/2.5 |
| IV | Is unable to carry on any physical activity without discomfort; discomfort increases with exercise; symptoms may be present at rest; >70% impairment | 1.5 | 1.0/1.0 | 2.0/1.6 |

\*MET calculated assuming 5 kcal·L $O_2^{-1}$ and a 70-kg person. MET, metabolic equivalents.

functional gains achieved to that point. The formal phase IV program should last for at least 6 months, and the phase IV patient should be encouraged to continue to make exercise a habitual part of their daily routine after that period by becoming involved in a home- or community-based exercise program. As with the healthy individual, the lifestyle pattern of exercise and risk factor modification should hopefully last the rest of the individual's life.

The New York Heart Association has established general guidelines for exercise rehabilitation of cardiopulmonary patients. This classification system is presented in *Table 21.3*. The table gives an estimate of patients' likely exercise capacity with reasonable targets for exercise during rehabilitation. These general guidelines, while helpful, should not replace the direct determination of functional capacity via graded exercise testing. *Table 21.4* presents general exercise prescription guidelines for patient groups common in cardiopulmonary rehabilitation.

*Figure 21.6* provides a scheme of how patients may progress from one phase of cardiopulmonary rehabilitation to the next. Although this scheme is generalized, the exercise prescription must be individualized to each patient to be optimally effective. The patient's response to the rehabilitation effort must be individually determined prior to being moved from one phase to the next. As can be seen in Figure 21.6, graduation from one phase to the next, beginning in phase II, should ideally be partially based on the results of a graded exercise test. This provides objective standards by which to judge satisfactory improvements in functional capacity. Regardless of the phase the individual

is in, the medical stability of the patient should be continually assessed. Patients may digress even in the later phases of cardiopulmonary rehabilitation. The unstable status may be warranted because of some of the following: ischemic pain, congestive heart failure, resting tachycardia, severe bradycardia. These conditions should limit participation in an exercise program on a given day, and a reevaluation of the patient would be warranted. Case Study 21.3 presents a patient who becomes unstable while in phase II.

▶ *INQUIRY SUMMARY.* Cardiopulmonary rehabilitation is divided into inpatient and outpatient phases, which are designed to track the patient's recovery starting from the moment the individual is stable and following through the subacute and chronic stages. The main focus of rehabilitation is the safe administration of an exercise prescription, which is designed to increase functional capacity. *Why is an increase in functional capacity of prime importance for the average cardiopulmonary patient?*

## The Exercise Session

Once a patient has been referred to cardiopulmonary rehabilitation, the rehabilitation team must work together to formulate a program that is comprehensive and individualized to the person's needs. Exercise is only one aspect of the total program. Other needs may involve health care personnel skilled in providing behavior modification sessions such as weight control and nutritional counseling, smoking

| Table 21.4 | GENERAL EXERCISE PRESCRIPTION GUIDELINES FOR SPECIFIC CLIENT/PATIENT GROUPS IN OUTPATIENT CARDIOPULMONARY REHABILITATION | | |
|---|---|---|---|
| **Dysfunction** | **Exercise Prescription** | **Progression** | **Precautions** |
| Pacemaker Dependent, chronotropically competent | 20–60 min·session$^{-1}$; 4–7 d·wk$^{-1}$; 50–85% HRR (or % $\dot{V}O_2R$) | Tied to increases in work rate as fitness improves | Limit upper body movements for 2–3 weeks following implantation |
| Pacemaker Dependent, chronotropically incompetent | 20–60 min·session$^{-1}$; 50–85% SBP rate with targeted $\dot{V}O_2$ and RPE limits | Training intensity reduced at initiation of session and increased gradually | Modify Karvonen THR formula to reflect SBP; limit upper body movements for 2–3 weeks following implantation; more extensive warmup and cooldown periods and SBP monitored throughout sessions |
| Congestive heart failure | 10–40 min·session$^{-1}$ with initial brief sessions and 2–6-minute intervals with 1–2 minutes of rest; 3–7 d·wk$^{-1}$; 40–75% HRR (or %$\dot{V}O_2R$); RPE and dyspnea scale may be preferentially used | 10–15-minute warmup and cooldown periods, lengthen training sessions as tolerated | Patients should have at least a 3-MET functional capacity |
| Cardiac transplant | 15–60 min·session$^{-1}$; 4–6 d·wk$^{-1}$; 50–70% HRR (or %$\dot{V}O_2R$) | Progressively lengthen training sessions | Monitoring should focus on resting and exercise BP, adverse immunosuppressive drug therapy effect, and evidence of rejection; angina symptoms are absent due to denervation; exercise ECG is insensitive in detecting myocardial ischemia; longer periods of warmup and cooldown are needed |
| Stable angina | 5–10 min·session$^{-1}$ for 2–3 times per day may be considered as an alternative to the more traditional format of longer sessions; 4–6 d·wk$^{-1}$; set THR ≥10 bpm below the ischemic ECG or anginal threshold | Warmup and cooldown ≥10 minutes; HR should be progressed gradually in each session | Exercise may be inappropriate for patients with an anginal threshold of 3 MET or less; goal is to increase ischemic ECG threshold by lowering submaximal exercise double product; patients should be taught to grade anginal episodes on a scale of 1–4 |
| Stable heart disease | 20–60 min·session$^{-1}$; 3–5 d·wk$^{-1}$; 40–50% $\dot{V}O_2R$ is threshold intensity for significant adaptations | Individualization is important to achieve because of the great disparity in functional capacities; patients should achieve a caloric expenditure of 1000 kcal·wk$^{-1}$ after 3–6 months of training | Training can be continuous or intermittent activity but duration is inversely related to intensity; exercise intensity should be above threshold required to produce physiologic adaptations but below that producing abnormal clinical signs or symptoms |
| Pulmonary disease | Exercise should be started for several minutes as tolerated for 3–5 d·wk$^{-1}$ at 50% $\dot{V}O_2R$ | Intermittent several times per day until endurance improves; then move to more traditional 3–5 d·wk$^{-1}$ scheme | Generally lower functional capacity patients require more frequent exercise exposure |
| Hypertension | 30 min·session$^{-1}$; 3–7 d·wk$^{-1}$; 40–70% $\dot{V}O_2R$ | Progress to about 700–2000 kcal·wk$^{-1}$ energy expenditure | Exaggerated pressor responses should be avoided; medication regimen should remain consistent around exercise |

| | **Table 21.4** | **GENERAL EXERCISE PRESCRIPTION GUIDELINES FOR SPECIFIC CLIENT/PATIENT GROUPS IN OUTPATIENT CARDIOPULMONARY REHABILITATION** (Continued) | | |

| Dysfunction | Exercise Prescription | Progression | Precautions |
| --- | --- | --- | --- |
| PVD | 20–40 min·session$^{-1}$; 3–7 d·wk$^{-1}$; 40–70% $\dot{V}O_2R$ | As exercise tolerance is increased and PVD is no longer as great a limiting factor, patients often manifest underlying coronary artery disease symptoms (i.e., angina) | Use of the claudication scale is indicated to judge leg pain during exercise intermittently to a score of 3 out of 4; weight-bearing exercise is preferred since greater functional adaptations will ensue. |
| Diabetes mellitus | 20–60-minute daily sessions at 40–70% $\dot{V}O_2R$ (use RPE scale as tolerated if HR response is blunted) | As tolerated | If obese (type II), caloric expenditure should be maximized; do not exercise when blood glucose >300 mg·dL$^{-1}$; as a novice exerciser, monitor blood glucose before, during, and after exercise if taking insulin or oral agents; do not inject insulin into the muscle groups to be exercised; consume carbohydrate snacks during exercise; insulin-dependent individuals should exercise on the lower end of the duration scale per session and make exercise a daily pattern; non-insulin-dependent people should exercise on the upper end and exercise only 4–5 days per week |

These guidelines are for aerobic (endurance) type activities. In all examples, the exercise prescription should be based on a recent symptom-limited exercise test with specific reference to workload achieved, ECG and hemodynamic response, perceived exertion, and symptoms. Patients should have no absolute contraindications and in the case of more debilitated patients (i.e., congestive heart failure) more definitive tests such as exercise echocardiogram, radionuclide studies, and gas analysis may help formulate workloads that avoid ischemic wall motion abnormalities, a drop in ejection fraction, excessive pulmonary wedge pressures, or that exceeds the ventilatory threshold. BP, blood pressure; ECG, electrocardiogram; HR, heart beat; HRR, heart rate reserve; MET, metabolic equivalents; PVD, peripheral vascular disease; RPE; rating of perceived exertion; SBP, systolic blood pressure; THR, target heart rate.

cessation, and stress reduction. Social and psychologic support is also important in cardiopulmonary rehabilitation because these factors enhance patient compliance with exercise training, the backbone of the program.

Of prime importance in the rehabilitative effort is exercise intervention. Therapeutic exercise training must be carefully managed for the individual patient. Referring back to the dosage limb of the exercise prescription intervention triad, factors such as sequence, environment, and feedback relate specifically to planning the exercise session for maximum effect. We now address these factors in order.

## SEQUENCING

Sequencing the cardiorespiratory exercise session consists of properly ordering the session by including for each phase of cardiopulmonary rehabilitation an active warmup period, a training period that applies the principles of specificity and overload, and an active cooldown period. In addition, some resistance exercise training may be applied when the patient has achieved chronic status (phases III and IV) and after a period of baseline cardiorespiratory conditioning has been achieved. The

warmup and cooldown periods of the exercise session slowly increase and decrease, respectively, metabolic rate to allow the individual to attain (during warmup) the overload stimulus and recover (during cooldown) safely from the overload stimulus. These periods should not be overlooked even with phase IV (or home- or community-based) patients who have been training habitually for some time. It is equally as dangerous to abruptly achieve the overload stimulus without a warmup as it is to abruptly cease exercise without a period of cool-down. Without a proper warmup, the patient may be placed needlessly in a state of anaerobic metabolism that may lead to excessive demands on the cardiovascular system (i.e., increased rate pressure product leading to myocardial ischemia). Also, an improper cooldown may lead to complications such as cardiac arrhythmias and the pooling of blood in the extremities, which may cause symptoms of vertigo, syncope, palpitations, or nausea. The length of the warmup and cooldown periods may vary, but some consideration should be given to making these periods last for an extended period of time. An extended period of time (e.g., 15 minutes) for the cooldown is probably more important than for warmup especially if strenuous exercise is employed.

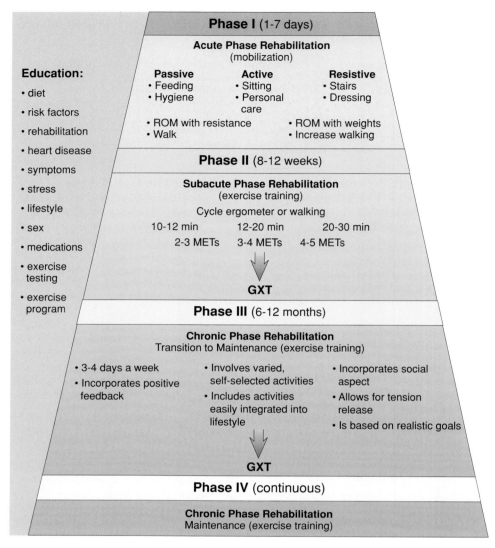

**FIGURE 21.6.** Cardiopulmonary rehabilitation progression over four phases covering the acute, subacute, and chronic states.

## ENVIRONMENT AND FEEDBACK

The environment in which exercise is performed should be quiet, controlled, and professional to ensure, as much as possible, that patient responses will not be adversely affected. The dosage limb category of environment extends to all aspects of the patient's experience in the clinical setting and not just the formalized exercise session. This includes instructions to follow prior to and after exercising. For example, exercise sessions should not be conducted within 2 hours of a heavy meal. Showering after should be brief, using moderate water temperature, and the individual should avoid standing in place too long. Extremes of heat and cold should be avoided, and patients should not exercise in high humidity. However, patients should be taught to modify their exercise prescription when they do exercise in hot environments. For example, work rates should be decreased so that they can remain within their prescribed HR training zone when exercising in heat and humidity. *Can you think of other environmental factors about which you should be concerned?*

Finally, the therapist should be concerned with the patient's ability to learn and adhere to instructions regarding exercise prescription. If the motor task is relatively difficult for the patient, dosage may have to be altered to not cause greater than normal physiologic responses. Feedback is an important factor of the dosage limb of the triad and is necessary to optimize performance.

*LINKUP: A series of research studies beginning in the mid-1990s and continuing today is clarifying the way in which exercise intensity prescriptions are written. One of the more recent studies is presented in* **Research Highlight: The Relationship Between Heart Rate Reserve and $\dot{V}O_2$ Reserve in Patients with Heart Disease,** *found at http://connection.lww.com/go/brownexphys and on the Student Resource CD-ROM.*

## CASE STUDY 21.3: OUTPATIENT CARDIOPULMONARY REHABILITATION

Henry is a retired 65-year-old business-man who had no history of heart disease, chest pain, or dyspnea with activity. However, he has a positive family history (mother and father with heart disease in their sixties). Henry was admitted to the emergency room where he was diagnosed with acute anterior myocardial infarction. Cardiac catheterization showed a total occlusion in the lower one-third of the left anterior descending (LAD) coronary artery and a normal right coronary artery. In recovery from this procedure, he experienced atrial fibrillation and multifocal premature ventricular contractions (PVCs). He was placed on a course of low-dose verapamil.

He spent 4 days in the coronary care unit and was then placed in the stepdown unit, where phase I cardiopulmonary rehabilitation commenced. Phase I was initiated with self-care monitoring during which he demonstrated several abnormal responses. While washing his face, he experienced an abnormally high heart rate and became hypotensive accompanied by syncope. The electrocardiogram (ECG) showed atrial fibrillation. He was returned to bed, self-care was discontinued, and his physician added digoxin to his medication regimen. This improved his ability to perform light activity (responses were normal). He was ob-

served for 2 more days and progressed well. Finally, 6 days after being admitted, he underwent a low-level treadmill test and completed 4.5 minutes of the modified Bruce protocol. There were no ECG ischemic changes, but he did experience multifocal PVCs. Two days after discharge, Henry entered a phase II cardiopulmonary rehabilitation program and was given a low-level exercise prescription (training heart rate of 100 beats per minute). Three weeks into phase II, he was doing 20 minutes of continuous ambulation. He then started to experience a junctional rhythm with frequent episodes of supraventricular tachycardia (rate = 170) and multifocal PVC with coupling. Lightheadedness accompanied these ECG changes. The referring cardiologist was immediately notified, and she increased his dosage of verapamil and scheduled him for a thallium stress test. Before this test could be performed, he presented again to the emergency room with chest pain. A catheterization study confirmed that his old LAD lesion needed to be dilated again. This procedure was successful. He was observed in the hospital for 3 days at the end of which he was given a thallium treadmill test, which demonstrated that a small segment of the left ventricle becomes ischemic under stress. He re-entered the phase II program and commenced with his former exercise prescription with no further problems.

▶ *INQUIRY SUMMARY.* The well-managed exercise session is the heart of the rehabilitative effort for cardiopulmonary patients. Important components of the session interact with the dosage limb of the exercise prescription triad. Safety is a chief concern. *Why should the exercise session be more strictly controlled in phase II, but not in phase III or IV?*

through several outpatient phases. The health care team carefully guides each phase of recovery with outcomes being improved medical and functional status. Physiologic rehabilitation is focused around the exercise session, and the exercise prescription is the guiding tool used to accomplish improved function.

## Summary

People should engage in lifelong exercise and physical activity to remain as healthy as possible as they age. When this is done, they will enjoy a lower risk of chronic disease and will maintain their functional abilities well into old age. When individuals develop a form of cardiopulmonary impairment, exercise prescription and intervention is an essential aspect of the recovery process. Exercise prescription for these patients is formalized based on the functional status of the cardiopulmonary system. Dosage and activity components of the exercise prescription guide the recovery process and allow the safe attainment of higher functional levels. In recovery, the patient undergoes a four-phase stepwise plan that begins in the hospital and continues

### SUMMARY KNOWLEDGE

1. What is the relative reduced risk of disease when adopting a lifestyle of physical activity compared with quitting smoking and controlling high blood pressure?
2. What is activity dosage?
3. If a gain in $\dot{V}O_{2max}$ is the desired outcome, what dosage factors must be of primary concern?
4. Mobilization versus therapeutic exercise training focuses on which aspect of the rehabilitation process during the course of cardiovascular disease?
5. What are the three primary functions of the exercise prescription?
6. What are the goals of outpatient cardiopulmonary rehabilitation?

### References

1. Leon AS, Richardson M. Exercise, health, and disease. In: Roberts SO, Robergs RA, Hanson P, eds. *Clinical exercise testing and prescription: theory and application.* New York: CRC Press, 1997:281–302.
2. Paffenbarger RS, Hyde RT, Wing AL. Physical activity, all-cause mortality, and longevity of college alumni. *N Engl J Med* 1986;314: 605–613.
3. Paffenbarger RS, Hyde RT, Wing AL. The association of changes in physical-activity level and other lifestyle characteristics with mortality among men. *N Engl J Med* 1993;328:538–545.
4. Blair SN, Kohl HW III, Paffenbarger RS. Physical fitness and all-cause mortality. *JAMA* 1989;262:2395–2401.
5. Franklin BA, ed. *ACSM's guidelines for exercise testing and prescription.* 6th ed. Baltimore: Lippincott Williams & Wilkins, 2000.

### Suggested Readings

Cooper CB. Exercise in chronic pulmonary disease: aerobic exercise prescription. *Med Sci Sports Exerc* 2001;33:S671–S679.

LeMura LM, von Duvillard SP, eds. *Clinical exercise physiology: applications and physiological principles.* Baltimore: Lippincott Williams & Wilkins, 2004.

Persinger R, Foster C, Gibson M, et al. Consistency of the talk test for exercise prescription. *Med Sci Sports Exerc* 2004;36:1632–1636.

Storer TW. Exercise in chronic pulmonary disease: resistance exercise prescription. *Med Sci Sports Exerc* 2001;33:S680–S686.

### On the Internet

Exercise Prescription on the Net. Available at: **http://www.exrx.net/**. Accessed August 10, 2005.

The University of York: Cardiac Rehabilitation. Available at: **http://www.cardiacrehabilitation.org.uk/**. Accessed August 10, 2005.

Cardiology.org. Available at: **http://www.cardiology.palo-alto.med.ca.gov/**. Accessed August 10, 2005.

## Writing to Learn

The history of cardiopulmonary rehabilitation is intertwined with the emergence of the use of clinical concepts of exercise physiology in the practice of medicine and allied health. Research and write a paper that investigates the beginning of the practice of cardiopulmonary rehabilitation in North America and answer the question: how has that practice changed the fields of nursing, physical therapy, and medicine? Resting $\dot{V}O_2$ has been assumed to be 3.5 $mL \cdot kg^{-1} \cdot min^{-1}$ for both healthy and clinical populations, and this value plays a large role in exercise prescription. Research and write a paper on why this value may be lower for patients with heart failure and respiratory diseases, and how this may affect the exercise prescription process.

# CHAPTER

# 22 Exercise for Obesity and Weight Control

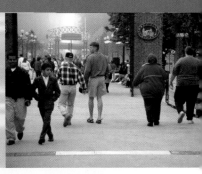

Society's view of overweight has changed dramatically over the past century. What was previously considered a protector against communicable diseases that led to early morbidity and mortality is now considered a risk for some of the biggest killers of modern society: cardiovascular disease, diabetes, and hypertension. As the 20th century unfolded, the medical sciences, as well as the fashion industry, shaped our perceptions about overweight and body fatness. Think of ways that different forms of media have shaped your perceptions about body fat and overweight.

Overweight and obesity are becoming more prevalent in the United States.

## CHAPTER OUTLINE

PROBLEMS WITH OBESITY
- The Prevalence of Obesity
- Obesity and Disease Risk
- Exercise, Body Weight, and Health
- Assessment of the Overweight Patient

ETIOLOGY OF OBESITY
- Genetics and Body Weight
- Energy Intake and Body Fatness
- Diet Composition and Body Composition
- Inactivity and Overweight
- Metabolic Rate and Overweight

PSYCHOLOGIC ASPECTS OF OBESITY
- The Psychologic Profile of the Obese Person
- Body Image Disparagement
- Emotional Distress and Weight Control

BARRIERS TO WEIGHT CONTROL

EFFECTIVENESS OF EXERCISE IN WEIGHT CONTROL
- Exercise and Metabolism
- Exercise Intensity and Substrate Use
- Exercise and Weight-Loss Success

THE EXERCISE PRESCRIPTION

RELAPSE PREVENTION

The prevalence of overweight and obesity has increased dramatically over the past decade in the United States and in many other developed countries. In fact, obesity has been called a modern-day epidemic. Consequently, recent campaigns against obesity have been initiated. Exercise programming is a key strategy used in these campaigns and has been claimed the most effective method a person can use to reduce body weight. The goal of this chapter is to provide insight into the magnitude of the obesity problem, to help you understand the barriers a person faces in weight control, and to outline guidelines for designing exercise prescriptions for the overweight population.

## Problems with Obesity

One of the first problems encountered with **obesity** is trying to define it. *Where does one draw the line between normal weight and* **overweight**, *and between overweight and obesity?*

The World Health Organization and other agencies use **body mass index** (BMI) to distinguish among different categories of body weight for adults (*Table 22.1*). However, for children and adolescents, only one classification is used to define both overweight and obesity (see Chapter 15 and below). Since overweight is simply defined as a less severe form of obesity in adults and both overweight and obesity are used to describe the same condition in children, both terms are often used interchangeably throughout the literature. In the context of this book, the terms overweight and obesity are also used interchangeably. Only when it is necessary to distinguish differences between the categories of overweight and obesity is careful word selection used. Otherwise the reader can assume that whatever parameter is being presented applies to people who are overweight and to those who are obese.

Weight gain and body fat storage have been viewed as signs of health and prosperity throughout most of human history. Today, however, as standards of living continue to

| Table 22.1 | **BMI CLASSIFICATIONS OF OVERWEIGHT AND OBESITY IN ADULTS WITH ASSOCIATED HEALTH RISKS** | |
|---|---|---|
| **Classification** | **BMI** | **Risk of Comorbidities** |
| Underweight | <18.5 | Low |
| Normal weight | 18.5–24.9 | Average |
| Overweight | 25.0–29.9 | Increased |
| Obesity class I | 30.0–34.9 | Moderate |
| Obesity class II | 35.0–39.9 | Severe |
| Obesity class III | ≥40.0 | Very Severe |

BMI = body mass index.

rise, as food production increases, as the percentage of family income spent on food decreases, and as food becomes more readily available, weight gain and obesity are posing a growing threat to public health all over the world. Obesity is a chronic disease that is prevalent in both developed and developing countries—it affects all ethnic groups, both genders, and all age groups, including children. Obesity has become so common that it is replacing more traditional health concerns such as undernutrition and infectious diseases. Despite recent progress in obesity research and treatment, the challenge to public health professionals in fighting the obesity epidemic is great. Obesity presents a problem to health care professionals for several reasons:

- The prevalence of obesity is rising throughout the world
- Obesity is associated with many other diseases or conditions
- Obesity has many **etiologies** and therefore is difficult to treat
- The costs for treating obesity are great
- Obesity hinders rehabilitation for accidents, injuries, and other conditions

## THE PREVALENCE OF OBESITY

It is well known that the prevalence of overweight and obesity in the United States has risen dramatically over the past several years. If a BMI of 25 is used as the criteria for overweight and a BMI of 30 as the criteria for obesity, 126 million Americans or 65% of the adult population is either overweight or obese (*Fig. 22.1*) (1). Although overweight pervades all segments of the population, certain groups present a higher incidence of overweight than others. Overweight is more common among African American and Hispanic women than among Caucasian women. Among African Americans, the proportion of women who are overweight is 80% higher than the proportion of men who are overweight. The same holds true for Hispanic women and men, but the percentage of Caucasian women and men who are overweight is about the same. Overweight is

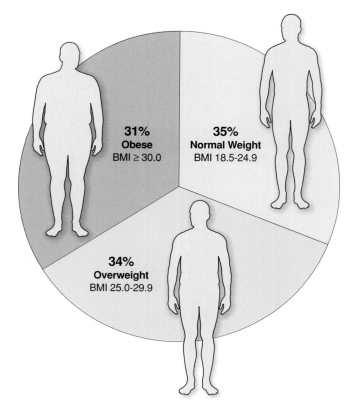

**FIGURE 22.1.** The prevalence of overweight and obesity in the United States adult population. Normal-weight: body mass index (BMI) = 18.5 to 24.9; overweight: BMI = 25.0 to 29.9; obese: BMI ≥30.0. (Data from Flegal KM, Carroll MD, Ogden CL, et al. Prevalence and trends in obesity among US adults, 1999–2000. *JAMA* 2002;288:1723–1727.)

particularly prevalent among women with lower incomes and less education.

The prevalence of overweight is also rising in children (*Fig. 22.2*). The definition of overweight among children is a statistical definition based on the year 2000 Centers for Disease Control and Prevention growth charts for children in the United States. Overweight is defined as at or above the 95th percentile of BMI. Accordingly, 10% of young children are overweight, and 15% of school-aged children and teenagers are overweight (2). Race and ethnicity appears to have no influence on childhood overweight until the ages of 12 to 19 years. At this point, more African American and Mexican American children become overweight compared with Caucasian children. The proportion of teenagers from poor households who are overweight is almost twice that of those from middle- and high-income households. Thus, at a time when it seems like the public has a heightened interest in physical activity and health, the prevalence of overweight continues to rise.

## OBESITY AND DISEASE RISK

Obesity itself is a medical condition in which excess body fat places a person at increased risk for other diseases. A disease that is strongly related to other diseases is called a

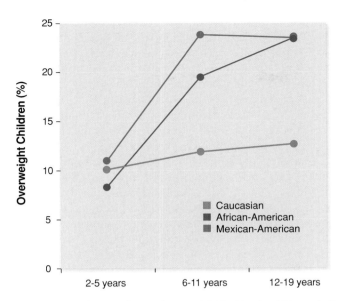

**FIGURE 22.2.** The prevalence of overweight is rising in children of all ages. (Data from Ogden CL, Flegal KM, Carroll MD, et al. Prevalence and trends in overweight among children and adolescents, 1999–2000. *JAMA* 2002;288:1728–1732.)

**comorbidity**. Obesity has been associated with several comorbidities, including heart disease, stroke, diabetes, hypertension, hyperlipidemia, gallbladder disease, kidney disease, liver malfunction, musculoskeletal disorders, arthritis, sleep disturbances, and cancer (*Fig. 22.3*). Most of the research shows that the complications associated with obesity can be improved or eliminated with weight loss, even with only a 5% to 10% reduction in body weight. Other research shows that even without a substantial weight loss, obese persons can significantly improve their health by participating in healthful behaviors. For example, obese persons who exercise regularly and eat a healthful diet report that their quality of life is improved, even though they have not lost weight.

 *LINKUP:* **Research Highlight: Quality of Life and Weight Loss,** *found at http://connection.lww.com/go/brownex phys and on the Student Resource CD-ROM, provides perspective into how the quality of life of the obese patient is affected by weight loss.*

## EXERCISE, BODY WEIGHT, AND HEALTH

A physical activity program should be an integral part of any type of intervention for the overweight individual,

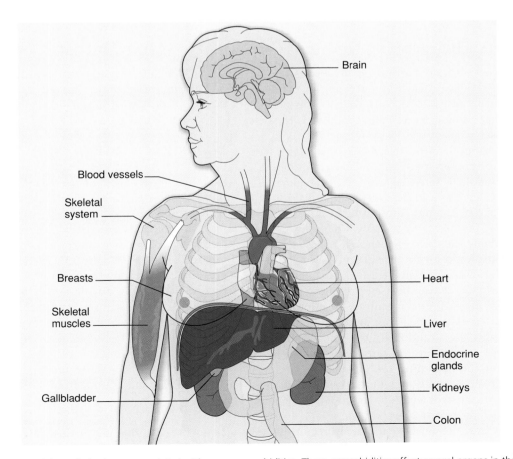

**FIGURE 22.3.** Overweight and obesity are associated with many comorbidities. These comorbidities affect several organs in the body.

whether the ultimate goal of the intervention is weight loss or not. Regular physical activity is associated with lower death rates for adults of any age, even when moderate levels of physical activity are performed. Furthermore, physical fitness, not body fatness, has been shown to be a strong predictor of premature mortality. For persons of any size, regular physical activity can reduce the risk and alleviate the symptoms associated with cardiovascular disease, diabetes and poor glucose control, hypertension, colon cancer, and depression. Children and adolescents need weight-bearing or strength exercises for normal skeletal development and achievement of optimal bone mass. Older adults can improve strength, increase cardiovascular fitness, and develop flexibility through regular exercise. This can decrease the risk of injury for older persons and help them maintain an independent living status.

The health benefits of exercise for persons of all ages and sizes are unquestionable. However, a paradox seems to exist—overweight people can reap tremendous benefits from exercise, but being overweight seems to impede people from being physically active. Imagine if you were overweight, a single parent of two middle-school–aged children, working full time, and without any apparent medical problems. *How much motivation and energy would you have to maintain a regular exercise program?* Imagine instead that you were obese and physical activity was exhausting. *Would you be able to maintain an exercise program even though you were at high risk for weight-related comorbidities?*

## ASSESSMENT OF THE OVERWEIGHT PATIENT

Although exercise is desired for people of all sizes, special considerations should be taken into account for the overweight patient because excess body weight is associated with many other chronic diseases and conditions. The first step in the assessment of the overweight patient is to determine the magnitude of overweight. People with a BMI $\geq$35 present a severe risk for obesity-related comorbidities. These people should be screened more carefully than those in lower BMI categories. Since cardiovascular disease, hypertension, diabetes, and musculoskeletal disorders are the most prevalent diseases associated with obesity, overweight individuals should be screened for these diseases prior to the initiation of an exercise program. The Physical Activity Readiness Questionnaire (PAR-Q; Chapter 20) is a good screening tool that can be used for this purpose. Information from the PAR-Q is useful in screening for cardiovascular disease, hypertension, and musculoskeletal disorders. In addition to the PAR-Q, a simple query regarding glucose control, insulin sensitivity, and diabetes will round out the screening for the major problems associated with excess body weight. A review of the patient's medical history will reveal the status of treatment for any obesity-related comorbidities.

At the same time the objective medical screening is being completed, a more subjective evaluation of the patient's condition can be made (see SOAP notes, Chapter 12). Specific items to look for in the subjective evaluation of the overweight patient are (a) the patient's perception of the overweight problem, (b) the patient's perception of exercise, (c) the patient's perceived barriers to exercise participation, (d) apparent barriers to healthful eating, (e) history of disordered eating or an eating disorder, and (f) the existence of a positive environment and social support system. Once the screening of the overweight patient is completed, an exercise prescription can be constructed.

Case Study 22.1 presents an overview of how an assessment of an obese woman is made prior to designing a weight-loss intervention. This case has been written as a continuation case study; as you read through the chapter, the case will be referred to repeatedly to show how the various concepts explained throughout the chapter are applied to the clinical setting. Each chapter reference to the case study will indicate where in the case the applied textual material can be found. Refer to Case Study 22.1 now to learn the case background, case description, and how the initial assessment of the patient was made. After reading these parts of the case, you can continue in the chapter text until the case is referred to again. You may also want to read through the case entirely first, and then refer back to it as it is referenced in different parts of the chapter.

▶ *INQUIRY SUMMARY.* The prevalence of overweight and obesity is rising in the United States to a point at which 65% of the adult population is considered overweight or obese. Obesity is associated with several chronic diseases including diabetes, hypertension, and cardiovascular disease. Exercise can help reduce body weight as well as improve health of all overweight individuals. *What are some reasons why the prevalence of obesity and its comorbidities are increasing in the United States?*

## *Etiology of Obesity*

Although obesity is often referred to as a disease, it is technically only a condition—the condition in which excess body fat is stored on the body. There are many factors that may contribute to excess body fat deposition. These factors can be divided into two categories: genetics or inherited factors and behavioral factors. However, a person's genetic expression can be altered by disease, accident, injury, mutation, radiation, etc. Furthermore, there are innumerable things that may affect a person's behavioral patterns. It is therefore understandable that the development of obesity in any one person and in populations can be caused by a multitude of interacting factors. Box 22.1 highlights the accomplishments of Albert Stunkard, the most prolific obesity researcher in the United States over the past 40 years.

### GENETICS AND BODY WEIGHT

The obese condition is a gradual culmination of many factors that promote the storage of body fat. Some of the factors that either directly or indirectly contribute to obesity are

## CASE STUDY 22.1: *ASSESSMENT OF AN OBESE PATIENT*

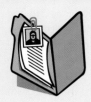

### CASE
Melissa is a 48-year-old Caucasian woman who comes to you for a weight-loss program. She is 6.0 feet tall and weighs 287 pounds. She wants to lose about 100 pounds and says that she has lost weight before but regained that weight, plus more, over a 2-year period. Melissa is single with no children, but she has been living with her boyfriend for the past 9 years. She says that she was a little overweight throughout high school and college but gained most of her excess weight the year after her husband died unexpectedly 13 years ago. She has been struggling with weight ever since.

### DESCRIPTION
The simplistic way to describe obesity is a positive energy balance in which more energy is consumed than expended. However, this simplistic view of obesity does not identify the specific factors that cause the positive energy balance. To help the obese lose weight and manage their condition, the factors that cause them to deposit excess body fat must be identified and dealt with systematically. More often than not, these factors are complex and interdependent. Moreover, some of the causative factors may not be manageable, such as genetics or medical causes. Nonetheless, the identification of all possible contributors to obesity, with intervention techniques for those contributors that can be controlled, provides the best prognosis for the obese person.

### Reference 1: Assessment
You calculate Melissa's body mass index (BMI) to be 39.0, which categorizes her as class II obese. With a BMI at this level Melissa is at severe risk for comorbidities. When Melissa completes the standard medical history form for the clinic where you work, you are surprised to find that she has no comorbidities nor is she taking any medications.

You probe further into Melissa's medical condition by using the Physical Activity Readiness Questionnaire. This questionnaire also indicates that Melissa does not have any comorbidities and that she is able to safely participate in a regular exercise program. You specifically ask if Melissa has a history of any metabolic problems such as diabetes, poor glucose control, or thyroid dysfunction. The response is negative.

### Reference 2: Genetics
There is no valid test to see if a person's obesity is caused by genetics. However, by asking the right questions, the professional can deduce if there is a propensity toward genetically induced obesity. Even though the genetic factor is uncontrollable, knowledge of a genetic contribution toward obesity helps the patient and professional understand that behavioral interventions are likely to be more difficult.

You ask Melissa about her family—her parents, grandparents, aunts, uncles, and siblings. She reports that her mother was overweight but not obese and that one of her three uncles was overweight. Her father, grandparents on both sides, four aunts, and brother were all normal weight. You conclude from this interview that genetics is probably not an influencing factor on Melissa's obesity.

### Reference 3: Energy Intake and Diet Composition
During the intake interview, you (or the dietitian) ask Melissa to complete a 24-hour dietary recall and a food frequency questionnaire. The subsequent diet analysis reveals that Melissa is consuming 3540 kcal·d$^{-1}$, of which 34% of the intake is fat and 50% of the carbohydrate intake is refined sugar.

### Reference 4: Psychologic Aspects
The initial intake interview with a new patient always provides much medical information and some behavioral history. The second and subsequent sessions with the patient are mostly devoted to behavioral issues and are when many of the psychologic aspects of obesity are uncovered.

The second session with Melissa is enlightening. She reports that after her husband's unexpected death, she went into a pattern of binge eating. She mentions that she was filled with anger, frustration, confusion, doubt, and abandonment. She gained most of her excess weight during the year or so of mourning over her husband's death. Four years after his death she entered into a relationship with her current boyfriend. She is brought to tears as she describes their relationship. According to Melissa's description, you are led to believe that her boyfriend is selfish, self-centered, controlling, and emotionally detached. She mentions herself that she should probably leave this relationship but just cannot right now. You suggest that Melissa seek some more qualified help for her relationship problems from her clergy or a clinical psychologist, but she refuses politely, stating that she is not ready to deal with those issues now. You reiterate that, as an exercise specialist, you are not qualified to counsel on relationship problems; when she becomes ready, you will help guide her to the professionals she needs. You do clearly explain to Melissa, however, that even though the two of you are not going to be working on solving her relationship issues, the emotional undertones of those issues will probably affect her attempts at changing her eating and exercise behaviors.

### Reference 5: Barriers to Weight Control
Your interview with Melissa reveals that she has the following barriers to healthy eating and exercise:
1. She eats when depressed, frustrated, or angry
2. She eats to avoid confrontation with her boyfriend
3. She eats because of romantic discord
4. She eats too many sweets, too much fat, and too many unhealthy snacks
5. She eats because she cannot express her feelings to her boyfriend

---

*Case Study 22.1, continued*

6. She eats for pleasure, comfort, security, and companionship
7. She does not exercise because she doesn't like exercise
8. She does not exercise because she feels so sluggish carrying all her extra weight

### INTERVENTION

- Fortunately Melissa does not have any comorbidities.
- Melissa does not present a strong genetic link to her obesity.
- Melissa consumes too much, and her overconsumption is probably due to eating too many foods that are high in fat and refined sugar.
- Melissa's poor eating patterns are based in emotional eating. This emotional eating stems from two periods of emotional turmoil in her life:
  - The unexpected death of Melissa's husband sent her into a pattern of emotional eating in which Melissa used food to deal with the negative emotions associated with her husband's death.
  - Melissa's current relationship is emotionally unhealthy; because of this emotional turmoil, Melissa continues to use food for emotional release.
- Melissa does not enjoy exercise and will probably not maintain an exercise program unless it becomes enjoyable and she achieves some weight-loss success.

### PROGNOSIS

The prognosis for this case may seem dismal to you as an exercise specialist with little experience. However, cases like these are the common reality for many people. The prognosis for Melissa would be much poorer than it is if you could not at least identify the strong emotional links to Melissa's eating behaviors. As illustrated in the case, you are not capable of solving Melissa's relationship problems, but also as illustrated, you can be a valued facilitator in Melissa's health care.

You start by setting Melissa up on a healthier eating and exercise plan. Melissa plays an integral part in structuring this plan. The plan takes into account Melissa's current environment, her willingness to change, how much restriction she wishes to place upon herself, and ways she can make physical activity more enjoyable. She starts on her new program immediately.

As the weeks of treatment proceed, you systematically begin to dismantle Melissa's barriers to exercise. For example, you teach Melissa that we participate in habits because habits meet needs. As an assignment, you ask Melissa to write down all her emotional needs and how she currently meets those needs. With your help, Melissa can now see that she meets many of her emotional needs with food. So you design ways in which she can meet her emotional needs without the use of food, such as talking to her close friend, spending time with her brother's family, and setting proper boundaries by learning to say NO. (Remember that she still refuses to talk about her boyfriend issues so emotional needs related to him cannot be dealt with directly.)

Another behavioral assignment you ask Melissa to perform is to write down the feelings she is experiencing every time she has a craving for food, does not want to exercise, or is tempted to disregard her healthy eating and exercise plan. This assignment identifies anger, frustration, and loneliness as the key emotions that set Melissa off into a lapse of behavior. Together you figure out healthier ways for Melissa to deal with these emotions.

You become pleasantly surprised when in one of your counseling sessions, Melissa asks you if you think she is ready for psychologic counseling to help her leave her unhealthy romantic relationship. You assure her that whenever she is ready to work on those relationship issues, you can direct her to the best people that can help her. Nothing more is said until three sessions later when she asks you for a referral. Melissa has lost 57 pounds in the 7 months she has been working with you. Melissa still has a lot of work to do, but her prognosis is now better than ever.

---

genetics, diet, inactivity, and emotional health. The influence of genetics is direct, regulating an individual's metabolic response to food intake and physical activity. The influence of diet and inactivity are also direct, contributing to a positive **energy balance** and an increase in body fat deposition. On the other hand, emotional health indirectly relates to obesity by affecting one's eating and exercise behaviors.

It is estimated that 55% of the variance in percent body fat or total fat mass is transmissible between generations (Fig. 22.4). This means that what is passed on from one generation to the next determines 55% of a person's body fatness. However, the genetic effect contributing to this transmissible component is only 25%; the cultural or environmental influences on the transmissible variation consti-

tute the other 30%. Nontransmissible variation (45%) and the behavioral portion of the transmissible variation (30%) add up to 75% of the variation in body fatness that is nongenetic. Based on these observations, the role of genetics on body fat content is significant but of limited value. Case Study 22.1, reference point 2, shows how hereditary information on obesity is obtained from a patient.

 *LINKUP:* **Perspective: Genetics and Obesity,** *which can be accessed at* **http://connection.lww.com/ go/brownexphys** *and on the Student Resource CD-ROM, describes the relationship between these elements.*

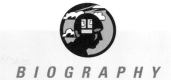

**Box 22.1**

## BIOGRAPHY

# Albert J. Stunkard

Albert J. Stunkard received a BS from Yale University in 1943 and a medical degree from Columbia University in 1945. Stunkard completed an internship in medicine at Massachusetts General Hospital and a residency in psychiatry at Johns Hopkins Hospital. He has been a faculty member at the University of Pennsylvania since 1957, except for an appointment as professor in the department of psychiatry at Stanford University from 1973 to 1976. Stunkard has served in several administrative positions at several hospitals and at the University of Pennsylvania. He has served as past president of the American Psychosomatic Society, Society of Behavioral Medicine, Association for Research in Nervous and Mental Disease, and American Association of Chairmen of Departments of Psychiatry. Stunkard has served as editor of several journals such as the *American Journal of Clinical Nutrition, Appetite, International Journal of Eating Disorders, International Journal of Obesity,* and *Obesity Research.* Several organizations have bestowed upon Stunkard their Distinguished Scientist award or Lifetime Achievement award.

Stunkard has been a leader in the study of obesity and eating disorders for the past 40 years. His name comes to mind immediately when obesity research is discussed. His more than 400 publications have contributed to our understanding of genetic, physiologic, psychologic, and sociologic determinants of obesity. He was a pioneer in the development of the behavioral treatment of obesity, and he has made significant contributions to its treatment by pharmacotherapy, surgery, psychoanalysis, self-help groups, work-site programs, and the geographical community. Stunkard is currently studying a relatively new eating disorder, the night eating syndrome.

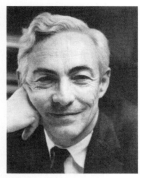

Albert J. Stunkard

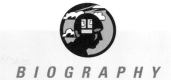

**FIGURE 22.4.** Genetic vs. nongenetic contributions to variations in body fat content. Although body fatness is affected by genetics, behavior plays a large role in body fat regulation. (Data from Bouchard C, Perusse L. Heredity and body fat. *Annu Rev Nutr* 1988;8:259–277.)

## ENERGY INTAKE AND BODY FATNESS

The traditional view of obesity is that the obese condition results from a chronic, positive energy balance. This positive energy balance can be due to excess energy intake, decreased energy expenditure, or a combination of both. Along this line of thinking, weight control is viewed as simply maintaining a balance between energy intake and expenditure, a view that has become widely accepted (*Fig.* 22.5). As is frequently recommended in the popular press, the first response to increased body weight is to reduce energy intake (i.e., dieting). Promotion of dieting as the first line of attack on obesity is also seen in the scientific literature. Rampone and Reynolds concluded:

*Calorie overconsumption must be regarded as the major contributor to body weight gain, and reduced consumption as the first line of defense. The simple algebraic relationship, which balances this single source of the body's energy supply against a multiplicity of energy expenditure forms, makes the conclusion inevitable (3).*

Although many would like to believe that weight loss can occur so easily, it most often does not. Long-term weight control after dieting may be as low as 5% (4). Nonetheless, some researchers are persistent in blaming the dieter for failure rather than the diet. Welle and colleagues (5) noted that "failure to lose weight on self-

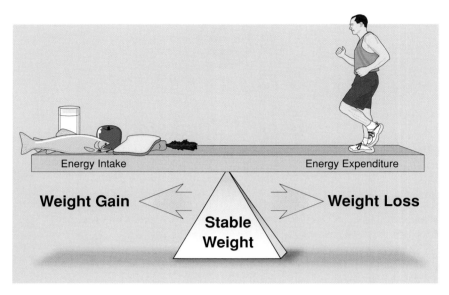

**FIGURE 22.5.** Traditional view of energy balance in weight control. A shift toward more energy expenditure triggers weight loss, and an imbalance toward energy intake leads to weight gain.

reported intakes of 1000 kilocalories per day or less should be attributed to the underestimation of caloric intake."

The preceding statement implies that obese people do not accurately record their eating behaviors. Although some studies show that obese subjects have inaccurately estimated their food quantity and energy intake by as much as 25% to 53%, other studies conclude that there is no difference between lean and obese individuals with respect to reported energy intake and measured or observed energy intake (1,6–10). The issue remains as to whether or not overweight individuals under- or over-report energy intake. It may be that all individuals under- or over-report to some extent. *How accurately do you think you would self-report your caloric intake?*

Assuming the inaccuracies in reporting dietary behavior apply to both the obese and nonobese, there are significant data to suggest that overeating is not the major factor contributing to body fat deposition in the average overweight adult. When direct observation of energy intake during a meal was compared with a 24-hour dietary recall of the same meal, overweight and normal-weight women both over-reported, but there was no difference between groups for total calories consumed or for protein, fat, and carbohydrate intake (8). Similarly, when the energy intake of 63 women in a metabolic unit was compared with their self-reported intake, there was no relationship between energy intake and body weight, BMI, or percent body fat (9). Under-reporting was positively related to energy intake in this study but not to body fatness. Other researchers have found no relationship between energy intake and body fatness in adult men and women of various ages and adiposity levels. When energy intake is expressed relative to body weight, obese men and women actually eat less than their lean counterparts.

The fact that the average overweight person does not consume more energy than the normal weight person does not negate the principle of energy balance. There are other factors that may disrupt the balance between intake and expenditure; including diet composition, hormone status, enzyme activity, metabolic adaptations, and inactivity. Moreover, it may be that if overeating promotes body fat deposition, then overeating is related to metabolic rate, activity level, or some macronutrient and not to absolute energy intake or some measure of body size.

## DIET COMPOSITION AND BODY COMPOSITION

Animal and human research has been conducted to examine the composition of the diet as a contributing factor in the development of obesity. Specifically the contributions of dietary fat, refined sugar, and dietary fiber to the promotion of obesity have been investigated. It has been hypothesized that dietary fat promotes body fat deposition because it is stored more efficiently than carbohydrate. In one report, the energy value of dietary fat was calculated to be $11.1$ kcal·$g^{-1}$ or about 24% greater than the expected value of 9 kcal·$g^{-1}$ (11). This efficiency factor for dietary fat has been shown to promote fat deposition in animals, even to the point of severe obesity, when their total energy intake was normal or even restricted.

Descriptive research on humans seems to coincide with that on animals. Several studies have shown no relationship between daily energy intake (kcal consumed) and adiposity, but a significant correlation has been found between dietary fat content and body fatness for both men and women. When men and women are classified into subgroups of lean and obese, individuals with obesity derive a greater portion of their daily energy intake from fat when compared with individuals who are lean (*Fig. 22.6*).

Carbohydrate intake, primarily in the form of refined sugar, has been implicated as a fat-promoting agent. It is

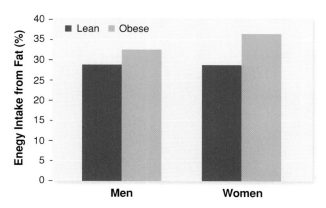

**FIGURE 22.6.** Dietary fat intake of lean and obese men and women. Obese men and women derive a greater portion of their energy intake from fat than do lean men and women. Many professionals believe dietary fat is a significant contributor to obesity. (Data from Miller WC, Lindeman AK, Wallace J, et al. Diet composition, energy intake, and exercise in relation to body fat in men and women. *Am J Clin Nutr* 1990;52:426–430.)

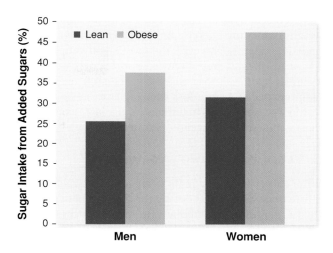

**FIGURE 22.7.** Added or refined sugar intake of lean and obese men and women. Obese men and women consume more added sugar than lean men and women. Many professionals believe that rising consumption of added sugar has contributed significantly to the obesity epidemic. (Data from Miller WC, Niederpruem MG, Wallace JP, et al. Dietary fat, sugar, and fiber predict body fat content. *J Am Diet Assoc* 1994;94:612–615.)

generally believed that since refined sugar is virtually void of vitamins and minerals, any energy derived from refined sugar would be excess energy contributing to body fat storage. Since the majority of evidence indicates either an inverse relationship or no relationship between body fatness and total carbohydrate intake, it seems unlikely that refined sugar contributes significantly to increased body fat storage, especially if overweight individuals do not overeat. Thus, the only way refined sugar could contribute substantially to the development of obesity is either in the absence of overeating or if overeating was specific to refined sugar intake only. Experiments with animals have shown that obesity can be induced by a high intake of sucrose even when total energy intake is below normal. Descriptive data on humans reveals that obese men and women derive a greater portion of their sugar energy from refined sugars than their lean counterparts, even though total sugar intake is similar between the groups (*Fig.* 22.7).

The physiologic role of dietary fiber includes reduced intestinal transit time, an increased rate of transit, increased **postprandial satiety**, and reduced glucose absorption. Another distinguishing characteristic between lean and obese adults is dietary fiber intake. Obese men and women have been found to consume less fiber than lean men and women (*Fig.* 22.8). Although a generous fiber intake may be advantageous for some individuals who are attempting to prevent weight gain or trying to lose weight, supplementing a diet that is already rich in fiber is not necessary. Refer to Case Study 22.1, reference point 3, to see how energy intake and diet intake information on a patient is collected and used.

## INACTIVITY AND OVERWEIGHT

If one remains faithful to the traditional view of weight control, then the only explanation for becoming over-

weight is overeating and/or inactivity. The opinion that prevails in the minds of many lean individuals is that individuals who are obese are lazy and that they have become obese because of this laziness. It is true that individuals with obesity are characteristically less active than those who are lean, but no cause and effect relationship has been established. Obese individuals themselves recognize the importance of exercise in weight control and credit their unsuccessful management of weight to the lack of a consistent exercise program. However, being overweight may be seen as a "two-edged sword" or a "catch 22"—inactivity can lead to overweight, but being overweight also makes it more difficult to be active. Thus, a person's propensity toward obesity is exacerbated by his/her inability to be active.

It is difficult to verify the preventive effect of exercise on obesity in humans. Animal research suggests that exercise can prevent obesity as well as negate the effect of dietary fat

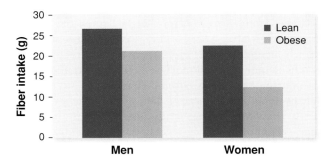

**FIGURE 22.8.** Dietary fiber intake of lean and obese men and women. A high dietary fiber intake may prevent or help reduce obesity. (Data from Miller WC, Niederpruem MG, Wallace JP, et al. Dietary fat, sugar, and fiber predict body fat content. *J Am Diet Assoc* 1994;94:612–615.)

on excess body fat deposition. From the standpoint of weight reduction, exercise has long been known to reduce body fat content. However, the most significant role of exercise in obesity treatment is its preventative effect on weight regain. Almost all of the research on long-term maintenance of weight loss shows that exercise is the critical key to successful maintenance. In fact, exercise is almost a guarantee for weight maintenance.

## METABOLIC RATE AND OVERWEIGHT

If the energy balance equation suggests that energy expenditure must be reduced during the development of obesity, then a depressed metabolic rate may contribute to a reduced energy expenditure. It is well established that obese individuals possess an elevated absolute **resting metabolic rate** (RMR) when compared with their lean counterparts. A greater **lean body mass** (LBM) in the obese person accounts for this increased RMR. When RMR is corrected for differences in LBM and total body mass, RMR levels in the obese are similar to the lean. Even though there is not a distinct difference in RMR between the lean and obese, an inherently low RMR may contribute to the development of obesity or put one at higher risk for gaining body weight.

Although logic seems to dictate that restrictive dieting should assist weight-control efforts, data now show that restrictive dieting may actually hinder attempts at weight control. Bray was the first to demonstrate that a reduction in energy intake results in a decline in RMR. Later, he found that this decrease in RMR was about 15% when subjects were removed from a maintenance diet of 3500 kcal·d$^{-1}$ and placed on a very–low-calorie diet of 450 kcal·d$^{-1}$ (12). These studies imply that restrictive dieting is somewhat detrimental to the weight-loss process.

The implication is that when an overweight individual attempts to lose weight by strict dieting and exercise, two opposing metabolic forces are working against each other that result in a hindrance of the weight-loss process. This conflict between the two opposing forces has been demonstrated by experimental design (*Fig. 22.9*). Metabolic measurements during treadmill exercise were taken in a group of mildly overweight (26% body fat) women who were cyclical dieters and compared with normal-weight (21% body fat) nondieting controls. Regardless of the workload examined, relative exercise energy expenditure was significantly lower in the dieters than the nondieters. These results demonstrate an increased efficiency of food utilization during exercise in chronic dieters.

The long-term effects of dieting on RMR are not currently known. However, daily exercise continued over a long period of time may reverse the detrimental effects of dieting on RMR. Additional research is necessary to determine how the interactions of diet and exercise affect metabolic rate over prolonged periods of time, how long a regimen of diet and exercise can safely be employed, and what mechanisms are responsible for the diet and exercise effects on metabolism.

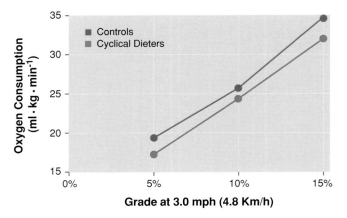

**FIGURE 22.9.** Exercise energy expenditure in cyclical dieters vs. nondieting controls during treadmill walking at various workloads. Cyclical dieters had a lower energy expenditure at each workload when compared with nondieters. Repeated dieting may hinder future attempts at weight loss. (Data from Manore MM, Berry TE, Skinner JS, et al. Energy expenditure at rest and during exercise in nonobese female cyclical dieters and in nondieting control subjects. *Am J Clin Nutr* 1991;54:41–46.)

The last factor contributing to energy expenditure is dietary-induced thermogenesis or the **thermic effect of food** (TEF). TEF is defined as the energy-requiring processes of digesting, absorbing, and assimilating the various nutrients in the diet. These processes cause a temporary increase in energy expenditure following a meal that may approach 10% to 15% of the total energy value of the digested food. Some scientists suggest that overweight people have a decreased TEF and that this contributes to obesity. Other scientists contend that there is no difference in the TEF between lean and overweight people. Until definitive data can be obtained relative to the TEF and obesity, one can assume that the TEF does not play a critical role in the development of obesity.

Considering all of the research regarding the physiologic aspects of obesity, it seems appropriate that a new, contemporary view of obesity development (*Fig. 22.10*) should replace the traditional view (see Fig. 22.7). This new perspective takes into consideration several factors that affect body fat deposition which have been overlooked traditionally.

The implications of this new perspective are several: (a) weight control is affected by a myriad of factors, (b) weight control is not as simple as balancing measured energy intake with calculated energy expenditure, (c) weight control is affected by factors other than behavior, (d) energy balance is specific to each individual and subject to change, (e) some aspects of weight control are beyond behavioral influence, and (f) the concept of ideal body weight for a given height may be impractical. This also means that exercise weight-loss programs will not be as effective as predicted if one is basing the effectiveness of the program solely on a theoretic negative energy balance

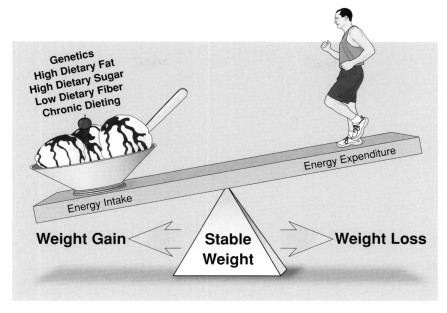

**FIGURE 22.10.** Contemporary theory on energy balance and weight control. This model considers contributors to the metabolic equation other than just calorie intake and expenditure.

between energy intake and calculated energy expenditure (e.g., kcal in vs. kcal out). Maximal success will only be obtained when the exercise program is coupled with an eating plan that alters the composition of the diet to favor weight loss. Moreover, certain metabolic factors that are beyond control will also affect the person's ability to lose weight. The unfortunate consequence of recognizing these facts is that it remains difficult to accurately predict weight-loss success in response to a prescribed program.

*LINKUP: Refer to Case Study:* **Obesity Treatment Plan for a Thyroid Patient,** *found at http://connection.lww.com/go/brownexphys and on the Student Resource CD-ROM, for an overview of how this patient was evaluated and how a treatment plan was designed.*

▶ *INQUIRY SUMMARY.* There are multiple factors that contribute to the deposition of excess body fat. *What are the factors that interact in either the promotion or prevention of obesity? Why is it such a difficult task to determine the cause of obesity for any one individual?*

## *Psychologic Aspects of Obesity*

The mind and body are not separate but are tightly connected. Accordingly, anything that affects the psyche of an individual can also affect his/her physical well-being. Obesity is one area in which psychology can play a major role in the prevention, promotion, and treatment of the

condition. Some questions that psychologists have asked in regard to obesity are:

1. *Do obese people have a psychologic profile different from normal-weight people?*
2. *How has the focus of modern culture on slimness factored into the obesity epidemic?*
3. *What psychologic burdens do obese people carry because of society's bias and prejudice against them?*
4. *Is obesity a natural result of emotional distress?*
5. *What emotional coping strategies are helpful in the treatment of obesity?*

Answers to questions such as these will undoubtedly help us understand the etiology and curative aspects of obesity.

### THE PSYCHOLOGIC PROFILE OF THE OBESE PERSON

One of the first questions to be asked relative to the psychologic aspects of obesity is: *Do obese people have a psychologic profile different from the nonobese?* The answer to this question depends on which psychologic aspects you examine. With respect to psychiatric disorders, most studies that have assessed conventional measures of psychopathology in obese persons have found little evidence of increased psychologic disturbances. Clinical studies that show elevated levels of psychopathology among obese people report levels no higher than those found among medical and surgical patients. The finding that obese persons generally are not psychologically disturbed does not preclude the possibility that obese individuals have a different psychologic makeup than nonobese people.

Obesity comes with a tremendous psychologic burden. Prejudice and discrimination against obese individuals begin in childhood and are probably magnified throughout adulthood. The obese person is often portrayed as being ugly, sloppy, dirty, and stupid. Professionally, obese people have a difficult time climbing the corporate ladder. Many employers will hot hire obese individuals at all, while others only hire them under special circumstances. Obese women find it difficult to compete in business because they feel they are evaluated according to appearance rather than performance. Surprisingly, the prejudice against obesity pervades the medical profession. Prejudice toward obese people is well documented among physicians, medical students, nurses, and mental health professionals. The result is that overweight people avoid routine health care (*Fig. 22.11*). One study showed that 32% of those with a BMI over 27 and 55% of those with a BMI over 35 delayed or canceled physician appointments because they knew they would be weighed (13). The most common reason women gave for delaying medical care was the embarrassment about their weight or avoidance of a weight-loss lecture by their physician.

In addition to the prejudice and discrimination, obese individuals also have the psychologic burden of literally fitting into a "thin" world. Imagine not being able to fit into a seat at the auditorium or ball game or on a bus or airline. Imagine not being able to purchase clothes at the local discount store or the feeling of being watched every time you eat an ice cream cone in public. The fact that obese persons show no higher levels of general psychopathology than do persons of normal weight is surprising when one considers the psychologic pressures obese people face. This conclusion is a remarkable testimony to the resilience of the human spirit.

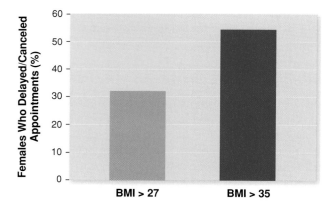

**FIGURE 22.11.** Many overweight people delay needed visits to their physicians because they are intimidated by the medical profession's view on obesity. Health professionals should make a conscious attempt to rid themselves of any bias toward obesity. Percentages represent the proportion of women who delayed or canceled doctor appointments because they knew they would be weighed. (Data from Olson CL, Schumaker HD, Yawn BP. Overweight women delay medical care. *Arch Fam Med* 1994;3:888–892.)

In spite of this resiliency, obese individuals often suffer from psychologic problems specific to obesity that cannot be measured by conventional personality and psychopathology inventories. Some of these problems include low self-esteem, loneliness, humiliation, and lack of self-confidence.

## BODY IMAGE DISPARAGEMENT

Most people have had the unsettling experience of having a mirror reveal an otherwise unnoticed disheveled appearance. Perhaps you have been at an amusement park and stepped in front of a distorted mirror to see a funny-looking body in the reflection. Fortunately, you can fix your makeup, straighten your hair, and jump away from the funny reflection in the mirror. What if this were not the case, and no matter where you were, there was always something about your body that did not appear acceptable.

One of the most common problems arising from being overweight or obese is that of **body image disparagement**. This disorder originates from the belief that one's body is ugly and loathsome. Body image disparagement manifests itself with an overwhelming preoccupation with body weight. The person sees their whole world in terms of his/her weight. The woman who, upon entering a crowded room, immediately seeks to verify that she is the fattest one in the room, whether she is or not, has a problem with body image disparagement. Most persons with body image disparagement will not look at themselves in the mirror and avoid any visual reflections of themselves such as those seen in large store windows. More severe cases of body image disparagement are manifested in people with anorexia who view themselves as fat even though they have starved themselves into an emaciated state.

Body image disparagement is an example of the distorted perception that afflicts many overweight individuals. This hatred for one's body often starts in childhood or adolescence when the person internalizes parental and/or peer criticism. Much of this distorted view has its roots in our culture and even the health care community. Rand and McGregor (14) employed a unique method to quantify how obese people perceive their obesity. This technique queried patients as to whether they would prefer their own disability to another. Normal-weight persons preferred their own disability when it was compared with other severe disabilities by a ratio of 62% to 95%. Obese individuals, however, were different. When 47 severely obese subjects who had successfully maintained a weight loss of 45 kg for 3 years were queried, 100% preferred being deaf, dyslexic, and diabetic to being severely obese. One hundred percent also preferred having heart disease or bad acne to being obese. Furthermore, 91.5% preferred having a leg amputated and 89.4% preferred being legally blind over severe obesity (*Fig. 22.12*) (14). The psychologic burden of being obese truly does exact a toll on the psyches of the obese.

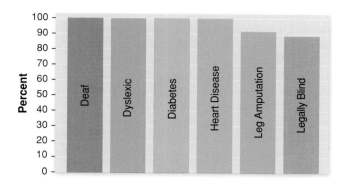

**FIGURE 22.12.** Preferences of previously obese persons for diseases other than obesity. Most people prefer their own set of health problems rather than another's. However for the obese person, a preference for any other disease than obesity seems dominant. This testifies to the presence of a "fat phobia" within our society. The percentages in the figure represent the proportion of previously obese individuals who would prefer having the indicated disease rather than being obese. (Data from Rand CSW, Macgregor AMC. Successful weight loss following obesity surgery and the perceived liability of morbid obesity. *Int J Obes* 1991;15:577–579.)

## EMOTIONAL DISTRESS AND WEIGHT CONTROL

To appreciate the psychologic distress that the obese person encounters when he/she is struggling with eating and exercise behaviors, one must understand some of the emotional histories that may have contributed to the obese condition as well as some of the barriers that may hinder weight control. Students of exercise science, physical therapy, and other allied health fields often wonder why they need to worry about all the emotional or psychologic variables when their job is only to treat or deal with the physical or physiologic aspects of the condition. The answer to this question was best given in a quote by Curry and Jaffe, two well-known authors and nutrition counselors.

*Today in the field of dietetics and nutrition, it is recognized that the reasons most people do not eat what they "should" have little to do with basic science, knowledge, or the information that is available (15).*

The same thing holds true for exercise. Most people admit that they should be exercising regularly, and many of them know how to go about exercising. Nonetheless, they continue in their sedentary lifestyles. It does not matter whether exercise is to be used for cardiac rehabilitation, diabetes management, hypertension, physical therapy, or fitness; the exercise scientist will encounter overweight patients on a regular basis. If the professional understands some of the psychology underlying behavior, he/she can be a much more effective member of the health care team.

It is very common for people struggling with weight to use food and sedentary behaviors as coping mechanisms to deal with emotional turmoil. Eating can be used as a way of expressing emotions. Eating soothes the "soul." People eat when they are depressed, discouraged, lonely, scared, anxious, tired, bored, and for many other reasons (*Fig. 22.13*).

Relieving the pain of negative emotions through eating can cause obesity as well as present a barrier to weight control once the client decides to lose weight.

A classic example of how overeating is used to deal with emotional turmoil is seen when food is used as a stress-relief technique. It is a common for a person under stress to turn to food for comfort, relief, and pleasure. This person will continue to have difficulty eating healthily until he/she finds another way to effectively deal with stress. A common example in which inactivity is used to deal with emotional turmoil is seen when a person remains inactive because of fears associated with exercising. Perhaps the person is ashamed of his/her body, feels uncomfortable exercising in a group, feels awkward, or feels intimidated by fitness professionals or the exercise environment. Unless these fears are dealt with, the individual will continue to prefer a sedentary lifestyle, regardless of what the physical consequences may be.

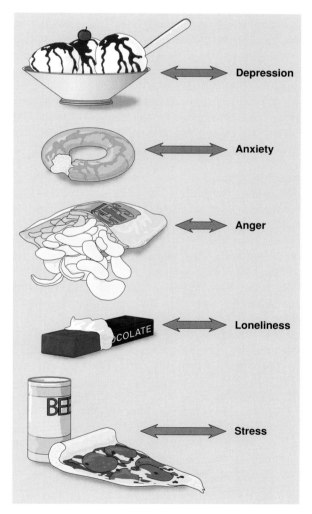

**FIGURE 22.13.** Emotional relationships with food. Most of us rely upon food to help us express our emotions. Our physical and emotional health becomes jeopardized when our emotional relationship with food becomes so distorted that food is our primary mechanism for dealing with emotions.

Often people hang on to their inappropriate or unhealthy eating behaviors because these behaviors fulfill the need people have to soothe or disperse their emotions. Food tastes good, makes us feel good, gives us pleasure, and is comforting. It is not inappropriate to use food to manage our emotions once in a while, but using food consistently for emotional release or eating as our only emotional expression is both physically and emotionally unhealthy. A specific example of how an assessment revealed possible emotional links to eating behavior is shown in Case Study 22.2. You may also want to refer to Case Study 22.1, reference point 4, to see how a more difficult emotional issue is handled by the exercise professional.

A skilled exercise professional will help the client express his/her negative emotions or deal with these emotions in an appropriate way. The professional will also help the client find more suitable behaviors that will meet the needs served by the noncompliant behaviors. Regardless of how food and sedentary behaviors are used to help a person deal with emotional turmoil, the professional who

---

## CASE STUDY 22.2: *EMOTIONAL LINKS TO EATING BEHAVIOR*

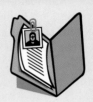

### CASE

Sandy is a 45-year-old mother and businesswoman. She reports that she has always struggled with weight control, but that over the past few years she has gained more than 30 pounds. Currently Sandy has a body mass index (BMI) of 36. She has hypertension, which is under control with medication. Sandy has been taking depression medication for 3 years. She reports that her mother is overweight but not obese and that nobody else in her family has a weight problem. Sandy had bad experiences in high school physical education and does not enjoy physical activity. She admits that her diet is unhealthy and does not understand why she cannot control her cravings for ice cream in the evenings.

### DESCRIPTION

Obesity is not technically a disease but a condition, which may be associated with chronic diseases such as diabetes, hypertension, or cardiovascular disease. The obese condition can be characterized, however, by measures of adiposity such as BMI or percent body fat. Treatment for the overweight person without comorbidities consists of interventions which will reduce body weight (fatness) and prevent the onset of associated diseases. Treatment for the overweight person with a related disease consists of interventions which will reduce body weight (fatness), as well as ameliorate symptoms of the related disease. Since the causes of obesity are multifactorial, treatment has to be individualized and multifaceted.

### INTERVENTION

1. Sandy presents with class II obesity (BMI = 36).
2. Although Sandy "has always struggled with weight control," it seems like the weight problem does not have a strong genetic link (nobody else in the family is obese). This suggests that behavior, rather than heredity, is the primary cause.
3. The fact that Sandy has gained a significant amount of weight in the past few years and that she started with depression medication a few years ago suggests a link between her depression and rapid weight gain.

4. The Physician's Desk Reference lists weight gain as a possible side effect from Sandy's medication.
5. A graded exercise test shows that Sandy's hypertensive medication is effective during exercise and that she can tolerate moderately intense aerobic exercise training without any adverse hypertensive response.
6. Sandy's diet is evaluated. Sandy is consuming 300 kcal a day more than the predicted intake for a person her gender, age, and size. She is consuming 36% of her intake as dietary fat.

### THERAPEUTIC RECOMMENDATIONS

1. Sandy and her doctor agree to try an alternative antidepressant medication that does not have weight gain as a possible side effect. She will monitor her weight closely as she switches medications.
2. Sandy begins to meet regularly with a clinical psychologist to explore ways to deal with her bad experiences with high school physical education, her depression, methods for mood control, and ice cream cravings (e.g., eating at the end of the day in response to stress, eating to control depression, and eating for pleasure). Strategies for cognitive restructuring and removing barriers to physical activity will also be employed.
3. Blood pressure will be monitored at rest and during exercise, and Sandy's blood pressure medication may be reduced as exercise training continues.
4. Adjustments in Sandy's diet are prescribed to produce a 300 to 500 kcal deficit in energy intake and reduce her dietary fat intake.
5. The long-term treatment goal is to develop a healthier lifestyle in which barriers to healthful eating and exercise are removed and skills for behavior maintenance are learned.
6. Other members of the health care team will work continuously and cooperatively to ameliorate the symptoms of Sandy's comorbidities of hypertension and depression as she begins her healthier lifestyle.
7. Continued follow-up through a long-term maintenance phase will be necessary to ensure lasting success for Sandy.

treats overweight and obesity must be alert to the possibility of emotional turmoil as an underlying cause of overweight. If the professional is not qualified to deal with the issues him/herself, the patient should be referred to the appropriate health care professional.

▶ *INQUIRY SUMMARY.* Obese persons do not generally show signs of serious psychiatric disorders, but they may have important emotional issues related to obesity. Obesity carries with it certain psychologic burdens that are imposed by our society. Emotional health is important for people of all sizes and shapes, but it is an important factor in the promotion or reduction of obesity for those who are predisposed. *What are some of the daily physiologic burdens with which overweight people struggle that may not be apparent to a normal-weight person?*

## Barriers to Weight Control

If one takes the philosophy that removal of the cause of obesity will cure obesity, then each one of the physiologic and psychologic aspects of obesity addressed previously could be a potential barrier to weight control. Additional environmental, social, and emotional factors that do not require psychotherapy per se can also become barriers to weight control. Unless these barriers are identified and conquered, long-term weight control is unlikely. A good weight-loss specialist will not only prescribe a prudent diet and exercise regimen for the client but will also help the client overcome individual barriers to weight control.

*Table 22.2* contains a checklist of common barriers to weight control. The therapist may wish to use this checklist with the client to identify some of the obvious barriers to weight control. In addition, the therapist may want to keep his/her own copy and mark some barriers that may not be obvious to the client at this time but may be suspicious to the therapist. The intervention should address specific ways to overcome or minimize each of the barriers to healthy weight management. It might be necessary to elicit help from other members of the health care team for assistance. For example, a psychologist or behavior specialist may be needed to help the patient overcome issues with emotional eating. Continual review and updating of this checklist will help the treatment process. Reference point 5 in the continuation case (Case Study 22.1) shows how the barriers to healthy weight management checklist was used to help a patient overcome some of her barriers.

It is not the intent of this checklist to infer that all eating is bad but to bring to the consciousness potential barriers to healthy weight management. For example, celebratory eating is a part of all cultures. Eating at parties and festivities is not bad per se, but it could be a potential barrier to healthy weight management if the person is celebrating with food several days a week. If *I eat when I am celebrating* is marked on the checklist, then this should be

explored further to see if this behavior is truly a barrier to healthy weight management. The same holds true for anything else that may be marked on the barriers checklist. *Is the marked item a frequent behavior and hence a true barrier to healthy weight management or is it an infrequent behavior that is inconsequential?*

Triumph in a weight-loss program is often associated with perceptions of body weight as well as expectations for successful weight management. Overweight individuals may have an inaccurate perception of body weight, demonstrate behavioral characteristics inconsistent with successful weight management, and/or have unrealistic expectations for weight loss. This presents an additional barrier to healthy weight management. While many researchers have sought to identify the reasons that people fail at weight management, these researchers have not examined carefully the reasons, perceived or real, for past failures of overweight people at the time they enter into a new weight-loss program.

Miller and Eggert (16) examined the weight-loss perceptions, characteristics, and expectations of overweight men and women who were previously unsuccessful at weight management and were about to enter a new weight-loss program. More women than men were currently dieting, women perceived having more difficulty dieting than men, more women than men reported that they had low self-control, women were dieting more frequently than men, and body weight of the women was fluctuating to a greater extent than men. Although these reported differences in weight-loss behavior between the sexes are probably due to society's obsession with slim, attractive women, the perceptions and past behaviors must be taken into account when strategizing for another weight-loss attempt.

It might seem a bit surprising, but both genders had an accurate perception of their body weight and a realistic expectation for rate of weight loss. The most common reasons reported for weight-control failure in both sexes were reverting back to old eating patterns (83%) and discontinuing exercise (82%) (Fig. 22.14) (16). This suggests that although overweight men and women may have a realistic understanding of their problem, their weight-loss behaviors are not always conducive to long-term weight management. Here again, a pretreatment assessment of the patient's history will help the therapist in strategizing for individual barriers to weight-loss success. *Table 22.3* lists some of the most likely pretreatment screening results that a clinician may find during a pretreatment evaluation, along with specific treatment recommendations that may enhance success rates for potential clients. Information about the integrity of commercial weight-loss programs and services as well as the Partnership for Healthy Weight Management can be found in Box 22.2.

▶ *INQUIRY SUMMARY.* All of us have things that discourage us from healthful eating and exercise. To maintain a long-term health plan, we need to overcome these obstacles or discouragements. *What are some of your own*

| Table 22.2 | BARRIERS TO HEALTHY WEIGHT MANAGEMENT |
|---|---|

Please mark any of the following that apply to your personal eating and activity patterns.

*I eat when I am . . .*
_____ depressed
_____ under stress
_____ frustrated
_____ angry
_____ nervous
_____ sad
_____ tired
_____ happy
_____ celebrating
_____ bored
other _____
_____

*I eat because of . . .*
_____ past failures at weight control
_____ fear of losing weight
_____ distrust of men (women)
_____ pressure from society
_____ lack of confidence
_____ low self-control
_____ guilt
_____ romantic discord
_____ no social support system
_____ food being accessible
other _____
_____

*I eat because I am (was) . . .*
_____ humiliated
_____ shamed
_____ expected to be perfect
_____ avoiding confrontations
_____ a victim of physical abuse
_____ a victim of sexual abuse
_____ a child of alcoholic parent(s)
_____ valued for my physical appearance
_____ not allowed to express my feelings
other _____
_____

*I eat . . .*
_____ too much sugar
_____ too much fat
_____ very little, but I am still fat
_____ few fruits and vegetables
_____ few grains or starches
_____ too many high-calorie drinks
_____ too many sweets
_____ too much "junk" food
_____ all the time
_____ when I am not hungry
_____ to please others
_____ too many fried foods

*I avoid exercise or physical activity because . . .*
_____ I don't like to exercise
_____ I don't know how to exercise
_____ I don't have time to exercise
_____ I don't like to get "sweaty"
_____ I have no place to exercise
_____ I am too tired to exercise
_____ I am embarrassed to exercise
_____ of a physical or medical reason
_____ of a bad experience with exercise
_____ I hate my body
other _____
_____

_____ for pleasure
_____ for security
_____ for comfort
_____ for fun
_____ to gain control
_____ for companionship
_____ until I am stuffed
_____ too much fast food
_____ unhealthy snacks
_____ in binges
_____ only what my diet allows
other _____
_____

barriers to eating healthy and exercising? *Do your barriers differ from those of a person whose body weight is different from yours? How?*

## Effectiveness of Exercise in Weight Control

Some people have touted exercise as the miracle cure for obesity, whereas others have given up on exercise in the treatment of obesity. It seems like claims related to exercise and weight loss reach both ends of the spectrum. *How much weight can be lost through exercise? Will exercise*

*maintain weight loss? Does exercise change metabolism? What type of exercise burns the most fat?* These and other questions are often raised by both the client and exercise specialist. In this section, we will uncover the realities of exercise and weight control.

### EXERCISE AND METABOLISM

The 24-hour energy expenditure can be broken down into three components, the RMR, TEF, and energy cost of physical activity. The RMR accounts for approximately 60% to 75% of the total daily energy expenditure, and therefore, anything that alters the RMR has the potential to significantly impact body weight. Since heavy exercise can

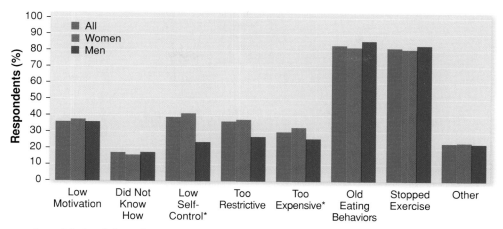

**FIGURE 22.14.** Reasons for weight-loss failure. The two most predominant reasons reported for weight-loss failure are returning to old eating behaviors and cessation of exercise. *Significant difference between genders. (Data from Miller WC, Eggert KE. Weight loss perceptions, characteristics, and expectations of an overweight male and female population. *Med Exerc Nutr Health* 1992;1:42–47.)

| Table 22.3 | PRETREATMENT SCREENING RESULT POSSIBILITIES AND RECOMMENDATIONS |
|---|---|

**Pretreatment result**

Return to old eating patterns: Patients who diet frequently, are currently dieting, do not understand how to diet, and/or report recent weight fluctuations due to previous diet attempts

**Recommendation**

Promote a conservative diet based on sound nutrition. The maintenance phase especially should promote realistic lifestyle changes in eating behaviors as well as skill competencies in areas of overeating and negative emotions.

**Pretreatment result**

Discontinue exercise: Patients who have stopped exercising or have never used exercise or physical activity for weight control

**Recommendation**

Initially prescribe an exercise or physical activity program of low intensity and low volume. Use motivational techniques and encourage increased physical activity within the client's lifestyle. Emphasize the health benefits of exercise other than just weight loss. As the patient becomes accustomed to regular physical activity and exercise, increase the volume of activity by adjusting intensity and duration.

**Pretreatment result**

Unrealistic expectations: Patients who report low motivation and low self-control, expect rapid weight loss, and/or expect to achieve an unhealthy body weight

**Recommendation**

Help the patient develop new cognitions about body weight, health, and lifestyle. Focus on a healthy lifestyle rather than just body weight or body image. Emphasize behavioral changes rather than temporary dieting. Probe further for a possible eating disorder.

**Pretreatment result**

Distorted perceptions: Patients who have an unrealistic view of their weight problem or an unrealistic view of their poor eating and inactivity patterns (patients in denial)

**Recommendation**

Take note of strong emotions associated with eating, exercise, diet, body size, weight, etc. If these emotional associations are apparent, the patient may have an eating disorder or a history of strong emotional trauma in which food has been used as a coping devise.

Remember that other members of the health care team should be alerted to and used as resources for any problem or difficulty that the exercise specialist is not adequately trained to handle.

*P E R S P E C T I V E*

# Partnership for Healthy Weight Management

The Partnership for Healthy Weight Management is a landmark effort to promote sound guidance on strategies for achieving and maintaining a healthy weight. Organized in 1998, it is composed of organizations and individuals from industry, public advocacy organizations, government agencies, scientific associations, and universities. The Partnership promotes methods for practicing healthy weight management. It has issued Voluntary Guidelines for Providers of Weight-Loss Products or Services to encourage weight-loss programs to provide basic information to consumers about their programs.

MISSION: to promote sound guidance to the general public on strategies for achieving and maintaining a healthy weight.

PRINCIPLES:

■ Following sensible and healthy guidelines for eating and physical activity is important for healthy weight management.

■ Obesity is a serious, chronic disease that is known to reduce lifespan, increase disability, and lead to many serious illnesses including diabetes, heart disease, and stroke.

■ Excess weight is caused by an interaction of genetic (inherited) and environmental (social and cultural) factors, which include metabolic (physical and chemical) and behavioral (psychologic and emotional) components. Because of the complexity of weight loss, gain, and maintenance, promises of quick and effortless weight loss are worthless.

■ A sedentary lifestyle is a significant barrier to successfully maintaining weight loss and preventing further weight gain.

■ Losing weight requires burning more calories than the body takes in, by either reducing caloric intake or increasing caloric expenditure, or preferably both.

■ Achieving and maintaining even a modest amount of weight loss can reduce the severity of illnesses associated with obesity.

■ Effective weight management involves behavior modification, which is a lifelong commitment and includes at least two components.

■ Healthful eating in accordance with the Dietary Guidelines for Americans, emphasizing a reduction in total calories, lowered fat consumption, and an increase in vegetables, fruits, and whole grains

■ Increased frequent and regular physical activity of at least moderate intensity

■ Medical, pharmacologic, and surgical interventions may be options for individuals with more serious cases of overweight and obesity. These interventions, used in conjunction with a plan for healthy eating and physical activity, should be utilized in conformance with applicable treatment guidelines.

■ The consumer is entitled to accurate, reliable, and non-deceptive information about methods for weight management. The Partnership encourages weight-loss providers to adopt the Partnership's Voluntary Disclosure Guidelines for Providers of Weight-Loss Products and Programs.

■ The Partnership opposes discrimination, including discrimination based upon size or weight.

■ The Partnership does not endorse any particular product or program for weight loss or weight management.

For more information on the Partnership for Healthy Weight Management, see http://www.consumer.gov/weightloss.

increase metabolic rate 20 times above resting levels, even short bouts of daily exercise may have a profound effect on body weight. Furthermore, it is well known that exercise increases the RMR, although the magnitude and duration of the increase are not well understood.

The most extensive review of how exercise affects RMR during weight loss was performed several years ago. This meta-analytical review pooled together data from 33 studies, which included 60 group means from weight-loss studies using either diet only or diet plus exercise interventions. The analysis revealed that there were no signifi-cant exercise or gender effects on RMR during dieting and weight loss. When diet-induced reductions in RMR were corrected for changes in body weight, RMR was reduced by less than 2%. These meta-analytical data indicate that aerobic exercise training does not differentially affect RMR during weight loss and that reductions in RMR normally seen during weight loss are proportional to the loss of the metabolically active tissue (17).

Since it is well accepted that strength training can increase muscle mass and that muscle mass is very active metabolically, investigators have recently examined how strength training may differentially affect RMR in comparison to aerobic exercise training. A cross-sectional study found that there was no significant difference in RMR among strength-trained, aerobically trained, and untrained women. In a randomized controlled clinical trial, moderately obese men and women were assigned to one of three groups: diet plus strength training, diet plus aerobic training, or diet only. The exercise protocols were designed to be isoenergetic, meaning that the energy balance for each protocol was calculated to be equal. The average weight loss among groups did not differ significantly after 8 weeks, but the strength-trained group lost less lean tissue mass than the other two groups. The RMR declined significantly in each group, with no difference among groups. These data indicate that neither strength training nor aerobic exercise training prevent the decline in RMR caused by restrictive dieting (18).

It is well known that metabolic rate is elevated immediately following an exercise session, but the metabolic rate declines back to pre-exercise levels within several hours of exercise cessation. It may be that in order to demonstrate a true exercise-induced elevation in RMR, which would enhance weight-loss success, the exercise stimulus must be repeated daily or several times per week. Accordingly, the incremental effects of the energy cost of exercise itself combined with the incremental effects of post-exercise elevations in metabolic rate may act synergistically to enhance weight-loss success and long-term reduced weight maintenance.

The increase in metabolic rate (measured as $O_2$ consumption) following exercise has been termed the excess post-exercise $O_2$ consumption (EPOC). Studies have shown that the magnitude of EPOC is linearly related to the duration and intensity of exercise and that EPOC following a moderate-intensity exercise bout (70% $\dot{V}O_{2max}$) accounts for about 15% of the total energy cost of the exercise. The time for metabolism to return to baseline following an acute exercise session can vary from as little as 20 minutes to 12 hours, depending on both the duration and intensity of exercise. Thus, one can see that over a period of months or more, increments of EPOC may play a contributing role in weight loss or reduced weight maintenance for the person struggling with body weight.

## EXERCISE INTENSITY AND SUBSTRATE USE

No significant relationship between body fatness and substrate utilization in response to the same relative exercise intensity (% $\dot{V}O_{2max}$) has been found. In other words, obesity or the degree of body fatness does not affect the metabolic response to exercise. The obese person exercising at 50% $\dot{V}O_{2max}$ derives the same amount of energy from fat as the normal-weight person (assuming both individuals are untrained). Moreover, the obese person responds to the training stimulus just the same as a normal-weight person. Therefore, if substrate utilization is a concern in exercise programming for overweight individuals, exercise proto-

cols need not be differentiated on the basis of the severity of obesity.

It is well established that the ratio of fat to carbohydrate-derived energy during exercise at low intensity is greater than that at high intensity. However, it has been suggested that with high-intensity exercise the total fat oxidation may be more than during low-intensity exercise because of the greater energy output required for high-intensity work. This theory has not been supported by the scientific data. The data show that fat oxidation at 65% $\dot{V}O_{2max}$ is greater than at 85% $\dot{V}O_{2max}$, while fat oxidation at 33% $\dot{V}O_{2max}$ is even greater than at 65% $\dot{V}O_{2max}$. Even with a higher total energy expenditure during a 15-minute exercise bout at 75% $\dot{V}O_{2max}$, more total fat-derived energy was expended during 15 minutes of exercise at 50% $\dot{V}O_{2max}$ (Fig. 22.15). Furthermore, peripheral lipolysis is maximally stimulated at lower exercise intensities. Since most obese individuals find it difficult to sustain an exercise session for 15 minutes when the intensity is above 70% $\dot{V}O_{2max}$, a more feasible exercise plan would be one of low to moderate exercise intensity (19).

## EXERCISE AND WEIGHT-LOSS SUCCESS

The National Heart Lung and Blood Institute (NHLBI) of the National Institutes of Health recently convened a panel to evaluate the effectiveness of exercise in weight control. The panel reported that weight-loss programs with exercise produced a greater weight loss than programs without exercise, but that the difference was only 2.4 kg (20). Other literature reviews have found the same thing—that exercise programs produce a weight loss of 1.5 to 3.0 kg or that exercise reduces weight at a rate of about 0.1 to 0.2 kg per week. The exercise regimen used in most research studies is one consisting of predom-

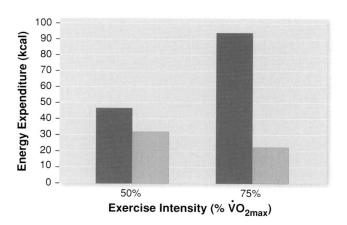

**FIGURE 22.15.** Exercise intensity and substrate use. Obese subjects burn more fat during a 15-minute continuous exercise bout at 50% $\dot{V}O_{2max}$ than at 75% $\dot{V}O_{2max}$, despite some theories that high-intensity exercise burns more total fat. (Data from Steffan HG, Elliott W, Miller WC, et al. Substrate utilization during submaximal exercise in obese and normal-weight women. *Eur J Appl Physiol Occup Physiol* 1999;80:233–239.)

inantly walking for 3 to 4 days a week for 20 to 40 minutes per session. Logic suggests that a more aggressive exercise intervention would produce larger weight losses. However, most obese persons are unable to tolerate such a rigorous exercise regimen.

Most experts recommend combining exercise with dietary restriction to produce a more substantial weight loss than with exercise alone. The NHLBI panel found that adding exercise to dietary restriction resulted in weight loss of only 1.9 kg greater than with diet alone (20). Other reviews show that although weight losses were greater in diet-plus-exercise groups, compared with diet alone, the differences were generally not statistically significant. The modest amount of extra weight loss seen when exercise is added to diet may be masked when the diet is severely restricted because the contribution of the diet to the energy deficit is much greater than that of the exercise.

Further masking of the exercise-induced weight-loss effect by restrictive dieting may be due to the fact that very–low-calorie diets can cause significant losses in water and lean body mass. Thus, a substantial amount of weight lost through very–low-calorie dieting can be lean tissue rather than fat mass. On the other hand, research studies have consistently shown that exercise will help an individual maintain lean body mass throughout the weight-loss process. The preservation of lean body mass during weight loss can help the individual retain their functional capacity, maintain their RMR, and sustain a reduced body weight.

Improving the maintenance of weight loss remains the central goal of obesity treatment, and for now, exercise seems to be the key to that goal. The importance of exercise during maintenance was illustrated in an early study in which body-weight changes of police officers who participated in an 8-week weight-loss program were analyzed. The officers were divided into four groups, each receiving a different type of very–low-calorie diet for 2 months. Each of the four groups was subsequently divided into an exercising subgroup. Follow-up measurements were taken at 6 and 18 months after treatment (8 and 20 months after the start of the intervention). As expected, diet plus exercise had a more pronounced effect upon body weight than dieting alone during the dieting phase (Fig. 22.16). There were no significant gains in body weight for those who exercised during the follow-up period. However, subjects who did not exercise following the diet gained approximately 60% of their weight back by the sixth month post-treatment and 92% back by the eighteenth month post-treatment.

Several other studies have found that individuals who are able to maintain a substantial amount of weight loss use exercise as a tool for weight maintenance. However, a cause and effect relationship cannot always be established in these studies. It is not definitive as to whether participants maintained their weight loss because they continued to exercise or continued to exercise because they maintained their weight loss. Patients who gain weight, despite reporting high levels of physical activity, may get discouraged and stop exercising. In these cases, the weight gain

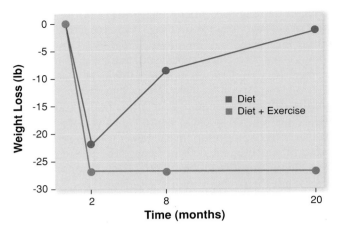

**FIGURE 22.16.** The importance of exercise in reduced weight maintenance. Exercise is the only factor that has been consistently demonstrated as effective for reduced body weight maintenance. Data in this figure represent a 2-month diet phase followed by an 18-month maintenance period. (Data extracted from Pavlou KN, Krey S, Steffee WP. Exercise as an adjunct to weight loss and maintenance in moderately obese subjects. *Am J Clin Nutr* 1989;49:1115–1123.)

may be due to a relapse in dietary behavior or other factors that precede the cessation of exercise. The false impression may therefore be that lack of exercise was responsible for weight regain.

Data from self-reports reveal that people who are unsuccessful at weight control blame the cessation of exercise for their failure. Adhering to an exercise program that requires daily exercise bouts of long duration may be problematic for many individuals. On the other hand, performing multiple short bouts of exercise during the day may be a feasible alternative. Obese people will lose comparable amounts of weight whether the energy expenditure through exercise is accumulated throughout the day or expended during one exercise bout during the day. The exercise professional should consider several alternatives to the traditional exercise prescription when working with people for whom exercise adherence may be an issue.

▶ *INQUIRY SUMMARY.* Exercise seems to be the most significant factor contributing to weight-loss maintenance. *What are some of the things a person can do to maximize the possibilities for maintaining their exercise behaviors?*

## The Exercise Prescription

The American College of Sports Medicine (ACSM) and the Centers for Disease Control have recommended that every adult accumulate 30 minutes or more of moderate-intensity physical activity on most, and preferably all, days of the week. Moderate-intensity activity in this recommendation means activity that elicits an energy expenditure of three to six times RMR or three to six **metabolic equivalents**. In layman's terms, this means simple activities such as walking, gardening, playing golf, and walking the dog, as well as incorporating more activity into one's lifestyle, like using the stairs instead of the elevator or parking the car at the far end of the lot. Those who follow these recommendations for activity can gain many of the health-related benefits of physical activity.

The overall objective of exercise participation for the overweight person is to bring about physiologic changes that will improve the health status of the individual, as well as reduce the risk of future disease. Health, however, is not a dichotomy but a continuum. Consistency, adherence, and enjoyment, rather than intensity or mode of exercise, are the goals of exercise for weight control. Once some of the barriers to physical activity are removed and activity starts to become part of one's lifestyle, higher levels of health and fitness can be achieved by participating in a more structured exercise program. Exercise professionals should work with patients to set reasonable short-term physical activity goals that contribute to achieving intermediate-term goals of consistent lifestyle activity coupled with regular bouts of moderate exercise. Thus, the art of exercise prescription is the successful integration of exercise science with behavior modification techniques that result in long-term program compliance and attainment of the individual's goals.

The Council of Scientific Affairs of the American Medical Association and the ACSM have given general guidelines for exercise in the treatment of overweight/obesity. As part of a weight-control program, the recommendation is that the exercise component should:

1. Promote increased energy expenditure
2. Promote fat loss and maintenance of lean tissue mass
3. Be safe for the participating individual
4. Promote increased activity levels within the individual's lifestyle

The ACSM specifies that the critical factor in exercise for weight control is a high-energy expenditure. Exercise professionals should manipulate the intensity and duration of exercise to promote a daily energy expenditure of 300 to 500 $kcal \cdot d^{-1}$ or 1000 to 2000 $kcal \cdot wk^{-1}$. The initial exercise prescription should be based upon low intensity and progressively longer durations of activity. This may require that the intensity of exercise be set at or below the intensity generally recommended for cardiorespiratory fitness (21). However, as the person responds to exercise training, the goal should be to bring the person into a target heart rate range at which cardiorespiratory fitness will be achieved. As intensity of exercise is increased, the duration can be decreased while maintaining a high-energy expenditure. For many patients, a walking or moderate-intensity exercise program will be all they desire, and movement toward a more intense program may not be warranted.

Accordingly, the exercise prescription for the overweight person should consist of the following.

■ Type or mode of exercise: aerobic, meaning continuous, rhythmic, and using the large-muscle groups; strength training may be used as an adjunct to aerobic training

■ Frequency: 5 days per week or daily
■ Duration: 40 to 60 minutes per session or split sessions of 20 to 30 minutes each
■ Intensity: 40% or 50% to 70% $\dot{V}O_{2max}$ or 40% or 50% to 70% of heart rate reserve; initially emphasize duration rather than intensity
■ Initially the volume of exercise should be large enough to expend 1000 $kcal \cdot wk^{-1}$; this should be gradually increased so that the client can safely expend 2000 or more $kcal \cdot wk^{-1}$ in physical activity

Adjustments in the exercise prescription should be made according to individual needs and any existing comorbidities or relative contraindications. The exercise session should be preceded by a warmup period and followed by a cooldown period, each consisting of several minutes of aerobic activity (e.g., walking). Medical parameters such as heart rate, blood pressure, or blood glucose may need to be monitored for patients with existing comorbidities.

The severely obese individual presents a different profile than the overweight or moderately obese individual. Severe obesity carries with it a greater prevalence of chronic diseases. The prevalence of diabetes, cardiovascular disease, hypertension, and musculoskeletal disorders runs particularly high in severe obesity. During exercise, severely obese subjects often demonstrate a higher cardiac output, absolute $O_2$ consumption ($L \cdot min^{-1}$), and minute ventilation at any given workload than normal-weight subjects. Heat dissipation is impaired for the severely obese person, exacerbating the physiologic strain during exercise in the heat. Other conditions that may limit exercise capacity for the severely obese include orthopedic pain, local muscle weakness, balance problems, movement restriction, and exercise anxiety. The practice then is to reduce the overall volume of exercise for the severely obese individual until he/she is accustomed to regular exercise. This can be done by initially reducing the frequency of exercise sessions, reducing the duration of the exercise bout, reducing the exercise intensity, or any combination of the three.

Severely obese persons cannot exercise at the same intensity as moderately obese people. High-impact exercises are more strenuous for the severely obese person than the moderately obese person. The risk of injury and pain can be diminished if high-impact exercises are avoided and exercise modalities that support the body weight are utilized. Activities such as swimming, water aerobics, cycling, rowing, and low-impact aerobic activities avoid the impact of the body mass on the ground and may be better tolerated by the severely obese. Modifications in equipment, such as wide seats on cycle ergometers, make the exercise experience more comfortable for the severely obese person and encourage continued participation.

 *Experiences in Work Physiology Lab Exercise 18: Assessment of the Overweight Patient takes you through the process of evaluating an overweight client and designing a behavioral intervention.*

▶ *INQUIRY SUMMARY.* The exercise prescription for the overweight or obese individual needs to be structured carefully. General guidelines have been given for exercise programming of the overweight person. However, individual differences, existing comorbidities, and severity of obesity must be considered when structuring the exercise program. As the person becomes accustomed to exercise, the volume of exercise can be increased. *Contrast the initial exercise prescription for a moderately obese individual with no existing comorbidities with that of a severely obese individual with chronic disease.*

## Relapse Prevention

Any weight-management program is not truly successful unless the weight loss is maintained or the other desired outcome variables from the program are maintained. The simplest way to maintain a healthy weight is to continue to participate in healthful behaviors. All of us lapse from our conditioned behaviors once in a while, either by choice or by force. However, we do not all have to relapse. The difference between lapse and relapse is subtle but critical. Relapse means to fall back to a former state or practice. Lapse, on the other hand, is a temporary decline or deviation from an expected or accepted state or practice. Any deviation from a newly accustomed behavior does not have to be permanent or bring the patient all the way back to his/her place of origin.

Several factors are characteristic of those people who successfully maintain their reduced body weight or healthy weight management behaviors. The three keys to successful weight maintenance are *exercise, self-monitoring,* and *emotional coping skills.* One group of scientists was able to make comparison measurements among three groups of women: those who successfully lost and maintained weight (maintainers), those who lost and regained weight (relapsers), and those who never had a weight problem (controls). The behavioral patterns of the three groups are outlined in *Table 22.4.* When one examines the table carefully, some behavioral patterns emerge. First of all, the maintainers tended to lose their weight through a personalized program that included self-monitoring of food intake and exercise, rather than dependence upon an external factor like their doctor, pills, or a weight-loss group. Another difference among groups was that the relapsers coped with problems by escaping and avoiding rather than problem solving and confronting. It is also interesting to note how similar the behaviors of the maintainers were to the controls, who always were at an average body weight.

The National Weight Control Registry contains self-reported data from formerly obese individuals who have been successful at weight maintenance for at least 1 year. Volunteers in the registry who have maintained a 13.6-kg

| **Table 22.4** | **DIET AND EXERCISE BEHAVIORS OF PREVIOUSLY OBESE WOMEN** | | |
|---|---|---|---|
| **How reduced** | **Relapsers** | **Maintainers** | **Controls** |
| Devised a personal eating plan | 39% | 73% | |
| Attended Weight Watchers | 43% | 10% | |
| Attended other programs or groups | 29% | 10% | |
| Exercised | 36% | 76% | |
| Followed doctor's orders | 34% | 20% | |
| Took pills or shots | 47% | 3% | |
| **How maintaining a healthy weight** | | | |
| Monitoring weight | | 87% | 76% |
| Exercising | | 83% | 88% |
| Eating less | | 83% | 73% |
| Watching food intake | | 60% | 50% |
| Reducing high-sugar food intake | | 57% | 50% |
| Reducing high-fat food intake | | 57% | 38% |
| Changing to good eating habits | | 57% | 29% |
| Changing attitude toward food | | 47% | 9% |
| Aware of body size by feel of clothes | | 23% | 29% |
| Not eating three meals a day | | 20% | 38% |
| **Coping with problems** | | | |
| Escape, avoidance, alcohol, pills | 70% | 33% | 35% |
| Seek social support (talk) | 38% | 70% | 80% |
| Self-control (no outside help) | 13% | 16% | 43% |
| Problem solving/confronting | 10% | 95% | 60% |
| Tension-reducing techniques | 2% | 17% | 42% |

Data from Kayman S, Bruvold W, Stern JS. Maintenance and relapse after weight loss in women: behavioral aspects. *Am J Clin Nutr* 1990;52:800–807.

weight loss for an average of 5 years reported substantial improvements in health and quality of life. Those same individuals also reported that their success was due to consuming 1381 to 1526 kcal·d$^{-1}$ and expending about 400 kcal·d$^{-1}$ in exercise (22).

People who are successful in weight maintenance have three things in common: exercise, self-monitoring, and emotional coping skills. Exercise itself is a healthy weight behavior that needs to be monitored, and so is emotional coping. So the three keys to maintenance really all consolidate into self-monitoring. To successfully maintain one's

newly established health behaviors then, one needs to self-monitor. There is not one specific set pattern for self-monitoring that works with each patient. The exercise professional needs to design a self-monitoring plan specific to individual patient needs. Some possible monitoring strategies can be taken from Table 22.4, while others might be taken from Table 22.3. Exercise logs, food diaries, journaling, goal setting, and reward systems are other examples of self-monitoring tools.

Box 22.3 contains information about a new approach to the treatment of overweight, called the Health At Any Size

**Box 22.3**

*P E R S P E C T I V E*

## *The Health At Every Size Paradigm for Obesity Treatment*

Traditionally health care professionals have used restrictive dieting and exercise intervention strategies in an effort to treat obesity. Despite these efforts, the prevalence of obesity continues to rise dramatically. This apparent ineffectiveness of diet and exercise programming to reduce obesity has caused both professionals and consumers to challenge the further use of diet and exercise for the sole purpose of reducing body weight in the obese and to suggest an alternative approach to obesity intervention—the health at every size (HAES) paradigm.

The HAES paradigm views obesity from the philosophy that dieting and weight obsession are contributing to the problem and that our societal obsession with thinness does not allow for diversity in body shapes. The HAES approach assumes that the overweight person wants to eat healthy food and be active and that once diet restrictions and barriers to activity have been removed, the individual will develop healthier eating and activity patterns which lead to a genetically determined healthy body weight. Under this new paradigm, the person is encouraged to stop dieting and exercising for weight loss and is taught skills to recognize what his or her body wants and needs. Quality of life and improved health are the goals of treatment, rather than reaching some predetermined body weight.

The fundamental belief of the HAES paradigm is that health is a result of behaviors that are independent of body weight. Therefore, supporters of the HAES philosophy propose that individuals have learned unhealthy behaviors that mask one's ability to eat healthily in response to internal cues and to participate in physical activity for enjoyment rather than weight loss. HAES supporters also believe that individu-

als who have engaged in restrained eating behaviors lack the coping skills necessary for situations that prompt emotional eating.

Accordingly, the HAES-based treatment is designed to enhance mind skills, body skills, and lifestyle skills. Under mind skills, persons are taught to identify feelings and needs, develop reasonable expectations, and develop positive cognitions. Body skills include the ability to honor and accept one's body, recognize resistance to losing weight, and attend to self-care and health-care. Lifestyle skills help the individual eat in response to hunger and without restraint and to participate in physical activity for fulfillment and restoration.

Although there is limited research available on the HAES approach, initial results show some promise in offering a more realistic and long-term approach to weight and lifestyle. Results showing improvement in psychologic states, eating pathology, and quality of life, as well as possibilities for long-term weight reduction and an increase in healthy behaviors, make the HAES paradigm more attractive than traditional weight-loss treatments that focus on restriction and deprivation. On the other hand, the liabilities of the HAES design include an underlying presumption of psychologic dysfunction (e.g., eating pathology and body image disparagement), of gender and culture bias (Caucasian women), and limited to persons capable of cognitive-behavior therapy. Furthermore, psychologic well-being is only one component of overall health, and if the HAES approach to overweight leads to decreased morbidity and mortality remains to be determined. Therefore, it is up to the medical community to further test the physiologic efficacy of this alternative method of weight management.

paradigm. The Health At Any Size approach assumes that the overweight person innately wants to eat healthy food and be active and that once diet restrictions and barriers to activity have been removed, the individual will develop healthier eating and activity patterns that lead to a genetically determined healthy body weight.

▶ *INQUIRY SUMMARY.* Self-monitoring must be individualized to be effective. A self-monitoring technique that works for one person may not work for another. The most effective self-monitoring techniques are those that take into account individual preferences, individual values, individual motivators, and individual coping skills. *What might be some other ways patients can self-monitor so that their chance for relapse is minimized?*

# Summary

The prevalence of overweight and obesity is increasing at a rapid rate. Obesity is associated with several chronic diseases including diabetes, cardiovascular disease, and hypertension. A multitude of factors are responsible for the promotion of obesity such as having a genetic predisposition toward obesity, a low metabolic rate, a positive energy balance, diet composition, and inactivity. Although overweight people present a psychologic profile that is similar to that of normal-weight people, the burden of being overweight brings unique emotional stressors. Healthful eating and regular exercise are the keys to successful weight control, but physical and emotional barriers often prevent obese persons from making lifestyle changes. The exercise specialist must design an appropriate exercise regimen for the overweight person and help the patient overcome barriers to behavior change. An individualized self-monitoring system is common to all persons who successfully maintain a reduced body weight. The lab experience for this chapter brings you through the process of interviewing and counseling an overweight patient.

## SUMMARY KNOWLEDGE

1. What are some of the diseases that are associated with overweight and obesity?
2. What can a person do if he/she has a genetic predisposition toward obesity?
3. What are some factors, other than just overeating, that may contribute to a positive energy balance?
4. What are some of the obstacles large people have to overcome to succeed in a society that values thinness?
5. What are some emotional links, positive or negative, people have with food and physical exercise?
6. Why is self-monitoring considered so important in maintaining weight loss, and how might exercise professionals assist patients in self-monitoring?

## References

1. Flegal KM, Carroll MD, Ogden CL, et al. Prevalence and trends in obesity among US adults, 1999–2000. *JAMA* 2002;288: 1723–1727.
2. Ogden CL, Flegal KM, Carroll MD, et al. Prevalence and trends in overweight among children and adolescents, 1999–2000. *JAMA* 2002;288:1728–1732.
3. Rampone AJ, Reynolds PJ. Obesity: thermodynamic principles in perspective. *Life Sci* 1988;43:93–110.
4. Kramer FM, Jeffery RW, Forster JL, et al. Long-term follow-up of behavioral treatment for obesity: patterns of weight regain among men and women. *Int J Obes* 1989;13:123–136.
5. Welle SL, Amatruda JM, Forbes GB, et al. Resting metabolic rates of obese women after rapid weight loss. *J Clin Endocrinol Metab* 1984;59:41–44.
6. Lansky D, Brownell KD. Estimates of food quantity and calories: errors in self-report among obese patients. *Am J Clin Nutr* 1982;35: 727–732.
7. Lichtman SW, Pasarska K, Berman ER, et al. Discrepancy between self-reported and actual caloric intake and exercise in obese subjects. *N Engl J Med* 1992;327:1893–1898.
8. Myers RJ, Klesges RC, Eck LH, et al. Accuracy of self-reports of food intake in obese and normal-weight individuals: effects of obesity on self-reports of dietary intake in adult females. *Am J Clin Nutr* 1988;48: 1248–1251.
9. Lissner L, Habicht JP, Strupp BJ, et al. Body composition and energy intake: do overweight women overeat and underreport? *Am J Clin Nutr* 1989;49:320–325.
10. Bray GA, Zachary B, Dahms WT, et al. Eating patterns of massively obese individuals. *J Am Diet Assoc* 1978;72:24–27.
11. Donato K, Hegsted DM. Efficiency of utilization of various sources of energy for growth. *Proc Natl Acad Sci USA* 1985;82:4866–4870.
12. Bray GA. The energetics of obesity. *Med Sci Sports Exerc* 1983;15: 32–40.
13. Olson CL, Schumaker HD, Yawn BP. Overweight women delay medical care. *Arch Fam Med* 1994;3:888–892.
14. Rand CSW, Macgregor AMC. Successful weight loss following obesity surgery and the perceived liability of morbid obesity. *Int J Obes* 1991;15:577–579.
15. Curry KR, Jaffe A. *Nutrition counseling and communication skills.* Philadelphia: WB Saunders, 1998:6.
16. Miller WC, Eggert KE. Weight loss perceptions, characteristics, and expectations of an overweight male and female population. *Med Exerc Nutr Health* 1992;1:42–47.
17. Ballor DL, Poehlman ET. A meta-analysis of the effects of exercise and/or dietary restriction on resting metabolic rate. *Eur J Appl Physiol Occup Physiol* 1995;71:535–542.
18. Geliebter A, Maher MM, Gerace L, et al. Effects of strength or aerobic training on body composition, resting metabolic rate, and peak oxygen consumption in obese dieting subjects. *Am J Clin Nutr* 1997;66: 557–563.
19. Steffan HG, Elliott W, Miller WC, et al. Substrate utilization during submaximal exercise in obese and normal-weight women. *Eur J Appl Physiol Occup Physiol* 1999;80:233–239.
20. National Institutes of Health. Clinical guidelines on the identification, evaluation, and treatment of overweight and obesity in adults— the evidence report. *Obes Res* 1998;6(Suppl 2):51S–209S.
21. Franklin BA, Whaley MH, Howley ET, eds. *ACSM's guidelines for exercise testing and prescription.* 6th ed. Baltimore: Lippincott Williams & Wilkins, 2000:214–216
22. Klem ML, Wing RR, McGuire MT, et al. A descriptive study of individuals successful at long-term maintenance of substantial weight loss. *Am J Clin Nutr* 1997;66:239–246.

### Suggested Readings

Miller WC. Effective diet and exercise treatments for overweight and recommendations for intervention. *Sports Med* 2001;31:717–724.

Miller WC, Jacob AV. The health at any size paradigm for obesity treatment: the scientific evidence. *Obes Rev* 2001;2:37–45.

Ross R, Janssen I. Physical activity, total and regional obesity: dose-response considerations. *Med Sci Sports Exerc* 2001;33(6 Suppl): S521–S527.

Thayer RE. *Calm energy: how people regulate mood with food and exercise.* New York: Oxford University Press, 2001.

### On the Internet

National Heart Lung, and Blood Institute: Obesity Education Initiative. Available at: **http://www.nhlbi.nih.gov/oei/**. Accessed June 28, 2005.

National Institute of Diabetes & Digestive & Kidney Diseases: Weight-Control Information Network. Available at: **http://win.niddk.nih.gov**. Accessed June 28, 2005.

Partnership for Healthy Weight Management. Available at: **http://www.consumer.gov/weightloss**. Accessed June 28, 2005.

Shape Up America! Available at: **http://www.shapeup.org**. Accessed June 28, 2005.

## Writing to Learn

*In this chapter, we have discussed the etiology of obesity and the interplay of several factors that affect treatment success. The foundation for the treatment plan is set primarily during the intake interview or the initial interview with the patient. Suppose Jane Doe has been referred to you by her physician. Jane is 55 years old and obese, and she desires to lose weight. Outline the types of information you would want to obtain from Jane which would help you structure her weight-loss program. In other words, what information would you gather during the initial interview? A possible outline format would be: Medical History, Behavioral History, Psychologic History, Patient Perceptions, Exercise Barriers, Social Support, and Barriers to Healthful Eating. What information would you seek under each of these headings?*

CHAPTER

# 23 *Exercise for Oncological and Neuromusculoskeletal Diseases*

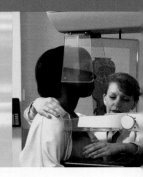

*Of the more than 2500 identified diseases in the world, only about 500 are curable. However, many of the incurable diseases are controllable. For example, there is no cure for diabetes, but the disease can be managed or controlled through proper medication and a healthy lifestyle. Exercise is used in the prevention and treatment of many cardiopulmonary and metabolic diseases such as hyperlipidemia, diabetes, heart disease, and obesity.* Are diseases that are not directly related to cardiopulmonary metabolism, such as cancers, stroke, Parkinson disease, and muscular dystrophy, positively influenced by exercise training?

A woman receiving a mammogram to screen for breast cancer. Early detection greatly increases the chances of surviving most forms of cancer.

## CHAPTER OUTLINE

Because exercise training can lessen or alleviate the symptoms associated with disease, the exercise prescription is often an integral part of the therapeutic or rehabilitative process for persons diagnosed with chronic diseases. Exercise has traditionally been used to prevent the onset of cardiopulmonary disease or in the rehabilitation of patients with these disorders; however, some diseases afflict the neuromusculoskeletal system itself. *Is exercise contraindicated for diseases such as muscular dystrophy or osteoarthritis, which seem to be aggravated by exercise?* Many diseases, like breast cancer, afflict organs of the body not directly involved in metabolic processes. *Does exercise have an effect on the disease itself or does exercise merely improve the quality of life for the person with the disease?* Answers to these and other questions about the relationship among exercise, oncology, and neuromusculoskeletal disorders are explored in this chapter.

## Brain and Nerve Disorders

As you already know, the brain, spinal cord, and nerves throughout the body make up the nervous system. The nervous system is divided into two distinct parts: the central nervous system, which comprises the brain and spinal cord, and the peripheral nervous system, consisting of a network of nerves that connect the brain and spinal cord to the rest of the body. When an area of the nervous system is abnormal or becomes damaged, a wide range of disorders may ensue. Many disorders of the central nervous system are manifest in the peripheral nervous system by way of motor dysfunction. For example, in **Parkinson disease**, an area deep within the brain degenerates, causing a lower production of the neurotransmitter **dopamine**. Low dopamine levels disallow proper communication among parts of the brain and peripheral nervous system, causing muscle tremors and/or jerky movements.

Disorders of the peripheral nervous system are also manifest through motor dysfunction. In **myasthenia gravis**, antibodies attack the acetylcholine receptors at the motor endplate, causing episodes of muscle weakness (see Chapter 9 for details on motor impulse transmission). Motor dysfunction can also be symptomatic of other diseases that affect the musculature itself, like muscular dystrophy (MD). Regardless of the cause, there are several types of disorders that directly affect neuromuscular function and the ability of an individual to exercise or respond to exercise training. Although it is beyond the scope of this book to investigate all of these brain and nerve disorders, several of the most common disorders seen by exercise professionals are discussed. These include *stroke, multiple sclerosis (MS), MD, epilepsy, Parkinson disease, and Alzheimer disease*. It is also common for exercise professionals to encounter clients with brain or nerve disorders included as **comorbidities** with cardiopulmonary disorders. Box 23.1 includes a biographic profile of Felix Bloch, one of the researchers who discovered magnetic resonance imaging, a diagnostic tool used to identify many of the diseases discussed in this chapter.

 **LINKUP: Perspective: Life Expectancy and Quality of Life**, *which can be accessed at http://connection.lww. com/go/brownexphys and on the Student Resource CD-ROM, is an interesting article on the fact that our life expectancy is rising, but our quality of life is deteriorating.*

## STROKE

**Stroke** is a leading cause of death and disability in the Western industrialized countries. One in 15 deaths in the United States is attributable to stroke, making it the third leading cause of death in this country. Approximately three quarters of a million new strokes occur each year with 4 million stroke survivors living in the United States. The

---

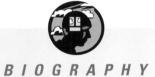

**Box 23.1**

*BIOGRAPHY*

## *Felix Bloch* (1905–1983)

Felix Bloch was born in Zurich, Switzerland on October 23, 1905. He attended elementary and secondary schools in Zurich and thereafter entered the Federal Institute of Technology. After 1 year of studying engineering, he switched his studies to mathematics and physics. Bloch received his PhD in physics from the University of Leipzig in 1928. Bloch left Germany in 1933, after Hitler's ascent to power, and 1 year later accepted a position at Stanford University in Palo Alto, California. Bloch studied the magnetic properties of neutrons for several years, and in 1945 he began studying neutron properties through electromagnetic procedures. In collaboration with William W. Hansen and Martin E. Packard, he developed a purely electromagnetic procedure for the study of nuclear properties in solids, liquids, and gases. A few weeks after his first successful experiments with the new magnetic resonance imaging (MRI), he received news that the same discovery was made independently by Edward M. Purcell at Harvard University. Bloch and Purcell were subsequently awarded the Nobel Prize for Physics in 1952.

MRI is an imaging technique used in medical settings to produce high-quality images of tissues in the body. MRI is based on the principles of nuclear magnetic resonance (NMR), a spectroscopic technique used by scientists to obtain microscopic and chemical information about molecules. The nucleus of each atom possesses a property called spin, which can be thought of as a small magnetic field with its own signal. An image can be constructed by mapping the NMR signal from the hydrogen atoms in a tissue. In medical MRI, radiologists are most interested in looking at the NMR signal from water and fat, the major hydrogen-containing components of the human body. MRI is a very sophisticated diagnostic tool in identifying neurologic legions, cancers, and tissue abnormalities related to some of the diseases discussed in this chapter.

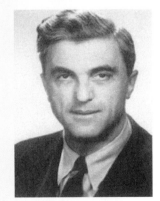
Felix Bloch

incidence of first stroke increases exponentially with age. Men have a greater risk for stroke than women earlier in life, while women have a greater risk later in life. Although the survival rate for stroke is 70%, many stroke survivors suffer from neurologic impairments that require rehabilitation programs of various durations. Consequently, it is quite common for clinical exercise physiologists and physical and occupational therapists to work with patients who have survived a stroke.

## Etiologies, Symptoms, and Prognosis

When stroke occurs, brain tissue dies because of lack of blood flow and insufficient $O_2$ delivery to a part of the brain. There are two possible types of stroke, **ischemic stroke** and **hemorrhagic stroke** (*Fig. 23.1*). In ischemic stroke, blood flow to a part of the brain is blocked either by atherosclerosis or a blood clot. The blockage does not have to be within the brain itself but can be in any blood vessel that leads to the brain. Hemorrhagic stroke occurs when a blood vessel bursts or is ruptured and the blood leaks into an area of the brain and destroys it. Most strokes begin suddenly, develop rapidly, and cause brain damage within minutes. A small number of strokes continue to worsen for up to a day or more as an enlarging part of the brain tissue dies. Strokes can cause swelling in the brain. Such swelling is dangerous because the resulting pressure within the skull furthers brain damage.

Several different symptoms and secondary conditions can occur, depending on which part of the brain is affected and the severity of the stroke. The major symptoms of stroke include weakness or paralysis and impaired balance. A major physiologic consequence of stroke is the loss of functional muscle mass. This generally manifests itself in a low $\dot{V}O_{2max}$ for stroke survivors with a severe reduction in muscular strength and muscular endurance. Comorbidities are also common for stroke patients. The most common comorbidities include coronary artery disease, hypertension, hyperlipidemia, diabetes mellitus, peripheral vascular disease, and obesity. Furthermore, more than 50% of stroke survivors suffer from depression.

A large negative consequence of stroke is muscle weakness due to loss of motor unit activation and changes in muscle fiber recruitment and firing. Additional muscle changes include stiffness, adaptive motor patterns, paralysis, and muscle imbalance. Muscle weakness, stiffness, and disordered motor control combine to cause functional movement disability. The stroke survivor consequently has a reduced fitness level and low energy level.

Many people who suffer from a stroke recover fully or regain most normal function. Others may retain some degree of paralysis and are left with only limited use of an

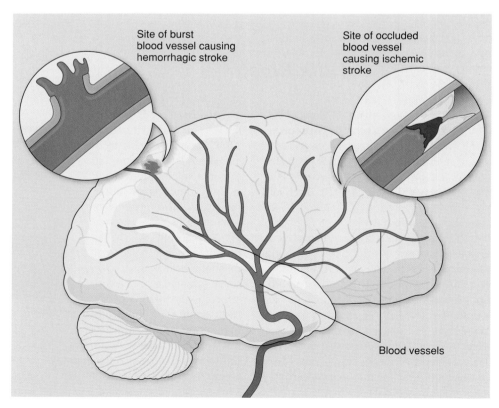

**FIGURE 23.1.** Hemorrhagic vs. ischemic stroke. Hemorrhagic stroke destroys brain tissue when the blood from a ruptured vessel enters the brain cavity and pollutes the surrounding area. Ischemic stroke destroys brain tissue because an occluded blood vessel disallows $O_2$ delivery to part of the brain.

affected arm or leg. Yet others become physically and/or mentally devastated and unable to move, speak, or eat normally. Outcome for stroke is particularly poor if the stroke causes unconsciousness or impairs breathing or heart function. Neurologic impairment that lasts longer than 6 months is generally permanent. Intensive rehabilitation can help those with disability learn to function despite their impairments.

Most stroke survivors have residual neurologic impairments that persistently limit function; one of the most common of these is **hemiparesis**, which is a paralysis or partial paralysis of only one side of the body. Persons with hemiparesis walk more slowly, are less capable of adjusting the speed of their walk, and possess a reduced range of walking speed. The hemiparesis walk requires increased energy expenditure, which is evidenced by a high $O_2$ consumption, heart rate, respiratory rate, and blood pressure response to exercise.

## Exercise Benefits and Prescription

Conditioning exercises, performed under proper supervision and within patient tolerance, have been found to be safe and effective for stroke survivors. Strength exercises have been shown to drive reorganization and adaptive processes in motor control. Aerobic exercise training on either a cycle ergometer or treadmill improves aerobic fitness and reduces energy expenditure for stroke survivors during a standardized walking task. Decreased exercise heart rate and blood pressure have also been seen in stroke survivors following aerobic exercise training. Flexibility training has been shown to improve function in the muscle groups of the hemiparetic side. Appropriate exercise training can improve functional capacity and reduce comorbidities for the stroke patient.

The stroke survivor should participate in daily exercise that is targeted at improving cardiovascular function, muscular strength and endurance, and muscular flexibility. The aerobic training program should consist of 30 minutes of continuous or discontinuous exercise performed 3 or more days per week. Participants should begin with intermittent exercise sessions during the first few weeks of the program and then progress to continuous exercise. The intensity of the exercise should begin at 40% $\dot{V}O_{2max}$ and then progress to 60% to 70%. The strength-training protocol should focus on performing one or more sets at 15 to 20 repetition maximum (RM). Individuals who cannot lift the minimal amount of weight on certain machines or free weights can start their strength-training program by using resistance bands or the person's own limb weight as the initial resistance. Blood pressure and rating of perceived exertion (RPE) should be recorded frequently during both the aerobic and strength-training session. It is suggested that RPE and blood pressure be recorded after each set of the strength-training session until a baseline is established and it is apparent that the performed exercise will not place the patient at risk. Case Study 23.1 provides information on how an exercise prescription is constructed for a stroke survivor.

## MULTIPLE SCLEROSIS

The incidence of MS is difficult to determine because physicians are not required to report newly diagnosed cases in the United States. The best estimates are 50 to 100 cases per 100,000 people. There are about 400,000 cases of MS in this country, and 2.5 million people worldwide suffer from the disease. It is also estimated that 200 Americans are newly diagnosed with multiple sclerosis each week. The disease attacks adults in the prime of life—most cases occur between the age of 20 and 50, with 70% of all diagnoses for individuals between 21 and 40. The prevalence of MS is greater in women than men, with twice as many women as men being afflicted. The majority of those afflicted with the disease do not become severely disabled and live to the normal lifespan.

## Etiologies, Symptoms, and Prognosis

As you learned in Chapter 9, nerve fibers inside and outside the brain are wrapped with layers of insulation called the myelin sheath. The myelin sheath permits the rapid transmission of nerve impulses along the nerve fiber. When the myelin sheath around the nerve loses its integrity, nerve impulse conduction is disrupted (*Fig. 23.2*). The result is that muscular movements become gross, jerky, and uncoordinated. MS is the most common disorder in which the myelin sheath of the central nervous system is destroyed. The cause of MS is unknown, but the theory is that a virus or some other agent triggers an autoimmune response in the body. The body then produces antibodies against its own myelin which cause inflammation and damage to the nerve.

In some people, MS may start with an isolated symptom, followed by months or years without further symptoms. In other people, symptoms become worse within weeks and months. Symptoms may intensify with heat, such as during hot weather, a hot bath, or fever. The disease may flare up spontaneously or may be triggered by an infection or influenza. The different courses of the disease within an individual or throughout the population differ in their timing, location of affliction, and severity. Despite the disability, most people with MS have a normal lifespan.

There are four different types of MS: relapsing/remitting, secondary progressive, progressive relapsing, and primary progressive (*Fig. 23.3*). Relapsing/remitting MS is characterized by intermittent periods of relapse and remission. During relapses, new symptoms appear or old ones resurface or worsen. A relapse can last for days, weeks, or months. Recovery from relapse can be instantaneous or slow. During remission, the person recovers either partially or fully. Most people presenting with MS are first diagnosed with this type. Many people who have relapsing/remitting MS will pass on to the secondary progressive phase. This is characterized by a gradual worsening of the

## CASE STUDY 23.1:  *EXERCISE PRESCRIPTION FOR STROKE SURVIVOR*

### CASE

You are a clinical exercise physiologist working for a cardiac rehabilitation center. A new patient who recently suffered an ischemic stroke due to atherosclerosis has been referred to the center. The patient, Keith, has worked with a physical therapist for 4 weeks and is now ready to begin a physical conditioning program.

### DESCRIPTION

Stroke is the third leading cause of death in the United States. In ischemic stroke, the blood supply to a part of the brain is cut off because of either atherosclerosis or a blood clot that has blocked a blood vessel. In either case, another stroke is likely to occur unless the underlying cause of the stroke is corrected. Rehabilitation, started as soon as the patient's vital signs have been stabilized, can help stroke victims overcome disability caused by impairment of brain tissue and can also help other parts of the brain assume tasks previously performed by the damaged part.

### EVALUATION/INTERVENTION

Keith has partial paralysis on one side of his body. The paralysis is noticeable when he walks but does not limit his activities of daily living. Your first step is to perform an assessment of functional aerobic capacity. Since Keith has a hemiparetic walk, you decide to administer a cycle ergometry test to measure $\dot{V}O_{2max}$. Keith performs the test without any complications, and his $\dot{V}O_{2max}$ value is 30.5 mL·kg$^{-1}$·min$^{-1}$. This score places him below the 30th percentile for a 55-year-old male. Keith's upper body strength ratio (0.64, bench press:body weight) places him in the lowest 20% of men his age, and his leg press-to-weight ratio of 1.40 places him in the 30th percentile for men his age. The last test you perform is the sit-and-reach, on which he scored in the 40th percentile.

The fitness assessment you administered to Keith shows that he has muscle weakness, muscle stiffness, and low aerobic capacity. You prescribe an aerobic exercise program for Keith, which includes exercising 4 to 5 days per week at 50% of his cycle ergometer $\dot{V}O_{2max}$ for 20 minutes. The exercise volume will increase as he progresses. In addition to the aerobic exercise training, Keith will strength train 2 to 3 days per week in a program designed to develop overall body strength and muscular endurance. You also design a flexibility program for Keith that particularly focuses on the stiff muscles of the partially paralyzed side. Keith will continue in his physical therapy once a week, and a reassessment of his functional capacities will be done in 2 months.

---

disease during relapses. As time progresses, the relapses merge into a general progression. People with secondary progressive MS experience good and bad days or weeks, with little remission and no real recovery. Fifty percent of those with relapsing/remitting MS pass on to secondary progressive MS within 10 years.

Progressive/relapsing MS follows a progressive course from the onset of the disease. There is some recovery after each relapse, but there is a gradual worsening of the symptoms between relapses. Unlike the other types of MS, primary progressive MS is characterized by a gradual progression of the disease without any remission. There may be periods of leveling off of the disease, but no real recovery or remission occurs. In spite of the debilitating effects of MS, two-thirds of those with the disease can still walk with use of an aid such as a cane.

### Exercise Benefits and Prescription

Patients with MS have shown improvements in aerobic capacity, muscular strength, body composition, and coordination following aerobic training and performing exercises focused on activities of daily living (ADL). The exercise prescription for the patient with MS must follow an assessment of physical abilities and limitations. Functional evaluation of the MS patient can be complicated by weakness, spasticity, **ataxia**, and lack of coordination. Moreover, an evaluation at rest may indicate normal function, whereas the patient may exhibit abnormal fatigue, spasticity, lack of coordination, or other symptoms after brief exercise or exposure to heat (1). Compounding the problem further is the fact that persons with MS are generally deconditioned; part of their decrement in muscle function can be attributed to their low fitness levels.

Petajan and White (1) classify physical activity for the MS patient in a pyramid fashion. For the purpose of exercise prescription, two pyramids are given, a physical activity pyramid (*Fig. 23.4*) and a muscular fitness pyramid (*Fig. 23.5*). Exercises that coincide with a given functional level in either pyramid can be incorporated into the exercise prescription. Although the pyramids are not necessarily mutually exclusive, the physical activity pyramid tends to focus on increasing energy expenditure through physical movement, while the muscle fitness pyramid tends to focus on muscular strength, flexibility, and endurance.

At the base of the physical activity pyramid are ADL. The completion of ADL may be the only physical activity for patients with severe motor deficiencies. To avoid further functional losses, the motor tasks for the completion of ADL should be done independently whenever possible. If the patient is able to complete ADL, he/she can move up to the next level of the pyramid, which increases energy expenditure by building inefficiencies into daily activities. For example, parking the car on the outskirts of the

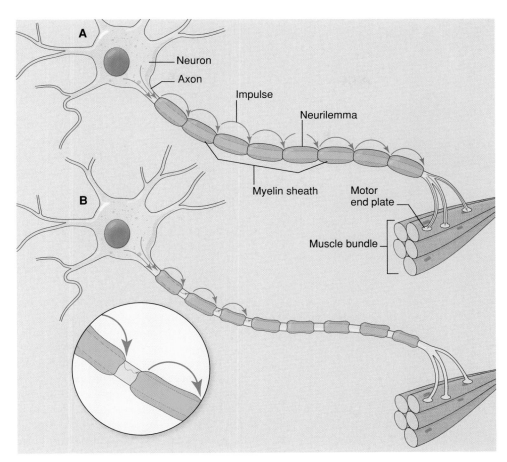

**FIGURE 23.2.** Demyelination of the nerve fiber in multiple sclerosis. **A.** The normal pathway of nerve impulse transmission where the impulse skips among the nodes of Ranvier as it travels along the myelinated nerve. **B.** Nerve impulse transmission is impeded when the myelin sheath degenerates, as in multiple sclerosis.

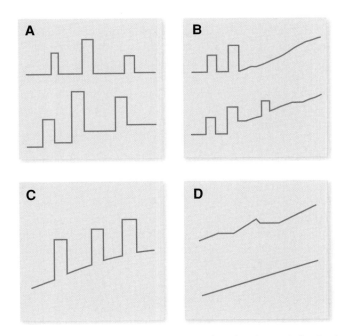

**FIGURE 23.3.** The four types of multiple sclerosis. **A.** Relapsing/remitting. **B.** Secondary progressive. **C.** Progressive relapsing. **D.** Primary progressive.

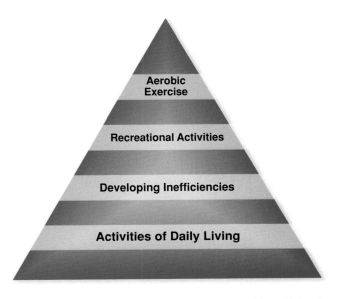

**FIGURE 23.4.** Physical activity pyramid for persons with multiple sclerosis. Data from Petajan JH, White AT. Recommendations for physical activity in patients with multiple sclerosis. *Sports Med* 1999;27: 179–191.

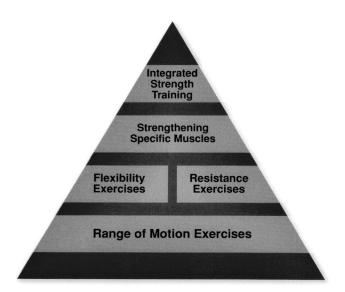

**FIGURE 23.5.** Muscular fitness pyramid for persons with multiple sclerosis. Data from Petajan JH, White AT. Recommendations for physical activity in patients with multiple sclerosis. *Sports Med* 1999;27: 179–191.

parking lot at the store can be used to increase walking activity. If the patient is capable, he/she should be encouraged to participate in active leisure. Research shows that patients are more willing to participate in leisure time physical activity than structured exercise programs. Patients who demonstrate adequate functional capabilities can participate in a more structured cardiorespiratory exercise program. The prescription should follow the guidelines of the American College of Sports Medicine for type, frequency, duration, intensity, and progression.

The base of the muscular fitness pyramid is the development of passive range of motion. Slow stretches should be performed that gradually increase in rate and extent until maximum range of motion is achieved. At the next level, active stretching and resistive exercises can be performed for muscles that are weak but still maintain some function. Initially no resistance or the resistance of gravity can be utilized, and then body-weight–resistance exercises can be performed. Specific muscle strengthening exercises can be prescribed for specific areas of weakness. Low-resistance exercises to develop muscle endurance should be implemented first. This can easily be done with stretch bands, small weights, or water-resistance exercises. For those patients with little or no motor deficit, major muscle groups can be strength trained following traditional strength-training methods that prescribe three sets of 10 to 12 repetitions until moderate fatigue occurs.

Body temperature increases can be problematic for the patient with MS. Temperature increases of as little as 0.5°C can slow and even block nerve impulse conduction in demyelinated muscle fibers, resulting in temporary clinical worsening. Pre-exercise cooling for 20 to 30 minutes in a water bath and cooling during physical activity by means of evaporative cooling methods can minimize the heat-related distress for the heat-sensitive patient. Case Study 23.2 shows how an exercise prescription was designed for a young woman with MS.

## MUSCULAR DYSTROPHY

Muscular dystrophy (MD) is a term used to describe a group of genetic diseases characterized by progressive weakness and degeneration of the skeletal muscles that control movement. The most common form of MD is **Duchenne MD**. The incidence and prevalence of this type of MD is 20 to 30 cases per 100,000 live male births. **Becker MD** is another common MD that is a less severe variant of Duchenne MD. Becker MD affects three of every 100,000 boys.

### Etiologies, Symptoms, and Prognosis

Both Duchenne and Becker MD are caused by defects in the X chromosome. Hence, females do not get the disease because they have a normal paired X chromosome that compensates for the recessive defective one. Both types of MD are the result of a mutation in the gene of the X chromosome that regulates the production of the protein **dystrophin**. The dystrophin protein is believed to be critical to the maintenance of the structure of muscle fibers (*Fig. 23.6*). The MD gene mutation causes a complete block in the production of dystrophin in Duchenne MD, whereas the dystrophin protein is produced but is oversized and does not function properly in Becker MD.

Duchenne MD affects boys between 3 and 7 years and is manifest early as muscular weakness around the pelvis. By school age, the boy may walk on his toes or the balls of his feet and may stick his belly out when walking to maintain balance. The disease progresses to the point at which weakness in the shoulders, arms, legs, and trunk develops. As the muscles become weaker, they enlarge but become less functional. Most boys with Duchenne MD lose the ability to walk by adolescence. By early teens, the boy's heart and respiratory muscles are affected. Duchenne MD usually causes death before age 20.

The symptoms of Becker MD are similar to those of Duchenne MD, but they do not appear until around adolescence or even early adulthood. As with Duchenne MD, the progression begins in the hip and pelvic area and spreads to the thighs, arms, and shoulders. The rate of muscle degeneration varies a great deal among individuals. Some men are confined to wheelchairs by age 30, while others manage for years beyond with the aid of canes. Ninety percent of those with Becker MD live beyond the age of 20.

### Exercise Benefits and Prescription

The effects of exercise training on functional capacity for patients with MD are minimal. Low-resistance strength training may improve strength slightly or retard muscle deterioration in boys with MD. However, the greatest

## CASE STUDY 23.2:  *EXERCISE PRESCRIPTION FOR PATIENT WITH MULTIPLE SCLEROSIS*

### CASE

You are an exercise physiologist working at a physical therapy clinic. One of the physical therapists asks you to assist in the exercise programming of a new patient with multiple sclerosis. The patient is a young women named Cindy, who is 23 years old and had been diagnosed with multiple sclerosis as a child. She has passed many years without any symptoms, but now she has increasingly more difficulty with motor control. She has come to the clinic for a physical assessment and for help in designing a fitness program that will help her maintain or gain functional capacity.

### DESCRIPTION

The cause of multiple sclerosis is not known, but the theory is that a virus or some other agent triggers an autoimmune response in the body—the body produces antibodies against its own myelin on the motor nerves. Multiple sclerosis may start with an isolated symptom for some people, followed by months or years without further symptoms. In other people, symptoms become worse within weeks and months. The person with multiple sclerosis is characterized by muscle weakness, **spasticity**, and lack of motor control. Symptoms may intensify with heat, such as during hot weather, a hot bath, or fever. The disease may flare up spontaneously or can be triggered by an infection or influenza. Despite disability, most people with multiple sclerosis have a normal lifespan.

### EVALUATION/INTERVENTION

The first part of your assessment is an intake interview with Cindy to determine her capacity for physical activity. You use the Physical Activity Pyramid for persons with multiple sclerosis (Fig. 23.4) as your assessment tool. Cindy reports that she does not have any trouble with her activities of daily living. She mentions that only once in a while she is not able to walk as quickly or as coordinated as she would like. As part of her physical activity program, you build in inefficiencies

when Cindy will be forced to walk more during her activities of daily living. For example, Cindy works on the third floor of her office building and has decided to take the stairs rather than the elevator. The stairs have a handrail for support, and eliminating the elevator will force Cindy to climb and descend four flights of stairs each day.

Cindy is not interested in recreational activities but would rather participate in a structured fitness program. So your next evaluation is a graded exercise test to determine Cindy's $\dot{V}O_{2max}$. The clinic does not have the capacity for gas analysis so you administer a treadmill test using the Bruce protocol. Cindy was able to go to maximal effort on the treadmill but with holding the handrail. By means of prediction equations, you calculate Cindy's $\dot{V}O_{2max}$ to be 35.1 mL·kg$^{-1}$·min$^{-1}$. This score places her in the 50th percentile for women her age. Cindy lives with a roommate, and they have a treadmill in their home. You prescribe a training program for Cindy in which she can do treadmill walking while holding the handrail at 50% of her $\dot{V}O_{2max}$.

You next prescribe a strength and flexibility program according to the Muscle Fitness Pyramid (Fig. 23.5). Cindy has a 15% loss in range of motion in her shoulders so you prescribe a series of flexibility exercises for her upper body, particularly the shoulder joint. As part of her flexibility training, you also give her some flexibility exercises to help with her legs. In addition, you prescribe a strength-training program for Cindy that focuses on developing strength in both the upper and lower body. The upper body strength training integrates exercises to strengthen the shoulder, while the lower body strength exercises are geared at helping her maintain strength and coordination in her legs.

Cindy is also taught how to monitor her exercise sessions and evaluate her level of symptoms. Special precautions are prescribed for Cindy so that she does not exercise in the heat and does not subject herself to overexertion. The three of you decide that Cindy will come to the clinic for the next four sessions to perform her exercise training before she is released to exercise independently at home.

effects are seen when the intervention is started early in the disease while there is still a substantial amount of trainable muscle tissue.

Muscle fibers that are deficient in dystrophin are more vulnerable to injury and less able to repair themselves than muscles that are not dystrophin deficient. Therefore, prudence suggests that exercise programs that invoke a high degree of mechanical stress may impose a high risk for the MD patient and should be avoided (2). Low-resistance training is also preferred because high-resistance training and eccentric exercises can lead to increased risk for muscle injury and death of myofibrils (2). Low-resistance

isotonic and isokinetic strength-training programs have demonstrated positive results without muscle deterioration, but when improvement in muscle function occurred, it was seen in individuals having the least amount of impairment and seen during the first weeks of training.

It is recommended that strength training of any specific muscle group be invoked no more frequently than every 48 hours. The intensity of resistance training should favor a higher number of repetitions at a lower percentage of 1 RM. A gradual increase in the percentage of 1 RM lifted can occur as the patient adapts to the training regimen. If the functional capacity of the individual allows, endurance

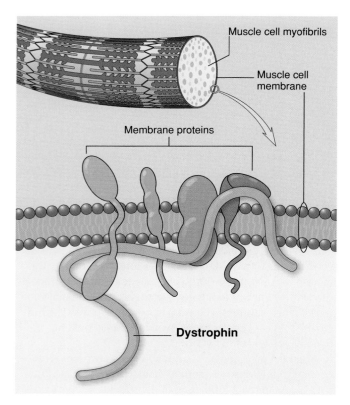

FIGURE 23.6. The dystrophin protein. Either inadequate amounts or the absence of the protein dystrophin cause the muscle to function improperly in muscular dystrophy.

exercise can be prescribed in the same manner as with otherwise healthy individuals.

It is very important that individuals with MD stretch and warm up prior to exercise. Flexibility exercises can be used as part of the warmup routine, but they should also be employed as a separate entity of the exercise program. Routine flexibility training can help prevent the muscles from contracting permanently around the joints.

Inspiratory muscle training by breathing against a resistive load may be beneficial for MD patients with moderate impairment of lung function. However, added inspiratory resistance for patients with advanced disease can be hazardous because the lungs and chest wall have a reduced compliance and added inspiratory resistance will cause the muscles to work closer to their fatigue threshold. Any exercise prescription for the patient with MD should be structured only after an assessment of specific physical abilities and limitations.

## EPILEPSY

Unlike the previously discussed brain and nerve disorders, which are all characterized by tissue structure abnormalities, **epilepsy** is a brain disorder with no apparent cause. More than 2.5 million Americans have epilepsy, and more than 180,000 new cases of epilepsy are diagnosed annually.

The prevalence of epilepsy is similar across both genders and across all races. Susceptibility to epilepsy is greater in children and older adults than adolescents and middle-aged adults.

### Etiologies, Symptoms, and Prognosis

Epilepsy is characterized by the tendency to have recurring seizures. These seizures result from abnormal electrical activity in the brain. Although some seizures can be caused by stroke, chemical imbalances, brain trauma, or tumors, most recurring seizures are **idiopathic**. People with idiopathic epilepsy usually have their first seizure during childhood or early adolescence.

Seizures can take on many forms and symptoms. Simple partial seizures begin with electrical discharges in a small area of the brain and are confined to that area. The afflicted person may have abnormal physical or psychologic sensations. Other seizures may begin by affecting one isolated part of the body, like a hand or foot, and then move up the limb as the electrical activity in the brain spreads. Psychomotor seizures begin with a few minutes of disorientation from the surroundings, and the person may stagger or move in purposeless ways. The patient remains confused for several minutes and then recovers fully. **Convulsive seizures**, or grand mal seizures, begin with abnormal electrical discharges in one part of the brain and then spread to the entire brain. The body reacts by going into a **convulsion**. During the convulsion, the person becomes unconscious, has severe muscle spasms throughout the body, clinches the teeth, and loses bladder control. Afterward the person feels confused and tired and may have a headache. In most cases, the patient does not remember what happened during the seizure.

Most persons with epilepsy can lead normal and productive lives. The disease is managed well with medications, and it does not progress or worsen with time. It is very unusual for a person to die during an epileptic seizure. The lifespan and quality of life for the person with epilepsy is generally the same as persons who are not afflicted with the disease.

### Exercise Benefits and Prescription

Most patients with epilepsy benefit from regular exercise. Experiments on electrical brain activity have shown that abnormal discharges which trigger epileptic seizures often disappear during exercise and return again at rest. Other studies have shown that people have fewer seizures during exercise than they do at rest. Furthermore, there is little evidence to show that contact and collision sports place persons with epilepsy at greater risk for injury than athletes without epilepsy. Therefore, persons with epilepsy can receive the same benefits from exercise as persons without the disease.

Persons with epilepsy can participate in any kind of exercise training without special consideration for their disorder. These persons will reap the same health and fitness benefits from exercise as do persons without epilepsy. Therefore, the exercise prescription for the person with epilepsy is unrestricted and may be structured the same way as the exercise prescription for any healthy individual.

### First Aid for Epileptic Seizures

It is very likely that the exercise professional will work with patients/clients who have epilepsy. On the other hand, it is less likely but still possible that the person with epilepsy will have a seizure in the presence of the exercise professional. The professional can best handle any incident if he/she is informed about how to give first aid during an epileptic seizure. The professional must recognize that he/she cannot do anything to prevent or terminate the attack, but if the professional remains calm, the person having the seizure will be reassured when he or she regains consciousness. When providing first aid to the person having an epileptic seizure, there are certain key things to remember:

- Remain calm and reassure others who may be nearby
- Time the length of the seizure
- Do not restrain the patient
- Cradle the patient's head or place something soft under the head
- Clear the surrounding area and loosen ties or anything around the neck
- Stay with the person until the seizure ends naturally
- At the end of the seizure, turn the person to his/her side and clear the mouth to provide an open airway for fluids and saliva to drain
- If repeated seizures occur, or the seizure lasts more than 5 minutes, take the person to a medical facility
- Reassure the patient when he/she regains consciousness

## PARKINSON DISEASE

Except for stroke, the brain and nerve disorders heretofore mentioned afflict primarily children and young adults. Parkinson and Alzheimer diseases, on the other hand, afflict the aging population. Parkinson disease is a degenerative disorder of the central nervous system that affects about 400 in every 100,000 people over 40 years old and 1000 in every 100,000 people over age 65. Approximately 1.5 million Americans suffer from Parkinson disease in this country, and 50,000 new cases are diagnosed each year. Studies differ in their statistics, but it seems like the prevalence of Parkinson disease is lower in women than men. African Americans and Asians appear to have lower prevalence rates than Caucasians. The ratio of African Americans to Caucasians with the disease is 1:4.

### Etiologies, Symptoms, and Prognosis

In healthy persons, the **basal ganglia**, which reside deep within the brain, transmit messages to other parts of the brain and rely on chemical substances as neurotransmitters. Dopamine appears to be the primary neurotransmitter. In Parkinson disease, the nerve cells of the basal ganglia degenerate and produce less dopamine. The lower production of dopamine affects communication among nerve cells (*Fig. 23.7*). The cause of nerve cell degeneration and dopamine loss in Parkinson disease is unknown. The disease usually begins subtly and progresses slowly. In most people, it begins with a tremor in a hand. Tremors may progress to the other hand, arms, or legs. Sometimes the tremor spreads to the jaw, tongue, forehead, and eyelids. Initiating movement is particularly difficult and muscle stiffness develops as well. Daily tasks such as buttoning a shirt, tying one's shoes, and even walking become increasingly more difficult. There are a variety of drugs used to treat Parkinson disease. The goal of drug treatment is to reduce tremor, which will allow patients to maintain mobility and independent living. Although medications can reduce the symptoms of the disease and prolong functional life, the disease is not curable.

### Exercise Benefits and Prescription

Mobility, posture, and balance are negatively affected by Parkinson disease. Progression of Parkinson disease results in a reduction in independent living. Exercise training is shown to be a positive factor in the development and maintenance of strength, flexibility, and aerobic capacity of the patient with Parkinson disease. The primary goals of the exercise training program for the patient with Parkinson disease are to increase joint range of motion, improve balance and gait, improve coordination, and increase mobility. Improvement in cardiorespiratory capacity is a secondary aim of the exercise program, focused upon only after enough motor capacity is gained to enable the patient to exercise at an intensity level that will increase cardiorespiratory endurance.

The physical activity pyramid and muscular fitness pyramid structures used for exercise prescription in MS can also be used for patients with Parkinson disease. Exercises that coincide with a given functional level in either pyramid can be incorporated into the exercise prescription. Although the pyramids are not necessarily mutually exclusive, the physical activity pyramid tends to focus on increasing energy expenditure through physical movement, while the muscle fitness pyramid tends to focus on muscular strength, flexibility, and endurance, making it more useful for most persons with Parkinson disease. Case Study 23.3 shows you how to help a client with Parkinson disease maintain a recreational sports program.

### ALZHEIMER DISEASE

**Alzheimer disease** is another degenerative brain disease that is incurable. Four million Americans have Alzheimer disease, and the numbers are increasing because the population is aging. Ten percent of those over age 65 have the disease and 50% of those over 85 have it. The prevalence of Alzheimer disease is greater in women than men,

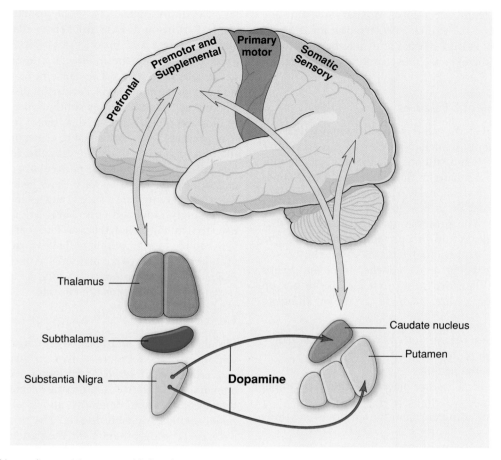

**FIGURE 23.7.** Parkinson disease. Motor control is largely regulated by communication between the motor centers of the brain and thalamus. In Parkinson disease, there is widespread destruction of the portion of the substantia nigra that sends dopamine-secreting nerve fibers to the caudate nucleus and putamen. The red arrows represent dopamine-secreting nerve fibers. The yellow arrows represent two-way communication between portions of the thalamus and cerebral cortex of the brain.

probably because the life expectancy of women is greater than that of men. Alzheimer disease is the most common reason for people entering nursing homes, and 50% of all nursing home beds are occupied by persons with Alzheimer disease.

## Etiologies, Symptoms, and Prognosis

The initiating cause of Alzheimer disease is unknown, but the disease progresses to the point at which some brain cells are destroyed and other cells become unresponsive to the chemical neurotransmitters necessary for nerve impulse transmission. Alzheimer disease also progresses slowly. The person may first find him/herself forgetting recent events. As the disease progresses, the person may talk differently by choosing simpler words, using words incorrectly, or being unable to express ideas coherently. Severe cases of Alzheimer disease render the person unable to remember names, places, and events, and make him/her socially dysfunctional. Alzheimer disease is the fourth leading cause of death in the United States, following heart disease, cancer, and stroke. The average life expectancy after diagnosis is 6 to 8 years.

## Exercise Benefits and Prescription

There is no evidence to show that exercise training has a positive effect on Alzheimer disease itself. People with Alzheimer disease can participate in any type of exercise as their age-matched controls. However, Alzheimer disease afflicts older individuals, and therefore the same exercise guidelines should be followed for persons with Alzheimer disease as for the healthy geriatric population. Persons with Alzheimer disease often become disoriented, forgetful, or confused. So it is wise for the person with Alzheimer disease to exercise with a companion or exercise specialist. In this way, the companion can monitor the exercise session for the patient so that the exercise prescription is followed properly.

▶ **INQUIRY SUMMARY.** Physical activity or regular exercise can have a tremendously positive effect on the treatment of certain diseases by eliminating or alleviating the symptoms associated with disease. Consequently, the exercise prescription is often an integral part of the therapeutic or rehabilitative process for persons diagnosed with a chronic disease. However, in some diseases, such as brain and nerve

## CASE STUDY 23.3:  *RECREATIONAL SPORTS FOR A CLIENT WITH PARKINSON DISEASE*

### CASE
You are an exercise physiologist working at a large wellness facility. Chuck is a 68-year-old man and long-time member of the facility who has developed Parkinson disease. The symptoms appeared gradually, and Chuck remained in denial for quite some time. He has now accepted the diagnosis and is receiving medication. Chuck is an avid badminton player and competed internationally when he was younger. He still enjoys playing once a week with a group of recreational players who come to the facility on Wednesday nights. He has come to you for help with an exercise program.

### DESCRIPTION
Dopamine is a primary neurotransmitter that is produced in the basal ganglia of the brain. In Parkinson disease, the nerve cells of the basal ganglia degenerate and produce less dopamine. The lower production of dopamine affects communication among nerve cells. The disease usually begins subtly and progresses slowly. The symptoms are tremors that start in the hand and then progress to the arms, legs, and face. Initiating movement is particularly difficult and muscle stiffness develops as well. Daily tasks such as buttoning a shirt, tying one's shoes, and even walking become increasingly more difficult.

### EVALUATION/INTERVENTION
You are well aware that mobility, posture, and balance are negatively affected by Parkinson disease and that Parkinson disease results in a reduction in independent living. You first do an intake interview with Chuck using the SOAP notes technique described in Chapter 12. Your notes tell you that Chuck is living independently and that he can perform all the functions of daily living. However, Chuck is slow to button his shirt or zip up a zipper. His gait is a little sluggish, and it appears that he has lost some flexibility in his hamstrings.

Since Chuck has been regularly active and is living independently without much impairment, you decide to structure his exercise program around the muscular fitness pyramid (Fig. 23.5). Prior to the exercise prescription, you ask Chuck to perform a complete fitness evaluation. You administer a submaximal cycle ergometer exercise test for determining aerobic capacity. Chuck has a $\dot{V}O_{2max}$ of 30.5 mL·kg$^{-1}$·min$^{-1}$, which places him in the 40th percentile for a man his age. Chuck's upper body strength ratio (0.58, bench press:body weight) places him in the lowest 20% of men his age, and his leg press-to-weight ratio of 1.31 places him in the 30th percentile for men his age. The last test you perform is the sit-and-reach. Chuck scored 18 cm, which places him in the 40th percentile.

The primary goals of the exercise training program for the patient with Parkinson disease are to increase joint range of motion, improve balance and gait, improve coordination, and increase mobility. Chuck's fitness evaluation shows that he has some muscle weakness, marked muscle stiffness, and a slightly less than average aerobic capacity. Since improvement in aerobic capacity is a secondary aim of the exercise program, you design a loosely structured walk/jog program for Chuck that will be coupled with his badminton activities. The walk/jog intensity is set as Chuck's preference so that he will not overextend himself and lose coordination or control to reach a predetermined target heart rate. His walk/jog exercises will be performed on the treadmill while holding the handrail. You design a strength-training program for the major muscle groups of the upper and lower body. A particular focus of the strength training will be shoulder strength. Chuck will do his strength training routine twice a week. The flexibility program you design for Chuck focuses on the legs and shoulders. Chuck will perform flexibility training daily. A reassessment of Chuck's fitness level will be performed in 3 months.

---

disorders, physical limitations may prevent the individual from being as physically active as they may wish. Stroke, MD, MS, Parkinson disease, and Alzheimer disease are examples of neuromuscular disorders in which the crippling effects of the disease itself can severely limit one's ability to exercise. Physical activity or exercise training for individuals with these brain and nerve disorders must be prescribed within the limits of functionality for each individual and must be implemented so as to not place the person at increased risk for worsening of the disorder.

Persons with the brain and nerve disorders presented in this section of the chapter have similar neuromuscular limitations. They present with muscle stiffness, mobility problems, poor motor control, imbalance, and poor posture. The exercise prescription for these individuals depends upon the severity of the disability. For example, in stroke victims with marked muscle weakness, the type of strengthening exercise prescribed may not matter, provided that it improves muscle force generation (3). In other words, when muscles are weak, methods such as electrical stimulation, weight-resistance exercises, isometric contractions, and machine-assisted exercises can be prescribed in the early stages simply as a means of improving the muscle's ability to contract (see Chapter 11). Once muscle strength reaches a certain threshold, prescribed exercise should be biomechanically similar to movement patterns that are weak in the individual. In this way, transfer of actions which are dynamically similar can occur. As an example, exercises that strengthen the lower limb extensor muscles can transfer to improved sit-to-stand movements and to improved speed of walking. *What are some of the specific precautions that should be taken when prescribing exercise for the person with stroke, MD, MS, Parkinson disease, or Alzheimer disease?*

## Cancers

Cancer is a disease in which a normal cell loses its control mechanisms and has unregulated growth. Cancer can develop in any tissue within any organ. A cancer by definition is **malignant**, meaning capable of spreading beyond its site of origin. As cancer cells grow and multiply, they form a mass of cancerous tissue that invades adjacent tissues and can spread or **metastasize** to different parts of the body (*Fig. 23.8*). The spread of cancer usually begins by infiltrating the tissue around its site of origin. The cancer can then spread to distant parts of the body via the lymph or circulatory system. Frequently cancer spreads to the lymph system that drains the tissue in which the cancer has arisen. A cancer that has spread beyond its tissue of origin and forms a new **tumor** is called a **metastasis**. The most common places for metastases to form are in the brain, bone, liver, and lungs. When metastases develop, the prognosis for survival dramatically decreases.

Cancer is the second leading cause of death in the United States, second only to cardiovascular disease. It affects middle-aged and older persons more often than children, and it is more likely to develop when the immune system is not functioning properly. Some cancers tend to run in families, while others are associated with certain behavioral risk factors (e.g., smoking). The sooner cancer is diagnosed and treated, the better is the chance for survival. Approximately two-thirds of those treated for cancer recover completely (>5-year survival). Prevention is a major key in managing cancer because the initiation of the cancer often begins with exposure to a chemical, virus, radiation, or sunlight (4). *Figures 23.9* and *23.10* show the incidence and death rates of selected cancers for men and women.

### ETIOLOGIES, SYMPTOMS, AND PROGNOSIS

Breast cancer accounts for approximately one-third of all cancers in this country and 15% of cancer deaths among women. Most breast cancers develop in women over age 30 and are thought to be related to an imbalance between the hormones **estrogen** and **progesterone**. These two hormones regulate the proper growth and development of the cells lining the ducts in breast tissue. It is postulated that an excess of estrogen, without the counterbalancing effects

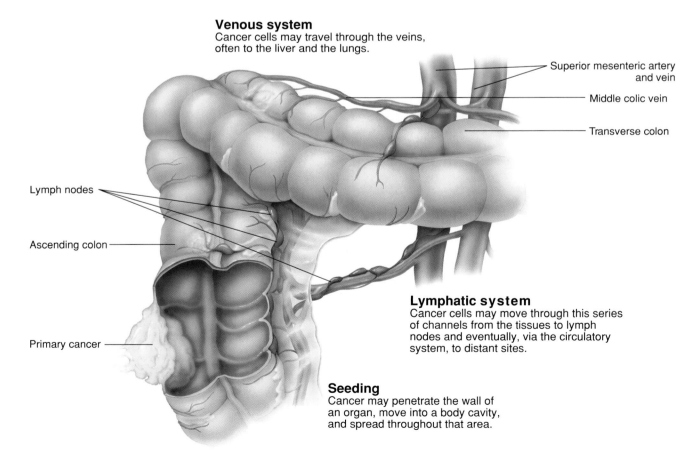

**Venous system**
Cancer cells may travel through the veins, often to the liver and the lungs.

Superior mesenteric artery and vein

Middle colic vein

Transverse colon

Lymph nodes

Ascending colon

Primary cancer

**Lymphatic system**
Cancer cells may move through this series of channels from the tissues to lymph nodes and eventually, via the circulatory system, to distant sites.

**Seeding**
Cancer may penetrate the wall of an organ, move into a body cavity, and spread throughout that area.

**FIGURE 23.8.** Cancer spreads by infiltrating the surrounding tissues or by being passed through the circulatory or lymphatic systems.

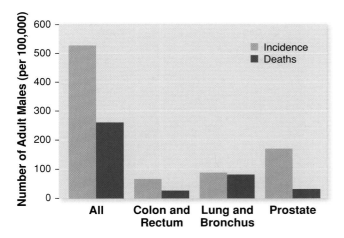

**FIGURE 23.9.** The incidence and mortality rates of selected cancers in men. Values are per 100,000. (Data from American Cancer Society. *Cancer facts and figures 2004*. Atlanta: American Cancer Society, 2004:1–56.)

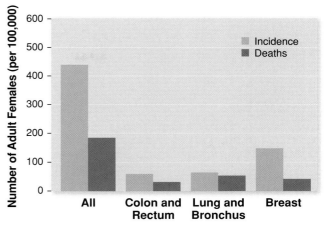

**FIGURE 23.10.** The incidence and mortality rates of selected cancers in women. Values are per 100,000. (Data extracted from American Cancer Society. *Cancer facts and figures 2004*. Atlanta: American Cancer Society, 2004:1–56.)

of progesterone, creates an environment more susceptible to the development of cancer.

Most breast cancers arise in two locations in the breast—at the outer and upper part of the breast that extends into the armpit, or directly underneath the nipple (*Fig. 23.11*). Initially the tumor cells grow within the ducts of the breast. Tumors that are diagnosed at this early stage of disease can

be treated effectively, and the 5-year survival rate is more than 90%. As the disease progresses, however, the cancer invades the surrounding fat and connective tissues of the breast. The cancer then continues to spread by entering the lymphatic and/or blood vessels. Prognosis during these latter stages of breast cancer is less optimistic than when the cancer is still limited to the linings of the ducts.

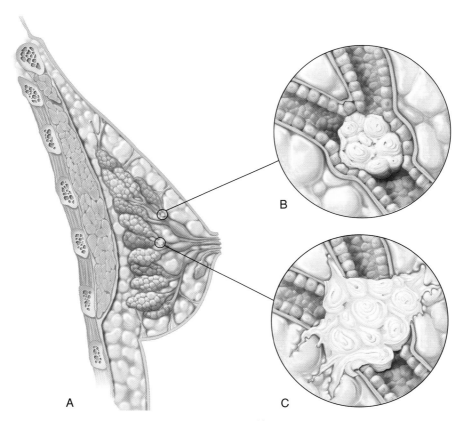

**FIGURE 23.11.** Location of breast cancer.

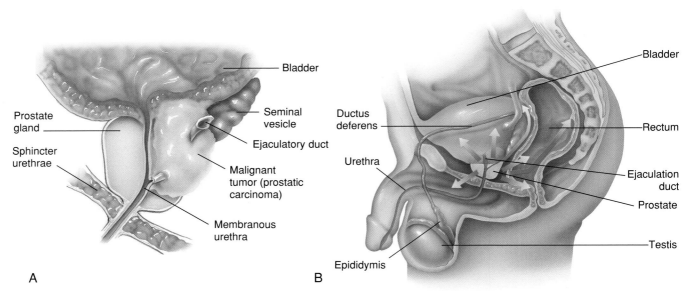

**FIGURE 23.12.** Location of prostate cancer.

Although breast cancer can develop in men, the biggest cancer risk for men is **prostate** cancer (*Fig. 23.12*). The prostate is a gland the size of a walnut that surrounds the neck of the bladder and **urethra** (Fig. 23.12). Secretions from the prostate gland contribute to the seminal fluid ejaculated during sexual orgasm. Prostate cancer, like breast cancer in women, typically occurs in older men. Very little is known about the development of prostate cancer, but it is thought that the growth of prostate cancer cells is in some way stimulated by the hormone **testosterone**. Unfortunately, there is no screening method that is 100% effective for the early detection of prostate cancer. Although a blood test is available, it is not considered sensitive enough to detect early prostate cancer. Rectal examination can sometimes, but not always, identify prostate cancer, and symptoms related to urinary outflow do not generally appear until later in the course of the disease. It is suggested that men over age 50 have yearly prostate exams because of the elusive nature of prostate cancer.

The colon is part of the large intestine that moves fecal material to the anus while absorbing salt and water. Colon cancer, like other cancers, develops when cells lining the colon become unable to control their growth. The specific causes of colon cancer may vary, but inevitably the underlying cause is that some type of **carcinogen** alters the genetic material in the cell so that a cancer develops. The most probable carcinogens for colon cancer are chemicals, preservatives, and substances found in our foods. A high-fat diet, for example, has been associated with colon cancer. On the other hand, dietary fiber seems to have a protective effect against colon cancer.

The **endometrium** is the mucus membrane lining of the uterus (*Fig 23.13*). It consists of tubular-shaped glands that undergo changes in thickness and composition as part of the woman's menstrual cycle. The endometrium is also where the **embryo** implants itself when a woman becomes pregnant. In post-menopausal women, hormonal support for the endometrium is lost and it becomes thinner and does not undergo cyclical changes. Cancer of the endometrium is almost exclusively limited to post-menopausal women. The most common symptom of endometrial cancer is vaginal bleeding after menopause. Diagnosing endometrial cancer involves taking a biopsy of the uterine wall and examining the tissue under a microscope.

Lung cancer is the second most common cancer for both men (after prostate cancer) and women (after breast cancer). Smoking is the primary contributor to lung cancer, followed by exposure to carcinogens such as asbestos, metal dusts, and industrial chemicals. Most lung cancers develop in the **endothelium** of the airways and then spread by infiltrating through the airway wall (*Fig. 23.14*). By the time symptoms of lung cancer become obvious enough for a diagnosis, the tumor has grown, invaded other structures, and spread to other parts of the body. Lung cancer is more aggressive than other cancers and is therefore the most common cause of cancer deaths. As with other cancers, early detection of lung cancer is difficult. There is no practical diagnostic test that can be used to screen the population for lung cancer.

## EXERCISE BENEFITS

There is no direct evidence to show that exercise or physical activity has any curative or therapeutic effect on cancer. Furthermore, there are no data to suggest that exercise training will increase cancer survival following diagnosis. However, there is consistent evidence to show that physical exercise has a positive effect on quality of

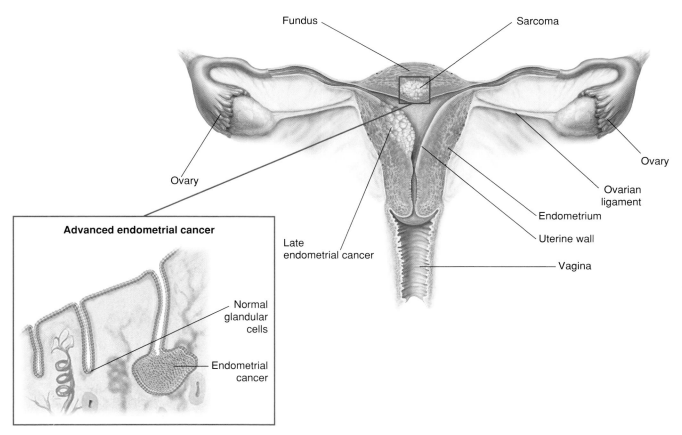

**FIGURE 23.13.** Location of endometrial cancer.

life after cancer diagnosis, including physical, functional, psychologic, and emotional well-being. Therefore, exercise should be encouraged as an adjunct to cancer treatment for those individuals who can tolerate the demands of physical activity.

Most of the research on cancer and exercise has focused on determining whether physical activity is a factor in the primary prevention of cancer. Since it has been estimated that environmental exposure or risk-associated behaviors cause of 80% to 90% of all cancers, the potential for exercise behaviors to reduce the incidence of cancer is significant. Accordingly, lack of exercise, along with tobacco use and poor dietary intake, has been cited as one of the three primary risk factors for cancer that can be modified through lifestyle change (*Fig. 23.15*).

The most definitive epidemiologic evidence for an association between physical activity and reduced incidence of cancer exists for colon cancer (5). Most of the studies performed to date show reductions in cancer risk for both men and women who are physically active. The average risk reduction was 40% to 50%, with reductions as high as 70% in some studies. There also seems to be a dose-response relationship, in that cancer risk was reduced the most in those who were the most physically active. The mechanism of effect may be that physical activity shortens fecal transit time and consequently shortens the period of contact between dietary carcinogens and mucosal cells of the colon. Physical activity may also positively affect the growth of colon cells through its influence on insulin, **prostaglandin**, and bile acid levels.

The evidence for an association between physical activity and breast cancer is also convincing. Most studies that examined this relationship showed that exercise reduced breast cancer risk by 30% to 40%, with a tendency toward a dose-response relationship. As mentioned earlier, the sex hormones estrogen and progesterone are strongly implicated in the etiology of breast cancer. Since physical activity can modulate the production, metabolism, and excretion of these hormones, protection against breast cancer through physical activity is possible. It has been suggested that estrogen levels decrease through mechanisms which reduce ovarian estrogen production, reduce fat-produced estrogens, and increase sex-hormone–binding globulins that render estrogen biologically inactive.

*LINKUP:* **Research Highlight: Physical Activity and Breast Cancer Risk,** *found at http://connection.lww. com/go/brownexphys and on the Student Resource CD-ROM, presents some interesting data about how exercise participation early in life can prevent breast cancer in women.*

**Right lung — Anterior view**

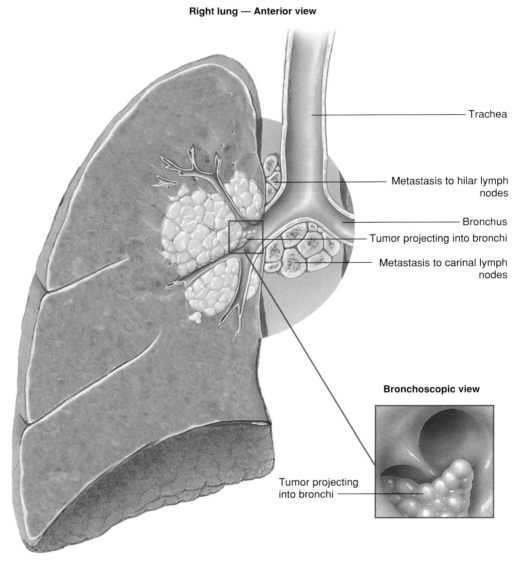

FIGURE 23.14. Development of lung cancer.

The risk reductions seen with increasing levels of physical activity and endometrial cancer have ranged from 0% to 90%, with an average of 30% to 40% (Fig 23.15). Since the etiologies of breast and endometrial cancers are similar, the prevalent thought is that exercise has a preventive effect for endometrial cancer that parallels that seen for breast cancer.

The evidence for an association between physical activity and prostate cancer is less consistent than that for colon or breast cancer. Only about half of the studies conducted on exercise and prostate cancer showed a positive exercise effect, whereas a few studies showed a negative effect and several studies demonstrated no effect. The lack of strong evidence to support the positive relationship between prostate cancer and exercise may be due to several factors, including: (a) a lack of understanding of the etiology of prostate cancer, (b) the elusive nature of prostate cancer

diagnosis, and (c) the inability to closely document how early life activity may affect prostate cancer development. Nonetheless, physical activity seems to produce a prostate cancer risk reduction ratio of about 10% to 30%. The most plausible mechanism for the protective effect of exercise on the prostate gland is that exercise increases the production of sex-hormone–binding globulins, which reduce the exposure of the prostate gland to testosterone.

The theory behind the protective effects of exercise on lung cancer centers on the well-established understanding that exercise improves ventilation and perfusion. When ventilation and perfusion are improved, the concentration of possible carcinogens in the airways of the lung is reduced as well as the duration of contact the airways may have with an airborne carcinogen. The bulk of research on exercise and lung cancer shows that cancer risk is reduced by an average of 30% to 40% with exercise training.

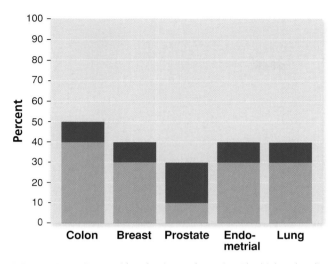

**FIGURE 23.15.** Cancer risk reduction and exercise. The high to low limits in the blue bars represent the average range of cancer reduction seen with exercise. For example, colon cancer is reduced by 40% to 50% with exercise. (Data from Friedenreich CM, Orenstein MR. Physical activity and cancer prevention: etiologic evidence and biological mechanisms. *J Nutr* 2002;132(11 Suppl):3456S–3464S.)

## EXERCISE PRESCRIPTION

Clearly exercise training can have a positive effect on persons suffering from cancer. The magnitude of effect depends upon the type of cancer and how much physical disability the cancer brings about. For example, persons with lung cancer generally have a decreased lung function. Thus, pulmonary function rather than metabolic factors or a low fitness level may limit their aerobic capacity. Nonetheless, the exercise prescription for the cancer patient with low pulmonary function is the same as that for any other person with a low capacity for cardiorespiratory exercise.

Persons with cancer may also be limited in their exercise capacity because of their cancer treatment. Since surgery is often the first line of treatment for most tumors, post-surgical patients may need a two-tiered exercise prescription. The first exercise prescription will be for rehabilitative purposes, to bring the person back to the presurgery level of functioning or to a level of functioning at which the patient can perform all ADL. The second tier of the exercise prescription is then formulated to increase physical fitness.

Cancer patients who receive **chemotherapy** may be suffering from treatment side effects that can limit their capacity for exercise such as extreme fatigue, anemia, nausea, pain, or muscle weakness. The exercise prescription for these patients can follow the guidelines for other patients, but the intensity, duration, and/or frequency should be set at the lower end of the spectrum and increased as the patient tolerates the exercise stress. It should also be stressed to these patients that the exercise prescription is flexible and that rigid compliance is not necessary if they are feeling the side effects of chemotherapy. In almost all cases, these side effects will subside once therapy is discontinued, and then they will be able to participate more fully in a physical fitness plan. The exercise prescription for the cancer patient is therefore only restricted by the limitations of the cancer itself or by the discomfort of treatment side effects. Case Study 23.4 illustrates how an exercise program can be adjusted and monitored for a woman with breast cancer who is receiving chemotherapy.

Since cancer is not a uniform disease with limited options that elicit predictable responses, the general guidelines for exercise prescription for the cancer patient presented in this chapter should be modified for each individual. There are more than 100 different types of cancers with a myriad of treatment protocols that produce a unique set of side effects and responses for each patient. Consequently, the type of cancer (e.g., breast, prostate, lung), the treatment protocol (e.g., specific drugs, surgery), the individual response to treatment (e.g., level of fatigue, nausea, pain), the baseline fitness level, and individual exercise preferences need to be evaluated as the exercise prescription is formulated.

For instance, just considering the site of metastases can impact the exercise prescription tremendously. Bone metastases are associated with an increased risk of pathologic bone fractures so weight-bearing activities should be carefully designed. Another example is that with liver metastases, the ability of the patient to mount a robust metabolic response to exercise will be impaired, resulting in undue and early fatigue. Kidney metastases may impair one's ability to maintain fluid balance or thermoregulate. Therefore, the optimal type, frequency, duration, intensity, and progression of exercise for the cancer patient is easily defined in general guidelines but must be patterned for each individual patient.

▶ *INQUIRY SUMMARY.* Cancer is a disease in which a normal cell loses its control mechanisms and has unregulated growth. Cancer can develop in any tissue or organ. Exercise has been shown to significantly reduce one's risk for colon, breast, prostate, endometrial, and lung cancers. Although exercise does not have any therapeutic effect on cancer per se, exercising cancer patients report a higher quality of life than those who do not exercise. The exercise prescription for the cancer patient can be structured similarly to that for a healthy individual, with considerations for the limitations imposed by the disease and treatment side effects. *Most cancer survivors do not have any exercise restrictions or limitations due to their cancer—can you explain why?*

## *Bone and Joint Disorders*

Unlike brain and nerve disorders that affect neuromusculoskeletal function by inhibiting motor impulse transmission, bone and joint disorders affect neuromusculoskeletal function by disabling the skeletal system. The two most common bone and joint disorders that exercise profession-

## CASE STUDY 23.4: *EXERCISE PRESCRIPTION FOR A CHEMOTHERAPY RECIPIENT*

### CASE

You are a personal trainer and exercise consultant who operates your own private business. Christy is a client of yours who has been exercising under your supervision for 8 months. She is a 32-year-old captain in the Air Force and has been diagnosed with breast cancer. Christy has just begun chemotherapy and will continue for several weeks. She has come to you to discuss how her breast cancer and treatment may affect her exercise program.

### DESCRIPTION

Cancer patients who receive chemotherapy may be suffering from treatment side effects that can limit their capacity for exercise such as extreme fatigue, anemia, nausea, pain, or muscle weakness. The exercise prescription for these patients can follow the guidelines for other patients, but the intensity, duration, and frequency should be set at the lower end of the spectrum. It should also be stressed to these patients that the exercise prescription is flexible and that rigid compliance is not necessary if they are feeling the side effects of chemotherapy. The exercise prescription for the cancer patient is therefore only restricted by the limitations of the cancer itself or by the discomfort of treatment side effects.

### EVALUATION/INTERVENTION

Christy is already participating in an exercise program in which she does aerobic exercises three to four times a week, strength training twice a week, and flexibility exercises 3 to 6 days a week. She is highly motivated and diligent in her exercise because of her military background. You explain to Christy that her cancer treatment may cause her to feel undue fatigue, muscle soreness, and/or nausea. You also explain to Christy that maintaining a rigorous exercise program during cancer treatment may exhaust her body too much and negatively affect the treatment. You stress to her that adequate nutrition and rest are just as important to her recovery from cancer as is maintaining physical fitness.

Your suggestion to Christy is to maintain her current exercise program with the following modifications. First, maintain her aerobic training but do not feel required to meet certain criteria for duration, frequency, or intensity. Duration and frequency can be reduced when she is feeling weak or ill. The intensity of exercise will be monitored strictly by ratings of perceived exertion (RPE), rather than a target heart rate, with the maximum RPE being set at 15. Second, Christy's strength training will be maintained, but the number of sets and repetitions can be reduced on days she is not feeling up to par. If she feels unusually fatigued, her strength training can be dropped for a day or until she feels less fatigued. Third, Christy is to maintain her flexibility training. You suggest to her that even on days when she is feeling fatigued or sore, she can perform flexibility exercises in an environment that will foster relaxation, such as in a hot bath or while listening to soft music. Fourth, you suggest that Christy keep a diary of how she feels physically and emotionally during her chemotherapy and exercise training. You will review this with her to look for times when exercise adjustments should be made.

---

als encounter are **osteoporosis** and **osteoarthritis**. These two pathologic conditions are related—osteoarthritis is characterized by disintegration of joint **cartilage**, while osteoporosis is characterized by disintegration of bone. Both conditions are degenerative and primarily afflict the aging population, and exercise has been advocated as an effective treatment for both conditions.

## ETIOLOGIES, SYMPTOMS, AND PROGNOSIS

Osteoporosis is a degenerative disease in which the density of bones progressively weakens and makes them more susceptible to fractures. To maintain bone density, the body needs an adequate supply of calcium and other minerals, proper hormonal balance, and an adequate supply of vitamin D. If the body cannot regulate the mineral composition of bones, they become less dense and more fragile, resulting in osteoporosis. Although there are several types of osteoporosis, the two common forms are **post-menopausal osteoporosis** and **senile osteoporosis**.

Women who are post-menopausal become more prone to developing osteoporosis because levels of the hormone estrogen, which helps incorporate calcium into bone, are reduced. Post-menopausal osteoporosis, therefore, afflicts women over 50 years of age. Senile osteoporosis, on the other hand, results from an age-related calcium deficiency, which is usually seen in individuals over 70 years of age. Senile refers only to the fact that the condition occurs in the elderly. Although senile osteoporosis occurs in both men and women, its prevalence in women is twice that in men. Women often develop both post-menopausal and senile osteoporosis.

Bone density decreases gradually in osteoporosis so that most people never manifest any symptoms. However, osteoporosis can be diagnosed with tests that assess bone density. The most accurate test is **dual-energy x-ray absorptiometry** (DXA). The DXA evaluation is simply an x-ray of either the lumbar spine or neck of the femur (*Fig. 23.16*). Bone density ($g\cdot cm^{-2}$) is measured and compared with normative data for 20- to 29-year-old adults. If

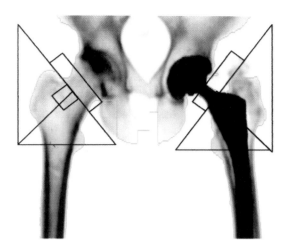

**FIGURE 23.16.** Dual-energy x-ray absorptiometry photo of an elderly woman who received a hip replacement because of osteoporosis Note the artificial structure in the hip replacement as compared with the bone structure in the natural hip.

the bone density of the patient falls more than 2.5 standard deviations below that seen for the average young adult, the diagnosis is osteoporosis.

Osteoarthritis, often called degenerative joint disease, is a chronic disorder characterized by degeneration of the joint cartilage and adjacent bone. Men and women are equally affected, but the disorder tends to develop at an earlier age in men. Osteoarthritis begins when the cells that synthesize the components of cartilage, such as collagen, develop an abnormality. The cartilage may grow too much, but eventually it thins and cracks develop on its surface. Tiny cavities form in the marrow of the bone beneath the cartilage, weakening the bone. The underlying bone sometimes overgrows at the edge of the joint, and this overgrowth interferes with joint movement. Soon the smooth, slippery surface of the cartilage becomes rough and pitted so that the joint no longer moves smoothly. Although osteoarthritis usually develops because of excessive use, long-distance runners are not at higher risk for developing the disease. It is still undetermined whether or not obesity is a major contributor to the development of osteoarthritis.

X-rays reveal some evidence of osteoarthritis in many adults by the age of 40, but few of these people manifest any symptoms. As the disease progresses, symptoms develop gradually and affect only one to a few joints. Common joints where symptoms of pain occur are joints of the hips, knees, feet, spine, and hands. These joints most commonly afflicted by osteoarthritis are also the weight-bearing joints of the body. Pain, worsened by exercise, is usually the first symptom of osteoarthritis.

## EXERCISE BENEFITS

It is widely accepted that exercise can increase bone density at specific locations in the body. Cross-sectional studies have shown that athletes have denser bones than nonexercising control subjects and that exercise-induced bone density may be specific to training (e.g., forearm bone density of tennis players). Just as loading the skeleton with exercise induces bone hypertrophy, lack of exercise can cause bone atrophy. If exercise is to be used as an intervention to gain or maintain bone density, the behavior must be continued to preserve the results achieved.

Even though most professionals agree that exercise is beneficial for bone health, the actual amount of bone gained or maintained seems to be modest. Several studies have investigated the cause and effect relationship between exercise and bone mineral content, with mixed results. Many studies show a positive effect, some studies show no effect, and a few studies show a negative effect. The inconsistent research results may be due to differences in training methods, exercise modes, intensity of exercise, nutrition, and exercise loading volume. In spite of these inconsistencies in research protocols, the main objective of an exercise intervention is to delay the age-related loss in bone mineral density.

Exercising early in life may build greater amounts of bone so that it takes longer to reach critically low levels of bone mineral density, whereas exercising later in life may provide an additional stimulus to maintain bone stock already present (6). Building bone mass in your younger years is probably a more realistic and beneficial method of preventing or delaying osteoporosis than trying to build or maintain bone mass later because most older people become less active as they age, even when they are aware of the health benefits of exercise.

Similar to bone, the health of cartilage depends upon the mechanical loading it experiences. High-impact loading of a joint may lead to joint degeneration, whereas too little loading can lead to disuse degeneration. Researchers who have studied the effects of exercise on osteoarthritis conclude that exercise training does not impact the pathologic process of osteoarthritis. They also agree that exercise training does not exacerbate pain but relieves pain and improves function in those suffering from osteoarthritis. The main functional benefit for patients with osteoarthritis who exercise is improved postural and gait stability that can reduce the risk of falls in this population. Other benefits of exercise training for the patient with osteoarthritis include increased joint mobility, increased strength, reduced reliance on medication, enhanced **proprioception**, enhanced activity performance, and reduced disability. These benefits of exercise are equally produced in either moderate aerobic or resistance training programs.

## EXERCISE PRESCRIPTION

The exercise prescription for persons with osteoporosis or osteoarthritis should focus on strategies to maintain bone and joint health as well as strategies to improve overall health. The first step in designing an exercise program for the patient with a bone or joint disorder is to understand which functional problems are most important to the patient. Once functional limitations have been inventoried and prioritized, both the patient and exercise professional can set short- and long-term goals, which will determine the exercises to be prescribed (7). The initial program should be constructed to elicit exercises that address the impairments previously prioritized (pain, limited range of motion, muscle weakness). As soon as these impairments begin to improve, a generalized fitness program designed to improve health and functional capacity should be started (7).

All exercise sessions should begin with a proper warmup because bone and joint disorders result in increased stiffness of the muscles and joints and reduced connective tissue compliance. The warmup should consist of 5 to 10 minutes of low-intensity aerobic exercise, similar to a warmup that would be prescribed in any cardiorespiratory training program. The warmup should be followed by 5 to 10 minutes of flexibility exercises. The flexibility portion of the exercise session should be increased for the patient with osteoarthritis and focus on reducing arthritic joint impairments as well as overall flexibility. Either a weight-bearing exercise program designed to increase cardiorespiratory endurance or resistance training can then follow flexibility

exercises. Resistance training should focus on muscle groups used in common everyday activities as well as muscles that support the affected joints in persons with osteoarthritis. Individuals with a limited range of motion should exercise within the part of the range that is not painful (6). Case study 23.5 illustrates how an exercise physiologist helped a woman with osteoporosis begin an exercise regimen.

▶ *INQUIRY SUMMARY.* Osteoporosis and osteoarthritis are the two most common bone and joint disorders that the exercise professional will encounter. These disorders afflict a large segment of the aging population. Physical activity can significantly improve the functional capacities of persons with bone and joint disorders. Contrary to popular belief, exercise does not exacerbate pain in patients with osteoarthritis. Persons with these bone and joint disorders can safely participate in aerobic, strength, and flexibility training programs. *What might be some ways in which you can help the hesitant patient with osteoarthritis overcome his/her hesitancy to begin an exercise program?*

## CASE STUDY 23.5: *EXERCISE PRESCRIPTION FOR A CLIENT WITH OSTEOPOROSIS*

### CASE
You are a recreational therapist working in a center for independent living that houses more than 100 older adults. Many of these individuals are older women who have varying degrees of osteoporosis. Rose is a new resident of the complex who has osteoporosis and received a hip replacement 1 year ago. Rose has come to you for the initial consultation that is required of all new residents before they begin any physical activity program.

### DESCRIPTION
One of the most common problems an exercise professional will encounter in older women is osteoporosis. Osteoporosis is a degenerative disease in which the density of bones progressively decreases and they become more susceptible to fractures. To maintain bone density, the body needs an adequate supply of calcium and other minerals, the proper hormonal balance, and an adequate supply of vitamin D. If the body cannot regulate the mineral composition of bones, they become less dense and more fragile, resulting in osteoporosis.

### EVALUATION/INTERVENTION
Rose is a post-menopausal woman with osteoporosis who has not participated in a regular exercise program throughout her life. Rose was diagnosed with osteoporosis 2 years ago and received a hip replacement 1 year ago. She is on estrogen replacement therapy and takes a calcium supplement. Rose's husband died a few months ago, and her

children thought it best for her to move to the independent living community where you work. Rose presents a positive self-efficacy about exercise and does not present with any psychologic disorders.

As a therapist, you have two main goals for Rose's physical activity programming: (a) increase cardiorespiratory fitness and (b) increase muscular fitness. Although walking is an excellent mode of training for cardiorespiratory fitness in older adults, it does not produce a stimulus strong enough to significantly improve bone mineral density. You begin by creating a walking program for Rose in which she will walk 5 days per week for 20 minutes at a rating of perceived exertion (RPE) of 11 to 13 (fairly light to somewhat hard). She will gradually increase the duration of walking to 30 minutes per session before she increases intensity to an RPE of 13 to 15 (somewhat hard to hard). Following this progression, Rose can increase her duration as she feels comfortable.

The strength program you suggest for Rose consists of a three-tiered approach. During the first 3 weeks of training, Rose will exercise using rubber bands to increase muscular strength, range of motion, and flexibility. Then she will be re-evaluated and another form of resistance training will be added to the rubber band exercises. The resistance exercises will consist of three sets of five to eight repetitions of rising from a chair, climbing a flight of stairs, and performing front lunges using a handrail. After 2 months of these exercises, Rose will begin to add resistance by wearing a weighted vest during the strength exercises. After 6 months of exercise training, Rose will receive a complete fitness evaluation and new exercise prescription.

## Summary

Exercise can have a tremendously positive effect in the treatment of certain diseases or conditions because exercise training can eliminate or alleviate the symptoms associated with disease. Consequently, the exercise prescription is often an integral part of the therapeutic or rehabilitative process for persons diagnosed with chronic diseases. Exercise presents a special challenge for persons with brain and nerve disorders because their motor abilities are often limited due to abnormalities in the neuromuscular system. Physical activity can, however, help retard the progression of these degenerative diseases.

The most significant effect physical activity has on cancer is preventative. Regular exercise is known to reduce the risk for developing colon, breast, prostate, lung, and endometrial cancer. Exercise restrictions for the cancer patient are few, and these are generally found only in patients in which the cancer has metastasized to the cardiorespiratory system. Exercise is also a preventative factor in bone and joint disorders and can be used to increase bone density and alleviate the pain and disability associated with osteoarthritis. If patient safety is considered and individual limitations recognized, exercise can be used as a tool for most patients suffering from oncologic and neuromuscular disorders.

### SUMMARY KNOWLEDGE

1. What are some of the benefits that could be expected for the stroke victim who begins to exercise regularly?
2. What difficulties might a person with muscular dystrophy or multiple sclerosis have when they begin an exercise program?
3. Would the exercise prescription differ for patients with breast, prostate, or colon cancer?
4. What are the similarities and differences in prescribing an exercise training program for the person with osteoporosis versus osteoarthritis?
5. Is there any evidence to show that exercise can cure any of the oncologic or neuromuscular diseases discussed in this chapter?

### References

1. Petajan JH, White AT. Recommendations for physical activity in patients with multiple sclerosis. *Sports Med* 1999;27:179–191.
2. Ansved T. Muscle training in muscular dystrophies. *Acta Physiol Scand* 2001;171:359–366.
3. Shepherd RB. Exercise and training to optimize functional motor performance in stroke: driving neural reorganization? *Neural Plast* 2002;8:121–129.
4. American Cancer Society. *Cancer facts and figures 2004.* Atlanta: American Cancer Society, 2004:1–56.
5. Friedenreich CM, Orenstein MR. Physical activity and cancer prevention: etiologic evidence and biological mechanisms. *J Nutr* 2002;132(11 Suppl):3456S–3464S.
6. Sharkey NA, Williams NI, Guerin JB. The role of exercise in prevention and treatment of osteoporosis and osteoarthritis. *Nurs Clin North Am* 2000;35:209–221.
7. American Geriatrics Society Panel on Exercise and Osteoarthritis. Exercise prescription for older adults with osteoarthritis pain: consensus practice recommendations. A supplement to the AGS Clinical Practice Guidelines on the management of chronic pain in older adults. *J Am Geriatr Soc* 2001;49:808–823.

### Suggested Readings

Eldar R, Marincek C. Physical activity for elderly persons with neurological impairment: a review. *Scand J Rehab Med* 2000;32:99–103.

Evenson KR, Stevens J, Cai J, et al. The effect of cardiorespiratory fitness and obesity on cancer mortality in women and men. *Med Sci Sports Exerc* 2003;35:270–277.

Poehlman ET, Dvorak RV. Energy expenditure, energy intake, and weight loss in Alzheimer disease. *Am J Clin Nutr* 2000;71:650S–655S.

Thune I, Furberg AS. Physical activity and cancer risk: dose-response and cancer, all sites and site-specific. *Med Sci Sports Exerc* 2001;33 (6 Suppl):S530–S550.

### On the Internet

HeartCenter Online: The Stroke Resource Center. Available at: **http://heart.healthcentersonline.com/stroke/**. Accessed June 30, 2005.

The National Multiple Sclerosis Society. Available at: **http://www.nmss.org/**. Accessed June 30, 2005.

Muscular Dystrophy Association. Available at: **http://www.mdausa.org/**. Accessed June 30, 2005.

National Institute of Neurological Disorders and Stroke: Epilepsy Information Page. Available at: **http://www.ninds.nih.gov/disorders/epilepsy/epilepsy.htm**. Accessed June 30, 2005.

Parkinson Disease Information. Available at: **http://www.parkinsons.org/**. Accessed June 30, 2005.

Alzheimer Disease Education and Referral Center. Available at: **http://www.alzheimers.org/**. Accessed June 30, 2005.

## Writing to Learn

*Select an oncologic or neuromusculoskeletal disorder that was not highlighted in this chapter and write a paper on the etiology of the disorder, how exercise affects the disorder, and what type of exercise prescription would be given to a person with this type of disorder.*

# Experiences in Work Physiology

*This part of the text presents a feature unique to exercise physiology texts – laboratory exercises. The best way to learn exercise physiology content is to get into the laboratory and experience these phenomena for yourself. These exercises, which are keyed to content within the text chapters (look for the Lab icon), allow you to systematically test some of the principles you have studied in the text and to correlate what you have learned in the classroom with laboratory data you generate yourself.*

# Tests and Measures Used in Exercise Physiology

Exercise physiology is the study of how the body responds and adapts to acute and chronic exercise. Physiologic measurement plays a key role by helping the scientist or clinician quantify these responses. The variables listed here appear throughout the text as each system is presented. The important categories within which these measures are made include the following:

1. Aerobic/anaerobic capacity
2. Circulatory status
3. Anthropometric measures
4. Muscle performance

The table below is meant to introduce key measurement areas that exercise physiology students will encounter during undergraduate preparation or while in a graduate or professional program. It is not meant to be a comprehensive list of all possible measurements, especially at the doctoral level of education.

**Table 1    KEY MEASUREMENT AREAS IN EXERCISE PHYSIOLOGY**

| Category | Variables Measured | Measurement Technique/Instrumentation | Data Gathered |
|---|---|---|---|
| Aerobic capacity (maximal and submaximal work tests) | $O_2$ consumption | Open-circuit spirometry, electrocardiograph, nomograms, regression equations | $O_2$ consumption (maximal and submaximal), 12-lead ECG, rhythm strips, respiratory exchange ratio |
| | Cardiopulmonary signs and symptoms | Pulse oximeters, sphygmomanometers, stethoscopes, spirometers, dyspnea and perceived exertion scales, anginal and claudication pain scales, palpation, observations | Arterial oxygenation, blood pressure, heart rate and rhythm, respiration (rate and rhythm), ventilation (flow, force, and volume) |
| | Physical work capacity | Ergometers, metronomes | Power output, ergometric workloads |
| | Blood lactic acid | Lactate analyzer | Blood lactate concentration |
| Circulatory status (rest) | Cardiopulmonary signs and symptoms | Electrocardiograph, sphygmomanometers, stethoscopes, observations, palpation, dyspnea scale, anginal and claudication pain scales | skin color, vital signs at rest (heart rate, respiration rate, temperature), presence and severity of abnormal body fluid distribution (edema) |
| Anthropometric | Percent body fat, fat-free mass, body density, body dimensions, somatotype | Calipers (skinfold and joint), electrical impedance device, weight scale, tape measure, hydrostatic weighing tank, nomograms, dual energy x-ray absorptiometry | Height, weight, body mass index, girth measures, skinfold thickness, rating of somatotype, bone density |
| Muscle performance | Electrophysiologic integrity | Electromyographs | Electrophysiologic response to stimulus |
| | Muscle strength, muscle power, muscle endurance | Dynamometers, muscle performance tests (i.e., isokinetic) | Muscle strength, power, endurance |

# Analyzing Your Diet

Many guidelines and recommendations have been given for nutritional planning. For example, the Food Guide Pyramid is an excellent guide for planning a healthy diet. However, it is often beneficial to know the exact composition of your diet to make it more compatible with what you desire. If a person has specific dietary goals (e.g., weight loss, reduced sodium, fat restriction, vegetarian diet), he/she may want to periodically analyze his/her diet to ensure the goals are being met.

In this lab you will have the opportunity to analyze your diet. Specifically you will complete a 3-day dietary recall, and then analyze your diet to evaluate its quality.

## OBJECTIVES

1. Complete a 3-day dietary recall.
2. Analyze the diet for nutrient content.
3. Evaluate the quality of the diet.

## PROCEDURES

The 3-day dietary recall is a standard method for analyzing a person's diet. Specific procedures vary, depending upon the nature of the recall, but the basic process is the same. Although the procedures used by a registered dietitian under clinical conditions or in a research setting provide the most accurate results, you can perform an analysis of your own diet and get a good estimate of your diet composition.

Record and describe everything you eat for 3 days on the Food Diary Form provided. Include at least one weekend day (Saturday or Sunday). Include all foods and beverages (including water) eaten at each meal and between meals. Please be as specific as possible and include (a) the brand name of the food, if possible; (b) whether the food was raw or cooked; (c) how the food was prepared (e.g., fried chicken, baked chicken, etc.); (d) the percentage of fat in milk and dairy products (e.g., 1% milk, 2% cottage cheese); (e) whether food (e.g., orange juice) was frozen, fresh, or canned; and (f) any other relevant specific information. Do not forget items such as gravy, jam, jelly, butter, margarine, salt, sauces, salad dressings, nuts, or sugar and milk added to cereal or beverages. Also include gums and mints and specify whether they are sugarless or not. Record any vitamin or mineral supplements.

Complete the diary after each meal or snack. Do not delay and rely on your memory. If you can, weigh the food; otherwise use household measurements such as: cup, slice, tablespoon, teaspoon, pat (pat of butter), package, etc. For example: a ham sandwich may be listed as 2 slices of bread, 3 ounces of ham, 1 pat butter, 1 teaspoon of mustard, 1 leaf iceberg lettuce, 1 slice tomato.

Since the purpose of this diary is to estimate the adequacy of your normal diet, reasonable diet records must be kept—that means no fasting or severely restricted diets. Try to select days that are most representative of your normal dietary intake. The accuracy of the assessment depends on the completeness of your diary. Please be specific in all your entries. Use one page of the form for each of the 3 days on which you record your eating.

## RESULTS

Upon completion of the 3-day food diary, you will need to analyze the results. If you have access to a diet analysis software program, use that program to analyze your diet. Some software programs have food codes that are used to enter the data. If you are using a software program that requires food codes, enter those codes in the appropriate column; otherwise ignore that column. If you do not have access to diet analysis software, there are several online programs that are available for free or minimal cost. Below is a list of some Internet locations where you can analyze your diet online.

- Nutrition Analysis Tools and System (NATS). Available at: http://www.nat.crgq.com/. Accessed June 07, 2005.
- The Diet Channel: Diet analysis tools, calorie and fat calculators, menus and more. Available at: http://www.thedietchannel.com/diettools.htm. Accessed June 07, 2005.
- dietsure.com. Available at: http://www.dietsure.com. Accessed June 07, 2005.

## ASSIGNMENT

Once you have analyzed your diet, review the results.

1. Do you think the results were accurate? Why or why not?
2. Did you consume the proper proportion of carbohydrate, fat, and protein?
3. If there were deficiencies for any nutrients, how might you change your diet to improve upon these deficiencies?
4. Did you consume the recommended number of servings according to the Food Guide Pyramid?

| Table 1 | UNITS OF MEASURE | |
|---|---|
| 1 cup = | 8 oz |
| 1 coffee cup = | 6 oz |
| 3 teaspoons = | 1 tablespoon |
| 16 tablespoons = | 1 cup |
| 2 cups = | 1 pint |
| 4 cups = | 1 quart |
| 3 oz of meat = | Size of a deck of cards |

Name: _____ Age: _____ Sex: _____

Date: _____ Day of week: _____

| SOFTWARE CODE (IF NECESSARY) | FOOD OR BEVERAGE CONSUMED | AMOUNT |
|---|---|---|
| | | |
| | | |
| | | |
| | | |
| | | |
| | | |
| | | |
| | | |
| | | |
| | | |
| | | |
| | | |
| | | |
| | | |
| | | |

# Temperature Regulation During Exercise

Humans are homeothermic, that is, despite extreme variance in environmental conditions, body temperature is regulated within a relatively narrow range. Active regulation is accomplished through cardiovascular adjustments, metabolic changes, and sweating. Passive control is through convection, conduction, radiation, and evaporation. Better understanding of temperature regulation by coaches, personal trainers, and health care professionals has reduced the number of heat-related deaths in young and old athletes. The purpose of this experiment is to examine basic aspects of temperature regulation during exercise.

## OBJECTIVES

1. Measure approximate heat production at rest and at three levels of exertion.
2. Calculate heat dissipation and make elementary efforts at partitioning heat loss into the four categories.
3. Relate cardiovascular adjustments to metabolic and thermal regulatory events.

## PROCEDURES

One subject will cycle continuously for 45 minutes (15 at 35% $\dot{V}O_{2max}$, 15 at 50% $\dot{V}O_{2max}$, and 15 at 75% $\dot{V}O_{2max}$). Heart rates are determined by ECG measurement or telemetry device at rest and every 5 minutes thereafter. Blood pressures will be taken during the same periods by standard auscultatory methods. Steady-state $O_2$ consumption will be determined by open-circuit spirometry, and heat production will be calculated by assuming 4.8 kcal of heat produced for each L of $O_2$ consumed. Steady-state temperatures will be determined for:

1. Core ($T°_C$): either rectal (inserted 10 cm) or tympanic
2. Chest ($T°_{CH}$): center of sternum
3. Forearm ($T°_A$): volar surface of flexors
4. Leg ($T°_L$): centered on gastrocnemius

Mean skin temperature will be estimated by:

$$T°_{SK} = 0.5(T°_{CH}) + 0.36(T°_L) + 0.14(T°_A)$$

Total body temperature will be determined by:

$$T°_B = 0.65(T°_C) + 0.35(T°_{SK})$$

Body heat content can be calculated as:

$$BHC = \text{Body mass (kg)} \times T°_B \times 0.83 \text{ (the specific heat of the human body)}$$

Heat dissipation is obtained by determining heat production over a specific period of time along with initial and final values of BHC. Partitioning into evaporative heat loss and other avenues can be done by obtaining body weights pre- and post-exercise and assuming that all sweat lost was evaporated (580 kcal for each L of sweat evaporated).

## RESULTS

Pre-exercise body weight: _____kg;
Post-exercise body weight: _____kg;
Lost: _____kg
Sweat evaporated: _____mL
kcal dissipated by evaporation: _____
kcal lost by radiation, conduction, and convection: _____

## STEADY-STATE THERMAL, CARDIOVASCULAR, AND METABOLIC DATA

| | $T°_C$ | $T°_{CH}$ | $T°_A$ | $T°_L$ | BHC | RPE | HR | SBP | DBP | $\dot{V}O_2$ | kcal |
|---|---|---|---|---|---|---|---|---|---|---|---|
| Resting: | | | | | | | | | | | |
| 25% max: | | | | | | | | | | | |
| 50% max: | | | | | | | | | | | |
| 75% max: | | | | | | | | | | | |

DBP, diastolic blood pressure; HR, heart rate; RPE, rating of perceived exertion; SBP, systolic blood pressure.

## ASSIGNMENT

1. Compare the steady-state values of $T°_C$ with published data. Comment.
2. Discuss differences to be expected if this experiment had been done in very cold or very hot and humid conditions.
3. How would the state of acclimatization affect results of this experiment?
4. Attach a neat copy of all data and all calculations for this experiment.

# Measuring Metabolic Transitions from Rest to Exercise

At rest, the body is in a state of homeostasis or energy balance. The power output of the muscles at rest is very low, and it is easy for the body to maintain this state of energy balance. The amount of energy (ATP) used to sustain cellular activity at rest is derived almost exclusively from aerobic metabolism, with a mixture of fat and carbohydrate fuels used to meet the energy demand. The instant exercise begins, the body has to adjust its metabolic rate so that enough ATP is available to support the energy demand of the exercise. At this point in time, the body adjusts how fast ATP supplies the exercising muscles according to exercise intensity. Low- to moderate-intensity exercise can be sustained primarily by aerobic metabolism of fat, while moderate- to high-intensity exercise will be sustained by aerobic metabolism of carbohydrate. A clear relationship exists between the power output of an energy system and the relative contribution of fat and carbohydrate to the fuel mix. The purpose of this lab is to measure the energy expenditure and the contribution of fat and carbohydrate to the fuel mix at rest and during increasing intensities of aerobic exercise.

## OBJECTIVES

1. Manually calculate the respiratory exchange ratio (RER) and energy expenditure for submaximal aerobic exercise to gain an understanding of how metabolic measurements are made in clinical and laboratory settings.
2. Measure $O_2$ consumption and $CO_2$ production during rest and at different intensities of steady-state exercise.
3. Measure energy expenditure at rest and at different intensities of steady-state exercise.

## PROCEDURES

### Manually calculating energy expenditure and RER

Although computer technology and automation have made metabolic measurements relatively easy for the exercise specialist, it is important to understand the principles underlying the procedures used in determining metabolic rate through indirect calorimetry. This portion of the lab will guide you through the basics of indirect calorimetry by providing data for you to use in metabolic calculations.

1. Your test subject is Kevin, a 43-year-old businessman who exercises regularly to maintain cardiorespiratory fitness. Kevin has come to you to determine his metabolic rate during his routine exercise bout. You have an indirect calorimeter that is only semiautomated, meaning it consists of gas analyzers for $O_2$ and $CO_2$ and a flow meter to measure ventilatory volume. Therefore, you will have to perform some manual calculations.

2. After a good warmup, Kevin steps on the treadmill and runs at the same pace he keeps during his training runs. Several minutes go by, and you begin to measure Kevin's gas exchange while he is at steady state. The monitors for the gas analyzers are shown in Table 1.

3. The change in concentration of $O_2$ going in and out of Kevin's lungs is 2.78% or 0.0278. Similarly the value for $CO_2$ is 2.50% or 0.0250. If you multiply the change in concentration of these gases by Kevin's ventilatory volume (amount of air going in and out of Kevin's lungs), you will obtain the $O_2$ consumption ($\dot{V}O_2$) and $CO_2$ production ($\dot{V}CO_2$).

Kevin's exercise $\dot{V}O_2$ = _____ L·min$^{-1}$

Kevin's exercise $\dot{V}CO_2$ = _____ L·min$^{-1}$

4. The exercise RER is calculated by dividing $\dot{V}CO_2$ by $\dot{V}O_2$.

Kevin's exercise RER = _____

5. Table 4.3 in your textbook presents the caloric equivalents of $O_2$ at specific RER values. Look in the table to find the caloric value for $O_2$ during Kevin's exercise bout.

Kevin's caloric equivalent for $O_2$ during exercise = _____ kcal·L$^{-1}$ $O_2$

6. Calculate Kevin's energy expenditure by multiplying his caloric equivalent for $O_2$ by his $\dot{V}O_2$ value.

Kevin's energy expenditure during exercise = _____ kcal·min$^{-1}$

7. What percentage of the exercise energy expenditure is derived from carbohydrate and what percentage from fat?

_____ % contribution to the exercise energy supply from fat

_____ % contribution to the exercise energy supply from carbohydrate

**Table 1  KEVIN'S GAS EXCHANGE WHILE RUNNING AT A STEADY PACE ON THE TREADMILL**

| Gas Concentration | $O_2$ | $CO_2$ |
|---|---|---|
| Inspired % | 20.93 | 0.03 |
| Expired % | 18.15 | 2.53 |
| Change % | 2.78 | 2.50 |

Ventilatory volume = 80 $L \cdot min^{-1}$

### Automated calculations of energy expenditure

In this section of the lab, you will obtain values for energy expenditure and RER at rest and increasing exercise intensities. The experiment can be performed on a treadmill or cycle ergometer. Select a lab partner to be the subject for this test. Calibrate and prepare your indirect calorimetry system (metabolic cart) to measure gas exchange during exercise according to the manufacturer's guidelines.

1. Measure the metabolic rate of your subject while he/she sits in a chair for 3 minutes.
2. Ask the subject to begin exercising at 4 $miles \cdot hr^{-1}$ on the treadmill or at a level of 100 watts on the cycle ergometer. Continue for 3 to 5 minutes. Measure the metabolic rate during the last minute of this stage.
3. Increase the workload to 6 $miles \cdot hr^{-1}$ on the treadmill or 200 watts on the cycle ergometer. Continue for 3 to 5 minutes. Measure the metabolic rate during the last minute of this stage.
4. Increase the workload to 8 $miles \cdot hr^{-1}$ on the treadmill or 300 watts on the cycle ergometer. Continue for 3 to 5 minutes. Measure the metabolic rate during the last minute of this stage.
5. Ask the subject to cool down at an intensity that is comfortable for him/her.

Record the data from the computer output into the table below. (You may have to perform some of the calculations yourself if your system is not fully automated. If you need to do this, simply follow the same procedures you did during the first section of this lab.)

| Exercise Intensity | $\dot{V}O_2$ | $\dot{V}CO_2$ | RER | $kcal \cdot min^{-1}$ | % Energy from Fat | % Energy from Carbohydrate |
|---|---|---|---|---|---|---|
| Resting | | | | | | |
| 100 watts or 4 $miles \cdot hr^{-1}$ | | | | | | |
| 200 watts or 6 $miles \cdot hr^{-1}$ | | | | | | |
| 300 watts or 8 $miles \cdot hr^{-1}$ | | | | | | |

How does the contribution to the fuel mix change as the exercise intensity increases?

# Measuring Cycling Efficiency

When you exercise, only part of your total energy expenditure is applied toward performing the work. That is, the exercising person is not 100% efficient. The physiologist usually defines exercise efficiency in the following terms:

Efficiency (%) = (Work output ÷ Energy expended) × 100

Since computation of work is not possible during most forms of exercise, this equation is considered applicable only to cycle ergometry. In practice, the energy expended is estimated by measuring the oxygen consumption ($\dot{V}O_2$) of the subject during exercise; $\dot{V}O_2$ is then converted into heat units (kcal) via the following conversion: 1.0 L $O_2$ = 5.0 kcal. Work output, which is measured in kg·m·min$^{-1}$ can be converted to kcal (i.e., 427 kg·m = 1 kcal). The purpose of this laboratory is to measure cycling efficiency at three separate power outputs.

## OBJECTIVES

1. Measure $O_2$ uptake and work performed.
2. Calculate cycling efficiency using four methods.
3. Compare cycling efficiency among subjects of different genders.

## PROCEDURES

1. Subjects (one male and one female) remain seated and quiet on the cycle ergometer for 5 minutes while resting $\dot{V}O_2$ is measured.
2. Subjects pedal at 60 rpm (no resistance) for 5 minutes. Determine $\dot{V}O_2$ for unloaded pedaling.

Subjects perform three 5-minute bouts of exercise (no rests between stages). Determine $\dot{V}O_2$ for each stage. The loads are as seen in Table 1.

| Table 1 | WORKLOADS | |
|---|---|---|
| **Bout** | **Resistance** | **Workload** |
| 1 | 1 kg | 60 W |
| 2 | 2 kg | 120 W |
| 3 | 3 kg | 180 W |

## ASSIGNMENT

1. Record (or calculate) $\dot{V}O_2$, respiratory exchange ratio, and kcal at rest, during unloaded pedaling, and at each workload.
2. Calculate gross, net, work, and delta efficiency from the following equations:
   a. Gross efficiency = (Work performed ÷ Energy used) × 100
   b. Net efficiency = Work performed ÷ (Energy used − Rest $\dot{V}O_2$) × 100
   c. Work efficiency = Work performed ÷ (Energy used − Unloaded pedaling $\dot{V}O_2$) × 100
   d. Delta (Δ) efficiency = (Change in work rate ÷ Change in energy used) × 100
3. *What happened to the cycling efficiency as the workload increases? Why? Is this pattern the same for all forms of cycling efficiency?*
4. Plot $\dot{V}O_2$ as a function of workload ($O_2$ cost of cycling curve). *Do you expect a straight line? Why/Why not?*
5. *What was the effect of body mass on cycling efficiency?*

## SUGGESTED READINGS

Berry MJ, Storsteen JA, Woodard CM. Effects of body mass on exercise efficiency and $\dot{V}O_2$ during steady-state cycling. *Med Sci Sports Exerc* 1993;25:1031–1037.

Nickleberry BL Jr, Brooks GA. No effect of cycling experience on leg cycle ergometer efficiency. *Med Sci Sports Exerc* 1996;28:1396–1401.

# Ventilatory Threshold

Minute ventilation is precisely geared to meet the body's need for $O_2$ during exercise up to the intensity at which significant anaerobic metabolism commences. This point has been traditionally termed the anaerobic threshold (AT) and is the point after which there is a loss in respiratory efficiency (the ventilatory threshold [VT]). The exact terminology used to describe these phenomena has been heavily debated due to experimental evidence that clearly shows adequate $O_2$ availability beyond the point of the AT and VT. Breathing frequency (f) and tidal volume ($T_v$) interact to determine inspired ($\dot{V}_I$) and expired ($\dot{V}E$) minute ventilation, which in turn react with $CO_2$ production and $O_2$ consumption in the tissues, differentially affecting fractions of expired $CO_2$ and $O_2$. These kinds of data are useful in determining relative fitness, examining physiologic mechanisms, and screening for normal pulmonary function. The purpose of this experiment is to measure the ventilatory threshold in high and low fit individuals.

## OBJECTIVES

1. Observe f, $T_v$, and minute ventilation responses to a wide range of work rates.
2. Analyze the $\dot{V}E$—workload relationship, seeking evidence of the VT.
3. Examine fractions of expired $CO_2$ and $O_2$.
4. Make inferences about respiratory efficiency from these and other data.

## PROCEDURES

Two subjects will exercise on the treadmill using the Bruce protocol set to 2-minute stages. The bout will be terminated after near maximal effort is achieved. Measurements will be taken at rest and during the last 30 seconds of each stage of exercise. They will include $\dot{V}E$, f, $T_v$, $FECO_2$, $FEO_2$, and $\dot{V}O_2$.

## RESULTS

| | | Respiratory Data at Rest and in Exercise<br>minutes | | | | | | | | | |
|---|---|---|---|---|---|---|---|---|---|---|---|
| | 0 | 2 | 4 | 6 | 8 | 10 | 12 | 14 | 16 | 18 | 20 |
| $\dot{V}E$ | | | | | | | | | | | |
| f | | | | | | | | | | | |
| $T_v$ | | | | | | | | | | | |
| $FECO_2$ | | | | | | | | | | | |
| $FEO_2$ | | | | | | | | | | | |
| $\dot{V}O_2$ | | | | | | | | | | | |

## ASSIGNMENT

1. Plot the ventilatory responses to increased workload.
2. Comment on the relationship between metabolic activity and $\dot{V}E$. Explain the mechanisms by which this relationship is maintained.
3. *How does break from linearity at the VT affect the efficiency of respiration?*
4. Ventilatory equivalent for $O_2$ ($\dot{V}E/\dot{V}O_2$) is defined as the minute ventilation per 100 mL of $O_2$ consumed. *How does this change after VT is reached? Can this be used as an index of respiratory efficiency?*
5. Discuss changes in $FECO_2$ and $FEO_2$ across workloads.

# Isometric Contractions and Cardiovascular Function

Activities that produce static or isometric muscular contractions are common in many aspects of everyday life and in some sports. In the 1950s isometrics were popularized as an effective and efficient means of developing strength, but more recent research has indicated that other procedures are generally preferable. Furthermore, because of the characteristic cardiovascular responses, isometrics and other resistance exercises are generally not recommended for some patient populations, i.e., individuals with hypertension, patients with heart failure, etc. However, over the last decade, the value of resistance exercise training for maintaining normal cardiovascular functioning in older adults and some patient groups has been recognized. The central cardiac and hemodynamic responses to resistance exercise are different than those seen with endurance exercise. As opposed to the volume overload imposed on the heart by endurance exercise, resistance (i.e., dynamic or static) exercise imposes a pressure overload. Accordingly, this form of exercise is characterized by a disproportional increase in heart rate (HR) and blood pressure (BP) for a given metabolic rate (i.e., $\dot{V}O_2$). The purpose of this experiment is to determine the cardiovascular responses to isometric and combined isometric and rhythmic exercise.

## OBJECTIVES

1. Observe the effect of duration of isometric contraction on HR and BP responses.
2. Note the effect of intensity of isometric contraction on HR and BP responses.
3. Evaluate the effect on HR and BP of adding isometric gripping exercise to cycle work.

## PROCEDURES

Assuming there is an adequate number of students, the class will be randomly divided into three groups with three subjects in each group. Group 1 will be used to examine the effect of duration of contraction on HR and BP. Group 2 will be used for evaluating the effects of intensity of contraction on HR and BP. Group 3 will carry out isometric contractions while cycling, providing data on effects of combining two kinds of exercises on HR and BP.

When several exercise tasks must be completed, there is the possibility of an effect controlled by the order of testing. This might be a result of cumulative fatigue or of learning to do the work more efficiently. To control for this source of variability, a rotational experimental design can be used for groups 1 and 2:

| Group 1 Trials | | | | Group 2 Trials | | |
|---|---|---|---|---|---|---|
| S1 | 60 sec | 120 sec | 180 sec | S1 | 25% | 50% | 75% |
| S2 | 120 sec | 180 sec | 60 sec | S2 | 50% | 75% | 25% |
| S3 | 180 sec | 60 sec | 120 sec | S3 | 75% | 25% | 50% |
| S, subject. | | | | | | |

### Group 1:

Each subject will grip the hand dynamometer at 50% maximum voluntary contraction (MVC) with HR taken during the last 5 seconds and BP taken during the last 20 seconds of work. Times of contraction are 60, 120, and 180 seconds. Include 5-minute rests between trials.

### Group 2:

Each subject will exert force on the hand dynamometer for a period of 60 seconds. Heart rate will be taken during the last 5 seconds and BP during the last 20 seconds. Contraction strengths will be 25%, 50%, and 75% MVC. Include 5-minute rests between trials.

### Group 3:

Each subject will ride the cycle ergometer for a total of 12 minutes. The load will be adjusted to give a steady-state pulse rate of 120 to 140 beats per minutes (bpm) within 5 minutes. During the last half of the sixth minute, HR and BP will be determined and recorded. Following collection of these data, at the beginning of the seventh minute, the subject will hold a 50% MVC with a hand dynamometer for 3 minutes. HR and BP measures will be taken during the last half of the ninth minute. The subject will continue to pedal at the same load for an additional 3 minutes without the isometric task. HR and BP measures will be taken again during the final 30 seconds.

## RESULTS

### Mean cardiovascular responses to different durations at 50% MVC

|  | 60 sec | 120 sec | 180 sec |
| --- | --- | --- | --- |
| Heart rate (bpm) |  |  |  |
| Systolic pressure (mm Hg) |  |  |  |
| Diastolic pressure (mm Hg) |  |  |  |
| Double product |  |  |  |

### Mean cardiovascular responses to 60 seconds at varying percentages of MVC

|  | 25% MVC | 50% MVC | 75% MVC |
| --- | --- | --- | --- |
| Heart rate (bpm) |  |  |  |
| Systolic pressure (mm Hg) |  |  |  |
| Diastolic pressure (mm Hg) |  |  |  |
| Double product |  |  |  |

### Mean responses to adding 50% MVC grip to cycle exercise

|  | Cycle work | Cycle work + Gripping | Cycle work |
| --- | --- | --- | --- |
| Heart rate (bpm) |  |  |  |
| Systolic pressure (mm Hg) |  |  |  |
| Diastolic pressure (mm Hg) |  |  |  |
| Double product |  |  |  |

## ASSIGNMENT

1. *Does there seem to be a trend in cardiovascular responses to increased duration of isometric contractions?* Discuss the observed and expected responses in terms of physiologic mechanisms.

2. *Do differing intensities of contractions affect HR and BP in a systematic manner?* Discuss the physiologic regulation involved.

3. *Were there measurable effects of superimposition of isometric on rhythmic work?* Give the theoretic basis for such responses.

4. Discuss in detail the practical importance of your findings in this series of experiments.

5. At a given HR, $\dot{V}O_2$ is lower during resistance exercise versus endurance exercise. Provide an explanation for this observation.

6. Research the current literature and discuss current findings regarding the principles in this laboratory assignment in relation to the older literature provided.

## SUGGESTED READINGS

Buck JA, Amundsen LR, Nielsen DH. Systolic blood pressure responses during isometric contractions of large and small muscle groups. *Med Sci Sports Exerc* 1980;12:145–147.

Falkel JE, Fleck SJ, Murray TF. Comparison of central hemodynamics between powerlifters and bodybuilders during resistance exercise. *J Appl Sci Res* 1992;6:24–35.

MacDougall JD, Tuxen D, Sale DG, et al. Arterial blood pressure response to heavy resistance exercise. *J Appl Physiol* 1985;58:785–790.

Sagiv M, Ben-Sira, D, Rudoy J. Cardiovascular response during upright isometric dead lift in young, older, and elderly healthy men. *Int J Sports Med* 1988;9:134–136.

Smith DL, Misner JE, Bloomfield DK, et al. Cardiovascular responses to sustained maximal isometric contractions of the finger flexors. *Eur J Appl Physiol Occup Physiol* 1993;67:48–52.

Van Loan MD, Massey BH, Boileau RA, et al. Age as a factor in the hemodynamic responses to isometric exercise. *J Sports Med Phys Fitness* 1989;29:262–268.

# Cardiovascular Adjustments to Exercising in the Heat or Cold

Exercising in a warm environment places added stress on the body because the metabolic heat from the exercising muscles must be dissipated to maintain the core temperature within the normal range. One of the major mechanisms for dissipating heat is an increase in blood flow to the skin surface. As a greater portion of the cardiac output is distributed to the skin, adjustments in the cardiovascular system must be made to maintain the $O_2$-rich blood flow to the exercising muscles. These adjustments include alterations in heart rate (HR) and blood pressure (BP).

## OBJECTIVE

1. Compare the cardiovascular adjustments that are made while a person exercises in a cold environment with those made while exercising in the heat.

## PROCEDURES

HR, BP, and body temperature will be recorded while a subject exercises on a cycle ergometer under two environmental conditions. The first condition mimics heat stress and the second condition mimics cold stress.

### Heat stress

1. Position the subject on the cycle ergometer that will be used for the exercise bout. The subject should be fully clothed in a sweat suit, full-length spandex, or other full-body exercise attire.
2. Be prepared to record HR (carotid or radial pulse, electrocardiogram [ECG], or HR monitor), BP (sphygmomanometer and stethoscope or automatic BP cuff), and body temperature (oral and/or skin surface).

3. Record resting HR, BP, and temperature(s).
4. Place a heat lamp above the subject.
5. Ask the subject to pedal the cycle ergometer at a work rate of 150 watts (900 kgm·min$^{-1}$) for 5 minutes.
6. Turn off the heat lamp at the completion of the 5-minute exercise bout.
7. Record HR, BP, and temperature(s) immediately post-exercise and at 1, 3, and 5 minutes into recovery.
8. Record the measurements for each of the variables in the table provided.

### Cold stress

1. Soak either a wet towel or t-shirt in very cold water. Squeeze the excess water from the towel or t-shirt just enough so that water will not be dripping from the cloth.
2. Be prepared to record HR (carotid or radial pulse, ECG, or HR monitor), BP (sphygmomanometer and stethoscope or automatic BP cuff), and body temperature (oral and/or skin surface).
3. Record resting HR, BP, and temperature(s).
4. Position the subject on the cycle ergometer that will be used for the exercise bout. The subject should be clothed in shorts, no shirt (men), sport bra (women), and either the wet t-shirt or wet towel. (Place towel over bare shoulders.)
5. Place one or two fans close to the subject.
6. Ask the subject to pedal the cycle ergometer at a work rate of 150 watts (900 kgm·min$^{-1}$) for 5 minutes.
7. Turn off the fan(s) and remove the wet clothing upon completion of the 5-minute exercise bout.

## WORK TABLE 1

| | REST | | POST-EXERCISE | | 1-MINUTE RECOVERY | | 3-MINUTE RECOVERY | | 5-MINUTE RECOVERY | |
|---|---|---|---|---|---|---|---|---|---|---|
| | HEAT | COLD | HEAT | COLD | HEAT | COLD | HEAT | COLD | HEAT | COLD |
| HR | | | | | | | | | | |
| Systolic BP | | | | | | | | | | |
| Diastolic BP | | | | | | | | | | |
| Esophageal temperature | | | | | | | | | | |
| Skin temperature | | | | | | | | | | |

8. Record HR, BP, and temperature(s) immediately post-exercise and at 1, 3, and 5 minutes into recovery.
9. Record the measurements for each of the variables in the table provided.

## ASSIGNMENT

1. Do heat and cold exposure affect exercise HR and BP?
2. Plot HR versus time for both the hot and cold conditions.
3. Plot BPs versus time for both the hot and cold conditions.
4. Plot temperature(s) versus time for both the hot and cold conditions.
5. How much difference is there in HR and BP for each degree difference in temperature between the hot and cold conditions?

# Nerve Conduction Velocity

The speed at which an action potential can be propagated down the length of a nerve can be calculated. To assess the speed or conduction velocity of a nerve, direct stimulation is applied to a motor or sensory nerve. This stimulation initiates an impulse, and the conduction velocity can be calculated by recording evoked potentials either from the sensory nerve or the muscle innervated by the motor nerve. Nerve conduction velocity tests can only be done on peripheral nerves that are superficial enough to be stimulated through the skin at two different points along the length of the nerve. This test is most commonly done on the ulnar, median, peroneal, and posterior tibial nerves. The results of this test, along with other diagnostic tests, can be used to diagnose nerve and muscle disorders.

## OBJECTIVE

1. Determine the conduction velocity of the ulnar nerve.

## PROCEDURES

Turn the equipment on and attach the three electrodes to the cable. Place electrode paste on the electrodes. Clean the lateral aspect and back of the hand to be tested and place the ground electrode to the back of the hand. Attach the active electrode to the muscle belly of the abductor digiti minimi and the reference electrode over the distal tendon. Set the stimulator to deliver 1 pulse per second (pps). Set the duration to 0.1 milliseconds, stimulus intensity to 100 to 150 V and gain to 2 k mV/div. Set the filter to 210. Now apply the stimulator to the skin over the ulnar nerve near the wrist. Move the stimulating electrode slightly to get the largest muscle action potential from the abductor digiti minimi. Measure the time in tenths of milliseconds between stimulus and rise of action potential. This time is called the distal latency. Decrease the amplitude to zero and remove the stimulation electrode and mark the position of where the stimulator elicited the largest action potential. Next place the stimulator over the ulnar nerve where the nerve passes under the medial epicondyle of the humerus. Move the stimulating electrode slightly to get the largest muscle action potential from the abductor digiti minimi. Measure the time between the stimulus and the rise of action potential to determine the proximal latency. Mark the site on the skin where this measure was obtained. Next measure the distance between the proximal and distal locations with a metric tape measure. Compute the nerve conduction velocity in meters/second.

## RESULTS

Distal latency _____

Proximal latency _____

Conduction distance _____

Nerve conduction velocity is calculated by dividing conduction distance by the difference between proximal latency and distal latency.

## ASSIGNMENT

1. Calculate nerve conduction velocity given the formula above.
2. Compare your results with the normal conduction velocity of the ulnar nerve (60 to 70 milliseconds).
3. What do you think you would observe if you did this test on a person who had an ulnar nerve compression?

# Muscle-Length Tension Relationship

The initial length of the muscle before the development of force is one factor that determines the amount of force that the muscle exerts. This concept is related to the amount of overlap that exists between actin and myosin. Understanding this relationship is important to allied health professionals as they prescribe exercise to increase strength and function.

## OBJECTIVE

1. Determine the relationship between muscle length and force output.

## PROCEDURES

Set the stirrup on the handgrip dynamometer so that the stirrup is closest to the body of the dynamometer and obtain grip strength. Then, move the stirrup to the next setting farther away from the body of the dynamometer and obtain grip strength. Continue increasing the grip width and measuring strength. At each setting, make sure to measure the width between the stirrup and dynamometer.

## RESULTS

**TABLE 1**

| Width of Dynamometer (cm) | Tension (kg) |
| --- | --- |
| | |
| | |
| | |
| | |

## ASSIGNMENT

1. Plot the width of the dynamometer versus the tension generated.
2. Comment on the relationship between length and force output. What does the graph tell you about the underlying physiology?
3. Why would knowledge of this relationship be important in the development of exercise programs?

## SUGGESTED READINGS

Burkholder TJ, Lieber RL. Sarcomere length operating range of muscles during movement. *J Experiment Biol* 2001;204:1529–1536.

Close RI. Dynamic properties of mammalian skeletal muscles. *Physiol Rev* 1972;52:129–197.

# Taking SOAP Notes to Evaluate Dietary Supplements

Subjective Objective Assessment Plan (SOAP) notes are a valuable tool for health care professionals in evaluating the efficacy and safety of products and promotional materials that claim to enhance exercise performance. The S or subjective part of the evaluation is the process by which you gather all the unscientific information about the supplement in question. The O or objective part of the evaluation is the process by which you gather factual scientific and medical information about the supplement in question. The A or assessment part of the evaluation is when an assessment of the gathered data must be made, relevant to using the supplement in question. Finally the P or plan part of the evaluation represents the plan of action for either using the supplement or eliminating it from consideration.

In this lab, you will use the SOAP notes method to evaluate a dietary supplement that is claimed to enhance exercise performance. You will be evaluating the supplement for personal use so any personal information relevant to age, height, weight, gender, lifestyle, anthropometrics, fitness, disease risk or symptoms, health status, etc. will be familiar to you and can easily be incorporated into the SOAP process. (Although the assignment is to evaluate a product for your own personal use, we are not suggesting that you need to consider a dietary supplement. Just imagine yourself as a potential client, patient, or customer.)

## OBJECTIVES

1. Select a dietary supplement that is claimed to enhance exercise performance (e.g., amino acid supplement, metabolic enhancer, weight loss product, herb).
2. Employ the SOAP process to make an evaluation of the supplement relevant to your own personal use.
3. Make a recommendation for use of the supplement in accordance with your SOAP evaluation.

## PROCEDURES

1. Search on the Internet for any dietary supplement that may be of interest to you. The search may start out general (e.g., *dietary supplements*), may be narrowed by subject (e.g., weight loss pills), or may be specific (e.g., creatine).
2. Find a single product in which you are interested in evaluating.
3. Evaluate the product in accordance with the SOAP outline below and in accordance with your own personal demographics. You may need to connect to links provided by the website of the supplement or go to sources of information that are not contained on the website.
4. Make a recommendation as to the appropriate use of the product or its elimination from consideration.

## SUBJECTIVE

What claims are being made for the supplement? Who is making the claims? Why are the claims being made? What is the motivation behind the claims? How is the supplement being marketed? Why would you be interested in taking the supplement? What have you been told about the supplement? What sources of information do you have about the supplement?

## OBJECTIVE

Is the supplement safe? Who produces the supplement? What is the producer's reputation? What is known about the efficacy of the supplement? Does the preparation method affect potency or safety? What is action of the main ingredient? What does the active ingredient do? What is the recommended dose? What is the medical or biologic need for the supplement? How might your condition affect the effectiveness and safety of this supplement? What is the likelihood of an adverse reaction to the supplement?

## ASSESSMENT

What is the validity of the effectiveness claims? What are the risks and benefits of taking the supplement? What other evidence is there to support the use of this supplement?

## PLAN

Should this supplement be eliminated from consideration? Why or why not? If the supplement is to be used, plan the following. How will potential side effects be monitored? How will side effects be reported? What dose will be administered? How long will the supplement be used? How will effectiveness be monitored? When and how will the supplement be discontinued if effectiveness is not demonstrated?

# Body Composition

Applied physiologists are often interested in determining an athlete's relative percentage of body fat. When percent body fat is known, proper advice on training techniques can then be given to help maintain ideal percent fat for a given sport. In addition, since obesity is a major health problem in our society, the capability to monitor the average individual's body composition is important from a preventive health standpoint. Currently the science of body composition assessment has progressed to the point at which the body can be divided into four distinct components, with the density of each component estimated. However, the two-component model (fat mass and fat-free mass) is still widely used as represented by the following commonly used techniques for assessing body composition: (a) hydrostatic weighing, (b) skinfold measurement, and (c) bioelectrical impedance analysis (BIA). Another common method, body mass index (BMI; the ratio of body mass in kg to height squared), while not technically estimating body composition, is nevertheless an index of obesity. Each of these methods used to measure body composition has advantages and disadvantages, with hydrostatic weighing still generally accepted as the "gold" standard. Other more sophisticated techniques that assess body composition based on three or four body components are: isotope dilution, photon absorptiometry, nuclear magnetic resonance, dual energy X-ray absorptiometry, total body electrical conductivity, radiography, and near-infrared interactance. The purpose of this experiment is to measure body composition (% fat) of male and female subjects.

## OBJECTIVES

1. Determine the % fat of male and female subjects using hydrostatic weighing, skinfold measurement, and bioelectrical impedance analysis.
2. Determine the BMI of these same subjects.
3. Correlate these findings using the Pearson Product-Moment correlation statistic.

## PROCEDURE

1. Select several male and female subjects for measurement. Record their heights in meters, body mass in kilograms, age in years, and activity level (needed for BIA assessment) as follows:

| Table 1 | ACTIVITY LEVELS |
|---|---|
| Inactive | No regular activity with a sit-down job |
| Light | No organized physical activity during leisure time, with 3 to 4 hours of walking or standing per day |
| Moderate | Sporadically involved in recreational activities such as weekend golf or tennis, occasional jogging, swimming, or cycling |
| Heavy | Consistent job activities of lifting or stair climbing or participating regularly in recreational/fitness activities such as jogging, swimming, or cycling at least three times a week for 30 to 60 minutes per session |
| Vigorous | Participation in extensive physical activity for 60 or more minutes at least 4 days per week |

2. Skinfold measurement: Using skinfold calipers and the correct technique (as demonstrated by the instructor), measure the specified seven anatomic sites on the right side of the body. Follow these simple procedures (ACSM 2005): (a) place calipers 1 cm away from the thumb and index finger, perpendicular to the skinfold, and halfway between the crest and base of the fold; (b) maintain the pinch while reading the calipers; (c) wait only 1 to 2 seconds before reading the calipers; (d) take duplicate measures at each site and retest if duplicate measures are not within 1 to 2 mm; and (e) rotate through measurement sites or allow time for the skin to regain normal texture and thickness between measurements. Calculate the percent body fat for each subject using the regression equations below.

Males: $1.112 - [4.35 \times 10^{-4} \times \text{Sum of seven sites}]$
$+ [5.5 \times 10^{-7} \times (\text{Sum of seven sites})^2]$
$- [2.88 \times 10^{-4} \times \text{Age}]$

Females: $1.097 - [4.70 \times 10^{-4} \times \text{Sum of seven sites}]$
$+ [5.6 \times 10^{-7} \times (\text{Sum of seven sites})^2]$
$- [2.28 \times 10^{-4} \times \text{Age}]$

*Note: For the umbilical and midaxillary sites use a vertical rather than horizontal skinfold.

## WORK TABLE 1

| | Males | Females |
|---|---|---|
| Iliac crest | mm | mm |
| Umbilical | mm | mm |
| Subscapular | mm | mm |
| Triceps | mm | mm |
| Pectoralis | mm | mm |
| Anterior thigh | mm | mm |
| Midaxillary | mm | mm |
| Sum | mm | mm |
| % Fat | % | % |

3. BIA: Follow these simple procedures (ACSM 2005): (a) No eating or drinking within 4 hours of the assessment; (b) no moderate or vigorous physical activity within 12 hours of the assessment; (c) void completely before the assessment; (d) no alcohol consumption within 48 hours of the assessment; (e) ingest no diuretic agents (i.e., caffeine, etc.) prior to the assessment unless prescribed by a physician. Follow the exact procedures from the manufacturers for electrode placement.

## WORK TABLE 2

| | Males | Females |
|---|---|---|
| Resistance | ohms | ohms |
| Reactance | ohms | ohms |

4. Hydrostatic weighing: Determining % body fat by this method makes use of the following equations:

$$TBV = [(Ma - Mw) \div Dw] - RV - VGI$$

TBV, Total body volume; Ma, Body mass in air (kg); VGI, Volume of gas in GI tract (estimated as 0.1 L); Mw, Body mass in water (kg); Dw, Water density at a given water temperature; RV, Residual lung volume in L (BTPS).

If measurement of residual volume is not possible, RV can be estimated with the following equations:

Males: $RV_{BTPS}$ (L) = (0.017 × Age) + (0.06858 × Height [inches]) − 3.477

Females: $RV_{BTPS}$ (L) = (0.009 × Age) + (0.08128 × Height [inches]) − 3.90

See the table for the density of water at a given temperature.

$$Db = Ma \div TBV$$

Db, body density.

$$\% \text{ body fat} = [(4.95 \div Db) - 4.5] \times 100$$

Exact techniques for measuring the variables in these equations will be introduced by your instructor.

## WATER DENSITY CORRECTION FACTORS

| Water TE | Dw | Water TE | Dw |
|---|---|---|---|
| 23°C | 0.997569 | 30°C | 0.995678 |
| 24°C | 0.997327 | 31°C | 0.995372 |
| 25°C | 0.997075 | 32°C | 0.995057 |
| 26°C | 0.996814 | 33°C | 0.994734 |
| 27°C | 0.996544 | 34°C | 0.994403 |
| 28°C | 0.996264 | 35°C | 0.994063 |
| 29°C | 0.995976 | 36°C | 0.993716 |

5. BMI: Since height and body mass have already been measured, simply calculate BMI using the following formula:

$$BMI \ (kg \cdot m^{-2}) = Body \ mass \ (kg) \div Height^2 \ (m)$$

Use the BMI table below to determine obesity.

## Table 3   BMI

| Classification | BMI |
|---|---|
| Nonobese | <25 |
| Moderately obese | 25–30 |
| Obese | >30 |

### ASSIGNMENT

1. Calculate (from data obtained in the experiment) the following masses: (a) Fat mass = % fat × Body mass, and (b) Fat-free mass = Total body mass − Fat mass.
2. Do you expect to find sex differences in body composition? Why or why not?
3. Based on research findings, what percentages of body fat (estimate) would you expect to find on the following individuals: (a) 25-year-old male distance runner, (b) 20-year-old female tennis player, (c) 25-year-old male professional boxer?
4. Determine the correlate coefficients for all % fat scores and BMI.

### SUGGESTED READINGS

Franklin BA, ed. *ACSM's guidelines for exercise testing and prescription.* 6th ed. Baltimore: Williams & Wilkins, 2005.

Brodie DA. Techniques of measurement of body composition. Part I. *Sports Med* 1988;5:11–40

Brodie DA. Techniques of measurement of body composition. Part II. *Sports Med* 1988;5:74–98.

Brozek J, Grande F, Anderson JT, et al. Densitometric analysis of body composition: revision of some quantitative assumptions. *Ann N Y Acad Sci* 1963;110:113–140.

Jequier E. Energy, obesity, and body weight standards. *Am J Clin Nutr* 1987;45:1035–1047.

Jackson AS, Pollock ML. Practical assessment of body composition. *Phys Sportsmed* 1985;13:76–90.

Lohman TG, Going SB. Multicomponent models in body composition research: opportunities and pitfalls. In: Ellis KJ, Eastman JD, eds. *Human body composition: in vivo methods, models, and assessment.* New York: Plenum Press, 1993:53–58.

# Fitness Testing and Activity Monitoring

Health professionals have always been concerned with the health status of our youth. Traditionally the biggest health threats to children were communicable diseases. However, advances in medicine have reduced and even eliminated the risk for most communicable diseases in children. The biggest health threat in modern times is that posed by unhealthy lifestyles. It is estimated that more than 50% of the health problems in the United States can be attributed to lifestyle. Physical fitness is a major lifestyle factor that can contribute to the health of our nation, and physical activity is what brings about physical fitness. The purpose of this experiment is to gain experience in fitness testing and activity monitoring in children.

## OBJECTIVES

1. Practice administering the tests included in the Presidential Health Fitness Award Program.
2. Compare different methods for monitoring physical activity in children.

## PROCEDURES

### Fitness testing

1. Select a partner from class. You will first test your partner and then your partner will test you.
2. Refer to Table 15.3 in the textbook for instructions on administering the evaluations for the Presidential Health Fitness Award Program.
3. Health Fitness Tests
   a. Muscular endurance, partial curlups: According to the instructions in Table 15.3, administer the partial curlups test to your partner. What difficulties did you encounter while administering the test? *What things could be done to ensure that the test is administered correctly? What difficulties might you encounter while giving this test to children of different fitness levels? What precautions could be taken prior to administering this test to a large number of children at once?*
   b. Body composition, body mass index (BMI): Determine the height and weight of your partner, and then calculate his/her BMI. The actual BMI value does not matter, but you need to practice so that you can make these calculations quickly. *How might knowledge of one's BMI affect a child's self-concept? How might the privacy of a child be protected when administering this test to a large number of children at once?*
   c. Flexibility, v-sit reach or sit & reach: According to the instructions in Table 15.3, administer either the

v-sit reach or sit & reach test to your partner. *What difficulties did you encounter while administering the test? What things could be done to ensure that the test is administered correctly? What could you do to make the administration of this test most efficient when giving this test to a large number of children at once?*
   d. Cardiorespiratory endurance, 1-mile run: Either you or your partner perform the 1-mile run. *What difficulties might you encounter while administering this test to many children at once? How might you encourage a child to give a maximal performance on this test?*
   e. Muscular strength, pullups or pushups: According to the instructions in Table 15.3, administer either the pullups or pushups test for muscular endurance to your partner. *What difficulties did you encounter while administering the test? What things could be done to ensure that the test is administered correctly? At what points might a child have a tendency to cheat on this test to obtain a higher score? What precautions could be taken prior to administering this test to a large number of children at once?*

   Although the actual test will not be valid for your partner because he/she is not a child, you can gain insight into how the test is administered while testing your partner.

### Activity monitoring

1. The class can be divided into working lab groups. One person in your group will be assigned to wear an activity monitor and pedometer for 3 days. Data from this individual can be used by the entire group.
2. Follow the manufacturer's instructions for setting up the activity monitor and pedometer for measuring.

   - Wear both of the monitors 24 hours per day. Only take the monitors off when you shower, swim, or where they might get submerged in water.
   - If you remove the monitors, make sure you reattach them to the same location and with the same firmness as previously.
   - Wear the monitors for two weekdays and one weekend day.
   - Follow the manufacturer's instructions to obtain (download) the data from each of the monitors.
3. Calculate the average energy expenditure for the physical activity in each day ($kcal \cdot day^{-1}$). (The manufacturer's instructions for the activity monitor will show you how to obtain this number. If the pedometer manufacturer

does not give instructions, estimate the energy expenditure by assuming that it costs 100 kcal to walk 1 mile.)

4. Compare the numbers for energy expenditure during physical activity from the two devices.

Activity monitor physical activity energy expenditure: _____ kcal·day$^{-1}$

Pedometer physical activity energy expenditure: _____ kcal·day$^{-1}$

# Comparison of Fitness Evaluations Between Genders

Morphological and physiological differences between men and women affect the way each gender responds to exercise training and to what level a man or woman may peak functionally. Fitness tests have been used to assess the level of functional capacity of the cardiorespiratory and musculoskeletal systems in both genders. Fitness scores between men and women may vary considerably, depending on how the test results are expressed.

## OBJECTIVES

1. Practice administering fitness tests for cardiorespiratory endurance, muscular strength, muscular endurance, and flexibility in men and women.
2. Compare fitness scores between men and women by expressing the test results in absolute and relative terms.

## PROCEDURE

1. Body Composition Assessment.

| | |
|---|---|
| Body Mass | _____kg |
| Age | _____yr |

- Using the appropriate three-site skinfold protocol, have your partner measure your skinfold thickness at the sites indicated. (See American College of Sports Medicine. *ACSM's Guidelines for Exercise Testing and Prescription*, 6th ed. Lippincott, Williams & Wilkins: Baltimore 2000;65–66.)

- Measure each skinfold site three times by rotating through each series of measurements sequentially.
- Using the Jackson & Pollock formula (*Physician & Sports Medicine* 1985;13:76–90), calculate your body fat. (See also ACSM's Guidelines, pp. 65–66.)

Go to the ACSM's Guidelines (American College of Sports Medicine. *ACSM's Guidelines for Exercise Testing and Prescription,* 6th ed. Lippincott, Williams & Wilkins: Baltimore 2000,62) and use the appropriate formula to calculate the percentage of body fat. (If you have the equipment and ability to use another method for determining body composition, such as hydrostatic weighing, bioelectrical impedance, or BOD POD, feel free to use that method rather than skinfolds.)

| | |
|---|---|
| Body Fat | _____% |
| Fat Tissue Mass | _____kg |
| Lean Tissue Mass | _____kg |

2. Cardiorespiratory Capacity ($\dot{V}O_{2max}$).

- Standard Bruce Treadmill Protocol: Administer a treadmill graded exercise test using the standard Bruce protocol, either with or without gas analysis. If you do not use gas analysis, calculate the estimated $\dot{V}O_{2max}$ using either the ACSM equation for handrail or no handrail holding (see ACSM's Guidelines, p. 305).

**Women**

| | | | | | |
|---|---|---|---|---|---|
| Triceps | _____mm | Suprailiac | _____mm | Abdominal | _____mm |
| Triceps | _____mm | Suprailiac | _____mm | Abdominal | _____mm |
| Triceps | _____mm | Suprailiac | _____mm | Abdominal | _____mm |
| Mean | _____mm | Mean | _____mm | Mean | _____mm |

Sum of Mean Skinfolds _____mm

**Men**

| | | | | | |
|---|---|---|---|---|---|
| Chest | _____mm | Triceps | _____mm | Subscapular | _____mm |
| Chest | _____mm | Triceps | _____mm | Subscapular | _____mm |
| Chest | _____mm | Triceps | _____mm | Subscapular | _____mm |
| Mean | _____mm | Mean | _____mm | Mean | _____mm |

Sum of Mean Skinfolds _____mm

| Stage (Time) | MPH | Grade (%) | Completed ✓ |
|---|---|---|---|
| 1 (0–3 Minutes) | 1.7 | 10 | |
| 2 (3–6 Minutes) | 2.5 | 12 | |
| 3 (6–9 Minutes) | 3.4 | 14 | |
| 4 (9–12 Minutes) | 4.2 | 16 | |
| 5 (12–15 Minutes) | 5.0 | 18 | |
| 6 (15–18 Minutes) | 5.5 | 20 | |

- Cycle Ergometer Protocol: Administer a graded cycle ergometer exercise test using the following protocol, either with or without gas analysis. If you do not use gas analysis, calculate the estimated $\dot{V}O_{2max}$ using the prediction equation (see ACSM's Guidelines, p. 306).

| Stage (Time) | Watts | Completed ✓ |
|---|---|---|
| 1 (0–1 Minute) | 25 | |
| 2 (1–2 Minutes) | 50 | |
| 3 (2–3 Minutes) | 75 | |
| 4 (3–4 Minutes) | 100 | |
| 5 (4–5 Minutes) | 125 | |
| 6 (5–6 Minutes) | 150 | |
| 7 (6–7 Minutes) | 175 | |
| 8 (7–8 Minutes) | 200 | |
| 9 (8–9 minutes) | 225 | |
| 10 (9–10 Minutes) | 250 | |

$\dot{V}O_{2max}$ _____ l·min⁻¹

$\dot{V}O_{2max}$ _____ mL·kg⁻¹·min⁻¹

$\dot{V}O_{2max}$ _____ mL·kg LBM⁻¹·min⁻¹

3. Upper Body Strength: Bench Press 1 RM.

- Warm up by bench-pressing approximately 50% of your body mass for several repetitions.
- Start the measure of 1 RM by pressing about 75% of your body mass.
- Increase the amount of weight until maximal amount of weight lifted is achieved.
- Rest 1 to 2 minutes between attempts.

Bench Press 1 RM _____ kg

Bench Press Strength-to-Body Mass Ratio _____

Bench Press Strength-to-Lean Body Mass Ratio _____

4. Lower Body Strength: Leg Press 1 RM.

- Set the chair position so the knee joint is at 90°.
- Warm up by leg pressing approximately 100% of your body mass for several repetitions.
- Start the measure of 1 RM by pressing about 125% of your body mass.
- Increase the amount of weight until maximal amount of weight lifted is achieved.
- Rest 1 to 2 minutes between attempts.

Leg Press 1 RM _____ kg

Leg Press Strength-to-Body Mass Ratio _____

Leg Press Strength-to-Lean Body Mass Ratio _____

5. Overall Body Strength: Hand Grip 1 RM.

- Assume the standing position with your head erect, facing forward.
- Adjust the grip dynamometer so that so that the middle finger's second phalanx opposes the gripping device at a 90° angle.
- Set your forearm at a 45° angle and rotate the forearm slightly outward.
- Squeeze the handgrip dynamometer quickly and maximally, taking no more than a few seconds to perform each trial. Do not move from your original body position.
- Perform two to three trials on each hand alternately with each hand. Rest about 20 to 60 seconds between trials.
- After each trial, record your results.

| Right Hand | Left Hand |
|---|---|
| _____kg | _____kg |
| _____kg | _____kg |
| _____kg | _____kg |
| _____Mean kg | _____Mean kg |
| **Sum of Left and Right Hand Mean Scores** _____ kg | |

Hand Grip-to-Body Mass Ratio _____

Hand Grip-to-Lean Body Mass Ratio _____

6. Overall Muscular Endurance: Handgrip Endurance.

- Calculate 50% of the maximal voluntary contraction (MVC) for each hand from the Grip Strength test. (Record below)
- Grip the dynamometer as in No. 5 above.
- Squeeze the dynamometer until the needle reaches the position of 50% maximal strength.
- Hold the muscular contraction at this position for as long as possible.
- Record the time to fatigue. (Fatigue is defined as not being able to hold the contraction at 50% maximal.)
- Repeat the test with the opposite hand.

| 50% MVC Left hand _____ kg | 50% MVC Right Hand _____ kg |
| --- | --- |
| Left Hand Time to Fatigue _____ | Right Hand Time to Fatigue _____ |

7. Flexibility: Trunk Flexion.
   - The subject sits with the legs fully extended and the soles of the feet against the box (shoes removed).
   - The subject reaches forward with both hands as far as possible, holding this position momentarily. Keep both hands parallel and do not lead with one hand. The fingers may overlap.
   - Ensure that the subject's knees remain extended.
   - The subject should lower the head and exhale as the test is performed.
   - Repeat this procedure three times.
   - Record the most distant point reached with the fingertips (cm).

Trunk Flexibility Score _____ (cm)

8. Flexibility: Shoulder Flexibility.
   - The subject attempts to clasp hands behind the back as one arm reaches down from over the shoulder and the other reaches up from behind and below.
   - The score is recorded as centimeters measured from joining hands behind the back. (The arm on top is the shoulder being tested.)
   - Test the left and right side of the body.

Flexibility Score Left Shoulder: _____ cm

Flexibility Score Right Shoulder: _____ cm

9. Gender Comparisons.
   - Make a tally of the scores for each test from all the members of the class.
   - Separate the scores by group, according to gender.
   - Calculate the average group score for each measure and record below.
   - Compare the scores. (Score comparison can be done by simply contrasting the group mean scores, calculating strength ratios between men and women for each score, and/or performing a statistical comparison, such as a $t$-test.)

**Fitness Scores for Men:**

| | |
| --- | --- |
| $\dot{V}O_{2max}$ | _____ $l \cdot min^{-1}$ |
| $\dot{V}O_{2max}$ | _____ $mL \cdot kg^{-1} \cdot min^{-1}$ |
| $\dot{V}O_{2max}$ | _____ $mL \cdot kg\ LBM^{-1} \cdot min^{-1}$ |
| Bench Press 1 RM | _____ kg |
| Bench Press Strength-to-Body Mass Ratio | _____ |

| | |
| --- | --- |
| Bench Press Strength-to-Lean Body Mass RatioLeg Press 1 RM | _____ kg |
| Leg Press Strength-to-Body Mass Ratio | _____ |
| Leg Press Strength-to-Lean Body Mass Ratio | _____ |
| Sum of Left and Right Hand Mean Scores | _____ kg |
| Hand Grip-to-Body Mass Ratio | _____ |
| Hand Grip-to-Lean Body Mass Ratio | _____ |
| Left Hand Time to Fatigue | _____ |
| Right Hand Time to Fatigue | _____ |
| Trunk Flexibility Score | _____ (cm) |
| Flexibility Score Left Shoulder | _____ (cm) |
| Flexibility Score Right Shoulder | _____ (cm) |

**Fitness Scores for Women:**

| | |
| --- | --- |
| $\dot{V}O_{2max}$ | _____ $l \cdot min^{-1}$ |
| $\dot{V}O_{2max}$ | _____ $mL \cdot kg^{-1} \cdot min^{-1}$ |
| $\dot{V}O_{2max}$ | _____ $mL \cdot kg\ LBM^{-1} \cdot min^{-1}$ |
| Bench Press 1 RM | _____ kg |
| Bench Press Strength-to-Body Mass Ratio | _____ |
| Bench Press Strength-to-Lean Body Mass Ratio | _____ |
| Leg Press 1 RM | _____ kg |
| Leg Press Strength-to-Body Mass Ratio | _____ |
| Leg Press Strength-to-Lean Body Mass Ratio | _____ |
| Sum of Left and Right Hand Mean Scores | _____ kg |
| Hand Grip-to-Body Mass Ratio | _____ |
| Hand Grip-to-Lean Body Mass Ratio | _____ |
| Left Hand time to fatigue | _____ |
| Right Hand time to fatigue | _____ |
| Trunk Flexibility Score | _____ (cm) |
| Flexibility Score Left Shoulder | _____ (cm) |
| Flexibility Score Right Shoulder | _____ (cm) |

# Discussing Differential Diagnosis of Chest Pain

Therapists monitoring exercise sessions should understand the differential diagnosis of chest pain. This laboratory exercise focuses on chest pain originating as anginal pain, pain from a myocardial infarction, and pain caused by pericarditis. Referring to Figures 18.10 through 18.12 the following descriptions should be thoroughly studied.

## Anginal Chest Pain Pattern

| | |
|---|---|
| Location | Substernal/Retrosternal |
| Referral | Neck, jaw, back, shoulder, or arms (more common in the left arm) |
| | Occasionally radiates to the abdomen |
| Description | Viselike pressure, squeezing, heaviness, burning indigestion |
| Intensity | Mild ot moderate (builds up gradually or may be sudden) |
| Duration | Usually less than 10 minutes (never more than 30 minutes) |
| Associated Signs and Symptoms | Extreme fatigue, lethargy, weakness, shortness of breath, nausea, diaphoresis, anxiety, belching, heartburn |
| Relieving Factors | Rest or Nitroglycerin |
| Aggravating Factors | Exercise or physical exertion, cold weather, heavy meals, emotional stress |

## Myocardial Infarction Chest Pain Pattern

| | |
|---|---|
| Location | Substernal, anterior chest |
| Referral | May radiate like angina, frequently down both arms |
| Description | Burning, stabbing, viselike pressure, squeezing, heaviness |
| Intensity | Severe |
| Duration | Usually at least 30 minutes, may last 1–2 hours |
| Associated Signs and Symptoms | None with a silent myocardial infarction |
| | Dizziness, feeling faint, nausea, vomiting, pallor, diaphoresis, severe anxiety, fatigue, sudden weakness, shortness of breath, |
| Relieving Factors | None (unrelieved by rest or nitroglycerin taken every 5 minutes for 20 minutes) |
| Aggravating Factors | Not necessarily anything, may occur at rest or may follow emotional stress or physical exertion |

## Pericarditis Chest Pain Pattern

| | |
|---|---|
| Location | Substernal or over the sternum, sometimes to the left of midline toward cardiac apex |
| Referral | Neck, upper back, upper trapezious muscle, left supraclavicular area, down the left arm, costal margins |
| Description | More localized than pain of myocardial infarction |
| Intensity | Moderate to severe |
| Duration | Continuous, may last hours or days with residual soreness following |
| Associated Signs and Symptoms | Usually medically determined associated symptoms (e.g., by chest auscultation using a stethoscope) |
| Relieving Factors | Sitting upright or leaning forward |
| Aggravating Factors | Muscle movement associated with deep breathing (e.g., laughter, inspiration, coughing), left lateral (side) bending of the upper trunk, trunk rotation (either to the right or to the left), supine position |

## LABORATORY EXERCISE

In groups of 3 to 5, perform mock cases of individuals presenting with any of the three patterns described above. One student serves as the patient and the others practice any of the following scenarios using one of the pain patterns:

1. An outpatient during cardiopulmonary rehabilitation doing ergometer exercise complains of chest pain.

2. An inpatient doing bedside range of motion exercise complains of chest pain.

3. A patient performing a prescribed home exercise routine calls in to the center complaining of chest pain.

## ASSIGNMENT

In round table discussion with the group, discuss your perceptions of the exercise in differential diagnosis. How has it made you ready for clinical practice?

# The Relationship Between $\dot{V}O_2$ and Heart Rate During Wheelchair Exercise

The relationship between $\dot{V}O_2$ and heart rate has been quantified for many modes of activity, such as running, walking, cycling, arm ergometry, and rowing. Knowledge of this relationship is vital for writing the exercise prescription. Given the popularity of the paralympics movement, many individuals who are either confined to a wheelchair for ambulatory purposes or for whom the wheelchair is their primary mode of ambulation now consider themselves to be "wheelchair athletes." For these individuals, and others who are less ambitious, the necessity of wheelchair ambulation is a way of life. For many, wheelchair ambulation in performing activities of daily living is their primary fitness activity. Therefore, knowledge of the relationship between heart rate and $\dot{V}O_2$ for wheelchair ambulation should provide a basis for prescribing exercise to individuals who rely heavily on this ambulatory mode. The purpose of this laboratory exercise is to establish the relationship between heart rate and $\dot{V}O_2$ for wheelchair ambulation in a group of healthy college-aged students. A secondary purpose is to gain practical experience formulating regression equations.

## METHODS

Five students (male and/or female) will volunteer for a modified graded exercise test (wheelchair on treadmill). Subjects should be well rested and at least 6 hours postprandial. The students should have at least two separate practice sessions ambulating with a wheelchair on the treadmill before testing. The test will be conducted over five treadmill speeds (stages): 26.8, 67.0, 93.8, 120.6 $m \cdot min^{-1}$ (1, 2.5, 3.5, 4.5 miles per hour, respectively). Speeds may be adjusted so that

all subjects can complete steady-state stages of 4 minutes. Steady state is defined as a difference in $\dot{V}O_2$ of less than 50 $mL \cdot min^{-1}$ from minute 3 to 4 of each stage. If needed, a fifth minute may be used to ensure steady-state. Each subject's heart rate should be continuously monitored by ECG leads and $\dot{V}O_2$ should be monitored continuously by the standard open circuit technique. Four pairs of data will be matched for the five subjects (20 pairs total). These data will be analyzed via regression using any standard statistical software. If need be, a handheld calculator with regression capability may be used to generate the slope and intercept for the relationship between heart rate and $\dot{V}O_2$.

## ASSIGNMENTS

1. Plot the data and generate a regression line with graphics software and explain any differences seen between your results and the same relationships for other modes of exercise.
2. Were the heart rate and $\dot{V}O_2$ responses to this graded exercise test linear? Explain.
3. How might the relationship be different if you used individuals with paraplegia or quadriplegia, instead of healthy individuals?
4. How close to maximal predicted heart rates were your subjects by the last stage of the test?

## SUGGESTED READINGS

Abel T, Kröner M, Vega SR, et al. Energy expenditure in wheelchair racing and handbiking—a basis for prevention of cardiovascular diseases in those with disabilities. *Eur J Cardiovas Prevention Rehabil* 2003;10: 371–376.

# Vector Analysis of the Mean QRS Axis

## PROCEDURES

There are many different electrical vectors produced during the course of a single cardiac cycle. When dealing with the mean QRS vector, it is important to realize that the activation sequence of ventricular depolarization starts with septal activation and then progresses to ventricular activation. Several vectors are produced in this sequence, but it is important to determine the mean of these vectors to have a clear understanding of the general direction in the frontal plane in which the QRS complex is predominantly pointed. To do this, an easy four-step method is followed.

Step 1 is to determine which half (left or right) of the hexaxial array the QRS complex is pointed toward. This is done by examining lead I. If the QRS complex is mostly positive in this lead, it is pointed toward the left. If it is mostly negative, the QRS is pointed toward the right. See *Figure 1* below which shows a sample electrocardiogram (ECG) and a demonstration hexaxial array. In this figure, lead I is positive, making it possible to determine the location of the vector as +90° to −90° and to the left. Remember that "left" presupposes that the array is superimposed onto your thorax. When this is done, the arrow points left, not "right," as the arrow appears on the page.

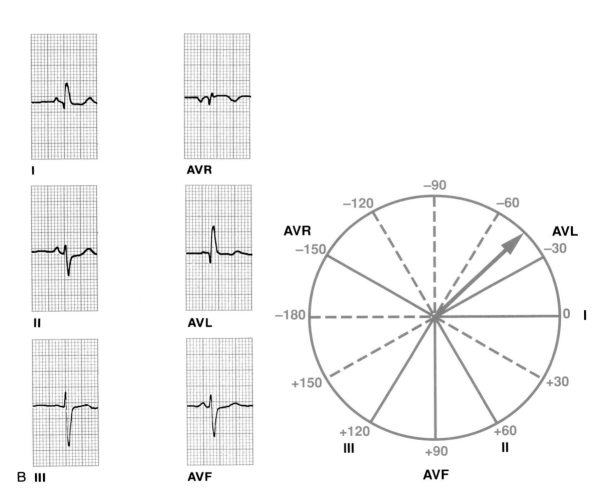

Step 2 is to determine which other half (top or bottom) of the array the QRS complex is pointed toward. To find this, examine lead aV$_F$; if positive, the QRS complex is pointed downward, and if negative, it is pointed upward. *In our example, lead aV$_F$ is negative; therefore, the QRS vector is upward, but in which quadrant?* To determine quadrant, simply notice the common quadrant identified by completing steps 1 and 2. In our example, the common quadrant is the upper left-hand quadrant. We have now determined the location of the mean QRS vector as between 0° and −90°. Also, *Figure 2* identifies this vector as representing left axis deviation.

*Is this the closest we can come to determining the mean QRS axis?* The answer is no. With the next step, you should be able to determine the axis to within ±15°. At this point, two general rules are important to keep in mind:

- The mean QRS axis is oriented at right angles to any lead showing a biphasic complex and toward leads showing tall R waves
- The mean QRS axis points midway between any two leads that show tall R waves of equal height

We can test these rules with our example by going to step 3, which is simply a consideration of these rules taken together.

In step 3, now that we know the quadrant, we can determine the vector to within ±15°. Look first for the most biphasic QRS complex. In our example, we do not have a biphasic complex, but AVR is closest.

*The question is: what if the most biphasic QRS complex is not exactly biphasic?* In that instance, you simply ask a rhetorical question: *what would the vector be if the most biphasic lead were exactly biphasic?* Answer the question by going through step 3 as demonstrated above. The answer in such an instance is critical.

In case the biphasic QRS complex is not exactly biphasic, determine the exact amplitude of the R and S waves as before. In our example, if R wave amplitude was 1 mm greater than S wave amplitude, then the vector would be "pulled" towards lead AVR (the opposite is also true). The question then becomes: *how much would the vector be moved off lead aV$_L$?* This should be fairly easy at this point because we are not going to try to get to the exact vector in this method without an exactly biphasic lead. Once you have the direction of movement, step 4 involves examining the tallest R waves. In our example, lead I and aV$_L$ are the tallest. Again, *if lead AVR was slightly more positive and if lead I and aV$_L$ were of equal amplitude, the vector would fall around −15°. If lead I was slightly more positive, the vector would be moved closer to lead I (about half the distance between −15° and 0°). You would simply keep examining key leads to make minor adjustments in your vector analysis. This is a fairly qualitative method of analysis that is simple and relatively easy to grasp.*

### ASSIGNMENT

To practice determining QRS vector and taking ECGs, record resting extremity lead ECGs on your classmates. In groups of two to three individuals, determine the mean electrical QRS axis on each ECG and determine if the heart has a normal axis or if it is deviated.

In our example, since AVL is the tallest R wave we can start with the vector directly on −30°. But, since AVR is more negative than positive, the vector is "pushed" off of −30°. But by how much? The rule of thumb in this approximation method is to come off 15°, making our final vector −45°.

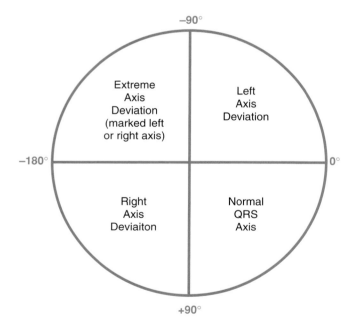

# Assessment of the Overweight Patient

Helping a person change their eating and exercise patterns is a difficult task. The undertaking becomes even more difficult for the overweight person, and especially difficult for the obese person with comorbidities. Nonetheless, behavior change is the key to generating the physiological outcomes we desire as exercise specialists. Regardless of whether we are normal weight, overweight, or obese, most of us can make behavioral changes to improve our health.

In this lab, you will pair up with a partner and perform an intake interview with that partner as if he/she were coming to you for assistance in changing eating and exercise behaviors. It does not matter whether your partner is overweight or not, the process of gathering information during the intake interview is the same.

## OBJECTIVES

1. Determine a client's risk of comorbidities according to their BMI.
2. Determine if a client has an inherited propensity toward obesity.
3. Identify a client's specific barriers to healthy eating and exercise.
4. Design some possible approaches that can be employed to help a client change his/her eating and exercise behaviors.

## PROCEDURES

If you have not already read Chapter 22 in the text completely, do so before completing this lab experience. You may want to pay special attention to Case Study 22.1, because it relates closely to the material that is covered in this lab. After reading the chapter, select a lab partner from class. You will interview your partner in order to obtain the information necessary to complete this lab, and then you will reverse roles and he/she will interview you. Complete the intake interview assignment as instructed in the following information.

1. Risk of comorbidities according to BMI.

| Name | | | |
|---|---|---|---|
| Height | _____ in | Height | _____ M |
| Weight | _____ lbs | Weight | _____ kg |
| | BMI | _____ | (BMI = kg ÷ M²) |
| Risk of Weight-Related Comorbidities _____ | | | |

2. Inherited propensity toward obesity.

Interview your client. If your client is overweight, ask how long he/she has been overweight. Determine whether the overweight condition came about at the onset of a significant life event (e.g., accident, medical condition, emotional trauma, change in environment). Regardless of whether your client is overweight or not, talk to him/her about his/her family. You might want to draw a family tree to identify which relatives are overweight. According to the family information gathered, what is the likelihood that your client has a genetic predisposition toward obesity?

Client predisposition toward obesity:
Low        Moderate        High

3. Specific barriers to healthy eating and exercise.

Use the Barriers to Healthy Weight Management checklist to identify specific barriers your client may have toward maintaining a healthy eating and exercise plan. Perform this exercise orally as you interact with your client. Your client may want to elaborate on anything he/she marks as a potential barrier.

4. Design some possible approaches that can be used to help your client change his/her eating and exercise behaviors.

First, review the Barriers to Healthy Weight Management checklist. Look for behavior patterns. Are your client's barriers related to emotional turmoil (e.g., stress, anger, boredom, embarrassment, need for comfort, pleasure, security)? Are your client's barriers related to emotional traumas from the past (e.g., abuse, humiliation, past bad experience)? Are your client's barriers physical or tangible (not enough time, facility availability, access to food)? If a pattern emerges, construct a behavioral plan that will help dismantle those barriers in the pattern. If no apparent pattern emerges, select two or three barriers to work on, and construct a specific plan to tackle those barriers.

As the professional, you should not construct the eating and exercise plan for the client. The client himself/herself should construct the plan. You should facilitate by helping the client see things that may not be apparent to him/her, by helping the client set realistic goals, by helping the client design behavioral strategies, by giving supportive suggestions, and by helping the client commit to the plan. Remember that as an integral part of the plan, you must have a measurable way to determine if the plan is working, and remember also that weight loss is only one measure of success. Don't forget to set time intervals for when the plan can be evaluated and when adjustments can be made.

## BARRIERS TO HEALTHY WEIGHT MANAGEMENT

**Identify any of the following that apply to your personal eating and activity patterns.**

*I eat when I am . . .*
_____ depressed
_____ under stress
_____ frustrated
_____ angry
_____ nervous
_____ sad
_____ tired
_____ happy
_____ celebrating
_____ bored
other _____
_____

*I eat because I am (was) . . .*
_____ humiliated
_____ shamed
_____ expected to be perfect
_____ avoiding confrontations
_____ a victim of physical abuse
_____ a victim of sexual abuse
_____ a child of alcoholic parent(s)
_____ valued for my physical appearance
_____ not allowed to express my feelings
other _____
_____

*I avoid exercise or physical activity because . . .*
_____ I don't like to exercise
_____ I don't know how to exercise
_____ I don't have time to exercise
_____ I don't like to get "sweaty"
_____ I have no place to exercise
_____ I am too tired to exercise
_____ I am embarrassed to exercise
_____ of a physical or medical reason
_____ of a bad experience with exercise
_____ I hate my body
other _____
_____

*I eat because of . . .*
_____ past failures at weight control
_____ fear of losing weight
_____ distrust of men/women
_____ pressure from society
_____ lack of confidence
_____ low self-control
_____ guilt
_____ romantic discord
_____ no social support system
_____ because food is accessible
other _____
_____

*I eat . . .*
_____ too much sugar
_____ too much fat
_____ very little, but I am still fat
_____ few fruits and vegetables
_____ few grains or starches
_____ too many high-calorie drinks
_____ too many sweets
_____ too much "junk" food
_____ all the time
_____ when I am not hungry
_____ to please others
_____ too many fried foods
_____ for pleasure
_____ for security
_____ for comfort
_____ for fun
_____ to gain control
_____ for companionship
_____ until I am stuffed
_____ too much fast food
_____ unhealthy snacks
_____ in binges
_____ only what my diet allows
other _____
_____

# Summary Knowledge Answers

## CHAPTER OUTLINE

## SUMMARY KNOWLEDGE ANSWERS CHAPTER 1

1. Technology will allow scientists to take a closer look at the molecular basis of health and disease. In this way, the influence of an active lifestyle will come under greater scrutiny as we continue to understand the molecular basis of movement.

2. Exercise science is the discipline that studies movement, including physical activity and exercise. Exercise physiology is one subdisciplinary field under exercise science in which the physiology and biochemical basis of movement is explored.

3. Exercise physiologists study acute and chronic exercise to better understand how the body responds to exercise stress and how the body adapts to this stress over time.

4. Applied research question: What is the best training program to rehabilitate a person who recently had a heart attack, an aerobic exercise program or aerobic exercise plus resistance exercise program?

   Basic research question: What is the physiologic basis for the reduction in resting heart rate seen in aerobic exercise training?

5. Exercise is a physical form of stress, i.e., exercise is one of many stressors. Stressors cause common physical responses to occur.

6. Movement: typing at a keyboard, turning your head, arm movements while eating; physical activity: bowling, driving a car, lifting crates; exercise: jogging, weightlifting, skipping rope.

7. The laws of health: fresh air, proper food, exercise, sleep, bowel movements, and emotional health. The rest of your answer must draw upon your own understanding of wellness.

8. Exercise physiology is gaining increasing recognition in the health care community because exercise is increasingly being seen as an important preventive health and rehabilitative measure.

## SUMMARY KNOWLEDGE ANSWERS CHAPTER 2

1. a. Carbohydrates
   b. Fats
   c. Proteins
   d. Vitamins
   e. Minerals
   f. Water

2. 1 g of carbohydrate = 4 kcal; 1 g of fat = 9 kcal; 1 g of protein = 4 kcal.

3. Monosaccharides are the single sugar units glucose, fructose, and galactose. Disaccharides are composed of two single sugars linked together. One of these is always glucose. There are three disaccharides: sucrose, maltose, and lactose. Polysaccharides are composed of three or more single sugars. The most common polysaccharide is starch. Glycogen is the polysaccharide form in which animals store carbohydrates in the tissues.

4. a. Simple fats (fatty acids and triglycerides)
   b. Compound fats (fats in combination with other chemical groups—phospholipids, lipoproteins, glycolipids)
   c. Derived fats (sterols)

5. Saturated fatty acids are saturated with hydrogens and do not contain any double bonds between carbons. Polyunsaturated fatty acids contain two or more double bonds between carbons and are the healthiest for you.

6. A complete protein contains all of the essential amino acids in the same proportions that are found in the body.

7. The primary role for carbohydrates is energy. The primary roles for fat are energy, structure, and cushioning. The primary roles for protein are regulatory and structural.

8. Fat-soluble vitamins are associated with fat, store well in the body tissues, and can be toxic if consumed in large amounts. Water-soluble vitamins dissolve in water, are easily excreted from the body, and can be deficient if not consumed regularly.

9. Vitamins act as cofactors for many of the chemical reactions in the body that release energy for energy production. Vitamins also play a major role in maintaining the functioning of tissues and organs of the body (e.g., vision).

10. No, the terms major and trace refer to the recommended amount of the mineral to be consumed, not its importance physiologically.

11. The trace minerals primarily serve metabolic functions, whereas the major minerals primarily serve regulatory and structural functions.

12. Water is the most critical nutrient because a person will die without consuming water within several days. Moreover, exercise-induced dehydration can cause death within 1 to 2 hours.

13. All water compartments in the body are in equilibrium with each other. When the body loses water due to sweating, water is drawn from all body compartments. This fluid shift can place the cardiovascular system at great risk if the fluid loss through sweating is great.

14. a. Grains, cereals, pastas
    b. Vegetables
    c. Fruits
    d. Meat, legumes, beans, nuts
    e. Dairy
    f. Sweets and treats

15. a. Aim for fitness
    b. Build a healthy base
    c. Choose sensibly

The ABCs relate to the Food Guide Pyramid in that they help an individual maintain or obtain health through sensible eating and physical activity.

## SUMMARY KNOWLEDGE ANSWERS CHAPTER 3

1. Potential energy is energy due to position; it is stored energy which can be used to do work. Kinetic energy is energy due to the motion of an object.

2. The first law of thermodynamics concerns conservation of energy; it is an important concept when dealing with the physiology of weight loss and obesity, two topics of interest in the study of exercise physiology. The second law states that entropy is constantly increasing. This can be viewed in exercise physiology by considering the heat loss from the body during exercise. Only a small part of the energy transductions that occur during exercise ends up as useful work, the rest is dissipated.

3. Metabolism is the sum of all the chemical processes occurring in the body. It is composed of anabolic and catabolic processes.

4. Some exercise is considered anaerobic and some aerobic because some forms of exercise use primarily anaerobic energy sources and others forms primarily aerobic energy sources.

5. Coupled reactions connect anabolic and catabolic processes.

6. Lactate is produced in intense, prolonged activity ($>$15 seconds) as the muscle draws upon its glycogen stores to make ATP. The production of ATP is necessary and therefore it is good to sustain intense activity beyond 10 to 15 seconds.

7. Glycogen serves as a ready glucose source during all forms of physical activity.

8. Power relates to the ability of a metabolic process to produce ATP rapidly, and capacity refers to the total amount of ATP capable of being produced by a metabolic process.

9. There are different ATP production totals from different catabolic pathways of skeletal muscles because of the inherent differences in the metabolic systems and the energy substrates utilized.

10. At the onset of exercise, ATP and CP are the preferred energy sources over carbohydrate and fat because both ATP and CP are stored at rest in the muscle cell and they are a source of ready energy whose liberation is directly used to power muscle contraction. CP replenishes ATP as ATP is depleted.

11. Aerobic respiration is $O_2$ utilization in mitochondria in the process of oxidative phosphorylation.

## SUMMARY KNOWLEDGE ANSWERS CHAPTER 4

1. a. ATP-PC system
   b. Rapid glycolysis
   c. Slow glycolysis
   d. Fat oxidation

2. a. Fat oxidation
   b. Slow glycolysis
   c. Rapid glycolysis
   d. ATP-PC system

3. As exercise intensity increases, the rate at which ATP needs to be produced also increases. The higher the exercise intensity, the less aerobic metabolism (fat oxidation, slow glycolysis) can contribute to the energy supply to sustain the exercise. The shift is from aerobic fat oxidation through slow and rapid glycolysis and on to the ATP-PC stores.

4. a. Glycogenolysis in the liver
   b. Gluconeogenesis through the glucose-alanine cycle and the Cori cycle

5. Insulin is the energy-storage hormone. When blood glucose levels are high, insulin promotes the uptake of glucose into the cells, lipogenesis, and glycogen formation. Glucagon is the energy-release hormone. When blood glucose levels are low, glucagon promotes liver glycogenolysis, gluconeogenesis, and lipolysis.

6. a. Rephosphorylation of phosphagen stores
   b. Restoration of depleted $O_2$ stores
   c. Conversion of glycolytic intermediates back to glucose
   d. Metabolic cost of elevated post-exercise cardiac output
   e. Metabolic cost of elevated post-exercise respiration
   f. Post-exercise elevated body temperature
   g. Elevated catecholamine actions
   h. Metabolic cost of ion redistribution

7. The rapid rise in blood lactic acid levels represents the point of increasing reliance on rapid glycolysis for energy supply during increasing exercise intensity.

## SUMMARY KNOWLEDGE ANSWERS CHAPTER 5

1. The treadmill uses speed and grade in work calculations, the cycle uses an external load, and the step device uses step height/frequency and body weight.

2. Power is work done per unit of time.

3. Direct calorimetry measures heat directly as a change in temperature of a fluid, while indirect calorimetry measures heat as a consequence of the level of $O_2$ consumption.

4. Haldane transformation is important in open-circuit spirometry measurement because without this calculation, both inspired and expired minute ventilation would have to be measured.

5. It is possible for $FEN_2$ to be different than $FIN_2$ because although $N_2$ is not consumed or produced in metabolism, the percentage of the expired $N_2$ changes solely as an artifact of changes in expired $CO_2$ and $O_2$. These three expired gases must equal 100% of the total air exhaled.

6. Charles' and Boyle's laws are important in gas volume measures because gas volumes fluctuate depending on the ambient temperature and barometric pressure even if the same number of absolute gas molecules are present.

7. Respiratory quotient is specific to respired cells or tissue beds while respiratory exchange ratio is specific to respiration at the level of the whole organism. However, the two variables are most often used interchangeably.

8. Basal refers to a metabolic rate that sustains life process and is measured under strict conditions—early morning to ensure a very restful state, 12-hour fast to ensure that nonshivering thermogenesis is not present, supine body position so that muscles are as relaxed as possible, thermoneutral environmental lab conditions, and metabolically active medications are not taken.

9. As workload increases, energy expenditure increases. This relationship becomes curvilinear as workloads move beyond the moderate level, which ultimately decreases efficiency of movement.

10. Gross $\dot{V}O_2$ = Net $\dot{V}O_2$ + Resting $\dot{V}O_2$. Calculating efficiency after first removing resting $\dot{V}O_2$ provides net efficiency.

11. Efficiency is a term that is specific to movements for which work can be quantified, while economy is the term used for movements for which work cannot be quantified.

12. Movement economy and efficiency are directly related to the $\dot{V}O_2$ response to specific activities of daily living. Therefore, patients' symptoms are often reflective of poor movement economy.

13. Efficiency declines as exercise intensity increases.

14. The relationship between $\%\dot{V}O_{2max}$ and $\%HR_{max}$ is linear, but the slope and intercept of this relationship are dependent on exercise mode.

15. The nature of the work being performed produces differences in the $O_2$ cost per unit of work or power for a particular exercise ergometer. For example, in cycle ergometry, there is a static component to the muscular action that increases the $O_2$ cost of work.

## SUMMARY KNOWLEDGE ANSWERS CHAPTER 6

1. The relationship of $PaO_2$ to $P_{AO_2}$ is due to the venous admixture.

2. Altitude affects breathing because as you ascend in altitude, the barometric pressure decreases which reduces the driving pressure that "pushes" $O_2$ into the lungs.

3. Too much $CO_2$ buildup in the blood can cause respiratory acidosis.

4. Partial pressure gradients are important in respiration because these gradients allow gas species to enter or leave the body.

5. Chest circumference increases during inspiration (the diaphragm moves downward, protruding into the abdominal cavity and rotating the lower ribs toward the horizontal plane, which increases the cross-sectional area of the thoracic cavity) and decreases during expiration (rib motion is away from the horizontal plane and the thoracic cavity reduces in size as the diaphragm and ribs rebound to their original positions).

6. Exercise improves $\dot{V}/\dot{Q}$ matching because during exercise, ventilation increases at a faster rate than does pulmonary blood flow.

7. Hemoglobin is more important than myoglobin in respiratory physiology partly because of *location*—hemoglobin is in the blood—but mostly because of *biochemistry*—hemoglobin holds much more $O_2$ and holds it tightly in some areas and loosely in others. This allows hemoglobin to take up and release $O_2$ readily.

8. $CO_2$ is transported from muscle tissue to the lungs in physical solution as dissolved gas, as bicarbonate ions, and as carbamino compounds.

9. Dissolved $CO_2$ regulates ventilation and dissolved $O_2$ regulates how much $O_2$ is bound to hemoglobin.

10. The $O_2$ content of blood is lower in females because females have less hemoglobin concentration in blood.

## SUMMARY KNOWLEDGE ANSWERS CHAPTER 7

1. Electrical impulses in the heart start in the sinoatrial node, travel through the atria, and next stimulate the atrioventricular node. Impulses then travel down the bundle of His, through the bundle branches and Purkinje fibers, and to the ventricular cells.

2. For the heart to function mechanically, electrical stimulation must occur first.

3. As a chamber fills with blood, intrachamber pressure increases.

4. Blood pressure = Cardiac output × Peripheral resistance.

5. Heart rate and stroke volume regulate cardiac output because of this relationship: Cardiac output = Heart rate × Stroke volume.

6. Heart rate is regulated by the interplay between parasympathetic and sympathetic input to the sinoatrial node, and stroke volume is regulated by intrinsic (preload) and extrinsic (neural and hormonal input) forces.

7. Resistance exercise should not be recommended for improving cardiorespiratory fitness because resistance exercise does not stress aerobic metabolism or the cardiovascular system in such a way as to produce significant gains in $\dot{V}O_{2max}$.

## SUMMARY KNOWLEDGE ANSWERS CHAPTER 8

1. The four ways in which the body can gain or lose heat are conduction, convection, radiation, and evaporation.

2. The more sweat that is vaporized, the more heat is dissipated. When the relative humidity is low, the vapor pressure in the air is low, and this favors rapid heat removal from the body through evaporation. When the relative humidity is high, the vapor pressure in the air is high, which is less favorable to heat loss from the body through evaporation.

3. When thermal receptors increase their firing, their surrounding temperature rises. The hypothalamus interprets this communication, and thermal effectors are stimulated to dilate the blood vessels of the skin and activate the sweat glands. When surrounding temperature drops, thermal effectors cause blood vessels in the skin to constrict to conserve heat.

4. As a person exercises in the heat, vasodilation of the blood vessels in the skin allow for greater blood flow to the skin surface. A greater portion of the cardiac output is directed to the skin. Constriction of the vessels supplying the digestive organs and kidney helps maintain the distribution of blood flow to the exercising muscles.

5. Adjustments to heat exposure during exercise include improved circulation, increased plasma volume, earlier onset of sweating, higher sweat rates, reduced salt loss in sweat, and a reduced skin blood flow during exercise. Adjustments to cold exposure include the ability to withstand a colder skin temperature before shivering and an intermittent blood flow to the hands and feet.

6. The circulatory system helps the body conserve heat when it is exposed to a cold environment through constriction of the blood vessels in the skin and an increased distribution of the blood flow to the core.

7. Children exposed to the heat should be encouraged to exercise at a lower intensity and shorter duration than when not exposed to the heat. Children should be given a long time to acclimatize to exercise in the heat and

should always be encouraged to consume fluids, even though they are not thirsty. Children exercising in the cold should wear protective clothing because their body surface area to body mass ratio is greater than adults.

8. The WB-GT or WBT takes into account the environmental heat stress imposed on a person exposed to the heat, rather than just the ambient temperature stress.

9. The wind chill factor is an index of the total cold stress imposed on a person exposed to a cold and windy environment and represents a better indicator of cold exposure than just the ambient temperature.

10.  a. Heat cramps: muscle spasms
    b. Heat syncope: faintness, weakness, and fatigue
    c. Heat exhaustion: increased skin and core temperature, dizziness, nausea, vomiting, and diarrhea
    d. Heat stroke: increased skin and core temperatures, muscle flaccidity, involuntary limb movement, seizures, vomiting, diarrhea, rapid shallow heartbeat, and coma

11. Preparations for exercising in the heat and cold should include alterations of intensity and duration of exercise, proper clothing, fluid consumption, awareness of signs and symptoms of exposure disorders, and acclimatization.

## SUMMARY KNOWLEDGE ANSWERS CHAPTER 9

1.  a. Cell body: contains a nucleus where mRNA is synthesized and then translated into protein for transport to parts of the cell
    b. Dendrites: bring information into the cell body
    c. Axons: carry information away from the cell body

2.  a. Resting phase: inside of cell is negative; has a charge of −50 to −55 mV
    b. Depolarization phase: sodium gates open, sodium rushes into cell: charge inside of cell is positive (~+80 mV)
    c. Repolarization phase: when sodium channel gates close and potassium channel gates open; negativity of inside of cell is re-established

3. When the cell is refractory to an action potential, that means that even if another stimulus is applied to the cell, the cell will not depolarize until repolarization is approximately one-third complete.

4. Temporal summation is when several excitatory postsynaptic potentials (EPSPs) occur simultaneously at the axon hillock and an action potential occurs. Spatial summation is when several EPSPs occur in rapid succession to generate an action potential. Inhibitory postsynaptic potentials and EPSPs engage in temporal and spatial summation; if the sum is less than the threshold potential, then no action potential is generated. If the sum is greater than the threshold potential, then an action potential is generated.

5. An action potential is transmitted to the axon terminal; vesicles containing the neurotransmitter move to the presynaptic membrane; the neurotransmitter is released into synaptic space; the neurotransmitter crosses the synaptic cleft and binds to the receptor on the postsynaptic membrane.

6.
   a. Frontal lobe: involved in ethical behavior, morality, initiative, motivation; responsible for voluntary movements and motor planning
   b. Parietal lobe: integrates sensory information and taste
   c. Occipital lobe: visual area
   d. Temporal lobe: auditory processing, equilibrium, interpretation of smell, long-term memory recall
   e. Basal ganglia: involved in execution, coordination, and initiation of movement
   f. Brainstem: controls autonomic functions such as respiration and cardiovascular control; site where major motor tracts cross from one side of the brain to other
   g. Cerebellum: coordinates movement necessary for posture and balance
   h. Thalamus: relay site for information in and out of motor cortex
   i. Hypothalamus: regulates body's internal homeostasis
   j. Epithalamus: regulates circadian rhythm
   k. Subthalamus: fine tunes movement

7. When a person suffers damage on the right side of the brain, they manifest movement difficulties on the left side of the body because the motor tracts cross from one side of the brain to the other at the level of the medulla. Therefore, damage to tracts originating on the left side of the brain will manifest movement difficulties on the right side of the body and vice versa.

8.
   a. Olfactory: smell
   b. Optic: vision
   c. Oculomotor: innervates eye muscles
   d. Trochlear: innervates eye muscles
   e. Trigeminal: innervates muscles of mastication, sensory information from forehead, eyes, upper lip, teeth, palate, jaw
   f. Abducens: innervates eye muscles
   g. Facial: innervates face muscles, sensory info from anterior two-thirds of tongue
   h. Vestibulocochlear: vestibular information
   i. Glossopharyngeal: innervates pharynx, sensory info from posterior one-third of tongue
   j. Vagus: sensory and motor information from internal organs
   k. Spinal accessory: innervates muscles of shoulder, larynx and neck
   l. Hypoglossal: innervates tongue muscles

9. The sympathetic nervous system consists of preganglionic neurons located in the thoracic and upper lumbar (T1-L2) regions of the spinal cord. Short preganglionic fibers secrete acetylcholine and long postganglionic fibers secrete norepinephrine. Functions include mobilizing resources in the body for "fight or flight." The parasympathetic nervous system consists of preganglionic neurons in cranial nerves III, VII, IX, X, and sacral regions of the spinal cord. Long preganglionic fibers secrete acetylcholine and short preganglionic fibers also secrete acetylcholine. Functions include conserving the body's resources and maintaining organ function during periods of physical inactivity.

10. The muscle spindle is located in muscle and is receptive to stretch. When it is activated, an action potential is generated in the sensory axon which then goes to the dorsal horn in the spinal cord, synapses on the alpha motor neuron, generates an action potential in the alpha motor neuron, and muscle contraction is generated. This process is called the monosynaptic stretch reflex. The Golgi tendon organ is located at the junction of muscle and tendon. It monitors the force of muscle contraction and therefore helps to protect muscle from being overloaded. When tension increases in the muscle, sensory neurons fire, which causes a synapse with interneurons to inhibit the alpha motor neuron and decreases muscle contraction. This process is called the reverse myotatic reflex.

11. The spinal reflexes allow sensory information from proprioceptors, muscle spindles, and pain receptors to be processed in the spinal cord and thus make modifications to muscle contraction before the information ever reaches the brain.

## SUMMARY KNOWLEDGE ANSWERS CHAPTER 10

1. Epimysium, which is composed of connective tissue, surrounds the entire muscle. Perimysium surrounds a bundle of muscle fibers (fascicle). Endomysium surrounds each individual muscle fiber.

2. Fusiform muscles contain fibers that run parallel to one another. They generate less force and power than pennate muscles. Anatomic arrangement facilitates rapid muscle shortening. Pennate muscles can be unipennate, bipennate, and multipennate. Because of pennation angle, the fibers are oblique to the muscle tendon and generate less force to the tendon as compared with fusiform muscles. However, pennate muscles have a larger physiologic cross-sectional area and a greater number of fibers so overall they generate more force than fusiform muscles. This is useful when high power/force output is necessary.

3. Action potential travels down the length of the nerve and stimulates synaptic vesicles that contain acetylcholine to move to nerve endplate. Acetylcholine is released in the synaptic cleft and binds to receptors on the sarcolemma of muscle fiber. The sarcolemma is invaginated which increases the surface area for the spread of an action potential. Once acetylcholine is bound to receptors, depolarization of the fiber occurs and the fiber contracts.

4. In the relaxed state, actin and myosin heads are in a "weakly bound" state. Once the fiber depolarizes, actin and myosin become "strongly bound." Myosin heads rotate, pulling actin along the length of the myosin. The myosin head detaches and reattaches to actin and then repeats the previous step.

5. Calcium, released from the terminal cisternae, binds to troponin. Inorganic phosphate on the myosin head is released and crossbridge movement can begin. ADP is released from the myosin head and crossbridges stop movement. ATP binds to the myosin head and is hydrolyzed, resulting in myosin being energized and ready for next wave of depolarization.

6. a. Histochemical: determines the reaction of myosin ATPase when tissue sections are exposed to different pH solutions
   b. Biochemical: succinate dehydrogenase is assayed on tissue sections to determine the oxidative status of a fiber; α-glycerophosphate dehydrogenase is assayed in tissue sections to determine the glycolytic potential of fibers
   c. Immunochemistry: assay antibodies that are made against various fiber types to tissue sections
   d. Gel electrophoresis: separate fiber types based upon mass in homogenized muscle; uses electrophoresis to move proteins from the top to bottom of a gel with the smallest proteins migrating the furthest and heavier proteins migrating the least distance

7. a. Maximum tension generation: on a whole-muscle level, muscle composed primarily of type IIb fibers generate the most tension; still unclear about differences between fiber types on the single fiber level
   b. Maximal velocity of shortening: (fastest) type IIb > type II d/x > type IIa > type I (slowest)

8. a. Aerobic exercise: increases the number of type IIa fibers at the expense of type IIb fibers; fibers become more oxidative
   b. Resistance training: shift of type IIb (type IId/x) fibers to type IIa fibers; functional implications are unknown, but the fibers hypertrophy and generate more force when they contract
   c. Aging: decrease in the number of fibers; therefore, muscle strength increases; atrophy of type IIb

fibers; appears to result in a decreased ability to do some activities of daily living
   d. Immobilization: conversion of slow fiber types to faster fiber types; causes muscle fiber atrophy, which leads to a decrease in strength

## SUMMARY KNOWLEDGE ANSWERS CHAPTER 11

1. Motor units consist of motor neurons and all the muscle fibers innervated by that motor neuron.

2. a. Slow-twitch motor units (type I motor units): slow-twitch development, low tension, fatigue resistant
   b. Fast-fatigue-resistant (type IIa): fast-twitch development, medium tension, fatigue resistant
   c. Fast-fatigable (type IIb): fast-twitch development, high tension, fast fatigue

3. The size principle is a key concept in motor unit recruitment. The smallest motor units recruit low levels of activity. As force increases, motor units with increasingly larger axons are recruited. As force decreases, reversal of the entire process occurs.

4. Sarcomere length describes the relationship between length of sarcomere and amount of force developed.

   1.25 μm: too much overlap between actin and myosin—no force generated

   1.65 μm: ~70% to 80% of maximum force generated

   2.0 to 2.25 μm: optimal length; maximal crossbridge interaction

   3.65 μm: no overlap of actin and myosin filament and no force development

5. Muscle fatigue is a temporary loss of force development that is divided into two categories: central and peripheral mechanisms. Examples of central fatigue include stimulation of inhibitor pathways and psychologic factors. Examples of peripheral fatigue include neuromuscular junction failure, mismatch of ATP supply/demand, and decreased pH.

6. a. Isometric: contraction of muscle and no movement of joint
   b. Concentric: muscle contraction that results in decreasing joint motion
   c. Eccentric: muscle contraction that results in limb lengthening

7. Neural changes occur first and lead to increased motor unit recruitment and improved synchronization of motor unit discharge. Muscle changes occur next; these changes are muscle hypertrophy secondary to increased protein synthesis and decreased protein degradation.

8.  a.  Manual muscle testing: assesses isometric muscle strength at the end of the range of motion; generally done in an acute care/rehab setting
    b.  Tensiometer: measure of isometric tension by exerting force through a cable; isometric strength is usually measured at various joint angles; used primarily in a sports setting
    c.  Dynamometer: force applied to a spring-loaded device that measures force; measures isometric strength; used primarily in a sports setting
    d.  One repetition maximum: assesses isotonic strength and is a measure of the maximal amount of weight that can be lifted; used in sports medicine, acute care, and rehab settings
    e.  Isokinetic dynamometer: assesses torque throughout the entire range of motion; used in sport medicine/rehab settings

## SUMMARY KNOWLEDGE ANSWERS CHAPTER 12

1.  Carbohydrate loading has the potential to enhance exercise performance when the individual will be exercising for more than 90 minutes at an intensity of approximately 75% of $\dot{V}O_{2max}$.

2.  Taper the training regimen the week before the event. Consume a mixed diet (50% of energy from carbohydrate) for 3 to 6 days prior to the event, and then increase carbohydrate intake to 70% the last 3 days before the event.

3.  Some of the biochemical or physiologic adaptations to a high-fat diet that spare glycogen and enhance endurance exercise performance are increased fatty acid availability to the exercising muscle, sparing of muscle glycogen during exercise, and increased capacity of key regulatory enzymes in aerobics and fatty acid metabolism.

4.  Excess protein intake or amino acid supplementation may be unhealthy because excess protein energy can be converted to body fat and excess protein intake can cause kidney problems, dehydration, metabolic disorders, and an increased risk for heart disease.

5.  The only condition under which vitamin supplements enhance exercise performance is when there is a deficiency of the vitamin initially.

6.  Two minerals that should be monitored closely and may require dietary supplementation are calcium and iron.

7.  Fluid replacement should be undertaken as follows: 500 mL should be taken 2 hours prior to the exercise event. Fluids should be taken every 15 to 20 minutes during the event, and a sports drink should be used if the event lasts more than 60 minutes.

8.  SOAP would be used to formulate questions about effectiveness claims for the supplement. What subjective evidence is there to support the claims? What objective evidence is there to support the claims? Specific questions may include: Is there a physiologic principle upon which the claims are based? What is the normal effect demonstrated in the average client? Who is making the claims? Are there any scientific reports on the product? Who produces the product? How can I tell if the product is working? Does the advertising rely heavily on testimonials?

## SUMMARY KNOWLEDGE ANSWERS CHAPTER 13

1.  Some reasons why a professional would want to assess body composition in his/her clients are to assess fitness, health, treatment success, or progress in rehabilitation.

2.  Many years ago professionals suggested an "ideal" body weight. However, professionals now understand that there is no "ideal" weight standard for everyone. Furthermore, body composition is a better standard of reference than body weight, but body composition alone does not determine health or fitness status. Body weight, body composition, and adiposity level all have to be interpreted within the genetic predisposition of any given individual, as well as within their realm of behavior.

3.  A high degree of adiposity is related to increased risk for several diseases. However, the relationship between disease and exercise behavior is stronger than between disease and adiposity.

4.  There is a good correlation between the body mass index (BMI) and adiposity, and since most large databases have values for height and weight but not true body composition, the BMI calculation becomes very useful.

5.  The pros and cons of each method of body composition analysis are based on the circumstances for which they will be used. The cost-to-benefit factors for each method, therefore, need to be based on several factors such as

    a.  Financial cost of the equipment
    b.  Financial cost for testing
    c.  Ease of administration for the technique
    d.  Reliability and validity of the method
    e.  Comfort level for the patient
    f.  Training requirements for the professional

6.  The model for body composition analysis which gives the professional the most usable information depends upon the need of the professional. For example, if only total body fat is needed, almost any technique can be used. If regional fat content is needed, then the DXA technique or skinfolds are the only methods that can be used to obtain that type of data.

## SUMMARY KNOWLEDGE ANSWERS CHAPTER 14

1. Specificity states that training must be specific to the performance task. If the bioenergetic system that is primarily utilized in a sport or event is known, training routines can be devised to stress a given bioenergetic system(s), thereby linking training to performance via specificity.

2. The activity continuum is important in exercise training because the timing of the sport performance or event helps us make training decisions so as not to violate specificity.

3. Different forms of exercise produce differences in the physiologic/bioenergetic responses to training. Knowing these differences aids our understanding of specificity.

4. Cross-training can be both good and bad, depending on the form of cross-training employed. For example, the power athlete who crosses his sport-specific power training with significant amounts of endurance training is probably hurting his/her power performance. This knowledge will help the athlete avoid this mistake and maximize his/her performance.

5. The development of strength is crucial to maximize power for those sports or events in which power performance is important. Even in strictly endurance sports or events, a certain baseline strength development may also be important.

6. Free-weight resistance training may be better than machine resistance training as an adjunct to sport-specific training routines because in free-weight training, the athlete can more closely mimic the actual performance, thereby maximizing specificity.

7. Overload is an important principle of training because training improvements cannot occur without applying periodic and progressive overload in a systematic fashion.

8. The $\%\dot{V}O_2R$ method for determining endurance exercise intensity is superior to the $\%\dot{V}O_{2max}$ method because it allows a better understanding of the match between heart rate and metabolism during exercise.

## SUMMARY KNOWLEDGE ANSWERS CHAPTER 15

1. The following questions should be considered when evaluating the appropriateness of a fitness test for children

   a. Does the test measure health-related fitness or athletic skills?
   b. Are the results from the test compared with population norms or criterion-based standards?
   c. Is the test valid and reliable?

2. Clinical exercise testing is usually reserved for children with symptoms of disease, established disease, or suspected medical abnormalities. Clinical exercise testing may provide data to help the health professional prescribe exercise for prevention or rehabilitation purposes.

3. Direct observation is a method that is highly reliable and valid for assessing physical activity in children, but it is also very expensive and labor intensive. No estimate of metabolic intensity can be derived by observation alone. Activity questionnaires are moderately reliable and accurate. Their weakness is the inability of children to accurately remember and estimate physical activity levels. Heart rate monitors, pedometers, and activity monitors are objective and highly reliable. Pedometers will just give an estimate of overall volume of activity, whereas heart rate monitors and activity monitors can give estimates of intensity of activity. Metabolic measures are most accurate but are time consuming and expensive.

4. Physiologic differences between children and adults can cause a child to be working at a higher relative reserve capacity than an adult even while working at the same relative capacity. Also children are at higher injury risk than adults when exercising.

5. In general, when providing an exercise or activity program for children, precautions should be taken to ensure adequate hydration for the child, to place the child at minimal risk, to ensure the physical safety of the child, to ensure that the child is participating at his/her own level, and to induce a minimal amount of stress.

6. Ensure that the child participates in activities that are fun, activities of his/her own selection, at the duration and intensity he/she selects, and under proper supervision.

7. Six- to 8-year-olds should be encouraged to participate in a wide variety of activities that are both aerobic and anaerobic, as well as activities that are weight bearing. The goal should be to accumulate 1 to 3 hours of physical activity a day at low to moderate levels of intensity. Young adolescents can be encouraged to participate in more vigorous activities for 30 minutes per day, three times per week for greater health and fitness benefits. Older adolescents can begin to specialize in sports if they so desire. Safety should always be prominent.

## SUMMARY KNOWLEDGE ANSWERS CHAPTER 16

1. Primary aging is the normal aging process that occurs independent of disease processes. Secondary aging refers to physical and physiologic deteriorations caused by pathologic processes. Both may occur simultaneously, although primary and secondary aging

may be more pronounced at any given chronologic age in some individuals.

2. Chronologic aging refers to body changes as a result of the passage of time without reference to biologic or pathologic components. Biologic aging is a measure of one's success for adaptation with the passage of time and is tied inextricably to functional abilities and capacities, which help explain why some individuals feel younger than their chronologic age, while others feel older than their chronologic age. Changes that occur as a result of disease processes define the concept of pathologic aging.

3. Regular exercise helps an individual maintain his/her functional capacities and abilities with age, allowing him/her to perform a greater range of activities of daily living and providing independence from caregivers.

4. Maximal heart rate declines as a function of the reduced sympathetic outflow to the heart. Aerobic power declines as a direct consequence of the reduced maximal heart rate.

5. Maintenance of strength is necessary in old age to help maintain independent living.

6. The process of sarcopenia is an important concept in the study of the physiology of aging because the loss of muscle mass with aging brings severe functional and pathologic consequences.

7. Blood volume expansion increases maximal stroke volume, allowing for a greater maximal cardiac output and maximal oxygen consumption.

8. The relationship between disability and independence is inverse—increasing disability brings decreasing independence.

9. Aging slows neuromuscular responses and if sedentary living is pursued, there is a concomitant loss of muscle mass with reduced maximal strength and muscular endurance.

10. Functional capacity of the cardiovascular system and therefore the aerobic fitness of individuals can be improved by improving the peripheral vascular function alone through an increase in the maximal arterial venous $O_2$ difference.

## SUMMARY KNOWLEDGE ANSWERS CHAPTER 17

1. a. Men are taller, heavier, and have more muscle mass and lower percent body fat than women
   b. Men have the greatest advantage over women in sports for which strength, power, and leverage are important
   c. Women can compete with men in sports or activities in which performance is relative to body size and composition

2. Some absolute contraindications for exercising during pregnancy are heart disease, ruptured membranes, premature labor, and a history of spontaneous abortions. Some relative contraindications are hypertension, diabetes, anemia, and excessive obesity.

3. Health outcomes resulting from exercise during perimenopause and menopause include maintaining metabolic rate, maintaining bone health, reduced risk of disease, and positive effects on psychologic health.

4. Osteoporosis is a condition in which the bones become thin and brittle due to loss of mineral content; these bones are more susceptible to fractures. The risk of osteoporosis is increased when a woman does not receive adequate nutrients in her diet and if she is sedentary.

5. A female athlete who presents amenorrhea should be evaluated for signs and symptoms of an eating disorder and obsessive exercise disorder. Inadequate nutrition and overtraining are also causes of amenorrhea. Her history of menstruation should be evaluated to see when amenorrhea first developed. Other health care professionals should be involved in the athlete's evaluation, and her training routine may have to be altered.

6. Signs and symptoms of an eating disorder include an obsessive concern over body weight, an intense fear of gaining weight, a distorted body image, and binge and purge behaviors.

7. Symptoms of iron-deficiency anemia are reduced energy levels and feelings of sluggishness and tiredness.

8. The female athlete triad is a highly destructive disorder because the health consequences can be severe and irreversible. Also the behaviors that lead to the female athlete triad are seen as positive so it is hard to determine when the behaviors have been taken to excess.

9. Exercising for hours each day, continuing to exercise when injured or exhausted, and becoming obsessed with exercising are all signs and symptoms of excessive exercise disorder.

## SUMMARY KNOWLEDGE ANSWERS CHAPTER 18

1. Pharmacodynamics is the mechanism by which a drug achieves its effect within the body, whereas pharmacokinetics is the movement of a drug within the body.

2. A regimen of overmedication can sometimes conflict with acute exercise if certain drugs cause physiologic adjustments that are either opposite in action to the exercise being performed or that add to the effect of the exercise.

3. Elderly individuals are often on a course of multiple medications, many of which can have physiologic effects that are opposite of those brought on by acute endurance exercise or effects that can be heightened when combined with acute exercise.

4. Knowledge of membrane receptors is important to understanding pharmacologic effects because the effects occur at the tissue level working through membrane receptors.

5. Chest pain radiating to the left shoulder and arm, and less commonly to the neck, jaw, teeth, upper back, and abdomen. Burning indigestion may be present, as well as nausea, dyspnea, and exercise intolerance. If the patient is experiencing angina pectoris, it may be relieved by rest and nitrates; if he/she is experiencing a heart attack, symptoms are not relieved by rest or nitrates. Syncope is common.

6. For asthma: dyspnea, wheezing, cough, pursed-lip breathing, flared nostrils, unusual pallor, hunched-over body posture, and cough occurring 5 to 10 minutes after exercise. For bronchitis: acute form involves mild fever, malaise, back and muscle pain, sore throat, and cough with sputum production; chronic form involves persistent cough with sputum production, reduced chest expansion, wheezing, fever, dyspnea, cyanosis, and decreased exercise tolerance. For emphysema: shortness of breath, dyspnea on exertion, orthopnea immediately after assumption of the supine position, chronic cough, barrel chest, weight loss, malaise, use of accessory respiratory muscles, prolonged expiratory period, wheezing, pursed-lip breathing, increased expiratory rate, and peripheral cyanosis.

7. Respiratory acidosis causes hypoventilation, which leads to an increase in $PaCO_2$ with renal compensation (increased $HCO_3$) and metabolic acidosis, which causes a decrease in $HCO_3$ with respiratory compensation in the form of an increase in ventilation and a decreased $PaCO_2$. In the case of alkalosis, the compensatory responses are opposite to those of acidosis. Respiratory alkalosis causes an increased pH, which is caused by a decrease in plasma $PaCO_2$ due to hyperventilation. There is also a reduction in plasma concentration of $HCO_3$. Metabolic alkalosis causes an increase in pH; compensation is in the form of hypoventilation, which increases $PaCO_2$.

8. Typical signs and symptoms of diabetes mellitus include increased urination, increased thirst, increased appetite and ingestion of food, weight loss, hyperglycemia, presence of glucose in the urine, presence of ketone bodies in the urine, fatigue, blurred vision, irritability, recurring infections, numbness in the hands and feet, and cuts and bruises that are difficult to heal.

## SUMMARY KNOWLEDGE ANSWERS CHAPTER 19

1. The prevalence of disability is not as high today as it could be because of improved management and treatment of chronic diseases, increased use of devices (e.g., canes, walkers, walk-in showers, support rails, and accessible facilities), and changes in health behavior.

2. The main pathway to disability is as follows: active pathology, impairment, functional limitation, disability.

3. The medical model of disability places emphasis on the impairment of the individual causing the disability and defines disability in terms of the disease process, while the social model of disability focuses on the environment and defines disability in a social context.

4. Current research has shown that physical symptoms and self-efficacy beliefs play a key role in the way individuals perceive their limitations.

5. Physical activity dosage prescription (intensity, frequency, and duration); adherence by the client; tolerance to the stimulus is noted and recorded; progression or digression is managed.

6. A plan of behavioral modification conducted with the intervention program is effective in increasing adherence.

7. The exercise prescription triad systematizes exercise parameters for better control of therapeutic intervention.

## SUMMARY KNOWLEDGE ANSWERS CHAPTER 20

1. $\dot{V}O_{2max}$ and $\dot{V}O_{2peak}$ are not synonymous terms because maximum refers to the absolute physiologic limit inherent in the person and peak refers to the value achieved at the point when the test ended. Peak values are always less than maximal values.

2. Both ST depression and elevation indicate ischemia, but elevation indicates that an acute transmural myocardial infarction (MI) is occurring, whereas depression accompanies anginal pain and is reversible or it indicates a subendocardial MI.

3. For a test to be useful in *ruling out* a disease, it must have a high sensitivity. For a test to be useful at *confirming* a disease, it must have a high specificity.

4. There are 12 leads in electrocardiography because 12 leads give a better electrical picture of the heart than any single lead.

5. The purpose of exercise electrocardiography is to stress the heart under control conditions and capture any resulting electrical abnormality via the electrocardiogram.

6. Mean QRS electrical axis is important because it is used to determine cardiac problems such as right or left ventricular hypertrophy.

7. Contraindication means that the person should avoid the behavior when the condition is present.

## SUMMARY KNOWLEDGE ANSWERS CHAPTER 21

1. The relative reduced risk of disease when adopting a lifestyle of physical activity is 50% compared with 40% when quitting smoking and 35% for controlling high blood pressure.

2. Activity dosage is type, duration, frequency, and intensity of activity.

3. If a gain in $\dot{V}O_{2max}$ is the desired outcome, intensity and type are the dosage factors that must be of primary concern.

4. Mobilization focuses on the acute phase of the disease and rehabilitation process, while therapeutic exercise training focuses on the subacute and chronic phases of the disease and rehabilitation process.

5. The three primary functions of exercise prescription are to increase functional capacity, improve health by reducing risk factors for chronic disease, and ensure safety during exercise.

6. The goals of outpatient cardiopulmonary rehabilitation are to improve functional capacity through an individualized exercise prescription, provide education so that the patient can understand the disease for better lifestyle management of risk factors, improve confidence and self-reliance to become independent in all areas of care, and teach behaviors that are consistent with attaining and maintaining good health.

## SUMMARY KNOWLEDGE ANSWERS CHAPTER 22

1. Obesity and overweight have been associated with several diseases including heart disease, stroke, diabetes, hypertension, hyperlipidemia, gallbladder disease, kidney disease, liver malfunction, musculoskeletal disorders, arthritis, sleep disturbances, and cancer.

2. A person with a genetic predisposition toward obesity should provide the best environment he/she can. This means eating healthy, exercising, taking care of one's emotional health, and doing all he/she can to maintain health, regardless of weight status.

3. Some factors that may contribute to a positive energy

balance are low activity levels, a high-fat diet, a diet high in refined sugar, a low dietary fiber intake, genetic predisposition, and chronic dieting.

4. Some of the obstacles large people have to overcome to succeed in a society that values thinness are overcoming the prejudice against fat people, overcoming a poor self image, overcoming body image disparagement, and overcoming preconceived notions about overweight.

5. Some emotional links people have with food and physical exercise are eating to soothe emotions, eating for pleasure, eating for comfort, eating when stressed, eating when depressed, eating to celebrate, and being inactive when experiencing negative emotions.

6. Self-monitoring has been one of the strongest factors associated with weight-loss maintenance. However, each person has self-monitoring techniques that work best for him/her. The professional needs to help the overweight patient discover which self-monitoring techniques are best for him/her.

## SUMMARY KNOWLEDGE ANSWERS CHAPTER 23

1. Strength and flexibility exercises can improve muscle function and motor control in a stroke victim. Aerobic exercises can improve $\dot{V}O_{2max}$ and decrease heart rate and blood pressure during physical activity.

2. Both multiple sclerosis and muscular dystrophy are characterized by muscle weakness, spasticity, abnormal fatigue, lack of coordination, and muscle stiffness. These factors contribute to an increased risk of injury during physical activity.

3. The basic exercise prescription would not need to differ among patients with breast, prostate, or colon cancer, but the exercise prescription would differ, depending on the state of the cancer and the patient's response to medication and therapy.

4. Exercise programs for osteoporosis and osteoarthritis should focus on maintaining bone and joint integrity. The patient with osteoporosis should participate in weight-bearing exercises if there are no contraindications, whereas the person with osteoarthritis should focus more on nonweight-bearing exercises. The person with osteoarthritis should also spend more time on flexibility exercises than the person with osteoporosis.

5. Exercise will not cure any of the oncologic or neuromuscular diseases discussed in this chapter, but exercise training may reduce symptoms, retard progression of disease, and improve the quality of life for the patient.

# Glossary

**A band:** the part of the sarcomere where the myosin heads are located; this portion of the sarcomere appears "dark" under a microscope

**absolute refractory period:** the period of time immediately following an action potential during which the cell will not depolarize even if another stimulus is applied to the cell

**actin:** one of the contractile proteins; also known as the "thin filament"; during contraction, the myosin heads attach to the actin and pulls it across the length of the myosin

**action potential:** the rapid sequence of changes in electrical potential that takes place across a cell membrane during depolarization and repolarization

**active pathology:** disease

**activities of daily living (ADL):** daily tasks that are associated with self-care, i.e., eating, dressing, and grooming

**acute:** immediate, as in the physiologic responses from an exercise session

**acute fetal hypoxia:** lack of adequate oxygen or low oxygen concentration delivery to the fetus

**acute heart failure:** sudden and short-lasting diminution of pumping effectiveness of the heart due to damage as happens, for instance, with myocardial infarction leading to lowered cardiac output

**acute state:** having a sudden onset, sharp rise, and short course; lasting a short time

**adaptations:** chronically altered anatomy and/or physiology that improves the functional capacity of the specific system trained

**adiposity rebound:** the normal drop and rise in body mass index during a child's growth and development that occurs at about age 4 to 6 years

**aerobic:** refers to metabolic processes that are a part of, or directly lead to, the oxidative phosphorylation of ADP to form ATP with $O_2$ serving as the final electron acceptor

**afferent:** refers to nerves that transmit sensory information into the central nervous system

**afterload:** the impedance to ejection of blood from the left ventricle

**age-specific life expectancy:** the average duration of life expected for an individual of a given age

**agility:** ability to start, stop, and move the body quickly in different directions

**agonist:** drug that interacts with receptors to initiate a response

**air displacement plethysmography:** method used to determine body volume by measuring the amount of air displaced by the body when a person enters an airtight chamber; regression equations are then used to estimate body fat content

**all-or-none phenomenon:** occurs when all muscle fibers in a motor unit contract in response to stimulation via the motor neuron

**allosteric:** the quality some proteins have that enable them to alter their conformations (shapes) and functional properties when a substrate is bound to them

**alveolar dead space:** the volume of gas in alveoli that are ventilated but not perfused with capillary blood

**alveolar ventilation:** the movement of gas into and out of the alveoli

**Alzheimer disease:** incurable, degenerative brain disease in which some brain cells are destroyed and other cells become unresponsive to the chemical neurotransmitters necessary for nerve impulse transmission

**amino acids:** small compounds that constitute the building blocks for proteins; there are 20 amino acids that can be combined in a number of ways to form a protein

**anabolism:** the synthesis of biologic substances or compounds

**anaerobic:** refers to the metabolic processes that do not ultimately utilize $O_2$

**anaerobic threshold:** the inflection point at which there is a rapid rise in blood lactate levels as exercise intensity increases

**anatomic dead space:** volume of gas that occupies the nonrespiratory conducting airways

**androgen:** substance producing or stimulating male characteristics, such as the hormone testosterone

**aneurysm:** sac formed by the dilatation of the wall of an artery, a vein, or the heart

**anorexia nervosa:** eating disorder characterized by severe dieting to lose or control weight in spite of the person already being underweight

**antagonist:** (1) drug that interacts with receptors to block or inhibit a response; (2) when the actions of a muscle oppose the actions of another muscle; the quadriceps muscle extends the knee and is the antagonist of the hamstring muscles that bend the knee

**anthropometry or anthropometric:** measurements having to do with body size and shape, such as weight, height, circumference, girth, and width

**antidiuretic hormone:** vasopressin lessens urine secretion and raises blood pressure

**antioxidant:** donates an electron or hydrogen ion to an electron-seeking compound and protects other molecules from being oxidized

**arrhythmia:** abnormal rhythm of the heart

**arterio-mix venous O₂ difference:** the measured difference in $O_2$ concentration of the blood between the arterial and venous sides of a sample tissue, more commonly termed the $O_2$ extraction rate

**articular cartilage:** the cartilage that lines the opposing surfaces of the bones at a joint

**asthma:** inflammatory disorder of the airways, characterized by periodic attacks of wheezing, shortness of breath, chest tightness, and coughing

**ataxia:** general term for muscular incoordination that is particularly manifested when voluntary muscular movements are attempted

**athletic amenorrhea:** cessation of menses that occurs in female athletes

**atrioventricular valves:** the valves between both the right atrium and right ventricle as well as the left atrium and left ventricle; the name of the valve between the right chambers of the heart is the tricuspid valve, and the name of the valve between the left chambers of the heart is the mitral valve

**atropine:** antimuscarinic drug that blocks cholinergic (acetylcholine) activity at effector organs

**automaticity:** the property of spontaneous impulse generation; the slow sodium channels are leaky and cause the polarity to spontaneously rise to threshold for action potential generation; the fastest of these cells, those in the sinoatrial node, set the pace for the heartbeat

**autonomic ganglion:** grouping of autonomic neurons located in the peripheral nervous system

**autoregulation:** the ability of the capillaries to open or close in response to $O_2$ demands of the local tissues

**autorhythmicity:** the natural rhythm of spontaneous depolarization; those with the fastest autorhythmicity act as the heart's pacemaker

**axon:** the part of the neuron that receives incoming information and impulses from other neurons

**β oxidation:** the catabolism of fatty acids to produce acetyl-CoA

**Babinski sign:** dorsiflexion of the big toe when the sole of the foot is stimulated; this sign indicates a lesion in the pyramidal tract

**barometric pressure:** the force per unit area exerted by the earth's atmosphere; at sea level, it is 14.7 pounds per square inch or 760 mm Hg

**baroreceptors:** sensory nerve endings in the walls of the atria of the heart, vena cavae, aortic arch, and carotid sinuses that are sensitive to stretch (resulting from increased pressure from within)

**basal ganglia:** four masses of gray matter located deep in the cerebral hemisphere of the brain

**Becker muscular dystrophy:** form of muscular dystrophy in which the protein dystrophin, which is needed for muscle structure, is oversized and does not function properly

**behavior carryover:** when behavior is modeled, mimicked, or transferred from one area or period into another

**bicarbonate (HCO₃⁻):** major buffer in blood

**bilateral:** both sides of the body

**binge-eating disorder:** psychologic disorder characterized by consuming large amounts of food in a discrete period of time

**bioavailability:** physiologic availability of a specific amount of a drug

**bioenergetics:** study of the energy exchange or the transformation of energy in living things

**biologic aging:** the post-maturational changes in physical appearance and capability involving a progressive loss of physiologic capacities

**blood doping:** the process of infusing red blood cells or plasma into an athlete in an effort to increase hemoglobin concentration and enhance exercise performance

**bodybuilding:** the sport of developing muscle fibers through the combination of weight training, increased caloric intake, and rest; bodybuilders display their physiques to a panel of judges, who assign points

**body composition:** relative amounts of various components in the body, such as percent body fat

**body image disparagement:** the belief that one's body is ugly and loathsome, or that a part of one's body is ugly, disfigured, or disproportionate

**body mass index (BMI):** ratio of weight to height that is calculated by dividing body weight in kilograms by the square of height in meters (BMI $= kg \cdot m^{-2}$)

**bolus:** a mass of food ready to be swallowed or already passing through the intestines

**bomb calorimeter:** device used to burn food substances to measure their heat of combustion or energy value

**Boyle's law:** the pressure of a gas is inversely related to its volume under conditions of constant temperature

**bronchitis:** inflammation of the bronchi with mucus secretion; in chronic bronchitis there is inflammation of the bronchi, the main air passages in the lungs, which persists for a long period or repeatedly recurs; the chronic condition is characterized by excessive bronchial mucus and a productive cough that produces sputum for at least 3 months in at least 2 consecutive years, without any other disease that could account for this symptom

**bulimia nervosa:** eating disorder characterized by consuming large amounts of food in a discrete period of time, followed by some type of purging behavior

**bundle branch:** specialized tissue in the heart that conducts the depolarization wave through the ventricles; both the right and left ventricles have a bundle branch, called the right bundle branch and the left bundle branch, respectively

**bundle of His:** specialized tissue that conducts the depolarization wave from the atria to the ventricles

**calorimetry:** the process of measuring heat release from metabolic processes

**capacitance vessels:** in the circulatory system, the ability to "store" large amounts of blood; the veins are considered to be capacitance vessels to the large amount of blood that they contain; however, upon the initiation of exercise, this "stored" blood can be rapidly mobilized to the working tissues (muscles) in the body

**carbohydrate loading:** the process of consuming a high-carbohydrate diet, with or without prior glycogen depletion, in an effort to augment muscle glycogen stores and enhance exercise performance

**carcinogen:** any substance or agent the produces or incites cancer

**cardiac cycle:** the mechanical process whereby blood flows from the atria through the atrioventricular valves into the ventricles and out of the ventricles through the semilunar valves; the mechanical processes of the cardiac cycle correlate with the electrical activity observed on an electrocardiogram that indicates atrial contraction, ventricle contraction, and ventricle relaxation

**cardiac output:** the volume of blood that is pumped from the heart each minute; cardiac output is the product of stroke volume and heart rate

**cardiorespiratory endurance:** the ability of the lungs and heart to take in and transport adequate amounts of $O_2$ to the working muscles

**cartilage:** dense connective tissue that protects bone from grinding on bone at a joint

**cartilaginous apophysis:** projection point of the bone such as a tuberosity or tubercle that is still not completely ossified in children and where the muscle tendon connects to the bone

**catabolic:** the breakdown or degradation of biologic compounds or substances

**catecholamines:** the hormones epinephrine and norepinephrine, which have a marked effect on the nervous system, cardiovascular system, metabolic rate, temperature, and smooth muscle

**cauda equina:** refers to the branching of nerve fibers that characterize the end of the spinal cord at the level of L1–L3

**cell body:** the main part of the neuron where the nucleus, mitochondria, and other cellular constituents are located

**cellular respiration:** the aerobic process that couples $O_2$ to the regeneration of ATP via oxidative phosphorylation

**central venous pressure:** the pressure within the superior vena cava, reflecting the pressure under which the blood is returned to the right atrium; a high central venous pressure indicates circulatory overload as in congestive heart failure, and a low central venous pressure indicates reduced blood volume as in hemorrhage or fluid loss

**cerebral cortex:** the outer layer of the brain

**Charles' law:** temperature and gas volume are directly related, as temperature increases or decreases (at constant pressure), a gas volume will expand or constrict, respectively

**chemoreceptor:** sense organ that is stimulated by and reacts to certain chemical stimuli and is located outside of the central nervous system

**chemotherapy:** treatment of cancer using specific chemical agents or drugs that are selectively destructive to malignant cells and tissues; the application of chemical reagents that have a specific and toxic effect on disease-causing microorganisms

**chordae tendinae:** collagenous strands which extend from the apical margin of papillary muscles of the heart and attach to atrioventricular valve cusps

**chronic:** long term, as in chronic disease or chronic exercise training

**chronic disease/aging disability:** disability due to the consequences of chronic disease, sometimes in conjunction with the aging process, but not necessarily so

**chronic heart failure:** the pumping effectiveness of the heart beyond the acute stage is still lower, but the body has partially compensated with sympathetic reflexes that increase the pumping action and increase cardiac output and increase fluid retention to increase venous return by increasing mean systolic filling pressure

***chronic obstructive pulmonary disease (COPD):*** the category of lung disease that is associated with airway blockage; includes bronchitis and emphysema

***chronic state:*** marked by long duration, frequent recurrence over a long time, and slowly progressing seriousness; suffering from a disease or ailment of long duration or frequent recurrence

***chronologic aging:*** age based on duration (in years) of life from birth

***chronotropic:*** the rate of ventricular contraction

***chylomicron:*** large lipoprotein particle formed in the intestinal cells that helps transport digested fats into the circulation

***claudication:*** symptom of chronic arterial occlusive disease caused by tissue ischemia as a result of blockages in the arteries leading to insufficient blood flow, especially leading to the legs; symptoms may include pain, ache, or cramping of the muscles

***client:*** well person seeking professional health care services for prevention and to enhance performance

***closed-circuit spirometry:*** indirect calorimetry method in which the subject breathes from a container of known gas concentrations, usually 99.9% $O_2$, and the rate of utilization of available $O_2$ is then determined; the breathing circuit is closed to atmospheric air

***community-acquired:*** contracting an infection in the community rather than in the hospital

***comorbidity :*** disease associated with another disease or condition

***complete protein:*** food that contains all of the essential amino acids in the same ratio that they are found in the body

***compliance:*** the distensibility of a structure, such as the lung, chest wall, or artery; i.e., a measure of the force required to distend the lungs

***concentric:*** refers to a shortening contraction by skeletal muscle that produces force

***conduction:*** the transfer of heat by direct contact between two objects

***contractility:*** cardiac muscular performance at any given preload and afterload

***contralateral:*** the opposite side of the body

***convection:*** the transfer of heat by the movement of a heated substance, usually air or water

***convulsion:*** involuntary muscular contractions and relaxations that result in severe muscle spasms throughout the body

***convulsive seizures:*** abnormal electrical discharges in the brain that spread to the entire brain and cause convulsions

***core temperature:*** the temperature of the center or core of the body

***corpus callosum:*** the part of the brain that connects the right and left cerebral hemispheres

***creatine phosphate (CP):*** a readily available source of energy because CP carries a high-energy phosphate group similar to ATP; CP acts as a phosphate donor during anaerobic metabolism (CP + ADP = C + ATP)

***crossbridge:*** the globular portion of the myosin that "sticks out" from the body of the myosin molecule; binds to actin during contraction and generates the force necessary to pull the actin molecule across the length of the myosin molecule

***crossed-withdrawal reflex:*** the postural reflex that allows for withdrawal of a body part from a noxious stimulus while maintaining balance

***curare:*** drug that blocks acetylcholine at the neuromuscular junction

***cyanosis:*** slightly bluish, grayish, slate-like, or dark purple discoloration of the skin caused by the presence of abnormal amounts of deoxyhemoglobin in the blood

***Dalton's law:*** in a mixture of gases, the total pressure is equal to the sum of the partial pressures of each gas

***deaminate:*** the process of removing the amino group (nitrogen) from an amino acid during metabolism

***deconditioning:*** the loss of physical fitness due to sedentariness brought on by pathology or lifestyle choice

***decussate:*** refers to the crossing of motor nerve fibers from one side of the brain to the other

***deficiency:*** when nutrient intake does not meet the vitamin or mineral needs of the body, resulting in a specific health-related problem

***dendrites:*** the part of the neuron that transmits impulses to other neurons

***dephosphorylation:*** chemical reaction that removes a phosphate moiety to a molecule or compound

***depolarization:*** the reversal of the resting membrane potential in excitable cells when stimulated or the tendency of a cell membrane to become positive with respect to the potential outside of the cell

***dermatome:*** the relationship of specific spinal nerves with the sensory innervation of the skin

***desaturation:*** less $O_2$ is in combination with the hemoglobin molecule

***development:*** differentiation of cells and tissues for specialized functions

**developmental disability:** severe, chronic disability of an individual that is attributable to mental or physical impairment or combination thereof that is manifested before the age of 22

**diabetic neuropathy:** the most common chronic complication of long-term diabetes mellitus in which there is abnormal fluid and electrolyte shifts and nerve cell dysfunction

**diaphoresis:** profuse perspiration

**diastasis:** relatively quiescent period of slow ventricular filling during the cardiac cycle; it occurs in mid-diastole, following the rapid filling phase and just prior to atrial systole

**diastole:** resting phase of the cardiac cycle

**diastolic function:** the ability of the heart to relax following systole; diastolic dysfunction occurs when the relaxation process after systole is prolonged, slowed, or incomplete with a concomitant higher than normal ventricular pressure

**diffusivity:** ability of a gas to traverse a membrane, related to the size of the diffusing molecule and its solubility in water (diffusion coefficient multiplied by solubility)

**digestible energy:** the amount of energy contained by a food once it is digested and absorbed

**dipeptide:** protein strand consisting of only two amino acids

**disability:** the inability, after a time period in which functional limitations become severe, to engage in age- and gender-specific roles in a particular social and physical environment

**disaccharide:** simple sugar formed when two monosaccharides are combined

**diuretic:** drug or other substance that causes the formation and excretion of urine, often prescribed for hypertension, edema, and congestive heart disease

**dopamine:** neurotransmitter that allows for proper communication among parts of the brain and peripheral nervous system

**dosage:** the amount of exercise prescribed to a patient or client

**dromotropic:** influencing the conduction velocity of a nerve or muscle fiber

**drug:** chemical that alters bodily function and may produce beneficial effects when taken in therapeutic doses

**dual-energy x-ray absorptiometry (DXA):** form of x-ray that is used to determine bone density, bone mineral content, and body composition

**Duchenne muscular dystrophy:** common form of muscular dystrophy in which a defective gene does not allow for the production of dystrophin, a protein critical to the maintenance of the structure of muscle cells

**duration:** length of time in minutes of each exercise session

**dynamic:** muscle contraction that results in movement about a joint; eccentric and concentric contractions are considered to be dynamic muscle contractions

**dynamic exercise:** exercise or activity producing movement of the skeleton; some types of dynamic exercises or activities may involve a significant static or isometric component, as in resistance exercise

**dysdiadochokinesia:** the inability to rapidly alternate movements usually as a result of a lesion in the cerebellum

**dyskinesis:** segmental cardiac wall motion abnormalities during systole

**dyspnea:** difficulty in breathing characterized as shortness of breath

**dystrophin:** protein found in muscle tissue that is necessary to maintain the structure and integrity of muscle cells

**eccentric:** lengthening contraction by the muscle that produces force

**ECG lead:** electrocardiographic cable with connections within the electronics of the electrocardiograph designated for an electrode placed at a particular point on the body surface

**economy:** the $O_2$ cost of performing various physical activities

**edema:** fluid retention

**effector:** refers to the target organ of a nerve

**efferent:** refers to the motor nerves that carry information out of the central nervous system

**efficiency:** work performed divided by energy expended

**elastance:** the tendency of a structure to return to its original form after removal of a deforming force; the reciprocal of capacitance (compliance)

**electrocardiograph:** instrument for recording the potential of the electrical currents that traverse the heart and initiate its contraction

**electrocardiography:** refers to the recording of electrical changes that occur in the heart during the mechanical events of the cardiac cycle

**electrodes:** any terminal that conducts an electric current into or away from various conducting substances in a circuit (such as the anode or cathode of a battery)

**electrolytes:** minerals that are electrically charged particles or ions

**electron transport chain:** series of chemical reactions in which electrons are passed from one carrier to another with the ultimate result being the oxidative phosphorylation of ADP to ATP

**electrophoresis:** molecular technique that allows for separation and identification of proteins or DNA by molecular weight

**embryo:** fetus that is in the stage of development between 2 and 8 weeks

**emphysema:** enlargement of the air spaces, destruction of lung parenchyma, loss of lung elasticity, and closure of small airways; in this lung disease, the air sacs (alveoli) are damaged and are unable to completely deflate (hyperinflation) and are therefore unable to fill with fresh air to ensure adequate $O_2$ supply to the body

**end-diastolic volume:** the maximum volume of the ventricles achieved at the end of ventricular diastole; this is the amount of blood the heart has available to pump; if this volume increases, the cardiac output increases in a healthy heart

**endergonic:** chemical reaction that absorbs energy

**endocardium:** smooth endothelial lining of the heart; this helps to reduce friction of blood flow and prevent clotting

**endometrium:** the mucus membrane lining of the uterus that consists of tubular-shaped glands that undergo changes in thickness and composition as part of the woman's menstrual cycle

**endomysium:** the connective tissue that surrounds an individual muscle fiber

**endothelium:** form of flat cells that line the blood vessels, lymph vessels, heart, and other body cavities

**end-systolic volume:** the minimum volume remaining in the ventricle after systole; if this volume increases, it means less blood has been pumped and the cardiac output is less

**endurance exercise:** activities involving large muscle masses (e.g., running, swimming, bicycling) performed over long periods of time

**energy balance:** the balance between energy intake and energy expenditure; a positive energy balance results in weight gain, while a negative energy balance results in weight loss

**energy charge:** index of the energy status of the cell, calculated as a ratio, i.e., $([ATP] + 0.5[ADP]) \div ([ATP] + [ADP] + [AMP])$; a high energy charge inhibits ATP production, while a low energy charge stimulates ATP production

**energy reserve:** the energy difference between resting and maximal levels, best viewed as maximal $O_2$ consumption; when $\dot{V}O_{2max}$ increases, so does the energy reserve; patients may impinge less on their energy reserves during exercise or activities of daily living by improving movement economy

**enteral:** intestinal route of administering a drug

**entropy:** quantitative measure of the disorder produced by the second law of thermodynamics, always increases in size

**epicardium:** the fibrous covering of the heart; this layer is the visceral layer of the pericardium

**epilepsy:** brain disorder of no apparent cause that is characterized by the tendency to have recurring seizures

**epimysium:** the connective tissue that surrounds the entire muscle

**epiphyseal plate:** see growth plate

**ergogenic aid:** any device, product, supplement, or regimen used to increase work output or exercise performance

**ergometer:** device that measures work rate and is used most extensively in clinical and research programs

**essential body fat:** the amount of body fat that is necessary to sustain health, generally 3% body fat for men and 12% body fat for women

**essential fatty acid:** fatty acid that must be consumed because it cannot be made in the body

**estrogen:** female sex hormone responsible for secondary sex characteristics and the changes occurring during the menstrual cycle

**etiology:** the cause of a disease

**evaporation:** the transfer of heat when a liquid is changed to a gas, usually water to water vapor

**exacerbation:** increase in severity or symptoms of a disease

**excess post-exercise $O_2$ consumption (EPOC):** the elevation in metabolic rate seen after exercise that is above the resting metabolism

**excessive exercise disorder:** disorder in which the individual becomes so addicted to exercise that he/she continues to exercise for prolonged periods of time in spite of injury or other contraindications

**excitatory postsynaptic potential:** excitation of the postsynaptic membrane

**exercise-induced hypoxemia:** condition found in elite male endurance athletes in which the amount of $O_2$ carried in arterial blood is severely reduced at near maximal or maximal work output

**exercise prescription:** plan for physical activity formulated to achieve specific beneficial outcomes while minimizing the accompanying risks associated with exercise

**exercise protocol:** the sequence of applying ergometric workloads to an individual in a timed and deliberate manner so as to elicit graded metabolic and physiologic responses

**exercise science:** any aspect of science applied to the phenomenon of exercise; also the academic discipline that studies movement and physical activities from biophysical, behavioral, and sociocultural perspectives

**exercise training:** the repeated use of exercise over an extended period of time (months, years) to effect physiologic change

**exergonic:** chemical reaction that gives up energy

**external respiration:** the exchange of gases between the lungs and the blood

**extrafusal fibers:** the muscle fibers of the muscle

**extrapyramidal:** refers to motor tracts coming from the motor cortex that do not decussate in the medulla

**fascicle:** bundle of muscle fibers

**fatigue index:** test designed to measure the fatigue of a motor unit in which an electrical stimulus is applied repetitively and the amount of force the motor unit can generate after 2 minutes is compared with the initial force; this ratio is called the fatigue index

**fat-soluble vitamin:** vitamin that is found in the fat and oils of foods, dissolves in fat, and is stored or associated with body fat

**female athlete triad:** disorder in which a female presents the symptoms of an eating disorder, amenorrhea, and osteoporosis

**fetal hypoglycemia:** low blood sugar in the fetus

**first law of thermodynamics:** energy can neither be created nor destroyed, thus the total energy in the universe is constant

**first-pass effect:** partial inactivation of a drug as a result of metabolic processes

**flavin adenine dinucleotide (FAD/FADH$_2$):** an electron carrier; FADH$_2$ is energy rich in that it contains two electrons that have a high energy potential

**free radical:** highly biochemically reactive molecule that contains at least one unpaired electron; accumulation of free radicals increases the risk for cellular damage due to oxidative stress

**frequency:** number of exercise bouts per unit time (usually per week)

**functional ability:** capacity to perform necessary activities

**functional (aerobic) capacity:** the ability or power to perform necessary activities, especially of an endurance nature

**functional limitation:** restrictions in the ability of individuals to perform their usual physical tasks, actions, or activities in an efficient, typically expected, or competent manner

**functional residual capacity:** the volume of gas in the lungs at the end of a normal expiration

**fusiform:** a muscle that has fibers which lie parallel to one another

**gait:** manner or style of walking

**ganglia:** clusters of nerve cell bodies in the peripheral nervous system

**gene-chip microarray:** in biotechnology, a component of a device for screening genomic or cDNA for mutations, polymorphisms, or gene expression; a chip is a small (a few centimeters on each side) standardized glass or other solid surface on which thousands of immobilized oligodeoxynucleotide probes have been synthesized or robotically deposited in a predetermined array so that automated recording of fluorescence from each of the spots may score successful hybridizations; a chip may be designed for the detection of all known genes of a species (human, mouse, yeast) or selected specific sequences

**gene cloning:** a gene in molecular biology is defined narrowly as a section of DNA that is expressed as RNA or, more widely, as a coding sequence of DNA and associated regulatory sequences; cloning involves the duplication of a gene from a single ancestral gene

**general adaptation syndrome:** stereotypical response to stress which involves vasoregulatory and endocrine mechanisms

**genotype:** the hereditary combination of genes of an individual

**geriatric medicine:** the branch of medicine that concerns itself with the aging process; the prevention, diagnosis, and treatment of health care problems in the aged; and the social and economic conditions that affect the health care of the elderly; arbitrarily, the aged, or elderly, population is defined as persons aged 65 years or older

**gerontologist:** individual who has formal training in gerontology, the study of aging

**gerontology:** the multidisciplinary study of all aspects of aging, including health, biologic, sociologic, economic, behavioral, and environmental

**glucocorticoid:** general classification of adrenal cortical hormones, which are primarily active in protecting against stress and in affecting protein and carbohydrate metabolism

**gluconeogenesis:** the formation of glucose from substances other than glucose

**glycemic index:** measure of the effect of food on blood glucose levels; it is the ratio of blood glucose value after eating a particular food to the value after eating the same amount of glucose

**glycogen:** polysaccharide that is the storage form for carbohydrate in the body

**glycolipids:** carbohydrate-bound lipids that are found in cell membranes that allow for transport of material across the membrane

**glycolysis:** 10- or 11-step process wherein glucose is catabolized to form either pyruvate (slow glycolysis) or lactate (fast glycolysis), respectively

**glycosidic bond:** the bond formed between two sugars where $O_2$ is the common link between the carbon of one sugar and the carbon of another

**glycosuria:** presence of glucose in the urine

**Golgi tendon organ:** structure at the muscle tendon junction that is sensitive to the force of muscle contraction

**gross energy:** energy liberated as heat of combustion when a food is completely burned to ashes

**gross motor movement:** refers to movement of the entire body

**growth:** increase in size of the body or any of its parts

**growth cartilage:** cartilage that is present at the growth plate of an immature bone; this type of cartilage is replaced by permanent mature cartilage when the bone matures

**growth plate:** the site of bone growth in long bones; the growth plate will harden (ossify) with calcium as the bone finishes growing

**Haldane transformation:** the use of equal inspired and expired nitrogen volumes to solve for either inspired or expired ventilatory volumes

**half-life:** the time it takes for the plasma concentration of a drug to be reduced to 50% of its peak value

**heart rate range:** the range in which the heart will beat for any given individual; calculated by subtracting the maximal heart rate from the resting heart rate

**heat acclimatization:** the physiologic adaptations that are made to make a person more tolerant to heat

**hematocrit:** percentage of the volume of a sample of blood occupied by cells

**hemiparesis:** paralysis or partial paralysis of only one side of the body

**hemoconcentration:** movement of water from plasma into the surrounding tissues

**hemodynamics:** physical factors governing blood flow within the circulatory system

**hemoglobin:** the $O_2$-carrying protein in red blood cells

**hemorrhagic stroke:** a stroke that occurs because a blood vessel bursts or is ruptured and the blood leaks into an area of the brain and destroys brain tissue

**hexokinase:** a rate-limiting or regulatory enzyme in glycolysis

**homeostasis:** the state of dynamic equilibrium of the internal environment of the body

**homothermal control:** the process of controlling or maintaining body temperature to within a few degrees of 37°C

**hydrolysis:** chemical process in which a molecule is cleaved into two parts by the addition of a molecule of water

**hydrostatic weighing:** method of determining body volume by measuring the volume of water displaced when a person is submerged underwater; regression equations are then used to estimate body fat content

**hyperandrogenism:** the abundance of androgens, which stimulate or produce male sex characteristics

**hypercapnia:** excess $CO_2$ in the blood

**hyperglycemia:** increased blood glucose concentration (fasting level >126 mg/dL)

**hyperprolactinemia:** abundance of the hormone prolactin, which initiates and sustains lactation

**hyperthermia:** increase in body temperature above 39°C

**hypertrophy:** increase in size of a tissue; most commonly used to refer to the increase in muscle as a consequence of strength training

**hypoglycemia:** low blood glucose concentration (<70 mg/dL)

**hypokalemia:** extreme potassium depletion in the circulation, often manifest as muscle weakness, muscle tetany, or hypotension upon standing

**hypokinetic diseases:** diseases caused by hypokinesis, i.e., decreased physical activity

**hypoproteinemia:** abnormal deficiency of protein in the blood

**hypothalamus:** lower portion of the brain that secretes hormones affecting metabolism

**hypothermia:** drop in body temperature to below 35°C

**hypotonic:** solution that contains a lower concentration of particles than a comparable solution

**hypoxemia:** low level of $O_2$ in the blood, often characterized by a $PaO_2$ of less than 80 mm Hg

**hypoxia:** lack of $O_2$

**H zone:** the center of the sarcomere where there is no overlap of actin and myosin filaments

**I band:** the portion of the sarcomere where the actin filaments are located; this area appears "light" underneath a microscope

**idiopathic:** referring to a disease without any apparent cause

**immunohistochemistry:** microscopic localization of specific antigens in tissues (e.g., muscle fiber types) by staining with antibodies labeled with fluorescent or pigmented material

**impairment:** the consequence of disease pathology that results in alterations in anatomic, physiologic, or psychologic structures or functions (occurs at the tissue, organ, and system level, and is indicated by signs and symptoms)

**indirect calorimetry:** the process of measuring energy expenditure through gas exchange, specifically $O_2$ consumption and $CO_2$ production

**inhibitory post-synaptic potential:** hyperpolarization of the post-synaptic membrane

**injury-related disability:** disability caused by traumatic injury

**innervation ratio:** refers to the number of muscle fibers contained within each motor unit

**inotropy:** contractile state of muscular tissue

**insoluble fiber:** indigestible polysaccharide that does not dissolve in water and is not acted upon by intestinal bacteria

**inspiratory capacity:** the maximal volume of gas that can be inhaled from the resting expiratory level

**instrumental activities of daily living (IADL):** daily tasks that are complex (i.e., cooking, cleaning, or using a telephone) and allow for greater independence

**intensity:** degree of difficulty of an exercise bout

**intercalated discs:** specialized junctions between the muscle fibers of the heart that allow depolarization to occur rapidly from fiber to fiber and throughout the heart

**intercept:** the intercept is the point at which a line crosses an axis; the Y intercept is the value of Y at which the line crosses the Y axis (i.e., the value of Y when X = 0)

**internal respiration:** the exchange of gases at the cellular level

**interventricular septum:** muscular wall dividing the right from the left ventricles of the heart

**intervertebral foramen:** the small opening in the vertebrae where the spinal nerves exit the spinal cord

**intrafusal fibers:** specialized muscle fibers that are located in the muscle spindle

**ion:** a particle that carries either a positive or negative charge

**iron-deficiency anemia:** disease in which the hemoglobin content in red blood cells becomes abnormally low, resulting from low iron intake and/or excess iron loss and characterized by a low energy state, pale complexion, and fatigue

**ischemic stroke:** a stroke that occurs because there is not enough blood flow to a part of the brain and cells in that area of the brain die

**isocapnia:** $CO_2$ maintained at a constant level

**isoelectric:** the baseline of the electrocardiogram

**isoforms:** used to refer to proteins with the same or similar functions but slightly different amino acid sequences (e.g., myosin has several isoforms)

**isokinetic:** refers to movement about a joint that occurs at constant speed throughout the movement

**isometric:** muscle contraction that produces force, but no movement occurs

**isoproterenol:** sympathomimetic beta-receptor stimulant similar to epinephrine but which does not vasoconstrict

**isovolumic contraction:** time period at the beginning of systole; the ventricles are contracting against closed atrioventricular and semilunar valves

**isovolumic relaxation:** time period when the ventricles are rapidly relaxing during ventricular repolarization; the atrioventricular and semilunar valves are closed

**joint flexibility:** ability of a joint to move through a full range of motion

**ketoacidosis:** acidosis resulting from the formation of excessive ketone bodies

**ketonuria:** presence of ketone bodies in the urine (byproduct of fat metabolism)

**kilocalorie:** the amount of heat energy necessary to raise the temperature of 1 kg of water 1°C

**kilogram meter:** unit of work in which 1 kg of force (1 kg mass accelerated at 1 G) is moved through a vertical distance of 1 meter

**kinetic energy:** energy that is performing work

**Krebs cycle:** metabolic pathway in which acetyl CoA is catabolized to produce NADH, $FADH_2$, ATP, and $CO_2$; the Krebs cycle and electron transport chain constitute aerobic metabolism

**lactate threshold:** the point during a graded exercise test when the blood lactate concentration increases abruptly

**lanugo:** fine downy hairs that cover the body

**lean body mass:** the total body mass minus the adipose tissue mass

**left ventricular assist device:** device attached to the left ventricle to assist it in its pumping function

**life expectancy:** the average number of years a person born today can expect to live under current mortality conditions

**lifespan:** the duration of life of an individual

**lipolysis:** the splitting of a triglyceride molecule into glycerol and fatty acids

**lipoproteins:** compounds that contain a high content of lipid; the protein in lipoprotein compounds helps make the lipid more soluble

**lower motor neuron:** the motor neuron that originates in the spinal cord and travels out to the muscles; sometimes called the alpha motor neuron

**macrovascular disease:** disease of the larger blood vessels such as the coronary arteries

**major mineral:** mineral that should be consumed in an amount of 100 mg·day$^{-1}$ or more

**malignant:** growing worse, spreading, resisting treatment, as with cancer

**manual muscle testing:** a way of assessing isometric muscle strength whereby the tester manually resists the motion being tested

**maturation:** the process of becoming a fully functional adult

**maximal minute ventilation:** the maximal amount of air that can be taken in and out of the lungs per minute

**maximal shortening velocity:** refers to the speed of contraction of muscle

**maximum voluntary contraction:** the maximal force (100%) that the muscle can exert

**M band:** the band in the sarcomere that bisects the middle of the H zone

**McArdle disease:** glycogen storage disease in which the enzyme phosphorylase is missing in the muscle and results in the inability of the muscle to metabolize glycogen

**mean arterial blood pressure:** the average blood pressure throughout the cardiac cycle; calculated as DBP + 0.33(SBP − DBP) in which DBP = diastolic blood pressure and SBP = systolic blood pressure

**mechanoreceptor:** receptor that receives mechanical stimuli

**medullary respiratory center:** the lowest part of the brainstem where functions such as heart rate, breathing, blood pressure, and other reflexes such as coughing, sneezing, swallowing, and vomiting are regulated

**menopause:** the period that marks the permanent cessation of menstrual activity

**metabolic acidosis:** decreased arterial plasma pH and bicarbonate concentrations as the result of metabolic pathology

**metabolic alkalosis:** increased concentration of arterial plasma bicarbonate as the result of metabolic pathology

**metabolic equivalent (MET):** the resting metabolic rate or the amount of energy expended while an individual is at rest; one MET is equivalent to one times the resting metabolic rate, which is approximately 35 mL·kg$^{-1}$·min$^{-1}$

**metabolic pathway:** series of chemical reactions that can be catabolic and/or anabolic

**metabolic specificity:** refers to the specific response in a metabolic pathway that results from a particular intervention

**metabolism:** biochemical reactions that are either catabolic or anabolic in nature

**metabolizable energy:** the amount of energy made available to the body to do work when an energy-yielding nutrient is digested, absorbed, and ready for use in the cell

**metastases:** cancer that has spread beyond its tissue of origin and forms a new tumor

**microvascular disease:** disease of the very fine blood vessels of the body such as the capillaries

**mineralocorticoid:** hormone secreted by the adrenal cortex affecting the retention or secretion of sodium or potassium

**minute ventilation:** total amount of air breathed in 1 minute

**mitochondria:** cell organelle wherein aerobic metabolism occurs

**mitral regurgitation:** backflow of blood from the ventricle into the atria; this occurs due the inability of the atrioventricular valves to completely close after blood has flowed into the ventricles from the atria

**molecular biology:** study of the molecular structures and events underlying biologic processes, including the relation between genes and the functional characteristics they determine

**monosaccharide:** the basic carbohydrate unit composed of a single sugar molecule

**mortality rate:** the death rate; the ratio of the number of deaths to a given population

**motor endplate:** the portion of the muscle fiber that interfaces with a nerve

**motor unit:** a motor neuron and all the fibers innervated by that motor neuron

**motor unit recruitment:** activation of motor units to produce force

**motor unit remodeling:** turnover of synaptic connections at the neuromuscular junction by the process of denervation, axonal sprouting, and reinnervation

**mucociliary:** pertaining to mucus and to the cilia of the epithelia cells in the airways

**multinucleated:** containing more than one nucleus

**multiparous:** bearing more than one child

**multiple sclerosis:** disease in which the myelin sheath of the central nervous system is destroyed, causing poor motor control

**muscle fibers:** also called a muscle cell; contains all the organelles of a cell as well as the contractile proteins, actin, and myosin

**muscle spindle:** the structure inside the muscle that is sensitive to stretch on the muscle

**muscle wasting:** age-related sarcopenia with commensurate changes in muscle quality (increased fat content of muscle and decreased protein content) of specific tension as strength per unit of muscle mass

**muscular dystrophy:** neuromuscular disease in which dystrophin, a protein necessary for muscle cell structure, is either not produced or nonfunctional

**muscular endurance:** the ability of a muscle or muscle group to perform repeated contractions against a light load for an extended period of time

**muscular strength:** the maximal force that can be exerted by a muscle or group of muscles in one effort

**myasthenia gravis:** muscle disease characterized by severe muscle weakness when a nerve impulse is unable to cross the neuromuscular junction to propagate a muscle impulse

**myocardial $O_2$ consumption:** the rate of $O_2$ metabolism of the heart

**myocardium:** the muscular walls of the heart

**myocytes:** isolated cardiac muscle cells

**myofibrillar adenosinetriphosphatase:** the enzyme that is responsible for hydrolyzing ATP to form ADP and inorganic phosphate; often called myosin ATPase

**myofibrils:** refers to the contractile proteins, actin and myosin

**myosin:** a contractile protein; also known as the "thick filament;" there are different types of myosin, called isoforms, and these refer to the various fiber types contained in muscle

**myotatic stretch reflex:** monosynaptic reflex mediated within the spinal cord

**myotome:** groups of muscles that are innervated by a particular ventral root

**neural plasticity:** refers to the ability of parts of the brain to assume functions of other parts of the brain that have been damaged; forms the basis of rehabilitation of patients with damage to the brain as a result of injury or disease

**neuromuscular junction:** the interface between the muscle and nerve where the depolarization signal from the nerve is transmitted to the muscle

**neurotransmitter:** chemicals in the nervous system that are used to communicate with neurons and post-synaptic membranes such as muscles and internal organs

**nicotinamide adenine dinucleotide (NAD⁺/NADH):** an electron carrier; NADH is energy rich in that it contains two electrons that have a high energy potential

**nodes of Ranvier:** the part of the neuron not covered by myelin; allows for rapid conduction of action potentials

**nuclei:** collection of cell bodies in the central nervous system

**nutrients:** substances obtained from food that are necessary for growth, maintenance, and repair of tissues; nutrients are essential to the diet to maintain health

**$O_2$ deficit:** the anaerobic contribution to the energy supply during the initial stages of aerobic exercise before steady state is reached

**obesity:** accumulation of excess body fat, generally defined as having a body mass index of $\geq 30$

**occupational therapy:** health profession concerned with self-care, work, and play activities to increase function, enhance development, and prevent disability; may include modification of tasks or the environment to enable the patient to achieve maximum independence and to enhance the quality of the patient's life

**oligopeptide:** protein strand consisting of between four and 10 amino acids

**one-repetition maximum (1 RM):** the largest amount of weight that can be lifted only once

**onset of blood lactate accumulation:** see anaerobic threshold

**open-circuit spirometry:** indirect calorimetry method in which either inspired or expired ventilation is measured and $O_2$ consumption and $CO_2$ production are calculated; the breathing circuit is open to atmospheric air, i.e., the subject breaths from the atmosphere

**orthostatic hypotension:** low blood pressure that occurs with rapid changes in body posture (i.e., going from supine to upright position)

**osmolality:** the characteristic of a solution determined by the ionic concentration of the dissolved substances

**osmotic pressure:** the pressure exerted on a semipermeable membrane by a fluid, usually water, as it passes from the side of low solute concentration to the side of high solute concentration

**osteoarthritis:** degenerative joint disease in which the joint cartilage deteriorates, causing pain in the joints

**osteoporosis:** degenerative bone disease in which the bone loses mineral density

**overtraining:** excess training that results in maladaptive responses and decreased physical performance

**overweight:** accumulation of excess body fat, generally defined as having a body mass index between 25 and 30

**oxidative phosphorylation:** the process whereby inorganic phosphate is joined to ADP to form ATP as electrons are stripped from hydrogen in the electron transport chain

**oxygen pulse:** measure of the respiratory efficiency of the heart, which is calculated by dividing the mL of $O_2$ consumed per heartbeat

**palpitation:** perceptible pulsation of the heart

**papillary muscles:** a column of myocardium projecting into the ventricular cavity which is continuous with the ventricular wall and attached to the chordae tendinae of the atrioventricular valves

**parasympathetic:** division of the autonomic nervous system that affects, among other things, heart rate and gland secretions

**parasympatholytics:** drugs that inhibit cholinergic receptors of the autonomic nervous system

**parasympathomimetics:** drugs that stimulate cholinergic receptors of the autonomic nervous system

**parenchyma:** the tissue of an organ (essential parts concerned with function) as distinguished from supporting or connective tissue of the organ (concerned with organ framework)

**parenteral:** route of administration of a drug through means other than the intestinal route

**Parkinson disease:** disorder in which an area deep within the brain degenerates, causing a lower production of the neurotransmitter dopamine and marked by tremor, weakness of resting muscles, and a shuffling gait

**partial pressure:** the pressure exerted by an individual gas and represented as a percentage of the total pressure of all gases in a container

**pathologic aging:** changes that occur as a result of disease processes

**patient:** person with a diagnosed impairment or functional limitation and who is undergoing medical treatment

**pennate:** refers to muscle in which fibers lie at oblique angles to one another and into the tendon of insertion

**pennation angle:** the angle of the orientation of muscle fibers to the tendon

**peptide bond:** bond that is formed when the carboxyl group ($-COOH$) from one amino acid joins with the amino group ($-NH$) from another amino acid and water is released

**perfusion:** the passage of blood through a specific organ or area of the body

**periarthritis:** arthritic shoulder (or other joints) condition due to microangiopathy common in patients with diabetes mellitus

**perimenopause:** a period of a few years before and 1 year after the permanent cessation of menses

**perimysium:** the connective tissue that surrounds a bundle of muscle fibers

**periodization:** pattern of exercise training in which training cycles (harder and easier training) are applied that make optimal use of Selye's general adaptation syndrome to achieve the greatest possible physiologic adaptation to achieve peak performance for competition

**pharmacodynamics:** mechanism by which a drug achieves its effect within the body

**pharmacokinetics:** movement of a drug within the body

**pharmacology:** science dealing with the interactions between living systems and molecules

**phenoxybenzamine:** drug that blocks adrenergic activity at the alpha receptors

**phenylketonuria:** hereditable disease in which the enzyme that processes the amino acid phenylalanine is missing

**phlegm:** viscid mucus secreted in abnormal quantity in the respiratory passages

**phosphagen system:** refers to the immediate energy system that utilizes stored ATP and creatine phosphate to obtain energy to perform work

**phospholipid:** class of lipid similar to a triglyceride, with a phosphate and choline moiety attached

**phosphorylase:** the key enzyme in the catabolism of glycogen

**phosphorylation:** chemical reaction that adds a phosphate group to a molecule or compound; e.g., the oxidative phosphorylation of ADP produces ATP

**physical education:** teaching of activities that promote physical fitness

**physical fitness:** the ability to tolerate exercise stress without developing undue fatigue while retaining enough energy to meet other physical demands

**physical therapy:** health profession concerned with the promotion of health, prevention of physical disability, evaluation and rehabilitation of patients disabled by pain, disease, or injury, and use of physical therapeutic measures as opposed to medical, surgical, or radiologic measures

**physiologic cross-sectional area (PSCA):** the amount of contractile protein available to generate force; calculated by muscle mass (g) $\times$ cosine $\theta$/muscle density ($g \cdot cm^{-3}$) $\times$ fiber length (cm) in which muscle density is 1.056 $g \cdot cm^{-3}$ and $\theta$ is the pennation angle

**physiologic dead space:** the sum of the anatomic and alveolar dead spaces

**plexus:** complicated complex of nerves in the peripheral nervous system formed from several spinal nerves

**plyometrics:** method of power training that involves an eccentric loading of muscles followed by a quickly timed all-out concentric contraction

**polarized state:** the resting phase of the action potential

**polydipsia:** increased thirst in response to polyuria

**polymer:** natural or synthetic substance formed by the combination of two or more smaller molecules of the same substance

**polypeptide:** protein strand that consists of more than 10 amino acids

**polyphagia:** increased appetite and ingestion of food

**polypharmacy:** excessive and unnecessary use of medication especially in elderly individuals for whom many hospital admissions are medication related

**polysaccharide:** large carbohydrate polymer, made up of many smaller carbohydrate units linked together

**polyuria:** increased urination caused by osmotic diuresis

**post-menopausal osteoporosis:** form of osteoporosis that occurs after menopause due to low levels of circulating estrogen

**post-prandial satiety:** the feeling of fullness or being satisfied (satiety) following a meal

**post-synaptic neuron:** the neuron that is after a synapse; this is the neuron that binds a neurotransmitter

**potential energy:** stored energy, ready at any moment to do work

**power:** the amount of work done per unit of time

**power lifting:** weightlifting competition involving the following lifts: squat, bench press, and dead lift; the term is actually a misnomer because the lifts are performed slowly, indicating that power generation is a key factor in the lift—a better term may be strength lifting

**preganglionic neuron:** refers to a neuron in the autonomic system that originates in the spinal cord and synapses in one of the ganglia in the periphery; first neuron in the pathway from the spinal cord to the effector organs

**preload:** the workload imposed on the ventricles just prior to contraction

**pressor response:** caused by mechanical and chemical receptors in contracting muscle which signals the cardiovascular control center to increase blood pressure in an attempt to perfuse ischemic tissue, i.e., muscle during resistance exercise

**pressure load exercise:** class of exercise characterized by drastically elevated blood pressure due to the mechanical occlusion of the vasculature; cardiac output and $O_2$ consumption levels are moderately elevated, while heart rate may be high; the stimulus for cardiac physiologic and structural (increased thickness of the left ventricular free wall) adaptations is periodic (resistance exercise training) high afterload states

**presynaptic neuron:** the neuron prior to a synapse; this is the neuron that releases a neurotransmitter into the synaptic cleft

**primary aging:** the normal aging process

**primary amenorrhea:** the delay of the onset of menarche beyond 16 years

**primary prevention:** prevention of disease in a population by general health promotion efforts

**primiparous:** the first pregnancy of a woman

**progesterone:** female sex hormone responsible for changes in the uterus during the second half of the menstrual cycle and for development of the mammary glands

**progressive overload:** the principle of exercise training which states that a stimulus requiring an organism to adapt is progressively given by increasing the volume of exercise over the course of the training program

**prolongevity:** the significant extension of the length of life by human action

**prophylactic:** to prevent illness or disease

**propranolol:** drug that blocks the beta adrenergic receptors

**proprioception:** the awareness of posture, movement, changes in equilibrium, and position of the body

**prostaglandin:** biologic substances that affect the cardiovascular system and smooth muscle and stimulate the uterus to contract

**prostate gland:** gland that surrounds the neck of the bladder and urethra in the male and secretes a fluid that forms part of the semen

**pulmonary circuit:** the vasculature that connects the heart to the lungs

**pulmonary vascular resistance:** resistance to blood flow in the pulmonary circuit

**pulmonary ventilation:** the process by which air is moved into the lungs

**pyramidal tract:** refers to motor tracts coming from the motor cortex that cross in the pyramid of the medulla oblongata

**pyruvate:** the end product of slow glycolysis resulting from the partial catabolism of glucose

**radiation:** process in which electromagnetic waves transfer heat down a temperature gradient that exists between two objects that are not in physical contact with each other

**rate-pressure product:** the product of heart rate and systolic blood pressure; serves as a useful index of the work of the heart

**rating of perceived exertion (RPE):** a perceptual evaluation of exercise intensity ranked in the traditional scale (6–20) or revised scale (1–10), in which the lowest number represents a very easy workload and the highest number represents maximal exertion

**reciprocal inhibition:** the process by which the antagonist muscle is relaxed so that the agonist muscle can contract and complete the desired joint motion

**recommended dietary allowance:** the recommended amount of a given nutrient that should be consumed daily for optimal health

**redox potential:** the ratio of oxidizing agent (e.g., $NAD^+$) to reducing agent (e.g., NADH)

**reduction potential:** measure of the affinity a molecule has for attracting electrons

**refractory:** the inability of tissue to depolarize despite an action potential

**regression equation:** equation that predicts or estimates the dependent (y) variable from a known independent (x) variable

**relative refractory period:** the part of the refractory period when an action potential may be generated only if a supermaximal stimulus is applied to the cell

**renin-angiotensin-aldosterone mechanism:** primary mechanism by which the kidneys regulate blood volume by adjusting the excretion of water and sodium into the urine

**repolarization:** the re-establishment of polarity, especially the return of cell membrane potential to resting potential after depolarization

**residual volume:** the volume of air left in the lungs at the end of a maximal expiration

**resistance exercise:** exercise involving the exertion of force against a load used to develop muscle strength and endurance, and/or muscle hypertrophy; force exertion is usually great enough to occlude or nearly occlude blood flow to the contracting muscles

**respiratory acidosis:** inadequate pulmonary ventilation that results in the retention of $CO_2$ and a decrease in blood pH

**respiratory alkalosis:** hyperventilation that results in an abnormal loss of $CO_2$ and an increase in blood pH

**respiratory exchange ratio (RER):** the ratio of whole-body $CO_2$ production to $O_2$ consumption

**respiratory quotient (RQ):** the ratio of $CO_2$ production to $O_2$ utilization measured at the cellular level

**resting membrane potential:** the same as a polarized state; the period during which the inside of the cell is negative as compared with the outside of the cell

**resting metabolic rate (RMR):** the amount of energy that is expended when a person is at rest, multiples of the RMR are expressed as metabolic equivalents

**restrictive lung disease:** the category of lung disease involving restriction of the lung parenchyma and characterized by stiffness (reduced compliance) and reduced lung volume

**reverse myotatic reflex:** protective spinal reflex that senses the force of muscle contraction and inhibits further motor input into the muscle

**risk factor:** an element in the environment or a chemical, psychologic, physiologic, or genetic element thought to predispose an individual to the development of a disease

**sarcolemma:** the membrane that lies directly underneath the endomysium; surrounds the entire muscle fiber

**sarcomere:** the individual unit of a myofibril

**sarcopenia:** the decrease in muscle mass that occurs as a result of aging

**sarcoplasm:** the cytoplasm of the muscle fibers; contains all the organelles of the muscle fiber

**sarcoplasmic reticulum:** network of membranous channels that stores calcium, releases it with muscle depolarization, and take it up once the depolarization signal has ceased

**saturation:** measure of the degree to which $O_2$ is bound to hemoglobin, given as the percentage calculated by dividing the maximum $O_2$ capacity into the actual $O_2$ content and multiplying by 100

**second law of thermodynamics:** energy and matter tends toward randomness or disorder; therefore, when energy is exchanged, the efficiency of the exchange is less than 100%

**secondary aging:** the age-related deterioration in functional capacity that results from diseases

**secondary amenorrhea:** when menses ceases in a woman who has previously been menstrual

**secondary conditions:** complications that are causally related to a primary disabling condition; may include complications such as decubitus ulcers, contractures, physical deconditioning, cardiopulmonary conditions, and mental depression

**secondary prevention:** work to decrease the duration and severity of disease by early diagnosis and intervention

**self-efficacy:** a person's perceived capability to perform a behavior; a person with a positive self-efficacy expects to succeed and will persevere in an activity until the task is completed, and a person with low self-efficacy anticipates failure and is less likely to attempt or persist in challenging activities

**semilunar valves:** valves between the right ventricle and pulmonary artery and between the left ventricle and aorta

**senile osteoporosis:** type of osteoporosis that results from age-related calcium deficiency

**sensitivity:** percentage of individuals with disease who have an abnormal test; for a test to be useful in ruling out a disease, it must have a high sensitivity

**size principle:** describes motor unit recruitment in terms of the size of the motor unit: small units are recruited first, medium-sized units are recruited next, and the largest motor units are recruited last

**skin temperature:** the temperature of the body just below the surface of the skin

**sliding filament theory:** describes the muscle contraction process of how myosin and actin generate force

**slope:** the steepness of a line, measured as the change in Y associated with a change of one unit on X

**soluble fiber:** dissolves or swells in water and is acted upon by intestinal bacteria

**somatotopically:** refers to the specific arrangement of tracts in the spinal cord

**spasticity:** increase in muscle above the normal resting tone

**spatial summation:** refers to the process in which several inhibitory post-synaptic potentials and excitatory post-synaptic potentials summate simultaneously at the axon hillock

**specific tension:** describes the force generated by either a muscle fiber or whole muscle as calculated by dividing the absolute force by the cross-sectional area of the fiber or muscle

**specificity:** (1) percentage of individuals free of disease who have a normal test; for a test to be useful at confirming a disease, it must have a high specificity (2) the training principle which states that the physiologic adaptations achieved are governed by the type of exercise or training program imposed

**sphygmomanometer:** the device used to obtain blood pressure; the pressure in the cuff is inflated until no sounds are heard through a stethoscope, then the pressure is slowly released, and the first sound heard with the release of pressure and the last sound heard constitute the blood pressure reading

**stadiometer:** instrument with a vertical rule used to measure body height

**static exercise:** exercise or activity that does not produce limb displacement or joint rotation and therefore no movement results; muscle contraction in static activity is of an isometric nature (no sarcomere shortening, i.e., no change in muscle fiber length)

**steady state:** the point during exercise at which the metabolic demand is met by aerobic metabolism

**sterols:** class of lipids that is derived from acetic acid and has a multi-ring structure

**stethoscope:** the instrument that is used to intensify Korotkoff sounds during the measurement of blood pressure

**storage fat:** consists of that fat which is stored in the fat cells of the adipose tissues and the fat surrounding the internal organs, resulting from excess energy intake

**stress:** physical or psychologic forces experienced by individuals that produce nonspecific physiologic responses

**stressor:** any social, environmental, physical, or psychologic stimulus which produces a demand for adaptation in the individual

**striated:** describes the dark and light areas of a muscle that are observed microscopically due to the location and overlap of actin and myosin in the sarcomeres

**stroke:** condition in which brain tissue has died because of lack of blood flow and insufficient $O_2$ delivery to a part of the brain

**stroke volume:** the amount of blood ejected by the left ventricle in one beat

**subacute state:** falling between acute and chronic in character especially when closer to acute; less marked in severity or duration than a corresponding acute state

**substrate:** in a chemical reaction, the compound that is acted upon

**summation:** refers to the process whereby repeated twitches are applied to muscle; each twitch generates greater tension

**sympathetic nervous system:** division of the autonomic nervous system that affects, among other things, the cardiovascular system and adrenal gland secretions

**sympatholytics:** drugs that inhibit adrenergic receptors of the autonomic nervous system

**sympathomimetics:** drugs that stimulate adrenergic receptors of the autonomic nervous system

**synapse:** the small gap between the presynaptic neuron and post-synaptic neuron

**synaptic cleft:** the space at the neuromuscular junction between the nerve and motor endplate where acetylcholine is transported from the nerve to the muscle

**synaptic terminal:** the part of presynaptic neuron where a neurotransmitter is released into the synapse

**syncope:** temporary loss of consciousness due to generalized cerebral ischemia

**systemic circuit:** the vasculature that connects the heart to all areas of the body except the lungs

**systole:** ventricular contraction

**systolic function:** the contractile ability of the left ventricle; dysfunction is defined in terms of ejection fraction, with normal ejection fraction equaling 50% or more and systolic dysfunction equaling less than 40%

**tachyarrhythmia:** irregular heart rhythm producing rates greater than 100 beats per minute

**temporal summation:** refers to the process in which several inhibitory post-synaptic potentials and excitatory post-synaptic potentials summate in rapid succession at the axon hillock

**tendon:** tough connective tissue that attaches muscle to bone

**terminal cisternae:** the enlarged portion of the sarcoplasmic reticulum that interfaces with the transverse tubules

**tertiary prevention:** work to decrease the degree of disability by rehabilitating patients with chronic diseases

**testosterone:** steroid hormone that is produced in the adrenal cortex of males and females and in the testicles of the male; responsible for secondary sex characteristics in the male and normal sexual functioning of the male

**tetanic tension:** the tension that is generated by muscle when twitches are applied so rapidly that no relaxation can occur between twitches and the muscle contraction appears smooth and sustained

**therapeutic exercise:** scientific supervision of exercise for the purpose of preventing muscle atrophy, restoring joint and muscle function, increasing muscle strength, and improving efficiency of cardiovascular and pulmonary functions

**thermal effectors:** tissues or organs that are stimulated to conserve or release body heat

**thermal receptors:** sensory nerves that provide information about temperature to the thermal regulatory center in the hypothalamus

**thermal regulatory center:** portion of the hypothalamus in the brain that receives, interprets, and responds to sensory input relative to temperature

**thermic effect of food:** the energy-requiring processes of digesting, absorbing, and assimilating the various nutrients in the diet

**threshold potential:** the membrane potential that is necessary for the generation of an action potential

**tidal volume:** the volume of air inspired and expired in each breath taken

**titration:** determining the quantity of added dosage of exercise given in a progressive manner over time as physiologic and anatomic adaptations occur

**total lung capacity:** the maximum volume to which the lungs can be expanded; the sum of all the pulmonary volumes

**total peripheral resistance:** the total force in the vascular system that serves as the opposition to the flow of blood

**toxicity:** being poisonous; vitamin or mineral toxicity occurs when a nutrient is consumed in excess, resulting in a specific health-related problem

**trace mineral:** mineral that should be consumed daily in an amount less than 100 mg

**transgenic animal model:** animal with a transgene (an artificial gene cloned in the lab by recombinant DNA technology and microinjected into the animal's fertilized eggs, which are then transferred into foster mothers for gestation) in addition to its normal complement of genes; transgenes integrate randomly into chromosomal DNA and are transmitted as Mendelian traits

**transit time:** the time that the red blood cell stays in the pulmonary or tissue capillary

**translung pressure:** the pressure gradient between the inside of the lung (alveolus) and the outside of the lung (pleural space)

**transverse tubules:** membranous channel system that conducts the depolarization potential deep within the muscle fibers to the triad so that calcium can be released

**triad:** composed of two terminal cisternae and a transverse tubule; the site where the depolarization potential from the transverse tubule causes release of calcium from the terminal cisternae

**triglyceride:** fat molecule consisting of a glycerol unit bound to three fatty acids

**tripeptide:** protein strand consisting of three amino acids

**tropomyosin:** protein that covers the active sites on the actin when the muscle is relaxed

**troponin:** calcium-binding protein; once calcium is bound to troponin, the troponin causes the tropomyosin molecule to uncover the active sites on actin so that myosin crossbridges can attach to actin

**tumor:** enlargement or abnormal growth in a tissue

**twitch tension:** the force that is generated when a single impulse is applied to muscle

**type I osteoporosis:** age-related osteoporosis that is seen in older, post-menopausal women

**upper motor neuron:** motor neuron that begins in the motor cortex and synapses in the ventral horn of the spinal cord

**urethra:** canal for the discharge of urine that extends from the bladder to the outside of the body

**Valsalva maneuver:** holding your breath against a closed glottis while exerting (as in weightlifting) and contracting the abdominal muscles increases intrathoracic pressure and afterload and can momentarily reduce venous return, cardiac output, and blood pressure, leading to syncope

**vasoactive:** exerting an effect on the caliber of blood vessels

**vasoconstriction:** narrowing of the blood vessels resulting from contracting of the muscular wall of the vessels; usually evoked by impulses in sympathetic nerve fibers

**vasodilation:** widening of blood vessels resulting from relaxation of the muscular wall of the vessels

**vector:** magnitude and direction of an electrocardiogram lead or mean electrical axis

**venous blood:** blood that has moved through peripheral tissue from the systemic or coronary arterial tree and has given off $O_2$ to the tissues and taken up $CO_2$ from the tissues

**ventilation:** process by which gases are moved into and out of the lungs

**ventilatory equivalent for $O_2$:** ratio of minute ventilation to $O_2$ consumption

**ventilatory threshold:** breakpoint at which pulmonary ventilation and $CO_2$ output begin to increase exponentially during an incremental exercise test

**venule:** tiny vein continuous with the capillary

**vital capacity:** measurement of the amount of air that can be expelled at the normal rate of exhalation after maximal inspiration

**volume load exercise:** class of exercise characterized by graded levels of cardiac output in response to incremental exercise; blood pressure increases are moderate; the stimulus for cardiac physiologic and structural (increased internal diameter of the left ventricle) adaptations is periodic (endurance exercise training) high preload states

**water-soluble vitamin:** vitamin that dissolves in water, while excess amounts are excreted rather than stored in the body

**wet-bulb globe temperature:** index that is used to determine environmental heat stress by taking into account ambient temperature, humidity, and radiation

**windchill:** index that is used to determine environmental cold stress by taking into account ambient temperature and convection properties of the wind

**work:** the product of a given force acting through a given vertical distance

**X-linked recessive disorder:** refers to a defective gene that is located on the X chromosome; if a male receives the X chromosome that contains the defective gene, he will manifest the pathology caused by the defective gene

**Z line:** defines the boundaries of a single sarcomere

# Index

## A

AAAPE. *See* American Association for the Advancement of Physical Education
ABI. *See* Ankle-brachial index
Absolute refractory period, 220
Accelerometers, 376, *376,* 377
ACE. *See* Angiotensin-converting enzyme inhibitors
Acetylcholine, 223, 224*t,* 258
Acidosis, 156, 157*b*
  metabolic, 454
ACSM. *See* American College of Sports Medicine
ACTH. *See* Adrenocorticotropic hormone
Actins, 249, *250,* 255
Action potentials, 165, 167, *168, 169,* 614, 615
  development of, 220, *222*
  generation of, 223
"Active Living Policy and Environmental Studies," 366*b*
Active pathology, 459
Activities of daily living (ADL), 10, 11*t,* 13–14, 98, 391
Adaptations, 466
Adenosine diphosphate (ADP), 54, 92–93, 258
Adenosine monophosphate (AMP), 53, 93. *See also* Cyclic 3′,5′ adenosine monophosphate (cyclic AMP)
Adenosine triphosphate (ATP), 51–53, *52,* 258, 611
  capacity/power and, 56–57
  CP and, 54–55, *55, 59,* 59–60, *60*
  hydrolysis, 84, *85*
  muscles and, 75
  pathways, 56–59, *58,* 68*t*
  production of, *69,* 72
    from different energy systems, 76, *76,* 76*t,* 77
  tally, *70, 73,* 73*t*
Adenosine triphosphate-phosphocreatine (ATP-PC), 75. *See also* Phosphagen system
  ratio, 76, 78*b*
  regeneration of, 94, *95*
  system, 76*t,* 77, *77*
Adenylate cyclase, 82
Adipocytes, 28, 64
Adiposity rebound, 331, 616
ADL. *See* Activities of daily living
ADP. *See* Adenosine diphosphate
Adrenocorticotropic hormone (ACTH), 83, 84, *85*
Aerobic endurance training, 352, 352*t*
  exercise dosage in, *336,* 353–354, 355*t*

exercise intensity in, 354–358, 355*t, 356, 357t, 358*
  inquiry summary on, 359
  techniques, 358–359
Affymetrix. *See* GeneChip technology
Afterload, 162, 183
Agility, 351
Aging, 4–5, 387, 388*t,* 572, 617–618, 619
  biologic, 388, 389
  cardiovascular system and, 394–397, *395, 396*
  chronologic, 388–389
  definition of, 388–389, 390*t*
  disability/physical inactivity and, 390–393, *391,* 393*b*
  exercise physiologic changes with, 393–400, 394*t, 395, 396, 398*
  exercise training and, *400,* 400–403, *401, 402*
  neuromuscular system and, 397–400
  pathologic, 388, 389
  physiologic, 7*b*
  primary, 391
  pulmonary system and, 394*t,* 397
  -related changes, 264–266, *266, 267*
  secondary, 391
  summary on, 403
  theories of, 389–390
Air-displacement plethysmography (BOD POD), 314, *318,* 318–320, 319*b*
Aldosterones, 84
Alkalosis, 156, 157*b*
All-or-none phenomenon, 272
Allosteric compounds, 146
ALS. *See* Amyotrophic lateral sclerosis
Alveolar dead space, 135
Alveolar-capillary interface
  gas diffusion at, 129, *130*
  respiratory gas exchanges at, 128–134, *129, 130, 131, 132, 133*
Alzheimer disease, 563–566, *564*
Ambient temperature and pressure (ATPS), 112–113, 113*t*
Ambulation, 120, *120*
American Academy of Pediatrics, 383
American Alliance of Health, 366*b*
American Association for the Advancement of Physical Education (AAAPE), 18
American College of Obstetricians and Gynecologists, 416
American College of Sports Medicine (ACSM), 103, 210*b,* 295*b,* 482, 549
  *Guidelines for Exercise Testing and Prescription,* 357, 385
  recommendations, 306, 373, 400–401
  *Resource Manual for Guidelines for Exercise Testing and Prescription,* 385

American Heart Association, 482
*American Journal of Clinical Nutrition,* 535*b*
American Physiological Society, 18
American Psychiatric Association, 421
American Psychological Association, 366*b*
Amino acid(s), 32
  metabolism, 94, *94*
  peptide bonds of, 32–33
  processing disorders of, 33
  radicals, 93
  structure of, 32, *33*
  supplements, 298*b*
AMP. *See* Adenosine monophosphate
Amyotrophic lateral sclerosis (ALS), 273, 274*b*
Anabolism, 51, 52–53, *53*
Anaerobic thresholds, 89
Anatomic dead space, 135
Androgens, 409
Anemia, 40, 41, 618
Aneurysms, 444
Angina, *509*
Angiotensin-converting enzyme inhibitors (ACE), *442,* 442–443
Animal models, transgenic, 4
Ankle-brachial index (ABI), 179
Anorexia, 421–422
ANRT. *See* Atrioventricular re-entrant tachycardia
Anthropometric data, 315
Antiarrhythmia prescription, 431
Anti-inflammatory agents, 443
Antioxidants, 36
Antitussives, 444
*Appetite,* 535*b*
Arrhythmias, 165, 441
  cardiac, 165
  recognition of, 499–506, *500, 501, 502, 503, 504, 505, 506, 507*
  ventricular, 503–506, *504, 505, 506, 507*
Arthritis, 10, 267
Arthrokinematics, 13
Articular cartilage, 380
Asthma, 443, 451, 619
Astrand, Per-Olof, *104,* 105, 106*b,* 488
Ataxia, 229
Athletes, 89, 133
  movement of, 244
  performance of, 312–313
  pre-event meals of, 291
  SV of, 190*b*
Athletic amenorrhea, 413
ATP. *See* Adenosine triphosphate
ATP-PC. *See* Adenosine triphosphate-phosphocreatine
ATPS. *See* Ambient temperature and pressure
Atrial fibrillation, 165, 503, *504*